## COMMUNITY NURSING DEFINITIONS

**Community-Oriented Nursing Practice** is a philosophy of nursing service delivery that involves the generalist or specialist public health and community health nurse providing "health care" through community diagnosis and investigation of major health and environmental problems, health surveillance, and monitoring and evaluation of community and population health status for the purposes of preventing disease and disability and promoting, protecting, and maintaining "health" in order to create conditions in which people can be healthy.

**Public Health Nursing Practice** is the synthesis of nursing theory and public health theory applied to promoting and preserving health of populations. The focus of practice is the community as a whole and the effect of the community's health status (resources) on the health of individuals, families, and groups. Care is provided within the context of preventing disease and disability and promoting and protecting the health of the community as a whole. Public Health Nursing is population focused, which means that the population is the center of interest for the public health nurse. *Community Health Nurse* is a term that is used interchangeably with *Public Health Nurse.*

**Community-Based Nursing Practice** is a setting-specific practice whereby care is provided for "sick" individuals and families where they live, work, and go to school. The emphasis of practice is acute and chronic care and the provision of comprehensive, coordinated, and continuous services. Nurses who deliver community-based care are generalists or specialists in maternal–infant, pediatric, adult, or psychiatric–mental health nursing.

## Select Examples of Similarities and Differences Between Community-Oriented and Community-Based Nursing

| | COMMUNITY-ORIENTED NURSING | | COMMUNITY-BASED NURSING |
|---|---|---|---|
| | PUBLIC HEALTH NURSING: POPULATION FOCUSED/ POPULATION CENTERED | | |
| **Philosophy** | PRIMARY focus is on "health care" of communities and populations | SECONDARY focus is on "health care" of individuals, families, and groups in community to unserved clients by health care system | Focus is on "illness care" of individuals and families across the life span |
| **Goal** | Prevent disease; preserve, protect, promote, or maintain health | Prevent disease; preserve, protect, promote, or maintain health | Manage acute or chronic conditions |
| **Service context** | Community and population health care "the greatest good for the greatest number" | Personal health care to unserved clients | Family-centered illness care |
| **Community type** | Varied: local, state, nation, world community | Varied, usually local community | Human ecological |
| **Client characteristics** | • Nation<br>• State<br>• Community<br>• Populations at risk<br>• Aggregates<br>• Healthy<br>• Culturally diverse<br>• Autonomous<br>• Able to define problem<br>• Client primary decision maker | • Individuals/families at risk if unserved by health care system<br>• Usually healthy<br>• Culturally diverse<br>• Autonomous<br>• Able to define own problem<br>• Client primary decision maker | • Individuals<br>• Families<br>• Usually ill<br>• Culturally diverse<br>• Autonomous<br>• Client able to define own problem<br>• Client involved in decision making |
| **Practice setting** | • Community<br>• Organization<br>• Government<br>• Community agencies | • May be organization<br>• May be government<br>• Community agencies<br>• Home<br>• Work<br>• School<br>• Playground | • Community agencies<br>• Home<br>• Work<br>• School |
| **Interaction patterns** | • Governmental<br>• Organizational<br>• Groups<br>• May be one-to-one | • One-to-one<br>• Groups<br>• May be organizational | • One-to-one |
| **Type of service** | • Indirect<br>• May be direct care of populations | • Direct care of at-risk persons<br>• Indirect (program management) | • Direct illness care |
| **Emphasis on levels of prevention** | • Primary | • Primary<br>• Secondary: screening<br>• Tertiary: maintenance and rehabilitation | • Secondary<br>• Tertiary<br>• May be primary |

| | COMMUNITY-ORIENTED NURSING | | COMMUNITY-BASED NURSING |
|---|---|---|---|
| | **PUBLIC HEALTH NURSING: POPULATION FOCUSED/ POPULATION CENTERED** | | |
| **Roles** | **Client and delivery oriented: community/ population** | **Client and delivery oriented: individual, family, group** | **Client and delivery oriented: individual, family** |
| | • Educator | • Individual/family oriented— as needed | • Caregiver |
| | • Consultant | • Caregiver | • Educator |
| | • Advocate | • Social engineer | • Counselor |
| | • Planner | • Educator | • Advocate |
| | • Collaborator | • Counselor | • Care manager |
| | • Data collector/evaluator | • Advocate | **Group Oriented** |
| | • Health status monitor | • Case manager | • Leader, disease management |
| | • Social engineer | **Group Oriented** | • Change agent, managed care services |
| | • Community developer/partner | • Leader, personal health management | |
| | • Facilitator | • Change agent, screening | |
| | • Community care agent | • Community advocate | |
| | • Assessor | • Case finder | |
| | • Policy developer/maker | • Community care agent | |
| | • Assuror of health care | • Assessment | |
| | • Enforcer of laws/compliance | • Policy developer | |
| | • Disaster responder | • Assurance | |
| | **Population oriented** | • Enforcer of laws/compliance | |
| | • Program manager, aggregates | | |
| | • Health initiator | | |
| | • Program evaluator | | |
| | • Counselor | | |
| | • Change agent—population health | | |
| | • Educator | | |
| | • Population advocate | | |
| **Priority of nurses' activities** | • Community development | • For individual and family clients—as needed | • Care management, direct care |
| | • Community assessment/ monitoring | • Case finding | • Patient education |
| | • Health policy/politics | • Client education | • Individual and family advocacy |
| | • Community education | • Community education | • Interdisciplinary practice |
| | • Interdisciplinary practice | • Interdisciplinary practice | • Continuity of care provider |
| | • Program management | • Case management, direct care | |
| | • Community/population advocacy | • Program planning, implementation | |
| | | • Individual and family advocacy | |

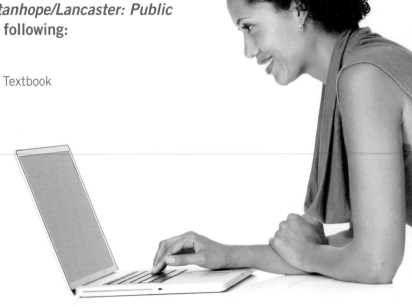

9TH EDITION

# PUBLIC HEALTH NURSING

Population-Centered Health Care in the Community

**Marcia Stanhope**, PhD, RN, FAAN
Education and Practice Consultant
*and*
Professor Emerita
College of Nursing
University of Kentucky
Lexington, Kentucky

**Jeanette Lancaster**, PhD, RN, FAAN
Professor and Dean Emerita
School of Nursing
University of Virginia
Charlottesville, Virginia

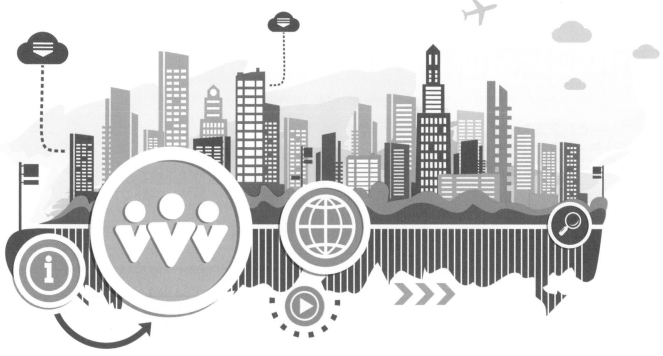

ELSEVIER

# ELSEVIER

3251 Riverport Lane
St. Louis, Missouri 63043

PUBLIC HEALTH NURSING: POPULATION-CENTERED          ISBN: 978-0-323-32153-2
HEALTH CARE IN THE COMMUNITY, EDITION NINE

---

### Notices

Knowledge and best practice in this field are constantly changing. As new research and experience broaden our understanding, changes in research methods, professional practices, or medical treatment may become necessary.

Practitioners and researchers must always rely on their own experience and knowledge in evaluating and using any information, methods, compounds, or experiments described herein. In using such information or methods they should be mindful of their own safety and the safety of others, including parties for whom they have a professional responsibility.

With respect to any drug or pharmaceutical products identified, readers are advised to check the most current information provided (i) on procedures featured or (ii) by the manufacturer of each product to be administered, to verify the recommended dose or formula, the method and duration of administration, and contraindications. It is the responsibility of practitioners, relying on their own experience and knowledge of their patients, to make diagnoses, to determine dosages and the best treatment for each individual patient, and to take all appropriate safety precautions.

To the fullest extent of the law, neither the Publisher nor the authors, contributors, or editors, assume any liability for any injury and/or damage to persons or property as a matter of products liability, negligence or otherwise, or from any use or operation of any methods, products, instructions, or ideas contained in the material herein.

---

Previous editions copyrighted 2014, 2008, 2004, 2000, 1996, 1992, 1988, 1984

Library of Congress Cataloging-in-Publication Data
Public health nursing (Stanhope)
   Public health nursing : population-centered health care in the community / [edited by] Marcia Stanhope,
Jeanette Lancaster.—9th edition.
      p. ; cm.
   Includes bibliographical references and index.
   ISBN 978-0-323-32153-2 (pbk. : alk. paper)
   I. Stanhope, Marcia, editor. II. Lancaster, Jeanette, editor. III. Title.
   [DNLM: 1. Community Health Nursing. 2. Public Health Nursing. WY 106]
   RT98
   610.73′43—dc23
                                                                      2015007429

*Content Strategist:* Jamie Randall
*Content Development Manager:* Laurie Gower
*Content Development Specialist:* Lisa Newton
*Publishing Services Manager:* Jeff Patterson
*Senior Project Manager:* Anne Konopka
*Design Direction:* Margaret Reid

Printed in Canada

Last digit is the print number:   9   8   7   6   5   4   3   2

Working together
to grow libraries in
developing countries

www.elsevier.com • www.bookaid.org

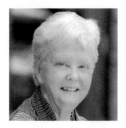

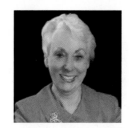

## Marcia Stanhope, PhD, RN, FAAN

Marcia Stanhope is currently an education consultant with Berea College, Berea Kentucky, as in Berea, Kentucky an Associate with Tuft and Associate Search Firm, Chicago, Illinois, and Professor Emerita from the University of Kentucky, College of Nursing, Lexington, Kentucky. In recent years she received the Provost Public Scholar award for contributions to the communities of Kentucky. She was appointed to the Good Samaritan Endowed Chair in Community Health Nursing 12 years ago. She has practiced community and home health nursing, has served as an administrator and consultant in home health, and has been involved in the development of a number of nurse-managed centers. She has taught community health, public health, epidemiology, primary care nursing, and administration courses. Dr. Stanhope was the former Associate Dean and formerly directed the Division of Community Health Nursing and Administration at the University of Kentucky. She has been responsible for both undergraduate and graduate courses in population-centered, community-oriented nursing. She has also taught at the University of Virginia and the University of Alabama, Birmingham. Her presentations and publications have been in the areas of home health, community health and community-focused nursing practice, nurse-managed centers, and primary care nursing. Dr. Stanhope holds a diploma in nursing from the Good Samaritan Hospital, Lexington, Kentucky, and a bachelor of science in nursing from the University of Kentucky. She has a master's degree in public health nursing from Emory University in Atlanta and a doctorate of science in nursing from the University of Alabama, Birmingham. Dr. Stanhope is the co-author of four other Elsevier publications: *Handbook of Community-Based and Home Health Nursing Practice, Public and Community Health Nurse's Consultant, Case Studies in Community Health Nursing Practice: A Problem-Based Learning Approach,* and *Foundations of Community Health Nursing: Community-Oriented Practice.*

## Jeanette Lancaster, PhD, RN, FAAN

Jeanette Lancaster is Professor and Dean Emerita at the University of Virginia, School of Nursing in Charlottesville, Virginia. She served as Dean of the School of Nursing at the University of Virginia from 1989 until 2008. From 2008 to 2009 she served as a visiting professor at the University of Hong Kong where she taught courses in public health nursing and worked with faculty to develop their scholarship programs. She then taught at the University of Virginia from 2010 until 2012. She also taught at Vanderbilt University and is an Associate with Tuft & Associates, Inc, an executive search firm. She has practiced psychiatric nursing and taught both psychiatric and community health nursing. She formerly directed the master's program in community health nursing at the University of Alabama, Birmingham, and served as Dean of the School of Nursing at Wright State University in Dayton, Ohio. Her publications and presentations have been largely in the areas of community and public health nursing leadership and change and the significance of nurses to effective primary health care. Dr. Lancaster is a graduate of the University of Tennessee Health Science Center Memphis. She holds a master's degree in psychiatric nursing from Case Western Reserve University and a doctorate in public health from the University of Oklahoma. Dr. Lancaster is the author of another Elsevier publication, *Nursing Issues in Leading and Managing Change,* and the co-author with Dr. Marcia Stanhope of *Foundations of Community Health Nursing: Community-Oriented Practice.*

# ACKNOWLEDGEMENTS

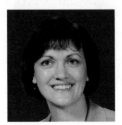

Dr. Hale holds a BSN from the University of Wisconsin-Milwaukee, an MSN and FNP from the University of Virginia, and a PhD from the University of Maryland.

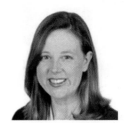

Dr. Turner holds a BSN and MSN from the University of Virginia and a PhD from the University of Kentucky.

## INTRODUCING DRS HALE AND TURNER

In this edition, we are pleased to have Professor Patty Hale, RN, FNP, PhD, FAAN, Graduate Program Director, Department of Nursing, at James Madison University, Harrisburg, Virginia, and Lisa Turner, PhD, RN, PHCNS-BC, Assistant Professor of Nursing, Berea College, Berea, Kentucky, join us in this edition of the text as Assistant Editors.

## A SPECIAL THANKS TO CONTRIBUTORS

Each edition our goal has been to offer special thanks to those who contributed to past editions of the text. To continue that tradition we want to extend heartfelt thanks to those who contributed to the 8th edition. They are Jean Bokinskie, Bonnie Jerome D'Emili, Diane Downing, James Fletcher, Karen Landenburger, Robert McKeown, Susan Patton, Molly Rose, Juliann Sebastian, Mary Silva, and Jeanne Sorrell.

*Jeanette Lancaster and Marcia Stanhope*

DEDICATIONS:
It has been my special privilege to be advised and mentored by a number of exemplary professionals and to be loved and supported by numerous friends, big and small. Their contributions have made significant differences to my life and career. This edition of the text is dedicated to the memory of Charlotte Denny and Lois Merrill, University of Kentucky; Mary Hall, Emory University; Atlanta, Dorothy Carter, my community partner, Pikeville, Kentucky, and Norma Mobley, University of Alabama, Birmingham; as well as to two special friends, John C. and CiCi.

*Marcia Stanhope*

I would like to dedicate my work on this 9th edition to my late husband, I. Wade Lancaster. He supported and encouraged me through the first eight editions of the text, and I am deeply grateful for his love, support, and encouragement.

*Jeanette Lancaster*

# CONTRIBUTORS

**Swann Arp Adams, MS, PhD**
Associate Professor
College of Nursing and the
Dept. of Epidemiology and Biostatistics
Associate Director
Cancer Prevention and Control Program
University of South Carolina
Columbia, South Carolina
*Chapter 12: Epidemiology*

**Mollie Aleshire, DNP, FNP-BC, PPCNP-BC**
Assistant Professor
University of Kentucky
College of Nursing
Lexington, Kentucky
*Chapter 28: Family Health Risks*

**Jeanne L. Alhusen, PhD, CRNP, RN**
Assistant Professor
Department of Community and Public Health
Johns Hopkins University School of Nursing
Baltimore, Maryland
*Chapter 38: Violence and Human Abuse*

**Debra Gay Anderson, PhD, PHCNS-BC**
Associate Professor
University of Kentucky
College of Nursing
Lexington, Kentucky
*Chapter 28: Family Health Risks*

**Dyan A. Aretakis, RN, FNP, MSN**
Project Director and APN3
University of Virginia Teen Health Center
Charlottesville, Virginia
*Chapter 35: Teen Pregnancy*

**Tina Bloom, PhD, MPH, RN**
Assistant Professor and Robert Wood Johnson Foundation Nurse Faculty Scholar, Sinclair School of Nursing
Columbia, Missouri
*Chapter 38: Violence and Human Abuse*

**Nisha Botchwey, PhD, MCRP, MPH**
Associate Professor of City and Regional Planning,
Georgia Institute of Technology
Affiliated Faculty,
Center for Geographic Information Systems,
Georgia Institute of Technology
Director, Research Committee, National Academy of Environmental Design
Member, Centers for Disease Control and Prevention Advisory Committee to the Director
Atlanta, Georgia
*Chapter 17: Building a Culture of Health through Community Health Promotion*

**Kathryn H. Bowles, RN, PhD, FAAN**
vanAmeringen Professor in Nursing Excellence; Director of the Center for Integrative Science in Aging; Beatrice Renfield Visiting Scholar Visiting Nurse Service of New York
Philadelphia, Pennsylvania
*Chapter 41: The Nurse in Home Health, Palliatire Care, and Hospice*

**Angeline Bushy, PhD, RN, FAAN, PHCNS-BC**
Professor & Bert Fish Chair
University of Central Florida
College of Nursing
Daytona Beach, Florida
*Chapter 19: Population-Centered Nursing in Rural and Urban Environments*

**Jacquelyn C. Campbell, PhD, RN, FAAN**
Professor
Anna D. Wolf Chair
National Program Director, Robert Wood Johnson Foundation Nurse Faculty Scholars
Department of Community-Public Health
The Johns Hopkins University
Baltimore, Maryland
*Chapter 38: Violence and Human Abuse*

**Ann H. Cary, PhD, MPH, RN, FNAP**
Professor and Dean; School of Nursing and Health Studies, University of Missouri Kansas City; Robert Wood Johnson Foundation Executive Nurse Fellow
Kansas City, Missouri
*Chapter 22: Case Management*

**Ann Connor, DNP, MSN, RN, FNP-BC**
Assistant Professor, School of Nursing
Emory University
Atlanta, Georgia
*Chapter 33: Poverty and Homelessness*

**Lois A. Davis, RN, MSN, MA**
Public Health Nursing Manager
Lexington—Fayette County Health Department in Lexington, Kentucky
*Chapter 46: Public Health Nursing at Local, State, and National Levels*

**Cynthia E. Degazon, RN, PhD**
Professor Emerita
Hunter College of the City University of New York
New York, New York
*Chapter 7: Cultural Diversity in the Community*

**Janna Dieckmann, PhD, RN**
Clinical Associate Professor
School of Nursing, University of North Carolina at Chapel Hill
Chapel Hill, North Carolina
*Chapter 2: History of Public Health and Public and Community Health Nursing*

**Sharon L. Farra, PhD, RN**
Assistant Professor of Nursing,
Wright State University
Dayton, Ohio
*Chapter 23: Public Health Nursing Practice and the Disaster Management Cycle*

**Hartley Feld, RN, MSN, PHCNS-BC**
University of Kentucky, College of Nursing
Lecturer/Clinical Instructor, Public and Community Health Nursing
University of Kentucky
Lexington, Kentucky
*Chapter 28: Family Health Risks*

**Mary E. Gibson, PhD, RN**
Associate Professor in Nursing
Assistant Director, Bjoring Center for Nursing Historical Inquiry
University of Virginia School of Nursing
Charlottesville, Virginia
*Chapter 18: Community as Client: Assessment and Analysis*

**Rosa M. Gonzalez-Guarda, PhD, MPH, RN, CPH**
Assistant Professor, Robert Wood Johnson
  Foundation Nurse Faculty Scholar,
  University of Miami School of Nursing
  and Health Studies
Coral Gables, Florida
*Chapter 38: Violence and Human Abuse*

**Monty Gross, PhD, RN, CNE, CNL**
Clinical Nurse Educator
Veterans Administration
North Las Vegas, Nevada
*Chapter 30: Major Health Issues and Chronic
  Disease Management of Adults Across the
  Life Span*

**Patty J. Hale, RN, FNP, PhD, FAAN**
Professor and Graduate Program Director
James Madison University
Harrisonburg, Virginia
*Chapter 14: Communicable and Infectious
  Disease Risks*

**Susan B. Hassmiller, PhD, RN, FAAN**
Robert Wood Johnson Foundation Senior
  Advisor for Nursing, and Director,
  Future of Nursing: Campaign for Action
Princeton, New Jersey
*Chapter 23: Public Health Nursing Practice
  and the Disaster Management Cycle*

**Anita Thompson-Heisterman, MSN, PMHCNS-BC, PMHNP-BC**
Assistant Professor
University of Virginia School of Nursing
Claude Moore Nursing Education Building
Charlottesville, Virginia
*Chapter 36: Mental Health Issues*

**DeAnne K. Hilfinger Messias, PhD, RN, FAAN**
Professor
College of Nursing and Women's and
  Gender Studies
University of South Carolina
Columbia, South Carolina
*Chapter 12: Epidemiology*

**Linda Hulton, PhD, RN**
Professor of Nursing
Coordinator of Doctor of Nursing Practice
  Program
James Madison University
Harrisonburg, Virginia
*Chapter 30: Major Health Issues and Chronic
  Disease Management of Adults Across the
  Life Span*

**Anita Hunter, PhD, APRN-CPNP**
Executive Board Member, Holy Innocents
  Children's Hospital, Inc., Mbarara, Uganda
Adjunct Professor, Washington State University
Vancouver, Washington
*Chapter 4: Perspectives in Global Health Care*

**Joanna Rowe Kaakinen, PhD, RN**
Professor, School of Nursing
Linfield College-Portland Campus
Portland, Oregon
*Chapter 27: Working with Families in the
  Community for Healthy Outcomes*

**Linda Olson Keller, DNP, CPH, APHN-BC, RN, FAAN**
Clinical Associate Professor
University of Minnesota School of Nursing
Minneapolis, Minnesota
*Chapter 9: Population-Based Public Health
  Nursing Practice: The Intervention Wheel*

**Loren Kelly, RN, MSN**
Clinical Educator Undergraduate Faculty at
  University of New Mexico College of
  Nursing
Interprofessional Education Coordinator,
  UNM College of Nursing
Albuquerque, New Mexico
*Chapter 20: Promoting Health Through
  Healthy Communities and Cities*

**Katherine K. Kinsey, PhD, RN, FAAN**
Nurse Administrator
Philadelphia Nurse-Family Partnership
Mabel Morris Family Home Visit Program
Early Childhood Initiatives
Sponsored by the National Nursing Centers
  Consortium
Philadelphia, Pennsylvania
*Chapter 21: The Nurse-led Health Center: A
  Model for Community Nursing Practice*

**Pamela A. Kulbok, DNSc, RN, PHCNS-BC, FAAN**
Theresa A. Thomas Professor of Primary
  Care Nursing and Professor of Public
  Health Sciences
Chair, Family Community, and Mental
  Health Systems
Coordinator of Public Health Nursing
  Leadership
Robert Wood Johnson Executive Nurse
  Fellow 2012-2015
University of Virginia School of Nursing
Charlottesville, Virginia
*Chapter 17: Building a Culture of Health
  through Community Health Promotion*

**Jeanette Lancaster, PhD, RN, FAAN**
Professor and Dean Emerita
School of Nursing
University of Virginia
Charlottesville, Virginia
*Chapter 11: Genomics in Public Health Nursing*

**Susan C. Long-Marin, DVM, MPH**
Epidemiology Manager
Mecklenburg County Health Department
Charlotte, North Carolina
*Chapter 13: Infectious Disease Prevention and
  Control*

**Karen S. Martin, RN, MSN, FAAN**
Health Care Consultant
Martin Associates
Omaha, Nebraska
*Chapter 41: The Nurse in Home Health,
  Palliative Care, and Hospice*

**Mary Lynn Mathre, RN, MSN, CARN**
Addictions Nurse Consultant
President, Patients Out of Time
President, American Cannabis Nurses
  Association
Howardsville, Virginia
*Chapter 37: Alcohol, Tobacco, and Other
  Drug Problems*

**Natalie McClain, PhD, RN, CPNP**
Clinical Associate Professor
Boston College
William F. Connell School of Nursing
Chestnut Hill, Massachusetts
*Chapter 44: Forensic Nursing in the Community*

**Mary Ellen T. Miller, PhD, RN**
Assistant Professor
DeSales University
Center Valley, Pennsylvania
*Chapter 21: The Nurse-led Health Center:
  A Model for Community Nursing Practice*

**Marie Napolitano, PhD, RN, FNP**
Director—Doctor of Nursing Practice
  Program
University of Portland
Portland, Oregon
*Chapter 34: Migrant Health Issues*

**Bobbie J. Perdue, RN, PhD**
Professor—Nursing
South Carolina State University
Orangeburg, South Carolina
*Chapter 7: Cultural Diversity in the Community*

**Bonnie Rogers, DrPH, COHN-S, LNCC, FAAN**
North Carolina Occupational Safety and
  Health Education and Research Center
  and the
Occupational Health Nursing Program
School of Public Health
University of North Carolina, Chapel Hill
Chapel Hill, North Carolina
*Chapter 43: The Nurse in Occupational Health*

**Cynthia Rubenstein, PhD, RN, CPNP-PC**
James Madison University
Undergraduate Program Director
Assistant Professor
Harrisonburg, Virginia
*Chapter 29: Child and Adolescent Health*

**Barbara Sattler, RN, DrPH, FAAN**
Professor, Masters of Public Health
 Program, School of Nursing and Health
 Professions, University of San Francisco
San Francisco, California
*Chapter 10: Environmental Health*

**Erika Metzler Sawin, PhD, RN**
Assistant Professor
Department of Nursing
James Madison University
Harrisonburg, Virginia
*Chapter 14: Communicable and Infectious
 Disease Risks*

**Kellie A. Smith, RN, EdD**
Assistant Professor
Thomas Jefferson University
School of Nursing
Philadelphia, Pennsylvania
*Chapter 39: The Advanced Practice Nurse in
 the Community*

**Sharon A.R. Stanley, PhD, RN, FAAN**
Visiting Professor, Wright State University
Robert Wood Johnson Executive Nurse
 Fellow, 2011-2014
Dayton, Ohio
*Chapter 23: Public Health Nursing Practice
 and the Disaster Management Cycle*

**Sharon Strang, RN, DNP, APRN, FNP-BC**
Associate Professor and Graduate Faculty
James Madison University
Dept of Nursing
Harrisonburg, Virginia
*Chapter 30: Major Health Issues and Chronic
 Disease Management of Adults Across the
 Life Span*

**Sue Strohschein, MS, RN/PHN, APRN, BC**
*Culture of Excellence* Project Coordinator
University of Minnesota
School of Nursing
Minneapolis, Minnesota
*Chapter 9: Population-Based Public Health
 Nursing Practice: The Intervention Wheel*

**Melissa Sutherland, PhD, FNP-BC**
Associate Professor
Boston College
William F. Connell School of Nursing
Chestnut Hill, Massachusetts
*Chapter 44: Forensic Nursing in the Community*

**Francisco S. Sy, MD, PhD**
Editor, *AIDS Education and Prevention—An
 Interdisciplinary Journal*; Director, Office
 of Extramural Research Administration,
 National Institute on Minority Health
 and Health Disparities, National
 Institutes of Health
Bethesda, Maryland
*Chapter 13: Infectious Disease Prevention and
 Control*

**Esther J. Thatcher, PhD, RN, APHN-BC**
Postdoctoral Fellow
School of Nursing
University of North Carolina at Chapel Hill
Chapel Hill, North Carolina
*Chapter 18: Community as Client:
 Assessment and Analysis*

**Lisa Pedersen Turner, PhD, RN, PHCNS-BC**
Assistant Professor
Berea College Nursing Program
Berea, Kentucky
*Chapter 40: The Nurse Leader in the
 Community*
*Chapter 42: The Nurse in the Schools*

**Lynn Wasserbauer, RN, FNP, PhD**
Nurse Practitioner
Behavioral Health Partners
University of Rochester Medical Center
Rochester, New York
*Chapter 31: Disability Health Care Across the
 Life Span*

**Jacqueline F. Webb, FNP-BC, MS, RN**
Assistant Professor
Linfield College School of Nursing
Portland, Oregon
*Chapter 27: Working with Families in the
 Community for Healthy Outcomes*

**Carolyn A. Williams, RN, PhD, FAAN**
Professor and Dean Emeritus
College of Nursing
University of Kentucky
Lexington, Kentucky
*Chapter 1: Community and Prevention-
 Oriented, Population-Focused Practice:
 The Foundation of Specialization in
 Public Health Nursing*

**Lisa M. Zerull, PhD, RN**
Academic Liaison and Program Manager,
 Winchester Medical Center, Valley
 Health System
Adjunct Clinical Faculty, Shenandoah
 University (Winchester, VA)
Editor, Perspectives out of the Church
 Health Center (Memphis, TN)
*Chapter 45: The Nurse in the Faith
 Community*

**Elke Jones Zschaebitz, DNP, FNP-BC**
Family Nurse Practitioner
Pediatric Primary Care Provider
Wilkerson Pediatric Clinic, Kenner Army
 Health Clinic
Ft. Lee, Virginia
And Adjunct Faculty:
Clinical Faculty Advisor, Family Nurse
 Practitioner Program
Georgetown University School of Nursing
 and Health Sciences
Washington, DC
*Chapter 11: Genomics in Public Health
 Nursing*

## ANCILLARY AUTHORS

**Patty Bollinger, MSN, APRN-CNS**
Bryan College of Health Sciences
Lincoln, Nebraska
*TEACH/Powerpoint reviewer*

**Joanna E. Cain, BSN, BA, RN**
President and Founder of Auctorial
 Pursuits, Inc.
Atlanta, Georgia
*Student Case Studies*
*Review Questions*
*Answer Key for Review Questions*

**Linda Turchin, RN, MSN, CNE**
Assistant Professor of Nursing
Fairmont State University
Fairmont, West Virginia
*Test Bank Reviewer*

**Anna K. Wehling Weepie, DNP, RN, CNE**
Associate Professor
Allen College
Waterloo, Iowa
*Test Bank Writer*

**Linda Wendling, MS, MFA**
Learning Theory Consultant
University of Missouri—St. Louis
St. Louis, Missouri
*TEACH for Nurses*
*Power Point Lecture Slides*

# PREFACE

Since the last edition of this text, many changes have occurred in society as well as in health care. The rapid and often startling changes in society are influencing the amount and ways in which health care is delivered. Many of the industrialized nations around the world are engaged in health care reform, and a major driver for reform is the enormous cost of providing health care to citizens. The human, financial, infrastructure, and other costs associated with war, natural and human-made diseases, and civil uprising continue to affect many nations, including the United States. The world, as many people know, has changed dramatically in the past few decades because of such disruptions as war, hurricanes and tsunamis, terrorism, earthquakes, floods, and tornados that have cost lives, homes, and livelihoods. These destructive events have had enormous costs in terms of money and the damage to individuals, families, and communities. The need for stronger public health resources has grown as these disruptions have occurred in the United States and many other countries. Public health professionals play a key role in helping communities deal with both emergency and non-emergency aspects of their lives.

As is explained in Chapter 1 and discussed in other chapters throughout the text, there are three core functions of public health: assessment, policy development, and assurance. The Centers for Disease Control and Prevention (CDC, 2014, p. 1) have developed 10 essential public health services, and the list below aligns these services with the core functions:

## ASSESSMENT

1. Monitor health status to identify and solve community environmental health problems.
2. Diagnose and investigate health problems and health hazards in the community.

## POLICY DEVELOPMENT

3. Inform, educate, and empower people about health issues.
4. Mobilize community partnerships and actions to identify and solve health problems.
5. Develop policies and plans that support individual and community health efforts.

## ASSURANCE

6. Enforce laws and regulations that protect health and ensure safety.
7. Link people to needed health services and assure the provision of health services when otherwise unavailable.
8. Assure competent public and personal health care workforce.
9. Evaluate effectiveness, accessibility, and quality of personal and population-based health services.
10. Research for new insights and innovative solutions to health problems (CDC, 2014, p. 1).

Chapters in this text include all of the critical roles listed above as well as guidance in how to deal with other major issues, including the quality of care, the cost of care, and access to care. The growing shortage of nurses and other health care providers will only increase the concerns about these issues. One of the ways in which quality of care could be improved would include new uses of technology to manage an information revolution. Great improvements in quality would require a restructuring of how care is delivered, a shift in how funds are spent, changing the workplace, and using more effective ways to manage chronic illness. There will be costs associated with these quality improvements.

The United States' health care spending has slowed in recent years due to the economy. In 2013, the health care costs were at about 1.2 trillion dollars, or 16.7% of the gross domestic product. After the implementation of the Affordable Care Act, the numbers of unisured dropped from 48 million to 41 million by 2013 (KFF 2014). However, the cost burden to employers and consumers needs to be explored to see if there has been any change. This number of uninsured is larger than the population of either Canada or Australia. Despite spending more money per person in the United States for illness care than any other country, Americans are not the healthiest of all people. The infant mortality and life expectancy rates—indexes of health care—while improving, are not close to what they should be given the amount spent on health care. Some of the most important factors leading to the high health care costs are diagnostic and treatment technologies, drugs, an aging population, more chronic illness, shortages in health care workers, and medical-legal costs. Lifestyle continues to play a big role in morbidity and mortality. It is embarrassing that, overall, citizens in the United States are the most obese citizens in any industrialized nation. In addition, half of all deaths are still caused by tobacco, alcohol, and illegal drug use; diet and activity patterns; microbial agents; toxic agents; firearms; sexual behavior; and motor vehicle accidents.

In the past two decades the greatest improvements in population health have come from public health achievements such as immunizations leading to eliminating and controlling infectious diseases, motor vehicle safety, safer workplaces, lifestyle improvements reducing the risk of heart disease and strokes, safer and healthier foods through improved sanitation, clean water and food fortification programs, better hygiene and nutrition to improve the health of mothers and babies, family planning, fluoride in drinking water, and recognition of tobacco as a health hazard. Continued changes in the public health system are essential if death, illness, and disability resulting from preventable problems are to continue to decline.

The need to focus attention on health promotion, lifestyle factors, and disease prevention led to the development of a major public policy about health for the nation. This policy was designed by a large number of people representing a wide range of groups interested in health. The policy, first introduced in

1979, was updated in 1990 and in 2000; it is reflected in the most recent document updated in 2010, titled *Healthy People 2020*. These four documents have identified a set of national health promotion and disease prevention objectives for each of four decades. Examples of these objectives are highlighted in chapters throughout the text.

The most effective disease prevention and health promotion strategies designed to achieve the goals and objectives of *Healthy People 2020* are developed through partnerships between government, businesses, voluntary organizations, consumers, communities, and health care providers. According to *Healthy People 2020*, the partners who join a newly established consortium will work to achieve the goals and objectives of *Healthy People 2020*.

*Healthy People 2020* emphasizes the concept of social determinants of health—that is, the belief that health is affected by many social, economic, and environmental factors that extend far beyond individual biology of disease. This means that improving health requires a broad approach to including the concept of health in all policies and creating environments where the healthy choice is the easy choice. To develop healthy communities, individuals, families, communities, and populations must commit to these approaches. Also, society, through the development of health policy, must support better health care, the design of improved health education, and new ways of financing strategies to alter health status.

The regrettable fact is that few health indicators have been substantially improved since *Healthy People 2010* was released in 2000. *Healthy People 2020* retains many of the original objectives and adds new ones. What does this mean for nurses who work in public health? Because people do not always know how to improve their health status, the challenge of nursing is to create change. Nursing takes place in a variety of public and private settings and includes disease prevention, health promotion, health protection, surveillance, education, maintenance, restoration, coordination, management, and evaluation of care of individuals, families, and populations, including communities.

To meet the demands of a constantly changing health care system, nurses must have vision in designing new and changing current roles and identifying their practice areas. To do so effectively, the nurse must understand concepts, theories, and the core content of public health, the changing health care system, the actual and potential roles and responsibilities of nurses and other health care providers, the importance of health promotion and disease orientation, and the necessity of involving consumers in the planning, implementation, and evaluation of health care efforts.

Since its initial publication in 1984, this text has been widely accepted and is popular among nursing students and nursing faculty in baccalaureate, BSN-completion, and graduate programs. The text was written to provide nursing students and practicing nurses with a comprehensive source book that provides a foundation for designing population-centered nursing strategies for individuals, families, aggregates, populations, and communities. The unifying theme for the book is the integrating of health promotion and disease prevention concepts into the many roles of nurses. The prevention focus emphasizes traditional public health practice with increased attention to the effects of the internal and external environment on health of communities. The focus on interventions for the individual and family emphasizes the aspects of population-centered practice with attention to the effects of all of the determinants of health, including lifestyle, on personal health.

## CONCEPTUAL APPROACH TO THIS TEXT

The term *community-oriented* has been used to reflect the orientation of nurses to the community and the public's health. In 1998, the Quad Council of Public Health Nursing comprised of members from the American Nurses Association Congress on Nursing Practice, the American Public Health Association Public Health Nursing section, the Association of Community Health Nursing Educators, and the Association of State and Territorial Directors of Public Health Nursing developed a statement on the *Scope of Public Health Nursing Practice*. Through this statement, the leaders in public and community health nursing attempted to clarify the differences between public health nursing and the newest term introduced into nursing's vocabulary during health care reform of the 1990s, *community-based nursing*. The Quad Council recognized that the terms *public health nursing* and *community health nursing* have been used interchangeably since the 1980s to describe population-focused, community-oriented nursing and community-focused practice. They decided to make a clearer distinction between community-oriented and community-based nursing practice. In 2007, the definitions were further refined, and nurses once referred to as *public health nurses* and *community health nurses* are now referred to only as *public health nurses* in the revised standards of practice.

In this textbook, two different levels of care in the community are acknowledged: community-oriented care and community-based care. Two role functions for nursing practice in the community are suggested: public health nursing (community health nursing) and community-based nursing. This text focuses only on public health nursing (community health nursing), using the term *community-oriented nursing*, which encompasses a focus on populations within the community context or *population-centered nursing practice*.

For the fifth edition of this text, with consultation from C. A. Williams (author) and June Thompson (Mosby editor), Marcia Stanhope developed a conceptual model for community-oriented nursing practice. This model was influenced by a review of the history of community-oriented nursing from the 1800s to today. Marcia Stanhope studied Betty Neuman's model intensively while in school, which influenced this model.

The model itself is presented as a caricature of reality—or an abstract—with a description of the characteristics and the philosophy on which community-oriented nursing is built. The *model* is shown as a flying balloon (see inside front cover of this book). The balloon represents community-oriented nursing and is filled with the knowledge, skills, and abilities needed in this practice to carry the world (the basket of the balloon) or the clients of the world who benefit from this practice.

The *subconcepts* of public health nursing with the community and populations as the center of care are the *boundaries* of the practice. The public health foundation pillars of assurance, assessment, and policy development hold up the world of communities, where people live, work, play, go to school, and worship. The ribbons flying from the balloon indicate the interventions used by nurses. These ribbons (interventions) serve to provide lift and direction, tying the services together for the clients who are served. The intervention names and the services are listed on the inside cover of this book. The *propositions* (statements of relationship) for this model are found in the definitions of practice, public health functions, clients served, specific settings, interventions, and services. Many *assumptions* have served as the basis for the development of this model. Community-oriented nursing is a specialty within the nursing discipline. The practice has evolved over time, becoming more complex. The practice of nursing in public health is based on a philosophy of care rather than being setting specific. It is different from community-based nursing care delivery. The development of community-oriented nursing has been influenced by public health practice, preventive medicine, community medicine, and shifts in the health care delivery system. Community-oriented nursing requires nurses to have specific competencies to be effective providers of care.

The definition of community-oriented nursing appears on the inside front cover of this book. This practice involves public health nurses. Community-based nurses differ from community-oriented nurses in many ways. These differences are described in the table following the definitions. The differences are described as they relate to philosophy of care, goals, service, community, clients served, practice settings, ways of interacting with clients, type of services offered to clients, prevention levels used, goals, and priority of nurses' activities.

The four concepts of nursing, person (client), environment, and health are described for this model. These concepts appear in many works about nursing and in almost every educational curriculum for undergraduate students. Each of the four concepts may be defined differently in these works because of the beliefs of the persons writing the definitions.

In this text *nursing* is defined as community-oriented with a focus on providing health care through community diagnosis and investigation of major health and environmental problems. Health surveillance, monitoring, and evaluating community and population status are done to prevent disease and disability and to promote, protect, preserve, restore, and maintain health. This in turn creates conditions in which clients can be healthy. The person, or client, is the world, nation, state, community, population, aggregate, family, or individual.

The boundaries of the client *environment* may be limited by the world, nation, state, locality, home, school, work, playground, religion, or individual self. *Health,* in this model, involves a continuum of health rather than wellness, with the best health state possible as the goal. The best possible level of health is achieved through measures of prevention as practiced by the nurse.

The nurse engages in autonomous practice with the client, who is the primary decision maker about health issues. The nurse practices in a variety of environments, including, but not limited to, governments, organizations, homes, schools, churches, neighborhoods, industry, and community boards. The nurse interacts with diverse cultures, partners, other providers in teams, multiple clients, and one-to-one or aggregate relationships. Clients at risk for the development of health problems are a major focus of nursing services. Primary prevention–level strategies are the key to reducing risk of health problems. Secondary prevention is done to maintain, promote, or protect health, whereas tertiary prevention strategies are used to preserve, protect, or maintain health.

The community-oriented nurse has many roles related to community clients and roles that relate specifically to practice with populations (or population-centered). Community-oriented nurses engage in activities specific to community development, assessment, monitoring, health policy, politics, health education, interdisciplinary practice, program management, community/population advocacy, case finding, and delivery of personal health services when these services are otherwise unavailable in the health care system. This conceptual model is the framework for this text.

## ORGANIZATION

The text is divided into seven sections:

- **Part 1, Influencing Factors in Health Care and Population-Centered Nursing,** describes the historical and current status of the health care delivery system and public health nursing practice, both domestically and internationally.
- **Part 2, Forces Affecting Health Care Delivery and Population-Centered Nursing,** addresses the economics, ethics, policy, and cultural issues that affect public health, nurses, and clients.
- **Part 3, Conceptual and Scientific Frameworks Applied to Population-Centered Nursing Practice,** provides conceptual models and scientific bases for public health nursing practice. Selected models from nursing and related sciences are also discussed.
- **Part 4, Issues and Approaches in Population-Centered Nursing,** examines the management of health care, quality and safety, and populations in select community environments and groups, as well as issues related to managing cases, programs, and disasters.
- **Part 5, Health Promotion with Target Populations Across the Life Span,** discusses risk factors and population-level health problems for families and individuals throughout the life span.
- **Part 6, Promoting and Protecting the Health of Vulnerable Populations,** covers specific health care needs and issues of populations at risk.
- **Part 7, Nurses' Roles and Functions in the Community,** examines diversity in the role of public health nurses and describes the rapidly changing roles, functions, and practice settings.

## NEW TO THIS EDITION

New content has been included in the ninth edition of *Public Health Nursing: Population-Centered Health Care in the Community* to ensure that the text remains a complete and comprehensive resource:

- **NEW!** In each chapter, content is applied to Quality and Safety Education for Nurses (QSEN).

## PEDAGOGY

Other key features of this edition are detailed below. Each chapter is organized for easy use by students and faculty.

### Additional Resources

Additional Resources listed at the beginning of each chapter direct students to chapter-related tools and resources contained in the book's Appendixes or on its Evolve website.

### Objectives

Objectives open each chapter to guide student learning and alert faculty to what students should gain from the content.

### Key Terms

Key Terms are identified at the beginning of the chapter and defined either within the chapter or in the glossary to assist students in understanding unfamiliar terminology.

### Chapter Outline

The Chapter Outline alerts students to the structure and content of the chapter.

### How To Boxes

How To boxes provide specific, application-oriented information.

### Evidence-Based Practice Boxes

Evidence-Based Practice boxes in each chapter illustrate the use and application of the latest research findings in public health, community health, and community-oriented nursing.

### Practice Application

At the end of each chapter a case situation helps students understand how to apply chapter content in the practice setting. Questions at the end of each case promote critical thinking while students analyze the case.

### Key Points

Key Points provide a summary listing of the most important points made in the chapter.

### Clinical Decision-Making Activities

Clinical Decision-Making Activities promote student learning by suggesting a variety of activities that encourage both independent and collaborative effort.

### Appendixes

The **Appendixes** provide additional content resources, key information, and clinical tools and references.

## EVOLVE STUDENT LEARNING RESOURCES

Additional resources designed to supplement the student learning process are available on this book's website at http://evolve. elsevier.com/Stanhope, including:

- **Additional Resources for Students** in select chapters
- **Answer Key to Review Questions** with suggested solutions to the Practice Application questions at the end of each chapter
- **Audio Glossary** with complete definitions of all key terms and other important community and public health nursing concepts
- **Review Questions** questions with answers
- **Student Case Studies** with questions and answers

## INSTRUCTOR RESOURCES

Several supplemental ancillaries are available to assist instructors in the teaching process:

- **TEACH for Nurses lesson plans** provided for each chapter, with Nursing Curriculum Standards, Teaching Strategies and Learning Activities, Case Studies, and more
- **Test Bank** with 1200 NCLEX®-style questions and answers
- **PowerPoint Lecture Slides** for each chapter
- **Image Collection** with illustrations from the text
- **Answers to Practice Application Questions**
- **Audio Glossary**

## REFERENCES

Centers for Disease Control and Prevention: *Ten Great Public Health Achievements in the 20th Century.* Retrieved from: www.cdc.gov/about/history/tengpha.htm. 10/28/14.

Centers for Disease Control and Prevention, 2014, p. 1. *The public health system and the 10 essential public health services.* Available at http://www.cdc.gov/nphpsp/

essentialservices.html. Retrived 4/28/15.

Centers for Medicare and Medicaid Services (CMS): *Office of the Actuary: National Health Expenditure Projections 2011-2021.* Baltimore, MD, 2012a, U.S.Department of Health and Human Services. Retrieved from: http://www.cms

.gov/NationalHealthExpendData/. December 2014.

DeNavas-Walt C, Proctor BD, Smith JC: *Income, Poverty, and Health Insurance Coverage in the United States, 2012.* U.S. Census Bureau, Current Population Reports. Washington, DC, 2013, U.S. Government Printing Office, pp P60–P245.

Kaiser Family Foundation: *The unisured a primer: key facts about Americans without health insurance.* Menlo Park Calif. 2012a.

U.S. Department of Health and Human Services (USDHHS): *Healthy People 2020: A Roadmap to Improve All American's Health.* Washington, DC, 2010, USDHHS, Public Health Service.

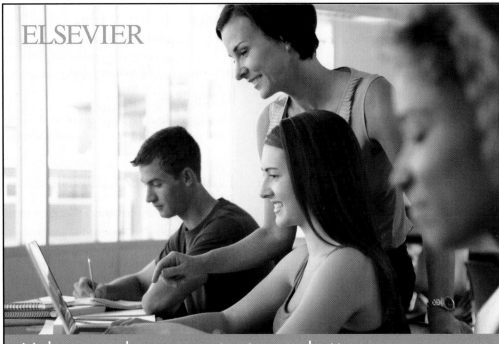

# CONTENTS

# PART 1

# Influencing Factors in Health Care and Population-Centered Nursing

Population-centered nursing emphasizes the community where nursing is based in the population providing care on-site to individuals or group members of the population. It also emphasizes a focus on a defined population whereby the nurse seeks knowledge about the health issues or problems facing the total population so the nurse can then find ways to resolve the issues and problems for all members of the population. The focused approach seeks to improve health for all within the community's population. In this section information emerges to show how community-based nursing and community oriented (focused) nursing are different in approach but similar in the goal to improve health for the populations served.

Since the late 1800s, public health nurses have been leaders in making improvements in the quality of health care for individuals, families, and aggregates, including populations and communities. As nurses around the world collaborate with one another, it is clear that, from one country to another, population-centered nursing has more similarities than differences.

Important changes in health care have been taking place since the early 1990s, and there is data to show that changes are occurring as a result of the health care reform work in the United States. Although considerable controversy surrounded the implementation of the Patient Protection and Affordable Care Act of 2010, it is clear that change is providing more access to care and reductions in hospitalization. It is also reducing cost and providing more preventive care.

The areas in health care that have posed the greatest problems for persons over the years have been access, quality, and cost. These problems are being addressed but are still present. A number of people still have either no insurance or inadequate insurance, access to quality care is unevenly distributed across the country, and the cost of health care remains high for consumers, employers, insurers, and state and federal governments. Changes in the health care system and delivery are attempting to address these issues.

Some of the key areas of emphasis in the current efforts to reform health care include preventing disease, coordinating care, and shifting care from the hospital to the home or community facilities where possible. In the coming years, a large growth in the number of nurses employed in home health care and in nursing care facilities is expected. An area targeted for growth is that of the federal community health centers. Nurses comprise the largest category of employees in those centers. It is also expected that more new graduates will go directly into community health work rather than working for a few years in the hospital before making that transition. This trend supports the recommendations that nurses need to be prepared at the baccalaureate level.

Over the years, funding for public health has decreased, or remained neutral, while the needs for population-centered services have increased. The key question is whether health care reform will provide what is needed for population-centered care in America's communities. There is much discussion about the new emphasis on prevention, community-oriented care, continuity, and the important role that nurses will play in health care. With anticipation that many of these projections will become a reality and that nurses will become increasingly key practitioners in promoting the health of the people, they must understand the history of public health nursing and the current status of the public health system.

Part One presents information about significant factors affecting health in the United States. Changing the level and quality of services and the priorities for funding requires that nurses be involved, informed, courageous, and committed to the task. The chapters in Part One are designed to provide essential information so that nurses can make a difference in health care by understanding their own roles and their functions in population-centered practice. Understanding how the public health system differs from the primary care system is described as well as the movement to integrate public health and primary care.

There is a core of knowledge known as "public health" that forms the foundation for population-centered public health nursing. This core has historically included epidemiology, biostatistics, environmental health, health services administration, and social and behavioral sciences. In recent years, new areas of focus within public health have included informatics, genomics, communication, cultural competence, community-based participatory research, evidence-based practice, policy and law, global health, ethics, and forensics. This book covers both the traditional and the newer content either in a full chapter or as a section in one or more chapters.

# Community and Prevention–Oriented, Population-Focused Practice: The Foundation of Specialization in Public Health Nursing

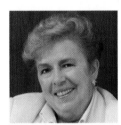

## Carolyn A. Williams, RN, PhD, FAAN

Dr. Carolyn A. Williams is Dean Emeritus and Professor at the College of Nursing at the University of Kentucky, Lexington, Kentucky. Dr. Williams began her career as a public health nurse. She has held many leadership roles, including President of the American Academy of Nursing; membership on the first U.S. Preventive Services Task Force, Department of Health and Human Services; and President of the American Association of Colleges of Nursing. She received the Distinguished Alumna Award from Texas Woman's University in 1983. In 2001 she was the recipient of the Mary Tolle Wright Founder's Award for Excellence in Leadership from Sigma Theta Tau International, and in 2007 she received the Bernadette Arminger Award from the American Association of Colleges of Nursing. In 2011 she was awarded an Honorary Doctorate of Public Service from the University of Portland, Portland, Oregon. In 2014 she received the honor of being conducted into the University of Kentucky College of Public Health Hall of Fame for international, national, state and local contributions to public health and nursing.

## ADDITIONAL RESOURCES

- ⓔ **Evolve Website http://evolve.elsevier.com/Stanhope**
- Healthy People 2020
- WebLinks—Of special note, see the link for this site:
  - Guide to Community Preventive Services
- Quiz
- Case Studies
- Glossary
- Answers to Practice Application

- Resource Tools
  - Resource Tool 5.A: Schedule of Clinical Preventive Services
  - Resource Tool 46: Core Competencies and Skill Levels for Public Health Nursing
- Appendixes
  - Appendix G.1: Examples of Public Health Nursing Roles and Implementing Public Health Functions

## OBJECTIVES

*After reading this chapter, the student should be able to do the following:*

1. State the mission of and core functions of public health and the essential public health services and the quality performance standards program in public health.
2. Describe specialization in public health nursing and other nurse roles in the community and the practice goals of each.
3. Contrast clinical nursing practice with population focused practice in the community.
4. Describe what is meant by community and prevention–oriented, population-focused practice.
5. Name barriers to acceptance of community and prevention–oriented, population-focused practice.
6. State key opportunities for community and prevention–oriented, population-focused practice.

## KEY TERMS

The second decade of the twenty-first century finds the United States entering an era when more public attention is being given to efforts to protect and improve the health of the American people and the environment. Despite what many see as a failure to make fundamental changes in the delivery and financing of health care, significant change has occurred. Federal and state initiatives, private market forces, the development of new scientific knowledge and new technologies, and the expectations of the public are bringing about changes in the health care system. With the national legislation that passed in 2010—the Patient Protection and Affordable Care Act (ACA) (www.hhs.gov/opa/affordable-care-act)—which in part was designed to increase access to care; concerns have been raised about the availability of adequate numbers of professional personnel to provide services, particularly in primary care and strained health care facilities. Despite initial turbulence in implementation of the legislation, including difficulties with enrollments due to technological problems, initial reports are that good progress has been made in enrolling people and the Congressional Budget Office projected that by 2014 the number of uninsured people will decrease by 12 million and by 26 million by 2017 (Blumenthal and Collins, 2014). Blumenthal and Collins (2014) also reported that the Urban Institute projected that the proportion of uninsured people adults in the United States fell from 18% in the third quarter of 2013 to 13.4% in May of 2014. Before the passage of the ACA many at the national level were seriously concerned about the growing cost of medical care as a part of federal expenditures (Orszag, 2007; Orszag and Emanuel, 2010). The concern with the cost of medical care remains a national issue and Blumenthal and Collins (2014) argue that the sustainability of the expansions of coverage provided by the ACA will depend on whether the overall costs of care in the United States can be controlled. If costs are not controlled the resulting increases in premiums will become increasingly difficult for all—consumers, employers, and the federal government. Other health system concerns focus on the quality and safety of services, warnings about bioterrorism, and global public health threats such as infectious diseases and contaminated foods. Because of all of these factors, the role of public health in protecting and promoting health, as well as preventing disease and disability, is extremely important.

Whereas the majority of national attention and debate surrounding national health legislation has been focused primarily on insurance issues related to medical care, there are indications of a renewed interest in public health and in population-focused thinking about health and health care in the United States. For example, incorporated into the Patient Protection and Affordable Care Act are provisions that address health promotion and prevention of disease and disability. These include (1) establishment of the National Prevention, Health Promotion, and Public Health Council to coordinate federal prevention, wellness, and public health activities and to develop a national strategy to improve the nation's health (www.surgeongeneral.gov/initiatives/prevention/about), and (2) as indicated in Chapter 3 and 5, creation of a Prevention and Public Health Fund to expand and sustain funding for prevention and public health programs (Trust for America's Health, 2013), and (3) improvement of preventive efforts by covering only proven preventive services and eliminating state cost sharing for preventive services, including immunizations recommended by the U.S. Preventive Services Task Force (USPHS 2000) (www.uspreventiveservicestaskforce.org). Also, grants and technical assistance will be available to employers who establish wellness programs (www.dol.gov/ebsa/newsroom/2013/13).

Although populations have historically been the focus of public health practice, specifically defined populations are becoming a focus of the "business" of managed care; therefore more managed care executives are joining public health practitioners in becoming population oriented. Increasingly, managed care executives and program managers are using the basic sciences and analytic tools of the field of public health. However, their focus is on using such epidemiological and statistical strategies to develop databases and analytical approaches to making decisions at the level of a defined population or subpopulation enrolled in a particular care delivery organization or those covered by a particular insurance company. A population-focused approach to planning, delivering, and evaluating various aspects of care delivery is increasingly being used in an effort to achieve better outcomes in the population of interest and has never been more important.

Where is public health nursing in all of the changes swirling around in the world of health and health care? This is a crucial

*Lifespan Aug ↓*

time for public health nursing, a time of opportunity and challenge. The issue of growing costs together with the changing demography of the U.S. population, particularly the aging of the population, is expected to put increased demands on resources available for health care. In addition, the threats of bioterrorism, highlighted by the events of September 11, 2001, and the anthrax scares, will divert health care funds and resources from other health care programs to be spent for public safety. Also important to the public health community is the emergence of modern-day epidemics (such as the mosquito-borne West Nile virus, the H1N1 influenza virus, and the emerging Ebola virus crisis) and globally induced infectious diseases such as avian influenza and other causes of mortality, many of which affect the very young (see Chapters 3 and 5). Most of the causes of these epidemics are preventable. What has all of this to do with nursing?

Understanding the importance of community-oriented, population-focused nursing practice and developing the knowledge and skills to practice it will be critical to attaining a leadership role in health care regardless of the practice setting. The following discussion explains why those who practice community-based, prevention-oriented, population-focused nursing will be in a very strong position to affect the health of populations and decisions about how scarce resources will be used.

## PUBLIC HEALTH PRACTICE: THE FOUNDATION FOR HEALTHY POPULATIONS AND COMMUNITIES

During the last 25 years, considerable attention has been focused on proposals to reform the American health care system. These proposals focused primarily on containing cost in medical care financing and on strategies for providing health insurance coverage to a higher proportion of the population. In the national health legislation that passed in 2010, the Patient Protection and Affordable Care Act, the majority of the provisions and the vast majority of the discussion of the bill focused on those issues (www.hhs.gov/opa/affordable-care-act).

Because physician services and hospital care combined account for over half of the health care expenditures in the United States, it is understandable that changes in how such services would be paid for would receive much attention (kaiserEDU.org, 2010). However, as stated in the Public Health Functions Steering Committee Report on the Core Functions of Public Health (1998), while it was important to make reforms in the medical insurance system there is a clear understanding among those familiar with the history of public health and its impact that such reforms alone will not be adequate to improve the health of Americans.

Historically, gains in the health of populations have come largely from public health efforts. Safety and adequacy of food supplies, the provision of safe water, sewage disposal, public safety from biological threats, and personal behavioral changes, including reproductive behavior, are a few examples of public health's influence. In 2008 Fielding and colleagues argued that

there is incontrovertible evidence that public health policies and programs were primarily responsible for increasing the average life span from 47 in 1900 to 78 in 2005, an increase of 66% in just a little over a century. They asserted that most of that increase was through improvements in sanitation, clean water supplies, making workplaces safer, improving food and drug safety, immunizing children, and improving nutrition, hygiene, and housing (Fielding et al, 2008).

In an effort to help the public better understand the role public health has played in increasing life expectancy and improving the nation's health, in 1999 the Centers for Disease Control and Prevention (CDC) began featuring information on the Ten Great Public Health Achievements in the $20^{th}$ Century. The areas featured include Immunizations, Motor Vehicle Safety, Control of Infectious Diseases, Safer and Healthier Foods, Healthier Mothers and Babies, Family Planning, Fluoridation of Drinking Water, Tobacco as a Health Hazard, and Declines in Deaths from Heart Disease and Stroke (CDC, 2014). A case can be made that the payoff from public health activities is well beyond the resources directed to the effort. For example, recent data reported by the Centers for Medicare and Medicaid Services (CMS) showed that in 2012 only 3% (up from 1.5% in 1960) of all national expenditures supported by governmental entities supported public health functions (CMS, 2012). The expeditures in 2014 were the same.

Unfortunately, the public is largely unaware of the contributions of public health practice. After the passage of Medicare and Medicaid, federal and private monies in support of public health dwindled, public health agencies began to provide personal care services for persons who could not receive care elsewhere, and the health departments benefited by getting Medicaid and Medicare funds. The result was a shift of resources and energy away from public health's traditional and unique prevention-oriented, population-focused perspective to include a primary care focus (U.S. Department of Health and Human Services [USDHHS], 2002).

One consequence of a successful implementation of the Affordable Care Act might actually be that the majority of the population would be covered by insurance and public health agencies will not need to provide direct clinical services in order to assure that those who need them can receive them. If this occurs public health organizations can refocus their efforts on the core functions and emphasize community-oriented, population-focused health promotion and preventive strategies, if ways can be found to finance such efforts. An Institute of Medicine report, *For the Public's Health: Investing in a Healthier Future*, released in 2012, began with presentation of data showing that in comparison with other wealthy Western countries the United States lags well behind its peers on health status while outspending every country in the world on health. However, a key message was that health-related spending in the United States is primarily expended on clinical care costs for medical and hospital services; very little spending is for public health activities.

A central conclusion of the report was that "to improve health outcomes in the United States, there will need to be a transforming of the way the nation invests in health to pay more attention to population-based prevention efforts; remedy the dysfunctional manner in which public health funding is allocated, structured, and used; and ensure stable funding for public health departments." Further, the committee recommended that "a minimum package of public health services—those foundational and programmatic services needed to promote and protect the public's health" be developed. The report concluded by recommending that "Congress authorize a dedicated, stable, and long-term financing structure—a national tax on all health care transactions—to generate the enhanced federal revenue required to deliver the minimum package of public health services in every community" (Institute of Medicine [IOM], 2012a).

## Definitions in Public Health

In 1988 the Institute of Medicine published a report on the future of public health, which is now seen as a classic and influential document. In the report, public health was defined as "what we, as a society, do collectively to assure the conditions in which people can be healthy" (IOM, 1988, p. 1). The committee stated that the mission of public health was "to generate organized community efforts to address the public interest in health by applying scientific and technical knowledge to prevent disease and promote health" (IOM, 1988, p. 1; Williams, 1995).

It was clearly noted that the mission could be accomplished by many groups, public and private, and by individuals. However, the government has a special function "to see to it that vital elements are in place and that the mission is adequately addressed" (IOM, 1988, p. 7). To clarify the government's role in fulfilling the mission, the report stated that assessment, policy development, and assurance are the public health core functions at all levels of government.

- **Assessment** refers to systematically collecting data on the population, monitoring the population's health status, and making information available about the health of the community.
- **Policy development** refers to the need to provide leadership in developing policies that support the health of the population, including the use of the scientific knowledge base in making decisions about policy.
- **Assurance** refers to the role of public health in ensuring that essential community-oriented health services are available, which may include providing essential personal health services for those who would otherwise not receive them. Assurance also refers to making sure that a competent public health and personal health care workforce is available. Fielding (2009) subsequently made the case that assurance also should mean that public health officials should be involved in developing and monitoring the quality of services provided.

Because of the importance of influencing a population's health and providing a strong foundation for the health care system, the U.S. Public Health Service and other groups strongly advocated a renewed emphasis on the population-focused essential public health functions and services that have been most effective in improving the health of the entire population.

As part of this effort, a statement on public health in the United States was developed by a working group made up of representatives of federal agencies and organizations concerned about public health. The list of essential services presented in Figure 1-1 represents the obligations of the public health system to implement the core functions of assessment, assurance, and policy development. The How To Box further explains these essential services and lists the ways public health nurses implement them (U.S. Public Health Service, 1994 [updated 2008]).

## Public Health Core Functions

The Core Functions Project (U.S. Public Health Service, 1994 [updated 2008]) developed a useful illustration, the Health Services Pyramid (Figure 1-2), which shows that population-based public health programs support the goals of providing a foundation for clinical preventive services. These services focus on disease prevention; on health promotion and protection; and on primary, secondary, and tertiary health care services. All levels of services shown in the pyramid are important to the health of the population and thus must be part of a health care system with health as a goal. It has been said that "the greater the effectiveness of services in the lower tiers, the greater is the capability of higher tiers to contribute efficiently to health improvement" (U.S. Public Health Service, 1994 [updated 2008]). Because of the importance of the basic public health programs, members of the Core Functions Project argued that all levels of health care, including population-based public health care, must be funded or the goal of health of populations may never be reached.

Several new efforts to enable public health practitioners to be more effective in implementing the core functions of assessment, policy development, and assurance have been undertaken at the national level. In 1997 the Institute of Medicine published *Improving Health in the Community: A Role for Performance Monitoring* (IOM, 1997). This monograph was the product of an interdisciplinary committee, cochaired by a public health nursing specialist and a physician, whose purpose was to determine how a performance monitoring system could be developed and used to improve community health.

The major outcome of the committee's work was the Community Health Improvement Process (CHIP), a method for improving the health of the population on a community-wide basis. The method brings together key elements of the public health and personal health care systems in one framework. A second outcome of the project was the development of a set of 25 indicators that could be used in the community assessment process (see Chapter 18) to develop a community health profile (e.g., measures of health status, functional status, quality of life, health risk factors, and health resource use) (Box 1-1). A third product of the committee's work was a set of indicators for specific public health problems that could be used by public health specialists as they carry out their assurance function and monitor the performance of public health and other agencies.

In 2000 the CDC established a Task Force on Community Preventive Services, which is in place and works to provide evidence-based findings and recommendations about a variety of community preventive services, programs, and policies to prevent morbidity and mortality (CDC, 2014b). The result

PUBLIC HEALTH IN AMERICA

**Vision:**
Healthy people in healthy communities

**Mission:**
Promote physical and mental health and
prevent disease, injury, and disability

**Public health**
- Prevents epidemics and the spread of disease
- Protects against environmental hazards
- Prevents injuries
- Promotes and encourages healthy behaviors
- Responds to disasters and assists communities in recovery
- Ensures the quality and accessibility of health services

**Essential public health services by core function**
*Assessment*
1. Monitor health status to identify community health problems
2. Diagnose and investigate health problems and health hazards in the community

*Policy Development*
3. Inform, educate, and empower people about health issues
4. Mobilize community partnerships to identify and solve health problems
5. Develop policies and plans that support individual and community health efforts

*Assurance*
6. Enforce laws and regulations that protect health and ensure safety
7. Link people to needed personal health services and assure the provision of health care when otherwise unavailable
8. Assure a competent public health and personal health care workforce
9. Evaluate effectiveness, accessibility, and quality of personal and population-based health services

*Serving All Functions*
10. Research for new insights and innovative solutions to health problems

**FIG 1-1** Public health in America. (From U.S. Public Health Service: *The Core Functions Project.* Washington, DC, 1994/update 2000, DC, Office of Disease Prevention and Health Promotion. Update 2008.)

is *The Community Guide: What Works to Promote Health*, a versatile set of resources available electronically at www.thecommunityguide.org/index.html that can be used by public health specialists and others interested in a community-level approach to health improvement and disease prevention. Information is available on 22 topics, which include health problems/issues such as obesity, mental health, asthma, cancer, diabetes, and concerns such as violence, tobacco, nutrition, vaccination, excessive consumption of alcohol, motor vehicle injury, emergency preparedness, and worksite initiatives (CDC, 2014b). The materials, which include systematic reviews of research, can be used to help make choices about policies and programs that have been shown to be effective (CDC, 2014b). Community Preventive Services are important because they provide tools for

public health practitioners, many of whom are public health nursing specialists, to enable them to be more effective in dealing with the core functions.

## Core Competencies of Public Health Professionals

To improve the public health workforce's abilities to implement the core functions of public health and to ensure that the workforce has the necessary skills to provide the 10 essential services listed in Figure 1-1, a coalition of representatives from 17 national public health organizations (the Council of Linkages) began working in 1992 on collaborative activities to "assure a well-trained, competent workforce and a strong, evidence-based public health infrastructure" (U.S. Public Health Service, 1994 [updated 2008]). In the spring of 2010 the Council,

**HOW TO** **Participate, as a Public Health Nurse, in the Essential Services of Public Health**

1. Monitor health status to identify community health problems.
   - Participate in community assessment.
   - Identify subpopulations at risk for disease or disability.
   - Collect information on interventions to special populations.
   - Define and evaluate effective strategies and programs.
   - Identify potential environmental hazards.
2. Diagnose and investigate health problems and hazards in the community.
   - Understand and identify determinants of health and disease.
   - Apply knowledge about environmental influences of health.
   - Recognize multiple causes or factors of health and illness.
   - Participate in case identification and treatment of persons with communicable disease.
3. Inform, educate, and empower people about health issues.
   - Develop health and educational plans for individuals and families in multiple settings.
   - Develop and implement community-based health education.
   - Provide regular reports on health status of special populations within clinic settings, community settings, and groups.
   - Advocate for and with underserved and disadvantaged populations.
   - Ensure health planning, which includes primary prevention and early intervention strategies.
   - Identify healthy population behaviors and maintain successful intervention strategies through reinforcement and continued funding.
4. Mobilize community partnerships to identify and solve health problems.
   - Interact regularly with many providers and services within each community.
   - Convene groups and providers who share common concerns and interests in special populations.
   - Provide leadership to prioritize community problems and development of interventions.
   - Explain the significance of health issues to the public and participate in developing plans of action.
5. Develop policies and plans that support individual and community health efforts.
   - Participate in community and family decision-making processes.
   - Provide information and advocacy for consideration of the interests of special groups in program development.
   - Develop programs and services to meet the needs of high-risk populations as well as broader community members.
   - Participate in disaster planning and mobilization of community resources in emergencies.
   - Advocate for appropriate funding for services.
6. Enforce laws and regulations that protect health and ensure safety.
   - Regulate and support safe care and treatment for dependent populations such as children and frail older adults.
   - Implement ordinances and laws that protect the environment.
   - Establish procedures and processes that ensure competent implementation of treatment schedules for diseases of public health importance.
   - Participate in development of local regulations that protect communities and the environment from potential hazards and pollution.
7. Link people to needed personal health services and ensure the provision of health care that is otherwise unavailable.
   - Provide clinical preventive services to certain high-risk populations.
   - Establish programs and services to meet special needs.
   - Recommend clinical care and other services to clients and their families in clinics, homes, and the community.
   - Provide referrals through community links to needed care.
   - Participate in community provider coalitions and meetings to educate others and to identify service centers for community populations.
   - Provide clinical surveillance and identification of communicable disease.
8. Ensure a competent public health and personal health care workforce.
   - Participate in continuing education and preparation to ensure competence.
   - Define and support proper delegation to unlicensed assistive personnel in community settings.
   - Establish standards for performance.
   - Maintain client record systems and community documents.
   - Establish and maintain procedures and protocols for client care.
   - Participate in quality assurance activities such as record audits, agency evaluation, and clinical guidelines.
9. Evaluate effectiveness, accessibility, and quality of personal and population-based health services.
   - Collect data and information related to community interventions.
   - Identify unserved and underserved populations within the community.
   - Review and analyze data on health status of the community.
   - Participate with the community in assessment of services and outcomes of care.
   - Identify and define enhanced services required to manage health status of complex populations and special risk groups.
10. Research for new insights and innovative solutions to health problems.
    - Implement nontraditional interventions and approaches to effect change in special populations.
    - Participate in the collecting of information and data to improve the surveillance and understanding of special problems.
    - Develop collegial relationships with academic institutions to explore new interventions.
    - Participate in early identification of factors that are detrimental to the community's health.
    - Formulate and use investigative tools to identify and impact care delivery and program planning.

## BOX 1-1    Indicators Used to Develop a Community Health Profile

**Sociodemographic Characteristics**
- Distribution of the population by age and race/ethnicity
- Number and proportion of persons in groups such as migrants, homeless, or the non–English speaking, for whom access to community services and resources may be a concern
- Number and proportion of persons aged 25 and older with less than a high school education
- Ratio of the number of students graduating from high school to the number of students who entered ninth grade 3 years previously
- Median household income
- Proportion of children less than 15 years of age living in families at or below the poverty level
- Unemployment rate
- Number and proportion of single-parent families
- Number and proportion of persons without health insurance

**Health Status**
- Infant death rate by race/ethnicity
- Numbers of deaths or age-adjusted death rates for motor vehicle crashes, work-related injuries, suicide, homicide, lung cancer, breast cancer, cardiovascular diseases, and all causes, by age, race, and sex as appropriate
- Reported incidence of AIDS, measles, tuberculosis, and primary and secondary syphilis, by age, race, and sex as appropriate
- Births to adolescents (ages 10 to 17) as a proportion of total live births
- Number and rate of confirmed abuse and neglect cases among children

**Health Risk Factors**
- Proportion of 2-year-old children who have received all age-appropriate vaccines, as recommended by the Advisory Committee on Immunization Practices
- Proportion of adults aged 65 and older who have ever been immunized for pneumococcal pneumonia; proportion who have been immunized in the past 12 months for influenza
- Proportion of the population who smoke, by age, race, and sex as appropriate
- Proportion of the population aged 18 and older who are obese
- Number and type of U.S. Environmental Protection Agency air quality standards not met
- Proportion of assessed rivers, lakes, and estuaries that support beneficial uses (e.g., approved fishing and swimming)

**Health Care Resource Consumption**
- Per capita health care spending for Medicare beneficiaries—the Medicare-adjusted average per capita cost (AAPCC)

**Functional Status**
- Proportion of adults reporting that their general health is good to excellent
- Average number of days (in the past 30 days) for which adults report that their physical or mental health was not good

**Quality of Life**
- Proportion of adults satisfied with the health care system in the community
- Proportion of persons satisfied with the quality of life in the community

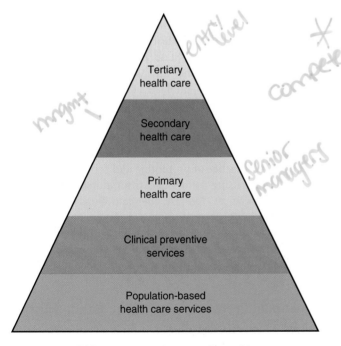

**FIG 1-2** Health Services Pyramid.

## BOX 1-2    Categories of Public Health Workforce Competencies

- Analytic/assessment
- Policy development/program planning
- Communication
- Cultural competency
- Community dimensions of practice
- Basic public health sciences
- Financial planning and management
- Leadership and systems thinking

Compiled from Centers for Disease Control and Prevention: Genomics and disease prevention: Frequently asked questions, 2010. Accessed 1/11/11 from http://www.cdc.gov/genomics/faq.htm; Centers for Disease Control and Prevention: Genomics and disease prevention.

different stages of a career. Specifically, Tier 1 applies to entry level public health professionals without management responsibilities. Tier 2 competencies are expected in those with management and/or supervisory responsibilities, and Tier 3 is expected of senior managers and/or leaders in public health organizations. It is recommended that these categories of competencies be used by educators for curriculum review and development and by agency administrators for workforce needs assessment, competency development, performance evaluation, hiring, and refining of the personnel system job requirements. A detailed listing of the 2014 competencies can be found at www.phf.org/corecompetencies.

Using an earlier version of the Council on Linkage's Core Competencies as a starting point, a coalition of public health nursing organizations called the Quad Council developed levels

funded by the CDC and USDHHS, adopted an updated set of Core Competencies ("a set of skills desirable for the broad practice of public health") for all public health professionals, including nurses. In 2014 the Core Competencies were updated again (Council on Linkages, 2010/2014). The 72 Core Competencies are divided into 8 categories (Box 1-2). In addition, each competency is presented at three levels (tiers), which reflect the of skills to be attained by public health nurses for each of the competencies. Skill levels are specified and have been updated for the generalist/staff nurse and the specialist in public health nursing (Quad Council, 2003). (See Resource Tool 45.A on the Evolve website for the Public Health Nursing Core Competencies.)

## Quality Improvement Efforts in Public Health

In 2003, the Institute of Medicine released a report, "Who Will Keep the Public Healthy?" that identified eight content areas in which public health workers should be educated—informatics, genomics, cultural competence, community-based participatory research, policy, law, global health, and ethics—in order to be able to address the emerging public health issues and advances in science and policy.

Two broad efforts designed to enhance quality improvement efforts in public health have been developed within the last 20 years: the National Public Health Performance Standards Program and the accreditation process for local and state health departments. The National Public Health Performance Standards Program is a high-level partnership initiative started in 1998 and led by the Office of Chief of Public Health Practice, CDC. The collaborative partners are the American Public Health Association, Association of State and Territorial Health Officials, National Association of County and City Health Officials, National Association of Local Boards of Health, National Network of Public Health Institutes, and the Public Health Foundation. The National Public Health Performance Standards (NPHPS) "provide a framework to assess capacity and performance of public health systems and public health governing bodies." The program is "to improve the practice of public health, the performance of public health systems, and the infrastructure supporting public health actions" (CDC, 2014a). The performance standards, collectively developed by the participating organizations, set the bar for the level of performance that is necessary to deliver essential public health services. Four principles guided the development of the standards. First, they were developed around the 10 Essential Public Health Services (see the How To Box on page 8). Second, the standards focus on the overall public health system rather than on single organizations. Third, the standards describe an optimal level of performance. Finally, they are intended to support a process of quality improvement.

States and local communities seeking to assess their performance can access the Assessment Instruments developed by the program and other resources such as training workshops, on-site training, and technical assistance to work with them in conducting assessments (CDC, 2014a).

## PUBLIC HEALTH NURSING AS A FIELD OF PRACTICE: AN AREA OF SPECIALIZATION

Most of the preceding discussion has been about the broad field of public health. Now attention turns to public health nursing. What is public health nursing? Is it really a specialty, and if so, why? Public health nursing is a specialty because it has a distinct focus and scope of practice, and it requires a special knowledge

base. The following characteristics distinguish public health nursing as a specialty:

- *It is population-focused.* Primary emphasis is on populations whose members are free-living in the community as opposed to those who are institutionalized.
- *It is community-oriented.* There is concern for the connection between the health status of the population and the environment in which the population lives (physical, biological, sociocultural). There is an imperative to work with members of the community to carry out core public health functions.
- *There is a health and preventive focus.* The primary emphasis is on strategies for health promotion, health maintenance, and disease prevention, particularly primary and secondary prevention.
- *Interventions are made at the community or population level.* Target populations are defined as those living in a particular geographic area or those who have particular characteristics in common and political processes are used as a major intervention strategy to affect public policy and achieve goals.
- *There is concern for the health of all members of the population/community, particularly vulnerable subpopulations.*

In 1981 the public health nursing section of the American Public Health Association (APHA) developed *The Definition and Role of Public Health Nursing in the Delivery of Health Care* to describe the field of specialization (APHA, 1981). This statement was reaffirmed in 1996 (APHA, 1996). In 1999 the American Nurses Association, with input from three other nursing organizations—the Public Health Nursing Section of the APHA, the Association of State and Territorial Directors of Public Health Nursing, and the Association of Community Health Nurse Educators—published the *Scope and Standards of Public Health Nursing Practice* (Quad Council, 1999 [revised 2005]). In that document, the 1996 definition was supported. Since 1999 the scope and standards have been revised twice. In the latest version Public Health Nursing continues to be defined as "the practice of promoting and protecting the health of populations using knowledge from nursing, social, and public health sciences" (APHA, 1996 and Quad Council, 1999 [revised 2005], 2011) but the following statement was added in 2011: "Public Health Nurses engage in population-focused practice, but can and do often apply the Council of Linkages concepts at the individual and family level" (see Quad Council, 2011, p. 9).

## Educational Preparation for Public Health Nursing

Targeted and specialized education for public health nursing practice has a long history. In the late 1950s and early 1960s, before the integration of public health concepts into the curriculum of baccalaureate nursing programs, special baccalaureate curricula were established in several schools of public health to prepare nurses to become public health nurses. Today it is generally assumed that a graduate of any baccalaureate nursing program has the necessary basic preparation to function as a beginning staff public health nurse.

Since the late 1960s, public health nursing leaders have agreed that a specialty in public health nursing requires a master's

## BOX 1-3   Areas Considered Essential for the Preparation of Specialists in Public Health Nursing

- Epidemiology
- Biostatistics
- Nursing theory
- Management theory
- Change theory
- Economics
- Politics
- Public health administration
- Community assessment
- Program planning and evaluation
- Interventions at the aggregate level
- Research
- History of public health
- Issues in public health

From Consensus Conference on the Essentials of Public Health Nursing Practice and Education, Rockville, MD, 1985, U.S. Department of Health and Human Services, Bureau of Health Professions, Division of Nursing.

## BOX 1-4   Eight Principles of Public Health Nursing

1. The client or "unit of care" is the population.
2. The primary obligation is to achieve the greatest good for the greatest number of people or the population as a whole.
3. The processes used by public health nurses include working with the client(s) as an equal partner.
4. Primary prevention is the priority in selecting appropriate activities.
5. Selecting strategies that create healthy environmental, social, and economic conditions in which populations may thrive is the focus.
6. There is an obligation to actively reach out to all who might benefit from a specific activity or service.
7. Optimal use of available resources to assure the best overall improvement in the health of the population is a key element of the practice.
8. Collaboration with a variety of other professions, organizations, and entities is the most effective way to promote and protect the health of the people.

Sources: Quad Council of Public Health Nursing Organizations: Scope and standards of public health nursing practice, Washington, DC, 1999, revised 2005, 2007 with the American Nurses Association

degree. Today, a master's degree in nursing is necessary to be eligible to sit for a certification examination. In the future, a Doctor of Nursing Practice (DNP) degree will probably be required to sit for certification. the American Association of Colleges of Nursing has proposed the DNP should be the expected level of education for specialization in an area of nursing practice (AACN, 2004, 2006). The educational expectations for public health nursing were highlighted at the 1984 Consensus Conference on the Essentials of Public Health Nursing Practice and Education sponsored by the USDHHS Division of Nursing. The participants agreed "that the term 'public health nurse' should be used to describe a person who has received specific educational preparation and supervised clinical practice in public health nursing" (USDHHS, 1985, p. 4). At the basic or entry level, a public health nurse is one who "holds a baccalaureate degree in nursing that includes this educational preparation; this nurse may or may not practice in an official health agency but has the initial qualifications to do so" (USDHHS, 1985, p. 4). Specialists in public health nursing are defined as those who are prepared at the graduate level, with either a master's or doctoral degree, "with a focus in the public health sciences" (USDHHS, 1985, p. 4) (Box 1-3). The consensus statement specifically pointed out that the public health nursing specialist "should be able to work with population groups and to assess and intervene successfully at the aggregate level" (USDHHS, 1985, p. 11).

The Association of Community Health Nursing Educators reaffirmed the results of the 1984 Consensus Conference (ACHNE, 2003). The educational requirements were reaffirmed by ACHNE (2009) and in the revised *Scope and Standards of Public Health Nursing Practice* and include both clinical specialists and nurse practitioners who engage in population-focused care as advanced practice registered nurses in public health (Quad Council, 1999 [revised 2005]). The latest iteration of the *Scope and Standards of Practice for Public Health Nursing* was published by the American Nurses Association in 2013 (ANA, 2013).

## Population-Focused Practice versus Practice Focused on Individuals

The key factor that distinguishes public health nursing from other areas of nursing practice is the focus on populations, a focus historically consistent with public health philosophy. Box 1-4 lists principles on which public health nursing is built. Although public health nursing is based on clinical nursing practice, it also incorporates the population perspective of public health. It may be helpful here to define the term *population*.

A population, or aggregate, is a collection of individuals who have one or more personal or environmental characteristics in common. Members of a community who can be defined in terms of geography (e.g., a county, a group of counties, or a state) or in terms of a special interest or circumstance (e.g., children attending a particular school) can be seen as constituting a population. Often there are subpopulations within the larger population, such as high-risk infants under the age of 1 year, unmarried pregnant adolescents, or individuals exposed to a particular event such as a chemical spill. In population-focused practice, problems are defined (by assessments or diagnoses), and solutions (interventions), such as policy development or providing a particular preventive service, are implemented for or with a defined population or subpopulation (examples are provided in the Levels of Prevention Box). In other nursing specialties, the diagnoses, interventions, and treatments are usually carried out at the individual client level.

Professional education in nursing, medicine, and other clinical disciplines focuses primarily on developing competence in decision making at the individual client level by assessing health status, making management decisions (ideally *with* the client), and evaluating the effects of care. Figure 1-3 illustrates three levels at which problems can be identified. For example, community-based nurse clinicians, or nurse practitioners, focus on individuals they see in either a home or a clinic setting. The focus is on an individual person or an individual family in a

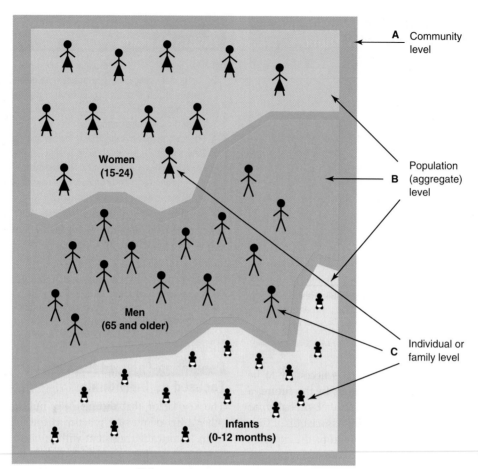

**FIG 1-3** Levels of health care practice.

## LEVELS OF PREVENTION

### Examples in Public Health Nursing

**Primary Prevention**

Using general and specific measures in a population to promote health and prevent the development of disease (incidence) and using specific measures to prevent diseases in those who are predisposed to developing a particular condition.

*Example:* The public health nurse develops a health education program for a population of school-age children that teaches them about the effects of smoking on health.

**Secondary Prevention**

Stopping the progress of disease by early detection and treatment, thus reducing prevalence and chronicity.

*Example:* The public health nurse develops a program of toxin screenings for migrant workers who may be exposed to pesticides and refers for treatment those who are found to be positive for high levels.

**Tertiary Prevention**

Stopping deterioration in a patient, a relapse, or disability and dependency by anticipatory nursing and medical care.

*Example:* The public health nurse develops a diabetes clinic in which nursing care including educational programs for nutrition and self-care are provided for a defined population of adults in a low-income housing unit of the community.

subpopulation (the *C* arrows in Figure 1-3). The provider's emphasis is on defining and resolving a problem for the individual; the client is an individual.

In Figure 1-3 the individual clients are grouped into three separate subpopulations, each of which has a common characteristic (the *B* arrows in Figure 1-3). Public health nursing specialists often define problems at the population or aggregate level as opposed to an individual level. Population-level decision making is different from decision making in clinical care. For example, in a clinical, direct care situation, the nurse may determine that a client is hypertensive and explore options for intervening. However, at the population level, the public health nursing specialist might explore the answers to the following set of questions:

1. What is the prevalence of hypertension among various age, race, and sex groups?
2. Which subpopulations have the highest rates of untreated hypertension?
3. What programs could reduce the problem of untreated hypertension and thereby lower the risk of further cardiovascular morbidity and mortality for the population as a whole?

Public health nursing specialists are usually concerned with more than one subpopulation and frequently with the health of the entire community (in Figure 1-3, arrow *A*: the entire box containing all of the subgroups within the community). In reality, of course, there are many more subgroups than those in Figure 1-3. Professionals concerned with the health of a whole community must consider the total population, which is made up of multiple and often overlapping subpopulations. For example, the population of adolescents at risk for unplanned pregnancies would overlap with the female population 15 to 24 years of age. A population that would overlap with infants under 1 year of age would be children from 0 to 6 years of age. In addition, a population focus requires considering those who may need particular services but have not entered the health care system (e.g., children without immunizations or clients with untreated hypertension).

## Public Health Nursing Specialists and Core Public Health Functions: Selected Examples

The core public health function of *assessment* includes activities that involve collecting, analyzing, and disseminating information on both the health status and the health-related aspects of a community or a specific population. Questions such as whether the health services of the community are available to the population and are adequate to address needs are considered. Assessment also includes an ongoing effort to monitor the health status of the community or population and the services provided. Excellent examples of assessment at the national level are the efforts of the USDHHS to organize the goal setting, data collecting and analysis, and monitoring necessary to develop the series of publications describing the health status and health-related aspects of the U.S. population. These efforts began with *Healthy People: The Surgeon General's Report on Health Promotion and Disease Prevention* in 1980 and continued with *Promoting Health/Preventing Disease: Objectives for the Nation, Healthy People 2000,* and *Healthy People 2010,* and are now moving forward into the future with *Healthy People 2020* (U.S. Department of Health, Education, and Welfare, 1979; USDHHS, 1980, 1979, 1991, 2000, 2010; *Healthy People 2020* retrieved at www.healthypeople.gov).

Many states and other jurisdictions have developed publications describing the health status of a defined community, a set of communities, or populations. Unfortunately, it is difficult to find published descriptions of health assessments on particular communities unless they demonstrate new methods or reveal unusual findings about a community. Such working documents and data sets should be available in specific settings, such as a county or state health department, and should be used by public health practitioners to develop services.

In 2009 Turnock described a survey conducted to determine the extent to which local health departments were performing the core public health functions. The questions asked about *assessment* included the following:

1. Whether there was a needs assessment process in place that described the health status of the community and community needs
2. Whether there had been a survey of behavioral risk factors within the last 3 years
3. Whether an analysis had been done of "the determinants and contributing factors of priority health needs, adequacy of existing health resources, and the population groups most affected"

The results were disappointing and suggested that in 1993 less than 40% of the population in the United States were served by a health department that was effectively addressing the core function of public health. In this study, compliance with the performance measures was highest for practices related to the assurance function and lowest for practices related to policy development (Turnock, 2012). It should be part of the public health nurse specialist's role within a local health department to participate in and provide leadership for assessing community needs, the health status of populations within the community, and environmental and behavioral risks; looking at trends in the health determinants; identifying priority health needs; and determining the adequacy of existing resources within the community (see Evidence-Based Practice Box 1), and engaging in policy development efforts.

## EVIDENCE-BASED PRACTICE

This study used a randomized controlled design to evaluate the effectiveness of a community participatory research-grounded intervention among women with chronic health conditions who were receiving Temporary Assistance for Needy Families (TANF). Previous descriptive studies noted that women receiving TANF were likely to experience poor physical, mental, and general health. The 432 participants were assigned to either the intervention group or the wait-control group. Outcomes were assessed at baseline and at 3, 6, and 9 months. The intervention sought to (1) increase rates of health care visits for mental health and chronic health conditions, (2) increase the ability to navigate the Medicaid system, and (3) improve functional and health status over time among this group of women, using 9 months of public health nursing (PHN) case management and a one-time 2-hour Medicaid knowledge and skills training program. The PHN case management focused on health care access; care coordination; health education; health and social service referrals; obtaining preventive services, screening, and routine care; and assistance in meeting health goals that the participants had set for themselves. A Community Advisory Group consisting of diverse academic researchers, agency representatives, and lay community members guided the research team in developing the intervention. Furthermore, three women who were recently in the Welfare Transition Program were hired onto the research team and participated in personal and community capacity building.

Both groups showed improvement in Medicaid knowledge and skills. Those in the intervention group were more likely to have a new mental health visit as well as improvement in depression and functional status over time. No differences existed between the groups in routine or preventive care or general health.

### Nurse Use

The results of this study suggest that public health interventions can improve health outcomes among women receiving Temporary Assistance for Needy Families. The intervention was developed with input from the community and used community members on the research team. The researchers noted that trust between the public health nurse and the client was crucial to the success of the intervention.

Modified from Kneipp SM, Kairalla JA, Lutz BJ, et al: Public health nursing case management for women receiving Temporary Assistance for Needy Families: a randomized controlled trial using community-based participatory research. *Am J Public Health* 101:1759–1768, 2011.

*Policy development* is both a core function of public health and a core intervention strategy used by public health nursing specialists. Policy development in the public arena seeks to build constituencies that can help bring about change in public policy. In an interesting case study of her experience as director of public health for the state of Oregon, Christine Gebbie (1999), a nurse, describes her experiences in developing a constituency for public health. This enabled her to mobilize efforts to develop statewide goals for *Healthy People 2000* as well as to update Oregon's disease- reporting laws. Gebbie's experiences as a state director of public health illustrate how a public health nursing specialist can provide leadership at a very broad level. Gebbie left Oregon to go to Washington, DC, to serve in the federal government as President Clinton's key official in the national effort to control acquired immunodeficiency syndrome (AIDS). Clearly, Gebbie is an example of an individual who has provided leadership in policy development at both state and national levels. Another public health nursing specialist who has and continues to provide strong policy leadership is Ellen Hahn, PhD, director of the Kentucky Center for Smoke-Free Policy (www.mc.uky.edu/tobaccopolicy/), which is based at the University of Kentucky's College of Nursing. Through her research Dr. Hahn has developed considerable evidence to support important policy changes (antismoking ordinances) to reduce exposure to tobacco smoke in Kentucky, a state that has a long tradition of a tobacco culture, both in production of tobacco and in use. A number of studies conducted by Hahn and her colleagues can be found on the website identified above. Two particularly interesting ones are listed in the references at the end of this chapter (Hahn et al, 2010, 2011).

The third core public health function, *assurance*, focuses on the responsibility of public health agencies to make certain that activities have been appropriately carried out to meet public health goals and plans. This may result in public health agencies requiring others to engage in activities to meet goals, encouraging private groups to undertake certain activities, or sometimes actually offering services directly. Assurance also includes the development of partnerships between public and private agencies to make sure that needed services are available and that assessing the quality of the activities is carried out. A recent report suggested that much more attention should be paid by public health officials to the quality of direct care services provided by clinicians in their communities (Fielding, 2009). It is important to point out that when personal services to individuals are offered by public health agencies to ensure that they can get care they might not receive without the intervention of the official agency, the goal is to "promote knowledge, attitudes, beliefs, practices and behaviors that support and enhance health with the ultimate goal of improving... population health" (Quad Council, 1999 [revised 2005]; and see Evidence-Based Practice Box 2).

## PUBLIC HEALTH NURSING VERSUS COMMUNITY-BASED NURSING

The concept of public health should include all populations within the community, both free-living and those living in

### HEALTHY PEOPLE 2020

In 1979 the surgeon general issued a report that began a 30-year focus on promoting health and preventing disease for all Americans. The report, entitled *Healthy People,* used morbidity rates to track the health of individuals through the five major life cycles of infancy, childhood, adolescence, adulthood, and older age.

In 1989 *Healthy People 2000* became a national effort of representatives from government agencies, academia, and health organizations. Their goal was to present a strategy for improving the health of the American people. Their objectives were being used by public and community health organizations to assess current health trends, health programs, and disease prevention programs.

Throughout the 1990s, all states used *Healthy People 2000* objectives to identify emerging public health issues. The success of the program on a national level was accomplished through state and local efforts. Early in the 1990s, surveys from public health departments indicated that 8% of the national objectives had been met, and progress on an additional 40% of the objectives was noted. In the mid-course review published in 1995, it was noted that significant progress had been made toward meeting 50% of the objectives.

In light of the progress made in the past decade, the committee for *Healthy People 2010* proposed two goals. The hope was to reach these goals by such measures as promoting healthy behaviors, increasing access to quality health care, and strengthening community prevention.

The major premise of *Healthy People 2010* was that the health of the individual cannot be entirely separate from the health of the larger community. Therefore the vision for *Healthy People 2010* was "Healthy People in Healthy Communities."

The vision for *Healthy People 2020* is: A society in which all people live long, healthy lives(see Chapter 8 for a listing of the goals for each of the decades and highlighting of the policy implications of *Healthy People*).

In contrast to previous years, *Healthy People 2020* has a web-accessible database that is searchable, multilevel, and interactive to be more useful. A progress report as of March 2014 on the leading indicators is available on the website: www.healthpeople.gov/2020//hi//hi-progressreport-execsum.pdf

### EVIDENCE-BASED PRACTICE

The purpose of this study was to evaluate whether a brief nurse home-visiting intervention offered postnatally would be beneficial in preventing emergency health care services and promote positive parenting. The participants were the parents of infants and infants who were delivered in one of the two hospitals in Durham, North Carolina between July 1, 2009 and December 31, 2010 and randomly assigned to either the intervention group or to a control group. The project was aimed at alleviating parental stress and improving parent-child interaction among parents who attended an inner-city clinic. Participants were 199 parents of children 1 through 36 months of age. Serious life stress including poverty, low social support, personal histories of childhood maltreatment, and substance abuse defined the parents at risk. Program effects were evaluated in terms of improvement in self-reported parenting stress and observed parent-child interaction. Positive effects were documented for the group as a whole and within each of three subgroups: two community samples and a group of mothers and children in a residential drug treatment program. Program attendance and the amount of gain in observed parenting skills were the factors related to a positive outcome.

#### Nurse Use

This program was offered in partnership with academic researchers and the public clinic. The nurses in this agency can ensure better outcomes in parenting by providing a long-term program for high-risk parents.

Dodge K, Goodman B, Murphy R. et al: Implementation and randomized controlled trial evaluation of universal postnatal nurse home visiting, AJPJ 104(Suppl 1) S136-143m 2014.

institutions. Furthermore, the public health specialist should consider the match between the health needs of the population and the health care resources in the community, including those services offered in a variety of settings. Although all direct care providers may contribute to the community's health in the broadest sense, not all are primarily concerned with the population focus—the big picture. All nurses in a given community, including those working in hospitals, physicians' offices, and health clinics, may contribute positively to the health of the community. However, the special contributions of public health nursing specialists include looking at the community or population as a whole; raising questions about its overall health status and associated factors, including environmental factors (physical, biological, and sociocultural); and *working with the community* to improve the population's health status.

Figure 1-4 is a useful illustration of the arenas of practice. Because most nurses working in the community and many staff public health nurses, historically and at present, focus on providing direct personal care services—including health education—to persons or family units outside of institutional settings (either in the client's home or in a clinic environment), such practice falls into the upper right quadrant (section *B*) of Figure 1-4. However, specialization in public health nursing is population-focused and focuses on clients living in the community and is represented by the box in the upper left quadrant (section *A*).

There are three reasons, in addition to the population focus, that the most important practice arena for public health nursing is represented by section *A* of Figure 1-4, the population of free-living clients:

1. Preventive strategies can have the greatest impact on free-living populations, which usually represent the majority of a community.
2. The major interface between health status and the environment (physical, biological, sociocultural, and behavioral) occurs in the free-living population.

3. For philosophical, historical, and economic reasons, prevention-oriented population-focused practice is most likely to flourish in organizational structures that serve free-living populations (e.g., health departments, health maintenance organizations, health centers, schools, and workplaces).

What roles in the health care system do public health nursing specialists (those in section *A* of Figure 1-4) have? Options include director of nursing for a health department, director of the health department, state commissioner for health, director of maternal and child health services for a state or local health department, director of wellness for a business or educational organization, and director of preventive services for an integrated health system. Nurses can occupy all of these roles, but, with the exception of director of nursing for a health department, they are in the minority. Unfortunately, nurses who occupy these roles are often seen as "administrators" and not as public health nursing specialists. However, those who work in such roles have the opportunity to make decisions that affect the health of population groups and the type and quality of health services provided for various populations.

Where does the staff public health nurse or nurse working in the community fit on the diagram in Figure 1-4? That depends on the focus of the nurse's practice. In many settings, most of the staff nurse's time is spent in community-based direct care activities, where the focus is on dealing with individual clients and individual families, in which case the practice falls into section *B* of Figure 1-4. Although a staff public health nurse or a nurse practicing in the community may not be a public health nurse specialist, this nurse may spend some time carrying out core public health functions with a population focus, and thus that part of the role would be represented in section *A* of Figure 1-4. In summary, the field of public health nursing can be seen as primarily encompassing two groups of nurses:

- Public health nursing specialists, whose practice is community-oriented and uses population-focused strategies

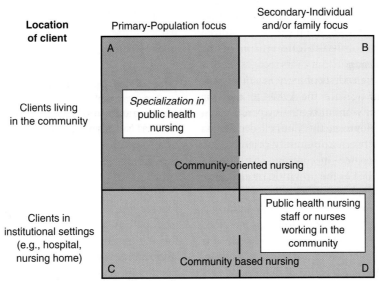

**FIG 1-4** Arenas for health care practice.

for carrying out the core public health functions (section *A* of Figure 1-4)

- Staff public health nurses or clinical nurses working in the community nurses, who are community-based, who may be clinically oriented to the individual client, and who combine some primary preventive population-focused strategies and direct care clinical strategies in programs serving specified populations (section *B* of Figure 1-4)
- Sections *C* and *D* of Figure 1-4 represent institutionalized populations. Nurses who provide direct care to these clients in hospital settings fall into section *D*, and those who have administrative/managerial responsibility for nursing services in institutional settings fall into section *C*.

Figure 1-4 also shows that specialization in public health nursing, as it has been defined in this chapter, can be viewed as a specialized field of practice with certain characteristics within the broad arena of community. This view is consistent with recommendations developed at the Consensus Conference on the Essentials of Public Health Nursing Practice and Education (USDHHS, 1985). One of the outcomes of the historical conference was consensus on the use of the terms *community health nurse* and *public health nurse*. It was agreed that the term *community health nurse* could apply to all nurses who practice in the community, whether or not they have had preparation in public health nursing. Thus nurses providing secondary or tertiary care in a home setting, school nurses, and nurses in clinic settings (in fact, any nurse who does not practice in an institutional setting) could fall into the category of community health nurse. Nurses with a master's degree or a doctoral degree who practice in community settings could be referred to as *community health nurse specialists,* regardless of the area of nursing in which the degree was earned. According to the conference statement: "The degree could be in any area of nursing, such as maternal/child health, psychiatric/mental health, or medical-surgical nursing or some subspecialty of any clinical area" (USDHHS, 1985, p. 4). The definitions of the three areas of practice have changed, however, over time.

In 1998 the Quad Council began to develop a statement on the scope of public health nursing practice (Quad Council, 1999 [revised 2005]). The council attempted to clarify the differences between the term *public health nursing* and the term introduced into nursing's vocabulary during health care reform of the 1990s: community-based nursing. The authors recognized that the terms *public health nursing* and *community health nursing* had been used interchangeably since the 1980s to describe population-focused, community-oriented nursing practice and community-based practice. However, the Council decided to make a clearer distinction between community-oriented and community-based nursing practice. In contrast, community-based nursing care was described as the provision or assurance of personal illness care to individuals and families in the community, whereas community-oriented nursing was the provision of disease prevention and health promotion to populations and communities. It was suggested that there be two terms for the two levels of care in the community: *community-oriented care* and *community-based care.* (see the list of definitions presented in Box 1-5).

---

**BOX 1-5   Definitions of the Key Nursing Areas in the Community**

- *Community-oriented nursing practice* is a philosophy of nursing service delivery that involves the generalist or specialist public health and community health nurse. The nurse provides health care through community diagnosis and investigation of major health and environmental problems, health surveillance, and monitoring and evaluation of community and population health status for the purposes of preventing disease and disability and promoting, protecting, and maintaining health to create conditions in which people can be healthy.
- *Community-based nursing practice* is a setting-specific practice whereby care is provided for clients and families where they live, work, and attend school. The emphasis of community-based nursing practice is acute and chronic care and the provision of comprehensive, coordinated, and continuous services. Nurses who deliver community-based care are generalists or specialists in maternal/infant, pediatric, adult, or psychiatric/mental health nursing.

---

There is a need and a place for a nursing specialty in the community; the nurse in this specialty is more than a clinical specialist with a master's degree who practices in a community-based setting, as was suggested by the Consensus Conference more than 25 years ago. Although in 1984 these nurses were referred to as community health nurses, today they are referred to as nurses in community-based practice (see definitions in the inside cover of this text). Those who provide community-oriented service to specific subpopulations in the community and who provide some clinical services to those populations may be seen as nurse specialists in the community. Although such practitioners may be community-based, they are also community-oriented as public health specialists but are usually focused on only one or two special subpopulations. Preparing for this specialty includes a master's or doctoral degree with emphasis in a direct care clinical area, such as school health or occupational health, and ideally some education in the public health sciences. Examples of roles such specialists might have in direct clinical care areas include case manager, supervisor in a home health agency, school nurse, occupational health nurse, parish nurse, and a nurse practitioner who also manages a nursing clinic.

## ROLES IN PUBLIC HEALTH NURSING

In community-oriented nursing circles, there has been a tendency to talk about public health nursing from the point of view of a role rather than the functions related to the role. This can be limiting. In discussing such nursing roles, there is a preoccupation with the direct care provider orientation. Even in discussions about how a practice can become more population focused, the focus is frequently on how an individual practitioner, such as an agency staff nurse, can adopt a population-focused practice philosophy. Rarely is attention given to how nurse administrators in public health (one role for public health nursing specialists) might reorient their practice toward a population focus, which is particularly important and easier for an administrator to do than for the staff nurse. This is because many agencies' nursing administrators, supervisors, or others (sometimes program directors who are not nurses) make the key decisions about how staff nurses will spend their time and what types of clients will be seen and under what circumstances. Public health nursing administrators who are prepared to practice in a population-focused manner will be more effective than those who are not prepared to do so.

Although their opportunities to make decisions at the population level are limited, staff nurses benefit from having a clear understanding of population-focused practice for three reasons:

- First, it gives them professional satisfaction to see how their individual client care contributes to health at the population level.
- Second, it helps them appreciate the practice of others who are population-focused specialists.
- Third, it gives them a better foundation from which to provide clinical input into decision making at the program or agency level and thus to improve the effectiveness and efficiency of the population-focused practice.

A curriculum was proposed by representatives of key public health nursing organizations and other individuals that would prepare the staff public health nurse or generalist to function as a community-oriented practitioner (Association of State and Territorial Directors of Nursing, 2000). The AACN developed a supplement to the document "The Essentials of Baccalaureate Education for Professional Nursing Practice," which highlights this organization's recommendations for public health nursing (AACN, 2013).

Unfortunately, nursing roles as presently defined are often too limited to include population-focused practice, but it is important not to think too narrowly. Furthermore, roles that entail population-focused decision making may not be defined as nursing roles (e.g., directors of health departments, state or regional programs, and units of health planning and evaluation; directors of programs such as preventive services within a managed care organization). If population-focused public health nursing is to be taken seriously, and if strategies for assessment, policy development, and assurance are to be implemented at the population level, more consideration must be given to organized systems for assessing population needs and managing care. Clearly, public health nurse specialists must move into positions where they can influence policy formation. This means, however, that some nurses will have to assume positions that are not traditionally considered nursing.

Redefining nursing roles so that population-focused decision making fits into the present structure of nursing services may be difficult in some circumstances at the present time, but future needs will require that nurses be prepared to make such decisions (IOM, 2010). At this point, it may be more useful to concentrate on identifying the skills and knowledge needed to make decisions in population-focused practice (see Appendix G.1), to define where in the health care system such decisions are made, and then to equip nurses with the knowledge, skills, and political understanding necessary for success in such positions. Although some of these positions are in nursing settings (e.g., administrator of the nursing service and top-level staff

nurse supervisors), others are outside of the traditional nursing roles (e.g., director of a health department).

## CHALLENGES FOR THE FUTURE

### Barriers to Specializing in Public Health Nursing

One of the most serious barriers to the development of specialists in public health nursing is the mindset of many nurses that the only role for a nurse is at the bedside or at the client's side (i.e., the direct care role). Indeed, the heart of nursing is the direct care provided in personal contacts with clients. On the other hand, two things should be clear. First, whether a nurse is able to provide direct care services to a particular client depends on decisions made by individuals within and outside of the care system. Second, nurses need to be involved in those fundamental decisions. Perhaps the one-on-one focus of nursing and the historical expectations of the "proper" role of women have influenced nurses to view other ways of contributing, such as administration, consultation, and research, less positively. Fortunately, things are changing. Within and outside of nursing, women have taken on every role imaginable. Further, the number of male nurses is steadily growing; nursing can no longer be viewed as a profession practiced by women exclusively. These two developments have opened doors to new roles that may not have been considered appropriate for nurses in the past.

A second barrier to population-focused public health nursing practice consists of the structures within which nurses work and the process of role socialization within those structures. For example, the absence of a particular role in a nursing unit may suggest that the role is undesirable or inaccessible to nurses. In another example, nurses interested in using political strategy to make changes in health-related policy—an activity clearly within the domain of public health nursing—may run into obstacles if their goals differ from those of other groups. Such groups may subtly but effectively lead nurses to conclude that their involvement in political effort takes their attention away from the client and it is not in their own or in the client's best interest to engage in such activities.

A third barrier is that few nurses receive graduate-level preparation in the concepts and strategies of the disciplines basic to public health (e.g., epidemiology, biostatistics, community development, service administration, and policy formation). As mentioned previously, master's level programs for public health nursing do not give the in-depth attention to population assessment and management skills that other parts of the curriculum receive, such as the direct care aspects receive. In 1995 Josten and colleagues noted that with few exceptions, graduate programs in public health nursing have not aggressively developed the population-focused skills that are needed. For individuals who want to specialize in public health nursing, these skills are as essential as direct care skills, and they should be given more attention in graduate programs that prepare nurses for careers in public health. Fortunately, the curricular expectations for academic programs leading to the Doctor of Nursing Practice (DNP) degree include serious attention to preparing nurses to develop a population perspective as well as the analytical, policy, and leadership skills necessary to be successful as a specialist in public health nursing (AACN, 2006).

## Developing Population-Focused Nurse Leaders

The massive organizational changes occurring in the health delivery system present a unique opportunity to establish new roles for nurse leaders who are prepared to think in population terms. In a book that is now viewed as a classic, Starr (1982) described the trend toward the use of private capital in financing health care, particularly institution-based care and other health-related businesses. The movement can be thought of as the "industrialization" of health care, which operated very much like a cottage industry or a small business for a very long time. The implications and consequences of this movement are enormous. First, the goal was to provide investors a return on their investment. Other aspects included more attention to the delivery of primary and community-based care in a variety of settings; less emphasis on specialty care; the development of partnerships, alliances, and other linkages across settings in an effort to build integrated systems, which would provide a broad range of services for the population served; and in some situations adoption of capitation, a payment arrangement in which insurers agree to pay providers a fixed sum for each person per month or per year, independent of the costs actually incurred. With the spread of capitation, health professionals have become more interested in the concept of populations, sometimes referred to by financial officers and others as *covered lives* (i.e., individuals with insurance that pays on a capitated basis). For public health specialists, it is a new experience to see individuals involved in the business aspects of health care, and frequently employed by hospitals, thinking in population terms and taking a population approach to decision making.

This new focus on populations, coupled with the integration of acute, chronic, and primary care that is occurring in some health care systems, is likely to create new roles for individuals, including nurses, who will span inpatient and community-based settings and focus on providing a wide range of services to the population served by the system. Such a role might be director of client care services for a health care system, who would have administrative responsibility for a large program area. There will also be a demand for individuals who can design programs of preventive and clinical services to be offered to targeted subpopulations and those who can implement the services. Who will decide what services will be given to which subpopulation and by which providers? How will nurses be prepared for leadership in the emerging and future structures for health care delivery and health maintenance?

Physician leaders are recognizing that physicians need to be prepared to use population-focused methods, such as epidemiology and biostatistics, to make evidence-based decisions in the development of programs and protocols. The attention being given to preparing nurses for administrative decision making seems to be declining. This may be a result of (1) the recent lack of federal support for preparing nurse

administrators, and (2) the growing popularity of nurse practitioner programs. However, it is time that nurse leaders give more attention to preparing nurses for leadership in the area of population-focused practice. Perhaps it is time to combine the specialty in public health nursing and nursing administration. As suggested some time ago by Williams (1985), some DNP programs are combining much of the preparation for specialization in public health nursing and administration into a systems-oriented curriculum with differentiation in the application to practice. This is the approach that is being taken in the DNP program in the College of Nursing at the University of Kentucky (www.uknursing.uky.edu). This makes sense because regardless of how the population is defined, there will be a growing need for nurses with population-level assessment, management, and evaluation skills to assume leadership roles as urged in the Institute of Medicine's report on the Future of Nursing (IOM, 2010).

The primary focus of the health care system of the future will be on community-oriented strategies for health promotion and disease prevention, and on community-based strategies for primary and secondary care. Directing more attention to developing the specialty of public health nursing as a way to provide nursing leadership may be a good response to the health care system changes. Preparing nurses for population-focused decision making will require greater attention to developing programs at the doctoral level that have a stronger foundation in the public health sciences, while providing better preparation of baccalaureate-level nurses for community-oriented as well as community-based practice.

Some observers of public health have anticipated that if access to health care for all Americans becomes more of a reality, public health practitioners can turn over the delivery of personal primary care services to other providers such as health maintenance organizations and integrated health plans, and return to the core public health functions. However, assurance (making sure that basic services are available to all) is a core function of public health. Thus even under the condition of improved access to care, there will still be a need to monitor subpopulations in the community to ensure that necessary care is available and that its quality is at an acceptable level. When these conditions are not met, public health practitioners will have to find a solution. If the Affordable Care Act is successful in enrolling the vast majority of the population and access to basic health services is available to them, public health organizations will be in a position to focus the majority of their attention on community-oriented and population-focused health promotion and primary prevention.

## Shifting Public Policy toward Creating Conditions for a Healthy Population

In 2012 the Institute of Medicine published a report (IOM, 2012B), on shifting public policy from a primary focus of supporting medical care to creating conditions for a healthy population. A major challenge for the future is the need for public health nursing specialists to be more aggressive in their practice of the core public health function of policy development, one of the major ways public health specialists intervene, with the focus on actively engaging in influencing public decisions that will create conditions for a healthy population. This is necessary at the local, state, and national levels and encompasses a wide range of concerns from the availability of adequate nutrition to the maintenance of a healthy and safe environment in schools, to the reduction of secondhand smoke, to assuring access to needed health services. Policy development is not a solitary activity; it involves working with many groups and coalitions. Also, policy development is not just the responsibility of public health specialists; it is important that all professional nurses become more serious and adept in the process of policy development.

In the just released report, *The Future of Nursing: Leading Change, Advancing Health* (IOM, 2010), a key message is that "Nurses should be full partners, with physicians and other health professionals, in redesigning health care in the United States" (IOM, 2010, pp. 1-11). In discussing this message, the report states that "to be effective in re-conceptualized roles, nurses must see policy as something they can shape rather than something that happens to them" (IOM, 2010, pp. 1-11). In other words, nurses need to be key actors. However, the report also makes clear that nurses need to be prepared for leadership in that area.

The history of public health nursing shows that a common attribute of leaders is to move forward to deal with unresolved problems in a positive, proactive way. This is the legacy of Lillian Wald at the Henry Street Settlement, and many others who have met a need by being innovative. Within the context of the core public health function of policy-making, public health nursing clearly has an opportunity to affect public decisions that will help create conditions for a healthy population and influence the provision of needed services to populations in the community, particularly those that are most vulnerable. As a specialty, public health nursing can have a positive impact on the health status of populations, but to do so "it will be necessary to have broad vision; to prepare nurses for leadership roles in policy making and in the design, development, management, monitoring, and evaluation of population-focused health care systems and to develop strategies to support nurses in these roles" (Williams, 1992, p. 268). With the focus on quality and safety education for nurses, public health nursing education will want to reflect this renewed focus and assist nurses who are population focused to develop the competencies noted in the QSEN box.

## LINKING CONTENT TO PRACTICE

In this chapter emphasis is placed on defining and explaining public health nursing practice with populations. The three essential functions of public health and public health nursing are assessment, policy development, and assurance. The Council on Linkages "Core Competencies for Public Health Professionals" revised in 2014 describes the skills of public health professionals, including nurses. In assessment function, one skill is assessment of the health status of populations and their related determinants of health and illness. For policy development, one of the skills is development of a plan to implement policy and programs. For the assurance function, one skill that public health nurses will need is to incorporate ethical standards of practice as the basis of all interactions with organizations, communities, and individuals. These skills can also be linked to the 10 essential services of public health nursing found on page 8. Assessment of health status is a skill needed for implementing essential service 1, the monitoring of health status to identify community problems. Development of a plan for policy and program implementation is a skill needed for essential service 5, to support individual and community health efforts. Incorporating ethical standards is done in essential service 3 when informing, educating, and empowering people about health issues.

## QSEN  FOCUS ON QUALITY AND SAFETY EDUCATION FOR NURSES

| QSEN Competency | Competency Definition |
| --- | --- |
| Client-Centered Care | Recognize the client or designee as the source of control and full partner in providing compassionate and coordinated care based on respect for client preferences, values, and needs |
| Teamwork and Collaboration | Function effectively within nursing and interprofessional teams, fostering open communication, mutual respect, and shared decision making to achieve quality care |
| Evidence-Based Practice | Integrate best current evidence with clinical expertise and client/family preferences and values for delivery of optimal health care |
| Quality Improvement | Use data to monitor the outcomes of care processes and use improvement methods to design and test changes to continuously improve the quality and safety of health care systems |
| Safety | Minimize risk for harm to clients and providers through both system effectiveness and individual performance |
| Informatics | Use information and technology to communicate, manage knowledge, mitigate error, and support decision making |

Prepared by Gail Armstrong, PhD(c), DNP, ACNS-BC, CNE, Associate Professor, University of Colorado Denver College of Nursing.

## PRACTICE APPLICATION

Population-focused nursing practice is different from clinical nursing care delivered in the community. If one accepts that the specialist in public health nursing is population-focused and has a unique body of knowledge, it is useful to debate where and how public health nursing specialists practice. How does their practice compare with that of the nurse specialist in community or community-based nursing?

A. In your public health class, debate with classmates which nurses in the following categories practice population-focused nursing:
1. School nurse
2. Staff nurse in home care
3. Director of nursing for a home care agency
4. Nurse practitioner in a health maintenance organization

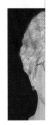

His
Co

AD

ⓔ Ev
• Hea
• Web
• Qui

OB

After re
followi
1. Inte
   thro
2. Trad
   pub
3. Disc
   soci
   prac

KE

Ameri
Ameri
Ameri
distric
distric
Floren
Fronti
Lillian
Metro
Nation

understand, and control disease. Their ability to preserve health and treat illness has depended on the contemporary level of science, use and availability of technologies, and degree of social organization.

In the early years of America's settlement, as in Europe, the care of the sick was usually informal and was provided by household members, almost always women. The female head of the household was responsible for caring for all household members, which meant more than nursing them in sickness and during childbirth. She was also responsible for growing or gathering healing herbs for use throughout the year. For the increasing numbers of urban residents in the early 1800s, this traditional system became insufficient.

American ideas of social welfare and community-based care of the sick were strongly influenced by the traditions of British settlers in the New World. Just as American law is based on English common law, colonial Americans established systems of care for the sick, poor, aged, mentally ill, and dependents based on England's Elizabethan Poor Law of 1601. In the United States, as in England, local poor laws guaranteed medical care for poor, blind, and "lame" individuals, even those without family. Early county or township government was responsible for the care of all dependent residents, but provided almshouse charity carefully, economically, and only for local residents. Travelers and wanderers from elsewhere were returned to their native counties for care. In 1751, Pennsylvania Hospital was founded in Philadelphia, the first hospital in what would become the United States. Yet until much later, hospitals were few and found only in large cities.

Early colonial public health efforts included the collection of vital statistics, improvements to sanitation systems, and control of communicable diseases introduced through seaports. Colonists lacked an organized and on-going means to ensure support and enforcement of public health efforts. Epidemics intermittently taxed the limited local organization for health during the seventeenth, eighteenth, and nineteenth centuries (Rosen, 1958).

After the American Revolution, the threat of disease, especially yellow fever epidemics, encouraged public support for new government-sponsored, official boards of health. New York City, with a population of 75,000 by 1800, established basic public health services, which included monitoring water quality, constructing sewers and a waterfront wall, draining marshes, planting trees and vegetables, and burying the dead (Rosen, 1958).

Increased urbanization and early industrialization in the new United States contributed to increased incidence of disease, including epidemics of smallpox, yellow fever, cholera, typhoid, and typhus. Tuberculosis and malaria remained endemic at a high incidence rate, and infant mortality was about 200 per 1000 live births (Pickett and Hanlon, 1990). American hospitals in the early 1800s were generally unsanitary and staffed by poorly trained workers; institutions were a place of last resort. Physicians received a limited education through proprietary schools or simple apprenticeship. Medical care was difficult to secure, although public dispensaries (similar to outpatient clinics) and private charitable efforts attempted to address gaps in the availability of sickness services, especially for the urban poor and working classes. Environmental conditions in urban neighborhoods, including inadequate housing and sanitation, were additional risks to health. Table 2-1 presents milestones of public health efforts that occurred from 1601 to the present.

| TABLE 2-1 | Milestones in the History of Public Health and Community Health Nursing: 1601 to 2014 |
|---|---|
| Year | Milestone |
| 1601 | The Act for the Relief of the Poor (the Elizabethan Poor Law) passed |
| 1751 | Pennsylvania Hospital founded in Philadelphia |
| 1793 | Baltimore Health Department established |
| 1798 | Marine Hospital Service established; in 1912 renamed the U.S. Public Health Service |
| 1813 | Ladies' Benevolent Society of Charleston, South Carolina, founded |
| 1815 | Sisters of Mercy established in Dublin, Ireland, where nuns visited the poor |
| 1836 | Lutheran deaconess movement founded in Kaiserswerth, Germany |
| 1851 | Florence Nightingale visits Kaiserswerth for 3 months of nurse training |
| 1859 | District nursing established in Liverpool, England, by William Rathbone |
| 1860 | Florence Nightingale Training School for Nurses established at St. Thomas Hospital in London, England |
| 1866 | New York Metropolitan Board of Health established |
| 1872 | American Public Health Association established |
| 1873 | New York Training School opens at Bellevue Hospital, New York City, as first Nightingale-model nursing school in the United States |
| 1877 | Women's Board of the New York Mission hires nurse Frances Root to visit the sick poor |
| 1881 | Clara Barton and a circle of her acquaintances found the American Red Cross in Washington, DC on May 21, 1881 |
| 1885 | Visiting Nurse Association established in Buffalo, NY |
| 1886 | Visiting nurse agencies established in Philadelphia and Boston |
| 1892 | First organized movement against tuberculosis |
| 1893 | Lillian Wald and Mary Brewster organize a visiting nursing service for the poor of New York, which later became the famous Henry Street Settlement and the Visiting Nurse Service of New York |
|  | Society of Superintendents of Training Schools of Nurses in the United States and Canada established (in 1912 it became known as the National League of Nursing Education) |

**TABLE 2-1   Milestones in the History of Public Health and Community Health Nursing: 1601 to 2014—cont'd**

| Year | Milestone |
| --- | --- |
| 1896 | Associated Alumnae of Training Schools for Nurses established (in 1911 it became the American Nurses Association) |
| 1902 | School nursing started in New York City, by Nurse Lina Rogers of Henry Street Settlement |
| 1903 | First Nurse Practice Acts passed |
| 1908 | National Association of Colored Graduate Nurses founded |
| 1909 | Metropolitan Life Insurance Company provides first insurance reimbursement for nursing care |
| 1910 | Public health nursing program instituted at Teachers College, Columbia University, NYC |
| 1912 | National Organization for Public Health Nursing formed; Lillian Wald is first president |
| 1916 | *Public Health Nursing* textbook by Mary Sewall Gardner published |
| 1918 | Vassar Training Camp for Nurses organized |
| | U.S. Public Health Service (USPHS) establishes division of public health nursing to work in the war effort |
| | Worldwide influenza epidemic begins |
| 1921 | Maternity and Infancy Act (Sheppard-Towner) passed; 2978 Prenatal and Child Health Centers |
| 1925 | Frontier Nursing Service using nurse-midwives established in Kentucky |
| 1933 | Pearl McIver is first nurse employed by the U.S. Public Health Service |
| 1935 | Social Security Act passed |
| | Association of State and Territorial Directors of Nursing founded |
| 1941 | United States enters World War II |
| 1943 | Bolton Act provides $5 million for nursing education; establishes Cadet Nurse Corps, with Lucille Petry as chief; 124,000 nurses graduate by 1948 when Corps ends |
| | USPHS Division of Nurse Education begun; becomes Division of Nursing in 1946 |
| 1944 | First basic program in nursing accredited as including sufficient public health content |
| 1946 | Nurses classified as professionals by U.S. Civil Service Commission |
| | Hill-Burton Act approved, providing funds for hospital construction in underserved areas and requiring these hospitals to provide care for poor people |
| | Passage of National Mental Health Act |
| 1950 | 25,091 nurses employed in public health |
| 1951 | National organizations recommend that college-based nursing education programs include public health content |
| 1952 | National Organization for Public Health Nursing merges into the new National League for Nursing |
| | Closure of Metropolitan Life Insurance Nursing Program |
| 1964 | Passage of Civil Rights Act and Economic Opportunity Act |
| | Public health nurse defined by the American Nurses Association (ANA) as a graduate of a BSN program |
| 1965 | ANA position paper recommends that nursing education take place in institutions of higher learning |
| 1966 | Medicare and Medicaid (Titles 18 and 19, of the Social Security Act) are implemented on July 1 (legislation passed in 1965) |
| 1977 | Passage of Rural Health Clinic Services Act, which provided indirect reimbursement for nurse practitioners in rural health clinics |
| 1978 | Association of Graduate Faculty in Community Health Nursing/Public Health Nursing founded (later, Association of Community Health Nursing Educators) |
| 1979 | Publication of *Healthy People: The Surgeon General's Report on Health Promotion and Disease Prevention* |
| 1980 | Medicaid amendment to the Social Security Act to provide direct reimbursement for nurse practitioners in rural health clinics |
| | ANA and APHA develop statements on the role and conceptual foundations of community and public health nursing, respectively |
| 1983 | Beginning of Medicare prospective payment system |
| 1985 | National Center for Nursing Research established in the National Institutes of Health |
| 1988 | Institute of Medicine reports on *The Future of Public Health* |
| 1990 | *Essentials of Baccalaureate Nursing Education*, from Association of Community Health Nursing Educators |
| 1991 | More than 60 nursing organizations join in support of health care reform; publish *Nursing's Agenda for Health Care Reform* |
| 1993 | American Health Security Act of 1993: blueprint for national health care reform; legislation fails; states and the private sector left to design own programs |
| 1994 | National Institute of Nursing Research, as part of the National Institutes of Health (was NCNR) |
| 1996 | *The Definition and Role of Public Health Nursing*, updated: Public Health Nursing Section, American Public Health Association |
| 1998 | *The Public Health Workforce: An Agenda for the 21st Century*, U.S. Public Health Service; examines current workforce in public, health, and educational needs, and the use of distance learning strategies to prepare future public health workers |
| 1999 | The Public Health Nursing Quad Council works with American Nurses Association on new *Scope and Standards of Public Health Nursing Practice*; differentiates between community-oriented and community-based nursing practice |
| 2001 | Public health gains a national presence in addressing concerns about biological and other terrorism, following September 11 attacks |
| 2002 | Department of Homeland Security established to provide leadership to protect against intentional threats to the health of the public |

*Continued*

| Year | Milestone |
|---|---|
| **TABLE 2-1** | **Milestones in the History of Public Health and Community Health Nursing: 1601 to 2014—cont'd** |
| 2003 | *Public Health Nursing Competencies* finalized by the Quad Council of Public Health Nursing Organizations |
| 2003–2005 | Multiple natural disasters including earthquakes, tsunamis, and hurricanes demonstrate the weak infrastructure for managing disasters in the United States and other countries and emphasize the need for strong public health programs that included disaster management |
| 2007 | An entirely new *Public Health Nursing: Scope and Standards of Practice* is released through the ANA, reflecting the efforts of the Quad Council of Public Health Nursing Organizations |
| 2010 | The Patient Protection and Affordable Care Act is signed by President Barack Obama |
| 2012 | The Association of State and Territorial Directors of Nursing (ASTDN) becomes the Association of Public Health Nurses (APHN) |
| 2013 | The revised *Public Health Nursing: Scope and Standards of Practice,* prepared by representatives of the Quad Council of Public Health Nursing Organizations, is released by the American Nurses Association |

*APHA,* American Public Health Association; *BSN,* Bachelor of Science in Nursing; *NCNR,* National Center for Nursing Research; *NYC,* New York City.

The federal government's early efforts for public health aimed to secure America's maritime trade and major coastal cities by providing health care for merchant seamen and by protecting seacoast cities from epidemics. The U.S. Public Health Service, still the most important federal public health agency in the twenty-first century, was established in 1798 as the Marine Hospital Service. The first Marine Hospital opened in Norfolk, Virginia, in 1800. Additional legislation to establish quarantine regulations for seamen and immigrants was passed in 1878.

During the early 1800s, experiments in providing nursing care at home focused on moral improvement and less on illness intervention. The Ladies' Benevolent Society of Charleston, South Carolina, provided charitable assistance to the poor and sick beginning in 1813. In Philadelphia, following a brief training program, lay nurses cared for postpartum women and newborns in their homes. In Cincinnati, Ohio, the Roman Catholic Sisters of Charity began a visiting nurse service in 1854 (Rodabaugh and Rodabaugh, 1951). Although these early programs provided services at the local level, they were not adopted elsewhere, and their influence on later public health nursing is unclear.

During the mid-nineteenth century, national interest increased for addressing public health problems and improving urban living conditions. New responsibilities for urban boards of health reflected changing ideas of public health, and these boards began to address communicable diseases and environmental hazards. Soon after it was founded in 1847, the American Medical Association (AMA) formed a hygiene committee to conduct sanitary surveys and to develop a system to collect vital statistics. The Shattuck Report, published in 1850 by the Massachusetts Sanitary Commission, called for major innovations: The establishment of a state health department and local health boards in every town; sanitary surveys and collection of vital statistics; environmental sanitation; food, drug, and communicable disease control; well-child care; health education; tobacco and alcohol control; town planning; and the teaching of preventive medicine in medical schools (Kalisch and Kalisch, 2004). However, these recommendations were not implemented even in Massachusetts until 1869, and in other states much later.

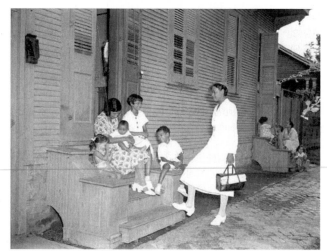

**FIG 2-1** A New Orleans nurse visiting a family on the doorstep of their home. (Courtesy of the New Orleans Public Library WPA Photograph Collection.)

In some areas, charitable organizations addressed the gap between known communicable disease epidemics and the lack of local government resources. For example, the Howard Association of New Orleans, Louisiana, responded to periodic yellow fever epidemics between 1837 and 1878 by providing physicians, lay nurses, and medicine. The Association established infirmaries and used sophisticated outreach strategies to locate cases (Hanggi-Myers, 1995)(Figure 2-1).

## NIGHTINGALE AND THE ORIGINS OF TRAINED NURSING

The origins of professional nursing are found in the work of Florence Nightingale in nineteenth-century Europe. With tremendous advances in transportation, communication, and other forms of technology, the Industrial Revolution led to deep social upheaval. Even with the advancement of science, medicine, and technology during the two previous centuries, nineteenth-century public health measures continued to be unsophisticated. Organization and management of cities

← Nightingale →

improved slowly, and many areas lacked systems of sewage disposal and depended on private enterprise for water supply. Previous caregiving structures, which relied on the assistance of family, neighbors, and friends, became inadequate in the early nineteenth century because of human migration, urbanization, and changing demand. During this period, a few groups of Roman Catholic and Protestant women provided nursing care for the sick, poor, and neglected in institutions and sometimes in the home. For example, Mary Aikenhead, also known by her religious name Sister Mary Augustine, organized the Irish Sisters of Charity in Dublin (Ireland) in 1815. These sisters visited the poor at home and established hospitals and schools (Kalisch and Kalisch, 2004).

In nineteenth-century England, the Elizabethan Poor Law continued to guarantee medical care for all. This minimal care, provided most often in almshouses supported by local government, sought as much to regulate where the poor could live as to provide care during illness. Many women who performed nursing functions in almshouses and early hospitals in Great Britain were poorly educated, untrained, and often undependable. As the practice of medicine became more complex in the mid-1800s, hospital work required skilled caregivers. Physicians and hospital administrators sought to advance the practice of nursing. Early innovations yielded some improvement in care, but Florence Nightingale's efforts were revolutionary.

Florence Nightingale's vision for trained nurses and her model of nursing education influenced the development of professional nursing and, indirectly, public health nursing in the United States. In 1850 and 1851, Nightingale had carefully studied nursing "system and method" by visiting Pastor Theodor Fliedner at his School for Deaconesses in Kaiserswerth, Germany. Pastor Fliedner also built on the work of others, including Mennonite deaconesses in the Netherlands who were engaged in parish work for the poor and the sick, and Elizabeth Fry, the English prison reformer. Thus mid-nineteenth century efforts to reform the practice of nursing drew on a variety of interacting innovations across Europe.

The Kaiserswerth Lutheran deaconesses incorporated care of the sick in the hospital with client care in their homes, and their system of district nursing spread to other German cities. American requests for the deaconesses to respond to epidemics of typhus and cholera in Pittsburgh provided only temporary assistance because local women were uninterested in joining the work. The early efforts of the Lutheran deaconesses in the United States ultimately focused on developing systems of institutional care (Nutting and Dock, 1935).

Nightingale also found a way to implement her ideas about nursing practice. During the Crimean War (1854–1856) between the alliance of England and France against Russia, the British military established hospitals for sick and wounded soldiers at Scutari (now Üsküdar, in modern Istanbul). The care of sick and wounded soldiers was severely deficient, with cramped quarters, poor sanitation, lice and rats, insufficient food, and inadequate medical supplies (Palmer, 1983; Kalisch and Kalisch, 2004). When the British public demanded improved conditions, Nightingale sought and received an appointment to address the chaos. Because of her wealth, social and political

connections, and knowledge of hospitals, the British government sent her 40 ladies, 117 hired nurses, 15 paid servants, and extensive supplies for patient care.

In Scutari, Nightingale progressively improved soldiers' health outcomes, using a population-based approach that strengthened environmental conditions and nursing care. Using simple epidemiological measures, she documented a decreased mortality rate from 415 per 1000 men at the beginning of the war to 11.5 per 1000 at the end (Palmer, 1983; Cohen, 1984). Paralleling Nightingale's efforts, public health nurses typically identify health care needs that affect the entire population, mobilize resources, and organize themselves and the community to meet these needs.

Nightingale's fame was established even before she returned to England in 1856 after the Crimean War. She then reorganized hospital nursing practice and established hospital-based nursing education to replace untrained lay nurses with trained Nightingale nurses. Nightingale also emphasized public health nursing: "The health of the unity is the health of the community. Unless you have the health of the unity, there is no community health" (Nightingale, 1894/1984, p. 455). She differentiated "sick nursing" from "health nursing." The latter emphasized that nurses should strive to promote health and prevent illness. Nightingale (1859/1946, p. v) wrote that the task of nurses is to "put the constitution in such a state as that it will have no disease, or that it can recover from disease." Proper nutrition, rest, sanitation, and hygiene were necessary for health. Nurses continue to focus on the vital role of health promotion, disease prevention, and environment in their practice with individuals, families, and communities.

Nightingale's contemporary and friend, British philanthropist William Rathbone, founded the first district nursing association in Liverpool, England. Rathbone's wife had received outstanding nursing care from a Nightingale-trained nurse during her terminal illness at home. He wanted to offer similar care to relieve the suffering of poor persons unable to afford private nurses. With Rathbone's advocacy and economic support between 1859 and 1862, the Liverpool Relief Society divided the city into nursing districts and assigned a committee of "friendly visitors" to each district to provide health care to needy people (Kalisch and Kalisch, 2004). Building on the Liverpool experience, Rathbone and Nightingale recommended steps to provide nursing in the home, leading to the organization of district nursing throughout England. Florence Sarah Lees Craven shaped the profession through her book *A Guide to District Nurses*, which highlighted, for example, that nursing care during the illness of one family member provided the nurse with influence to improve the entire family's health status (Craven, 1889/1984).

## AMERICA NEEDS TRAINED NURSES

As urbanization increased during the Industrial Revolution in the 1800s, the number of occupations for American women rapidly increased. Educated women became elementary school teachers, secretaries, or saleswomen. Less educated women worked in factories of all kinds. The idea of becoming a trained nurse increased in popularity when Nightingale's successes became known across the United States. During the 1870s, the first nursing schools based on the Nightingale model opened in the United States.

Trained nurse graduates of the early schools for nurses in the United States usually worked in private duty nursing or held the few positions as hospital administrators or instructors. Private duty nurses might live with families of clients receiving care, to be available 24 hours a day. Although the trained nurse's role in improving American hospitals was very clear, the cost of private duty nursing care for the sick at home was prohibitive for all but the wealthy.

The care of the sick poor at home was made more economical by using home-visiting nurses who would attend several families in a day, rather than only one patient as the private duty nurse did. In 1877 the Women's Board of the New York City Mission hired Frances Root, a graduate of Bellevue Hospital's first nursing class, to visit sick poor persons to provide nursing care and religious instruction (Bullough and Bullough, 1964). In 1878 the Ethical Culture Society of New York hired four nurses to work in dispensaries, a type of community-based clinic. In the next few years, visiting nurse associations (VNAs) were established in Buffalo, New York (1885), Philadelphia (1886), and Boston (1886). Wealthy people interested in charitable activities funded both settlement houses and VNAs. Upper-class women, freed of some of the social restrictions that had previously limited their public life, participated in the charitable work of creating, supporting, and supervising the new visiting nurses.

Public health nursing in the United States began with organizing to meet urban health care needs, especially for the disadvantaged. The public was interested in limiting disease among all classes of people, not only for religious reasons as a form of charity, but also because the middle and upper classes feared the impact of communicable diseases believed to originate in the large communities of new European immigrants. In New York City in the 1890s, about 2.3 million people lived in 90,000 tenement houses. Deplorable environmental conditions for immigrants in urban tenement houses and sweatshops were common across the northeastern United States and upper Midwest. People living in poor housing conditions were ravaged by epidemics of communicable diseases, including typhus, scarlet fever, smallpox, and typhoid fever; in the nineteenth century, tuberculosis was the leading cause of infectious disease mortality (Kalisch and Kalisch, 2004). From the beginning, nursing practice in the community included teaching and prevention.

For example, in 1886 two Boston women approached the Women's Education Association to seek local support for district nursing. To increase the likelihood of financial support, they used the term *instructive district nursing* to emphasize the relationship of nursing to health education. The Boston Dispensary provided support in the form of free outpatient medical care. In 1886 the first district nurse was hired, and in 1888 the Instructive District Nursing Association became incorporated as an independent voluntary agency. Sick poor persons, who paid no fees, were cared for under the direction of a trained physician (Brainard, 1922).

Nursing interventions, improved sanitation, economic improvements, and better nutrition were credited with reducing the incidence of acute communicable disease by 1910. New scientific explanations of communicable disease suggested that preventive education would reduce illness. Through home visits and well-baby clinics, the visiting nurse became the key to communicating this prevention campaign. Visiting nurses worked with physicians, gave selected treatments, and kept temperature and pulse records. Visiting nurses emphasized education of family members in the care of the sick and in personal and environmental prevention measures, such as hygiene and good nutrition. Most public health nursing practice in the early twentieth century was generalized practice with diverse responsibilities. Only a few public health nurses had a specialized practice, such as caring only for patients with tuberculosis or working only in an occupational health practice. Public health nurses also established settlement houses—neighborhood centers that became hubs for health care, education, and social welfare programs. For example, in 1893 Lillian Wald and Mary Brewster, both trained nurses, began visiting the poor on New York's Lower East Side. The nurses' settlement they established became the Henry Street Settlement and later the Visiting Nurse Service of New York City. By 1905 the public health nurses had provided almost 48,000 visits to more than 5000 clients (Kalisch and Kalisch, 2004). Other settlement houses influenced the growth of public health nursing including the Richmond (Virginia) Nurses' Settlement, which became the Instructive Visiting Nurse Association; the Nurses' Settlement in Orange, New Jersey; and the College Settlement in Los Angeles, California. See the box below for a photo of Lillian Wald (Figure 2-2).

Lillian Wald emerged as the key leader of public health nursing during its early decades. Wald took steps to increase access to public health nursing services nationally through insightful innovations: She persuaded the American Red Cross to sponsor rural health nursing services across the country, which stimulated local governments to sponsor public health nursing through county health departments. Beginning in 1909, Wald worked with Dr. Lee Frankel of the Metropolitan Life Insurance Company (MetLife) to implement the first insurance payment for nursing services. She argued that keeping working people and their families healthier would increase their productivity. MetLife found that nursing care for communicable diseases, injuries, and mothers and children reduced mortality and saved money for this life insurance company. MetLife nursing services continued for 44 years, with successes such as (1) providing home nursing services on a fee-for-service basis, (2) establishing an effective cost-accounting system for visiting nurses, and (3) reducing mortality from infectious diseases.

Convinced that environmental conditions as well as social conditions were the causes of ill health and poverty, Wald became actively involved in using epidemiological methods to campaign for health-promoting social policies. She advocated for creation of the U.S. Children's Bureau as a basis for improving the health and education of children nationally. She fought for better tenement living conditions in New York City, city recreation centers, parks, pure food laws, graded classes for mentally handicapped children, and assistance to immigrants.

WWI y

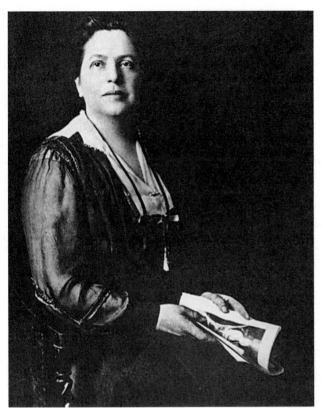

**FIG 2-2** Lillian Wald. (Courtesy of the Visiting Nurse Service of New York.)

She firmly believed in women's suffrage and considered its acceptance in 1917 in New York State to be a great victory. Wald supported efforts to improve race relations and championed solutions to racial injustice. She wrote *The House on Henry Street* (Wald, 1915) and *Windows on Henry Street* (Wald, 1934) to describe this public health nursing work.

Many public health nurses contributed to the development of the profession, including Jessie Sleet (Scales), a Canadian graduate of Provident Hospital School of Nursing (Chicago), who was the first African-American public health nurse; Ms. Sleet was hired by the New York Charity Organization Society in 1900. Although it proved difficult for her to find an agency willing to hire her as a district nurse, she persevered and was able to provide exceptional care for her clients until she married in 1909. At the Charity Organization Society in 1904 to 1905, she studied health conditions related to tuberculosis among African-American people in Manhattan, using interviews with families and neighbors, house-to-house canvases, direct observation, and speeches at neighborhood churches. Sleet reported her research to the Society board, recommending improved employment opportunities for African-Americans and better prevention strategies to reduce the excess burden of tuberculosis morbidity and mortality among the African-American population (Thoms, 1929; Hine, 1989; Mosley, 1994; Buhler-Wilkerson, 2001).

In 1909 Yssabella Waters published her survey, *Visiting Nursing in the United States,* which documented the concentration of visiting nurse services in the northeastern quadrant of the nation (Waters, 1909). In 1901 New York City alone had 58 different organizations with 372 trained nurses providing care in the community. Despite the numbers, 68% of visiting nurses nationally were employed in single-nurse agencies. In addition to VNAs and settlement houses, a variety of other organizations sponsored visiting nurse work, including boards of education, boards of health, mission boards, clubs, churches, social service agencies, and tuberculosis associations. With tuberculosis then responsible for at least 10% of all mortality, visiting nurses contributed to its control through gaining "the personal cooperation of patients and their families" to modify the environment and individual behavior (Buhler-Wilkerson, 1987, p. 45). Most visiting nurse agencies depended financially on the philanthropy and social networks of metropolitan areas. As today, fund-raising and service delivery in less densely populated and rural areas was challenging.

The American Red Cross, through its Rural Nursing Service (later the Town and Country Nursing Service), provided a framework to initiate home nursing care in areas outside larger cities. Wald secured initial donations to support this agency, which provided care of the sick and instruction in sanitation and hygiene in rural homes. The agency also improved living conditions in villages and isolated farms. The Town and Country nurse dealt with diseases such as tuberculosis, pneumonia, and typhoid fever with a resourcefulness born of necessity. The rural nurse might use hot bricks, salt, or sandbags to substitute for hot water bottles; chairs as back-rests for the bedbound; and boards padded with quilts as stretchers (Kalisch and Kalisch, 2004). In the two years after World War I, the 100 existing Red Cross Town and Country Nursing Services expanded to 1800, and eventually to almost 3000 programs in small towns and rural areas. This service demonstrated the importance and feasibility of public health nursing across the country at local and county levels. Once established, ongoing responsibilities for these new agencies were passed on to local voluntary agencies or local government support.

Occupational health nursing began as industrial nursing and was a true outgrowth of early home-visiting efforts. In 1895 Ada Mayo Stewart began work with employees and families of the Vermont Marble Company in Proctor, Vermont. As a free service for the employees, Stewart provided obstetric care, sickness care (e.g., for typhoid cases), and some postsurgical care in workers' homes. Although her employer provided a horse and buggy, she often made home visits on a bicycle. Unlike contemporary occupational health nurses, Stewart provided few services for work-related injuries. Before 1900 a few nurses were hired in industry, such as in department stores in Philadelphia and Brooklyn. Between 1914 and 1943, industrial nursing grew from 60 to 11,220 nurses, reflecting increased governmental and employee concerns for health and safety in the workplace (American Association of Industrial Nurses, 1976; Kalisch and Kalisch, 2004).

## SCHOOL NURSING IN AMERICA

In New York City in 1902, more than 20% of children might be absent from school on a single day. The children suffered from the common conditions of pediculosis, ringworm, scabies, inflamed eyes, discharging ears, and infected wounds. Physicians began to make limited inspections of school students in 1897, but they focused on excluding sick children from school rather than on providing or obtaining medical treatment to enable children to return to school. Familiar with this community-wide problem from her work with the Henry Street Nurses' Settlement, Lillian Wald sought to place nurses in the schools and gained consent from the city's health commissioner and the Board of Education for a 1-month demonstration project.

Lina Rogers, a Henry Street Settlement resident, became the first school nurse. She worked with the children in New York City schools and made home visits to instruct parents and to follow up on children excluded or otherwise absent from school. The school nurses found that "many children were absent for lack of shoes or clothing, because of malnourishment, or because they were serving their families as babysitters" (Hawkins et al, 1994, p. 417). The school nurse experiment made such a significant and positive impact that it became permanent, with 12 more nurses appointed 1 month later. School nursing was soon implemented in Los Angeles, Philadelphia, Baltimore, Boston, Chicago, and San Francisco.

## THE PROFESSION COMES OF AGE

Established by the Cleveland Visiting Nurse Association in 1909, the *Visiting Nurse Quarterly* initiated a professional communication medium for clinical and organizational concerns. In 1911 a joint committee of existing nurse organizations convened to standardize nursing services outside the hospital. Under the leadership of Lillian Wald and Mary Gardner, the committee recommended forming a new organization to address public health nursing concerns. Eight hundred agencies involved in public health nursing were invited to send delegates to a June 1912 organizational meeting in Chicago. After a heated debate on its name and purpose, the delegates established the National Organization for Public Health Nursing (NOPHN) and chose Wald as its first president (Dock, 1922). Unlike other professional nursing organizations, the NOPHN membership included both nurses and their non-nurse supporters. The NOPHN sought "to improve the educational and services standards of the public health nurse, and promote public understanding of and respect for her work" (Rosen, 1958, p. 381). With greater administrative resources than other contemporary national nursing organizations, the NOPHN was soon the dominant force in public health nursing (Roberts, 1955).

The NOPHN also sought to standardize public health nursing education. Visiting nurse agencies found that hospital training school graduates were unprepared for home visiting. Hospital training schools emphasized hospital care of sick patients, but public health nurses required additional educational preparation to provide services through home-visiting and population-focused programs. In 1914, in affiliation with the Henry Street Settlement, Mary Adelaide Nutting began the first post–training-school course in public health nursing at Teachers College in New York City (Deloughery, 1977). The

American Red Cross provided scholarships for training school graduates to attend the public health nursing course. Its success encouraged the development of other programs, using curricula that might seem familiar to today's nurses. During the 1920s and 1930s, many newly hired public health nurses had to verify completion or promptly enroll in a certificate program in public health nursing. Others took leave for a year to travel to an urban center to obtain this further education.

Public health nurses were also active in the American Public Health Association (APHA), which had been established in 1872 to facilitate interprofessional efforts and promote the "practical application of public hygiene" (Scutchfield and Keck, 1997, p. 12). The APHA targeted reform efforts toward contemporary public health issues, including sewage and garbage disposal, occupational injuries, and sexually transmitted diseases. In 1923 the Public Health Nursing Section was formed within the APHA to provide a forum for nurses to discuss their concerns and strategies within the larger APHA. The PHN Section continues to serve as a focus of leadership and policy development for public health nursing in the twenty-first century.

## PUBLIC HEALTH NURSING IN OFFICIAL HEALTH AGENCIES AND IN WORLD WAR I

Public health nursing in voluntary agencies and through the Red Cross grew more quickly than public health nursing in official agencies, those sponsored by state, local, and national government. By 1900, 38 states had established state health departments; however, these early state boards of health had limited impact. Only three states—Massachusetts, Rhode Island, and Florida—annually spent more than 2 cents per capita for public health services (Scutchfield and Keck, 1997).

The federal role in public health gradually expanded. In 1912 the federal government redefined the role of the U.S. Public Health Service, empowering it to "investigate the causes and spread of diseases and the pollution and sanitation of navigable streams and lakes" (Scutchfield and Keck, 1997, p. 15). The NOPHN loaned a nurse to the U.S. Public Health Service during World War I to establish a public health nursing program for military outposts. This led to the first federal government sponsorship of nurses (Shyrock, 1959; Wilner et al, 1978).

During the 1910s, public health organizations began to target infectious and parasitic diseases in rural areas. The Rockefeller Sanitary Commission, a philanthropic organization active in hookworm control in the southeastern United States, concluded that concurrent efforts for all phases of public health were necessary to successfully address any individual public health problem (Pickett and Hanlon, 1990). For example, in 1911, efforts to control typhoid fever in Yakima County, Washington, and to improve health status in Guilford County, North Carolina, led to the establishment of local health units to serve local populations. Public health nurses were the primary staff members of local health departments. These nurses assumed a leadership role on health care issues through collaboration with local residents, nurses, and other health care providers.

The experience of Orange County, California, during the 1920s and 1930s illustrates the role of the public health nurse in these new local health departments. Following the efforts of a private physician, social welfare agencies, and a Red Cross nurse, the county board created the public health nurse's position, which began in 1922. Presented with a shining new Model T car sporting the bright orange seal of the county, the nurse focused on the serious communicable disease problems of diphtheria and scarlet fever. Typhoid became epidemic when a drainage pipe overflowed into a well, infecting those who drank the well water or raw milk from an infected dairy. Almost 3000 residents were immunized against typhoid. Weekly well-baby conferences provided an opportunity for mothers to learn about care of their infants, and the infants were weighed and given communicable disease immunizations. Children with orthopedic disorders and other disabilities were identified and referred for medical care in Los Angeles. At the end of a successful first year of public health nursing work, the Rockefeller Foundation and the California Health Department recognized the favorable outcomes and provided funding for more public health professionals.

The personnel needs of World War I in Europe depleted the ranks of public health nurses, at the same time the NOPHN had identified a need for more public health nurses within the United States. Jane Delano of the Red Cross (which was sending 100 nurses a day to the war) agreed that despite the sacrifice, the greatest patriotic duty of public health nurses was to stay at home. In 1918 the worldwide influenza pandemic swept the United States from coast to coast within 3 weeks, and was met by a coalition of the NOPHN and the Red Cross. Houses, churches, and social halls were turned into hospitals for the immense numbers of sick and dying. Some of the nurse volunteers died of influenza as well (Shyrock, 1959; Wilner et al, 1978).

## PAYING THE BILL FOR PUBLIC HEALTH NURSES

Inadequate funding was the major obstacle to extending nursing services in the community. Most early VNAs sought charitable contributions from wealthy and middle-class supporters. Even poor families were encouraged to pay a small fee for nursing services, reflecting social welfare concerns against promoting economic dependency by providing charity. In 1909, as a result of Wald's collaboration with Dr. Lee Frankel, the Metropolitan Life Insurance Company began a cooperative program with visiting nurse organizations that expanded availability of public health nursing services. The nurses assessed illness, taught health practices, and collected data from policyholders. By 1912, 589 Metropolitan Life nursing centers provided care through existing agencies or through visiting nurses hired directly by the Company. In 1918 Metropolitan Life calculated an average decline of 7% in the mortality rate of policyholders and almost a 20% decline in the mortality rate of policyholders' children under age 3. The insurance company attributed this improvement and their reduced costs to the work of visiting nurses. Voluntary health insurance was still decades in the future; public and professional efforts to secure compulsory health insurance seemed promising in 1916, but had evaporated by the end of World War I.

Nursing efforts to influence public policy bridged World War I, including advocacy for the Children's Bureau and the Sheppard-Towner Program. Responding to lengthy advocacy by Wald and other nurse leaders, the Children's Bureau was established in 1912 to address national problems of maternal and child welfare. Children's Bureau experts conducted extensive scientific research on the effects of income, housing, employment, and other factors on infant and maternal mortality. Their research led to federal child labor laws and the 1919 White House Conference on Child Health.

Problems of maternal and child morbidity and mortality spurred the passage of the Maternity and Infancy Act (often called the Sheppard-Towner Act) in 1921. This act provided federal matching funds to establish maternal and child health divisions in state health departments. Education during home visits by public health nurses stressed promoting the health of mother and child as well as seeking prompt medical care during pregnancy. Although credited with saving many lives, the Sheppard-Towner Program ended in 1929 in response to charges by the AMA and others that the legislation gave too much power to the federal government and too closely resembled socialized medicine (Pickett and Hanlon, 1990). Federal funding during the 1930s and 1940s established maternal-child health programs that continued some of the successes of Sheppard-Towner.

Some nursing innovations were the result of individual commitment and private financial support. In 1925 Mary Breckinridge established the Frontier Nursing Service (FNS), based on systems of care used in the Highlands and islands of Scotland. The unique pioneering spirit of the FNS influenced the development of public health programs geared toward improving the health care of the rural and often inaccessible populations in the Appalachian region of southeastern Kentucky (Browne, 1966; Tirpak, 1975). Breckinridge introduced the first nurse-midwives into the United States when she deployed FNS nurses trained in nursing, public health, and midwifery. Their efforts led to reduced pregnancy complications and maternal mortality, and to one-third fewer stillbirths and infant deaths in an area of 700 square miles (Kalisch and Kalisch, 2004). The early efforts of the Frontier Nursing Service are recorded in the book, *Wide Neighborhoods* (Breckinridge, 1952). Today the FNS continues to provide comprehensive health and nursing services to the people of that area and sponsors Frontier Nursing University, which provides advanced practice nursing education for midwifery and other specialties.

## AFRICAN-AMERICAN NURSES IN PUBLIC HEALTH NURSING

African-American nurses seeking to work in public health nursing faced many challenges. Nursing education was absolutely segregated in the South until at least the 1960s, and elsewhere was also generally segregated or rationed until mid-century. Even public health nursing certificate and graduate education programs were segregated in the South; study outside the South for southern nurses was difficult to afford and study leaves from the workplace were rarely granted. The situation improved somewhat in 1936, when collaboration between the U.S. Public Health Service and the Medical College of Virginia (Richmond) established a certificate program in public health nursing for African-American nurses, with tuition provided by the federal government. Discrimination continued during nurses' employment: African-American nurses in the American South were paid significantly lower salaries than their white counterparts for the same work. In 1925 just 435 African-American public health nurses were employed in the United States, and in 1930 only 6 African-American nurses held supervisory positions in public health nursing organizations (Thoms, 1929; Hine, 1989; Buhler-Wilkerson, 2001).

African-American public health nurses had a significant impact on the communities they served. The National Health Circle for Colored People was organized in 1919 to promote public health work in African-American communities in the South. One approach provided scholarships to assist African-American nurses to pursue university-level public health nursing education. Bessie B. Hawes, the first recipient of the scholarship, completed the Columbia University program in New York City. The Circle sent Hawes to Palatka, Florida, a small, isolated lumber town. Hawes' first project recruited local school girls to promote health by dressing as nurses and marching in a parade while singing community songs. She conducted mass meetings, led mother's clubs, provided school health education, and visited the homes of the sick. Eventually she gained the community's trust, overcame opposition, and built a health center for nursing care and treatment (Thoms, 1929).

## BETWEEN THE TWO WORLD WARS: ECONOMIC DEPRESSION AND THE RISE OF HOSPITALS

The economic crisis during the Depression of the 1930s deeply influenced the development of nursing. Not only were agencies and communities unprepared to address the increased needs and numbers of the impoverished, but decreased funding for nursing services reduced the number of employed nurses in hospitals and in community agencies. The NOPHN's tenacious effort to ensure inclusion of public health nursing in federal relief programs secured success after a flurry of last-minute telegrams and lobbying efforts. Federal funding led to a wide variety of programs administered at the state level, including new public health nursing programs.

The Federal Emergency Relief Administration (FERA) supported nurse employment through increased grants-in-aid for state programs of home medical care. FERA often purchased nursing care from existing visiting nurse agencies, thus supporting more nurses and preventing agency closures. The FERA program varied among states; the state FERA program in New York emphasized bedside nursing care, whereas in North Carolina, the state FERA prioritized maternal and child health, and school nursing services. Some Depression-era federal programs built new services; public health nursing programs of the Works Progress Administration (WPA) were sometimes later incorporated into state health departments. In West Virginia, as

elsewhere, the Relief Nursing Service had a dual purpose—to assist unemployed nurses and to provide nursing care for families on relief. Fundamental services included "(1) providing bedside care and health supervision for the family in the home; (2) arranging for medical and hospital care for emergency and obstetric cases; (3) supervising the health of children in emergency relief nursery schools; and (4) caring for patients with tuberculosis" (Kalisch and Kalisch, 2004, p. 283).

In another Depression-era program, more than 10,000 nurses were employed by the Civil Works Administration (CWA) and assigned to official health agencies. "While this facilitated rapid program expansion by recipient agencies and gave the nurses a taste of public health, the nurses' lack of field experience created major problems of training and supervision for the regular staff" (Roberts and Heinrich, 1985, p. 1162).

A 1932 survey of public health agencies found that only 7% of nurses employed in public health were adequately prepared (Roberts and Heinrich, 1985). Basic nursing education focused heavily on the care of individuals, and students received limited information on groups and the community as a unit of service. Thus in the 1930s and early 1940s, new hospital training school graduates continued to be inadequately prepared to work in public health and required considerable remedial orientation and education from the hiring agencies (NOPHN, 1944).

Public health nurses continued to weigh the relative value of preventive care compared with bedside care of the sick. They also questioned whether nursing interventions should be directed toward groups and communities, or toward individuals and their families. Although each nursing agency was unique and services varied from region to region, voluntary VNAs tended to emphasize care of the sick, whereas official public health agencies provided more preventive services. Compared with nursing in VNAs, nurses in official agencies may have had less control over their practice roles because physicians and politicians often determined services and personnel assignments in public health departments. See Figure 2-1 for a photo of a nurse making a home visit to a family in New Orleans.

Not surprisingly, the conflicting visions and splintering of services between "visiting" and "public health" nurses further impeded development of comprehensive population-centered nursing services (Roberts and Heinrich, 1985). In addition, some households received services from several community nurses representing several agencies, for example, visits to the same home (1) for a postpartum woman and new baby, (2) for a child sick with scarlet fever, and (3) for an older adult sick in bed. Nurses believed that multiple caregivers and agencies confused families and duplicated scarce nursing resources. Interest grew in the "combination service"—the merger of sick care services and preventive services into one comprehensive agency, administered jointly between a voluntary agency and an official health agency.

## INCREASING FEDERAL ACTION FOR THE PUBLIC'S HEALTH

Expansion of the federal government during the 1930s affected the structure of community health resources. Credited as "the beginning of a new era in public nursing" (Roberts and Heinrich, 1985, p. 1162), Pearl McIver in 1933 became the first nurse employed by the U.S. Public Health Service. In providing consultation services to state health departments, McIver was convinced that the strengths and ability of each state's director of public health nursing would determine the scope and quality of local health services. Together with Naomi Deutsch, director of nursing for the federal Children's Bureau, and with the support of nursing organizations, McIver and her staff of nurse consultants influenced the direction of public health nursing. Between 1931 and 1938, greater than 40% of the increase in public health nurse employment was in local health agencies. Even so, nationally more than one-third of all counties still lacked local public health nursing services.

The Social Security Act of 1935 was designed to prevent reoccurrence of the problems of the Depression. Title VI of this act provided funding for expanded opportunities for health protection and promotion through education and employment of public health nurses. More than 1000 nurses completed educational programs in public health in 1936. Title VI also provided $8 million to assist states, counties, and medical districts in the establishment and maintenance of adequate health services, as well as $2 million for research and investigation of disease (Buhler-Wilkerson, 1985, 1989; Kalisch and Kalisch, 2004).

A categorical approach to federal funding for public health services reflected the U.S. Congress's preference for funding specific diseases or specific groups, rather than providing dollar allocations to local agencies. In categorical funding, resources are directed toward specific priorities rather than toward a comprehensive community health program. When funding is directed by established national preferences, it becomes more difficult to respond to local and emerging problems. Even so, local health departments shaped their programs according to the pattern of available funds, including maternal and child health services and crippled children (in 1935), venereal disease control (in 1938), tuberculosis (in 1944), mental health (in 1947), industrial hygiene (in 1947), and dental health (in 1947) (Scutchfield and Keck, 1997). Categorical funding continues to be a preferred federal approach to address national health policy objectives.

## WORLD WAR II: EXTENSION AND RETRENCHMENT IN PUBLIC HEALTH NURSING

The U.S. involvement in World War II in 1941 accelerated the need for nurses, both for the war effort and at home. The Nursing Council on National Defense was a coalition of the national nursing organizations that planned and coordinated activities for the war effort. National interests prioritized the health of military personnel and workers in essential industries. Many nurses joined the Army and Navy Nurse Corps. Through the influence and leadership of U.S. Representative Frances Payne Bolton of Ohio, substantial funding was provided by the Bolton Act of 1943 to establish the Cadet Nurse Corps, supporting increased enrollment in schools of nursing at undergraduate and graduate levels. Under management by

the U.S. Public Health Service, the Nursing Council for National Defense received $1 million to expand facilities for nursing education. Additional programs that expanded both the total number of nurses and the number of nurses with preparation in public health nursing included the Training for Nurses for National Defense, the GI Bill, the Nurse Training Act of 1943, and Public Health and Professional Nurse Traineeships (McNeil, 1967).

As more and more nurses and physicians left civilian hospitals to meet the needs of the war, responsibility for client care was shifted to families, non-nursing personnel, and volunteers. "By the end of 1942, over 500,000 women had completed the American Red Cross home nursing course, and nearly 17,000 nurse's aides had been certified" (Roberts and Heinrich, 1985, p. 1165). By the end of 1946, more than 215,000 volunteer nurse's aides had received certificates.

In some cases, public health nursing expanded its scope of practice during World War II. For example, nurses increased their presence in rural areas, and many official agencies began to provide bedside nursing care (Buhler-Wilkerson, 1985; Kalisch and Kalisch, 2004). The federal Emergency Maternity and Infant Care Act of 1943 (EMIC) provided funding for medical, hospital, and nursing care for the wives and babies of servicemen. Health services seeking EMIC funds were required to meet the high standards of the U.S. Children's Bureau, which resulted in increased quality of care for all. In other situations, nursing roles were constrained by wartime and postwar nursing shortages. For example, the Visiting Nurse Society of Philadelphia ceased home birth services, drastically reduced industrial nursing services, and deferred care for the long-term chronically ill client.

Reflecting the complex social changes that had occurred during the war years, in the late 1940s local health departments faced sudden increases in client demand for care of emotional problems, accidents, alcoholism, and other responsibilities new to the domain of official health agencies. Changes in medical technology offered new possibilities for screening and treatment of infectious and communicable diseases, such as antibiotics to treat rheumatic fever and venereal diseases, and photofluorography for mass case finding of pulmonary tuberculosis. Local health departments expanded, both to address underserved areas and to expand types of services, and they often fared better economically than voluntary agencies.

Job opportunities for public health nurses grew because they continued to constitute a large proportion of health department personnel. Between 1950 and 1955, the proportion of U.S. counties with full-time local health services increased from 56% to 72% (Roberts and Heinrich, 1985). With more than 20,000 nurses employed in health departments, VNAs, industry, and schools, public health nurses at the middle of the twentieth century continued to have a crucial role in translating the advances of science and medicine into saving lives and improving health.

In 1946, representatives of agencies interested in community health met to improve coordination of various types of community nursing and to prevent overlap of services. The resulting guidelines proposed that a population of 50,000 be required to support a public health program and that there should be 1 nurse for every 2200 people. Nursing functions should include health teaching, disease control, and care of the sick. Communities were encouraged to adopt one of the following organizational patterns (NOPHN, 1946):

- Administration of all community health nurse services by the local health department;
- Provision of preventive health care by health departments, and provision of home visiting for the sick by a cooperating voluntary agency; or
- A combination service jointly administered and financed by official and voluntary agencies with all services provided by one group of nurses.

## THE RISE OF CHRONIC ILLNESS

Between 1900 and 1955, the national crude mortality rate decreased by 47%. Many more Americans survived childhood and early adulthood to live into middle and older ages. Although in 1900 the leading causes of mortality were pneumonia, tuberculosis, and diarrhea/enteritis, by mid-century the leading causes had become heart disease, cancer, and cerebrovascular disease. Nurses helped to reduce communicable disease mortality through immunization campaigns, nutrition education, and provision of better hygiene and sanitation. Additional factors included improved medications, better housing, and innovative emergency and critical care services. Studies such as the National Health Survey of 1935-1936 had documented the national transition from communicable to chronic disease as the primary cause of significant illness and death. However, public policy and nursing services were diverted from addressing the emerging problem, first by the 1930s Depression and then by World War II.

As the aged population grew from 4.1% of the total in 1900, to 9.2% in 1950, so did the prevalence of chronic illness. Faced with a client population characterized by extended life spans and increased longevity after chronic illness diagnosis, nurses addressed new challenges related to chronic illness care, long-term illness and disability, and chronic disease prevention. In official health agencies, categorical programs focusing on a single chronic disease emphasized narrowly defined services, which might be poorly coordinated with other community programs. Screening for chronic illness was a popular method of both detecting undiagnosed disease and providing individual and community education.

Some VNAs adopted coordinated home care programs to provide complex, long-term care to the chronically ill, often after long-term hospitalization. These home care programs established a multidisciplinary approach to complex client care. For example, beginning in 1949, the Visiting Nurse Society of Philadelphia provided care to clients with stroke, arthritis, cancer, and fractures using a wide range of services, including physical and occupational therapy, nutrition consultation, social services, laboratory and radiographic procedures, and transportation services. During the 1950s, often in response to family demands and the shortage of nurses, many visiting nurse agencies began experimenting with auxiliary nursing personnel,

variously called housekeepers, homemakers, or home health aides. These innovative programs provided a substantial basis for an approach to bedside nursing care that would be reimbursable by commercial health insurance (such as Blue Cross) and later by Medicare and Medicaid.

The increased prevalence of chronic illness also encouraged a resurgence in combination agencies—the joint operation of official (city or county) health departments and voluntary visiting nurse agencies by a unified staff. The nursing profession preferred that services be provided in a coordinated, cost-effective manner respectful to the families served, as well as to avoid duplication of care. Where nursing services were specialized, one household might simultaneously receive care from three different agencies for postpartum and newborn care, tuberculosis follow-up, and stroke rehabilitation. In cities with combination agencies, a minimal number of nurses provided improved services, ensuring continuity of care at a cheaper price. No longer would an agency "pick up and drop a baby," but instead would follow the child through infancy, preschool, school, and into adulthood as part of one public health nursing program using one client record. The "ideal program" of the combination agency proved difficult to fund and administer, and many of the combination services implemented between 1930 and 1965 later retrenched into their former divided, public and private structures.

During the 1950s, public health nursing practice, like nursing in general, increased its focus on the psychological elements of client, family, and community care. To be more effective as helping professionals, nurses sought improved understanding of their own behavior, as well as the behavior of their clients and their coworkers. The nurse's responsibility for health and human needs expanded to include stress and anxiety reduction associated with situational or developmental stressors, such as birth, adolescence, and parenting. Public health nurses sought a comprehensive approach to mental health that avoided dividing persons into physical components and emotional components (Abramovitz, 1961). The following Evidence-Based Practice example traces the development of nursing and home health care in the United States.

## DECLINING FINANCIAL SUPPORT FOR PRACTICE AND PROFESSIONAL ORGANIZATIONS

During the 1930s and 1940s hospitals became the preferred place for illness care and childbirth. Improved technology and the concentration of physicians' work in the acute care hospital were influential, but the development of health insurance plans such as Blue Cross provided a means for the middle class to seek care outside the traditional arena of the home. Federal health policy after World War II supported the growth of institutional care in hospitals and nursing homes rather than community-based alternatives. Figure 2-3 depicts a public health nurse speaking with a family on their porch. Home visiting although valuable to health care was not consistently supported by insurance companies.

## EVIDENCE-BASED PRACTICE

*No Place Like Home: A History of Nursing and Home Care in the United States* (Buhler-Wilkerson, 2001) is a book-length analysis of the development of nursing care for those at home. Buhler-Wilkerson traces how the care of the sick moved from a domestic function to a charitable or public responsibility provided through visiting nurse associations and official health agencies. The central dilemma she raises is, "why, despite its potential as a preferred, rational, and possibly cost-effective alternative to institutional care, home care remains a marginalized experiment in caregiving" (p. xi).

Buhler-Wilkerson follows the origins of home care from its beginnings in Charleston, South Carolina, to its expansion into northern cities at the end of the nineteenth century. She interprets the founding of public health nursing by Lillian Wald "as a new paradigm for community-based nursing practice within the context of social reform" (p. xii), and she particularly analyzes the effects of ethnicity, race, and social class. She traces the difficulties of organizing and financing care of the sick in the home, including the work of private duty nurses and the role of health insurance in shaping home services. The concluding section of the book highlights contemporary themes of "chronic illness, hospital dominance, financial viability, and struggles to survive" (p. xii) and projects the future of home care.

Buhler-Wilkerson brings to bear the stories of patients' needs and nurses' work against the financial challenges that have characterized home care. While focusing on one element, this book raises important questions for nurses' work across elements of community/public health nursing. Clearly identified need does not by itself open the doors to adequate financing for nursing care of the sick, for public health nursing, or for population care for health promotion.

### Nurse Use

This book points out the complex issues involved in trying to provide the most effective care to patients. The needs of patients and their families may not entirely correlate with what is financially available. A lesson for each of us to learn is the following: Identified need does not always influence the availability of funds to provide the desired care.

From Buhler-Wilkerson K: *No Place Like Home: A History of Nursing and Home Care in the United States*. Baltimore, 2001, Johns Hopkins Press.

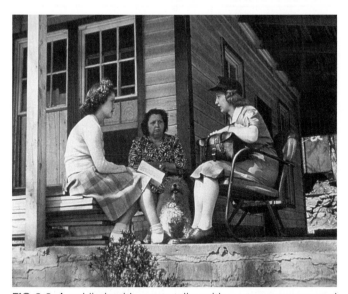

**FIG 2-3** A public health nurse talks with a young woman and her mother about childbirth, as they sit on a porch. (U.S. Public Health Service photo by Perry, Images from the History of Medicine, National Library of Medicine, Image ID 157037.)

Financing for voluntary nursing agencies was greatly reduced in the early 1950s when both the Metropolitan and John Hancock Life Insurance Companies stopped funding visiting nurse services for their policyholders. The life insurance companies had found nursing services financially beneficial when communicable disease rates were high in the 1910s and 1920s, but reductions in communicable disease rates, improved infant and maternal health, and the increased prevalence of expensive chronic illnesses reduced sponsor interest in financing home visiting. The American Red Cross also discontinued its programs of direct nursing service by the mid-1950s.

The NOPHN had long sought additional approaches for funding public health nursing. Beginning in the 1930s, the NOPHN collaborated with the American Nurses Association (ANA) through the Joint Committee on Prepayment. Both organizations had identified the growth potential of early health insurance innovations. Voluntary nursing agencies developed a variety of initiatives to secure health insurance reimbursement for nursing services, including demonstration projects and educational campaigns directed toward nurses, physicians, and insurers. Blue Cross and other hospital insurance programs gradually adopted a formula that exchanged unused days of hospitalization coverage for postdischarge nursing care at home. Unlike organized medicine and hospital associations, nursing organizations contributed substantially to securing federal medical insurance for the aged, which was implemented as the Medicare program in 1966. The support of the ANA, so integral to the passage of Medicare legislation, was publicly recognized by President Lyndon Baines Johnson at the 1965 ceremony to sign the bill.

Despite the successes and importance of the NOPHN, by the late 1940s its membership had declined and financial support was weak. At the same time, the nursing profession as a whole sought to reorganize its national organizations to improve unity, administration, and financial stability. Three existing organizations—the NOPHN, the National League for Nursing Education, and the Association of Collegiate Schools of Nursing—were dissolved in 1952. Their functions were distributed primarily to the new National League for Nursing. The American Nurses Association, which merged with the National Association of Colored Graduate Nurses, continued as the second national nursing organization. Occupational health nursing and nurse-midwifery organizations declined to join the consolidation, and both nursing specialties have continued to set their own course. School nurses also soon established a separate specialty organization. Despite the optimism of the national reorganization and its success in some areas, the subsequent loss of independent public health nursing leadership and focus resulted in a weakened specialty.

## PROFESSIONAL NURSING EDUCATION FOR PUBLIC HEALTH NURSING

The National League for Nursing enthusiastically adopted the recommendations of Esther Lucile Brown's 1948 study of nursing education, reported as *Nursing for the Future* (Brown, 1948). Her recommendation to establish basic nursing preparation in colleges and universities was consistent with the NOPHN's goal of including public health nursing concepts in all basic baccalaureate programs. The NOPHN believed that this would remedy the preparation problems found among many nurses new to the practice and would thus upgrade the public health nursing profession. Unfortunately, the implementation of the plan fell short, and training programs in public health nursing for college and university faculty were very brief and inadequate. The population focus of public health nursing toward groups and the larger community was compromised and became less distinct in the hands of educators who themselves lacked education and practice in public health nursing.

During the 1950s, public health nursing educators carefully considered steps to enhance undergraduate and graduate education. Educational programs for public health nurses were then found in schools of nursing, schools of public health, and other university departments. Although all claimed legitimacy, collegiate education for nurses gradually moved completely into schools of nursing. The Haven Hill Conference (NOPHN, 1951) and Gull Lake Conference (Robeson and McNeil, 1957) clarified roles and definitions, built expectations for graduate education, and set standards for undergraduate field experiences. As public health nursing education drew closer to university schools of nursing, it adopted and applied broad principles characteristic of general nursing education. For example, rather than have the education director of the placement agency teach nursing students as done previously, collegiate programs themselves hired faculty who provided direct student supervision at community placements (NOPHN, 1951; Robeson and McNeil, 1957). The How To box describes the way to conduct an oral history interview in order to preserve vital information about public health nursing.

> **HOW TO**
>
> *Nurse historians are increasingly using oral history methodology to uncover and preserve the history of public health nursing and individual nurses on audio files and written transcripts.*
>
> **Conduct an Oral History Interview**
> 1. *Identify an issue or event of interest.*
> 2. *Research the issue or event, using a variety of written and/or photographic materials.*
> 3. *Locate a potential oral history interviewee or narrator.*
> 4. *Obtain the agreement of the narrator to be interviewed. Arrange an interview appointment.*
> 5. *Research the narrator's background and the time period of interest.*
> 6. *Write an outline of questions for the narrator. Open-ended questions are especially helpful.*
> 7. *Meet with the narrator. Bring an audio recorder to the interview.*
> 8. *Interview the narrator. Ask one brief question at a time. Give the narrator time to consider your question and answer it.*
> 9. *Ask clarifying questions. Ask for examples. Give encouragement. Allow the narrator to tell his or her story without interruption.*
> 10. *After the interview, transcribe the interview tape and prepare a written transcript (some digital programs can immediately produce a written transcript).*
> 11. *Carefully compare the written transcript with the narrator's recorded interview. It may be appropriate to have the narrator review and edit the written transcript.*
> 12. *If you have made written arrangements with the narrator, place the oral history audio and transcripts in an appropriate archive or library (highly recommended).*
>
>   **Keep In Mind**: *Oral history is a type of nursing research. Please consider that oral history interviews may require formal consent by the interviewee or narrator before the interview, as well as prior approval of the research from an institutional review board.*
>
>   **Consult the Literature:** *An example of oral history is presented in an article on the Michigan Oral History Project (Gates et al, 1994).*

## NEW RESOURCES AND NEW COMMUNITIES: THE 1960s AND NURSING

Beginning in earnest in the late 1940s but on the basis of advocacy begun in the late 1910s, policymakers and social welfare representatives sought to establish national health insurance. In 1965 Congress amended the Social Security Act to include health insurance benefits for older adults (Medicare) and increased care for the poor (Medicaid). Unfortunately, the revised Social Security Act did not include coverage for preventive services, and home health care was reimbursed only when ordered by a physician. Nevertheless, this latter coverage prompted the rapid proliferation of home health care agencies, with for-profit agencies responding to new financial opportunities. Many local and state health departments rapidly changed their policies to include reimbursable home health care as bedside nursing. This could result in reduced health promotion and disease prevention activities, as funding for these activities was less stable. From 1960 to 1968, the number of official agencies providing home care services grew from 250 to 1328, and the number of for-profit agencies continued to grow (Kalisch and Kalisch, 2004).

## COMMUNITY ORGANIZATION AND PROFESSIONAL CHANGE

Social changes during the 1960s and 1970s influenced both nursing and public health. "The emerging civil rights movement shifted the paradigm from a charitable obligation to a political commitment to achieving equality and compensation for racial injustices of the past" (Scutchfield and Keck, 1997, p. 328). New programs addressed economic and racial differences in health care services and delivery. Funding was increased for maternal and child health, mental health, mental retardation, and community health training. Beginning in 1964, the federal Economic Opportunity Act provided funds for neighborhood health centers, Head Start, and other community action programs. Neighborhood health centers increased community access for health care, especially for maternal and child care. The work of Nancy Milio in Detroit, Michigan, is an example of this commitment to action with the community. Milio built a dynamic decision-making process that included neighborhood residents, politicians, the Visiting Nurse Association and its board, civil rights activists, and church leaders. The Mom and Tots Center emerged as a neighborhood-centered service to provide maternal and child health services and a day-care center. Milio (1971) recorded this story in her book, *9226*

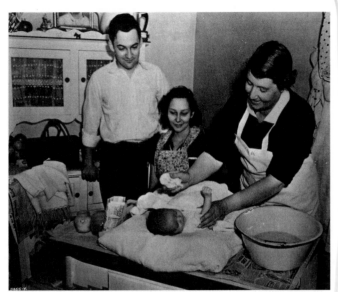

**FIG 2-4** A Visiting Nurse Association nurse demonstrates proper infant care and bathing techniques to the parents. (Images from the History of Medicine, National Library of Medicine, Image ID 144048.)

*Kercheval: The Storefront That Did Not Burn.* As shown in Figure 2-4 visiting nurses provided vital services to families.

New personnel also added to the flexibility of the public health nurse to address the needs of communities. Beginning in 1965 at the University of Colorado, the nurse practitioner movement opened a new era for nursing involvement in primary care that affected the delivery of services in community health clinics. Initially, the nurse practitioner was often a public health nurse with additional skills in the diagnosis and treatment of common illnesses. Although some nurse practitioners chose to practice in other clinical areas, those who continued in public health settings made sustained contributions to improving access and providing primary care to people in rural areas, inner cities, and other medically underserved areas (Roberts and Heinrich, 1985). As evidence of the effectiveness of their services grew, nurse practitioners became increasingly accepted as cost-effective providers of a variety of primary care services.

## PUBLIC HEALTH NURSING FROM THE 1970s INTO THE TWENTY-FIRST CENTURY

During the 1970s, nursing was viewed as a powerful force for improving the health care of communities. Nurses made significant contributions to the hospice movement, the development of birthing centers, day care for older adult and disabled persons, drug abuse programs, and rehabilitation services in long-term care. Federal evaluation of the effectiveness of care was emphasized (Roberts and Heinrich, 1985).

By the 1980s, concern grew about the high costs of health care in the United States. Programs for health promotion and disease prevention received less priority as funding was shifted to meet the escalating costs of acute hospital care, medical procedures, and institutional long-term care. The use of ambulatory services including health maintenance organizations was

encouraged, and the use of nurse practitioners increased. Home health care weathered several threats to adequate reimbursement and, by the end of the decade, had secured favorable legal decisions that increased its impact on the care of the sick at home. Individuals and families assumed more responsibility for their own health because health education, always a part of nursing, became increasingly popular. Advocacy groups representing both consumers and professionals urged the passage of laws to prohibit unhealthy practices in public such as smoking and driving under the influence of alcohol. Sophisticated media campaigns contributed to changing health behaviors and improving health status. As federal and state funds grew scarce, fewer nurses were employed by official public health agencies. Committed and determined to improve the health care of Americans, nurses continued to press for greater involvement in official and voluntary agencies (Roberts and Heinrich, 1985; Kalisch and Kalisch, 2004).

The National Center for Nursing Research (NCNR), established in 1985 within the federal National Institutes of Health near Washington, DC, had a major impact on promoting the work of nurses. Through research, nurses analyze the scope and quality of care provided by examining the outcomes and cost-effectiveness of nursing interventions. With the concerted efforts of many nurses, the NCNR gained official institute status within the National Institutes of Health in 1993, becoming the National Institute of Nursing Research (NINR).

By the late 1980s, public health as a whole had declined significantly in its effectiveness in accomplishing its mission and in shaping the public's health. Significant reductions in local and national political support, financing, and outcomes were vividly described in a landmark report by the Institute of Medicine, *The Future of Public Health* (Institute of Medicine [IOM], 1988). The IOM study group found America's public health system in disarray and concluded that, although there was widespread agreement about what the mission of public health should be, there was little consensus on how to translate that mission into action. Not surprisingly, the IOM reported that the mix and level of public health services varied extensively across the United States (Williams, 1995).

*The Future of Public Health* (IOM, 1988) determined that "contemporary public health is defined less by what public health professionals know how to do than by what the political system in a given area decides is appropriate or feasible" (p. 4). Nurses working in health departments saw underfunding reduce the breadth and depth of their role. When local public health departments provided insufficient care, voluntary agencies such as VNAs stepped in to assist vulnerable groups. However, without adequate funding for care of the poor, VNAs and other voluntary home health agencies faced hard economic choices, and some closed their doors.

America's *Healthy People* initiative has influenced goals and priority setting in both public health and nursing, beginning in 1979 (U.S. Department of Health, Education, and Welfare, 1979), with the current objectives detailed in *Healthy People 2020* (U.S. Department of Health and Human Services [USDHHS], 2010). Evidence-based practice recommendations that complement the Healthy People initiative are detailed for health promotion, disease prevention, and screening in primary care through the clinical guidelines from the U.S. Preventive Services Task Force, *Guide to Clinical Preventive Services* (2014), and for groups and communities, through *The Guide to Community Preventive Services*, now known also as *The Community Guide* (Community Preventive Services Task Force, 2014). Implementation of these strategies has influenced the work of public health nurses through their employment in health agencies and through participation in state or local health coalitions. See the Healthy People box that follows and that traces the development of this important series of documents.

The health care debate in the 1990s focused on cost, quality, and access to direct care services. Despite considerable interest in health care reform and securing universal health insurance coverage, the core economic debate—who will pay for what—emphasized reform of medical care rather than comprehensive changes in health promotion, disease prevention, and health care. In 1993, the American Health Security Act received insufficient Congressional support. Reflecting the weakness of public health, the aims of public health were never clearly considered in the proposed program. Proposals to reform existing services also failed to apply the lesson learned from the *Healthy People* initiative—that health promotion and disease prevention appear to yield reductions in costs and illness/injury incidence while increasing years of healthy life.

In 1991 the ANA, the American Association of Colleges of Nursing, the National League for Nursing, and more than 60 other specialty nursing organizations joined to support health care reform. The coalition of nursing organizations emphasized key health care issues of access, quality, and cost, and proposed a range of interventions designed to build a healthy nation through improved primary care and public health efforts. Professional nursing's continued support for improved health care access and reduced cost was rewarded in 2010 with the passage of the federal Patient Protection and Affordable Care Act. These successes emphasize that public health nursing must continue to advocate for extension of public health services to prevent illness, promote health, and protect the public.

The Quad Council of Public Health Nursing Organizations was founded in the early 1980s, and is composed of representatives from four organizations that include public health nurses: The Association of State and Territorial Directors of Nursing (ASTDN, established in 1935), known since 2012 as the Association of Public Health Nurses (APHN); the Association of Community Health Nursing Educators (ACHNE, established in 1977); the Public Health Nursing Section of the American Public Health Association (PHN-APHA; the Section was formed in 1923); and the American Nurses Association Council on Nursing Practice and Economics (ANA).

 **HEALTHY PEOPLE 2020**

### History of the Development of *Healthy People*

In 1979 the groundbreaking *Healthy People: The Surgeon General's Report on Health Promotion and Disease Prevention* asserted that "the health of the American people has never been better" (U.S. Department of Health, Education, and Welfare [USDHEW], 1979, p. 3). But this was only the prologue to deep criticism of the status of American health care delivery. Between 1960 and 1978, health care spending increased 700%—without related improvements in mortality or morbidity. During the 1950s and 1960s, evidence had accumulated about chronic disease risk factors, particularly cigarette smoking, alcohol and drug use, occupational risks, and injuries. But these new research findings were not systematically applied to health planning and to improving population health.

In 1974 the Government of Canada published *A New Perspective on the Health of Canadians* (Lalonde, 1974), which found death and disease to have four contributing factors: inadequacies in the existing health care system, behavioral factors, environmental hazards, and human biological factors. Applying the Canadian approach, in 1976 U.S. experts analyzed the 10 leading causes of U.S. mortality and found that 50% of American deaths were the result of unhealthy behaviors, and only 10% were the result of inadequacies in health care. Rather than just spending more to improve hospital care, clearly prevention was the key to saving lives, improving the quality of life, and saving health care dollars.

A multidisciplinary group of analysts conducted a comprehensive review of prevention activities. They verified that the health of Americans could be significantly improved through "actions individuals can take for themselves" and through actions that public and private decision makers could take to "promote a safer and healthier environment" (p. 9). Similar to Canada's *New Perspectives*,

America's *Healthy People* (USDHEW, 1979) identified priorities and measurable goals. *Healthy People* grouped 15 key priorities into three categories: key preventive services that could be delivered to individuals by health providers, such as timely prenatal care; measures that could be used by governmental and other agencies, as well as industry, to protect people from harm, such as reduced exposure to toxic agents; and activities that individuals and communities could use to promote healthy lifestyles, such as improved nutrition.

In the late 1980s, success in addressing these priorities and goals was evaluated, new scientific findings were analyzed, and new goals and objectives were set for the period from 1990 to 2000 through *Healthy People 2000: National Health Promotion and Disease Prevention Objectives* (U.S. Department of Health and Human Services [USDHHS], 1991). This process was repeated 10 years later to develop goals and objectives for the period 2000 to 2010 (USDHHS, 2000), and for the current decade of 2010 to 2020—*Healthy People 2020: Improving the Health of Americans* (USDHHS, 2010). Recognizing the continuing challenge to using emerging scientific research to encourage modification of health behaviors and practices, *Healthy People 2020* addresses health equity, elimination of disparities, and improved health for all groups across the life span through disease prevention, improved social and physical environments, and healthy development and health behaviors.

Just as the public health nurse in the early twentieth century spread the "gospel of public health" to reduce communicable diseases, today's population-centered nurse uses *Healthy People* to reduce chronic and infectious diseases and injuries through health education, environmental modification, and policy development.

Lalonde M: *A New Perspective on the Health of Canadians.* Ottawa, Canada, 1974, Information Canada; U.S. Department of Health and Human Services: *Healthy People 2010: Understanding and Improving Health,* ed 2. Washington, DC, 2000, U.S. Government Printing Office; U.S. Department of Health and Human Services: *Healthy People 2020: The Road Ahead.* Available at: http://www.healthypeople.gov/hp2020/. Accessed December 2, 2010; U.S. Department of Health, Education, and Welfare: *Healthy People: The Surgeon General's Report on Health Promotion and Disease Prevention.* DHEW Publication No. 79-55071, Washington, DC, 1979, U.S. Government Printing Office; U.S. Public Health Service: *Healthy People 2000: National Health Promotion and Disease Prevention Objectives.* Washington, DC, 1991, U.S. Government Printing Office.

During the 1990s and 2000s the Quad Council of Public Health Nursing Organizations supported the efforts of its organizational members and public health organizations to establish mechanisms to improve quality of care and to advance the public health nursing profession in the twenty-first century. For example, the certification of public health nurses with graduate degrees was reinforced through collaborative agreements with the American Nurses Credentialing Center (ANCC). The Quad Council also revised its *Competencies for Public Health Nurses* in 2011. The competencies are separated into three tiers: Tier 1 for generalist public health nurses who conduct clinical, home visiting and population-based services; Tier 2 for public health nurses with management and/or supervisory responsibilities; and Tier 3 for public health nurses at executive, senior management, or leadership levels in public health nursing organizations. Under Domain #6, a public health nurse "Describes the historical foundation of public health and public health nursing" (Quad Council, 2011, p. 17).

In addition to the actions of the Quad Council itself, the four constituent members of the Council have also worked in their areas of expertise to link content to the practice of public health nursing through their development of standards and competencies that influence practice in various ways.

The Association of Community Health Nursing Educators developed important position papers, including *Graduation Education for Advanced Practice Public Health Nursing* (ACHNE, 2007) and *Academic Faculty Qualifications for Community/ Public Health Nursing* (ACHNE, 2009). The Association of State and Territorial Directors of Nursing asserted the importance of public health nurses within public health systems through the publication of *Every State Health Department Needs a Public Health Nurse Leader* (ASTDN, 2008). And the Association of Public Health Nurses revised the ASTDN position paper on *The Role of the Public Health Nurse in Disaster Preparedness, Response, and Recovery* (APHN, 2014).

The Council on Linkages between Academia and Public Health Practice provides exchanges and collaborations among all public health disciplines, including public health nursing. The Council's *Core Competencies for Public Health Professionals* (2014) features a core competency under the domain of public health sciences skills: "Identifies prominent events in the history of the public health profession" (p. 17).

The American Nurses Association's *Scope and Standards of Public Health Nursing Practice* (ANA, 2013) is a key guide for the practice of public health nursing. Periodically revised, the *Scope and Standards* is developed by a group of public health nursing leaders representing the major public health nursing organizations and reflects the central ideas of public health nursing. As there is substantial agreement about the characteristics and goals of public health nursing across organizations, it is not surprising that the ANA *Scope and Standards* and the Quad Council's *Public Health Nursing Competencies* both includes the processes of assessment, analysis, and planning. Each also incorporates the importance of communication, cultural competency, policy, and public health skills in their recommendations for effective public health nurse practice. The Linking Content to Practice box describes how historically public health nursing journals have preserved the history of public health nursing.

 **LINKING CONTENT TO PRACTICE**

*Public Health Nursing*, a major journal in the field of public health nursing, publishes articles that very broadly reflect contemporary research, practice, education, and public policy for population-based nurses. Begun in 1984, *Public Health Nursing (PHN)* was published quarterly through 1993, and has been a bimonthly journal since 1994. Marilyn G. King, DNSc, RN, is the historical editor and Patricia J. Kelly, PhD, MPH, APRN, is the journal's current editor (2014).

More than any other journal, *PHN* has assumed responsibility for preserving the history of public health nursing and for publishing new historical research on the field. The contemporary *Public Health Nursing* shares its name with the official journal of the National Organization for Public Health Nursing in the period 1931 to 1952 (earlier names were used for the official journal from 1913 to 1931, which built on the *Visiting Nurse Quarterly*, published 1909 to 1913).

The contemporary *Public Health Nursing* presents a wide variety of articles, including both new historical research and reprints of classic journal articles that deserve to be read and reapplied by modern public health nurses. One historical article reprinted in *PHN* addressed a nurse's 1931 work on county drought relief that underscores continuing professional themes of case-finding, collaboration, and partnership (Wharton, 1999). Another historical reprint recalled the important 1984 dialogue between two public health nurse leaders, Virginia A. Henderson and Sherry L. Shamansky, with an added contextual introduction from Sarah Abrams (Abrams, 2007). Original historical research presented in *PHN* is extremely varied, from public health nursing education, to public health nurse practice in Alaska's Yukon, to excerpts from the oral histories of public health nurses.

Contemporary nurses find inspiration and possibilities for modern innovations in reading the history of public health nursing in the pages of *PHN*.

Abrams SE: Nursing the community, a look back at the 1984 dialogue between Virginia A. Henderson and Sherry L. Shamansky. *PHN* 24:382, 2007; reprinted from PHN 1:193, 1984; Wharton AL: County drought relief: a public health nurse's problem. *PHN* 16(4):307–308, 1999; reprinted from PHN 23, 1931.

## PUBLIC HEALTH NURSING TODAY

In the last decades, new and continuing challenges have triggered growth and change in nursing. Where existing organizations have been unable to meet community and neighborhood needs, nurse-managed health centers provide a diversity of nursing services, including health promotion and disease/injury prevention. New populations in communities continue to challenge schools of nursing, health departments, rural health clinics, and migrant health services to provide the range of services to meet specific needs, including the needs of new immigrants. Transfer of official health services to private control has sometimes reduced professional flexibility and service delivery. Nurses also make the difficult choice to leave public health nursing to work in acute care, where the salaries are often higher. This is even more prominent in times of a nursing shortage. The Association of Community Health Nurse Educators calls for increased graduate programs to educate public health nurse leaders, educators, and researchers. Natural disasters (such as floods, hurricanes, and tornados) and human-made disasters (including explosions, building collapses, and airplane crashes) require innovative and time-consuming responses. Preparation for future disasters and potential bioterrorism demands the presence of well-prepared nurses. Many of these stories are detailed in the chapters that follow.

Some states have heard renewed persuasion to deploy school nurses in every school; a new recognition of the link between school success and health is again making the school nurse essential. Evidence from cost-benefit research on school nursing services underscores modern financial advantages for families and communities (Wang et al, 2014). Renewed evidence is also available from research on the use of nurses for prenatal and infant/toddler home visits to reduce "all-cause mortality among mothers and preventable-cause mortality in their first-born children living in highly disadvantaged settings" (Olds et al, 2014, p. E1). Even though both of these research inquiries have related precedents in the history of nursing, contemporary public health nurses must seek research approaches to demonstrate the outcomes of this work.

Today, public health nurses' past contributions ground twenty-first century public health nurses in a narrative that explains and gives importance to contemporary work. Nurses look to their history for inspiration, explanation, and prediction. Information and advocacy are used to promote a comprehensive approach to address the multiple needs of the diverse populations served. In the twenty-first century, public health nursing both reflects the past and builds on and beyond it.

Nurses will seek to learn from the past and to avoid known pitfalls, even as they seek successful strategies to meet the complex needs of today's vulnerable populations. As plans for the future are made, and as the public health challenges that remain unmet are acknowledged, it is this vision of what nursing can accomplish that sustains these nurses. In public health nursing as in all other specialty areas, quality and safety are key issues. The box below outlines the six Quality and Safety in Nursing Education (QSEN) competences and describes the development of these competences.

---

## QSEN FOCUS ON QUALITY AND SAFETY EDUCATION FOR NURSES

Although the scope and responsibilities of public health nurses have changed over time, the commitment to quality and safety has remained constant. Since the beginning of population-centered nursing in the United States, the nurses who worked in this specialty have been committed to preserving health and preventing disease. They have focused on environmental conditions such as sanitation and control of communicable diseases, education for health, prevention of disease and disability, and at times care of the sick and aged in their homes. This long-standing commitment to quality and safety is consistent with the work of *Quality and Safety Education for Nurses* (QSEN), a national initiative designed to transform nursing education by including in the curriculum content and experiences related to building knowledge, skills and attitudes for six quality and safety initiatives (Cronenwett, Sherwood, and Gelmon, 2009). The QSEN work, led by Drs. Linda Cronenwett and Gwen Sherwood at the University of North Carolina, has made great progress in bridging the gap between quality and safety work in both practice and academic settings (Brown, Feller, and Benedict, 2010). The six QSEN competencies for Nursing are:

1. **Patient-centered care:** Recognizes the client or designee as the source of control and as a full partner in providing compassionate and coordinated care that is based on the preferences, values, and needs of the client.
2. **Teamwork and collaboration:** Refers to the ability to function effectively with nursing and interprofessional teams and to foster open communication, mutual respect, and shared decision making to provide quality client care.
3. **Evidence-based practice:** Integrates the best current clinical evidence with client and family preferences and values to provide optimal client care.
4. **Quality improvement:** Uses data to monitor the outcomes of the care processes and uses improvement methods to design and test changes to continually improve quality and safety of health care systems.
5. **Safety:** Minimizes the risk for harm to clients and provides through both system effectiveness and individual performance.
6. **Informatics:** Use information and technology to communicate, manage knowledge, mitigate error, and support decision making (Brown et al, 2010, p. 116).

Of the six QSEN competencies, all but safety were derived from the Institute of Medicine report, *Health Professions Education* (2003). The QSEN team added safety because this competency is central to the work of nurses. Articles have been published to teach educators about QSEN, and national forums have been held. Also the American Association of Colleges of Nursing (AACN) has held faculty development institutes for faculty and academic administrators using a train-the-trainer model, and safety and quality objectives have been built in the AACN essentials for nursing education. Similarly, the National League for Nursing has incorporated the "NLN Educational Competencies Model" into their educational summits. The six QSEN competencies will be integrated in the chapters throughout the text to emphasize the importance of quality and safety in public health nursing today. *NOTE:* The terms *patient* and *care* will be changed to *client* and *intervention* to reflect a public health nursing approach.

Specifically related to the history of nursing, the following targeted competency can be applied:

- **Targeted Competency: Safety**—Minimizes risk for harm to clients and providers through both system effectiveness and individual performance.
Important aspects of safety include:
  - **Knowledge:** Discuss potential and actual impact of national client safety resources initiatives and regulations
  - **Skills:** Participate in analyzing errors and designing system improvements
  - **Attitudes:** Value vigilance and monitoring by clients, families, and other members of the health care team

### Safety Question

Updated definitions around client safety include addressing safety at the individual level and at the systems level. The history of public health nursing demonstrates the myriad ways that public health nurses have addressed client safety in their evolving practice. Public health nurses support safety through caring for individuals and providing care for communities and groups. Historically, how have public health nurses addressed safety at the individual client level? How have public health nurses addressed client safety at the systems level? How have public health nurses been involved in system improvements?

**Answer:** *Individual level: A rich part of public health nursing's history has been the development of home visitation, in which clients are cared for in their own environment. Similarly, public health nurses have improved client outcomes by pioneering new models of interventions for maternal–child health and individuals in rural communities.*

**Systems level:** *Through their work with communities, public health nurses were an integral part of reducing the incidence of communicable diseases by the mid-twentieth century. More recently, public health nursing has contributed to health care system improvements through the development of the hospice movement, birthing centers, day care for elderly and disabled persons, and drug-abuse and rehabilitation services. These initiatives have updated the health care system to provide targeted care for previously overlooked populations.*

Prepared by Gail Armstrong, PhD(c), DNP, ACNS-BC, CNE, Associate Professor, University of Colorado Denver College of Nursing.

## PRACTICE APPLICATION

Mary Lipsky has worked for the county health department in a major urban area for almost 2 years. Her nursing responsibilities include a variety of services, including consultations at a senior center, maternal/newborn home visits, and well-child clinics. As she leaves work each evening and returns to her own home, she keeps thinking about her clients. Why was it so difficult today to qualify a new mother and her baby to receive WIC (Women, Infants, and Children) nutrition services? Why must she limit the number of children screened for high lead levels, when last year the health department screened twice as many children? Several children last month seemed asymptomatic, but the laboratory found lead levels that were high enough

to cause damage. One of the mothers Ms. Lipsky is acquainted with is having a difficult time emotionally. Why is it so difficult to find a behavioral health provider for her? And the health department still cannot find a new staff dentist! And families on welfare cannot find a private dentist to care for their children.

A. Why might it be difficult to solve these problems at the individual level, on a case-by-case basis?
B. What information would you need to build an understanding of the policy background for each of these various populations?

**Answers can be found on the Evolve site.**

## KEY POINTS

- A historical approach can be used to increase understanding of public health nursing in the past, as well as its current dilemmas and future challenges.
- The history of public health nursing can be characterized by change in specific focus of the specialty but continuity in approach and style of the practice.
- Public health nursing, referred to in this text as population-centered nursing, is a product of various social, economic, and political forces; it incorporates public health science in addition to nursing science and practice.
- Federal responsibility for health care was limited until the 1930s, when the economic challenges of the Depression permitted reexamination of local responsibility for care.
- Florence Nightingale designed and implemented the first program of trained nursing, and her contemporary, William Rathbone, founded the first district nursing association in England.
- Urbanization, industrialization, and immigration in the United States increased the need for trained nurses, especially in public health nursing.
- Increasing acceptance of public roles for women permitted public health nursing employment for nurses, as well as public leadership roles for their wealthy supporters.
- In 1887 the Women's Board of the New York City Mission hired Frances Root, a trained nurse, to provide care to sick persons at home.
- The first visiting nurses' associations were founded in 1885 and 1886 in Buffalo, Philadelphia, and Boston.
- Lillian Wald established the Henry Street Settlement, which became the Visiting Nurse Service of New York City, in 1893. She played a key role in innovations that shaped public health nursing in its first decades, including school nursing, insurance payment for nursing, national organization for public health nurses, and the United States Children's Bureau.
- Founded in 1902 with the vision and support of Lillian Wald, school nursing sought to keep children in school so that they could learn.
- The Metropolitan Life Insurance Company established the first insurance-based program in 1909 to support community health nursing services.

- The National Organization for Public Health Nursing (founded in 1912) provided essential leadership and coordination of diverse public health nursing efforts; the organization merged into the National League for Nursing in 1952.
- Official health agencies slowly grew in numbers between 1900 and 1940, accompanied by a steady increase in public health nursing positions.
- The innovative Sheppard-Towner Act of 1921 expanded community health nursing roles for maternal and child health during the 1920s.
- Mary Breckinridge established the Frontier Nursing Service in 1925, which influenced provision of rural health care.
- African-American nurses seeking to work in public health nursing faced many challenges, but ultimately had significant impact on the communities they served.
- Tension between the nursing role of caring for the sick and the role of providing preventive care, and the related tension between intervening for individuals and intervening for groups, have characterized the specialty since at least the 1910s.
- As the Social Security Act attempted to remedy some of the setbacks of the Depression, it established a context in which public health nursing services expanded.
- The challenges of World War II sometimes resulted in extension of nursing care and sometimes in retrenchment and decreased public health nursing services.
- By the mid-twentieth century, the reduced prevalence of communicable diseases and the increased prevalence of chronic illness, accompanied by large increases in the population more than 65 years of age, led to examination of the goals and organization of public health nursing services.
- Between the 1930s and 1965, organized nursing and community health nursing agencies sought to establish health insurance reimbursement for nursing care at home.
- Implementation of Medicare and Medicaid programs in 1966 established new possibilities for supporting community-based nursing care but encouraged agencies to focus on services provided after acute care rather than on prevention.
- Efforts to reform health care organization, pushed by increased health care costs during the last 40 years, have

## KEY POINTS—cont'd

focused on reforming acute medical care rather than on designing a comprehensive preventive approach.

- The 1988 Institute of Medicine report documented the reduced political support, financing, and impact that increasingly limited public health services at national, state, and local levels.

- In the late 1990s, federal policy changes dangerously reduced financial support for home health care services, threatening the long-term survival of visiting nurse agencies.
- *Healthy People 2000* (USDHHS, 1991), *Healthy People 2010* (USDHHS, 2000), and recent disasters and acts of terrorism have brought renewed emphasis on prevention to nursing.

## CLINICAL DECISION-MAKING ACTIVITIES

1. Interview nurses at your clinical placement about the changes they have seen during their years in a population-centered nursing practice. How do these changes relate to the changing needs of the community or the population?

2. Identify the visible record of nursing agencies in your community. Note the buildings, plaques, and display cases that document the past provision of nursing care in community settings. What forces have influenced these agencies over time? Which factors do they wish to make known publicly, and which factors are less apparent?

3. Secure a copy of your clinical agency's recent annual report. How is the history of the agency presented? How does this agency's history fit in with the points made in this chapter? What are your conclusions about how this agency's past influences its present?

4. Interview older relatives for their memories of public health nursing care received by them, their families, and their friends. When they were younger, how was the public health nurse perceived in their community? What interventions were used by the public health nurse? How was the public health nurse dressed? How has the position of the public health or community health nurse changed?

5. Of what element or aspect of the history of public health nursing would you like to learn more? At your nursing library, review a period of 10 years of one journal from the past to identify trends in how this element or aspect was addressed. What conclusions do you reach?

6. The work and impact of several nursing leaders is reviewed or noted in this chapter. Of these leaders, which one strikes you as most interesting? Why? Locate and read further articles or books about this leader. What personal strengths do you note that supported this nurse's leadership?

# REFERENCES

Abramovitz AB, editor: *Emotional Factors in Public Health Nursing: A Casebook.* Madison, WI, 1961, University of Wisconsin Press.

American Association of Industrial Nurses (AAIN): *The Nurse in Industry: A History of the American Association of Industrial Nurses, Inc.* New York, 1976, AAIN.

American Nurses Association (ANA): *Public Health Nursing: Scope and Standards of Practice,* ed 2. Washington, DC, 2013, ANA.

Association of Community Health Nursing Educators (ACHNE): *Graduate Education for Advanced Practice Public Health Nursing: At the Crossroads,* 2007. Retrieved November 2014 from: http://achne. org/file/ublic/ GraduateEducationDocument.pdf.

Association of Community Health Nursing Educators (ACHNE): *Position paper: Academic Faculty Qualifications for Community/Public Health Nursing,* 2009. Retrieved November 2014 from: https:// www.resourcecenter.net/mages/ Achne/files/2009/Faculty QualificationsPositionPape.pdf.

Association of Public Health Nurses (APHN): *The Role of the Public Health Nurse in Disaster Preparedness, Response, and*

*Recovery,* 2014. Retrieved November 2014 from: http://www. phnurse.org/images/docs/ APHN_Role%20of%20PHN%20 in%20Disaster%20PRR _FINALJan14.pdf.

Association of State and Territorial Directors of Nursing (ASTDN): *Every State Health Department Needs a Public Health Nurse Leader,* 2008. Retrieved November 2014 from: http://www.phnurse. org/docs/Every_State_Health _Dept._Needs_a_PHN_Leader _2008.pdf.

Brainard A: *Evolution of Public Health Nursing.* Philadelphia, 1922, WB Saunders.

Breckinridge M: *Wide Neighborhoods: A Story of the Frontier Nursing Service.* New York, 1952, Harper.

Brown EL: *Nursing for the Future: A Report Prepared for the National Nursing Council.* New York, 1948, Russell Sage Foundation.

Brown, Feller, and Benedict, 2010

Browne H: A tribute to Mary Breckinridge. *Nurs Outlook* 14:54, 1966.

Brown R, Feller L, Benedict L: Reframing nursing education: the Quality and Safety Education for Nurses Initiative. *Teach Learn Nurs* 5:115–118, 2010.

Buhler-Wilkerson K: Public health nursing, in sickness or in health? *Am J Public Health* 75:1155, 1985.

Buhler-Wilkerson K: Left carrying the bag: experiments in visiting nursing, 1877–1909. *Nurs Res* 36:42–45, 1987.

Buhler-Wilkerson K: *False Dawn: The Rise and Decline of Public Health Nursing, 1900–1930.* New York, 1989, Garland.

Buhler-Wilkerson K: *No Place Like Home: A History of Nursing and Home Care in the United States.* Baltimore, 2001, Johns Hopkins Press.

Bullough V, Bullough B: *The Emergence of Modern Nursing.* New York, 1964, Macmillan.

Cohen IB: Florence Nightingale. *Sci Am* 250:128, 1984.

Community Preventive Services Task Force: *The Community Guide,* 2014. Retrieved November 2014 from: http://www. thecommunityguide.org/.

Council on Linkages between Academia and Public Health Practice: *Core Competencies for Public Health Professionals* [revised 2014], Retrieved November 2014 from: http://www.phf.org/ resourcestools/Documents/Core

_Competencies_for_Public _Health_Professionals_2014June .pdf.

Craven FSL: *A Guide to District Nurses,* 1889. Reprint, New York, 1984, Garland.

Cronenwett L, Sherwood G, Gelmon SB: Improving quality and safety education: the QSEN learning collaborative. *Nurs Outlook* 57:304–312, 2009.

Deloughery GL: *History and Trends of Professional Nursing,* ed 8. St. Louis, 1977, Mosby.

Dock LL: The history of public health nursing. *Public Health Nurs* 14:522, 1922.

Gates MF, Schim SS, Ostrand L: Uniting the past and the future in public health nursing: the Michigan Oral History Project. *Public Health Nurs* 11:3, 1994.

Hanggi-Myers L: The Howard Association of New Orleans: precursor to district nursing. *Public Health Nurs* 12:78, 1995.

Hawkins JW, Hayes ER, Corliss CP: School nursing in America: 1902–1994: a return to public health nursing. *Public Health Nurs* 11:416, 1994.

Hine DC: *Black Women in White: Racial Conflict and Cooperation in the Nursing Profession,*

*1890–1950*. Bloomington, IN, 1989, Indiana University Press.

Institute of Medicine (IOM): *The Future of Public Health*. Washington, DC, 1988, National Academies Press.

Kalisch PA, Kalisch BJ: *American Nursing: A History*, ed 4. Philadelphia, 2004, Lippincott Williams & Wilkins.

Lalonde M: *A New Perspective on the Health of Canadians*. Ottawa, Canada, 1974, Department of Supply and Services. Retrieved November 2014 from: http://www. phac-aspc.gc.ca/ph-sp/pdf/ perspect-eng.pdf.

McNeil EE: *Transition in Public Health Nursing: John Sundwall Lecture*. Ann Arbor, February 27, 1967, University of Michigan.

Milio N: *9226 Kercheval: The Storefront That Did Not Burn*. Ann Arbor, MI, 1971, University of Michigan Press.

Mosley MOP: Jessie Sleet Scales: first black public health nurse. *ABNF J* 5:45, 1994.

National Organization for Public Health Nursing (NOPHN): Approval of Skidmore College of Nursing as preparing students for public health nursing. *Public Health Nurs* 36:371, 1944.

National Organization for Public Health Nursing (NOPHN): Desirable organization for public health nursing for family service. *Public Health Nurs* 38:387, 1946.

National Organization for Public Health Nursing (NOPHN): *Proceedings of Work Conference: Collegiate Council on Public Health Nursing Education*. New York, 1951, NOPHN.

Nightingale F: *Notes on Nursing: What It Is, and What It Is Not*. 1859. Reprint, Philadelphia, 1946, Lippincott.

Nightingale F: *Sick Nursing and Health Nursing*. 1894. Reprint. In Billings JS, Hurd HM, editors: *Hospitals, Dispensaries, and Nursing*. New York, 1984, Garland.

Nutting MA, Dock LL: *A History of Nursing*. New York, 1935, Putnam.

Olds DL, Kitzman H, Knudtson MD, et al: Effect of home visiting by nurses on maternal and child mortality: results of a 2-decade follow-up of a randomized clinical trial. *JAMA Pediatr* [serial online]. 2014. Retrieved November 2014 from: http://www.ncbi.nlm.nih.gov/ pubmed/25003802.

Palmer IS: *Florence Nightingale and the First Organized Delivery of Nursing Services*. Washington, DC, 1983, American Association of Colleges of Nursing.

Pickett G, Hanlon JJ: *Public Health: Administration and Practice*. St. Louis, 1990, Mosby.

Quad Council of Public Health Nursing Organizations: *Competencies for Public Health Nursing Practice*. Washington DC, 2003 [revised 2011], Association of State and Territorial Directors of Nursing. Retrieved November 2014 from: http://www.resourcenter.net/ images/ACHNE/Files/ QuadCouncilCompetencies ForPublicHealthNurses _Summer2011.pdf.

Roberts M: *American Nursing: History and Interpretation*. New York, 1955, Macmillan.

Roberts DE, Heinrich J: Public health nursing comes of age. *Am J Public Health* 75:1162–1165, 1985.

Robeson KA, McNeil EE: *Report of Conference on Field Instruction in Public Health Nursing*. New York, 1957, National League for Nursing.

Rodabaugh JH, Rodabaugh MJ: *Nursing in Ohio: A History*. Columbus, OH, 1951, Ohio State Nurses' Association.

Rosen G: *A History of Public Health*. New York, 1958, MD Publications.

Scutchfield FD, Keck CW: *Principles of Public Health Practice*. Albany, NY, 1997, Delmar.

Shyrock H: *The History of Nursing*. Philadelphia, 1959, WB Saunders.

Thoms AB: *Pathfinders: A History of the Progress of Colored Graduate Nurses*. New York, 1929, Kay Printing House.

Tirpak H: The Frontier Nursing Service: fifty years in the mountains. *Nurs Outlook* 33:308, 1975.

U.S. Department of Health, Education, and Welfare (USDHEW): *Healthy People: The Surgeon General's Report on Health Promotion and Disease Prevention*. DHEW (PHS) Publication No. 79-55071. Washington, DC, 1979, U.S. Government Printing Office.

U.S. Department of Health and Human Services (USDHHS): *Healthy People 2000: National Health Promotion and Disease Prevention Objectives*. DHHS Publication No. 91-50212. Washington, DC, 1991, U.S. Government Printing Office. Retrieved November 2014 from: http://odphp.osophs.dhhs.gov/pubs/ hp2000/.

U.S. Department of Health and Human Services (USDHHS): *Healthy People 2010: Understanding and Improving Health*, ed 2. Washington, DC, 2000, U.S. Government Printing Office.

U.S. Department of Health and Human Services (USDHHS): *Healthy People 2020: Improving the Health of Americans*. 2010. Retrieved November 2014 from: http://www.healthypeople. gov/2020/default.aspx.

U.S. Preventive Services Task Force: *Guide to Clinical Preventive Services, 2014*. Retrieved November 2014 from: http:// www.ahrq.gov/professionals/ clinicians-providers/guidelines -recommendations/guide/index .html.

Wald LD: *The House on Henry Street*. New York, 1915, Holt.

Wald LD: *Windows on Henry Street*. Boston, 1934, Little, Brown.

Wang LY, Vernon-Smiley M, Gapinski MA, et al: Cost-benefit study of school nursing services. *JAMA Pediatr* 168:642–648, 2014. Retrieved November 2014 from: http://www.msno.org/wp-content/ uploads/2014/05/Cost-Benefit -Study-of-School-Nursing-Services .pdf.

Waters Y: *Visiting Nursing in the United States*. New York, 1909, Charities Publication Committee.

Wharton, 1999.

Williams CA: Beyond the Institute of Medicine report: a critical analysis and public health forecast. *Fam Community Health* 18:12, 1995.

Wilner DM, Walkey RP, O'Neill EJ: *Introduction to Public Health*, ed 7. New York, 1978, Macmillan.

# 3

# The Changing U.S. Health and Public Health Care Systems

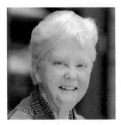

## Marcia Stanhope, PhD, RN, FAAN

Dr. Marcia Stanhope is currently an Associate of the Tufts and Associates Search Firm, Chicago, Ill. She is also a consultant for the nursing program at Berea College, Kentucky. She has practiced community and home health nursing, has served as an administrator and consultant in home health, and has been involved in the development of two nurse-managed centers. At one time in her career, she held a public policy fellowship and worked in the office of a U.S. Senator. She has taught community health, public health, epidemiology, policy, primary care nursing, and administration courses. Dr. Stanhope formerly directed the Division of Community Health Nursing and Administration and served as Associate Dean of the College of Nursing at the University of Kentucky. She has been responsible for both undergraduate and graduate courses in population-centered nursing. She has also taught at the University of Virginia and the University of Alabama, Birmingham. During her career at the University of Kentucky she was appointed to the Good Samaritan Foundation Chair and Professorship in Community Health Nursing, and was honored with the University Provost's Public Scholar award. Her presentations and publications have been in the areas of home health, community health and community-focused nursing practice, as well as primary care nursing.

## ADDITIONAL RESOURCES

**Evolve Website http://evolve.elsevier.com/Stanhope**
- NCLEX Review Questions
- Case Study, with questions and answers
- Community Assessment Applied
- *Healthy People 2020*

**Appendixes**
- Appendix A.3: Declaration of Alma-Ata
- Appendix E.3: The Health Insurance Portability and Accountability Act (HIPAA): What Does It Mean for Public Health Nurses?

## OBJECTIVES

*After reading this chapter, the student should be able to do the following:*

1. Describe the events and trends that influence the status of the health care system.
2. Discuss key aspects of the private health care system.
3. Compare the public health system to primary care.
4. Explain the model of primary health care.
5. Assess the effects of health care and insurance reform on health care delivery.
6. Evaluate the changes needed in public health and primary care to have an integrated health care delivery system.

## KEY TERMS

advanced practice nursing (APN), p. 47
Affordable Care Act, p. 48
community participation, p. 54
Declaration of Alma-Ata, p. 45
disease prevention, p. 45
electronic health record (EHR), p. 47
health, p. 45
health promotion, p. 45

managed care, p. 50
primary care, p. 50
primary health care (PHC), p. 54
public health, p. 50
U.S. Department of Health and Human Services (USDHHS), p. 50
*—See Glossary for definitions*

## CHAPTER OUTLINE

**Health Care in the United States**
**Forces Stimulating Change in the Demand for**
  **Health Care**
    Demographic Trends
    Social and Economic Trends
    Health Workforce Trends
    Technological Trends

**Current Health Care System in the United States**
  Cost
  Access
  Quality
**Organization of the Health Care System**
  Primary Care System
  Public Health System

A special thanks to Bonnie Jerome-D-Emilia for the many contributions to this chapter in edition 8 of the text.

As is known, the U.S. government began providing public health services in the 1700s, and public health nursing was first recognized 125 years ago (see Chapter 2). Although there were physicians in England in the 1600s and 1700s and in the United States since the 1700s, official recognition of the general practitioner (GP) occurred in England only in 1844. In the 1950s and 1960s in the United States, discussions were held to elevate the GP to a specialty practice in medicine. Thus family practice medicine became a reality in the 1960s (ABFM, 2005). After this development in medicine the first nurse practitioner program was begun in 1965 (Medscape, 2000). Then, in September 1978, an international conference was held in the city of Alma-Ata, which at that time was the capital of the Soviet Republic of Kazakhstan. During this conference, the Declaration of Alma-Ata and the primary health care model emerged (Appendix A.3). This declaration states that health is a human right and that the health of its people should be the primary goal of every government. One of the main themes of this declaration was the involvement of community health workers and traditional healers in a new health system (World Health Organization [WHO], 1978).

It was through this conference that the concept of primary health care (PHC) was introduced, defined, and described. In 2008, the WHO renewed its call for health care improvements and reemphasized the need for public policymakers, public health officials, primary care providers, and leadership within countries to improve health care delivery. The WHO said: "Globalization is putting the social cohesion of many countries under stress, and health systems … are clearly not performing as well as they could and should. People are increasingly impatient with the inability of health services to deliver. … Few would disagree that health systems need to respond better—and faster—to the challenges of a changing world. PHC can do that" (WHO, 2008; and see Chapter 4).

As defined by the WHO, PHC reflects and evolves from the economic conditions and sociocultural and political characteristics of the country and its communities, and is based on the application of social, biomedical, and health services research and public health experience. It addresses the main health problems in the community, providing for health promotion, disease prevention, and curative and rehabilitative services (WHO, 1978).

Defined differently than primary care or public health, PHC promotes the integration of all health care systems within a community to come together to improve the health of the community, including primary care and public health.

## HEALTH CARE IN THE UNITED STATES

Despite the fact that health care costs in the United States are the highest in the world and comprise the greatest percentage of the gross domestic product, the indicators of what constitutes good health do not document that Americans are really getting their money's worth. In the first decade of the twenty-first century there have been massive and unexpected changes to health, economic, and social conditions as a result of terrorist attacks, hurricanes, fires, floods, infectious diseases, and an economic turndown in 2008. New systems have been developed to prevent and/or deal with the onslaught of these horrendous events. Not all of the systems have worked, and many are regularly criticized for their inefficiency and costliness. Simultaneously, new, nearly miraculous advances have been made in treating health-related conditions. Organs and joints are being replaced and medicines are keeping people alive who only a few years ago would have suffered and died. These advances and "wonder drugs" save and prolong lives, and a number of deadly and debilitating diseases have been eliminated through effective immunizations and treatments. In addition, sanitation, water supplies, and nutrition have been improved, and animal cloning has begun.

However, attention to all of these advances may overshadow the lack of attention to public health and prevention. Several of the most destructive health conditions can be prevented either through changes in lifestyle or interventions such as immunizations. The increasing rates of obesity, especially among children; substance use; lack of exercise; violence; and accidents are alarmingly expensive, particularly when they lead to disruptions in health.

This chapter describes a health care system in transition as it struggles to meet evolving global and domestic challenges. The overall health care and public health systems in the United States are described and differentiated, and the changing priorities are identified. Nurses play a pivotal role in meeting these needs, and the role of the nurse is described.

## FORCES STIMULATING CHANGE IN THE DEMAND FOR HEALTH CARE

In recent years, enormous changes have occurred in society, both in the United States and most other countries of the world. The extent of interaction among countries is stronger than ever, and the economy of each country depends on the stability of other countries. The United States has felt the effects of rising labor costs as many companies have shifted their production to other countries with lower labor costs. It is often less expensive to assemble clothes, automobile parts, and appliances and to have call distribution centers and call service centers in a less industrialized country and pay the shipping and other charges involved than to have the items fully assembled in the United States. In recent years the vacillating cost of fuel has affected almost every area of the economy, leading to both higher costs of products and layoffs as some industries have struggled to stay solvent. This has affected the employment rate in the United States. The economic downturn of 2008 left many people unemployed, and many lost their homes because they could not pay their mortgages. When the unemployment rate is high, more people lack comprehensive insurance coverage, since in the United States this has been typically provided by employers. In late November 2008, the U.S. unemployment rate was 6.7%. This represented an increase from 4.6% in 2007. In July 2012 the unemployment rate had increased to 8.2%, close to double the rate in 2007. In recent years the economy has begun to recover. In 2014, for example, the unemployment rate decreased to 6.1%—down by 2.1 percentage points from 2012 (Bureau of Labor Statistics [BLS], 2014a). Also, health care services and the ways in which they are financed are changing, with the continuing implementation of the Patient Protection and Affordable Care Act (ACA, enacted in 2010).

## Demographic Trends

The population of the world is growing as a result of increased fertility and decreased mortality rates. The greatest growth is occurring in underdeveloped countries, and this is accompanied by decreased growth in the United States and other developed countries. The year 2000, however, marked the first time in more than 30 years that the total fertility rate in the United States was above the replacement level. *Replacement* means that for every person who dies, another is born (Hamilton et al, 2010). Both the size and the characteristics of the population contribute to the changing demography.

Seventy-seven million babies were born between the years of 1946 and 1963, giving rise to the often discussed baby boomer generation (Office of National Statistics, 2014) The oldest of these boomers reached 65 years of age in 2011, and they are expected to live longer than people born in earlier times (see Chapter 5). The impact on the federal government's insurance program for people 65 years of age and older, Medicare, is expected to be enormous, and this population is expected to double between the years 2000 and 2030, representing 20% of the total population (CDC, 2013a).

In 2014, the U.S. population was 318,804 million people, representing the third most populated country in the world. From 1990 to 2012, the U.S. foreign-born immigrant population grew from about 19 million to about 41 million and is continuing to increase every year (US Census Bureau, 2014).

At the time of the 1990 census, African Americans were the largest minority group in the United States (U.S. Census Bureau, 1996). However, in 2014, the U.S. Census Bureau announced that Hispanic persons outnumbered African Americans, with non-Hispanic whites being the largest single ethnic group in the

United States (Office of National Statistics [ONS], 2014). The nation's foreign-born population is growing, and it is projected that from now until 2050 the largest population growth will be due to immigrants and their children. States with the largest percentage of foreign-born populations are California, New York, Hawaii, Florida, and New Jersey. The states with the fastest-growing immigrant populations in 2012 were Nevada, Texas, Maryland, Illinois, and Arizona (Migration Policy Institute, 2014; Pew Research Center, 2012).

The composition of the U.S. household is also changing (see Chapter 25 for changes in families). From 1935 to 2010, mortality for both genders in all age groups and races declined (Hoyert, 2012) as a result of progress in public health initiatives, such as antismoking campaigns, AIDS prevention programs, and cancer screening programs. The leading causes of death have changed from infectious diseases to chronic and degenerative diseases (NCHS, 2014). New infectious diseases are emerging, such as Ebola virus, which affected the United States in 2014 with the first case in Dallas, Texas (CDC, 2014a). New treatments for infectious diseases have resulted in steady declines in mortality among children, as long as parents participate in immunization programs. A recent measles outbreak in Orange County, California shows that continuous focus on control of infectious diseases is essential (Orange County Health Care Agency, 2014). The mortality for older Americans has also declined. However, people 50 years of age and older have higher rates of chronic and degenerative illness and they use a larger portion of health care services than other age groups.

## Social and Economic Trends

In addition to the size and changing age distribution of the population, other factors also affect the health care system. Several social trends that influence health care include changing lifestyles, a growing appreciation of the quality of life, the changing composition of families and living patterns, changing household incomes, and a revised definition of quality health care.

Americans spend considerable money on health care, nutrition, and fitness (Bureau of Labor Statistics, 2012), because health is seen as an irreplaceable commodity. To be healthy, people must take care of themselves. Many people combine traditional medical and health care practices with complementary and alternative therapies to achieve the highest level of health. Complementary therapies are those that are used in addition to traditional health care, and alternative therapies are those used instead of traditional care. Examples include acupuncture, herbal medications, and more (National Center for Complementary and Alternative Medicine, 2014). People often spend a considerable amount of their own money for these types of therapies because few are covered by insurance. In recent years, some insurance plans have recognized the value of complementary therapies and have reimbursed for them. State offces of insurance are good sources to determine whether these services are covered and by which health insurance plans.

About 65 years ago, income was distributed in such a way that a relatively small portion of households earned high incomes; families in the middle-income range made up a somewhat larger proportion and households at the lower end of the income scale made up the largest proportion. By the 1970s, household income had risen, and income was more evenly distributed, largely as a result of dual-income families.

Since 1970 and to 2008, two trends in income distribution have emerged. The first is that the average per-person income in America has increased. Income of households in the top 1% of earners grew by 275%, compared with 65% for the next 19%, just under 40% for the next 60%, and 18% for the bottom fifth of households (Congressional Budget Office [CBO], 2011). However, as a result of what is being called the Great Recession, which began in 2008, and in recent years with layoffs, outsourcing, and other economic forces, many families are seeing decreases in wages. The second trend is that the gap between the richest 25% and the poorest 25% is widening because of the percent wage increase in the higher income levels (CBO, 2011). Chapter 5 provides a detailed discussion of the economics of health care and how financial constraints influence decisions about public health services.

## Health Workforce Trends

The health care workforce ebbs and flows. The early years of the twenty-first century saw the beginning of what is expected to be a long-term and sizable nursing shortage. Similarly, most other health professionals are documenting current and future shortages. Historically, nursing care has been provided in a variety of settings, primarily in the hospital. Approximately 56% of all registered nurses (RNs) continue to be employed in hospitals (American Nurses Association, 2012). A few years ago hospitals began reducing their bed capacity as care became more community based. Now they are expanding, including building for both acute and longer term chronic care. This growth is due to the factors previously discussed: the ability to treat and perhaps cure more diseases, the complexity of the care and the need for inpatient services, and the growth of the older age group.

The nursing shortage has been discussed in recent years, yet new graduates often have difficulty finding positions on graduation (American Association of Colleges of Nursing [AACN], 2014). Participating in a nurse internship program and being a bachelor of science in nursing (BSN) graduate or higher provides more opportunities for the new graduate. By 2016 there are expected to be 527,000 new nursing positions (BLS, 2014b). In addition, 55% of nurses reported in a recent survey that they intended to retire between 2011 and 2020, which will open positions for others (Fears, 2010).

There tend to be periodic shortages, especially in the primary care workforce in the United States, as providers choose to be specialists in fields such as medicine and nursing. Primary care providers include generalists who are skilled in diagnostic, preventive, and emergency services. The health care personnel trained as primary care generalists include family physicians, general internists, general pediatricians, nurse practitioners (NPs), clinical nurse specialists (CNSs), physician assistants, and certified nurse-midwives (CNMs) (Steinwald, 2008).

NPs, CNSs, and CNMs, considered advanced practice nursing (APN) specialties, are vital members of the primary care teams (see Chapter 39). Although there is a shortage of primary care physicians, nurse practitioners may or may not be able to fill the gap because of state nurse practice acts and medical practice acts, which influence the practice of both groups.

In terms of the nursing workforce, increasing the number of minority nurses remains a priority and a strategy for addressing the current nursing shortage. In 2013 minority nurses represented about 22% of the registered nurse population. It is thought that increasing the minority population will help close the health disparity gap for minority populations (AACN, 2014). For example, persons from minority groups, especially when language is a barrier, often are more comfortable with and more likely to access care from a provider from their own minority group.

## Technological Trends

The development and refinement of new technologies such as telehealth have opened up new clinical opportunities for nurses and their clients, especially in the areas of managing chronic conditions, assisting persons who live in rural areas, and in providing home health care, rehabilitation, and long-term care. On the positive side, technological advances promise improved health care services, reduced costs, and more convenience in terms of time and travel for consumers (see Chapter 5). Reduced costs result from a more efficient means of delivering care and from replacement of people with machines. It also reduces paperwork, gets accurate information to providers and clients and agencies, assists with care coordination and safety, and provides direct access to health records between agencies and to clients (HealthIT.gov, 2013). Contradictory as it may seem, cost is also the most significant negative aspect of advanced health care technology. The more high-technology equipment and computer programs become available, the more they are used. High-technology equipment is expensive, quickly becomes outdated when newer developments occur, and often requires highly trained personnel. There are other drawbacks to new technology, particularly in the area of home health care. These include increased legal liability, the potential for decreased privacy, too much reliance on technological advances, and the inconsistent quality of resources available on the Internet and other places (Palma, 2014).

Advances in health care technology will continue. One example of an effective use of technology is the funding provided by the U.S. Department of Health and Human Services, Health Resources and Services Administration (HRSA) to health centers so they can adopt and implement electronic health records (EHRs) and other health information technology (HRSA, 2008). HRSA's Office of Health Information Technology (HIT) was created in 2005 to promote the effective use of HIT as a mechanism for responding to the needs of the uninsured, underinsured, and special-needs populations (HRSA, 2014). Specifically, in December 2012, an award of $18 plus million through the Affordable Care Act was announced to expand health information technology in 600 health centers (HRSA, 2012). One innovative use of the EHR in public health is to embed reminders or guidelines into the system. For

ACA

example, the CDC published health guidelines that contain clinical recommendations for screening, prevention, diagnosis, and treatment. To find and keep current on these guidelines, clinicians must visit the CDC website. The availability of an EHR system allows the embedding of reminders so that the clinician can have access to practice guidelines at the very point of care. Some additional benefits in public health (and these are some of the uses health centers make of such records) include the following:

- 24-hour availability of records with downloaded laboratory results and up-to-date assessments
- Coordination of referrals and facilitation of interprofessional care in chronic disease management
- Incorporation of protocol reminders for prevention, screening, and management of chronic disease
- Improvement of quality measurement and monitoring
- Increased client safety and decline in medication errors

Two federal programs, Medicaid and the State Children's Health Insurance Program (SCHIP), have effectively used health information technology (HIT) in several key functions including outreach and enrollment, service delivery, and care management, as well as communications with families and the broader goals of program planning and improvement. In early 2009, the surgeon general's office reopened a web site that had been tried first in 2004, and then closed: an electronic family tree for your health (National Institutes of Health [NIH], 2010). This is described as an easy-to-use computer application for people to keep a personal record of their family health history (https://familyhistory.hhs.gov/FHH/html/index.html). Before the initiative described above, the CDC began a family history public health initiative through the Office of Public Health Genomics to increase awareness of family history as an important risk factor for common chronic diseases. This initiative had four main activities:

1. Research to define, measure, and assess family history in populations and individuals
2. Development and evaluation of tools for collecting family history
3. Evaluation of how family history-based strategies work
4. Promotion of evidence-based applications of family history to health professionals and the public (CDC, 2013b).

## CURRENT HEALTH CARE SYSTEM IN THE UNITED STATES

Despite the many advances and the sophistication of the U.S. health care system, the system has been plagued with problems related to cost, access, and quality (see more discussion in Chapters 5, 21, and 26). These problems are different for each person and have been affected by the ability of individuals to obtain health insurance. Most industrialized countries want the same things from their health care system. Several give their government a greater role in health care delivery and eliminate or reduce the use of market forces to control cost, access, and quality. Seemingly, there is no one perfect health care system in the world.

### Cost

Beginning in 2008, a historic weakening of the national and global economy—the "Great Recession"—led to the loss of 7 million jobs in the United States (Economic Report, 2010). Even as the gross domestic product (GDP), an indicator of the economic health of a country, declined in 2009, health care spending continued to grow and reached $2.5 trillion in the same year (Truffer et al, 2010). In the years between 2010 and 2019, national health spending is expected to grow at an average annual rate of 6.1%, reaching $4.5 trillion by 2019, for a share of approximately 19.3% of the GDP. This translates into a projected increase in per capita spending (see Chapter 5).

In Chapter 5, additional discussion illustrates how health care dollars are spent. The largest share of health care expenditures goes to pay for hospital care, with physician services being the next largest item. The amount of money that has gone to pay for public health services is much lower than for the other categories of expenditures. Other significant drivers of the increasingly high cost of health care include prescription drugs, technology, and chronic and degenerative disease.

Following the "Great Recession," the economic rebound will likely coincide with the burgeoning Medicare enrollment of the aging baby boomer population. It was projected that these new Medicare enrollees will increase Medicare expenditures for the foreseeable future. Medicaid recipients can be expected to decline as jobs are added to the economy, and the percentage of workers covered by employer-sponsored insurance should rise to reflect that growth. Although workers' salaries have not kept pace, employer-sponsored insurance premiums have grown 119% since 1999 (Kaiser Family Foundation, 2009a), and the inability of workers to pay this increased cost has led to a rise in the percentage of working families who are uninsured. It is essential to read about the changes in the above facts as the American Affordable Care Act is implemented.

### Access

Another significant problem is poor access to health care (case study in Box 3-1). The American health care system is described as a two-class system: private and public. People with insurance or those who can personally pay for health care are viewed as receiving superior care; those who receive lower quality care are

---

**BOX 3-1  Case Study**

Public health nurses who worked with local Head Start programs noted that many children had untreated dental caries. Despite qualifying for Medicaid, only two dentists in the area would accept appointments from Medicaid patients. Dentists asserted that Medicaid patients frequently did not show up for their appointments and that reimbursement was too low compared with other third-party payers. They also said the children's behavior made it difficult to work with them. So the waiting list for local dental care was approximately 6 years long. Although some nurses found ways to transport clients to dentists in a city 70 miles away, it was very time consuming and was feasible for only a small fraction of the clients. When decayed teeth abscessed, it was possible to get extractions from the local medical center. The health department dentist also saw children, but he, too, was booked for years.

Created by Deborah C. Conway, Assistant Professor, University of Virginia School of Nursing.

(1) those whose only source of care depends on public funds or (2) the working poor, who do not qualify for public funds either because they make too much money to qualify or because they are illegal immigrants. Employment-provided health care is tied to both the economy and to changes in health insurance premiums. By 2009, 61% of the nonelderly population continued to obtain health insurance through their employer as a benefit; however, employment did not guarantee insurance (Rowland et al, 2009). This became clear when considering that 9 in 10 (91%) of the middle-class uninsured came from families with at least one full-time worker in jobs that did not offer health insurance or where coverage was unaffordable (Rowland et al, 2009).

In 2012, the total number of uninsured persons in the United States was 48 million. As discussed, there was a strong relationship between health insurance coverage and access to health care services. Insurance status determines the amount and kind of health care people are able to afford, as well as where they can receive care. During this same year 15% of the total population was uninsured and 48% were covered by employer health insurance. All but 5% of the remaining, or 32%, were covered by government insurance programs (Kaiser Health News 2012; Kaiser Family Foundation, 2014).

The uninsured receive less preventive care, are diagnosed at more advanced disease states, and once diagnosed tend to receive less therapeutic care in terms of surgery and treatment options. There is a safety net for the uninsured or underinsured. As discussed later in this chapter, there are more than 1300 federally funded community health centers throughout the country. Federally funded community health centers provide a broad range of health and social services, using nurse practitioners and RNs, physician assistants, physicians, social workers, and dentists. Community health centers serve primarily in medically underserved areas, which can be rural or urban. These centers serve people of all ages, races, and ethnicities, with or without health insurance.

## Quality

The quality of health care leaped to the forefront of concern following the 1999 release of the Institute of Medicine (IOM) report *To Err Is Human: Building a Safer Health System* (IOM, 2000). As indicated in this groundbreaking report, as many as 98,000 deaths a year could be attributed to preventable medical errors. Some of the untoward events categorized in this report included adverse drug events and improper transfusions, surgical injuries and wrong-site surgery, suicides, restraint-related injuries or death, falls, burns, pressure ulcers, and mistaken client identities. It was further determined that high rates of errors with serious consequences were most likely to occur in intensive care units, operating rooms, and emergency departments. Beyond the cost in human lives, preventable medical errors result in the loss of several billions of dollars annually in hospitals nationwide. Categories of error include diagnostic, treatment, and prevention errors as well as failure of communication, equipment failure, and other system failures. Significant to nurses, the IOM estimated the number of lives lost to preventable errors in medication alone represented more than 7000 deaths annually, with a cost of about $2 billion nationwide.

Although the IOM report made it clear that the majority of medical errors today were not produced by provider negligence, lack of education, or lack of training, questions were raised about the nurse's role and workload and its effect on client safety. In a follow-up report, *Keeping Patients Safe: Transforming the Work Environment of Nurses,* the IOM (2003) stated that nurses' long work hours pose a serious threat to patient safety, because fatigue slows reaction time, saps energy, and diminishes attention to detail. The group called for state regulators to pass laws barring nurses from working more than 12 hours a day and 60 hours a week—even if by choice (IOM, 2003). Although this information is largely related to acute care, many of the patients who survive medical errors are later cared for in the community.

The culture of quality improvement and safety has made providers and consumers more conscious of safety, but medical errors and untoward events continue to occur. As a means to improve consumer awareness of hospital quality, the Centers for Medicare and Medicaid Services (CMS) began publishing a database of hospital quality measures, Hospital Compare, in 2005. Hospital Compare, a consumer-oriented website that provides information on how well hospitals provide recommended care in such areas as heart attack, heart failure, and pneumonia, is available through the CMS website (www.cms.gov). In a further effort, the CMS, in 2008, announced that it will no longer reimburse hospitals, under Medicare guidelines, for care provided for "preventable complications" such as hospital-acquired infections. This reimbursement policy was extended to Medicaid reimbursement in 2011 (Galewitz, 2011; CMS, 2009).

The accreditation process for public health is new and the impact of quality and safety monitoring has not yet been determined. The ability of a public health agency or a community to respond to community disasters is one event that will be monitored. In December 2014, 60 of 303 local, tribal, and state centralized integration systems, and multijurisdictional health departments, have received accreditation in this new process. The accredited health departments served a 111 million population base. The purpose of this process is to

- Assist and identify quality health departments to improve performance and quality, and to develop leadership
- Improve management
- Improve community relationships (Public Health Accreditation Board [PHAB], 2014)

## ORGANIZATION OF THE HEALTH CARE SYSTEM

An enormous number and range of facilities and providers make up the health care system. These include physicians' and dentists' offices, hospitals, nursing homes, mental health facilities, ambulatory care centers, freestanding clinics and clinics inside stores such as drugstores, as well as free clinics, public health, and home health agencies. Providers include nurses, advanced practice nurses, physicians and physician assistants, dentists and dental hygienists, pharmacists, and a wide array of essential allied health providers such as physical, occupational, and recreational therapists; nutritionists; social workers; and a range of technicians. In general, however, the American health care system is divided into the following two, somewhat distinct, components: a private or personal care component and a public health component, with some overlap, as discussed in the following sections. It is important to discuss primary health care and examine the interest in developing such a system.

## Primary Care System

Primary care, the first level of the private health care system, is delivered in a variety of community settings, such as physicians' offices, urgent care centers, in-store clinics, community health centers, and community nursing centers. Near the end of the past century, in an attempt to contain costs, managed care organizations grew. Managed care is defined as a system in which care is delivered by a specific network of providers who agree to comply with the care approaches established through a case management approach. The key factors are a specified network of providers and the use of a gatekeeper to control access to providers and services. This form of care has not become as prominent as the original concept outlined.

The government tried to reap the benefits of cost savings by introducing the managed care model into Medicare and Medicaid, with varying levels of success. The traditional Medicare plan involves Parts A and B. Part C, the Medicare Advantage program, incorporates private insurance plans into the Medicare program including HMO (health maintenance organization) and PPO (preferred provider organization) managed care models and private fee-for-service plans. In addition, Medicare Part D has been added to cover prescriptions (see Chapter 5).

## Public Health System

The public health system is mandated through laws that are developed at the national, state, or local level. Examples of public health laws instituted to protect the health of the community include a law mandating immunizations for all children entering kindergarten and a law requiring constant monitoring of the local water supply. The public health system is organized into many levels in the federal, state, and local systems. At the local level, health departments provide care that is mandated by state and federal regulations.

## The Federal System

The U.S. Department of Health and Human Services (USDHHS; or simply HHS) is the agency most heavily involved with the health and welfare concerns of U.S. citizens. The organizational chart of the HHS (Figure 3-1) shows the office of the secretary, 11 agencies, and a program support center (USDHHS, 2014a). Ten regional offices are maintained to provide more direct assistance to the states. Their locations are shown in Table 3-1. The HHS is charged with regulating health care and overseeing the health status of Americans. See Box 3-2 for the goals and objectives of the HHS strategic plan for fiscal years 2010-2015. Newer areas in the HHS are the Office of Public Health Preparedness, the Center for Faith-Based and Neighborhood Partnerships and the Office of Global Affairs. The Office of Public Health Preparedness was added to assist the nation and states to prepare for bioterrorism after September 11, 2001. The Faith-Based Initiative Center was developed by President George W. Bush to allow faith communities to compete for

**TABLE 3-1   Regional Offices of the U.S. Department of Health and Human Services**

| Region | Location | Territory |
|---|---|---|
| 1 | Boston | Connecticut, Maine, Massachusetts, New Hampshire, Rhode Island, Vermont |
| 2 | New York | New Jersey, New York, Puerto Rico, Virgin Islands |
| 3 | Philadelphia | Delaware, District of Columbia, Maryland, Pennsylvania, Virginia, West Virginia |
| 4 | Atlanta | Alabama, Florida, Georgia, Kentucky, Mississippi, North Carolina, South Carolina, Tennessee |
| 5 | Chicago | Illinois, Indiana, Michigan, Minnesota, Ohio, Wisconsin |
| 6 | Dallas | Arkansas, Louisiana, New Mexico, Oklahoma, Texas |
| 7 | Kansas City | Iowa, Kansas, Missouri, Nebraska |
| 8 | Denver | Colorado, Montana, North Dakota, South Dakota, Utah, Wyoming |
| 9 | San Francisco | Arizona, California, Hawaii, Nevada, American Samoa, Commonwealth of the Northern Mariana Islands, Federated States of Micronesia, Guam, Republic of the Marshall Islands, Republic of Palau |
| 10 | Seattle | Alaska, Idaho, Oregon, Washington |

U.S. Department of Health and Human Services: *HHS Regional Offices.* Retrieved December 2014 from http://www.hhs.gov/about/regions/

federal money to support their community activities. The goal of the Office of Global Affairs is to promote global health by coordinating HHS strategies and programs with other governments and international organizations (USDHHS, 2014a).

The U.S. Public Health Service (USPHS; or simply PHS) is a major component of the Department of Health and Human Services. The PHS consists of eight agencies: Agency for Healthcare Research and Quality, Agency for Toxic Substances and Diseases Registry, Centers for Disease Control and Prevention, Food and Drug Administration, Health Resources and Services Administration, Indian Health Service, National Institutes of Health, and Substance Abuse and Mental Health Services Administration. Each has a specific purpose (see Chapter 8 for relevancy of the agencies to policy and providing health care). The PHS also has a Commissioned Corps, which is a uniformed service of more than 6500 health professionals who serve in many HHS and other federal agencies. The surgeon general is head of the Commissioned Corps. The corps fills essential services for public health, clinic and provides leadership within the federal government departments and agencies to support the care of the underserved and vulnerable populations (USPHS, 2014).

An important agency and a recent addition to the federal government, the U.S. Department of Homeland Security (USDHS, or simply DHS), was created in 2003 (USDHS, 2014). The mission of the DHS is to prevent and deter terrorist attacks and protect against and respond to threats and hazards to the nation. The goals for the department include awareness, prevention, protection, response, and recovery. The DHS works with first responders throughout the United States, and through the development of programs such as the Community

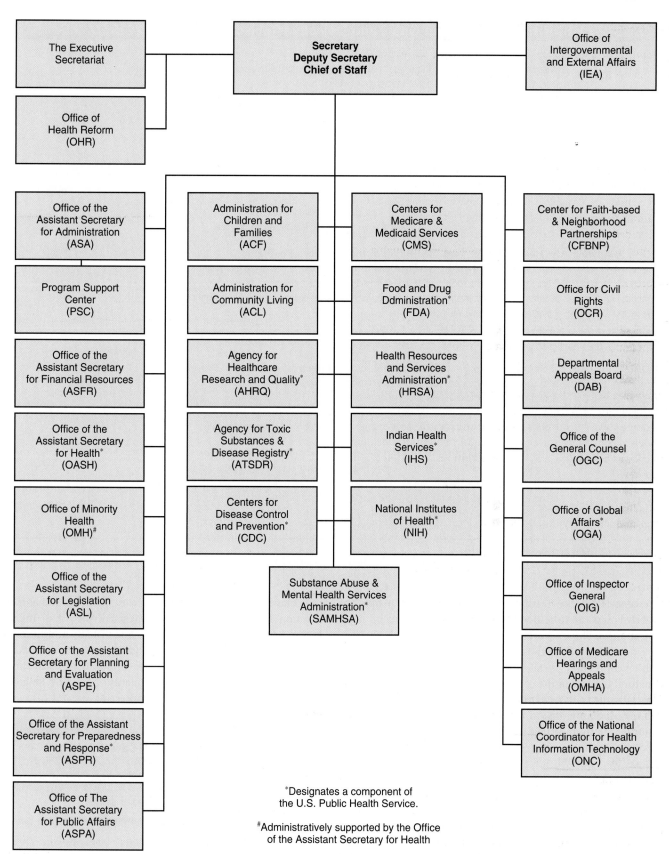

**FIG 3-1** Organization of the U.S. Department of Health and Human Services. (From U.S. Department of Health and Human Services; Available at http://www.hhs.gov/about/orgchart/.)

## BOX 3-2   USDHHS Strategic Plan Goals and Objectives—Fiscal Years 2010-2015*

**GOAL 1: Strengthen Health Care**

| | |
|---|---|
| Objective A | Make coverage more secure for those who have insurance, and extend affordable coverage to the uninsured. |
| Objective B | Improve health care quality and patient safety. |
| Objective C | Emphasize primary and preventive care linked with community prevention services. |
| Objective D | Reduce the growth of health care costs while promoting high-value, effective care. |
| Objective E | Ensure access to quality, culturally competent care for vulnerable populations. |
| Objective F | Promote the adoption and meaningful use of health information technology. |

**GOAL 2: Advance Scientific Knowledge and Innovation**

| | |
|---|---|
| Objective A | Accelerate the process of scientific discovery to improve patient care. |
| Objective B | Foster innovation to create shared solutions. |
| Objective C | Invest in the regulatory sciences to improve food and medical product safety. |
| Objective D | Increase our understanding of what works in public health and human service practice. |

**GOAL 3: Advance the Health, Safety, and Well-Being of the American People**

| | |
|---|---|
| Objective A | Promote the safety, well-being, resilience, and healthy development of children and youth. |
| Objective B | Promote economic and social well-being for individuals, families, and communities. |
| Objective C | Improve the accessibility and quality of supportive services for people with disabilities and older adults. |
| Objective D | Promote prevention and wellness. |
| Objective E | Reduce the occurrence of infectious diseases. |
| Objective F | Protect Americans' health and safety during emergencies, and foster resilience in response to emergencies. |

**GOAL 4: Increase Efficiency, Transparency, Accountability and Effectiveness of HHS Programs**

| | |
|---|---|
| Objective A | Ensure program integrity and responsible stewardship of resources. |
| Objective B | Fight fraud and work to eliminate improper payments. |
| Objective C | Use HHS data to improve the health and well-being of the American people. |
| Objective D | Improve HHS environmental, energy, and economic performance to promote sustainability. |

**GOAL 5: Strengthen the Nation's Health and Human Service Infrastructure and Workforce**

| | |
|---|---|
| Objective A | Invest in the HHS workforce to meet America's health and human service needs today and tomorrow. |
| Objective B | Ensure that the Nation's health care workforce can meet increased demands. |
| Objective C | Enhance the ability of the public health workforce to improve public health at home and abroad. |
| Objective D | Strengthen the Nation's human service workforce. |
| Objective E | Improve national, state, local, and tribal surveillance and epidemiology capacity. |

*In process of being updated for 2014-2018.
From the U.S. Department of Health and Human Services, 2014. Retrieved July 2, 2014, from http://www.hhs.gov/secretary/about/priorities.html.

Emergency Response Team (CERT) program trains people to be better prepared to respond to emergency situations in their communities. Nurses working in state and local public health departments as well as those employed in hospitals and other health facilities may be called on to respond to acts of terrorism or natural disaster in the course of their careers, and the DHS, along with the Food and Drug Administration (FDA) and CDC, is developing programs to ready nurses and other health care providers for an uncertain future (USDHS, 2014).

## The State System

When the United States faced a pandemic flu outbreak in 2009, the federal government and the public health community quickly prepared to meet the challenge of educating the public and health professionals about the H1N1 flu and making vaccinations available. In 2014 public health within the states was responding to an enterovirus affecting large numbers of children with systems of upper respiratory disease and weakness in arms and legs. The virus was considered life-threatening (CDC, 2014b). In addition to standing ready for disaster prevention or response, state health departments have other equally important functions, such as health care financing and administration for programs such as Medicaid, providing mental health and professional education, establishing health codes, licensing facilities and personnel, and regulating the insurance industry. State systems also have an important role in direct assistance to local health departments, including ongoing assessment of health needs (see Chapter 46).

### LEVELS OF PREVENTION

#### Related to the Public Health Care System

**Primary Prevention**
Implement a community-level program such as walking for exercise to assist citizens in improving health behaviors related to lifestyle.

**Secondary Prevention**
Implement a family-planning program to prevent unintended pregnancies for young couples who attend the local community health center.

**Tertiary Prevention**
Provide a self-management asthma program for children with chronic asthma to reduce their need for hospitalization.

*focal*

Nurses serve in many capacities in state health departments; they are consultants, direct service providers, researchers, teachers, and supervisors. They also participate in program development, planning, and the evaluation of health programs.

## The Local System

The local health department has direct responsibility to the citizens in its community or jurisdiction. Services and programs offered by local health departments vary depending on the state and local health codes that must be followed, the needs of the community, and available funding and other resources. For example, one health department might be more involved with public health education programs and environmental issues, whereas another health department might emphasize direct client care. Local health departments vary in providing sick care or even primary care (see Chapter 46). More often than at other levels of government, public health nurses at the local level provide population level or direct services. Some of these nurses deliver special or selected services, such as follow-up of contacts in cases of tuberculosis or venereal disease or providing child immunization clinics. Others provide more general care, delivering services to families in certain geographic areas. This method of delivery of nursing services involves broader needs and a wider variety of nursing interventions. The local level often provides an opportunity for nurses to take on significant leadership roles, with many nurses serving as directors or managers.

Since the tragedy of September 11, 2001, state and local health departments have increasingly focused on emergency preparedness and response. In case of an event, state and local health departments in the affected area will be expected to collect data and accurately report the situation, to respond appropriately to any type of emergency, and to ensure the safety of the residents of the immediate area, while protecting those just outside the danger zone. This level of knowledge—to enable public health agencies to anticipate, prepare for, recognize, and respond to terrorist threats or natural disasters such as hurricanes or floods—has required a level of interstate and federal-local planning and cooperation that is unprecedented for these agencies. Whether participating in disaster drills or preparing a local high school for use as a shelter, nurses play a major role in meeting the challenge of an uncertain future.

## FORCES INFLUENCING CHANGES IN THE HEALTH CARE SYSTEM

Although most people are personally satisfied with their own physicians or nurse practitioners, at present few people are satisfied with the health care system in general. Costs have been high and have continued to rise while quality and access have been uneven across the country and within communities, depending on the ability to pay. What, then, were some of the factors that might influence health care to change? First, as a nation, citizens must decide what has to be provided for all people, who will be in charge of the system, and who will pay for what. In recent years, federal and state services have been reduced and more responsibility for health care delivery has been moved to the private sector. Health care has become big business. Health care

company stocks are now traded by major stock exchanges, directors receive benefits when profits are high, and the locus of control had shifted from the provider to the payer. Many competing forces have influenced the changing design of the health care system, some of which are consumers, employers (purchasers), care delivery systems, and state and federal legislation.

First, consumers want lower costs and high-quality health care without limits and with an improved ability to choose the providers of their choice. Second, employers (purchasers of health care) want to be able to obtain basic health care plans at reasonable costs for their employees. Many employers have seen their profits diminish as they put more money into providing adequate health care coverage for employees. Third, health care systems want a better balance between consumer and purchaser demands. Thus they continually watch their own budget and expenses. To maintain a profit while providing quality care, many health care delivery groups have downsized and created alliances, mergers, and other joint ventures. Finally, legislation, especially concerning access and quality, continues to be enacted, thus creating one more force helping shape a health care system. The goal of "evidence-based care" is to ensure quality.

Many have said that solving the health care crisis requires the institution of a rational health care system that balances equity, cost, and quality. The fact that millions of people have been uninsured, that wide disparities have existed in access, and that a large proportion of deaths each year seem attributable to preventable causes (errors as well as tobacco, alcohol abuse, preventable injuries, and obesity) has indicated that the American system is currently not serving the best interests of the American population. The WHO has suggested that integrating primary care and public health into a primary health care system will be the basis for better health for all world citizens (WHO, 1986a).

## Integration of Public Health and the Primary Care Systems

Although primary care and public health share a goal of promoting the health and well-being of all people, these two disciplines historically have operated independently of one another. Problems that stem from this separation have long been recognized, but new opportunities are emerging for bringing these systems together to promote lasting improvements in the health of individuals, communities, and populations (IOM, 2012).

In recognition of this potential, the Centers for Disease Control and Prevention (CDC) and the Health Resources and Services Administration (HRSA), both agencies of the Department of Health and Human Services (HHS), asked the Institute of Medicine (IOM) to convene a committee of experts, including input from nursing, to examine the integration of primary care and public health (IOM, 2012).

To recognize the differences in these two systems, definitions were used to guide the work of the experts. Primary care was defined as "the providing of integrated, accessible health care services by clinicians who are accountable for addressing a large majority of personal health care needs, while developing partnerships with patients and practicing in the context of family and community" (IOM, 1996, p. 1). Public health was defined as "fulfilling society's interest in assuring conditions in which people can be healthy" (IOM, 1988, p. 140). The purpose of the integration is to achieve the WHO goal of primary health care.

## Potential Barriers to Integration

Contrasting the two systems, primary care, which can be either a public or a private entity, is person focused, provides a point of first contact for individuals to address health problems, and is considered comprehensive and provides coordination of individual care; public health can also be delivered through public and private entities to contribute to the health of society, but government plays a major role in public health. Health departments are legally bound to provide essential public health services, and to work with the total community and multiple stakeholders to address community-level health problems. Public health also has specific functions of assurance, assessment, and policy development to address community-level health issues and has a charge to create healthy communities (see Chapter 1).

In addition to differing roles and functions and issues related to funding, different clients and different foci will need to be addressed to form a solid foundation for a partnership. Primary care is largely funded through individual client payments, health insurance, and sometimes through federal grants. Public health is largely funded through tax dollars, federal and state grants, and sometimes health insurance payments through Medicare and Medicaid. Primary care serves the individuals who present to the practice while public health serves to assess the health problems of the population. Both focus on meeting the most prevalent health needs of the population. Primary care focuses more on the curative aspect of care while public health focuses more on the prevention of health problems (Levesque et al, 2013).

The common goal of public health and primary care, although these systems operate independently, is to ensure a healthier population. Integration of these two systems has the potential to produce a greater impact on the health of populations than either could have working alone, said the committee of experts convened by the IOM (2012).

The Healthy People initiatives, beginning with the U.S. surgeon general's 1979 report, indicate the long-standing desire to improve population health in the United States.

## Primary Health Care

Primary health care (PHC), the goal of the integration of public health and primary care, includes a comprehensive range of services including public health and preventive, diagnostic, therapeutic, and rehabilitative services. This system is composed of public health agencies, community-based agencies and primary care clinics, and health care providers. From a conceptual point of view, PHC is essential care made universally accessible to individuals, families, and the community. Health care is made available to them with their full participation and is provided at a cost that the community and country can afford. This care is not uniformly available and accessible to all people in many countries including the United States. Full community participation means that individuals within the community

help in defining health problems and in developing approaches to address the problems. The setting for primary health care is within all communities of a country and involves all aspects of society (WHO, 1978).

The primary health care movement officially began in 1977 when the 30th World Health Organization (WHO) Health Assembly adopted a resolution accepting the goal of attaining a level of health that permitted all citizens of the world to live socially and economically productive lives. At the international conference in 1978 in Alma-Ata, in the former Soviet Union (Russia), it was determined that this goal was to be met through PHC. This resolution, the Declaration of Alma-Ata, became known by the slogan "Health for All (HFA) by the Year 2000," which captured the official health target for all the member nations of the WHO. In 1998 the program was adapted to meet the needs of the new century and was deemed "Health for All in the 21st Century."

In 1981 the WHO established global indicators for monitoring and evaluating the achievement of HFA. In the *World Health Statistics Annual* (WHO, 1986b), these indicators are grouped into the following four categories: health policies, social and economic development, provision of health care, and health status. The indicators suggest that health improvements are a result of efforts in many areas, including agriculture, industry, education, housing, communications, and health care. Because PHC is as much a political statement as a system of care, each United Nations member country interprets PHC according to its own culture, health needs, resources, and system of government. Clearly, the goal of PHC has not been met in most countries including the United States.

## Promoting Health/Preventing Disease: Year 2020 Objectives for the Nation

As a WHO member nation, the United States has endorsed primary health care as a strategy for achieving the goal of "Health for All in the 21st Century." However, the PHC emphasis on broad strategies, community participation, self-reliance, and a multidisciplinary health care delivery team is not the primary strategy for improving the health of the American people. The national health plan for the United States identifies disease prevention and health promotion as the areas of most concern in the nation. Each decade since the 1980s has been measured and tracked according to health objectives set at the beginning of the decade. The U.S. Public Health Service of the HHS publishes the objectives after gathering data from health professionals and organizations throughout the country.

*Healthy People 2020*, which was officially launched in December 2010 (USDHHS, 2010a), is composed of a large number of objectives related to 42 topic areas. These objectives are designed to serve as a road map for improving the health of all people in the United States during the second decade of the twenty-first century. These objectives are described by four main goals (USDHHS, 2010b):

- Attain high-quality, longer lives free of preventable disease, disability, injury, and premature death
- Achieve health equity, eliminate disparities, and improve the health of all groups

• Create social and physical environments that promote good health for all
• Promote quality of life, healthy development, and healthy behaviors across all life stages

These goals provide the framework with which measurable health indicators can be tracked. The emphasis on the social and physical environment moves *Healthy People 2020* from the traditional disease-specific focus to a more holistic view of health consistent with a public health frame of reference (Healthy People 2020, 2012). This in turn will encourage public health nurses to broaden their scope to all aspects of their clients' lives that may need assessment and intervention, including where they live, the condition of their home, and how the

appropriateness of their environment may change as the client ages. The Healthy People 2020 box presents indicators of *Healthy People 2020* related to the strengthening of the public health infrastructure. These objectives will assist nurses in having data to show that their assessments and interventions are changing practice.

## HEALTH CARE DELIVERY REFORM EFFORTS—UNITED STATES

Over the centuries, both health insurance and health care reform have been the focus of numerous discussions and political battles. As can be seen in Chapter 2, the first health insurance plan, established in about 1798 in the United States, was for the Merchant Marines to assist in treating infectious diseases and protecting the ports of entry into the United States. The United States has discussed national health care reform since the 1900s (see Chapter 5). In 1912 Theodore Roosevelt campaigned on a health insurance proposal for industry. Then in 1915 the "progressive reformers" campaigned for a state-based system of compulsory health insurance. In the 1920s, the Committee on the Costs of Medical Care suggested group medicine and voluntary insurance, and this movement was labeled as promoting "socialized medicine." Since the 1930s, through surveys, Americans have generally shown support of the goals of guaranteed access to health care and health insurance, and a governmental role in financing of care. Some strides were made in improving access and defining the role of government financing through

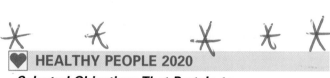

### HEALTHY PEOPLE 2020

#### Selected Objectives That Pertain to Strengthening the Public Health Infrastructure

• **PHI-7** (Developmental): Increase the proportion of population-based *Healthy People 2020* objectives for which national data are available for all major population groups.
• **PHI-8:** Increase the proportion of *Healthy People 2020* objectives that are tracked regularly at the national level.

From U. S. Department of Health and Human Services. Healthy People 2020. Available at http://www.healthypeople.gov/2020topics objectives2020/default.aspx. Accessed December 27, 2010.

### EVIDENCE-BASED PRACTICE

It is often said that the states are the laboratories of democracy. One state, Massachusetts, began an experiment in health reform in 2006. Two years after health reform legislation became effective, only 2.6% of Massachusetts residents were uninsured, the lowest percentage ever recorded in any state (Dorn et al, 2009). However, the program became one of the most successful and a model for the Affordable Care Act. After 5 years approximately 98% to 99% of all of the commonwealth's citizens were covered by the plan.

Although other states have experimented with various programs to decrease the number of uninsured, the Massachusetts plan has had the most success. The health reform plan rests on an individual mandate that requires everyone who can afford insurance to purchase coverage. Those unable to afford insurance receive subsidies that allow low-income individuals and families to purchase coverage. A new state-run program, Commonwealth Care (CommCare), provides benefits to adults who are not eligible for Medicaid but whose incomes fall below 300% of the federal poverty level.

To understand how the state was so successful in this effort toward universal coverage, a group of evaluators met with 15 key informants representing hospitals, community health centers, insurance companies, Medicaid, and CommCare. Several factors, it was found, have contributed to the historic level of coverage seen in the state. Rather than requiring consumers to complete separate applications for programs such as Medicaid, the Children's Health Insurance Program (CHIP), or CommCare, a single application system provides entry to all the state programs. If an uninsured client was admitted to a hospital or visited a community

health center, his or her eligibility was automatically evaluated and, if eligible, the client would be automatically converted to CommCare coverage, even without completing an application. A "Virtual Gateway" has been developed through which staff of community-based organizations have been trained to complete online applications on behalf of consumers, and to provide education and counseling about insurance options to underserved communities. By holding back reimbursement to providers who do not help consumers sign up for one of the available insurance options, hospitals and health centers are motivated to dedicate staff to provide education and counseling to the formerly uninsured. The result is that at least half of the new enrollees in Medicaid and CommCare have been enrolled without filling out any forms on their own. In addition to these efforts, shortly after the reform legislation was enacted, the state financed a massive public education effort to inform consumers about their new options.

#### Nurse Use
As health reform begins on the national level, nurses can play a crucial role in driving down the number of uninsured. Nurses should educate themselves so that they can encourage clients to apply and take advantage of all available coverage options. Taking an active role in consumer educational programs is a natural extension of a nurse's role as a client advocate. Nurses can promote legislation to simplify enrollment processes and encourage the development of shared databases for community health care providers, thus preventing consumers from falling through the cracks in our fragmented health care system.

Dorn S, Hill I, Hogan S: *The secrets of Massachusetts' success: why 97 percent of state residents have health coverage: state health access reform evaluation, Rommneycare-The truth about Massachusetts health care.* 2014, accessed at mittromneycentral.com/resources/romneycare. 9/25/20142009, Robert Wood Johnson Foundation. Available at http://www.urban.org/uploadedpdf/411987_massachusetts_success_brief.pdf. Accessed September 19, 2012.

the passing of Medicare in 1965, with Medicaid as a part of the proposal for social security amendments, and the Children's Health Insurance Program bill passed in 1996. Many proposals have been put forward over the decades for health care reform, as well as health insurance reform. Beginning in the 1970s Senator Ted Kennedy, President Richard Nixon, President Gerald Ford, and President Jimmy Carter all made health-related proposals, all followed by the Health Security Act of President Bill Clinton. None were accepted by Congress (Kaiser Family Foundation, 2009b).

Nurses and the American Nurses Association have been involved in the debates about health care reform over time. In its 2005 Healthcare System Reform Agenda, the American Nurses Association (American Nurses Association, 2008) promoted a blueprint for reform that includes the following:

• Health care is a basic human right, and so a restructured health care system with universal access to a standard package of essential health care services for all citizens and residents must be assured.
• The development and implementation of health policies that reflect the aims put forth by the Institute of Medicine (safe, effective, patient centered, timely, efficient, equitable) and are based on outcomes research will ultimately save money.
• The overuse of expensive, technology-driven, acute, hospital-based services must give way to a balance between high-tech treatment and community-based and preventive services, with emphasis on the latter.
• A single-payer mechanism is the most desirable option for financing a reformed health care system.

In 2010 the Affordable Care Act (ACA) was passed, after introduction by the Obama team and after much debate. This act reflects many of the tenets offered by the ANA in its Health System Reform Agenda and puts into place comprehensive health insurance reforms that are to be implemented by 2014 and beyond. The act was passed to improve quality and lower health care costs, provide access to care, and provide for consumer protection. Table 3-2 provides an overview of the key features of the act by year. The ACA has a major focus on prevention. This focus is designed to improve the health of Americans, but also help to reduce health care costs and improve quality of care. Through the Prevention and Public Health Fund, the ACA will address factors that influence health—housing, education, transportation, the availability of quality affordable food, and conditions in the workplace and the environment. By concentrating on the causes of chronic disease, the ACA will move the nation from a focus on sickness and disease to one based on wellness and prevention.

To improve the health of Americans, ways to make the healthy choice in each community an easy and affordable choice must be found. In addition, within the law there are specific benefits for women, young adults, and families. It strengthens Medicare and holds insurance companies accountable (USDHHS, 2014b).

Since the close of the first enrollment period for the ACA in early 2014, the numbers of uninsured have declined (see Chapter 1). Because of a lag in data, the effects of the health care reform will not be known until 2015.

Discussions and debates will continue about the impact of the ACA, and the IOM's discussions of integrating public health and primary care, reducing cost, increasing quality, and access for all Americans. It is important not to lose sight of the goal: to protect and improve the health of all populations. After spending 18 months in a public policy fellowship and working with the Ways and Means Committee in Congress, Nancy Ridenour, PhD, RN and dean of the College of Nursing at the University of New Mexico, described her opportunity to work with others as the ACA was being developed. At a board of nursing celebration in Kentucky in the summer of 2014, Dr. Ridenour explained to the audience that it would be important for nurses to be involved in the implementation of the ACA to promote the success of the health care changes proposed. It is all about the influence of nurses and the nursing profession! (Kentucky Board of Nursing, 2014).

---

**QSEN FOCUS ON QUALITY AND SAFETY EDUCATION FOR NURSES**

**Targeted Competency: Informatics**—Use information and technology to communicate, manage knowledge, mitigate error, and support decision making.

Important aspects of Informatics include the following:

**Knowledge:** Identify essential information that must be available in a common database to support interventions in the health care system.

**Skills:** Use information management tools to monitor outcomes of intervention processes.

**Attitudes:** Value technologies that support decision making, error prevention, and case coordination.

**Informatics Question:** Updated informatics definitions focus on having access to the necessary client and system information at the right time, to make the best clinical decision. In the U.S. Department of Health and Human Services (USDHHS) Strategic Plan for 2010 to 2015, there are five overarching goals.

*Goal 1, Objective C* focuses on "Emphasizing primary and preventive care linked with community prevention services." Which community data would a public health nurse assess to determine the work that needs to be done in a community related to this USDHHS strategic goal?

**Answer:** To assess future work that could be done to effectively address Goal 1, Objective C, public health nurses might gather data in the following areas:

• How informed are members of the community about existing community services that support health promotion (e.g., exercise classes, educational classes, self-management training, and nutrition counseling)?
• How relevant are the services offered by health centers to the needs of a community?
• Do payment or insurance barriers exist for individuals to access preventive health services?
• How accessible is entry to care for vulnerable populations such as pregnant women and infants?
• What community-based prevention programs exist for individuals with and at risk for chronic diseases and conditions?
• How available are substance abuse screening and intervention programs?
• How linked are primary care and health promotions and wellness programs in a community?

Prepared by Gail Armstrong, PhD(c), DNP, ACNS-BC, CNE, Associate Professor, University of Colorado Denver College of Nursing.

## TABLE 3-2    Overview of Key Features of the Affordable Care Act by Year

**2010**

**New Consumer Protections**

- Putting information for consumers online.
- Prohibiting denying coverage of children based on pre-existing conditions.
- Prohibiting insurance companies from rescinding coverage.
- Eliminating lifetime limits on insurance coverage.
- Regulating annual limits on insurance coverage.
- Establishing consumer assistance programs in the states.

**Improving Quality and Lowering Costs**

- Providing small business health insurance tax credits.
- Offering relief for 4 million seniors who hit the Medicare prescription drug "donut hole."
- Providing free preventive care.
- Preventing disease and illness.
- Cracking down on health care fraud.

**Increasing Access to Affordable Care**

- Providing access to insurance for uninsured Americans with pre-existing conditions.
- Extending coverage for young adults.
- Expanding coverage for early retirees.
- Rebuilding the primary care workforce.
- Holding insurance companies accountable for unreasonable rate hikes.
- Allowing states to cover more people on Medicaid.
- Increasing payments for rural health care providers.
- Strengthening community health centers.

**2011**

**Improving Quality and Lowering Costs**

- Offering prescription drug discounts.
- Providing free preventive care for seniors.
- Improving health care quality and efficiency.
- Improving care for seniors after they leave the hospital.
- Introducing new innovations to bring down costs.

**Increasing Access to Affordable Care**

- Increasing access to services at home and in the community.

**Holding Insurance Companies Accountable**

- Bringing down health care premiums.
- Addressing overpayments to big insurance companies and strengthening Medicare Advantage.

**2012**

**Improving Quality and Lowering Costs**

- Linking payment to quality outcomes.
- Encouraging integrated health systems.
- Reducing paperwork and administrative costs.
- Understanding and fighting health disparities.

**Increasing Access to Affordable Care**

- Providing new, voluntary options for long-term care insurance.

**2013**

**Improving Quality and Lowering Costs**

- Improving preventive health coverage.
- Expanding authority to bundle payments.

**Increasing Access to Affordable Care**

- Increasing Medicaid payments for primary care doctors.
- Open enrollment in the health insurance marketplace begins.

**2014**

**New Consumer Protections**

- Prohibiting discrimination due to pre-existing conditions or gender.
- Eliminating annual limits on insurance coverage.
- Ensuring coverage for individuals participating in clinical trials.

**Improving Quality and Lowering Costs**

- Making care more affordable.
- Establishing the health insurance marketplace.
- Increasing the small business tax credit.

**Increasing Access to Affordable Care**

- Increasing access to Medicaid.
- Promoting individual responsibility.

**2015**

**Improving Quality and Lowering Costs**

- Paying physicians based on value, not volume.

For more detail about each of the bulleted statements please refer to HHS.gov/HealthCare (Key Features of the Affordable Care Act, 2014: http://www.hhs.gov/healthcare/facts/timeline/).

## PRACTICE APPLICATION

During a well-child clinic visit, Jenna Wells, RN, met Sandra Farr and her 24-month-old daughter, Jessica. The Farrs had recently moved to the community. Mrs. Farr stated that she knew that Jessica needed the last in a series of immunizations and because they did not have health insurance, she brought her daughter to the public health clinic. On initial assessment, Mrs. Farr told the nurse that her husband would soon be employed, but the family had no health care coverage for the next 30 days. The Farrs also needed to decide which health care package they wanted. Mr. Farr's company offers a preferred provider organization (PPO), a health maintenance organization (HMO), and

a community nursing clinic plan to all employees. Neither Mr. nor Mrs. Farr has ever used an HMO or a community nursing clinic, and they are not sure what services are provided.

Mrs. Farr asks Nurse Wells what she should do.

Nurse Wells should do which of the following?

A. Encourage Mrs. Farr to choose the HMO because it will pay more attention to the family's preventive needs, and direct Mrs. Farr to other sources of health care should the family need to see a provider while they are uninsured.

B. Encourage Mrs. Farr to choose the PPO because it will have a greater number of qualified providers from which to

TABLE 4-1    Top 20 DALY Conditions

| | | | 2011 | | |
|---|---|---|---|---|---|
| Rank | GHE Code | Cause | DALYs (000s) | % DALYs | DALYs per 100,000 Population |
| 1 | 39 | Lower respiratory infections | 164804 | 6.0 | 2375 |
| 2 | 113 | Ischaemic heart disease | 159659 | 5.8 | 2301 |
| 3 | 114 | Stroke | 135369 | 4.9 | 1951 |
| 4 | 11 | Diarrhoeal diseases | 118789 | 4.3 | 1712 |
| 5 | 50 | Preterm birth complications | 110688 | 4.0 | 1595 |
| 6 | 10 | HIV/AIDS | 95226 | 3.5 | 1372 |
| 7 | 118 | Chronic obstructive pulmonary disease | 89605 | 3.3 | 1291 |
| 8 | 153 | Road injury | 78792 | 2.9 | 1136 |
| 9 | 51 | Birth asphyxia and birth trauma | 78199 | 2.8 | 1127 |
| 10 | 83 | Unipolar depressive disorders | 75002 | 2.7 | 1081 |
| 11 | 140 | Congenital anomalies | 57697 | 2.1 | 832 |
| 12 | 80 | Diabetes mellitus | 56402 | 2.1 | 813 |
| 13 | 22 | Malaria | 55414 | 2.0 | 799 |
| 14 | 138 | Back and neck pain | 52692 | 1.9 | 759 |
| 15 | 58 | Iron-deficiency anaemia | 46244 | 1.7 | 667 |
| 16 | 3 | Tuberculosis | 42240 | 1.5 | 609 |
| 17 | 155 | Falls | 40782 | 1.5 | 588 |
| 18 | 161 | Self-harm | 39787 | 1.4 | 573 |
| 19 | 68 | Trachea, bronchus, lung cancers | 37252 | 1.4 | 537 |
| 20 | 123 | Cirrhosis of the liver | 34925 | 1.3 | 503 |

From ChildInfo: Monitoring the situation of children and women. Available at http://www.childinfo.org/maternal_mortality.html. Accessed March 20, 2014.

TABLE 4-2    Top 10 DALYs in Broad Categories

| | | 2011 | | |
|---|---|---|---|---|
| Rank | Broad Cause | DALYs (000s) | % DALYs | DALYs per 100,000 Population |
| 1 | Infectious diseases (incl. respiratory infections) | 624141 | 22.7 | 8996 |
| 2 | Cardiovascular diseases | 378875 | 13.8 | 5461 |
| 3 | Injuries | 296836 | 10.8 | 4278 |
| 4 | Neonatal conditions | 231581 | 8.4 | 3338 |
| 5 | Cancers | 223539 | 8.1 | 3222 |
| 6 | Mental and behavioral disorders | 198370 | 7.2 | 2859 |
| 7 | Respiratory diseases | 134246 | 4.9 | 1935 |
| 8 | Neurological and sense organ conditions | 128613 | 4.7 | 1854 |
| 9 | Musculoskeletal diseases | 108401 | 4.0 | 1562 |
| 10 | Endocrine, blood, immune disorders, diabetes mellitus | 88211 | 3.2 | 1271 |

http://www.who.int/healthinfo/global_burden_disease/estimates_regional/en/index1.html

children under age 5 died during the same year in less developed countries. If these children could face the same risks as those in developed nations, the deaths would decrease by 90%. This example demonstrates the importance of having accessible and affordable disease prevention programs for children around the world (WHO, 2014e). Infections and parasitic diseases remain a threat to the health of the majority of the world and are diseases seen in the United States in newly arriving immigrants. Studies demonstrate the continuing need for intervention for infectious and other kinds of communicable diseases. Conditions that contribute to one fourth of the GBD throughout the world include diarrheal disease, respiratory tract infections, worm infestations, malaria, and childhood diseases such as measles and polio. Sub-Saharan Africa demonstrated a GBD of 43% DALYs lost, largely because of preventable diseases among children (WHO, 2014e).

According to the U.S. Global Health Policy fact sheet published by the Kaiser Family Foundation (2010), globally there were 33 million people living with HIV in 2007, up from 29.5 million in 2001, the result of continuing new infections, people living longer with HIV, and general population growth. HIV is a leading cause of death worldwide and the number one cause of death in Africa. An estimated 8 in 10 people infected with HIV do not know it. HIV has led to a resurgence of TB, particularly in Africa, and TB is a leading cause of death for people with HIV worldwide. Women represent half of all people living with HIV worldwide, and more than half (60%) in sub-Saharan Africa. Globally, there were 2.5 million children living with HIV in 2009, 370,000 new infections among children, and 260,000 AIDS deaths. There are approximately 16.6 million AIDS orphans today (children who have lost one or both parents to HIV), most of whom live in sub-Saharan Africa (89%).

Uganda's emphasis on ameliorating HIV/AIDS is a model for all African nations; however, there are still too many Ugandan children under 5 years old who are AIDS orphans. Unfortunately, despite the efforts of advocates, donors, and affected countries, there needs to be greater attention given to the long overdue effort to expand access to antiretroviral therapy, which is still available to less than 10% of those who urgently require it.

Determining the total amount of loss, even using the GBD, is difficult because it does not address the many consequences of disease and injury such as post–trauma and infectious physical disabilities. Nor can it measure the short- or long-term effects of familial and marital dysfunction, family violence, or war. The following further elaborates on selected communicable diseases that still contribute substantially to the worldwide disease burden (TB, AIDS, and malaria) and other health problems such as maternal and women's health, diarrheal disease in children, nutrition, natural and man-made disasters.

## Communicable Diseases

Prevention of communicable diseases is through immunization and improving environmental conditions. One example of the long-term benefits of immunizing children against communicable diseases is the successful campaign against smallpox that the WHO conducted during the 1960s and 1970s. Smallpox has been virtually eliminated throughout the world, with only occasional and incidental reporting from laboratory accidents and inoculation complications. The systematic and planned smallpox program formed the basis for a series of worldwide efforts that are now being implemented to control and eradicate other infectious and communicable diseases.

In 1974 the WHO formed the Expanded Program on Immunization, which sought to reduce morbidity and mortality from diphtheria, pertussis, tetanus, TB, measles, and poliomyelitis throughout the world (WHO, 2010). In the 2010 State of the World Report on immunizations and vaccines, the WHO noted that for the first time in documented history the number of children dying every year had fallen below 10 million. This appears to be the result of improved access to clean water and sanitation, increased immunization coverage, and the integrated delivery of essential health interventions. Unfortunately, almost 20% of the children born each year do not get the complete routine immunizations scheduled for their first year of life. This is most prevalent in developing countries and for those children born in the very rural communities. In developing countries, more vaccines are available and more lives are being saved; however, death from pertussis in developing countries is 40 per 1000 infants, and 10 per 1000 in older children. It still occurs in industrialized countries but at less than 1 per 1000 cases. Although free vaccination clinics are brought to the people, they are often not used because of lack of knowledge, fear propagated by the traditional healers, and suspicion of anything offered by the government. Reaching these vulnerable children—typically in poorly served remote rural areas, deprived urban settings, fragile states, and strife-torn regions—is essential in order to meet the Millennium Development Goals (MDGs; United Nations, 2013b).

The WHO has estimated that if all the vaccines now available against childhood diseases were widely adopted, and if countries could raise vaccine coverage to a global average of 90%, by 2015 an additional 2 million deaths a year could be prevented among children under age 5. This level of vaccination would reduce child deaths by two thirds and achieve one of the MDG goals. It would also greatly reduce the burden of illness and disability from vaccine-preventable diseases and contribute to improving child health and welfare, as well as reducing hospitalization costs (WHO, Immunizations, 2010b).

As discussed in Chapter 10, environmental sanitation is critical to the well-being of people around the globe. Many of the major health risks relate to interactions between people and their environment. For example, in developing nations, community drinking water sources can be contaminated by agricultural runoffs containing toxic pesticides and fertilizers, but they can also be contaminated by naturally occurring elements in the earth such as arsenic and fluoride. This author and her colleagues have found gross heavy metal (primarily arsenic) contamination of the water sources in Uganda including the government filtered water, bottled water from clean water bottling companies in Uganda, bore holes (wells), river, swamps, and springs (Bolender et al, 2012, 2013; Jameel et al, 2012). Efforts are underway to assess the extent of this problem across Uganda and to assess the effects on the population. We have already discovered unexplained neurological symptoms in the adults and persistent anemia in the children; which could have its causative origin in the arsenic-contaminated water consumed by the people. Long-term absorption of arsenic in humans has been associated with skin cancer, cancer of the bladder and lungs, developmental effects, neurotoxicity, diabetes, and cardiovascular disease (Global Poverty Project, 2013; WHO, Fact Sheet on Arsenic, 2012c).

In developing nations, it is not uncommon for hospitals and HIV testing centers to dump waste products into the local rivers that often supply the local household water. Worldwide, environmental factors play a role in more than 80% of adverse outcomes reported by the WHO, including infectious diseases, injuries, mental retardation, and cancer, to name a few. Globalization and industrialization in the developing world have increased daily exposure to pollution and a wide array of chemicals in air, water, and food. At the same time, fecal pollution of drinking water sources caused by a lack of basic sanitation still exists. The effects of environmental risk factors are magnified by conditions often prevalent in poorer, undeveloped countries such as poor nutrition, poverty, lack of education about risks, and conflicts. Children are particularly susceptible to environmental risks because their systems are still developing. It is estimated that about one quarter of global disease is caused by avoidable environmental exposures; for young children in the developing world, causes of environmentally related deaths are acute respiratory infections, related to poor air quality; and diarrhea, related to poor drinking water quality. Annually, about 3 million children under the age of 5 die of environment-related diseases. There are projects that train and give technical assistance, data collection and analysis, laboratory analyses, research, surveillance, and emergency responses to international communities (American Society of Hematology, 2013; WHO, Fact Sheet on Child Deaths, 2013b).

As of 2013, 783 million people still do not have access to clean water, and their water sources are often far away, unclean, and unaffordable; 2.5 billion people or 40% of the world's population lack an adequate toilet or latrine. Getting hold of clean water is not good enough if the water is being made dirty because there are no toilets, and toilets are not good enough if there is no hygiene promotion to persuade whole communities to change the habits of generations and use the latrines. Estimates by the Joint Monitoring Program of UNICEF and the WHO predict that at the current rate of progress, approximately 2 billion people will still lack access to a clean environment by 2015. In sub-Saharan Africa 50% of people lack this basic human right, and their need may not be met until 2072 if the current rate continues (UNICEF, Water, Sanitation and Hygiene, 2010).

### Tuberculosis

In 2012, according to the WHO (Tuberculosis Fact Sheet, 2012d) about 8.6 million people fell ill with tuberculosis and 1.3 million died of the disease. Ninety-five percent of TB deaths occur in low to middle income countries, and TB is one of the top three causes of death for women ages 15-44. Children are not immune to this bacterium, as the WHO report indicates that more than 530,000 children diagnosed with the disease and 74,000 HIV-negative children died of TB. It is a leading killer of people with HIV, and up to 80% of TB clients are HIV positive in countries with a high prevalence of HIV. People with HIV are much more likely to develop TB; as are those infected with malaria, especially children, because of the physiological damage to the liver, spleen, and hematological systems. A child or adult with any one of the three diseases mentioned is more prone to the other two, and this triad is the new scourge of impoverished nations. The WHO estimates that more than one third of infectious disease deaths are due to this deadly triad of AIDS, TB, and malaria (WHO, Tuberculosis Fact Sheet, 2012d).

It is expected that at least one third of the world's population, or 1.7 billion people, harbor the TB pathogen *Mycobacterium tuberculosis*. The Stop TB Partnership, engaging nearly 300 governments and agencies, has brought consensus on approaches to global control of this disease, galvanized support, and launched new support mechanisms, such as the Global TB Drug Facility, an initiative to increase access to high-quality TB drugs. The Working Group on Tuberculosis recommends seven priorities to meet the MDG targets for this disease for 2015. All this effort has resulted in some good news. It has been shown that the number of people falling ill with tuberculosis each year is declining, although very slowly. The world appears to be on track to achieve the Millennium Development Goal to reverse the spread of TB by 2015, especially given that the TB death rate dropped 45% between 1990 and 2010.

Two factors are a threat to TB control and eradication. The first is the AIDS virus. The appearance of HIV has added to the difficulty of treatment programs in both developed and less developed countries. More important, HIV-positive individuals with infectious TB have an increased likelihood of transmitting TB to their families and to the community, further increasing the prevalence of this condition.

The second is the growing multidrug resistance of the TB bacillus to isoniazid and rifampin, the two drugs used to treat it. Resistance to these drugs is already evident around the world, including in the Mexico-Texas border communities. The WHO and other organizations maintain that a high priority should be given to TB control and eradication programs around the world. They advocate a short-term chemotherapy regimen for smear-positive clients as being one of the most cost-effective health interventions available (Forman et al, 2012; WHO, Tuberculosis Fact Sheet, 2012d). The bacille Calmette-Guérin (BCG) vaccine, which has been available since the 1920s, was promoted as an effective vaccine to induce active immunity against TB, especially among children living in TB-endemic or high-risk TB areas that are impoverished and crowded. The BCG vaccine has a documented protective effect against meningitis and disseminated TB in children. It does not prevent primary infection and, more importantly, does not prevent reactivation of latent pulmonary infection, the principal source of bacillary spread in the community. The impact of BCG vaccination on transmission of TB is therefore limited (WHO, 2012d). The standard chemotherapeutic agents used in many countries for TB are isoniazid, thioacetazone, and streptomycin, and they are effective at converting sputum-positive cases to noninfectivity. The drugs and the combinations that are used vary from country to country. To be effective, however, treatment must be carried out on a consistent basis, and many less developed countries have difficulty persuading clients to purchase the medications and to adhere to any treatment regimen. In 1990 the WHO Global Tuberculosis Program (GTB) promoted the revision of national TB programs to focus on short-course chemotherapy (SCC), with directly observed treatment (DOT). DOT programs have been successful in the United States and in several less developed countries, including Malawi, Mozambique, Nicaragua, and Tanzania, producing a cure rate of approximately 80%. The SCC program involves aggressive administration of chemotherapeutic drugs combined with short-term hospitalization. The key to the program lies in a well-managed system with a regular supply of anti-TB drugs to the treatment centers, follow-up care, and rigorous reporting and analysis of client information (IOM, 2011).

Lasting control of AIDS, TB, and/or malaria will depend on strengthening the health, economic, political, education, and other infrastructure necessary to sustain life and promote the well-being of the people. It will require sustained investment in physical infrastructure, drug distribution systems, management at all levels, and, most importantly, human resources such as the training and appropriate use of community health workers to deliver some essential services and education. Unfortunately, the failure of developed countries to fulfill their pledges of more development aid, and the failure of developing countries themselves to invest in health, are overarching barriers to health systems development. HIV/AIDS, TB, and malaria are only three of the challenges facing poor people. Only stronger, integrated health systems can provide a platform to sustain a successful fight against these diseases while advancing the other health priorities of developing countries, including child and maternal health and chronic disease.

It is important, when conducting a health assessment interview, always to ask whether the client has recently traveled out of the United States or to one of the border areas along the United States–Mexico perimeter. People who travel abroad may bring back diseases that are difficult to diagnose. In addition, people often cross the border into Mexico to fill a prescription for medicine because it is often less expensive than in the United States. Unfortunately, many times the medications brought back have been relabeled and are out of date.

## Acquired Immunodeficiency Syndrome

As discussed in Chapter 14, AIDS remains a major cause of morbidity and mortality throughout the world. More than 70 million people have been infected with HIV since the beginning of the epidemic; approximately 35 million people have died of AIDS. At the end of 2011, 34.0 million people globally were living with HIV with an estimated 0.8% of the adult population aged 15-49 years infected. The burden of the epidemic continues to vary considerably between countries and regions; however, sub-Saharan Africa remains most severely affected, with nearly 1 in every 20 adults (4.9%) living with HIV and accounting for 69% of the global population infected with this virus (IOM, 2012; WHO, HIV/AIDS, 2014f). For more information, go to http://www.who.int/gho/hiv/hiv_013.jpg?ua=1 (WHO, Global Health Observatory—HIV/AIDS, 2014f).

The Kaiser Family Foundation report (2013a) stated that approximately 35.3 million people were living with HIV in 2012, up from 29.4 million in 2001. This rise appears to be the result of continuing new infections (averaging 6300 per day), people living longer with HIV, and general population growth. When comparing the population growth with the HIV incidence rates, overall new HIV infections have declined by 33% since 2001. Of interest is that 1.6 million people died of AIDS in 2012, which was a 30% decrease since 2005. Such results appear to be the result of antiretroviral treatment (ART) scale-up.

The majority of new infections are being transmitted heterosexually, placing women and children at increased risk for acquiring the infection. Gender inequalities, lack of access to services, and sexual violence against women and children increase their vulnerability to HIV. Women represent about half (52%) of all people living with HIV worldwide and younger women are biologically more susceptible to HIV. Unfortunately, young people often believe the disease can be cured with drugs and thus they can be less cautious; in addition, cultural practices exist whereby older men marry virgins to cure them of AIDS or to prevent them from getting AIDS.

By 2012, there were 3.3 million children globally living with HIV, with 260,000 new infections identified and 210,000 children who lost their lives to AIDS. Sadly, there are approximately 17.3 million children with AIDS who have lost one or both parents to HIV; most of these children live in sub-Saharan Africa (88%) and will either die from the disease or be treated as social outcasts by the community at large (Kaiser Family Foundation, 2013a).

Worldwide prevention programs are important because failing to control this virulent disease will result in damaging and costly consequences for all countries in the future. Ideally, the goal is primary prevention of HIV. When prevention efforts fail at this level, the next goal is secondary prevention, or early diagnosis and treatment. Aggressive interventions in many African nations have begun to make a difference in the life potential for patients diagnosed with HIV.

Combination ART has contributed to the reduced morbidity and mortality rate since 2001 and in sub-Saharan Africa alone, the number of people receiving ART increased significantly from 50,000 in 2002 to 7.5 million in 2012. In 2012, ART covered 61% of individuals who were eligible for treatment, representing 65% of the 2011 U.N.General Assembly Special Session target of treating 15 million by 2015. New WHO guidelines recommend starting treatment of HIV earlier in the course of illness. Given these new recommendations, 25.9 million people are now eligible for treatment (Kaiser Family Foundation, 2013a). See the levels of prevention box below to learn about prevention of HIV.

### LEVELS OF PREVENTION

#### Global Health Care

**Primary Prevention**
Teach people how to avoid or change risky behaviors that might lead to contracting human immunodeficiency virus (HIV).

**Secondary Prevention**
Initiate screening programs for HIV.

**Tertiary Prevention**
Manage symptoms of HIV, provide psychosocial support, and teach clients and significant others about care and other forms of symptom management.

## Malaria

Malaria affects more than 50% of the world's population and hits tropical Africa the hardest. However, there have been major global efforts to control and eliminate malaria that have saved an estimated 3.3 million lives since 2000, reducing malaria mortality rates by 45% globally and by 49% in Africa, according to the "World Malaria Report 2013" published by the WHO (see http://www.who.int/malaria/publications/world_malaria_report_2013/en/).

The large majority of the 3.3 million lives saved between 2000 and 2012 were in the 10 countries with the highest malaria burden, and among children under 5 years of age, which is the group most affected by the disease. Over the same period, malaria mortality rates among children in Africa were reduced by an estimated 54%. An expansion of prevention and control measures has contributed to a consistent decline in malaria deaths and illness. Unfortunately, the new WHO report notes a slowdown in the expansion of interventions to control mosquitoes for the second successive year, particularly in providing access to insecticide-treated bed nets, because of lack of funds to procure bed nets. My experience in Uganda still finds that malaria and its sequelae are the number one cause of death in children less than 8 years of age.

Malaria is caused by the *Anopheles* mosquito and is the only mosquito-borne disease that can be prevented and cured by pharmacological management (WHO, Malaria Report, 2013e). It is caused by parasitic transmission from the infected female mosquito to its host. There are four parasite species that cause malaria, the most serious being *Plasmodium falciparum,* which causes microvascular sequestration and obstruction in the brain, kidney, and liver leading to cerebral malaria, anemia, kidney failure, hypoglycemia, disseminated intravascular coagulation (DIC), fluid-electrolyte imbalance, and death (CDC, 2013a). Symptoms vary and range from mild to severe physiological responses (mild fever and chills to temperatures of 106° F with prolonged chills, seizures, and dehydration).

A range of effective antimalarial interventions exists for the prevention, treatment, and control of malaria. These include the use of insecticide-treated bed nets (ITNs); indoor residual spraying; intermittent presumptive treatment during pregnancy; early diagnosis and prompt treatment with effective antimalarials; management of the environment to control mosquitoes; health education; and epidemic forecasting, prevention, and response (CDC, 2013a; WHO, 2013e). Methods of vector control vary widely, from using the larvae-eating fish tilapia to the use of insecticidal sprays and oils. Needless to say, the latter poses a potential threat to the environment in tropical areas where a delicate ecosystem is already threatened by other potential hazards such as lumbering and mining.

Countries that do not have strict environmental laws continue to use dichlorodiphenyltrichloroethane (DDT) sprays to control mosquito populations despite the advent of DDT-resistant mosquitoes. The non-DDT insecticide sprays, such as malathion, generally cost more, presenting an extra financial burden to less developed countries. Methods for control and eradication that are being considered by malaria-ridden countries are environmental management, reduction and control of the source, and elimination of the adult mosquito. There are significant global efforts being made to "blanket" endemic communities with insecticide-treated mosquito nets. A multitude of NGO projects are distributing ITNs to contribute to this initiative: Project Mosquito Net in Kenya (www.projectmosquitonet.org), Nothing But Nets (www.nothingbutnets.net/), Global Giving for Africa (www.globalgiving.org/projects/mosquito-nets-for-africa-families), Angola Mosquito Net Project (https://angolamosquitonetproject.wordpress.com/) and Holy Innocents Children's Hospital Uganda (www.holyinnocentsuganda.org) are examples of organizations actively engaged in preventing malaria and saving lives.

However, coverage levels are inadequate in endemic countries, especially in poor communities. Without adequate and predictable funding, the progress against malaria is also threatened by emerging parasite resistance to artemisinin, the core component of artemisinin-based combination therapies (ACTs), and mosquito resistance to insecticides. Artemisinin resistance has been detected in four countries in Southeast Asia, and insecticide resistance has been found in at least 64 countries.

Although chemotherapeutic agents can be used for both protection and treatment of the disease, they are expensive and often cause side effects. However, evidence suggests that the *Plasmodium* sporozoites are becoming resistant to both treatment and preventive chemotherapeutic agents, especially chloroquine and its derivatives. Alternative therapies and/or combinations of medications such as sulfadoxine/pyrimethamine (Fansidar), amodiaquine, artemisinin, artemether, and atovaquone/proguanil (Malarone) are somewhat effective in treating malaria. Recent reports indicate that drug manufacturers in these endemic countries are diluting the drugs so that clients, especially children, are not receiving therapeutic levels of the medications. Many children suffer the effects of partially treated malaria, and once hospitalized, IV quinine is the drug of choice. Unfortunately, quinine has significant neurotoxic and cardiovascular side effects that need monitoring (CDC, 2013a). Efforts are underway to develop an antimalarial vaccine and one candidate vaccine, known as RTS,S/AS01, has been shown to almost halve the number of malaria cases in young children (aged 5 to 17 months at first vaccination) and to reduce by about one fourth the malaria cases in infants (aged 6 to 12 weeks at first vaccination) (Malaria Vaccine Initiative, 2013). As discussed in Chapter 13, persons who live or travel to *Anopheles*-infested areas should protect themselves with mosquito netting, clothing that protects vulnerable parts of the body, repellents for both their bodies and their clothes, and antimalarial medications such as Malarone or doxycycline.

## Diarrheal Disease

The normal intestinal tract regulates the absorption and secretion of electrolytes and water to meet the body's physiological needs. More than 98% of the 10 L of fluid per day entering the adult intestines is reabsorbed (Ahs et al, 2010; Alexander and Blackburn, 2013). The remaining stool water, related primarily to the indigestible fiber content, determines the consistency of normal feces from dry, hard pellets to mushy, bulky stools, varying from person to person, day to day, and stool to stool. This variation complicates the definition of *diarrhea.* For adults diarrhea is present when three or more liquid stools are passed in 24 hours. The frequent passage of formed stool is not diarrhea. Although young nursing infants tend to have five or more bowel movements per day, stools that are liquid without any formation and/or are more than what is normal for the child constitute diarrhea (Ahs et al, 2010; Farthing et al, 2012). Definitions are complicated by the observable presence of blood, mucus, or parasites and the age of the affected person.

Diarrhea, one of the leading causes of illness and death in children less than 5 years of age throughout the world, is most prominent in the less developed countries despite recent initiatives by the WHO to correct this problem. Each year there are 760,000 diarrhea deaths in children under five; there are 1.7 billion cases of diarrheal disease every year related to unsafe water, sanitation, and hygiene; and it is the leading cause of malnutrition in children under five (WHO, Diarrhea Fact Sheet, 2013f). Causes of diarrhea are just as varied and diverse as its definitions and perceptions. Some of the causes include (1) viruses such as the rotavirus and Norwalk-like agents, (2) bacteria, including *Campylobacter jejuni, Clostridium difficile, Escherichia coli, Salmonella,* and *Shigella,* (3) environmental toxins, (4) parasites such as *Giardia lamblia* and *Cryptosporidium,* and (5) worms. Nutritional deficiencies can also cause diarrhea and are most often a result of infectious agents. Of these, the rotavirus has emerged as a major world concern, hospitalizing 55,000 American children and killing 1 million children in the world each year (Farthing et al, 2012; WHO, Diarrhea Fact Sheet, 2013f). Three major diarrhea syndromes exist:

- Acute watery diarrhea, which results in varying degrees of dehydration and fluid losses that quickly exceed total plasma and interstitial fluid volumes and is incompatible with life unless fluid therapy can keep up with losses. Such dramatic dehydration is usually due to rotavirus, enterotoxigenic *E. coli,* or *Vibrio cholerae* (the cause of cholera), and it is most dangerous in the very young.
- Persistent diarrhea, which lasts 14 days or longer, and is manifested by malabsorption, nutrient losses, and wasting; it is typically associated with malnutrition, either preceding or resulting from the illness itself. Even though persistent diarrhea accounts for a small percentage of the total number of diarrhea episodes, it is associated with a disproportionately increased risk of death.
- Bloody diarrhea, which is a sign of the intestinal damage caused by inflammation. Bloody diarrhea, defined as diarrhea with visible or microscopic blood in the stool, is associated with intestinal damage and nutritional deterioration, often with secondary sepsis. Mild dehydration and fever may be present. Bloody diarrhea should not be confused with dysentery, because dysentery is a syndrome consisting of the frequent passage of characteristic, small-volume, bloody mucoid stools, abdominal cramps, and tenesmus (a severe pain that accompanies straining to pass stool). Agents that cause bloody diarrhea or dysentery can also provoke a form of diarrhea that clinically is not bloody diarrhea, although mucosal damage and inflammation are present microscopically. The release of host-derived cytokines alters host metabolism and leads to the breakdown of body stores of protein, carbohydrate, and fat and the loss of nitrogen and other nutrients. Those losses must be replenished during the expected prolonged convalescence. For these reasons, bloody diarrhea calls for management strategies that are markedly different than those for watery or persistent diarrhea. New bouts of infection that occur before complete restoration of nutrient stores can initiate a downward spiral of nutritional status terminating in fatal protein-energy malnutrition (Farthing et al, 2012).

Diarrheal diseases are rampant among the impoverished. Poverty is associated with poor housing, crowding, dirt floors, lack of access to sufficient clean water or to sanitary disposal of fecal waste, cohabitation with domestic animals and zoonotic transmission of pathogens, and a lack of refrigerated storage for food. Unfortunately, even when the cause of the diarrhea is eliminated, poverty can restrict the ability to provide age-appropriate, nutritionally balanced diets or to modify diets so as to mitigate and repair nutrient losses. The lack of adequate, available and affordable medical care increases the problem. Children suffer from an apparently never-ending sequence of infections and rarely receive appropriate preventive care, and too often their parents seek health care only when the children have become severely ill.

Dehydration is an immediate result of diarrhea and leads to a loss of fluid and electrolytes. The loss of up to 10% of the body's electrolytes can lead to shock, acidosis, stupor, and failure of the body's major organs (e.g., kidneys, heart). Persistent diarrhea often leads to loss of body protein, an increased time-limited inability to digest and absorb dairy products, and increased susceptibility to infection. Every country should have as a major aim the prevention and control of diarrheal disease, especially in infants and children. Many countries have developed diarrhea control programs that improve childhood nutrition. These programs instruct in breastfeeding and weaning practices and promote oral rehydration therapy and the use of supplementary feeding programs (Farthing et al, 2012). However, all these programs must be considered in conjunction with improving the social and economic conditions that contribute to safe environmental, sanitary, and general living conditions of populations around the world. The following How To box provides useful resources for keeping well informed about public health issues including water quality.

---

**HOW TO** Stay Current about Global Health

*One way to stay current with the world's health problems and advances is by reading the newspaper daily. Examples of newspapers that cover international health on an ongoing basis include the* Wall Street Journal, USA Today, *the* Washington Post, *and the* New York Times. *The following websites are examples of sources that pertain to international or global health:*

- *U.S. Department of Health and Human Services: http://www.globalhealth.gov/*
- *Global Health Council: http://www.globalhealth.org/*
- *Centers for Disease Control and Prevention: http://www.cdc.gov/globalhealth/*
- *World Health Organization: http://www.who.int/en/*
- *Pan American Health Organization: http://new.paho.org/*
- *World Bank: http://www.worldbank.org/*
- *Institute of Medicine: http://www.iom.edu/*
- *Millennium Development Goals: http://www.undp.org/mdg/*

---

## Maternal and Women's Health

Maternal health is central to the health of women, as well as the well-being of their children and families, and the economic productivity of their countries. A woman's ability to survive pregnancy and childbirth is closely related to how effectively societies invest in and realize the potential of women not only as mothers, but as critical contributors to sustaining families and transforming nations. When investments in women—as mothers, as individuals, as family members, and as citizens—lag, the economic cost of maternal death and illness is enormous. Ostrowski (2010) stated that when women have better education and health, then mothers have greater household decision-making power and their children are better educated, becoming productive adults able to help build long-term economic growth. The World Bank found that during economic crises, poor families who sent women to work were better able to make ends meet.

Progress and investment in maternal health have lagged far behind estimates of what is needed to achieve MDG 5, Improve Maternal Health. Progress in the last 20 years on key maternal health indicators varies by outcome and region, but it has been uneven, inequitable, and inadequate overall. The two regions of the world with the worst maternal health status—South Asia and sub-Saharan Africa—show minimal signs of improvement largely because of poverty, disempowerment of women, and overall poor health status of women in developing countries. Women's reproductive health, especially their ability to control their fertility and avoid HIV infection, is also closely associated with their health as mothers. Although maternal death and disability represent a high burden of disease in the developing world, interventions to improve maternal health are available and cost-effective (Kaiser Family Foundation, 2013c; Kott, 2011; WHO, Family Planning Fact Sheet, 2013g).

In Uganda, Reproductive Health Uganda (RHU), formerly the Family Planning Association of Uganda (FPAU), provides services in 29 of the country's districts, targeting young people and marginalized groups to improve reproductive health. They offer family planning; HIV/AIDS testing and counseling; diagnosis and treatment of sexually transmitted infections (STIs); advocacy against female genital mutilation (FGM); and post-abortion care to high-risk constituencies such as internally displaced persons (IDPs), people at high risk of HIV/AIDS, young women in conflict-affected areas, sex workers, hawkers, saloonists, bicycle taxi drivers, maids—any group subject to violence and disempowerment (www.rhu.or.ug). Despite FPAU's intent to improve the reproductive health of Ugandan women, there are barriers to the success of this initiative: continued cultural practices related to submissiveness of women and dependency on men for well-being of self and the children; bride wealth practices that give ownership to the man and permit beatings and other abuses of his wife; kinship patterns in which widowed women belong to the oldest brother; the fact that child care and all work related to the home and the children are performed by the women and girls; the fact that a woman's worth is still dependent on her ability to reproduce, even knowing that the more pregnancies a woman incurs, the less healthy the newborn and mother; and the practice of polygamy, allowing for transmission of STIs and HIV/AIDS.

The WHO and UNICEF have continued their worldwide initiatives to reform the health care received by women and children in less developed countries (WHO, Maternal Health Fact Sheet, 2013h). However, studies on women's health indicate that more than one third (35%) of all maternal deaths around the world are due to severe bleeding, primarily postpartum hemorrhage; sepsis (8%); unsafe abortion (9%); hypertension (18%); and conditions that complicate pregnancy such as malaria, anemia, and HIV (20%). In developing nations there is a significant incidence of lack of prenatal care during pregnancy and high fertility rates, often due to a lack of access to contraception and other family planning and reproductive

health services, as well as cultural belief systems that increase the lifetime risk of maternal death.

Every year, more than half a million women die in pregnancy and childbirth around the world. This figure has altered little in the last 30 years. In sub-Saharan Africa, a number of countries have halved their levels of maternal mortality since 1990 but not in the more impoverished nations such as the Congo, Uganda, Ghana, and others. However, between 1990 and 2010, the global maternal mortality ratio declined by only 3.1% per year. This is far from the annual decline of 5.5% required to achieve MDG 5 (WHO, Maternal Mortality Fact Sheet, 2012e).

Equally distressing is the fact that worldwide, the ratio of maternal deaths to live births (the maternal mortality ratio) has remained essentially static during this period. Africa continues to have the highest maternal-child morbidity and mortality rate, with 51% of all maternal deaths occurring in sub-Saharan Africa. The maternal mortality ratio in developing countries is 240 per 100,000 births versus 16 per 100,000 in developed countries. The risk of maternal mortality is highest for adolescent girls under 15 years old. HIV currently accounts for 6.2% of maternal deaths in Africa and has reversed the progress made in maternal health in some countries.

In sub-Saharan Africa, infectious diseases, childhood illnesses, and maternal causes of death account for as much as 70% of the burden of disease. By comparison, these conditions account for only one third of the burden in South Asia and Oceania, and less than 20% in all other regions. In addition, whereas the average age of death throughout Latin America, Asia, and North Africa increased by more than 25 years between 1970 and 2010, it rose by less than 10 years in most of sub-Saharan Africa (WHO, Global Burden of Disease Report, 2012b). The WHO found that some of the sociocultural factors that prevent women and girls from benefiting from quality health services and attaining the best possible level of health include the following (WHO, Women's Health Fact Sheet, 2013h):

- Unequal power relationships between men and women
- Social norms that decrease education and paid employment opportunities
- An exclusive focus on women's reproductive roles
- Potential or actual experience of physical, sexual and emotional violence

Within Africa, the greatest disease burden remains from maternal health, child health, HIV, TB, and malaria; outside Africa the greatest disease burden is the rising incidence of noncommunicable diseases and rising life expectancy (Summers, 2013). Throughout the world, women between 15 and 44 years of age account for approximately one third of the world's disease burden, and women between 45 and 59 for one fifth of the burden. This burden comprises diseases and conditions that are either exclusively or predominantly found in women, including maternal mortality and morbidity, cervical cancer, anemia, STIs, osteoarthritis, and breast cancer, with HIV/AIDS leading the statistics (Mathers, 2009).

Although most of these conditions can be dealt with by cost-effective prevention and screening programs, many less

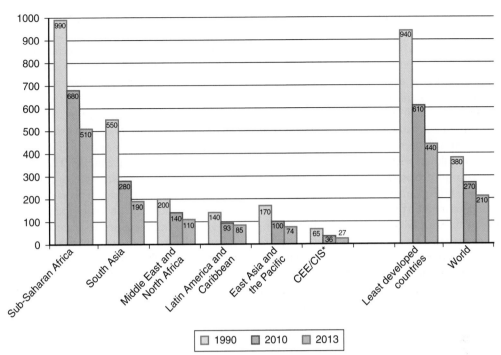

Lifetime Risk of Maternal Deaths in Sub-Saharan Africa versus Industrialized Nations. (From ChildInfo: Monitoring the situation of children and women. Available at http://www.childinfo.org/ maternal_mortality.html. Accessed March 20, 2014)

developed countries have ignored women's health issues other than those directly related to pregnancy and childbirth for two major reasons: (1) women are not seen as valued members of society, and (2) most of the afflicted women are poor, malnourished, and cannot pay for health care services.

Sub-Saharan Africa accounts for the majority of the world's births. Although all countries profess to offer prenatal services and safe birthing services, most are unavailable, inaccessible, and unaffordable by women (WHO, Maternal Health Fact Sheet, 2013h). An African woman's risk of dying from pregnancy-related causes is 1 in 20, followed by Bangladesh, Pakistan, and India. These three countries account for nearly half of the world's maternal deaths, but only 29% of the world's births; they have more maternal deaths each week than Europe has in a year. Still, an accurate reporting of maternal deaths is difficult to obtain because many of the women who die are poor and live in remote areas, and their deaths are considered by many to be unimportant (Mathers, 2009) (See table above).

Risk factors for maternal mortality include poor nutritional status, disease conditions, high parity, and age less than 20 years and greater than 35 years. To date, little attention has been paid to the problem of maternal mortality, even though the reported incidences are high throughout the world. The WHO and the UN are addressing this problem by calling for government initiatives and actions to address maternal morbidity and mortality from obstetrical deaths as well as those that arise from indirect causes. MDG 5 aims to reduce the maternal mortality ratio by three quarters, improve the proportion of births attended by skilled health personnel, promote universal access to reproductive health, improve contraceptive rates, decrease adolescent birth rates, provide antenatal care coverage, and

address the unmet need for family planning by 2015 (WHO, 2012c). In some countries it is difficult to counsel women on family planning and spacing their children so as to promote maternal and fetal health when a woman's value depends on her ability to reproduce and more than 50% of children die before they reach adolescence.

The result of poor maternal health accounts for the increase in premature births and the increased risk for high morbidity rates in children less than 5 years because of their own compromised nutritional and immune state. Low birth weight is a major risk factor for premature births, which account for more than one quarter (29%) of newborn deaths, followed by asphyxia (22%), sepsis (15%), pneumonia (10%), congenital abnormalities (7%), diarrhea (2%), and tetanus (2%). Undernutrition and lack of access to clean water and sanitation significantly increase children's vulnerability to death. Newborn deaths account for most child deaths (41%), followed by diarrhea (14%), pneumonia (14%), malaria (8%), injuries (3%), HIV/AIDS (2%), and other infectious or noncommunicable diseases (18%, including measles [1%]) (Kaiser Family Foundation, Global Health Policy, 2013b). In 2012 approximately 6.6 million children died before the age of 5 which is nearly one half the number that died in 1990 but still much too high a number of deaths (World Bank, 2013b).

Even though programs in many countries have been initiated, safe motherhood initiatives are still needed throughout the world. These programs and initiatives need to include providing accessible family planning services and prenatal and postnatal health care services, ensuring access to safe abortion procedures, and improving the nutritional status of all women.

## Nutrition and World Health

Many children around the world are underweight and have multiple micronutrient deficiencies such as for iron, zinc, and vitamin A. Poor nutrition by itself or that associated with infectious disease accounts for a large portion of the world's disease burden (Mathers, 2009; WHO, 2013d). Improved nutrition is related to stronger immune systems, decreased illness, better maternal and child health, longer life spans, and improved learning outcomes for children. Healthy protein balances are able to support major physiological stress with improved healing and ability to utilize protein-binding drugs; better nutrition is a prime entry point to ending poverty and a milestone to achieving better quality of life. Environmental and economic conditions related to poverty contribute to underconsumption of nutrients, especially those nutrients needed for protein building such as iodine, vitamin A, and iron. Worldwide, women and children suffer disproportionately from nutrition deficits, especially the micronutrients just mentioned (Mathers, 2009).

Children in Haiti die daily from hunger; more than 60% of the population is undernourished and children under the age of 5 suffer an even higher percentage. more than 800 million people (or one out of every five people in developing nations) are undernourished; and every few seconds, about every time one takes a breath, a child in the developing world dies of hunger and related diseases (Global Nutrition Alliance, 2010). Poor nutrition also leads to stunting, or low height and weight for a given age. Stunting often results from eating foods that do not provide adequate energy or protein. Because protein foods are usually more expensive than nonprotein food sources, many households reduce, or unconsciously eliminate, protein-rich foods to save money (Hunter, unpublished research, 2012). I have cared for and watched many children with marasmus (total caloric deprivation) and Kwashiorkor (protein deficiency starvation) die who could have been saved if affordable protein and nutritious food were available. Usually this condition begins because an infant has been weaned away from breastfeeding after a year to make room for the next baby, and the food used in its place is mainly sugar and water or a starchy gruel. Kwashiorkor symptoms are apathy, muscular wasting, edema, and pigmentation loss in the skin and hair. Marasmus is a wasting away of the body tissues and symptoms are like kwashiorkor with fretfulness and an appearance of "skin and bones."

Iron deficiencies are also common in less developed countries and severely affect women and children. When iron is low, fewer red blood cells are produced, and this reduces the capacity of the blood to transport oxygen. As a result, symptoms ranging from fatigue and inability to concentrate to impaired physical and cognitive development of children can occur. Iron deficiency anemia may also cause problems during pregnancy, particularly in developing countries where it can increase the risk of premature delivery, as well as the risk of maternal and fetal complications and death. Inadequate iron from food is the most common reason for iron deficiency anemia, especially among infants and children. Parasites, infections, stomach and digestive diseases, and blood loss during menstruation may also worsen anemia. A deficiency of iron in the diet can reduce appetite, physical productivity, the ability to learn, and growth.

The American Society of Hematology (2013) reported that while the global prevalence of anemia decreased between 1990 and 2010 (from 40.2% to 32.9%), the disease has demonstrated an increase in global YLDs from 65.5 million to 68.4 million. The DALY burdens associated with major depression (63.2 million YLDs), chronic respiratory diseases (49.3 million YLDs), and general injuries (47.2 million YLDs) are less than the DALY burden of anemia. This is due to the increased incidence of anemia in children <5 years. This age group accounted for more cases of anemia than any other age group and had the highest severity of disease in low- and middle-income regions. Unfortunately the data also demonstrated a widening gender gap in anemia burden over time with female prevalence rates remaining higher in most regions and age groups.

Other common dietary deficiencies include zinc, iodine, vitamin A, folic acid, and calcium. Zinc is important because it is an essential part of many enzymes and plays an important role in protein synthesis and cell division. The health consequences of zinc deficiency include poor immune system function, growth retardation, and delayed sexual maturity in children. Zinc deficiency is caused by low intake and/or low absorption of bioavailable zinc. Diets low in meat and fish increase the risk of zinc deficiency, because zinc is poorly bioavailable in cereals. Vitamin A is another essential nutrient in the human diet, contributing to the functioning of the retina, the growth of bone, and the immune response. Apart from preventable, irreversible blindness, vitamin A deficiency also causes reduced immune function, leading to an increased risk of severe infectious disease and anemia. It also increases the risk of death during pregnancy for both the mother and fetus and after birth for the newborn. An estimated 250 million preschool children in developing countries are affected by vitamin A deficiency, although severe deficiency that causes blindness is declining (Kaiser Family Foundation, 2013c; WHO, Global Prevalence of Vitamin A Deficiency, 2013i).

The impact of malnutrition and dietary deficiencies is significant. Any malnourished condition in a population can increase susceptibility to illness. For example, the principal causes of death among malnourished persons are measles, diarrheal and respiratory disease, TB, pertussis, and malaria. The loss of life from these diseases can be measured as 231 DALYs worldwide, with one fourth of the 231 being directly attributable to malnourishment and dietary deficiencies. Individual governments and organizations such as the International Red Cross, WHO, and many international religious and private foundations have been active in promoting better nutrition. Worldwide initiatives directed at overcoming nutritional deficits include the following (Global Nutrition Alliance, 2010): control of infectious diseases, nutritional education, control of intestinal parasites, micronutrient fortification of food, food supplementation, and food price subsidies.

Médecins sans Frontières (Doctors without Borders) was the first to use the life-saving supplement, invented in 2003 by a French scientist, called Plumpy'nut. Plumpy'nut requires no water preparation or refrigeration and has a 2-year shelf life, making it easy to deploy in difficult conditions to treat severe acute malnutrition. It is distributed under medical supervision, to humanitarian organizations for food aid distribution. The ingredients include peanut paste; vegetable oil; powered milk; powdered sugar; vitamins A, B-complex, C, D, E, and K; and minerals including calcium, phosphorus, potassium, magnesium, zinc, copper, iron, iodine, sodium, and selenium. These are combined in a foil pouch and each 92-g pack provides 500 kilocalories (kcal) or 2.1 megajoules (MJ).

## Natural and Man-Made Disasters

As discussed in Chapter 23, earthquakes, floods, drought, and other natural hazards continue to cause tens of thousands of deaths, hundreds of thousands of injuries, and billions of dollars in economic losses each year around the world. Disasters represent a major source of risk for the poor and wipe out development gains and accumulated wealth in developing countries. In 2012, only 357 natural triggered disasters were registered; a decrease from 394 observed in the years past. However, natural disasters still killed a significant number, even though there was a decline in deaths. Contrary to other indicators, economic damages from natural disasters did show an increase to above average levels (143 billion 2012 US$), with estimates placing the figure at US$ 157 billion. Over the last decade, China, the United States, the Philippines, India, and Indonesia together constitute the top five countries that are most frequently hit by natural disasters. In 2012, China had its fourth highest number of natural disasters over the last decade with 13 floods and landslides, 8 storms, 7 earthquakes, and 1 period of extreme temperature. The single deadliest disaster in 2012 was Typhoon Bopha, which killed 1901 people in the Philippines (Center for Research on the Epidemiology of Disaster, 2013).

Natural disasters such as earthquakes, tsunamis, and floods can often come at the least expected time. Others, such as hurricanes and cyclones, are increasing in severity and destruction. Droughts are increasing as the threat of global warming rises. Typically, the poor are the worst hit, for they have the least resources to cope and rebuild. Hurricane Katrina resulted in a 90,000 square mile disaster zone, equivalent to the area of Great Britain, and more than 1800 died. The Indonesian tsunami of 2005 killed at least 230,000 people, and the livelihoods of millions were destroyed in more than 10 countries affected by the tsunami. The earthquake in Haiti in 2010 destroyed a country and crushed the hopes of thousands of Haitians. Human activity is contributing to massive extinctions, from various animal species, to forests, and the ecosystems that support marine life. The costs associated with deteriorating or vanishing ecosystems are high. The World Resources Institute reports that there is a link between biodiversity and climate change, and rapid global warming can affect an ecosystem's chance to adapt naturally (World Resources Institute, 2012). The four worst types of natural disasters are as follows:

- *Earthquakes and tsunamis:* Examples are January 12, 2010—more than 230,000 people were killed when a 7.0-magnitude earthquake struck Haiti; May 12, 2008—about 70,000 people

were killed and 18,000 people were reported missing after a 7.9-magnitude earthquake struck Sichuan, China; October 8, 2005—at least 80,000 people were killed and 3 million left homeless after a quake struck the mountainous Kashmir district in Pakistan.
- *Volcanic eruptions:* Examples are July 15, 1991 when Mount Pinatubo on Luzon Island in the Philippines erupted, blanketing 750 square kilometers with volcanic ash and more than 800 died; November 13-14, 1985 when at least 25,000 were killed near Armero, Colombia, when the Nevado del Ruiz volcano erupted, triggering mudslides.
- *Hurricanes, cyclones, and floods:* Examples are July-August 2010, when monsoon rains hit northwest Pakistan and more than one fifth of the country was under water, more than 1700 people were killed, and 17.2 million people were victims; May 3, 2008, when Cyclone Nargis, with winds that exceeded 190 km/hour and waves six meters high, struck Myanmar, leaving as many as 100,000 dead, according to U.S. estimates; October 26-November 4, 1998, when Hurricane Mitch killed 11,000 in Honduras and Nicaragua and left 2.5 million homeless.
- *Pandemics and famines:* 1900-present, malaria has been the leading cause of death in the developing world, causing severe illness in 500 million people each year and killing more than 1 million annually; 1984-1985, the Ethiopian famine that killed at least 1 million in Ethiopia; and 1980-present, the toll from AIDS worldwide is estimated at 25 million, with 40 million others infected with HIV (http://www.cbc.ca/news/world/the-world-s-worst-natural-disasters-1.743208).

When poor countries face natural disasters, such as hurricanes, floods, earthquakes, and fires, the cost of rebuilding becomes even more of an issue when they are already burdened with debt. Often, poor countries suffer with many lost lives and/or livelihoods. Aid and disaster relief often do come in from international relief organizations, rich countries, and international institutions, but poor countries often pay millions of dollars a week back in the form of debt repayment.

The aftermath of a natural disaster may be as devastating as the disaster itself. Inadequate shelter, unclean water, and lack of security are some of the most commonly reported problems, even a year after the event. The physical force of a disaster not only causes immediate injury and death, but each type of disaster can result in its own combination of physical injuries. In earthquakes, buildings and the objects inside them can fall, injuring those who live or work there. Floods can result in drowning, and wildfires can cause burns and illness from smoke inhalation.

In addition to the direct injury and death caused by the disaster's force, there can be other serious adverse effects on the well-being of those living in the area. The large numbers of people who are suddenly ill or injured can exceed the capacity of the local health care system to care for them. In addition to the burden of increased numbers of clients, the system itself can become a victim of the disaster. Hospitals may be damaged, roads blocked, and personnel unable to perform their duties. The loss of these resources occurs at a time when they are most critically needed. The disaster can also hamper the ability to provide routine, nonemergency health services. Many people may be unable to obtain care and medications for their ongoing health problems. The disruption of these routine services can result in an increase in illness and death in segments of the population that might not have been directly affected by the disaster. The most serious consequences of natural disasters are related to mass population displacements, unsanitary conditions, lack of clean water, lack of nutritious foods, lack of safe housing, and the increased risk of diseases prevalent in crowded and unsanitary living conditions: typhoid fever, cholera, dysentery, TB, and infectious respiratory conditions (Petrucci, 2012).

Man-made disasters may include bioterrorism, chemical agents, pandemics and epidemics, radiation, and terrorism. The five worst man-made disasters in recent history are as follows:

- *Bhopal Gas Tragedy, India* in 1984 where more than 500,000 people were exposed to methyl isocyanine gas and other chemicals. Thousands of people died within the first hours of the leak, but over time estimates of 5000 to 16,000 deaths from the leak have been made.
- *Deepwater Horizon Oil Spill, Gulf of Mexico* in 2010 that killed 11; leaked anywhere from 40,000 to 162,000 barrels of oil a day; took 47,829 people 89 days to finally cap the well; and 3500 workers and volunteers on the clean-up site are suffering liver and kidney damage from their exposure to the 1.8 million gallons of toxic oil.
- *Chernobyl Meltdown, Ukraine* in 1986. Thirty-one volunteers died trying to shut the reactor down and nearly 4000 deaths so far have been thought to be attributable to the radiation poisoning people living near Chernobyl underwent. To this day, no one is sure what the final death toll from the Chernobyl meltdown will be.
- *Fukushima Meltdown, Japan* in 2011 with more than 100,000 people evacuated and displaced from the surrounding areas; 600 people dying during the evacuation; 300 cleanup workers receiving excessive exposure to radioactive waste; and the resulting unknown long-term health effects that could include people as far away from the meltdown as North America.
- *Global Warming* that impacts rising sea levels, desertification, animal extinction, and damage from intense superstorms such as Hurricane Katrina, Hurricane Sandy, and Typhoon Haiyan in the Philippines has already created some of the first groups of climate-change refugees, and some estimate that number will rise to 150 million by 2050 (http://www.policymic.com/articles/23620/5-worst-man-made-disasters-in-history).

Other man-made disasters are the bioterrorism attack and the deliberate release of viruses, bacteria, or other germs (agents) used to cause illness or death of people, animals, or plants, which may lead to pandemics and epidemics (anthrax, cholera, Ebola virus, Lassa fever, plague, and smallpox, to name a few). A pandemic is an epidemic of infectious diseases that spread through human populations across a large region such as a continent or the globe (e.g., HIV/AIDS, smallpox, TB, H1N1, SARS); whereas an epidemic is when new cases of a certain disease in a given human population exceed what is expected (cancer, heart disease, seasonal flu).

These agents are typically found in nature, but it is possible that they could be changed to increase their ability to cause disease, to make them resistant to current medicines, or to increase their ability to be spread into the environment in order to threaten a government or intimidate or coerce a civilian population (CDC, Bioterrorism, 2013b; Infectious disease: Global Challenges. Bioterrorism, 2013). Bioterrorism is a significant public health threat that could produce widespread, devastating, and tragic consequences, and it would impose particularly heavy demands on international public health and health care systems. Nurses and other health personnel need to be aware and vigilant to the health consequences of terrorism and the potential use of biological agents to instill fear and to spread disease.

A nation's capacity to respond to the threat of bioterrorism depends in part on the ability of health care professionals and public health officials to rapidly and effectively detect, diagnose, respond, and communicate during a bioterrorism event. The national health care community—including public health agencies, emergency medical services, hospitals, and health care providers—would bear the brunt of the consequences of a biological attack. Attacks with biological agents are likely to be covert, rather than overt (CDC, 2013b). Terrorists may prefer to use biological agents because they are difficult to detect; they do not cause illness for several hours to several days.

A chemical emergency occurs when a hazardous chemical has been released and the release has the potential to harm people's health. Chemical releases can be unintentional, as in the case of an industrial accident, or intentional, as in the case of a terrorist attack. Sarin and ricin are the two most recent notorious chemicals used; however, mustard gas, cyanide, and tear gas have existed for decades. Agent Orange was used by the American troops in Vietnam, and mustard gas was commonly used during World War I and even during the Gulf War (http://www.policymic.com/articles/62023/10-chemical-weapons-attacks-washington-doesn-t-want-you-to-talk-about; http://science.howstuffworks.com/mustard-gas4.htm).

Radiation poisoning occurs when an excess amount of radiation is released to harm people's health. These may be unintentional and intentional events. Intentional terrorist events are those designed to contaminate food and water with radioactive material; spread radioactive material into the environment by using conventional explosives (e.g., dynamite), called a dirty bomb, or by using wind currents or natural traffic patterns; bomb or destroy a nuclear reactor; cause a truck or train carrying nuclear material to spill its load; or explode a nuclear weapon.

The word genocide was developed by a jurist named Raphael Lemkin in 1944. By combining the Greek word *genos* (race) with the Latin word *cide* (killing), genocide was defined by the United Nations in 1948 to mean any of the following acts committed with intent to destroy, in whole or in part, a national, ethnic, racial, or religious group, including (1) killing members of the group, (2) causing serious bodily or mental harm to members of the group, (3) deliberately inflicting on the group conditions of life calculated to bring about its physical destruction in whole or in part, (4) imposing measures intended to prevent births within the group, and (5) forcibly transferring children of the group to another group (Genocide Watch, International Alliance to End Genocide, 2013; http://www.genocidewatch.org/). The most notable genocides were the *Al-Anfal genocide* of the Kurds in Iraq, with more than 280,000 killed and many thousands unaccounted for; the *Rwandan genocide*, where the Hutus slaughtered hundreds of thousands (possibly 1 million) of their Tutsi relatives; the *Irish potato famine*, where more than a million Irish died because of lack of intervention by the British to feed the starving populace; the Native American genocide, with the loss of more than 1 million indigenous people to intentional infections with smallpox, war, and starvation; the *Bosnian genocide* and the annihilation of the Bosnian Muslims and Serbs to ethnically cleanse the country; and the most notable, the *Holocaust*, in which more than 6 million Jews and other ethnically disenfranchised populations were lost (http://listverse.com/2013/05/03/10-atrocious-genocides-in-human-history/). Genocide continues today in Syria, Darfur, and the Central African Republic.

Following genocide, there are biopsychological changes such as physical stress reactions (cardiovascular, neurological) and mental stress responses, especially post-traumatic stress disorders and depression. Many people flee and become refugees or internationally displaced people. These refugees flee to neighboring countries, placing social, political, and economic burdens on these countries. I have been to the refugee camps in Uganda for refugees from Rwanda, the Congo, Kenya, and even northern Uganda, whose people have been victims of the Liberation Rebel Army (LRA) as political turmoil continues to plague the civilians in East Africa. The victims of genocide often face discrimination in refugee camps or in their new country of permanent residence if they do not return home. Individuals who return to their home countries are often plagued with uncertainty regarding lost property and other belongings.

The biological and psychosocial effects of genocide are not exclusive to the child and adult victims, but affect the perpetrators as well. Marginalization and dehumanization place a mental toll on the victims that often results in negative cognitive, behavioral, affective, relational, and spiritual effects. Many perpetrators are forced into committing these acts, and achieving desensitization is necessary for a nonviolent person to kill or to commit violent acts. This is evident in the boy soldiers of the LRA (some as young as 6 years old) who are forced to kill or be killed and become desensitized through the use of alcohol, drugs, and repeated exposure to death (Vollhardt and Bilewicz, 2013).

After genocidal conflicts have ceased, restoration of a country's infrastructure, as well as reconciliation, must begin. The ramifications of genocide are widespread, and community leaders must find the most effective ways of initiating the healing process. The United Nations has tried to develop strategies to prevent genocide from occurring and is encouraging initiatives that include appropriate comprehensive cultural competence in the delivery of services; supporting and organizing treatment and care that is fair and just to all members of specific societies, regardless of age, gender, race, cultural beliefs, religion, sexual orientation, affiliation, and civil status;

encouraging international organizations to make mental and behavioral health a priority in conflict assistance throughout the various stages of genocide; and encouraging its member organizations to emphasize the importance of social work in regard to genocide in their respective countries (Vollhardt and Bilewicz, 2013).

## Surveillance Systems

Surveillance systems, discussed in Chapter 24, are used to track potential risks for intentional harm to the people of the world. There are systems in place to assess the risks for man-made and natural disasters to prevent the atrocities to mankind discussed previously. These systems may be on-the-ground specialists who acquire information about the political stability of nations, or they may be satellite systems that track weather, volcanic, and earthquake activities.

How would a government find out that a deliberate outbreak had taken place? For the international system, the WHO monitors disease outbreaks through the Global Outbreak Alert and Response Network (Center for Research on the Epidemiology of Disaster, 2012; WHO, 2014g). This network, formally launched in April 2000, electronically links the expertise and skills of 72 existing networks from around the world, several of which were uniquely designed to diagnose unusual agents and handle dangerous pathogens. Its purpose is to keep the international community constantly alert to the threat of outbreaks and ready to respond. It has four primary tasks:

1. *Systematic disease intelligence and detection:* The first responsibility of the WHO network is to systematically gather global disease intelligence, drawing from a wide range of resources, both formal and informal. Ministries of Health, WHO country offices, government and military centers, and academic institutions all file regular formal reports with the Global Outbreak Alert and Response Network. An informal network scours world communications for rumors of unusual health events.

2. *Outbreak verification:* Preliminary intelligence reports from all sources, both formal and informal, are reviewed and converted into meaningful intelligence by the WHO Outbreak Alert and Response Team, which makes the final determination on whether a reported event warrants cause for international concern.

3. *Immediate alert:* A large network of electronically connected WHO member nations, disease experts, health institutions, agencies, and laboratories is kept continually informed of rumored and confirmed outbreaks. The network also maintains and regularly updates an Outbreak Verification List, which provides a detailed status report on all currently verified outbreaks.

4. *Rapid response:* When the Outbreak Alert and Response Team determines that an international response is needed to contain an outbreak, it enlists the help of its partners in the global network. Specific assistance available includes targeted investigations, confirmation of diagnoses, handling of dangerous biohazards (biosafety level IV pathogens), client care management, containment, and logistical support in terms of staff and supplies.

In summary, if health care professionals and emergency responders are to be prepared to manage natural or manmade disasters, it is critical that there be cooperative efforts at the international, national, state, and local levels (Box 4-5). Such disaster response is not the domain of any one specialty; nurses, doctors, mental health experts, first responders, EMTs, volunteers, engineers, and many more need to be part of the team that helps people overcome the physical, emotional, social, and economic devastation. Nurses need to have political, historical, social, medical, nursing, and public health knowledge in order to be more effective in finding the resources their clients need to recover successfully.

---

### BOX 4-5   What Can Nursing Do in the Event of a Disaster?

The International Council of Nursing (ICN, 2009) policy paper on disaster preparedness outlines actions, including risk assessment and multidisciplinary management strategies, as critical to the delivery of effective responses to the short-, medium-, and long-term health needs of a disaster-stricken population. These actions include the following:

**Help People to Cope with Aftermath of Terrorism**
- Assist people to deal with feelings of fear, vulnerability, and grief.
- Use groups that have survived terrorist attacks as useful resources for victims.

**Allay Public Concerns and Fear of Bioterrorism**
- Disseminate accurate information on the risks involved, preventive measures, use of antibiotics and/or vaccines, and reporting suspicious letters or packages to the police or other authorities.
- Address hoax messages, false alarms, and threats; any perceived threat to the public health must be investigated.

**Identify the Feelings That You and Others May be Experiencing**
- In the aftermath of terror, even health care professionals can feel bias, hatred, vengeance, and violence toward ethnic or religious groups that are associated with terrorism. These feelings can compromise their ability to provide care for these groups. Yet as the ICN *Code of Ethics for Nurses* affirms, nurses are ethically bound to provide care to all people. Explain that feelings of fear, helplessness, and loss are normal reactions to a disruptive situation.

- Help people remember methods they may have used in the past to overcome fear and helplessness.
- Encourage people to talk to others about their fears.
- Encourage others to ask for help and provide resources and referrals.
- Remember that those in the helping professions (e.g., nurses, physicians, social workers) may find it difficult to seek help.
- Convene small groups in workplaces with counselors/mental health experts.

**Assist Victims to Think Positively and to Move Toward the Future**
- Remind others that things will get better.
- Be realistic about the time it takes to feel better.
- Help people to recognize that the aim of terrorist attacks is to create fear and uncertainty.
- Encourage people to continue with the things they enjoy in their lives and to live their normal lives.

**Prepare Nursing Personnel to be Effective in a Crisis/ Emergency Situation**
- Incorporate disaster preparedness awareness in educational programs at all levels of the nursing curriculum.
- Provide continuing education to ensure a sound knowledge base, skill development, and ethical framework for practice.
- Network with other professional disciplines and governmental and nongovernmental agencies at local, regional, national, and international levels.

From ICN. Nursing Matters: Terrorism and bioterrorism: nursing preparedness. Available at http//www.icn.ch/publications/disaster-planning–and relief. Accessed December 27, 2010; International Council of Nurses (ICN): *Code of Ethics for Nurses*, Geneva, 2000, ICN.

---

### ⟩⟩ LINKING CONTENT TO PRACTICE

The role and involvement of nurses in global health relies heavily on nursing standards of practice and core competencies of both nurses and other public health professionals. The role also varies from country to country. It is not surprising to learn that nursing plays a more active role in health care delivery in the more technologically advanced countries. The more developed countries have a defined role for nurses, whereas the role is less well defined, if it is defined at all, in less developed countries. However, nurses need to remember that addressing the health of the people of the world is not restricted to meeting the physical health needs but, in order to be successful, must incorporate the concept of global health diplomacy. Physical, environmental, mental, political, fiscal, economic, safety, and educational "health" are intertwined in achieving the goals we all have for helping the people of the world obtain optimal well-being. Assessment of each of these areas is cited in standards of practice for nursing and public health professionals and is essential in the global nursing role. See the Quad Council on Nursing's competencies (Swider et al, 2014), which incorporate those of the Council on Linkages core competencies for public health professionals. Each set of competencies recommends analytic/assessment skills that are crucial to working in a global health arena. They also talk about the importance of cultural competence skills and communication skills that are relevant to the people with whom you are working.

During the last decade, some less developed countries have implemented primary health care programs directed at prevention and management of important public health problems. With the increasing migration between and within countries because of war and famine, a greater need for nursing expertise to alleviate suffering of refugees and displaced persons has emerged. Starvation, disease, death, war, and migration underscore the need for support from the wealthier nations of the world.

More than 30 million refugees and internally displaced persons in less developed countries currently depend on international relief assistance for survival. Death rates in these populations during the acute phase of displacement have been up to 60 times the expected rates. Displaced populations in Ethiopia and southern Sudan have suffered the highest death rates. In Afghanistan and in war-torn Iraq, infectious diseases accounted for one half of all admissions to the hospital—mostly malaria and typhoid fever. The greatest death rate has been in children 1 to 14 years old. The major causes of death have been measles, diarrheal diseases, acute respiratory tract infections, and malaria. In addition, poor sanitation in many hospitals and clinics and shortages of drugs and qualified health care workers produce huge gaps for needed health care services. Continued violence accounts for a population afraid to leave home to seek medical help.

Council on Linkages Between Academic and Public Health Practice: *Core Competencies for Public Health Professionals*. Washington, DC, 2010. Public Health Foundation/Health Resources and Services Administration. Quad Council of Public Health Nursing Organizations. Competencies for Public Health Nursing Practice, Washington, DC, 2003, ASTDN, revised 2009.

## LINKING CONTENT TO PRACTICE—cont'd

Nurses from more developed countries are recruited to combat the major mortality in refugee camps: malnutrition, measles, diarrhea, pneumonia, and malaria. Nurses, collaborating with other experts, are following the principles of primary health care and are promoting adequate food intake, safe drinking water, shelter, environmental sanitation, and immunizations. These life-saving practices have been implemented in the following countries: Thailand (Myanmar refugees), Rwanda, Zaire, Angola, Afghanistan, the Sudan, Uganda, and the former Yugoslavia. Nurses are making a difference; however, nurses involved in this work must be culturally astute and responsive, be well educated about the world and well versed in the tasks required to achieve positive outcomes, able to critically reason, able to make decisions, able to identify who are appropriate team members, and be able to collaborate with the team. They ought not be afraid of taking risks, they should be action-oriented, and they need to be flexible and altruistic. Global health work is a labor of love, it is a giving of self to make a difference in the lives of others less fortunate, and it is the most rewarding work in which many nurses have ever been engaged.

## PRACTICE APPLICATION

You are sent to a country ravaged by war, in which many people are refugees. You are asked to work side by side with other nurses, both foreign and native to the country.

A. What would you do first to develop this group of nurses into a functioning team?

B. Which health and environmental problems would you attempt to handle early in your work?

C. Identify second-stage interventions and prevention once the initial crisis stage is relieved.

**Answers can be found on the Evolve site.**

## KEY POINTS

- Global health is a collective goal of nations and is promoted by the world's major health organizations.
- Global health cannot be achieved without using the constructs of global health diplomacy: addressing and finding solutions to physical, environmental, fiscal, economic, political, safety, educational, and trade issues.
- As the political and economic barriers between countries fall, the movement of people back and forth across international boundaries increases. This movement increases the spread of various diseases throughout the world.
- Nurses play an active role in the identification of potential health risks at U.S. borders, with immigrant populations throughout the United States, and as participants in global health care delivery.
- Understanding a population approach is essential for understanding the health of specific populations.
- Universal access to health care for the world's populations relies on strong primary care.
- The major organizations involved in world health are (1) multilateral, (2) bilateral and nongovernmental or private voluntary, and (3) philanthropic.

- The health status of a country is related to its economic and technical growth. More technologically and economically advanced countries are referred to as *developed*, whereas those that are striving for greater economic and technological growth are termed *less developed*. Many less developed countries shift financial resources from health and education to other internal needs, such as defense or economic development, and this shift does not help the poor.
- The global burden of disease (GBD) is a way to describe the world's health. The GBD combines losses from premature death and losses that result from disability. The GBD represents units of disability-adjusted life-years (DALYs).
- Critical global health problems still exist and include communicable diseases such as tuberculosis, measles, mumps, rubella, and polio; maternal and child health; diarrheal diseases; nutritional deficits; malaria; and AIDS.
- Natural and man-made disasters have become global health concerns.

## CLINICAL DECISION-MAKING ACTIVITIES

1. In your class, divide into small groups and discuss how you might find out if there are immigrant communities in your area (you may need to contact your local health department, area social workers, or community social organizations and churches).
2. Discuss how you can gain access to one of these immigrant groups.
3. On gaining access, how would you go about determining what specific kinds of services the people need? What are their beliefs about health and health care? What customs regarding health were followed in their country of origin?

How does the American health care system differ from the health care system in their country?

4. As a nurse, what kinds of interventions can you implement with immigrant populations? What special skills or knowledge do you need to provide care to immigrant populations?
5. Write to one of the major international health organizations or visit their Internet web page and obtain their mission and goal statements. What is the focus of their health-related activities? Does the organization that you identified have a specific role defined for nurses? How can a nurse who is interested become involved in their programs and activities?

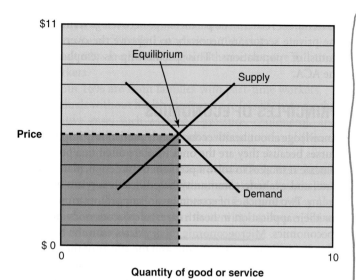

**FIG 5-1** Supply-and-demand curve.

Data from Curriculum Link, 2010.

---

## BOX 5-2   Efficiency versus Effectiveness

To illustrate the differences between efficiency and effectiveness, consider the case of a nurse who is designing a community outreach program to educate high-risk, first-time mothers about the importance of childhood immunizations. The most *efficient* method to disseminate the information to a large number of mothers might be to have the child health team from the public health department hold an evening educational session, open to the public, at the health department. The most *effective* means of offering the program might be to link public health nurses with new mothers for one-on-one, in-home counseling, demonstration, and follow-up. The goals of the program could be stated as follows:

- To change the behavior of the mothers regarding providing immunizations for their children
- To increase community mothers' knowledge and awareness of infectious diseases
- To reduce the incidence of preventable infections in the community
- To decrease the number of hospital admissions

---

## BOX 5-1   Principles of the Laws of Supply and Demand

**The Law of Supply**
- At higher prices, producers are willing to offer *more* products for sale than at lower prices.
- The supply increases as prices increase and decreases as prices decrease.
- Those already in business will try to increase production as a way of increasing profits.

**The Law of Demand**
- People will buy more of a product at a lower price than at a higher price, if nothing changes.
- At a lower price, more people can afford to buy more goods and more of an item more frequently than they can at a higher price.
- At lower prices, people tend to buy some goods as a substitute for more expensive goods.

good or service are available in the marketplace, the price tends to be higher than when larger quantities are available. The point on the curve where the supply and demand curves cross is the equilibrium, or the point where producer and consumer desires meet (See Box 5-1). Supply and demand curves can shift up or down as a result of the following factors (McPake et al, 2013):

- Competition for a good or service
- An increase in the costs of materials used to make a product
- Technological advances
- A change in consumer preferences
- Shortages of goods or services
  Provides a review of the laws of supply and demand.

Using the example of industry-offered health care, it was not likely that a small industry of fewer than 50 employees would be able to offer incentive-based on-site illness prevention services. The demand might be great to keep employees healthy and on the job. The supply has been limited by the cost and numbers of services available in the community. Therefore, the cost was likely to be higher for the small business than for the large

industry that offers its own services. The ACA proposes to offer preventive services free to the consumer, requiring insurance companies to cover these services (USDHHS, ACA, 2014a).

## Efficiency and Effectiveness

Two other terms are related to microeconomics: efficiency and effectiveness. Efficiency refers to producing maximal output, such as a good or service, using a given set of resources (or inputs), such as labor, time, and available money. Efficiency suggests that the inputs are combined and used in such a way that there is no better way to produce the service, or output, and that no other improvements can be made. The word *efficiency* often focuses on time, or speed in performing tasks, and the minimizing of waste, or unused input, during production. Although these notions are true, efficiency depends on tasks as well as processes of producing a good or service and the improvements made (Feldstein, 2012).

Effectiveness, on the other hand, refers to the extent to which a health care service meets a stated goal or objective, or how well a program or service achieves what is intended. For example, the effectiveness of a mass immunization program is related to the level of "herd immunity" developed to reduce the problem that the program was addressing (see Chapter 12). Box 5-2 illustrates the differences between efficiency and effectiveness (Feldstein, 2012).

## Macroeconomics

Microeconomics focuses on the individual or an organization, whereas macroeconomic theory focuses on the "big picture"—the total, or aggregate, of all individuals and organizations (e.g., behaviors such as growth, expansion, or decline of an aggregate). In macroeconomics, the aggregate is usually a country or nation. Factors such as levels of income, employment, general price levels, and rate of economic growth are important. This aggregate approach reflects, for example, the contribution of all organizations and groups within health care, or all industry within the United States, including health care, on the nation's economic outlook.

When the media refer to "the economy," the phrase is typically used as a macroeconomic term to describe the wealth and financial performance of the nation as an aggregate. Health care contributes to the economy through goods and services produced and employment opportunities.

The primary focuses of macroeconomics are the business cycle and economic growth. Business expands and contracts in cycles. These cycles are influenced by a number of factors, such as political changes (a new president is elected), policy changes (new legislation is implemented, such as the Patient Protection and Affordable Health Care Act of 2010), knowledge and technology advances (a new vaccine to treat H1N1/H5N1 is placed on the market), or simply the belief by a recognized business leader that the cycle is or should be shifting (e.g., when the head of the Federal Reserve Board changes interest rates).

The human capital approach is a measure of macroeconomic theory (Goodwin et al, 2014). In this approach improving human qualities, such as health, are a focus for developing and spending money on goods and services because health is valued; it increases productivity, enhances the income-earning ability of people, and improves the economy. Therefore, there is a positive rate of return on the "investment in human capital."

The individual, population, community, and nation all benefit. If the population is healthy, premature morbidity and mortality are reduced, chronic disease and disability are reduced, and economic losses to the nation are reduced. As an example, more people can work and be productive because they are healthy. The employing company makes more money because people are more productive. More taxes are paid into the local, state, and national economy, and more money is spent by individuals because they are productive, earning money, and taking advantage of the goods and services offered in their community.

## Measures of Economic Growth

Economic growth reflects an increase in the output of a nation. Two common measures of economic growth are the gross national product (GNP) and the gross domestic product (GDP). GNP is the total market value of all goods and services produced in an economy during a period of time (e.g., quarterly or annually). GDP is the total market value of the output of labor and property located in the United States (Strawser, 2014). GDP reflects only the national U.S. output, whereas GNP reflects national output plus income earned by U.S. businesses or citizens, whether within the United States or internationally. This discussion focuses on GDP, because U.S. health care spending reports are based on GDP (NCHS, 2010).

Nurses face microeconomic and macroeconomic issues every day. For example, they are influenced by microeconomics when referring clients for services, informing clients and others of the cost of services, assessing community need for a particular service, evaluating client access to services, and determining health provider and agency response to client needs. Nurses who work with aggregates of individuals and communities are faced with macroeconomic issues, such as health policies that make the development of new programs possible; local, state, and federal budgets that support certain programs; and the total effect that services will have on improving the health of the

community and reducing the poverty level of the population. In short, knowledge about health economics can enhance a nurse's ability to understand and argue a position for meeting population health needs.

## Economic Analysis Tools

The primary methods used to assess the economics of an intervention are cost-benefit analysis (CBA), cost-effectiveness analysis (CEA), and cost-utility analysis (CUA). CBA is considered the best of these methods. In simple form, CBA involves the listing of all costs and benefits that are expected to occur from an intervention during a prescribed time. Costs and benefits are adjusted for time and inflation. If the total benefits are greater than the total costs, the intervention has a *net positive value* (NPV). Future or continued funding is given to the intervention with the highest NPV. This technique provides a way to estimate overall program and social benefits in terms of net costs. A good example of using CBA would be the cost of an influenza vaccine mass immunization program in a community. If most people in the community are vaccinated and the rate of influenza is low or decreased from past years or in relation to the national average, the benefits are many. Citizens can work, play, go to school, participate in other community activities, and, again, be productive. The community is healthy. These are but a few of the benefits of this program.

CBA requires that all costs and benefits be known and quantifiable in dollars; herein lies the major problem with its use. Although it is fairly easy to estimate the direct dollar costs of a health care program, it is often very difficult to quantify the nondollar benefits and indirect costs. For example, benefits and costs could come in the form of increased income and expenses, which are fairly easy to measure. More difficult to measure are benefits such as improved community welfare resulting from a particular program, and the costs to the community that would result if the program did not exist. The value of *potential lives* lost because of lack of access to health care services is one example. The potential for a great number of lives lost from H1N1 resulted in the development of programs and monies invested with pharmaceutical companies in an attempt to reduce the risk of lives lost should the United States experience an epidemic from this disease risk. Although benefits could only be assumed from the cost investment, it was determined that the investment was essential (CDC, 2009).

CEA expresses the net direct and indirect costs and cost savings in terms of a defined health outcome. The total net costs are calculated and divided by the number of health outcomes. Although the data required for CEA are the same as for CBA, CEA does not require that a dollar value be put on the outcome (e.g., on an outcome such as quality of life). CEA is best used when comparing two or more strategies or interventions that have the same health outcome in the population. Both CEA and CBA are useful to nurses as they conduct community needs analyses and develop, propose, implement, and evaluate programs to meet community health needs. In both cases, the cost of a particular program or intervention is examined relative to the money spent and outcomes achieved. Using the same example of the mass immunization program, a comparison of number of bed days, work-loss days, and activity impairments. The most chronic medical condition was stroke.

## FINANCING OF HEALTH CARE

Against the backdrop of today's chronic conditions, it must be appreciated that health care financing has evolved through the twentieth and into the twenty-first century from a system supported primarily by consumers to a system financed by third-party payers (public and private). From 1980 to 2011, the percentage of third-party public insurance payments increased slightly while the percentage of out-of-pocket payments had declined. Combined state and federal governments paid the most in 2011 (CDC, 2014c).

### Public Support

The U.S. federal government became involved in health care financing for population groups early in its history. In 1798 the federal government created the Marine Hospital Service to provide medical care for sick and disabled sailors, and to protect the nation's borders against the importing of disease through seaports. The Marine Hospital Service is considered the first national health insurance plan in the United States (see Health Care Reform, Chapter 3). The National Health Board was established in 1879 and was later renamed the U.S. Public Health Service (PHS). Within the PHS, the federal government developed a public health liaison with state and local health departments for the purpose of controlling communicable diseases and improving sanitation. Additional health programs were also developed to meet obligations to federal workers and their families within the PHS, the Department of Defense, and the Veterans Administration (VA) (see Chapter 8).

Medicare and Medicaid, two federal programs administered by the CMS, account for the majority of public health care

spending. Table 5-3 compares these programs. The CMS is the federal regulatory agency within the U.S. Department of Health and Human Services (USDHHS) that is responsible for overseeing and monitoring Medicare and Medicaid spending. This agency routinely collects and reports actual health care use and spending and projects future spending trends. Through these programs, the federal government purchases health care services for population groups through independent health care systems, such as managed care organizations, private practice physicians, and hospitals.

### Medicare

The Medicare program, established in Title XVIII of the Social Security Act of 1965, provides hospital insurance and medical insurance to persons aged 65 and older, to permanently disabled persons, and to persons with end-stage renal disease—altogether approximately 46 million people in 2013 (CMS, 2014). Medicare has two parts: Part A (hospital insurance) covers hospital care, home care, hospice care, and skilled nursing care (limited); Part B (noninstitutional care insurance) covers "medically necessary" services such as health care provider services, outpatient care, home health, and other medical services such as diagnostic services, and physiotherapy. In 1999 a program called Medicare Advantage was added to the program (Part C). This is an option that can be chosen for additional coverage. This option includes both Part A and B services. The Part C plans are coordinated care plans that include health maintenance organizations (HMOs), private fee-for-service plans, and medical savings accounts (MSAs). Part C provides for all health care coverage costs after a high deductible (CMS, 2014).

Medicare Part A is primarily financed by a federal payroll tax that is paid by employers and employees. The proceeds from this tax go to the Hospital Insurance Trust Fund, which is managed by the CMS. If a person did not have federal payroll

| TABLE 5-3 | **Comparison of Medicare and Medicaid Program Features** | |
|---|---|---|
| **Feature** | **Medicare** | **Medicaid** |
| Where to obtain information | Local Social Security Administration office | State welfare office |
| Recipients | Client is 65 years or older, is disabled, or has permanent kidney failure | Specified low-income and needy, children, aged, blind, and/or disabled; those eligible to receive federally assisted income |
| Type of program | Insurance | Insurance |
| Government affiliation | Federal | Joint federal/state |
| Availability | All states | All states |
| Financing of hospital insurance | Medicare Trust Fund, mandatory payroll deduction, recipient deductibles, trust fund interest | Federal and state governments |
| Financing of medical insurance | Recipient premium payments; general revenue, U.S. Treasury | Federal and state governments |
| Types of coverage | Part A. Inpatient and outpatient hospital services, skilled nursing facilities (SNFs), limited nursing home care, home health services and hospice<br>Part B. Prevention and screening services<br>Part D. Prescription drugs from a formulary | Inpatient and outpatient hospital services; nursing facility services: home health, physician services, rural health clinic services, community health center services; laboratory and x-rays; family planning; advanced practice nurse services; free-standing birth center services; medical care transportation; tobacco cessation counseling for pregnant women, vaccines for children; many optional services are available by state's choice |

From U.S. Department of Health and Human Services, Centers for Medicare and Medicaid Services: *Medicare and You, and Medicaid Benefits,* Baltimore, MD, 2015, USDHHS.

deductions, Part A can be obtained by paying a monthly premium. Part A coverage is available to all persons who are eligible to receive Medicare, with older adults comprising the majority of these individuals. There is concern about the future of the Medicare Trust Fund, because projected expenses may be more than the trust fund resources. Payments to hospitals for covered services have been and continue to be higher than fund growth. Thus Medicare reimbursement policy has been changing in an attempt to control increasing hospital costs. Part A requires a deductible from recipients for the first 60 days of services with a reduced deductible for 61 to 90 days of service. The deductible has increased as daily hospital costs have increased. For skilled nursing facility (SNF) care, persons pay nothing for the first 20 days and a cost per day for days 21 through 100. After 100 days, persons must pay the total cost for care (CMS, 2013a). The person pays zero for hospice care and home health.

The medical insurance package, Part B, is a supplemental (voluntary) program that is available to all Medicare-eligible persons for a monthly premium ($99.90 minimum in 2012) (CMS, 2012a). The vast majority of Medicare-covered persons elect this coverage. Part B provides coverage for services other than hospital (physician care, outpatient hospital care, outpatient physical therapy, mental health, and home health care) that are not covered by Part A, such as laboratory services, ambulance transportation, prostheses, equipment, and some supplies. After a deductible, up to 80% of reasonable charges are paid for medical and other services. For mental health services, 55% of the costs are paid. Part B resembles the major medical insurance coverage of private insurance carriers. Figure 5-5 shows the total expenses of the Medicare program from 1966 to 2012.

Since the passing of the Medicare amendments to the Social Security Act in 1965, the cost of Medicare has increased dramatically. Hospital care continues to be the major factor contributing to Medicare costs. However, because of the shorter hospital stays, home health and nursing home costs have increased dramatically. As a result of rising health costs, Congress passed a law in 1983 that radically changed Medicare's method of payment for hospital services. In 1983 federal legislation (PL 98-21) mandated an end to cost-plus reimbursement by Medicare and instituted a 3-year transition to a prospective payment system (PPS) for inpatient hospital services (HCFA, 1998). The purpose of the new hospital payment scheme was to shift the cost incentives away from the providing of more care and toward more efficient services. The basis for prospective reimbursement is the 468 diagnosis-related groups (DRGs) (See Evidence-Based Practice Box). Also, the Balanced Budget Act of 1997 determined that payments to Medicare SNFs would be made on the basis of the PPS, effective July 1, 1998 (HCFA 1998). The PPS payment rates cover SNF services, including routine, ancillary, and capital-related costs (CMS, 2013b). In 2001 CMS developed a PPS for DRGs for home health with Health Insurance Prospective Payment System (HIPPS) codes.

## EVIDENCE-BASED PRACTICE

This retrospective study examined the incidence, costs, and factors associated with potentially avoidable hospitalizations (PAH) in dually eligible Medicare and Medicaid beneficiaries. This population was selected due to their complex clinical needs and high costs of care. Potentially avoidable hospitalizations were defined by an expert panel that identified conditions and associated Diagnostic Related Groups (DRGs) which can often be prevented or safely and effectively managed in a skilled nursing facility or home- and community-based services. Seventy-eight percent of the PAH were responsible from five conditions: pneumonia, congestive heart failure, urinary tract infections, dehydration, and chronic obstructive pulmonary disease. The total costs of these hospitalizations were $3 billion for Medicare beneficiaries and $463 million for Medicaid beneficiaries. A sensitivity analysis found that between 77,000 and 260,000 hospitalizations and between $625 million and $1.9 billion in expenditures could be avoided each year in this population.

**Nurse Use**

Community health nursing initiatives, such as health education and case management, could significantly reduce the amount of hospital admissions in this population. Such interventions could greatly reduce the negative health effects and quality of life for this population, as well as reduce the high health care costs for this group.

From Walsh EG, Wiener JM, Haber S, et al: Potentially avoidable hospitalizations of dually eligible Medicare and Medicaid beneficiaries from nursing facility and home- and community-based services waiver program. *J Am Geriatr Soc* 60:821–829, 2012.

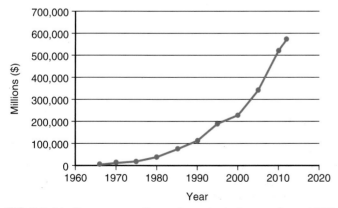

**FIG 5-5** Medicare expenditures for selected years from 1966 to 2012. (From Centers for Medicare & Medicaid Services: *National Health Expenditure Accounts: National Health Expenditure Data: Historical.* 2012. Retrieved December 2014 from http://www.cms.gov/Research-Statistics-Data-and-Systems/Statistics-Trends-and-Reports/NationalHealthExpendData/NationalHealthAccountsHistorical.html)

In 2009 the average amount spent for services for Medicare beneficiaries was approximately $8000 (Kaiser Family Foundation, 2012b). The average out-of-pocket spending is skewed to those beneficiaries who are older or have declining health. Approximately one in four Medicare beneficiaries spends 30% or more of their income on out-of-pocket health expenses (Kaiser Family Foundation, 2012b). This is because of the limits in Medicare coverage, including certain preventive care, and the limited number of physicians and agencies who accept

*MA: STATE & FED.*

Medicare and Medicaid payment. Older adults who do not have supplemental insurance must cover the difference between the Medicare payment and the additional costs for services.

## Medicaid

The Medicaid program, Title XIX of the Social Security Act of 1965, provides financial assistance to states and counties to pay for medical services for poor older adults, the blind, the disabled, and families with dependent children. The Medicaid program is jointly sponsored and financed with matching funds from the federal and state governments. In 2013, 55 million people were enrolled in Medicaid (Kaiser Family Foundation, 2014). Medicaid expenditures from 1966 to 2012 are shown in Figure 5-6. Since the beginning of Medicaid, full payment has been provided for five types of services (NCHS, 2012):

- Inpatient and outpatient hospital care
- Laboratory and radiology services
- Physician services
- Skilled nursing care at home or in a nursing home for people more than 21 years of age
- Early Periodic Screening, Diagnosis, and Treatment (EPSDT) programs for those less than 21 years of age

The 1972 Social Security amendments added family planning to the list of full-pay services. States can choose to add prescriptions, dental services, eyeglasses, intermediate care facilities, and coverage for the medically indigent as program options. By law, the medically indigent are required to pay a monthly premium.

Any state participating in the Medicaid program is required to provide the six basic services to persons who are below state poverty income levels. Optional programs are provided at the discretion of each state. In 1989 changes in Medicaid required states to provide care for children less than 6 years of age and to pregnant women under 133% of the poverty level. For example, if the poverty level were $12,000, a pregnant woman could have a household income as high as $16,000 and still be eligible to receive care under Medicaid. These changes also provided for pediatric and family nurse practitioner reimbursement.

In the 1990s states were allowed to petition the federal government for a waiver. If the waiver was approved, the states could use their Medicaid monies for programs other than the six basic services. The first waiver to be approved was given to Oregon for their health care reform plan. Other states have received waivers to develop Medicaid managed care programs for special populations. The 2010 health care reform plan provides for new approaches to offering Medicaid services and incentives for states to offer Medicaid services rather than through the waiver option as described previously (PL 111-148, 2010).

The major expense categories for the Medicaid program have historically been skilled and intermediate nursing home care and inpatient hospital care. When combined, these two categories account today for 3% of all costs to the program (NCHS, 2012).

## Public Health

Most public government agencies operate on an annual budget, and they plan for costs by estimating salaries, expenses, and costs of services for a year. Public health agencies, such as health departments and WIC (Women, Infants, and Children) programs, receive primary funding from taxes, with additional money for select goods and services through private third-party payers. Selected public health programs receive reimbursement for services as follows: through grants given by the federal

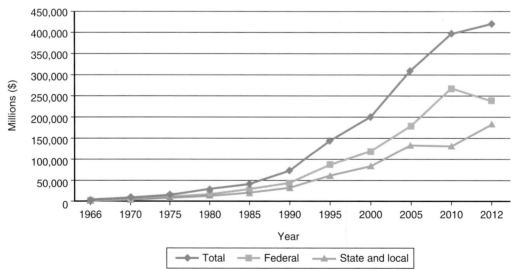

**FIG 5-6** Medicaid expenditures for selected years from 1987 to 2012. (From Centers for Medicare & Medicaid Services: *National Health Expenditure Accounts: National Health Expenditure Data: Historical.* 2012. Retrieved December 2014 from http://www.cms.gov/Research-Statistics-Data-and-Systems/Statistics-Trends-and-Reports/NationalHealthExpendData/NationalHealthAccountsHistorical.html)

government to states for prenatal and child health; through Medicare and Medicaid for home health, nursing homes, and WIC and EPSDT programs; and through collecting of fees on a sliding scale for select client services, such as immunizations. (Trust for America's Health, 2014).

In 2011 only 3% of all health care–related federal funds was expended for federal health programs such as WIC, versus 97% for other types of health and illness care (such as hospital and physician services). In addition to this 3% allotment, public health funds also come through states and territorial health agencies. State and local governments contributed 16% to public and general assistance, maternal and child health, public health activities, and other related services in 2010 (NCHS, 2013).

## Other Public Support

The federal government finances health services for retired military persons and dependents through TRICARE, the VA, and the Indian Health Service (IHS). These programs are very important in providing needed health care services to these populations (see Chapter 8).

## The Affordable Care Act: Public Health Support

The ACA provides for prevention and public health funds with emphasis on chronic disease. Funds are provided to states to implement these provisions. See Table 5-4 for more detail. Also check the state of interest to see what that state is doing to implement this provision in ACA.

## Private Support

Private health care payer sources include insurance, employers, managed care, and individuals. Although insurance and consumers have been prominent health care payment sources for some time, the role of employers, managed care, and consumers became increasingly prominent and powerful during the first decade of the twenty-first century, particularly as concerns grew about the use and changing nature of health insurance.

## Evolution of Health Insurance

Insurance for health care was first offered for the private sector in 1847 by a commercial insurance company. The purpose of the insurance was to provide security and protection when health care services were needed by individuals. The idea behind insurance was that it provided security, guaranteeing (within certain limits) monies to pay for health care services to offset potential financial losses from unexpected illness or injury related to accidents, catastrophic communicable diseases (such as smallpox and scarlet fever), and recurring (but unexpected) chronic illnesses.

A comprehensive study in the 1920s by the Committee on the Costs of Medical Care showed that a small portion of the population was paying most of the costs of medical care for the majority of the people. The Depression of the 1930s, rising medical costs, and the need to spread financial risk across communities spurred the development of the third-party payment system. The system began as a major industry in the 1930s with the Blue Cross system, which initially provided prepayment for hospital care. In 1939 Blue Shield created plans to provide physician payment. The Blue Cross plans began as tax-free, nonprofit organizations established under special enabling legislation in various states.

In the 1940s and 1950s, hospital and medical-surgical coverage increased. Employee group coverage appeared, and profit-making commercial insurance underwriters began offering health insurance packages with competitive premiums. The commercial insurance companies could offer lower premium rates because of the methods used to set rates. Insurance and premium setting, in general, are based on the notion of risk pooling (i.e., insurance companies were willing to risk the unlikely event that all or even a large portion of individuals covered under a plan would need payment for health services at any given time). Blue Cross used a *community rate*, establishing a similar premium rate for all subscribers regardless of illness potential. In contrast, the commercial companies used

---

### TABLE 5-4  The Affordable Care Act's Prevention and Public Health Fund in Your State

- **Prevention and Public Health Fund**
  - The fund is an unprecedented investment in promoting wellness, preventing disease, and protecting against public health emergencies

- **Much of this work is done in partnership with states and communities:**
  - To help control the obesity epidemic
  - Fight health disparities
  - Detect and quickly respond to health threats
  - Reduce tobacco use
  - Train the nation's public health workforce
  - Modernize vaccine systems
  - Prevent the spread of HIV/AIDS
  - Increase public health programs' effectiveness and efficiency
  - Improve access to behavioral health services

- **Preventing Chronic Disease: A Smart Investment**

- **Chronic diseases: The Prevention Fund helps states**
  - Tackle the leading causes of death and root causes of costly, preventable chronic disease:
    - Detect and respond rapidly to health security threats
    - Prevent accidents and injuries

Since the Affordable Care Act was passed in 2010, the U.S. Department of Health and Human Services has awarded $1.25 billion in Prevention Fund grants.
Check your state to see what is being done to promote the public's health.

3rd PARTY PAYER

an *experience rate,* in which the premium was based on an estimate of the illness *risk* or the number of claims to be made by the subscriber (Hicks, 2012).

Premium competition, the offering of health insurance as a fringe benefit, and the use of health insurance as a negotiable collective bargaining item led to an increase in covered benefits, first-dollar coverage for medical care expenses, and increased employer-paid premiums. In turn, these factors pushed up insurance premium costs and health care costs and enabled insurance plans to cover high-cost segments of the population (the aged, poor, or disabled) because of the number of low-risk enrollees.

The health needs of high-risk populations led to the passage of Medicare and Medicaid legislation. These and other national health programs targeted health care coverage for specific population groups. Because these programs directed additional money into the health care system to subsidize care, there were financial incentives to encourage the providing of services (i.e., the more services that were ordered, the greater the amount of money that would be received). Other incentives were related to the use of services by clients (i.e., the more available the payment was for services that might otherwise have gone unused, the more services that were requested).

Greater increases in health insurance premiums have occurred as a result of pressure from employers, consumers, and policymakers. Driving forces behind this pressure are quality of care, client dissatisfaction, clients' rights, and the concern that these areas are being compromised in the managed care system. Furthermore, the initial cost savings from managed care may have occurred already, and costs will have to be increased to simply maintain coverage, not to mention providing new services and technologies. Although managed care changed the structure of financing and delivery of care, it was soon recognized that managed care was not the solution to the health care system's problems (Shi and Singh, 2011).

## Employers

Since the beginning of Blue Cross and Blue Shield, health insurance has been tied to employment and the business sector. This tie was strengthened during World War II to compensate, attract, and retain employees. Since that time, employers have played the major role in determining health insurance benefits. However, with the economic downturn in 2008, employers began to reduce their health insurance benefits or return the cost of insurance. It is of interest that if a client has health insurance, the payment to the provider is less than the payment made by the client who does not have health insurance.

In 2005 approximately 70% of the population under 65 years of age had private health insurance, most of which was obtained through the workplace (NCHS, 2005). In 2009 the percentage had decreased to about 60% (Kaiser Family Foundation, 2009). In 2005, 87% of employers paid 50% to 100% of the insurance premium (Kaiser Family Foundation, 2005). In 2009 employees paid a minimum of 26% to 36% of the health insurance premium with the employee's share of a family premium doubling in cost since 2000. For employees of small firms, the percentage of payment increased for all premiums (Kaiser

Family Foundation, 2009). This substantial contribution to health care by the private business sector gave the employer considerable health care buying power in making policy about what services insurance would cover. Most older Americans were covered by Medicare; low-income children can now be covered by the Children's Health Insurance Program (CHIP) if enrolled by parents or guardians; and as previously described, some low-income adults were covered by Medicaid.

Before the growth of insurance (i.e., before 1930 and the beginning of Blue Cross), the health care consumer had more influence over health care costs because payment was out of pocket. Consumers made decisions about how they would spend their money, making certain tradeoffs—for example, about the type of health care they were willing to buy and how much they would pay. Entering the system was restricted in large part to those who could afford to pay for care, or to those few who could find care financed through charitable and philanthropic organizations. With the beginning of the insurance (or third-party payer) system, health care costs were set by payers, and they determined the type of care or service that would be offered and its price. This began to change somewhat in the 1980s with the increased use of managed care.

As the cost of health insurance has increased, some employers, in an effort to bypass the costs established by insurers, have found it less costly to self-insure. The employer does this by contracting directly with providers to obtain health care services for employees rather than going through health insurance companies. Some large businesses directly employ on-site providers for care delivery or offer on-site wellness programs. These programs within the private sector offer opportunities for nurses to provide wellness programs and health assessments to screen and monitor employees and their families. This move to self-insure resulted in savings to companies and reduced overall sick-care costs (Kovner et al, 2011).

In a truly competitive market, the consumer buys goods and services at will, knowing the costs and expected value of services bought and choosing the provider of those services. In the health system where a third party pays for the services, this transaction has less meaning. The third party makes decisions about the level and type of care that will be purchased for clients and determines how payment will be made. The service provider and client have no influence on how services will be reimbursed. However, the consumer may select the payer/plan and indeed may influence the system through political channels.

The average monthly cost for private health insurance has increased greatly through the years. Premiums reflect a shift of the health care cost burden from employers to employees as the percentage of employer contributions to health care declines. The decrease in employer contribution to health insurance premiums parallels the economic downturn of 2008, the move away from traditional insurance plans, and the move toward managed care plans or self-insurance plans by both small and large employers or toward dropping health insurance as a benefit. In 2008, 2 million people lost employer health insurance coverage (Kaiser Family Foundation, 2012a).

From an economic point of view, the shift in responsibility for the cost of health insurance is not bad. In theory, this shift makes consumers more knowledgeable about (sensitive to) the price of health services. This means that they have more information for health care decision making and may consider price in making the decision to access types of health care services. Satisfaction with the quality of service rests with the person buying the insurance and receiving health care. As with employers, employees may choose health insurance voluntarily. Therefore three factors—the shifting of responsibility for health insurance premiums to employees, the changing demographics of the workforce in general, and the loss of employment due to the economic downturn—have resulted in a decline in employee enrollment in health insurance plans. Employees are choosing to use their resources to meet basic needs and are assuming the risks of having an illness for which they may have to pay. A minor health problem can lead to major medical debt for someone without health insurance (Kaiser Family Foundation, 2013). PL 111-148 includes a mandate for all citizens and legal residents to have qualifying health coverage. Employers will be required to offer coverage also, except for employers with fewer than 50 employees. These two requirements were to be in effect by 2014 unless repealed by Congress.

Given that access to health insurance is tied to employment, there was growing concern in the late 1980s and early 1990s about the employment layoffs and downsizing occurring in private business. Those who lost their jobs lost their ability to pay for health insurance and to qualify to purchase insurance privately. The Health Insurance Portability and Accountability Act of 1996 (HIPAA) was enacted to protect health insurance coverage for workers and families after a job change or loss (Health Care Financing Administration [HCFA], 1999; Nichols and Blumberg, 1998). Although this has increased the number of people who have access to health insurance and health care, there are claims that individual premiums are high, that insurance companies have lost their ability to pool risks, and that HIPAA is just one more federal control mechanism undermining competitive market influences.

### Individuals

In 2011, individuals paid only approximately 14% of total health expenditures out of pocket (NCHS, 2014). However, these figures do not reflect the amount of money the consumer pays in taxes to finance government-supported programs such as Medicare and Medicaid, insurance premiums, and money paid for supplemental insurance to cover the gaps in a primary health insurance policy or Medicare.

### Managed Care Arrangements

Managed care is the term used for a variety of health care arrangements that integrate the financing and the delivery of health care. Managed care offers an array of services to purchasers, such as employers, Medicaid, or Medicare, for a set fee. These are called *risk-based plans*. This fee, in turn, is used to pay providers through preset arrangements for services delivered to individuals who are covered (NCHS, 2012). The concept of managed care is based on the notion that the use of costly care could be reduced if consumers had access to care and services that would prevent illness through consumer education and

health maintenance. Therefore, managed care uses disease prevention, health promotion, wellness, and consumer education (Kovner et al, 2011). In addition to risk-based plans, wherein the managed care organization accepts a set fee to cover all costs of care for the enrollee, there are cost-based plans. An example of such a managed care organization is the primary care case management (PCCM) organization often used by Medicaid programs. These PCCMs are composed of a variety of health care providers contracted with states to locate, coordinate, and monitor covered primary care and other services on a per client case management fee payment. Whereas HMOs assume risks for the costs of care, the PCCMs do not (NCHS, 2010).

Although they seem relatively new to many clients of care, HMOs have actually been around since the 1940s. The Health Maintenance Organization Act was enacted in 1972, and since that time, the number of individuals receiving care through HMOs and other types of managed care organizations has increased considerably. Managed care is based, in part, on the principles of managed competition. Managed competition was introduced in health care in the late 1980s and early 1990s to address the increasing costs of health care and to introduce quality into the forefront of discussions. Managed competition simply means that clients make decisions and choose the health care services they want on the basis of the quality or reputation of the service. To make decisions, they use knowledge and information about health care problems, care, and providers, and they look at the costs of care. However, health care is a complex market and not one in which information about health care, health problems, and the costs of care are easy to get. With the passing of the ACA (2010), Accountable Care Organizations are being introduced as a new approach to managing care.

### Medical Savings Accounts

Another insurance reform discussion at the political level concerns medical savings accounts (MSAs). These are also referred to as health savings accounts. MSAs are touted as a way of turning health care decision-making control over to the individuals receiving care. MSAs are tax-exempt accounts available to individuals who work for small companies, usually established through a bank or insurance company, that enable the individuals to save money for future medical needs and expenses (Internal Revenue Service [IRS], 2012). Money is contributed to an MSA by the employer, and the initial money put into an MSA does not come out of taxable income. Also, interest earned in MSAs is tax free, and unused MSA money can be held in the account from year to year until the money is used. MSAs, in theory, would allow individuals to make cost/quality tradeoffs and would require that individuals become knowledgeable about health care, become involved in health care decision making, and take responsibility for the decisions made. Providers, in turn, must be willing to provide and disclose information to individuals and give up control of health care decision making. The HIPAA and MSAs are examples of health insurance reform efforts, and these efforts will very likely remain in the forefront of political discussions for some time to come, especially with the health care reform discussions.

# HEALTH CARE PAYMENT SYSTEMS

Several methods have been used by public and private sources to pay health care providers for health care services. These include retrospective and prospective reimbursement for paying health care organizations, and fee-for-service and capitation for paying health care practitioners (Kovner et al, 2011).

## Paying Health Care Organizations

Retrospective reimbursement is the traditional reimbursement method, whereby fees for the delivery of health care services in an organization are set after services are delivered (Kovner et al, 2011). In this scenario, reimbursement is based on either organization costs or charges. The cost method reimburses organizations on the basis of cost per unit of service (e.g., home health visit, patient-day) for treatment and care. Costs include all or a percentage of added, allowable costs. Allowable costs are negotiated between the payer and provider and include items such as depreciation of building, equipment, and administrative costs (e.g., administrative salaries, utilities, and office supplies) (Kovner et al, 2011). For example, the unit of service in home health is the visit, and the agreed-on price is a set amount of money that the home health agency will be paid for a home visit in the region of the United States in which the home care agency is located.

The *charge method* reimburses organizations on the basis of the price set by the organization for delivering a service (Kovner et al, 2011). In this case, the organization determines a charge for providing a particular service, provides the service to a client, and submits a bill to the payer; the payer in turn provides payment for the bill. With this method, the charge may be greater than the actual cost to the agency to deliver the service. When the charge method is used, the client often has to pay the difference between what is paid and what is charged.

*Prospective reimbursement,* or payment, is a more recent method of paying an organization, whereby the third-party payer establishes the amount of money that will be paid for the delivery of a particular service before offering the services to the client (Kovner et al, 2011). Since the establishment of prospective payment in Medicare in 1983, private insurance has followed by requiring preapprovals before clients can receive certain services, such as hospital admission or mammograms more than once a year (Kovner et al, 2011). Under this payment scheme, the third-party payer reimburses an organization on the basis of the payer's prediction of the cost to deliver a particular service; these predictions vary by case mix (i.e., different types of clients, with different types, levels, and intensities of health problems), the client's diagnosis, and geographic location. This process is used in the DRG system of the hospital (Kovner et al, 2011).

Similarly, ambulatory care services received by Medicare recipients are classified into ambulatory payment classes (APCs), which reflect the type of ambulatory clinical services received and resources required (CMS, 2012b). Prospective payment to skilled nursing facilities is also adjusted for case mix and geographic variations (CMS, 2012c).

Positive and negative incentives are built into these reimbursement schemes. The retrospective method of payment encourages organizations to inflate prices in one area to offset agency losses in another. These losses can result from providing service to nonpaying clients or from providing care to clients covered under plans that do not cover the total costs of delivering a service (Kovner et al, 2011). The major disadvantage of this system is that little regard is given to the costs involved. This practice of charging a payer at a higher rate to cover losses in providing care is referred to as *cost-shifting.*

Prospective cost reimbursement encourages agencies to stay within budget limits and adds an incentive for providing less service to contain or reduce costs. If an organization provides care to a particular patient or group of patients and keeps the costs of delivering the service lower than the amount of reimbursement, the provider keeps the difference; however, if the provider's costs exceed the reimbursement, the provider must assume the risk and pay the difference. The major disadvantage of this method is that organizations tend to overemphasize controlling costs and sometimes compromise quality of care.

A growth in contracting, or competitive bidding, for health care services, intended to create incentives for providers to compete on price, has occurred as managed care has increased in health care markets. For example, contracting has been used by states to provide Medicaid services to eligible persons. Hospitals and other health care providers that do not have a contract with the state to provide services are not eligible to receive Medicaid payments for client care. Managed care organizations also use this approach to negotiate with health care organizations, such as hospitals, for coverage of services to be provided to covered enrollees, often called *covered lives.*

## Paying Health Care Practitioners

The traditional method of paying health care practitioners is known as fee for service (Kovner et al, 2011) and is like the retrospective method just described. The practitioner determines the costs of providing a service, delivers the service to a client, and submits a bill for the delivered service to a third-party payer; the payer then pays the bill. This method is based on usual, customary, and reasonable (UCR) charges for specific services in a given geographic region, determined by periodic regional evaluations of physician charges across specialties (Kovner et al, 2011). Historically, Medicare, Medicaid, and private insurance companies have used this method of reimbursing physicians.

A major effort to regulate and control the costs of physician fees was introduced in 1990 in the Omnibus Reconciliation Act. After a study by the Physician Payment Review Commission established by Congress, the *resource-based relative value scale* (RBRVS) was established. The RBRVS method reimburses physicians for specific services provided and the amount of resources required to deliver the service. Resources are defined broadly and include not only the costs of providing the service, but also the training that is required to provide a particular service and the time required to perform certain procedures, including client diagnosis and treatment. The RBRVS method of reimbursement, adopted by Medicare in 1991, acknowledges the breadth and depth of knowledge required by primary care physicians in the community to provide services aimed at prevention, health promotion, teaching, and counseling.

Capitation is similar to prospective reimbursement for health care organizations. Specifically, third-party payers determine the amount that practitioners will be paid for a unit of care, such as a client visit, before the delivery of the service, thereby placing a limit on the amount of reimbursement received per patient (Kovner et al, 2011). In contrast to a fee-for-service arrangement, where the practitioner determines both the services that will be provided to clients and the charges for those services, practitioners being paid through capitation are given the rate they will be paid for a client's care, regardless of specific services provided. Therefore, for example, physicians and nurse practitioners are aware in advance of the payment they will receive to perform a routine, uncomplicated physical examination or a more complex, detailed physical examination, diagnosis, and treatment (Kovner et al, 2011).

In capitated arrangements, physicians and other practitioners are paid a set amount to provide care to a given client or group of clients for a set period of time and amount of money. This arrangement, typically used by managed care organizations, is one whereby the practitioner contracts with the managed care organization to provide health care services to plan members for a preset and negotiated fee. The agreed-on fee is negotiated between the practitioner and the managed care organization before the delivery of services and is set at a discounted rate, and the practitioner and managed care organization come to a legal agreement, or contract, for the delivery and payment of services. The managed care organization pays the predetermined fee to the practitioner, often before the delivery of services, to provide care to plan members for a set period (Kovner et al, 2011).

### Reimbursement for Nursing Services

Historically, practitioners eligible to receive reimbursement for health care services included physicians only. However, nurses who function in certain capacities, such as NPs, CNSs, and midwives, also provide primary care to clients and receive reimbursement for their services. Being recognized as primary care providers and eligible to receive reimbursement has not been an easy achievement. There are currently more than 250 nurse-managed clinics in the United States providing population-based preventive services, primary care, or specific wellness programs. Most are receiving financial support through Medicare, Medicaid, contracts, gifts, grants, and private donations.

Hospital nursing care costs have traditionally been included as part of the overall patient room charge and reimbursed as such. Other agencies, such as home health care agencies, include nursing care costs with administrative costs, supplies, and equipment costs. Nursing organizations, such as the American Nurses Association (ANA), have long advocated that nursing care should become a separate budget item in all organizations so that cost studies can show the efficiency and effectiveness of the nursing profession.

Spurred by efforts to control the costs of medical care, effective January 1, 1998, NPs and CNSs were granted third-party reimbursement for Medicare Part B services only, under Public Law 105-33 (ANA, 1999). This new law set reimbursement for NPs and CNSs at 85% of physician rates for the same service, an extension of previous legislation that allowed the same reimbursement rate to NPs and CNSs practicing in rural areas (Buppert, 1999). This law was passed after years of work in this area, including research documenting NP and CNS contributions to health care delivery and client outcomes and after active lobbying efforts by professional nursing organizations. Reimbursement for these nurses has not changed to any extent since the 1990s.

In addition, data about the cost-to-benefit ratio, efficiency, and effectiveness of nursing care in general have been collected. Today, more than 250 nurse-managed clinics provide health care services to individuals in the United States who might not otherwise have access to health care, such as older adults, the homeless, and schoolchildren. All of these events have moved the discipline toward more autonomy in nursing practice and are serving as a means for evaluating and documenting nurses' contributions to health care delivery (Esperat et al, 2012).

---

### » LINKING CONTENT TO PRACTICE

The balance of interest within society and health care will continue to shift toward a focus on quality, safety, and elimination of health disparities through public and private sector partnerships. Health care system concerns of the twenty-first century are expected to focus on examining the quality of health care relative to the costs of care delivered, reduction in disparities, access to care, and health care reform. These changes will result from continued efforts of both the public and private sectors to reform the U.S. health care system. The current era of health care delivery will be noted as a time of vast changes in all sectors of health care delivery.

Nurses must plan for future changes in health care financing by becoming aware of the costs of nursing services, identifying aspects of care where cost savings can be safely achieved, and developing knowledge on how nursing practice affects and is affected by the principles of economics. Nursing must continue to focus on improving the overall health of the nation, defining its contribution to the health of the nation, deriving the value of nursing care, and ensuring its economic viability within the health care marketplace. Nurses must effect changes in the health care system by providing leadership in developing new models of care delivery that provide effective, high-quality care and by assuming a greater role in evaluating client care and nurse performance. It is through their leadership that nurses will contribute to improved decision making about allocating scarce health care resources, and promoting primary prevention as an answer to improve many of the current population level health outcomes.

## PRACTICE APPLICATION

Connie, a nursing student, has identified a caseload of five families in a chronic disease program offered by the local public health department. She is interested in assessing the costs of care to her clients and to the agency. Connie approaches the public health nurse administrator and asks the following questions:

A. How is the agency reimbursed for chronic disease management? Has the Affordable Care Act changed the way reimbursement occurs?

B. Does the client have a responsibility for paying for services?

C. Are nursing care costs known?

D. Are services rationed to clients? On what basis?

E. What effect will the chronic disease management program have on the community population?

**Answers can be found on the Evolve site.**

## KEY POINTS

- From 1800 to 2000, the U.S. health care delivery system experienced four developmental stages, with different emphases on health care economics. With the twenty-first century, the health care delivery system has changed the focus of the fourth developmental stage.
- Four basic components provide the framework for the development of delivery of health care services: service needs and intensity, facilities, technology, and labor (workforce).
- Three major factors have been associated with the growth of the health care delivery system: price inflation, changes in population demographics, and technology and service intensity.
- Chronic disease is becoming a major health factor affecting health care spending, with one in two Americans experiencing at least one chronic disease.
- Health care financing has evolved through the twentieth century from a system financed primarily by the consumer to a system financed primarily by third-party payers. In the twenty-first century, the consumer is being asked to pay more.
- To solve the problems of rising health care costs, the Affordable Care Act has been passed; this act also includes some form of rationing.
- Excessive and inefficient use of goods and services in health care delivery has been viewed as the major cause of rising health care costs.
- Economics is concerned with use of resources, including money, to fulfill society's needs and wants.
- Health economics is concerned with the problems of producing services and programs and distributing them to clients.
- The goal of public health economics is maximal benefits from services of public health providers, leading to health and wellness of the population.

- The goal of public health is to provide the most good for the most people.
- Nurses need to understand basic economic principles to avoid contributing to rising health care costs.
- The GNP reflects the market value of goods and services produced by the United States.
- The GDP reflects the market value of the output of labor and property located in the United States.
- Microeconomic theory shows how supply and demand can be used in health care.
- Macroeconomic theory helps one look at national and community issues that affect health care.
- Social issues, economic issues, and communicable disease epidemics mark the problems of the twenty-first century.
- Medicare and Medicaid are two government-funded programs that help meet the needs of high-risk populations in the United States.
- A majority of the U.S. population has had health insurance. It is now mandated by law and has a penalty if citizens are not covered.
- The uninsured segment represents millions of people, mostly the working poor, older adults, and children, and those who lost jobs in the economic downturn of 2008.
- Poverty has a detrimental effect on health.
- Health care rationing has always been a part of the U.S. health care system and will continue to be with health care reform.
- Nurses are cost-effective providers and must be an integral part of health care delivery.
- *Healthy People 2020* is a document that has established U.S. health objectives.
- Human life is valued in health economics, as is money. An emphasis on changing lifestyles and preventive care will reduce the unnecessary years of life lost to early and preventable death.

## CLINICAL DECISION-MAKING ACTIVITIES

1. Define the following terms in your own words: economics, health economics, public health economics, public health finance, gross national product, gross domestic product, consumer price index, and human capital. How do these terms relate to your work as a nurse?

2. Compare the advantages and disadvantages of applying economics to public health care issues. Be specific.

3. Compare and contrast efficiency and effectiveness of a public health program. What factors make these difficult to control?

## CLINICAL DECISION-MAKING ACTIVITIES—cont'd

4. Apply the concepts of supply and demand to an example from population health. Be precise in your answer.

5. Review Chapter 6. Debate in class the ethical implications of the goal of rationing. Focus your debate on the implications for nursing practice. What are some of the complexities of this question?

6. Invite a public health nurse administrator to meet with your class or clinical conference group. Ask how inflation, changes in population, and technology have changed the public health care delivery system and nursing practice. How could we check for ourselves to find the answers?

# REFERENCES

Affordable Care Act and Medicare: 2014. Retrieved December 2014 from: www.Medicare.gov.

Agency for Healthcare Research and Quality (AHRQ): *Guide to Clinical Preventive Services, 2014*. AHRQ Publication No. 14-05158. Rockville, MD, 2014, AHRQ.

American Association of Colleges of Nursing (AACN): *Nursing Shortage Fact Sheet*. Washington, DC, 2010, AACN.

American Nurses Association (ANA): *Medicare Reimbursement for NPs and CNSs*. Silver Spring, MD, 1999, ANA.

Buppert C: HEDIS for the primary care provider: getting an "A" on the managed care report card. *Nurse Pract* 24:84–94, 1999.

Centers for Disease Control and Prevention (CDC): *H1N1 Outbreaks*, 2009. Retrieved December 2014 from: http://www.cdc.gov.

Centers for Disease Control and Prevention (CDC): *Public Health Economists and Methods*, 2015. Retrieved January 2015from: http://www.cdc.gov.

Centers for Medicare and Medicaid Services (CMS), Office of the Actuary: *National Health Expenditure Projections 2011-2021*. Baltimore, MD, 2012a, U.S. Department of Health and Human Services. Retrieved December 2014 from: http://www.cms.gov/NationalHealthExpendData/.

Centers for Medicaid and Medicare Services (CMS): *Hospital Outpatient PPS*. Baltimore, MD, 2012b, U.S. Department of Health and Human Services. Retrieved December 2014 from: http://www.cms.gov/Medicare/Medicare-Fee-for-Service-Payment/HospitalOutpatientPPS/index.html?redirect=/HospitalOutpatientPPS/.

Centers for Medicaid and Medicare Services (CMS): *Skilled Nursing Facility PPS*. Baltimore, MD, 2012c, U.S. Department of Health and Human Services. Retrieved December 2014 from: http://www.cms.gov/Medicare/Medicare-Fee-for-Service-Payment/SNFPPS/index.html?redirect=/SNFPPS/.

Centers for Medicare and Medicaid Services (CMS): *MA Payment Guide for Out of Network Payments, 9/27/2013 Update*. Baltimore, MD, 2013a, U.S. Department of Health and Human Services. Retrieved December 2014 from: http://www.cms.gov/Medicare/Health-Plans/MedicareAdvtgSpecRateStats/Downloads/OONPayments.pdf.

Centers for Medicare and Medicaid Services (CMS): *Skilled Nursing Facility Prospective Payment System*. Baltimore, MD, 2013b, U.S. Department of Health and Human Services. Retrieved December 2014 from: http://www.cms.gov/Outreach-and-Education/Medicare-Learning-Network-MLN/MLNProducts/downloads/snfprospaymtfctsht.pdf.

Centers for Medicaid and Medicare Services (CMS): *CMS Fast Facts Overview*. 2014, U.S. Department of Health and Human Services. Retrieved December 2014 from: http://www.cms.gov/Research-Statistics-Data-and-Systems/Statistics-Trends-and-Reports/CMS-Fast-Facts/index.html.

Colander D: *Microeconomics*, ed 9. London, 2012, McGraw-Hill.

Community Preventive Services Task Force: *What Is the Task Force*. 2014. Retrieved December 2014 from: http://www.thecommunityguide.org/about/aboutTF.html.

Congressional Budget Office (CBO): *The Budget and Economic Outlook*. Washington, DC, 2010, U.S. Government Printing Office.

DeNavas-Walt C, Proctor BD, Smith JC: *Income, Poverty, and Health Insurance Coverage in the United States, 2012*. U.S. Census Bureau, Current Population Reports. Washington, DC, 2013, U.S. Government Printing Office, pp P60–P245.

Esperat MC, Hanson-Turton T, Richardson M, et al: Nurse-managed health centers: safety-net care through advanced nursing practice. *J Am Acad Nurse Pract* 24:24–31, 2012.

Feldstein PJ: *Health Care Economics*, ed 7. Clifton Park, NJ, 2012, Delmar Cengage Learning.

Flexner report. Birth of modern medical education. 1910, retrieved Jan 2015 at: MedicineNet.com.

Fortunato K, Sessions K: Philanthropy at the intersection of health and the environment. *Health Aff* 30:989–993, 2011.

Goodwin N, Harris J, Nelson J, et al: *Microeconomics in Context*, ed 3. New York, 2014, M.E. Sharpe, Inc.

Hall B: *A New Day: What the Patient Protection and Affordable Care Act Means to the Incentive Industry*. June/July 2010. Retrieved December 2014 from: www.incentivemag.com.

Health Care Financing Administration (HCFA): *Case Mix Prospective Payment for SNFs Balanced Budget Act of 1997*. Washington, DC, 1998, USDHHS.

Health Care Financing Administration (HCFA): *HIPAA: The Health Insurance Portability and Accountability Act of 1996*. Washington, DC, 1999, USDHHS.

Hicks L: *The Economics of Health and Medical Care*, ed 6. Boston, MA, 2012, Jones & Bartlett Learning.

Honoré PA: Measuring progress in public health finance. *J Public Health Manag Pract* 18:306–308, 2012.

Institute of Medicine: *The Future of the Public's Health in the 21st Century*. Washington, DC, 2003, National Academies Press.

Internal Revenue Service (IRS): *Health Savings Accounts and Other Tax-Favored Health Plans*. Publication No. 969. Washington, DC, 2012, IRS. Retrieved December 2014 from: http://www.irs.gov/pub/irs-pdf/p969.pdf.

Kaiser Family Foundation: *Medicare chart book*, ed 3. Menlo Park, CA, 2005, Kaiser Family Foundation.

Kaiser Family Foundation: *The Uninsured: A Primer: Key Facts about Americans without Health Insurance*. Menlo Park, CA, 2009, Kaiser Commission on Medicaid and the Uninsured.

Kaiser Family Foundation: *The Uninsured: A Primer: Key Facts about Americans without Health Insurance*. Menlo Park, CA, 2012a, Kaiser Commission on Medicaid and the Uninsured. Retrieved December 2014 from: http://kaiserfamilyfoundation.files.wordpress.com/2013/01/7451-08.pdf.

Kaiser Family Foundation: *Medicare Spending and Financing Fact Sheet*. Menlo Park, CA, 2012b, Kaiser Family Foundation. Retrieved December 2014 from: http://kff.org/medicare/fact-sheet/medicare-spending-and-financing-fact-sheet/.

Kaiser Family Foundation: *Employer Health Benefits Survey*. Menlo Park, CA, 2013, Kaiser Family Foundation.

Kaiser Family Foundation: *Medicaid Enrollment: June 2013 Data Snapshot, Jan 29, 2014*. Menlo Park, CA, 2014. Retrieved December 2014 from: http://kff.org/report-sectiuaryon/medicaid-enrollment-june-2013-data-snapshot-total-enrollment/.

Kovner AR, Knickman JR, Weisfeld VD: *Jonas and Kovner's Health Care Delivery in the United States*, ed 10. New York, 2011, Springer.

Lindemark F, Norheim OF, Johansson KA: Making use of equity sensitive QALYs: a case study on identifying the worse off across diseases. *Cost Eff Resour Alloc* 12:16, 2014.

Lockard CB, Wolf M: *Occupational Employment Projections to 2020*. 2012, Bureau of Labor Statistics. *Monthly Labor Review*. Retrieved December 2014 from: http://www.bls.gov/opub/mlr/2012/01/art5full.pdf.

McPake B, Normand C, Smith S: *Health Economics: An International Perspective*, ed 3. New York, 2013, Routledge.

National Center for Health Statistics (NCHS): *Health: United States, 2005, with Chartbook on Trends in the Health of Americans*. Hyattsville, MD, 2005, U.S. Government Printing Office.

National Center for Health Statistics (NCHS): *Health: United States, 2009, with Special Feature on Medical Technology*. Hyattsville, MD, 2010, U.S. Government Printing Office.

National Center for Health Statistics (NCHS): *Health: United States, 2011 with Special Feature on Socioeconomic Status and Health.* Hyattsville, MD, 2012, U.S. Government Printing Office.

National Center for Health Statistics (NCHS): *Health, United States, 2012: with Special Feature on Emergency Care.* Hyattsville, MD, 2013, U.S. Government Printing Office.

National Center for Health Statistics (NCHS): *Health, United States, 2013.* Hyattsville, MD, 2014, U.S. Government Printing Office.

Nichols LM, Blumberg LJ: A different kind of "new federalism"? The Health Insurance Portability and Accountability Act of 1996. *Health Aff* 17:25–42, 1998.

Patient Protection and Affordable Care Act (PL 111-148). March 2010. Retrieved December 2014 from www.healthcare.org.

Phelps CE: *Health Economics*, ed 5. Upper Saddle River, NJ, 2012, Prentice Hall.

Robert Wood Johnson Foundation (RWJF): *Cover the Uninsured,* 2009. Retrieved December 2014 from: www.covertheuninsured.org.

Robert Wood Johnson Foundation (RWJF): *Return on Investments in Public Health: Saving Lives and Money.* Princeton, NJ, 2012. Retrieved December 2014 from:

http://www.rwjf.org/content/dam/farm/reports/issue_briefs/2013/rwjf72446.

Robert Wood Johnson Foundation (RWJF): *Overcoming Obstacles to Health in 2013 and Beyond.* Princeton, NJ, 2013, RWJF. Retrieved December 2014 from: http://www.rwjf.org/content/dam/farm/reports/reports/2013/rwjf406474.

Shi L, Singh DA: *The Nation's Health,* ed 8. Sudbury, MA, 2011, Jones & Bartlett.

Strawser CJ: *Business Statistics of the United States, 2013: Patterns of Economic Change*, ed 18. Lanham, MD, 2014, Bernan Press.

Sturchio JL, Goel A: *The Private-Sector Role in Public Health: Reflections on the New Global Architecture in Health.* Washington, DC, 2012, Center for Strategic and International Studies. Retrieved December 2014 from: http://csis.org/files/publication/120131_Sturchio_PrivateSectorRole_Web.pdf.

Trust for America's Health: *Investing in America's Health: A State-by-State Look at Public Health Funding and Key Health Facts.* Washington, DC, 2013a, Trust for America's Health. Retrieved December 2014 from: http://healthyamericans.org/assets/files/

TFAH2013InvstgAmrcsHlth05%20FINAL.pdf.

Trust for America's Health: *A healthier America 2013: Strategies to Move from Sick Care to Health Care in the Next Four Years.* Washington, DC, 2013b, Trust for America's Health. Retrieved December 2014 from: http://healthyamericans.org/assets/files/TFAH2013HealthierAmericaFnlRv.pdf.

Trust for America's Health: *Key Health Data (by State): Public Health Funding Indicators.* 2014. Retrieved December 2014 from: http://healthyamericans.org/states/.

Turnock BJ: *Public Health: What It Is and How It Works*, ed 5. Boston, 2011, Jones & Bartlett.

U.S. Census Bureau: *Fueled by Aging Baby Boomers, Nation's Older Population to Nearly Double in Next 20 Years.* Census Report, 2014. Retrieved December 2014 from: http://www.census.gov/newsroom/press-releases/2014/cb14-84.html.

U.S. Department of Health and Human Services (USDHHS): *Healthy People 2020: A Roadmap to Improve All American's Health.* Washington, DC, 2010, USDHHS, Public Health Service.

U.S. Department of Health and Human Services (USDHHS):

*At Risk: Pre-Existing Conditions Could Affect 1 in 2 Americans: 129 Million People Could Be Denied Affordable Coverage without Health Reform,* 2011. Retrieved December 2014 from http://aspe.hhs.gov/health/reports/2012/pre-existing/.

U.S. Department of Health and Human Services (USDHHS): *2012 Medicare Costs.* Washington, DC, 2012. Retrieved July 2012 from: http://www.medicare.gov/cost/.

U.S. Department of Health and Human Services (USDHHS): *The ACA Prevention and Public Health Fund.* 2014a. Retrieved December 2014 from: HHS.gov.

U.S. Department of Health and Human Services (USDHHS): *HHS Federal Poverty Guidelines.* 2014b. Retrieved December 2014 from: HHS.gov.

U.S. Department of Health and Human Services (USDHHS): *Health, United States, 2013.* Publication No. 2014-1232. Rockville, MD, 2014c, Centers for Disease Control and Prevention, National Center for Health Statistics.

World Health Organization (WHO): *World Health Statistics, 2010.* Geneva, 2010, WHO.

# Application of Ethics in the Community

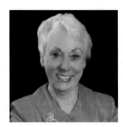

*Jeanette Lancaster, PhD, RN, FAAN\**

Dr. Lancaster is Professor and Dean Emerita of Nursing at the University of Virginia. She has edited this book with Dr. Marcia Stanhope through its previous eight editions.

## ADDITIONAL RESOURCES

Ⓔ **Evolve Website http://evolve.elsevier.com/Stanhope**
- *Healthy People 2020*
- WebLinks—Of special note, see the link for these sites:
  - International Council of Nurses Code of Ethics for Nurses
  - Nursing Ethics Column in Online Journal of Issues in Nursing
  - American Nurses Association Center for Ethics and Human Rights
- Kennedy Institute of Ethics: https://kennedyinstitute.georgetown.edu
- Bioethics Research Library at Georgetown University: https://bioethics.edu
- Bioethics Research at the Hastings Center
- Quiz
- Case Studies
- Glossary
- Answers to Practice Application

## OBJECTIVES

*After reading this chapter, the student should be able to do the following:*
1. Describe a brief history of the ethics of nursing practice.
2. Analyze ethical decision-making processes.
3. Compare and contrast ethical theories and principles, virtue ethics, caring and the ethic of care, and feminist ethics.
4. Comprehend the ethics inherent in the core functions of public health nursing.
5. Analyze codes of ethics for nursing and for public health.
6. Apply the ethics of advocacy to nursing practice.

## KEY TERMS

advocacy, p. 132
assessment, p. 129
assurance, p. 130
beneficence, p. 126
bioethics, p. 122
code of ethics, p. 123
communitarianism, p. 127
consequentialism, p. 125

deontology, p. 126
distributive justice, p. 126
ethical decision making, p. 123
ethical dilemmas, p. 124
ethical issues, p. 124
ethics, p. 125
feminine ethic, p. 129
feminist ethics, p. 129

---

\*Special thank you to Dr. Mary Silva who offered valuable guidance for the revision of this chapter.
A special thanks to James Fletcher, Mary Silva, and Jeanne Sorrell for the many contributions to this chapter in previous editions of the text.

The role of nurses who practice in the community is to focus on protecting, promoting, preserving, and maintaining health while preventing disease. These goals reflect the ethical principles of promoting good and preventing harm. In addition, nurses struggle with the rights of individuals and families versus the rights of local groups within a community. On the other hand, nurses struggle with the rights of a community or population versus the rights of individuals, families, and local groups within a community. These two types of struggle reflect the tensions among respect for autonomy, rights-based ethical theory, and community-based ethical theory.

Nurses also deal with consequence-based ethical theory, obligation-based ethical theory, and the ethical components of advocacy, justice, health policy, caring, women's moral experiences, and the moral character of health care practitioners. They are guided by codes of ethics and ethical decision-making frameworks. The purpose of this chapter, then, is to make explicit the preceding content as it relates to the ethics inherent in nursing.

## HISTORY

Chapter 2 discusses the history of public health nursing. The focus in this chapter is a brief history of nursing and public health ethics and the relationship between them and nursing.

Modern nursing has a rich heritage of ethics and morality, beginning with Florence Nightingale (1820 to 1910). Her values and the moral significance she inculcated into the profession have endured. She saw nursing as a call to service and viewed the moral character of persons entering nursing as important. She also viewed nursing within a broad social context, where

poor people mattered and where soldiers harmed in the Crimean War (1854 to 1856) did not have to endure unhealthy environments. Because of her commitment to poor individuals in communities, as well as her stances on primary prevention and on population-based evidence that healthy environments save soldiers' lives, she is seen as nursing's first enduring moral leader who defined the community as her client.

In 1860, Nightingale established the first nursing program in London. It was hospital based, but the curriculum contained not only care of the sick, but also public health concepts with their inherent ethical tenets. Many of these programs were associated with religious institutions. Students, therefore, often received ethics courses with a slant toward a particular religion's values. Soon thereafter in the United States, the notion of hospital-based nursing programs took hold, but nursing practice in the community was not a part of the curricula.

In the 1960s, two seminal events occurred. First, the American Nurses Association (ANA) recommended that all nursing education should occur in institutions of higher education. As this process slowly took place, ethics, as a course per se, was removed from many schools of nursing, although ethical values remained. Second, because of major advances in science and technology that affected health care, the field of bioethics began to emerge and was reflected in nursing curricula. Today, most nursing programs integrate bioethical content into their courses or have separate courses on this topic; some do both. Although some of these courses relate bioethics to community nursing, the emphasis has been primarily on acute care nursing.

Nurses' codes of ethics are important in the history of public health nursing practice. According to the American Nurses Association (ANA), the Nightingale Pledge is generally considered to be nursing's first code of ethics (ANA, 2001). After the Nightingale Pledge, a "suggested" code and a "tentative" code were published in the *American Journal of Nursing* but were not formally adopted. In 1950, the ANA House of Delegates formally adopted the *Code for Professional Nurses.* In 1956, 1960, 1968, 1976, 1985, and 2001 the code was amended or revised. After 5 years of work, the ANA House of Delegates adopted the Code of Ethics for Nurses with Interpretive Statements in 2001 (ANA, 2001). This code was revised in 2015 (ANA, 2015).

Nurses also should be familiar with the first known international code of ethics, developed by the International Council of Nurses (ICN) in 1953 (ICN, 1953). Like the ANA code, the ICN code has undergone various revisions and adoptions. The most recent version of the *ICN Code of Ethics for Nurses* was revised in 2012. This code makes it clear that nurses must respect human rights, including the right to life, to dignity, and to be treated with respect. The *ICN Code of Ethics for Nurses* has four principal elements that outline the standards of conduct. They are as follows: (1) nurses and people; (2) nurses and practice; (3) nurses and the profession; and (4) nurses and co-workers (ICN, 2012, pp. 2-4).

In addition to codes of ethics, the nursing literature and nursing associations have consistently reflected a commitment to ethics, as well as an awareness of nursing's ethical obligations to society. From the 1980s to the present, the number of centers for nursing and health care ethics has increased steadily. The majority of these centers are located in academic settings; however, in 1991 the ANA founded its Center for Ethics and Human Rights. The historical contributions of this center have affected the persistent ethicality of nursing. In 2008, the ANA published *Nursing and Health Care Ethics: A Legacy and a Vision,* which creatively assesses historical contributions of nursing scholars in ethics and explores a vision for the future scholarship of nursing ethics (Pinch and Haddad, 2008). Also in 2008, the ANA published *Guide to the Code of Ethics for Nurses: Interpretation and Application* (Fowler, 2008).

The bioethics movement of the late 1960s influenced not only nursing ethics, but also public health ethics. However, until recently, the relationship between public health and ethics was implicit rather than explicit (Callahan and Jennings, 2002; Petrini, 2010). The publication in 2015 of *Essentials of Public Health Ethics* by Bernheim and colleagues is a major contribution to describing the complex relationship between public health and ethics.

Finally, in 2000, public health professionals, individually and through their associations, initiated the writing of a code of ethics that was supported by the American Public Health Association (APHA). In 2001 the Public Health Code of Ethics was widely disseminated via the APHA website for critique (www.apha.org) and was adopted in 2002 (Olick, 2005). The code presents principles, rules, and ideals to guide public health practice but is not intended to provide a specific action plan for ethical decision making. Our language often programs us to think in terms of opposites, such as right or wrong, so that we think we need to choose one or the other. Often, there are more than two sides to an ethical issue. When we try to understand

## BOX 6-1 Key Ethical Terms

**Ethics** is a branch of philosophy that includes both a body of knowledge about the moral life and a process of reflection for determining what persons ought to do or be regarding this life.

**Bioethics** is a branch of ethics that applies the knowledge and processes of ethics to the examination of ethical problems in health care.

**Moral distress** is an uncomfortable state of self in which one is unable to act ethically.

**Morality** is shared and generational societal norms about what constitutes right or wrong conduct.

**Values** are beliefs about the worth or importance of what is right or esteemed.

**Ethical dilemma** is a puzzling moral problem in which a person, group, or community can envision morally justified reasons for both taking and not taking a certain course of action.

**Codes of ethics** are moral standards that delineate a profession's values, goals, and obligations.

**Utilitarianism** is an ethical theory based on the weighing of morally significant outcomes or consequences regarding the overall maximizing of good and minimizing of harm for the greatest number of people.

**Deontology** is an ethical theory that bases moral obligation on duty and claims that actions are obligatory irrespective of the good or harmful consequences that they produce. Because humans are rational, they have absolute value. Therefore, persons should always be treated as ends in themselves and never as mere means.

**Principlism** is an approach to problem solving in bioethics that uses the principles of respect for autonomy, beneficence, nonmaleficence, and justice as the basis for organization and analysis of ethical issues and dilemmas.

**Advocacy** is the act of pleading for or supporting a course of action on behalf of a person, group, or community.

the differing values of individuals and groups in a community, we find important points to consider on different sides of an ethical issue and focus not only on what we think is right, but also on what we should *respect* in each perspective of an ethical issue. As Bernheim and colleagues (2015, p. 3) point out, "Public health is an ethical enterprise, resting on moral foundations, yet some public health interventions appear to threaten or compromise other moral norms, such as liberty, privacy, and confidentiality." As is discussed later in this chapter, advances in social media pose ethical concerns about both privacy and confidentiality. Also, vulnerable or high-risk populations as discussed in Chapter 32 can pose ethical concerns and necessitate careful decision making by nurses. Gjengedal and colleagues (2013) point out that a key to acting ethically with vulnerable populations is to try to understand the clients from their perspective rather than from the perspective of the nurse that may be prejudiced.

Before discussing ethics related to nursing practice in the community, some key ethical terms are defined in Box 6-1. Other ethical terms are defined within the context of the chapter.

## ETHICAL DECISION MAKING

Ethical decision making is that component of ethics that focuses on the process of how ethical decisions are made. The process is the thinking that occurs when health care professionals must make decisions about ethical issues and ethical dilemmas. Ethical issues are moral challenges facing a person or a profession. In nursing, one such challenge is how to prepare an adequate and competent workforce for the future. In contrast, ethical dilemmas are human dilemmas and puzzling moral problems in which a person, group, or community can envision morally justified reasons for both taking and not taking a certain course of action. One example of an ethical dilemma is how to allocate resources to two equally needy populations when the resources are sufficient to serve only one of the populations. Ethical theories, principles, and decision-making frameworks help us think through these issues and dilemmas. In describing what ethics is, Bernheim and colleagues concentrate on normative ethics and say that in general terms, "normative ethics involves identifying and justifying moral norms regarding right and wrong, good and bad, and determining the meaning, range and strength of those moral norms for purposes of guiding human action" (2015, p. 4)

Ethical decision-making frameworks use problem-solving processes. They provide guides for making sound ethical decisions that can be morally justified. Many such frameworks exist in the health care literature, and some are presented in this chapter. A caveat, however, is in order. Weston (2006, p. 22) notes that the first requirement of ethics is to think appreciatively and carefully about moral matters. We should not simply obey rules or authorities without thinking for ourselves; thinking for ourselves is both a moral responsibility and a hard-won right.

Keeping the preceding caveat in mind, the following generic ethical decision-making framework is presented:
1. Identify the ethical issues and dilemmas.
2. Place them within a meaningful context.
3. Obtain all relevant facts.
4. Reformulate ethical issues and dilemmas, if needed.
5. Consider appropriate approaches to actions or options (such as utilitarianism, deontology, principlism, virtue ethics, caring and the ethic of care, feminist ethics).
6. Make a decision and take action.
7. Evaluate the decision and the action.

The steps of a generic ethics framework are often nonlinear, and, with the exception of step 5, they do not change substantially. The rationale for each of the seven steps is presented in Table 6-1. The six approaches to actions or options in the ethical decision-making framework (step 5) are outlined throughout the chapter in the How To Boxes.

Two factors affect this ethical decision-making framework: (1) the growing multiculturalism of the American society, and (2) moral distress. First, nurses often deal with ethical issues and dilemmas related to the diverse and at times conflicting values that result from ethnicity. From a moral perspective, what should the nurse do when facing ethnicity conflicts?

Callahan (2000) offers useful insights into these conflicts. He describes four situations in which ethnic diversity can be judged in relationship to cultural standards:
1. Situations that place persons at direct risk of harm, whether psychological or physical
2. Situations in which ethnic cultural standards conflict with professional standards

| TABLE 6-1 | **Rationale for Steps of Ethical Decision-Making Framework** |
|---|---|
| **Step** | **Rationale** |
| 1. Identify the ethical issues and dilemmas | Persons cannot make sound ethical decisions if they cannot identify ethical issues and dilemmas |
| 2. Place them within a meaningful context | The historical, legal, sociological, cultural, psychological, economic, political, communal, environmental, and demographic contexts affect the way ethical issues and dilemmas are formulated and justified |
| 3. Obtain all relevant facts | Facts affect the way ethical issues and dilemmas are formulated and justified |
| 4. Reformulate ethical issues and dilemmas if needed | The initial ethical issues and dilemmas may need to be modified or changed on the basis of context and facts |
| 5. Consider appropriate approaches to actions or options | The nature of the ethical issues and dilemmas determines the specific ethical approaches used |
| 6. Make decisions and take action | Professional persons cannot avoid choice and action in applied ethics |
| 7. Evaluate decisions and action | Evaluation determines whether or not the ethical decision-making framework used resulted in morally justified actions related to the ethical issues and dilemmas |

3. Situations in which the greater community's values are jeopardized by specific ethnic values
4. Situations in which specific ethnic community customs are annoying but not problematic for the greater community

Callahan (2000, p. 43) discusses how to judge diversity in the four situations. In situation 1, he says that "we in America imposed some standards on ourselves for important moral reasons; and there is no good reason to exempt [ethnic] subgroups from those standards." For situations 2 and 3, he suggests a thoughtful tolerance but also some degree of moral persuasion (not coercion) for ethnic groups to alter values so that they are more in keeping with what is normative in the American culture. However, Callahan says that "in the absence of grievous harm, there is no clear moral mandate to interfere with those values" (p. 43). Finally, regarding situation 4, he believes in moral tolerance of nonthreatening ethnic traditions, because there is no moral mandate to do otherwise.

Second, because decision making is central to the practice of nursing, and many decisions are difficult to make, it is useful to consider experience of ethical or moral distress. Moral or ethical distress occurs when a person is unable to act in a way that he or she thinks is right. You do not feel that you are able to act in a manner consistent with your own values, cultural expectations, and religious beliefs. When this conflict occurs, it can lead to a personal sense of failure in the kind of care you give and to subsequent performance issues and may lead to work and/or career dissatisfaction. However, there are ways to handle moral distress, as by (1) identifying the type(s) of situations that lead to distress; (2) communicating that concern to your manager and examining ways to work toward addressing the stressor; or (3) seeking support from colleagues. It is often useful to talk with colleagues. You may learn that they have similar concerns or that they have found ways to interrupt the stressful situation(s) (Carlock and Spader, 2007). Understanding both multiculturalism and moral distress aids in making ethical decisions.

Two cases are presented in later sections of the chapter. Examine each using the ethical decision-making processes outlined in the How To Boxes and the codes of ethics provided in the chapter. These cases provide an excellent opportunity to discuss with classmates your personal beliefs about the application of ethical processes and to assess your own thoughts, feelings, and possible actions. The cases deal with what the nurse's response should be when (1) the question arises about whether a parent can adequately care for a young child or the child should be removed from the mother, and (2) a client is not able or willing to take personal responsibility and does not want the nurse to report the situation. The Evidence-Based Practice box provides a summary of a research study that examined conflicting ethical concerns.

## EVIDENCE-BASED PRACTICE

Park (2013) developed and evaluated a case-based computer program to teach nursing students to effectively make ethical decisions. She used seven ethical cases chosen from 18 possible cases that were developed by practicing nurses and a six-step Integrated Ethical Decision-Making Model developed by the author. Interviews with the practicing nurses concerned ethical cases they had encountered as well as practical moral issues they had experienced. A total of 251 undergraduate students from three nursing schools used the program in their nursing ethics course. The program used in this study was based on *Principles of Biomedical Ethics* introduced by Beauchamp and Childress (2008). These principles are discussed in the chapter and they include autonomy, nonmaleficence, beneficence, justice, fidelity, veracity, and confidentiality. A goal of the program was for the students to learn to make an ethical decision justifiable in a real setting by applying ethical knowledge and critical thinking. The six steps of the Integrated Ethical Decision-Making Model were as follows: (1) the identification of an ethical program; (2) the collection of additional information to identify the problem and develop solutions; (3) the development of alternatives for analysis and comparison; (4) the section of the best alternatives and justification; (5) the development of diverse, practical ways to implement ethical decisions and actions; and (6) the evaluation of the effects and development of strategies to prevent a similar occurrence of the problem.

The study demonstrated that a case-based computer approach could successfully replicate real-world ethical case vignettes in a structured decision-making process. The users said the program was helpful to them in ethical decision making.

From Ulrich C, O'Donnell P, Taylor C, et al: Ethical climate, ethics stress, and the job satisfaction of nurse and social workers in the United States, Soc Sci Med 65(8):1708–1719, 2007.

## ETHICS

### Definition, Theories, Principles

Ethics is concerned with a body of knowledge that addresses questions such as the following: How should I behave? What actions should I perform? What kind of person should I be? What are my obligations to myself and to fellow humans? There

are general obligations that humans have as members of society. Among these general obligations are not to harm others, to respect others, to tell the truth, and to keep promises. Sometimes, however, a situation dictates that a person tell a lie or break a promise because the consequences of telling the truth or keeping the promise may bring about more harm than good. For example, as a nurse you have promised a family that you will visit them at a certain time, but your schedule has gone awry because of unexpected circumstances. One of the other families you visit is in a state of crisis—their adolescent child is suicidal—and your nursing intervention is needed. Most nurses would agree that this is not a good time to keep the original promise. You are morally justified in breaking your promise because you fear that more harm than good would be done if the promise were kept.

---

**HOW TO** Apply the Utilitarian Ethics Decision Process

1. *Determine moral rules that are important to society and that are derived from the principle of utility.**
2. *Identify the communities or populations that are affected or most affected by the moral rules.*
3. *Analyze viable alternatives for each proposed action based on the moral rules.*
4. *Determine the consequences or outcomes of each viable alternative on the communities or populations most affected by the decision.*
5. *Select the actions on the basis of the rules that produce the greatest amount of good or the least amount of harm for the communities or populations that are affected by the actions.*

*(Remember that the utilitarian ethics decision process is one of the approaches in step 5 of the generic ethical decision-making framework.)*

---

*\*Moral rules of action that produce the greatest good for the greatest number of communities or populations affected by or most affected by the rules.*

---

This example of promise breaking illustrates several things about ethical thinking. First, ethical judgments are concerned with values. The goal of an ethical judgment is to choose that action or state of affairs that is good or is right in the circumstances. Second, ethical judgments generally do not have the certainty of scientific judgments. For example, nurses diagnose an ethical situation on the basis of the best available information and then choose the course of action that seems to provide the best ethical resolution to the situation. In some situations, the decision is based on outcomes or consequences. That approach to ethical decision making is called consequentialism. It maintains that the right action is the one that produces the greatest amount of good or the least amount of harm in a given situation. Utilitarianism is a well-known consequentialist theory that appeals exclusively to outcomes or consequences in determining which choice to make.

In other situations, nurses touch on options open to fundamental beliefs. In such circumstances, these nurses may conclude that the action is right or wrong in itself, regardless of the amount of good that might come from it. This is the position known as **deontology**. It is based on the premise that persons should always be treated as ends in themselves and never as mere means to the ends of others. Deontological theory is often called nonconsequentialist. It is a "theory of duty holding that some features of actions other than or in addition to consequences make actions right or wrong" (Beauchamp and Childress, 2013, p. 361).

---

**HOW TO** **Apply the Deontological Ethics Decision Process**

1. *Determine the moral rules (e.g., tell the truth) that serve as standards by which individuals can perform their moral obligations.*
2. *Examine personal motives for proposed actions to ensure that they are based on good intentions in accord with moral rules.*
3. *Determine whether the proposed actions can be generalized so that all persons in similar situations are treated similarly.*
4. *Select the action that treats persons as ends in themselves and never as mere means to the ends of others.*
   *(Remember that the deontological ethics decision process is one of the approaches in step 5 of the generic ethical decision-making framework.)*

---

Members of the health professions have specific obligations that exist because of the practices and goals of the profession. These health care obligations have been interpreted in terms of a set of principles in bioethics. The primary principles are **respect for autonomy**, **nonmaleficence**, **beneficence**, and **distributive justice** as shown in Box 6-2. These principles are "general guidelines for the formulation of more specific rules" (Beauchamp and Childress, 2013, p. 13). This approach has been called **principlism**, and is clearly discussed in the seventh edition of *Principles of Biomedical Ethics* by Beauchamp and Childress (2013). This approach to ethical decision making in health care arose in response to life-and-death decision making in acute care settings, where the question to be resolved tended to concern a single localized issue such as the withdrawing or withholding of treatment (Holstein, 2001). In these circumstances, preserving and respecting a client's autonomy became the dominant issue. According to Beauchamp and Childress (2013), these four clusters of moral principles are central to the field of biomedical ethics. Principles are more general guides than are rules. Principlism is a "theory about how principles link to and guide practice" (Beauchamp and Childress, 2013, p. 25).

Despite its success as a basis for analysis in bioethics, principlism has come under attack (e.g., Callahan, 2000, 2003; Walker, 2009), and there are grounds for the criticism. First, the principles are said to be too abstract and narrow to serve as guides for action. Second, the principles themselves can conflict in a given situation, and there is no independent basis for resolving the conflict. Third, some persons claim that effective ethical problem solving must be rooted in concrete, individual experiences. Fourth, ethical judgments are alleged to depend more on the judgment of sensitive persons than on the application of abstract principles. The How To Box below can serve as a guide for how to use the principlism ethics decision process.

---

**HOW TO** **Apply the Principlism Ethics Decision Process**

1. *Determine the ethical principles (respect for autonomy, nonmaleficence, beneficence, justice) that are relevant to an ethical issue or dilemma.*
2. *Analyze the relevant principles within a meaningful context of accurate facts and other pertinent circumstances.*
3. *Act on the principle that provides, within the meaningful context, the strongest guide to action that can be morally justified by the tenets foundational to the principle.*
   *(Remember that the principlism ethics decision process is one of the approaches in step 5 of the general ethical decision-making framework.)*

---

**BOX 6-2** **Ethical Principles**

**Respect for autonomy:** Based on human dignity and respect for individuals, autonomy requires that individuals be permitted to choose those actions and goals that fulfill their life plans unless those choices result in harm to another.

**Nonmaleficence:** Nonmaleficence requires that we do no harm. It may be impossible to avoid harm entirely, but this principle requires that health care professionals act according to the standards of due care, always seeking to produce the least amount of harm possible.

**Beneficence:** This principle is complementary to nonmaleficence and requires that we do good. We are limited by time, place, and talents in the amount of good we can do. We have general obligations to perform those actions that maintain or enhance the dignity of other persons whenever those actions do not place an undue burden on health care providers.

**Distributive justice:** Distributive justice requires that there be a fair distribution of the benefits and burdens in society based on the needs and contributions of its members. This principle requires that, consistent with the dignity and worth of its members and within the limits imposed by its resources, a society must determine a minimal level of goods and services to be available to its members.*

Modified from Bateman N: *Advocacy Skills for Health and Social Care Professionals*. Philadelphia, PA, 2000, Jessica Kingsley, p 63.
*In public health nursing client may be a person, group, or community.

The dominance of the principle of respect for autonomy has been challenged by critics concerned about decision making in non–acute care settings, where the ethical decision is more likely to be about, for example, long-term care or access to health care for persons of diverse cultures (Callahan and Jennings, 2002; Walker, 2009). Thus, whereas autonomy may be stressed in acute care settings, an overemphasis on autonomy may inhibit ethical decisions in public health. In public health, beneficence and distributive justice are frequently a greater issue than autonomy. For this reason, it is useful to look at other models for ethical decision making, including models that expand the focus of nursing beyond the individual nurse-client relationship to the social environment and systems that impact health care (Bekemeier and Butterfield, 2005).

Utilitarianism and deontology were developed from the Age of Enlightenment's focus on universals, rationality, and isolated individuals. Each theory maintains that there is a universal first principle—the principle of utility for utilitarianism and the categorical imperative for deontology—that serves as a rational norm for our behavior and allows us to calculate the rightness or wrongness of each individual action. Both utilitarianism and deontology also follow the lead of classic liberalism in asserting that the individual is the special center of moral concern (Steinbock et al, 2008). Giving priority to individual rights and needs means that these should not be sacrificed for the interests of society (Steinbock et al, 2008). The focus on individual rights leads to complications in the interpretation of distributive or social justice.

Public health ethics rests on a set of general moral considerations. Bernheim and colleagues (2015, p. 21) identify nine moral considerations in public health: (1) producing benefits; (2) avoiding, preventing, and removing harms; (3) producing the maximal balance of benefits over harms and other costs (often called utility); (4) distributing benefits and burdens fairly (distributive justice); (5) respecting autonomous choices and actions, including liberty of actions; (6) protecting privacy and confidentiality; (7) keeping promises and commitments; (8) disclosing information as well as speaking honestly and truthfully (often grouped under transparency); and (9) building trust. These nine moral considerations in public health nursing are easy to apply. Distributive justice, or *social justice*, refers to the allocation of benefits and burdens to members of society. Benefits refer to basic needs, including material and social goods, liberties, rights, and entitlements. Wealth, education, and public services are benefits. Burdens include such things as taxes, military service, and the locations of incinerators and power plants. Justice requires that the distribution of benefits and burdens in a society be fair or equal. There is wide agreement that the distribution should be based on what one needs and deserves, but there is considerable disagreement as to what these terms mean. Three primary theories of distributive justice that are defended today include egalitarian, libertarian, and liberal democratic theories.

*Egalitarianism* is the view that everyone is entitled to equal rights and equal treatment in society. Ideally, each person has an equal share of the goods of society, and it is the role of government to ensure that this happens. The government has the authority to redistribute wealth if necessary to ensure equal treatment. Thus, egalitarians are supportive of welfare rights—that is, the right to receive certain social goods necessary to satisfy basic needs, including adequate food, housing, education, and police and fire protection. The weaknesses of egalitarianism are both practical and theoretical. It would be practically impossible to ensure the equal distribution of goods and services in any moderately complex society. Assuming that such a distribution could be accomplished, it would require a coercive authority to maintain it (Coursin, 2009; Hellsten, 1998). Further, egalitarianism is unable to provide any incentive for each of us to do our best, because there is no promise of our merit being rewarded.

The *libertarian* view of justice holds that the right to private property is the most important right. Libertarians recognize only liberty rights—the right to be left alone to accomplish our goals. Hellsten (1998, p. 822) notes, "The central feature of the libertarian view on distributive justice is that it is totally individualist. It rejects any idea that societies, states, or collectives of any form can be the bearers of rights or can owe duties." Libertarians see a limited role for government, namely, the protection of property rights of individual citizens through providing police and fire protection. While they also concede the need for jointly shared, publicly owned facilities such as roads, they reject the idea of welfare rights and view taxes to support the needs of others as coercive taking of their property. Given the libertarian rejection of the priority of the state, however, it is not clear where the right to property originates (Hellsten, 1998).

The work of John Rawls (2001) represents the *liberal democratic* theory. Rawls attempts to develop a theory that values both liberty and equality. He acknowledges that inequities are inevitable in society, but he tries to justify them by establishing a system in which everyone benefits, especially the least advantaged. This is an attempt to address the inequalities that result from birth, natural endowments, and historic circumstances. Imagining what he calls a "veil of ignorance" to keep us unaware of our actual advantages and disadvantages, Rawls would have us choose the basic principles of justice (p. 15). Once impartiality is guaranteed, Rawls (2001, p. 42) maintains that all rational people will choose a system of justice containing the following two basic principles:

> *Each person has the same indefeasible claim to a fully adequate scheme of equal basic liberties, which scheme is compatible with the same scheme of liberties for all; and social and economic inequalities are to satisfy two conditions: first, they are to be attached to offices and positions open to all under conditions of fair equality of opportunity; and second, they are to be to the greatest benefit of the least advantaged members of society (the difference principle).*

As the veil of ignorance and the justice principles indicate, Rawls and other justice theorists all assume the Enlightenment concept of isolated, atomic selves in competition for scarce resources. The significance of justice, then, becomes the assurance of fairness to individuals. Violating the dictates of distributive justice is an offense to the dignity of the collective preferences of autonomous, rational moral agents. The interests of the community may be in conflict with the interests of individuals; yet, confined to the Enlightenment ideal, the needs of society are not directly addressed, nor is society given any priority.

This Enlightenment assumption has been challenged by a number of ethical theories loosely grouped together under the heading communitarianism. The dominant themes of communitarianism are that individual rights need to be balanced with social responsibilities; individuals do not live in isolation but are shaped by the values and culture of their communities (Wringe, 2006). Among the theories with a communitarian focus are virtue ethics, caring and the ethic of care, and feminist ethics.

## Virtue Ethics

Virtue ethics is one of the oldest ethical theories; it belongs to a tradition dating back to the ancient Greek philosophers Plato and Aristotle. It is not concerned with actions, as utilitarianism and deontology are, but instead asks: What kind of person should I be? The goal of virtue ethics is to enable persons to flourish as human beings. According to Aristotle, virtues are acquired, excellent traits of character that dispose humans to act in accord with their natural good. During the seventeenth and eighteenth centuries, the Greek concept of the good as a principle of explanation went out of favor. In public health nursing the virtue of care, or caring, is central to professional ethics. "The ethics of care emphasizes traits valued in intimate personal relationships such as sympathy, compassion, fidelity and love" (Beauchamp and Childress, 2013, p. 35). Caring refers to the "emotional commitment to, and willingness to act on behalf of, persons with whom one has a significant relationship" (Beauchamp and Childress, 2013, p. 35). Beauchamp and Childress (2013) examine five focal virtues for health professionals. They are (1) compassion, which focuses on the pain, suffering, disability, and misery of another person; (2) discernment, which involves the ability to use sensitive insight, astute judgment, and understanding to make good decisions; (3) trustworthiness, which is essential in health care when clients put themselves in the hands of others; (4) integrity, with a differentiation between moral integrity and professional integrity; and (5) conscientiousness, which is the character trait of acting to achieve what one believes to be the right thing to do given the circumstances. The appeal to virtues results in a significantly different approach to moral decision making in health care (Olson, 2008). In contrast to moral justification via theories or principles, the emphasis is on practical reasoning applied to character development.

---

| **HOW TO**   Apply the Virtue Ethics Decision Process |

*1. Identify communities that are relevant to the ethical dilemmas or issues.*
*2. Identify moral considerations that arise from a communal perspective and apply the consideration to specific communities.*
*3. Identify and apply virtues that facilitate a communal perspective.*
*4. Modify moral considerations as needed to apply to the specific ethical dilemmas or issues.*
*5. Seek ethical community support to enhance character development.*
*6. Evaluate and modify the individual or community character traits that impede communal living.*
*(Remember that the virtue ethics decision process is one of the approaches in step 5 of the generic ethical decision-making framework.)*

---

Modified from Volbrecht RM: Nursing Ethics: Communities in Dialogue. *Upper Saddle River, NJ, 2002, Prentice Hall, p 138.*

## Caring and the Ethic of Care

Caring in nursing, the ethic of care, and feminist ethics are all interrelated and, historically, all converged between the mid-1980s and early 1990s. Seminal work in caring in nursing was done by nurse-scholars (e.g., Leininger, 1984; Watson, 2007), who wrote about caring as the essence of or the moral ideal of nursing. This conceptualization occurred as a response to the

technological advances in health care science and to the desire of nurses to differentiate nursing practice from medical practice. The discussion of the centrality of caring to nursing is reflected in Eriksson's (2002) work on a caring science theory, which she sees as ethical in its essence. Proponents of caring support its premises; its detractors believe that nursing is not the only essentially caring profession and that caring, when placed within a broader societal context, represents the use of a disempowering concept to identify the essence of nursing. However, most nurses, including those who work in the community, would agree that there is a relationship between caring and ethics or morality.

---

| **HOW TO**   Apply the Care Ethics Decision Process |

*1. Recognize that caring is a moral imperative.*
*2. Identify personally lived caring experiences as a basis for relating to self and others.*
*3. Assume responsibility and obligation to promote and enhance caring in relationships.*
*(Remember that the care ethics decision process is one of the approaches in step 5 of the generic ethical decision-making framework.)*

---

Carol Gilligan (1982) and Nel Noddings (1984) are often associated with the *ethic of care.* Gilligan (1982) speaks of a personal journey wherein, by listening and talking to people, she began to notice two distinct voices about morality and two ways of describing the interpersonal relationships between self and others. Contrary to what has been written about Gilligan and the two distinct voices (i.e., male and female) related to moral judgment, here is what she actually wrote: "The different voice I describe is characterized *not by gender* [italics added] but theme. Its association with women is an empirical observation, and it is primarily through women's voices that I trace its development. But this association is not absolute, and the contrasts between male and female voices are presented here to highlight a distinction between two modes of thought and to focus [on] a problem of interpretation rather than to represent a generalization about either sex" (Gilligan, 1982, p. 2). Her 1982 book is based on three qualitative studies about conceptions of morality and self and about experiences of conflict and choice. She discovered what she calls the "voice of care" through interviews with girls and women (Beauchamp and Childress, 2013). She identified two modes of moral thinking: an ethic of care and an ethic of rights and justice. Although she did not say that these two modes correlated with gender, she did maintain that men tended to be involved with the ethic of rights and justice whereas women were more likely to affirm an ethic of care centering on responsiveness in "an interconnected network of needs, care, and prevention of harm" (Beauchamp and Childress, 2013, p. 35). From these studies she formulated her basic premises about responsibility, care, and relationships. These premises, in Gilligan's (1982) own voice, are as follows:

- "Sensitivity to the needs of others and the assumption of responsibility for taking care lead women to attend to voices other than their own" (p. 16).

- "Women not only define themselves in a context of human relationships but also judge themselves in terms of their ability to care" (p. 17).
- "The truths of relationship, however, return in the rediscovery of connection, in the realization that self and other are interdependent and that life, however valuable in itself, can only be sustained by care in relationships" (p. 127).

Noddings' (1984) personal journey started at a point different from that of Gilligan's. Noddings noticed that ethics was described in the literature primarily on the basis of principles and logic. The goal for Noddings' book, therefore, was to express a feminine view that could be accepted or rejected by women or men.

The basic premises of Noddings (1984), in her own voice, are as follows:

- "The essential elements of caring are located in the relation between the one caring and the cared-for" (p. 9).
- "Caring requires me to respond with an act of commitment: I commit myself either to overt action on behalf of the cared-for or I commit myself to thinking about what I might do" (p. 81).
- "We are not 'justified'—we are obligated—to do what is required to maintain and enhance caring" (p. 95).
- "Caring itself and the ethical ideal that strives to maintain and enhance it guide us in moral decisions and conduct" (p. 105).

What both Gilligan and Noddings have in common has been called a feminine ethic, because they believe in the morality of responsibility in relationships that emphasize connection and caring. To them, caring is not a mere nicety but a moral imperative. Nevertheless, a long-term healthy debate has surrounded their premises.

---

**❚ HOW TO  Apply the Feminist Ethics Decision Process**

*1. Identify the social, cultural, legal, political, economic, environmental, and professional contexts that contribute to the identified problem (e.g., underrepresentation of women in clinical trials).*

*2. Evaluate how the preceding contexts contribute to the oppression of women.*

*3. Consider how women's lives are defined by their status in subordinate social groups.*

*4. Analyze how social practices marginalize women.*

*5. Plan ways to restructure those social practices that oppress women.*

*6. Implement the plan.*

*7. Evaluate the plan and restructure it as needed.*

*(Remember that the feminist ethics decision process is one of the approaches in step 5 of the generic ethical decision-making framework.)*

Modified from Volbrecht RM: Nursing Ethics: Communities in Dialogue. *Upper Saddle River, NJ, 2002, Prentice Hall, p 219.*

---

## Feminist Ethics

Although feminist ethics finally has entered nursing, for many years, nurses appeared reluctant to embrace feminism and its ethics (Silva, 2008). According to Rogers (2006), the tenets of feminist ethics are relevant to public health. Rogers notes that a feminist perspective leads us to think critically about connections among gender, disadvantage, and health, as well as the distribution of power in public health processes. Because these issues affect health, feminist perspectives and approaches are important for nursing practice.

What is meant by feminists and feminist ethics? **Feminists** are women and men who hold a worldview advocating economic, social, and political equality for women that is equivalent to that of men. Consequently, feminists reject the devaluing of women and their experiences through systematic oppression based on gender. In analyzing the common good, feminists pay careful attention to power relations that constitute a community, to the rules that regulate it, and to who pays and who benefits from membership in the community (Rogers, 2006). Feminists also can ascribe to the ethic of care.

**Feminist ethics** encompasses the tenets that women's thinking and moral experiences are important and should be taken into account in any fully developed moral theory, and that the oppression of women is morally wrong. Study of feminist ethics entails knowledge about and critique of classical ethical theories developed by men as well as ethical theories developed by women. Study of feminist ethics includes knowledge about the social, cultural, political, legal, economic, environmental, and professional contexts that insidiously and overtly oppress women as individuals, or within a family, group, community, or society. Feminists and persons who ascribe to feminist ethics are not passive; they demand social justice and political action, preferably at the societal level and through legislation.

## ETHICS AND THE CORE FUNCTIONS OF POPULATION-CENTERED NURSING PRACTICE

The three core functions of public health nursing (i.e., assessment, policy development, and assurance) are discussed in Chapter 1. This discussion, however, did not stress the basic assumption that public health nursing is an ethical endeavor, with moral leadership at its core. Now the links of these three core functions to ethics are described.

### Assessment

To review, "**assessment** refers to systematically collecting data on the population, monitoring the population's health status, and making information available about the health of the community" (see Chapter 1). Three ethical tenets underlie this core function. The first relates to competency related to knowledge development, analysis, and dissemination. An ethical question related to competency is: Are the persons assigned to develop community knowledge adequately prepared to collect data on groups and populations? This question is important because the research, measurement, and analysis techniques used to gather information about groups and populations usually differ from the techniques used to assess individuals. Wrong research techniques can lead to wrong assessments, which in turn may hurt rather than help the intended group or population. A startling example of this is the case of Henrietta Lacks, whose cancerous cervical cells were taken without her or her family's knowledge or permission and have now launched a medical revolution and a multimillion-dollar industry as the HeLa cells used in countless medical experiments (Skloot, 2010).

The second ethical tenet relates to virtue ethics or moral character. An ethical question related to moral character is: Do the persons selected to develop, assess, and disseminate community knowledge possess integrity? Beauchamp and Childress (2013) define integrity as the holistic integration of moral character. The importance of this virtue is self-evident: without integrity, the core function of assessment is endangered. Persons with compromised integrity are easy prey for potential or real scientific misconduct. An example of a failure of integrity for nurses would be bias in collecting or reporting based on racism or homophobic grounds.

The third ethical tenet relates to "do no harm." An ethical question related to "do no harm" is: Is disseminating appropriate information about groups and populations morally necessary and sufficient? The answer to "morally necessary" is yes, but to "morally sufficient," it is no. The fallacy with dissemination is that there is no built-in accountability that what is disseminated will be read or understood. If not read or understood, harm could come to groups and populations regarding their health status.

## Policy Development

To review, "policy development refers to the need to provide leadership in developing policies that support the health of the population, including the use of the scientific knowledge base in making decisions about policy" (see Chapter 1). At least three ethical tenets underlie this core function. First, an important goal of both policy and ethics is to achieve the public good (Silva, 2002). Denhardt and Denhardt (2000), Rogers (2006), and Ruger (2008) among others say that the concept of "the public good" is rooted in citizenship. For example, Denhardt and Denhardt (2000) view citizenship, or what they call "democratic citizenship" (p. 552), as a stance in which citizens play a more substantial role in policy development. For this to occur, citizens must be willing to be both informed about policy, and to do what is in the best interests of the community. The approach is basically one in which the voice of the community is the foundation on which policy is developed, rather than the voice of community and public health administrators.

The second ethical tenet purports that service to others over self is a necessary condition of what is "good" or "right" policy (Silva, 2002). Denhardt and Denhardt (2000) offer three perspectives on this matter:

- *Serve rather than steer.* An increasingly important role of the public servant (e.g., nurses and administrators) is to help citizens articulate and meet their shared interests rather than to attempt to control or steer society in new directions (p. 553).
- *Serve citizens, not customers.* The public interest results from a dialogue about shared values rather than the aggregation of individual self-interests. Therefore, public servants do not merely respond to the demands of "customers" but focus on building relationships of trust and collaboration with and among citizens (p. 555).
- *Value citizenship and public service above entrepreneurship.* The public interest is better advanced by public servants and

citizens committed to making meaningful contributions to society rather than by entrepreneurial managers acting as if public money were their own (p. 556).

Service is at the core of these three perspectives, and service has always been one of the enduring values of nursing.

The third ethical tenet holds that what is ethical is also good policy (Silva, 2002). What is ethical should be the singular foundational pillar on which nursing is based. Moral leadership is critical to policy development because it is the highest human standard and therefore should result in ethical health care policies.

## Assurance

To review, "assurance refers to the role of public health in ensuring that essential community-oriented health services are available, which may include providing essential personal health services for those who would otherwise not receive them. Assurance also refers to making sure that a competent public health and personal health care workforce is available" (see Chapter 1). At least two ethical tenets underlie this core function.

The first purports that all persons should receive essential personal health services or, put in terms of justice, "to each person a fair share" or, reworded, "to all groups or populations a fair share." This is an egalitarian perspective of justice. This perspective does not mean that all persons in a society should share all of society's benefits equally, but that they should share at least those benefits that are essential. People who see justice as fairness often think that basic health care for all is essential for social justice within a society. The case in Box 6-3 provides an example where the nurse needs to balance the client's right to autonomy and the principle of distributive justice.

The second ethical tenet purports that providers of public health services be competent and available. Although the Public Health Code of Ethics (Public Health Leadership Society [PHLS], 2002) does not speak directly to workforce availability, it does speak directly to ensuring professional competency of public health employees. In addition to the Public Health Code of Ethics, the *Healthy People 2020* objectives (U.S. Department of Health and Human Services [USDHHS], 2010) addresses competencies and workforce needs; a new objective (HP 2020-6) calls for an increased number of health care professionals certified in geriatrics.

The *Healthy People 2020* objectives address the need for all public health workers not only to have knowledge of public health, but also to have additional competencies as needed to fulfill their job responsibilities. Specific areas of knowledge include information technology, biostatistics, environmental health, cultural and linguistic competence, and genomics. The objectives also address needs of future public health leaders, who must be educated to meet new challenges in health care. Emphasis is also given to the availability and provision of lifelong learning opportunities for public health employees.

## NURSING CODE OF ETHICS

As noted in the history section of this chapter, the Code of Ethics for Nurses with Interpretive Statements was adopted by

Amelia Lewis, a 31-year-old African American woman with multiple mental health diagnoses, has been monitored in the local mental health system for over 10 years. She is the mother of Tyesha, who is 3 years old. Multiple agencies have monitored Ms. Lewis and her little girl, who live in a sparsely furnished apartment in subsidized housing. A guardian handles all of Ms. Lewis's financial affairs. Ms. Lewis's relationship with the father of Tyesha has deteriorated, and he does not live with her.

Ms. Lewis has issues of trust, and she is often suspicious of the care providers who come to her home. She does rely on some of the professionals with whom she interacts on a weekly or biweekly basis. She is both cognitively delayed and suffers from schizophrenia. Her developmental level places her at a stage at which her own needs are her primary focus, and this is not expected to change; her interaction with Tyesha is perfunctory, involving little outward affection. She is unable to understand that Tyesha is not capable of self-care and that her 3-year-old child will not always obey when Ms. Lewis instructs her to do something. Tyesha's needs, level of functioning, and cognitive development are quickly surpassing her mother's ability to cope. Frustration and misunderstanding ensue when Ms. Lewis thinks that Tyesha does not listen to her, and encouragement and parent education have done little to improve the situation as Tyesha gets older and more assertive. This has made toilet training, provision of an appropriate diet, and other aspects of normal child care problematic.

Many services besides those for mental health are involved to help this family of two cope. There is concern about abuse or neglect of Tyesha due to Ms. Lewis's lack of understanding of how to be a parent. Supplemental Security Income provides monetary support because of her mental disability and they have Medicaid coverage for their health care needs, as well as food stamps and modest financial assistance through Temporary Assistance for Needy Families (TANF). Ms. Lewis cannot currently work and take care of her child due to her mental disability. Before Tyesha's birth, Ms. Lewis held a job and maintained self-care, but the care of Tyesha has precluded her managing employment at this time. Child Protective Services are also monitoring Ms. Lewis's situation to determine to what extent she can meet the needs of her child. Ms. Lewis attends a local program to complete her General Education Development (GED), which provides child care during the day. Though Ms. Lewis is not expected to complete her GED, this program provides structured time for Tyesha three times a week. The child is considered developmentally normal at this time, and an infant development program monitors her progress on developmental issues. The Child Health Partnership, an agency that addresses the needs of challenged families, provides regular visits, family support, and parenting education, and the GED teachers make regular home visits to check on Ms. Lewis and Tyesha. Ms. Lewis thinks things are going just fine.

The Child Health Partnership nurse is concerned about this family and thinks that some permanent resolution of the situation is inevitable. There is minimal coordination of services and there is no "lead agency" in the family's care. Choose one of the ethical decision processes or one set of code of ethics discussed in the chapter and discuss and debate these questions:

1. Should the nurse involved in the Child Health Partnership program initiate any action to try to coordinate the work of the many agencies involved with this family?
2. Who has a professional responsibility to determine when the mother can no longer cope with the developing child?
3. Whose needs, Ms. Lewis's or Tyesha's, should take precedence?
4. Using one of the ethics decision processes, analyze the role of the nurse in this situation. For example, considering the utilitarian ethics decision process, decide if it is morally right for you to take the child away from the mother? If you do this, what are the implications for the mother, the child, and the community? What would be the possible consequences of removing the child? Of not removing the child? What principles can best guide your decision making? What possible moral dilemmas will you experience?
5. Safety is a core concept of public health nursing. Using two of the six quality and safety competences (patient-centered care and safety) for nurses identified in the *Quality and Safety Education for Nurses (QSEN)* work, develop a plan of action for the nurse who is caring for this family.

Created by Mary E. Gibson, Assistant Professor, School of Nursing, University of Virginia.

the ANA House of Delegates in 2001. The Code was revised in 2015 and consists of nine provisions and the accompanying interpretive statements. The Code provides the following:

- A succinct statement of the ethical values, obligations and duties of every individual who enters the nursing profession
- Serves as the profession's nonnegotiable ethical standard
- Expresses nursing's own understanding of its commitment to society (p. 5)

These purposes are reflected in the nine provisional statements of the code. The Code of Ethics for Nurses and its interpretive statements apply to population-centered nurses, although the emphasis for each type of nursing sometimes varies (for the ANA Code of Ethics for Nurses, see http://www.nursingworld.org/MainMenuCategories/Ethics Standards/CodeofEthicsforNurses.aspx).

As previously noted, the American Nurses Association has produced a *Guide to the Code of Ethics for Nurses: Interpretation and Application*, which serves as a companion reader to the 2001 Code of Ethics for Nurses (Fowler, 2008). This reader contains specific applications to nursing practice for each of the code's nine interpretive statements.

Whereas provisions 1 through 3 focus on the recipients of nursing care, provisions 4 through 6 focus on the nurse. This focus addresses nurses' accountability, competency, and contributions to their employment conditions.

Provisions 7 through 9 focus on the bigger picture of both the nursing profession and national and global health concerns. Regarding the nursing profession, the emphasis is on professional standards, active involvement in nursing, and the integrity of the profession. All nurses have a responsibility to meet these obligations. Regarding national and global health concerns, the emphasis is on social justice and reform. According to the ANA code (2015, p xi), The Code specifies that the patients and clients of nurses can be "individuals, families, communities or populations." The Code also specifies that health is a universal right and this right has economic, political, social and cultural dimensions. Many of the components of the Code support and help to elaborate on the ethical responsibilities related to chapters and content throughout the text such as genomics, social determinants of health, cultural uniqueness and so forth, the Levels of Prevention box presents actions related to ethics.

## PUBLIC HEALTH CODE OF ETHICS

The Public Health Code of Ethics (PHLS, 2002) mentioned in the history section of this chapter consists of a preamble; 12

## 📄 LEVELS OF PREVENTION

### *Ethics*

**Primary Prevention**

Use the Code of Ethics for Nurses to guide your nursing practice.

**Secondary Prevention**

If you are unable to behave in accordance with the Code of Ethics for Nurses (e.g., you speak in a way that does not communicate respect for a client), take steps to correct your behavior. You could explain to the client your error and apologize.

**Tertiary Prevention**

If you have treated a client or staff member in a way that is inconsistent with ethics practices, seek guidance on other choices you could have made.

## 💙 HEALTHY PEOPLE 2020

There are two new objectives outlined in *Healthy People 2020* related to access to health services:

- AHS-1: Increasing the proportion of persons who receive appropriate evidence-based clinical preventive services
- AHS-4: Increasing the proportion of practicing primary care providers, including nurse practitioners.

Both of these objectives relate to access to care and reflect important ethical considerations for nurses.

From U.S. Department of Health and Human Services: *Healthy People 2020*. Retrieved December 2014 from http://www.healthypeople.gov.

principles related to the ethical practice of public health (Box 6-4); 11 values and beliefs that focus on health, community, and action; and a commentary on each of the 12 principles. The preamble asserts the collective and societal nature of public health to keep people healthy. The 12 principles incorporate the ethical tenets of preventing harm; doing no harm; promoting good; respecting both individual and community rights; respecting autonomy, diversity, and confidentiality when possible; ensuring professional competency; manifesting trustworthiness; and promoting advocacy for disenfranchised persons within a community. Examples of values and beliefs include a right to health care resources, the interdependency of humans living in the community, and the importance of knowledge as a basis for action. The Healthy People box cites two new objectives that relate to ethics.

When the Code of Ethics for Nurses and the Public Health Code of Ethics are assessed, some commonalities emerge. These codes provide general ethical principles and approaches that are both enduring and dynamic. They guide nurses and public health personnel in thinking about the underlying ethics of their profession. Although the two codes do not specify

(nor should they specify) details for every ethical issue, other mechanisms such as standards of practice, ethical decision-making frameworks, and ethics committees help work out the details. Nevertheless, the preceding two codes address most approaches to ethical justification, including traditional and emerging ethical theories and principles, humanist and feminist ethics, virtue ethics, professional-individual and/or community relationships, and advocacy. Many websites provide further information on codes of ethics and other ethical concerns in public health; all can be accessed through the WebLinks section of this book's Evolve website. Some of them are noted in the Additional Resources feature at the beginning of the chapter.

## ADVOCACY AND ETHICS

**Advocacy** is an important concept in nursing that embodies an ethical focus grounded in quality of life. The American Public Health Association (APHA) represents a powerful voice for public health advocacy, focusing on finding ways to involve health care professionals in influencing policies related to protection of all Americans and their communities from preventable, serious health threats and helping to ensure access to health care and eliminating health disparities (APHA, 2014).

---

### BOX 6-4    Principles of the Ethical Practice of Public Health*

1. Public health should address principally the fundamental causes of disease and requirements for health, aiming to prevent adverse health outcomes.
2. Public health should achieve community health in a way that respects the rights of individuals in the community.
3. Public health policies, programs, and priorities should be developed and evaluated through processes that ensure an opportunity for input from community members.
4. Public health should advocate and work for the empowerment of disenfranchised community members, aiming to ensure that the basic resources and conditions necessary for health are accessible to all.
5. Public health should seek the information needed to implement effective policies and programs that protect and promote health.
6. Public health institutions should provide communities with the information they have that is needed for decisions on policies or programs and should obtain the community's consent for their implementation.
7. Public health institutions should act in a timely manner on the information they have, within the resources and the mandate given to them by the public.
8. Public health programs and policies should incorporate a variety of approaches that anticipate and respect diverse values, beliefs, and cultures in the community.
9. Public health programs and policies should be implemented in a manner that most enhances the physical and social environment.
10. Public health institutions should protect the confidentiality of information that can bring harm to an individual or community if made public. Exceptions must be justified on the basis of the high likelihood of significant harm to the individual or others.
11. Public health institutions should ensure the professional competencies of their employees.
12. Public health institutions and their employees should engage in collaborations and affiliations in ways that build the public's trust and the institution's effectiveness.

*A section of the Public Health Code of Ethics is presented.

Reprinted with permission from the Public Health Leadership Society: Public Health Code of Ethics, American Public Health Association (APHA), 2002. Available at http://phls.org/CMSuploads/Principles-of-the-Ethical-Practice-of-PH-Version-2.2-68496.pdf.

## BOX 6-5   Case #2: Applying Virtue Ethics, Truth Telling, and the Deontological Ethical Decision-Making Process

Because finding affordable housing was difficult, 26-year-old Terry White lived with her 6-month-old son, Tommy, and his father, Billy Smith, in one room of the landlord's own house. Ms. White was morbidly obese and was diagnosed with bipolar disease; Mr. Smith had served time for drug dealing and was out on parole and staying straight. Neither had finished high school. Mr. Smith's past drug use had rendered him unable to do much manual labor because of heart damage, but on occasion he would work in construction to support the family.

Public health nurse Jim Lewis had received a referral on Tommy when he was diagnosed with failure to thrive (FTT) 2 months earlier. Ms. White, who had had two children removed from her custody by Child Protective Services (CPS) in the past, and Mr. Smith seemed to adore their baby, so much so that Ms. White would hold the baby all day long. In the past 2 months, the nurse had taught Ms. White about infant nutrition and gotten her enrolled in the Women, Infants, and Children (WIC) nutrition program; as a result, Tommy had increased his rate of physical growth and was above the 5% level of his growth percentile. Yet he was not meeting his gross motor milestones per Denver Developmental Screening Test II (DDST II) testing. Mr. Lewis thought that Tommy was not allowed to play on the floor enough to progress in sitting, pushing his shoulders up, or crawling. Most of their small room was taken up with the bed and the boxes that stored their belongings. There wasn't really space for "tummy time" or play. When not in the room, the family would take the bus to a discount store and spend the day walking around to get a change of scene.

One week Ms. White told the nurse she was not taking her medications for bipolar disease anymore because they caused her to gain weight. The next week she confided that Mr. Smith had had a "dirty" urine specimen check and would have to return to prison in the near future. The following week Mr. Lewis found

the family living in a run-down motel since their landlord evicted them following a disagreement. Ms. White was agitated and told the nurse that they had only $100. Mr. Smith was going to have to return to prison that week, and the motel bill was already $240. Ms. White knew she would be homeless soon without Mr. Smith's support but refused to talk with her social worker about her needs. She asked the nurse not to tell anyone about her situation because she was afraid CPS would take Tommy from her. It was clear to Mr. Lewis that Ms. White might not know what would happen to Tommy after they left this motel.

1. Considering the principle of truth telling, what are Mr. Lewis' professional responsibilities to Ms. White, to Tommy, and to the social worker assigned to this family?
2. Using the generic ethical decision-making framework discussed earlier in the chapter and considering the deontological ethical decision-making process, answer the following questions.
   A. How should Mr. Lewis respond to Ms. White's request to not tell anyone about their situation?
   B. What communication, about truth telling, if any, should the nurse initiate with the social worker? With others?
   C. Consistent with the principle of truth telling, how can the nurse involve Mr. Smith in the ongoing support and involvement with his family?
3. Using virtue ethics, what actions would you take to resolve any moral dilemmas you have about the safety of Tommy in this family situation? If you do not tell anyone about the possible dangers to the child, what moral principles come into play? If you do tell the social worker about the situation and the child is removed from the mother, what moral principles come into play for you?
4. What ethical dilemmas may you experience if you are the nurse in this case? How can you deal effectively with these potential dilemmas?

Created by Deborah C. Conway, Assistant Professor of Nursing, School of Nursing, University of Virginia.

The APHA notes the critical need to shift from a nation focused on treating individual illness to one that also promotes population-based health services that encourage preventive and early intervention practices. Also, the field of genetics has increasingly become an important ethical focus in public health; two new *Healthy People 2020* objectives relate to genomics (G HP2020-1, G HP2020-2). The clinical case in Box 6-5 discusses the applicatioin of virtue ethics, truth telling and the deontological ethical decision-making process.

### Codes and Standards of Practice

Several codes and standards of practice address advocacy. Four are noted here. Advocacy is addressed in codes of ethics put forth by the ANA (2015) and the Public Health Leadership Society (PHLS, 2002), as well as by the ANA (2013) in Standard 17, Public Health Nursing: Scope & Standards of Practice and the PHLS Skills for the Ethical Practice of Public Health (Thomas, 2004). The American Association of Colleges of Nursing (AACN) has developed a document entitled *Recommended Baccalaureate Competencies and Curricular Guidelines for Public Health Nursing* that added specific public health nursing education competences to their competencies for baccalaureate education. Several of the competencies include a recommendation to include specific content related to ethics and public health nursing (AACN, 2013).

According to the ANA (2015) Code of Ethics for Nurses, "The nurse promotes, advocates for, and protects the rights, health, and, safety of the patient" (p. 9). The focus of the interpretive statements regarding advocacy is the nurse's responsibility to take action when the client's best interests are jeopardized by questionable practice on the part of any member of the health team, the health care system, or others.

The Public Health Code of Ethics (PHLS, 2002) and the PHLS Skills for the Ethical Practice of Public Health (Thomas, 2004) state that public health should advocate for disenfranchised community members, aiming to ensure that the basic resources necessary for health are accessible to all. The PHLS's code addresses two important issues: that the voice of the community should be heard and that the marginalized or underserved in a community should receive "a decent minimum" (p. 4) of health resources.

According to the ANA Public Health Nursing: Scope & Standards of Practice (2013), public health nurses have a moral mandate to establish ethical standards when advocating for health care policy. Specifically, Standard 7 says that public health nurses should practice ethically.

### Conceptual Framework for Advocacy

One framework that can be used to define helpful behaviors for advocacy is to contrast social justice and market justice

## (QSEN) FOCUS ON QUALITY AND SAFETY EDUCATION FOR NURSES

One of the six tenets of Quality and Safety Education for Nurses (QSEN) is patient-centered care (Barton et al, 2009). This chapter has discussed many ways in which an understanding of basic principles of ethics can guide safe and effective nursing practice. Some key aspects of patient-centered care in public health nursing include being certain that the information provided to individuals, families, and communities is accurate and reflects the most current evidence, and that it is presented in a timely fashion. Community health education should take into account the age, gender, and cultural and religious backgrounds of those who receive the information. Giving health information that does not meet these criteria can be unsafe and clearly does not reflect attention to quality nursing care. One of the QSEN competencies related to patient-centered care is as follows: Recognize the patient or designee as the source of control and full partner in providing compassionate and coordinated care based on respect for patient's preferences, values, and needs. Specific aspects of patient-centered care related to communication are as follows:

- **Knowledge:** Integrate understanding of multiple dimensions of patient-centered care: information, communication, and education.
- **Skills:** Communicate patient values, preferences, and expressed needs to other members of the health care team.

- **Attitudes:** Respect and encourage individual expression of patient values, preferences, and expressed needs (Barton et al, 2009, p. 315).

Specific aspects of patient-centered care related to the public health dilemma of serving the good of the population versus serving the good of the individual are as follows:

- **Knowledge:** Explore ethical and legal implications of patient-centered care.
- **Skills:** Recognize the boundaries of therapeutic relationships (Barton et al, 2009, p. 315).
- **Attitudes:** Acknowledge the tension that may exist between patient rights and the organizational responsibility for professional ethical care.

*Patient-centered ethical activity:* Public health is more concerned about the good of the collective group than of the individual. In order to think more closely about quality and safety, debate with a classmate about whether children should be required to have all of the Centers for Disease Control and Prevention vaccines before they can enter school or remain the school. At the present time, some parents are choosing not to give their children all the recommended immunizations because of fear of side effects of the vaccines. To support your argument see http://www.cdc.gov/vaccines/schedules/index.html for what is required. See web articles such as www.responsibility-project.libertymutual.com for the parents' point of view.

Park EJ: The development and implications of a case-based computer program to train ethical decision-making. *Nurs Ethics* 20:943–956, 2013.

## TABLE 6-2   Contrast of Social Justice and Market Justice as an Advocacy Framework

| Market Justice Values | Social Justice Values |
|---|---|
| Self-determination and self-discipline | Shared responsibility |
| Individual values and self-interest | Interconnection and cooperation among individuals in a community |
| Personal efforts key to desired benefits | Community shares responsibility for providing basic benefits |
| Limited responsibilities for good of the community | Important obligations for the collective good |
| Limited government intervention | Government involvement is necessary |
| Voluntary focus on individual moral behavior | Community well-being supersedes individual focus on well-being |

Adapted from Dorfman L, Wallack L, Woodruff K: More than a message: framing public health advocacy to change corporate practices. *Health Educ Behav* 32:320–336, 2005.

## BOX 6-6   Ethical Principles for Effective Advocacy

1. Act in the client's best interests.
2. Act in accordance with the client's wishes and instructions.
3. Keep the client properly informed.
4. Carry out instructions with diligence and competence.
5. Act impartially and offer frank, independent advice.
6. Maintain client confidentiality.

skills to compete effectively with adversaries in public debate and learn to frame their advocacy initiatives.

### Practical Framework for Advocacy

Bateman (2000) takes a practical approach to advocacy. He places the advocate's core skills (i.e., interviewing, assertiveness and force, negotiation, self-management, legal knowledge and research, and litigation) within the context of six ethical principles for effective advocacy, as shown in Box 6-6. His focus is on the individual client, although the focus could also apply to groups and communities.

Regarding the first ethical principle, Bateman (2000) is sensitive to the ethical conflict between clients' best interests and the best interests of groups, communities, or societies but does not elaborate on this conflict. The second ethical principle, which puts the client in charge, works in tandem with the first principle. It goes like this: "This is what I think we can do. What do you want me to do?" (Bateman, 2000, p. 51). Of course, the advocate can refuse the request if self or others may be harmed. By following the third ethical principle, the client is empowered to make knowledgeable decisions. The fourth ethical principle addresses standards of practice. The fifth ethical principle addresses fairness and respect for persons (population-centered

(Dorfman et al, 2005). As noted earlier in this chapter, it is important to recognize the potential conflict of individuals versus society. With communitarianism, individual rights need to be balanced with social responsibilities. When using a framework that contrasts social justice and market justice, the biggest barrier to achieving social justice is the competing concept of market justice. Market justice is grounded in the assumption that the best way to meet the needs of individuals in a society is to avoid regulations. The focus is on individual, not shared, needs (Table 6-2). A focus on market justice, rather than social justice, influences public dialogue about public health needs. It is important that existing values and beliefs in the society be understood in order to frame the public health message appropriately in terms of social justice values that relate to changes that they seek. Health care professionals must develop media nursing is more collaborative in nature than independent nursing). The last ethical principle, confidentiality, ensures that information will be shared only on a need-to-know basis.

## Advocacy: Issues that Have Ethical Implications
### Advocacy and Bioterrorism

Before the terrorist attacks in the United States on September 11, 2001, the subject of terrorism was not a major focus in philosophical discussions (*terrorism*, in Stanford Encyclopedia of Philosophy, 2007). The September 11th attack, however, brought a frightening new awareness of the vulnerability of individuals and groups in our society and the need for advocacy. Although some countries have been forced to live with the knowledge of this type of vulnerability for years, today's reality of global terrorism means that nurses must thoughtfully reflect on and debate ethical issues that arise with the threat, action, and aftermath of terrorism. They also must carefully consider their own responsibilities in terms of moral obligation to respond and make themselves available in a crisis that threatens the well-being of a community.

As noted at the beginning of this chapter, population-centered nursing is concerned with protecting, promoting, preserving, and maintaining health while preventing disease. These goals that address the promotion of good and prevention of harm are intimately related to ethics and bioterrorism. It is often difficult to balance goals for the protection of the public and protection of the individual, as evidenced by an incident in which airport security personnel ordered a 4-year-old disabled child to remove his leg braces to go through a metal detector, even though his mother told the screeners that the child could not walk without the braces (Rubin, 2010). As a nurse, it is often hard when confronted with terrorism or a disaster to determine whether the needs of one's family or the needs of one's clients predominate. Silva and Ludwick (2003) provide a helpful framework related to the need for advocacy in bioterrorism, using the principles of nonmaleficence, beneficence, and distributive justice. These principles can guide nurses as they learn to speak out against violence and terrorism, work with agencies in the community for short-term and long-term efforts to do good and avoid harm, and participate in policy debates that attempt to determine fair distribution of scarce resources to fight terrorism globally. The ANA Center for Ethics and Human Rights maintains a helpful list of resource information addressing biodefense at http://www.nursingworld.org/MainMenuCategories/ThePracticeofProfessionalNursing/EthicsStandards/CEHR.aspx.

### Advocacy and Health Care Reform

In the current focus on health care reform, it is critical that nurses advocate for reform that embodies ethical considerations that have been discussed in this chapter. Dr. Mary Wakefield, Administrator of the Health Resources and Services Administration (HRSA), noted that not only should nurses participate in implementing new directions for health care, but that it is important that they help to envision these new directions (Wakefield, 2008). Nurses can be an important voice in advocating for access to consistent, effective, efficient health care for all in our society. Wakefield says that educating the public can be a unique challenge because clever sound bites and attack ads in the media can lure consumers into thinking that the status quo is the best option. Nurses are an important part of the health care industry and are respected by the public; they can make meaningful contributions toward health care reform through advocating for clients and families. The signing of the 2010 health care bill by President Obama, after many years of controversial attempts at health care reform, provides an excellent opportunity for nurses to advocate for tying health care for all to ethics and social justice.

### Ethical Use of Social Media

As the trend for using social media grows in both personal and professional arenas the implications for establishing boundaries for its use by health care professionals also grow. As Baker (2013, p. 501) says, "If the risks (of using social media) are managed well, social media can be a positive force for patient advocacy and education, as well as a resource for evidence-based practice and research." She points out that nurses should practice within defined professional boundaries that center around four key elements: (1) promoting the dignity of the clients, (2) seeking client independence and working for their best interests, (3) abstaining from inappropriate involvement with clients, and (4) refraining from personal gain at the expense of the client. Ethical dilemmas arise when nurses act in ways that are not consistent with their professional boundaries. Baker (2013) points out that it is important to think through ethical concerns that are associated with social networking. This can be especially important when the nurse lives and works in a small community. For example, consider the public health nurse who goes to church with clients, attends the same parent-teacher meetings, and shops at the same stores as they do. Is it appropriate for her to then "friend" these clients on a social media site? Chapter 19 discusses rural health, and the issue of close relationships between nurses and clients is described there.

## ⨠ LINKING CONTENT TO PRACTICE

Throughout this chapter, there has been application of the content related to ethics in public health nursing and the many documents that influence the role of public health nurses. These include the ANA Scope and Standards of Public Health Nursing, the ANA Code of Ethics, the core functions of public health as outlined by the Institute of Medicine, and the *Healthy People 2020* objectives. Ethics is also an integral part of the Core Competencies for Public Health Professionals. Skill 8 in the section on analytic/assessment skills says that a public health professional uses "ethical principles in the collection, maintenance, use, and dissemination of data and information" and skill 2 under leadership and systems thinking says a professional "incorporates ethical standards of practice as the basis of all interactions with organization, communities, and individuals" (Council on Linkages between Academic and Public Health Practice, 2010).

Council on Linkages Between Academic and Public Health Practice: Core competencies for public health professionals, Washington, DC, 2010. Public Health Foundation/Health Resources and Services Administration.

## PRACTICE APPLICATION

The retiring director of the division of primary care in a state health department had recently hired Ann Green, a 34-year-old nurse with a master's degree in public health, to be director of the division. Ms. Green's work involved the monitoring of millions of dollars of state and federal money as well as the supervising of the funded programs within her division.

Ms. Green received many requests for funding from a particular state agency that served a poor, large district. The poor people of the district primarily consisted of young families with children and homebound older adults with chronic illnesses. Over the past 3 years, the federal government had allocated considerable money to the state agency to subsidize pediatric primary care programs, but no formal evaluation of these programs had occurred.

The director of the state agency was a physician who had been in this position for over 20 years. He was good at obtaining funding for primary care needs in his district, but the statistics related to the pediatric primary care program seemed implausible—that is, few physical examinations were performed on the children, which had resulted in extra money in the budget. This unspent federal money was being used to supplement home health care services for the indigent homebound older adults in his district. The thinking of the physician was that he was doing good by providing some needed services to both indigent groups in his district. Ms. Green felt moral discomfort because she did not have either the money or the personnel to provide both services. What should she do?

A. What facts are the most relevant in this scenario?
B. What are the ethical issues?
C. How can Ms. Green resolve the issues?

(The preceding case and answers are adapted and paraphrased from a real practice application shared by J.L. Chapin on the inappropriate distribution of primary health care funds [in Silva M, editor: *Ethical Decision Making in Nursing Administration.* Norwalk, CT, 1990, Appleton & Lange].)

**Answers can be found on the Evolve site.**

## KEY POINTS

- Nursing has a rich heritage of ethics and morality, beginning with Florence Nightingale.
- During the late 1960s, the field of bioethics began to emerge and influence nursing.
- Ethical decision making is the component of ethics that focuses on the process of how ethical decisions are made.
- Many different ethical decision-making frameworks exist; however, underlying each of them is the problem-solving process.
- Ethical decision making applies to all approaches to ethics: utilitarianism, deontology, principlism, virtue ethics, caring and the ethic of care, and feminist ethics.
- Cultural diversity makes ethical decision making more challenging.
- Moral distress can lead to a personal sense of failure in providing nursing care and may lead to work and/or career dissatisfaction.
- Classical ethical theories are utilitarianism and deontology.
- Principlism consists of respect for autonomy, nonmaleficence, beneficence, and justice.
- Other approaches to ethics include virtue ethics, caring and the ethic of care, and feminist ethics.
- The core functions of public health nursing (i.e., assessment, policy development, and assurance) are all grounded in ethics.
- *Healthy People 2020* objectives address workforce competencies, training in essential public health services, and continuing education.

- The 2015 Code of Ethics for Nurses contains nine statements that address the moral standards that delineate nursing's values, goals, and obligations.
- The 2002 Public Health Code of Ethics contains 12 statements that address the moral standards that delineate public health's values, goals, and obligations.
- Advocacy is the act of pleading for or supporting a course of action on behalf of a person, group, or community.
- Effective advocacy incorporates ethical principles and concepts.
- The Code of Ethics for Nurses, the Public Health Code of Ethics, Skills for the Ethical Practice of Public Health, and Public Health Nursing: Scope & Standards of Practice all address advocacy.
- Public health advocacy is composed of both products and processes.
- The products of advocacy are decreased morbidity and mortality.
- The processes of public health advocacy include, but are not limited to, identifying problems, collecting data, developing and endorsing regulations and legislation, enforcing policies, and assessing the policy process.
- Advocacy related to bioterrorism, health care reform, and ethical use of social media is important for community and public health nurses.

# CLINICAL DECISION-MAKING ACTIVITIES

1. Think about the differences in duties between a nurse working in a critical care facility and a nurse working in a community care or public health setting. How might these differences lead to differences in ethical problems and decision making?

2. Interview a long-retired nurse about the most important ethical issues that this nurse faced when practicing in the community. Next, interview a nurse actively practicing in the community about the most important ethical issues that this

nurse is now facing. Compare and contrast the ethical issues in the two interviews and place each within a historical context.

3. In a local or national newspaper, read one or more articles that discuss health care public policy with which you agree or disagree. Compose a letter to the editor analyzing why you agree or disagree with the policy but only after you take into account any of your own biases or vested interests.

# REFERENCES

American Association of Colleges of Nursing (AACN): *Recommended Baccalaureate Competencies and Curricular Guidelines for Public Health Nursing*. Washington, DC, 2013, AACN.

American Nurses Association (ANA): *Code of Ethics for Nurses with Interpretive Statements*. Silver Spring, MD, 2015, Nursebooks.org.

American Nurses Association (ANA): *Public Health Nursing: Scope & Standards of Practice*. Washington, DC, 2013, American Nurses Publishing.

American Public Health Association: *Advocacy and Policy, 2014*. Retrieved December 2014 from: www.apha.org/policies-and-advocacy/advocacy-for-public-health.

Baker JD: Social networking and professional boundaries. *AORN J* 97:501–506, 2013.

Barton AJ, Armstrong G, Preheim G, et al: A national Delphi to determine developmental progression of quality and safety competencies in nursing education. *Nurs Outlook* 57:313–322, 2009.

Bateman N: *Advocacy Skills for Health and Social Care Professionals*. Philadelphia, 2000, Jessica Kingsley.

Beauchamp TL, Childress JF: *Principles of Biomedical Ethics*, ed 6. New York, 2008, Oxford University Press.

Beauchamp TL, Childress JF: *Principles of Biomedical Ethics*, ed 7. New York, 2013, Oxford University Press.

Bekemeier B, Butterfield P: Unreconciled inconsistencies: a critical review of the concept of social justice in 3 national nursing documents. *ANS Adv Nurs Sci* 28:152–162, 2005.

Bernheim RG, Childress JF, Bonnie RJ, et al: *Essentials of Public Health Ethics*. Burlington, MA, 2015, Jones & Bartlett.

Callahan D: Universalism and particularism fighting to a draw. *Hastings Cent Rep* 30:37, 2000.

Callahan D: Principlism and communitarianism. *J Med Ethics* 29:287–291, 2003.

Callahan D, Jennings B: Ethics and public health: forging a strong relationship. *Am J Public Health* 92:169, 2002.

Carlock C, Spader C: Communication and understanding: best vs distress. *Nurs Spectr*, October 8, 2007. Retrieved December 2014 from: http://news.nurse.com/apps/pbcs. dll/article?AID= 2007710080311.

Council on Linkages between Academic and Public Health Practice: *Core Competencies for Public Health Professionals*. Washington, DC, 2010, Public Health Foundation/Health Resources and Services Administration.

Coursin CC: Inequalities affecting access to healthcare: a philosophical reflection. *Int J Hum Caring* 13:7–15, 2009.

Denhardt RB, Denhardt JV: The new public service: serving rather than steering. *Public Admin Rev* 60:549–552, 2000.

Dorfman L, Wallack L, Woodruff K: More than a message: framing public health advocacy to change corporate practices. *Health Educ Behav* 32:320–336, 2005.

Eriksson K: Caring science in a new way. *Nurs Sci Q* 15:61, 2002.

Fowler MDM, editor: *Guide to the Code of Ethics for Nurses: Interpretation and Application*. Silver Spring, MD, 2008, American Nurses Association.

Gilligan C: *In a Different Voice: Psychological Theory and Women's Development*. Cambridge, MA, 1982, Harvard University Press.

Gjengedal E, Ekra EM, Hol H, et al: Vulnerability in health care— reflections on encounters in every

day practice. *Nurs Philos* 14:127–138, 2013.

Hellsten S: Theories of distributive justice. In Chadwick R, editor: *Encyclopedia of Applied Ethics*, vol 1. New York, 1998, Academic Press, pp 815–827.

Holstein MB: Bringing ethics home: a new look at ethics in the home and the community. In Holstein MB, Mitzen PB, editors: *Ethics in Community-Based Elder Care*. New York, 2001, Springer.

International Council of Nurses (ICN): *ICN Code of Ethics for Nurses*. Geneva, 1953, ICN.

International Council of Nurses (ICN): *ICN Code of Ethics for Nurses*. Geneva, 2012, ICN.

Leininger M: *Care: The Essence of Nursing and Health*. Thorofare, NJ, 1984, Slack.

Noddings N: *Caring: A Feminine Approach to Ethics & Moral Education*. Berkeley, CA, 1984, University of California Press.

Olick RS: From the column editor: ethics in public health. *J Public Health Manag Pract* 11:258–259, 2005.

Olson LL: Provision Six. In Fowler MDM, editor: *Guide to the Code of Ethics for Nurses: Interpretation and Application*. Silver Spring, MD, 2008, American Nurses Association, pp 72–88.

Park EJ: The development and implications of a case-based computer program to train ethical decision-making. *Nurs Ethics* 20:943–956, 2013.

Petrini C: Theoretical models and operational frameworks in public health ethics. *Int J Environ Res Public Health* 7:189–202, 2010.

Pinch WJE, Haddad AM, editors: *Nursing and Health Care Ethics: A Legacy and a Vision*. Silver Spring, MD, 2008, American Nurses Association.

Public Health Leadership Society: *Public Health Code of Ethics*. 2002,

American Public Health Association (APHA). Retrieved December 2014 from: www.phls.org/home/ section/3-26.

Rawls J, Kelly E, editors: *Justice as Fairness: A Restatement*. Cambridge MA, 2001, Harvard University Press.

Rogers WA: Feminism and public health ethics. *J Med Ethics* 32:351–354, 2006.

Rubin D: Another case of TSA overkill. *Philadelphia Inquirer*, February 15, 2010. Retrieved December 2014 from: http://www.philly.com/philly/news/20100215_Daniel_Rubin_Another_case_of_TSA_overkill.html.

Ruger JP: Ethics in American health. 2. An ethical framework for health system reform. *Am J Public Health* 98:1756–1763, 2008.

Silva MC: Ethical issues in health care, public policy, and politics. In Mason D, Leavitt J, Chaffee M, editors: *Policy and Politics in Nursing and Health Care*, ed 4. Philadelphia, 2002, Saunders.

Silva MC: Provision Eight. In Fowler MDM, editor: *Guide to the Code of Ethics for Nurses: Interpretation and Application*. Silver Spring, MD, 2008, American Nurses Association, pp 72–88.

Silva MC, Ludwick R: Ethics and terrorism: September 11, 2001 and its aftermath. *Online J Issues Nurs* January 31, 2003. Retrieved December 2014 from: http://www.nursingworld.org/MainMenu Categories/ANAMarketplace/ ANAPeriodicals/OJIN/ TableofContents/Volume82003/ No1Jan2003/EthicsandTerrorism .html.

Skloot R: *The Immortal Life of Henrietta Lacks*. New York, 2010, Crown Publishers.

Stanford Encyclopedia of Philosophy: *Terrorism*, October 22, 2007 [revised August 8, 2011]. Retrieved December 2014 from: http:// plato.stanford.edu/entries/terrorism.

Steinbock B, Arras J, London AJ, editors: *Ethical Issues in Modern Medicine*, ed 7. Boston, 2008, McGraw-Hill.

Thomas J: *Skills for the Ethical Practice of Public Health*. 2004, Public Health Leadership Society. Retrieved December 2014 from: http://phls.org/CMSuploads/Skills-for-the-Ethical-Practice-of-Public-Health-68547.pdf.

U.S. Department of Health and Human Services: *Healthy People 2020*. Retrieved January 2015 from: www.healthypeople.gov.

Volbrecht RM: *Nursing Ethics: Communities in Dialogue*. Upper Saddle River, NJ, 2002, Prentice Hall.

Wakefield MK: Envisioning and implementing new directions for health care. *Nurs Econ* 26:49–51, 2008.

Walker T: What principlism misses. *J Med Ethics* 35:229–231, 2009.

Watson J: *Nursing: Human Science and Human Care*, revised edition. Norwalk, CT, 2007, Jones & Bartlett.

Weston A: *A Practical Companion to Ethics*, ed 3. New York, 2006, Oxford University Press.

Wringe C: Communitarianism. In *Philosophy & Education*, vol 14, Moral Education: Beyond the Teaching of Right and Wrong. New York, 2006, Springer, pp 74–82.

# 7

# Cultural Diversity in the Community

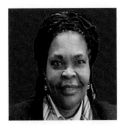

### Cynthia E. Degazon, RN, PhD

Dr. Cynthia E. Degazon is professor emerita at Hunter College, City University of New York. She received a BS in nursing from Long Island University, and an MA in Community Health nursing and a PhD from New York University. For 20 years she has prepared undergraduate and graduate nurses to provide culturally competent care to ethnically diverse populations. Dr. Degazon has given many national and international presentations, authored several scholarly publications, and served on the editorial board of the *Journal of Cultural Diversity*.

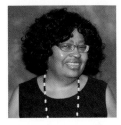

### Bobbie J. Perdue, RN, PhD

Dr. Bobbie Perdue is Professor of Nursing at South Carolina State University in Orangeburg, South Carolina. She is professor emerita at Syracuse University. Her teaching career in nursing spans 43 years and includes the teaching of associate degree, baccalaureate, and master degree nursing students. She received a BSN from Vanderbilt University, an MSN in child-psychiatric mental health nursing from Wayne State University, and a PhD in nursing research and theory development from New York University.

## ADDITIONAL RESOURCES

ⓔ **Evolve Website http://evolve.elsevier.com/Stanhope**
- Healthy People 2020
- WebLinks
- Quiz

- Case Studies
- Glossary
- Answers to Practice Application

## OBJECTIVES

*After reading this chapter, the student should be able to do the following:*

1. Describe the process for developing cultural competence to meet the health care needs of culturally diverse individuals, communities, and organizations.
2. Describe major facilitators and barriers to providing quality health care for diverse populations.
3. Identify culturally competent nursing interventions to promote positive health outcomes for culturally diverse clients.

4. Evaluate the role of the public health nurse in providing culturally competent nursing care.
5. Use a case scenario to chart the five elements of cultural competence as described by Campinha-Bacote.
6. Use electronic resources to locate current databases about culturally competent practices that reduce health disparities.

## KEY TERMS

biological variations, p. 143
communication, p. 145
cultural accommodation, p. 159
cultural awareness, p. 154
cultural blindness, p. 157
cultural competence, p. 151
cultural conflict, p. 157
cultural desire, p. 155
cultural diversity, p. 142

cultural encounter, p. 155
cultural imposition, p. 157
cultural knowledge, p. 154
cultural nursing assessment, p. 161
cultural preservation, p. 158
cultural relativism, p. 157
cultural repatterning, p. 159
cultural skill, p. 154
culture, p. 141

Caring for culturally diverse groups has been a focus of nursing from its beginning. As early as 1893, under the leadership of Lillian Wald, nurses in New York City started public health nursing and provided home care to inner city people, particularly immigrants, who could neither read nor write the English language (Anderson and McFarlane, 2010). Because nurses were not from the same cultural background as the immigrants, they had to deal with the cultural differences between themselves and the persons in their care. Today, the U.S. culture reflects a greater diversity of cultures from all over the world and assuring that individuals from these diverse cultures receive equity in health care is as much a challenge for nurses as it was during Lillian Wald's era. Such assurance is viewed as a moral imperative to reduce health disparities.

Data from the U.S. Census Bureau (2010) showed that (72.4%) of the U.S. population defined themselves as a member of a non-Hispanic white ethnic group followed by African Americans (12.6%), Asian Americans (4.8%), American Indians/Alaskan Natives (0.9%), Native Hawaiian and other Pacific Islanders (0.2%), some other race (6.2%), and two or more races (2.9%). Hispanic origin was considered to be a separate concept from race but accounted for 16.4% of the population with those predominantly identified as white or as some other race. Data also showed a decrease from the 2000 census when the white population accounted for 75.1%. This pattern of a decreasing white population is attributed to rapidly growing Hispanic populations, a strong increase in the Asian populations, a modest increase in Americans of African descent, and an increase in persons who identify as white in combination with another race.

Culture and language have a significant influence on health, belief systems, health practices, and health outcomes. As social determinants of health, they affect how clients and nurses perceive illness, and causes of and treatment of diseases. They contribute to the behaviors and attitudes that clients have about health care and the providers who care for them. As a result of this diversity, significant differences in beliefs and practices about health and illness have become apparent in health care systems. Nurses who want to incorporate their client's beliefs of health and illness when intervening to promote and maintain wellness face many challenges.

Nurses need to understand the sociocultural views that affect perceptions of an illness, as well as the pathophysiology of the illness. According to the American Association of Colleges of

Nursing (2014), the nursing workforce is overwhelmingly white (83%): African Americans account for 6%, Asian or Pacific Islanders 6%, Hispanics 3%, American Indian/Alaskan Natives 1%, Native Hawaiian/Pacific Islanders 1%, and 1% "other" nurses. There is also a small cadre of minority students enrolled in nursing schools (Phillips and Malone, 2014) even though clients are often more satisfied with nursing care when they have an ethnic connection with the provider of that care. Minority clients, in contrast to their white counterparts, are at greater safety risk in health care facilities as measured by the incidence of medical errors, length of hospital stay for a specific illness, and the number of laboratory tests ordered (Beacham et al, 2009; Smedley et al, 2002).

This chapter provides nurses with strategies to use in providing culturally competent care to diverse clients (individuals, aggregates, families, and communities) who may not share the nurse's culture. Although the chapter is population-focused, it emphases knowledge development in the care of clients from five culturally diverse marginalized groups: African Americans, Asian Americans, Hispanic Americans, Native American/Alaskan Natives, and immigrants.

There is much cultural and ethnic diversity present within and among these marginalized groups; they are consistently identified in the literature as more vulnerable, have less access to health care, receive a poorer quality of health care, have higher rates of chronic illnesses, and shorter life expectancies than Anglo-white groups (Agency for Healthcare Research & Quality, 2014; Agency for Healthcare Research & Quality, 2012). Many groups other than racial and ethnic groups also differ from the expected norms relative to place of origin, sexual orientation, gender identity, educational background, literacy, income, and language. Individuals who are members of these subcultures are marginalized by the dominant health care culture as well. However, evidence is beginning to show a narrowing of the health gap among these groups for some of the access and quality measures.

## CULTURE, RACE, AND ETHNICITY

### Culture

Culture is a set of beliefs, values, and assumptions about life that are widely held among a group of people and is transmitted intergenerationally (Leininger, 2002a). The term *culture* encompasses a broad range of concepts. It is an individual concept, a group phenomenon, and an organizational reality. Culture pervades all aspects of life and of health care. Culture determines how health care information is processed, received, and distributed; how rights and protections are exercised; what is considered to be a health problem; how symptoms and concerns of the problem are expressed; who provides treatment for the problem; and what type of treatment should be given (Giger, 2012; Purnell and Paulanka, 2012; Spector, 2012). Culture is applicable not only to minority groups, but also to majority groups such as white Americans of European descent (i.e. Irish, Italian, and Russian). Individuals are usually members of more than one culture. Each individual should be viewed as a unique human being with differences that are respected. Box 7-1

| BOX 7-1   **Factors Influencing Individual Differences Within Cultural Groups** |
| --- |
| • Age |
| • Religion |
| • Dialect and language spoken |
| • Gender identity roles |
| • Socioeconomic background |
| • Geographic location in the country of origin |
| • Geographic location in the current country |
| • History of the subcultural group with which clients identify in their current country of residence |
| • History of the subcultural group with which clients identify in their country of origin |
| • Amount of interaction between older and younger generations |
| • Degree of assimilation in the current country of residence |
| • Immigration status* |
| • Conditions under which migration occurred |

Except where noted with an asterisk, from Orque M: Orque's ethnic/cultural system: a framework for ethnic nursing care. In Orque MS, Bloch B, Monrroy LSA, editors: *Ethnic Nursing Care. A Multicultural Approach*. St. Louis, 1983, Mosby.

summarizes factors that may influence individual differences within cultural groups.

In response to the needs of its members and the environment, culture provides tested solutions to life's problems and guides our thinking, discourse, attitudes, and actions. In the present health care system, nurses have the chief responsibility for translating health information so that clients can understand it and engage in more effective strategies to achieve positive health outcomes. Understanding the beliefs and practices these clients bring to the clinical setting, their responses to health and illness, and the type of health care they expect to receive are important data that nurses should draw on when developing a plan of care for clients.

Individuals learn about their culture during the process of socialization and language development (Box 7-2). Parents and other family members are the primary sources for the transfer of traditions and teaching explicit and implicit behaviors of the culture. Schools, community, and cultural organizations are secondary sources of socialization. Explicit behaviors are straightforward and do not leave room for misinterpretation of what the person wants to communicate. Implicit behaviors are less exact and include the use of body language to communicate rather than persons saying verbally what is on their mind. An example of an explicit message is "No smoking is permitted" and an implicit message is: "Thank you for not smoking" (Figures 7-1 and 7-2).

### Race

Concepts of race and ethnicity within American society play a strong role in understanding human behavior and health. In everyday language, these two concepts are often used interchangeably. Nurses are expected to understand and appreciate the meaning of each concept as each relates to providing culturally competent health care to persons of diverse cultures.

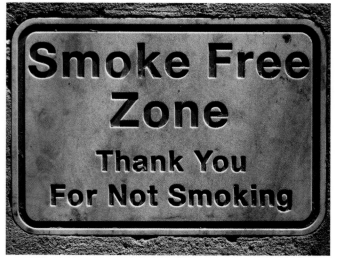

FIG 7-2 The sign is from a culture that values indirectness in communication. (© 2012 Photos.com, a division of Getty Images. All rights reserved. Image 122153579.)

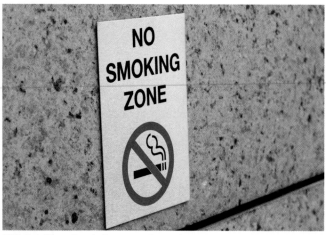

FIG 7-1 The sign is from a culture that values directness in communication. (© 2012 Photos.com, a division of Getty Images. All rights reserved. Image 91883504.)

Race is a biological variation within population groups based on physical markers derived from genetic ancestry such as skin color, physical features, and hair texture. It is a characteristic that allows for some groups to be separated, treated as superior, and given access to power and other valued resources, while others are treated as inferior and have limited access to power and resources. Race differences include areas of growth and development, skin color, enzymatic differences, susceptibility to disease, and laboratory test findings. Individuals may be of the same race but of different cultures. For example, African Americans, who may have been born in Africa, the Caribbean, North America, or elsewhere, are a heterogeneous group, but they may be considered culturally homogeneous by persons who think of African Americans as one group. Monolithic thinking means that the many cultural differences of individuals from these diverse geographic regions may be overlooked because of the similar racial characteristics (Degazon, 1994).

Individuals who belong to the Caucasian race also experience this same over-generalization of individuals along racial/ethnic lines.

## Ethnicity

Ethnicity, in contrast to race, is the shared feeling of peoplehood among a group of individuals and relates to cultural factors such as nationality, geographic region, culture, ancestry, language, beliefs, and traditions (Giger, 2012) (Figure 7-3). These ethnicity and racial patterns have been developed in a socioeconomic context with historical and political underpinnings. They are equally influenced by education, income, and cross-cultural experiences. Race and ethnicity account for much of the health disparities in the United States. Members of an ethnic group are likely to give up aspects of their identity and society when they adopt characteristics of another group's identity. However, when there is a strong ethnic identity, the individual maintains the values, beliefs, behaviors, practices, and ways of thinking of their group. Ethnic disparities in health care are explained largely by differences in English fluency whereas racial disparities in health care are best explained by delayed care due to a lack of knowledge by caregivers about culture and ethnic values, norms and thinking outside of their reference group, lack of insurance, and lack of transportation.

## CULTURAL DIVERSITY

Cultural diversity refers to the degrees of variation that is represented among populations based on lifestyle, ethnicity, race, interest, across place, and place of origin across time. It includes other aspects of variation among people, such as social class, gender identity, sexual orientation, physical abilities/disabilities and care beyond multiculturalism. Cultural diversity also refers to the changing populations of the world as it becomes more of a global village. It is about understanding and embracing each other's differences and similarities.

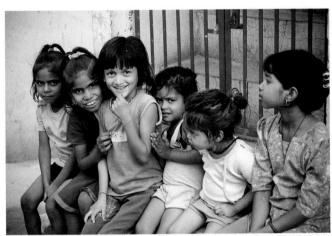

FIG 7-3 In countries around the world, there are distinct differences in people who represent the same cultural group. (Copyright © 2013 Thinkstock. All rights reserved. Image # 117003112).

## Cultural Variations among Selected Groups

Each culture has an organizational structure that distinguishes it from others and provides the direction for what members of the cultural group determine is appropriate or inappropriate behavior. The organizational elements of health culture have been described in nursing by Andrews and Boyle (2012), Giger (2012), Leininger (2002b), Purnell and Paulanka (2012), and Spector (2012). As part of the nursing process, nurses are expected to accurately assess a client's health needs based on information about seven primary cultural elements: biological variations, personal space, time, environmental control, social organizations, communication patterns, nutrition, and religion (Table 7-1). Usually, the assessment takes place in the initial nurse–client interview. It is important that nurses use this information to develop a client-centered care plan. Once this information is gathered, the nurse should schedule a second interview with the client to determine ways to individualize culturally congruent care so that it is acceptable to the client.

## Biological Variations

Biological variations are the physical, biological, and physiological characteristics that exist between racial groups and distinguish one race from another. These characteristics occur in areas of growth and development, skin color, enzymatic differences, susceptibility to disease, and laboratory test findings (Andrews and Boyle, 2012; Giger, 2012). For example, Western-born neonates are slightly heavier at birth than those born in non-Western cultures. Variations in growth and development may be influenced by environmental conditions such as nutrition, climate, and disease. Mongolian spots are bluish discolorations that are sometimes present on the skin of African American, Asian, Hispanic, and Native American/Alaskan Native babies. These spots may be mistaken for bruises. When nurses encounter situations involving unfamiliar biological variations, they may create embarrassing situations. Consider the following scenario: The school nurse observed a bluish discoloration on the thigh of a Filipino child that she mistook for a bruise. The nurse reported her observation to the child

protective agency in her state. The mother had to disprove the allegation to the agency's social worker before her child could be released into her care. Other common and obvious variations include eye shape, hair texture, adipose tissue, shape of earlobes, thickness of lips, and body configuration. A common enzyme deficiency is glucose-6-phosphate dehydrogenase (G6PD), which is responsible for lactose intolerance in many ethnic groups (Giger, 2012).

The findings that DNA composition for any two humans across race is 99.9% genetically identical and that difference between races occur only in 1 in 1000 people diminishes the ethnocentric debate about the importance of race. Another factor making race less important is the increasing numbers of interracial marriages that result in interracial children whose physical and genetic pool dilute the racial characteristics of their parents. Racial categories originated from a shared genealogy due to geographic isolation. In today's global village, this isolation has been broken down and there are more mixed groups. In the United States, children of biracial parents are usually assigned the race of the mother. The Levels of Prevention Box gives examples of cultural strategies for primary, secondary, and tertiary levels of prevention.

### 📄 LEVELS OF PREVENTION

#### Hypertension, Stroke, and Heart Disease Related to Cultural Differences

**Primary Prevention**
Provide health teaching about balanced diet and exercise. Based on the details of the individual's culture, the teaching should include members of the family and identification of culturally appropriate foods and the means for preparing them.

**Secondary Prevention**
Teach clients and/or family to monitor blood pressure. Teach about diet, keeping in mind the client's cultural preferences. Talk about health beliefs and cultural implications, such as the use of alternative therapies; make sure alternative therapies are compatible with any medications that may be prescribed.

**Tertiary Prevention**
If blood pressure cannot be controlled by diet and/or exercise, refer the client to a culturally appropriate medical practitioner for medication and supervision; advise the client to engage in a cardiac program that will oversee diet and exercise.

## Personal Space

Personal space is the physical distance maintained between individuals during an interaction (Giger, 2012). The amount of space varies among individuals and between cultures. When this space is violated, the nurse or the client may experience discomfort. There are four zones of interpersonal space—intimate space (direct contact to 1.5 feet), personal distance (1.5 to 4 feet), social distance (4 to 12 feet), or public distance (greater than 12 feet)—that may be observed when nurses care for clients. Cultural groups also have spatial preferences. To illustrate, Hispanic cultures tend to be comfortable with less space because individuals like to touch some persons with whom they

## TABLE 7-1   Cultural Variations among Selected Groups

| | African Americans | Asians | Hispanics | American Indian/ Native Alaskans |
|---|---|---|---|---|
| Verbal Communication | Asking personal questions of someone that you have met for the first time is seen as improper and intrusive. | High level of respect for others, especially those in positions of authority. | Expression of negative feelings is considered impolite. | Speak in a low tone of voice and expect the listener to be attentive. |
| Nonverbal Communication | Direct eye contact in conversation is often considered rude. | Direct eye contact with elders and authority figures may be considered disrespectful. | Avoidance of eye contact is usually a sign of attentiveness and respect. | Direct eye contact is often considered disrespectful. Avoidance of eye contact should not be interpreted as inattentiveness or evasiveness. |
| Touch | Very affectionate and expressive. Touching of one's hair by another is often considered offensive. | It is not customary to shake hands with persons of the opposite sex. | Very affectionate and use hand, face, and body gestures to express self. Touching is often observed between two persons in conversation. | Modesty. A light touch of the person's hand instead of a firm handshake is often used when greeting a person. |
| Family Organization | Usually have close extended family networks; women play key roles in health care decisions. | Usually have close extended family ties; emphasis may be on family needs rather than individual needs. | Usually have close extended family ties; all members of the family may be involved in health care decisions. | Usually have close extended family; emphasis tends to be on family rather than on individual needs. Decision making may vary among tribes. |
| Time Perception | Often present oriented. | Often present oriented. | Often present oriented. | Often past oriented |
| Environmental Control | Harmony of mind, health, body, and spirit with nature. | Balance between the "yin" and "yang" energy forces. | Balance and harmony among mind, body, spirit, and nature. | Harmony of mind, body, spirit, and emotions with nature. |
| Alternative Healers | "Granny," "root doctor," voodoo priest, and spiritualist. | Acupuncture, acupressure, acumassage, herbalist, moodang. | Curandero, espiritualista, Santero priest, yerbero, faith healers. | Medicine man, shaman. |
| Self-care Practices | Poultices, herbal medicine, oils, teas, massage, hot baths, and roots. | Hot and cold foods, herbal medicine, teas, soups, cupping, burning, rubbing, pinching. | Hot and cold foods, herbal teas. | Herbs, corn meal, medicine bundle. |
| Biological Variations | Sickle cell anemia, Mongolian spots, keloid formations, inverted "T" waves, lactose intolerance, skin color. | Thalassemia, alcohol intolerance, drug interactions, Mongolian spots, lactose intolerance, skin color. | Mongolian spots, lactose intolerance, skin color. | Cleft uvula, lactose intolerance, skin color, lumbar pigmented spots, and epicanthal eye folds, Mongolian spots. |

From Office of Immigration Statistics, Office of Management, Department of Homeland Security: 2008 yearbook of immigration statistics, Washington, DC, 2008, U.S. Government Printing Office.
*Australia, New Zealand, and the nearby islands.

are speaking. In the Filipino culture individuals may view touching strangers as inappropriate; therefore, nurses who wish to be culturally appropriate may elect to stand farther away from Filipinos than from Hispanics. On the other hand, clients who are comfortable with closer distances may experience discomfort when nurses stand farther away, interpreting the behavior as rejecting. Nurses should take cues from clients to place themselves in the appropriate spatial zone and avoid misinterpretation of clients' behavior as they handle their spatial needs.

### Perception of Time

Perception of time refers to past, present, and future time as well as to the duration of and period between events. Some cultures assign greater or lesser value to events that occur in the past, the

present, or the future. If members of a cultural group tend to be future oriented, they often will delay immediate gratification until future goals are accomplished. For example, some future-oriented persons who value longevity may engage in health promotion activities to moderate their dietary intake and engage in exercise activities to minimize future health risks. In contrast, some present-oriented cultural groups may place greater emphasis on the here and now and view information about their present set of circumstances as more important than what will happen in the future. Other cultures believe that their ancestral lineage determines their current health status. When nurses discuss health promotion and disease prevention strategies with persons who have a present orientation, they should focus on the immediate benefits these clients will gain rather than emphasizing future outcomes. That is not to say that clients cannot or will not learn about preventing future complications of illness, but nurses need to connect their teaching to the "here and now." It is important to listen carefully to what the clients say in order to gather information about their time orientation. In cultures that focus on a past orientation (e.g., the Vietnamese culture), individuals may be less concerned about planning ahead and focus more on wishes and memories of their ancestors (Giger, 2012). In a past-oriented culture, time is viewed as being more flexible than in a present-oriented culture. It has less of a fixed point, and individuals may not be offended by being late or early for appointments. Nurses socialized in the Western culture may view time as money and equate punctuality with correctness and being responsible. Working with clients who have a different time perception than the nurse can pose a dilemma for the nurse who wishes to be culturally competent and accountable for helping her client receive adequate health care. Nurses should clarify the clients' perceptions to avoid misunderstanding; however, nurses should explain the importance of keeping appointments from the Western perspective. For example, the nurse can communicate a willingness to be flexible in scheduling appointments and explain to clients that the time will be set aside, specifically for them. Along with culture, socioeconomic status and religion may influence the client's perception of time.

## Environmental Control

Environmental control refers to the person's relationship with nature and efforts to plan and direct factors in the environment that affect them. Different cultures can be distinguished on the basis of one of three views of nature and the role of environment in everyday life: (1) nature controls the environment, (2) nature and the environment work in harmony to promote health and wellness, and (3) the environment has mastery over nature. In cultures that perceive individuals as having mastery over the environment, one can expect that a client with the diagnosis of cancer will be willing to engage in a rigorous treatment, include chemotherapy, radiation, and laser therapy to beat the disease. Persons who value harmony with the environment (e.g., African Americans, Asians, and American Indian/Alaskan Natives) may perceive cancer as disharmony with other forces and that medicine can only relieve the symptoms rather than cure the disease. They would look to the mind, body, and spirit connection, for healing comes from within, to find treatments for the malignancy. Naturalistic solutions, such as herbs, acupuncture, and hot and cold treatments would be their treatment of choice to resolve the suffering associated with the cancerous condition. Individuals from cultures that view the environment as dominant over nature (e.g., Hispanics) may believe that they have little or no control over the serious illness for which they have been diagnosed. These individuals are less likely to engage in illness management interventions that are harsh and that they cannot trust to yield a positive health outcome.

## Social Organization

Social organization refers to the way in which families are structured to carry out role functions. Members depend on the extended family and kinship networks for emotional, social, and financial support in times of crises. The significance of kinship in the formation of family relations varies across cultures. Some cultures adopt individuals who are unrelated or remotely related as family members. Some Hispanic and Asian cultures place the needs of the family above those of the individual. In the American Indian/Alaskan Native family, members honor and respect their elders and look to them for leadership, believing that wisdom comes with increasing age. When working with clients who prefer family decision making over individual choice, nurses should be aware that it may be counterproductive to exclude family involvement—particularly mothers and grandmothers—in the health care decision making. At the same time, nurses should advocate for the individual, making sure that when families make decisions, the individual's needs have been considered.

## Communication

Communication is the means by which culture is shared. Both verbal and nonverbal communications are learned in one's culture. Communication is the most significant problem that presents itself in working with cross-cultural groups. Cross-cultural variations in verbal style can range from pronunciation, word meaning, voice quality, and humor, to nonverbal communication with eye contact, gesture, touch, body posture, facial expression, and silence. In all forms of communication, maintain respect for individuals. Often in cultures where the elderly are held in high esteem, they are addressed in a formal manner. Communicating trust is also important because it facilitates the nurse–client interaction and determines the extent to which the client will share information with the nurse (Morgan et al, 2006).

The following example involving a nurse giving instructions to Asian clients about taking anti-tuberculin drugs illustrates the need to understand cultural communication. The clients responded with a smile and a nod. The nurse interpreted this response to mean that the clients understood the instructions and had accepted the treatment protocol. A week later, when the clients returned for a follow-up visit, the nurse discovered that the medications had not been taken. The nurse knew that acceptance by and avoidance of confrontation or disagreement with those in authority are important behaviors in Asian culture. Interventions were adjusted accordingly: the nurse repeated the medication instructions and gave the clients an opportunity to raise questions and concerns and to repeat the instructions that were given; the nurse also discussed the cultural meaning and treatment of tuberculosis. Other factors influencing communication include forms of address such as the use of first names or surnames, and whether it is polite to wait until a person finishes speaking or to talk over each other.

## Nutrition

For many cultures, the preparation and eating of food is a social activity and members of the group come together to celebrate life and comfort with one another. Almost all family rituals, including birth, baptisms, graduations, marriages, retirements, and deaths, include food as part of the ceremony. Many of these practices may have their origin in religious (for example, Muslims avoid pork and foods cooked with alcohol) as well as cultural (for example, African Americans may have a large meal with family and friends after church on Sunday) traditions. The culture domain of nutrition includes much more than having adequate food to sustain dietary requirements.

Efforts to understand dietary patterns of clients should go beyond relying on membership in a defined group. Knowing the client's nutritional practices enables nurses to develop dietary regimens that do not conflict with their cultural food requirements. Health care teams that prescribe an American diet to a Hispanic or an Asian client whose mealtime and food choices may be different from American food patterns may be negligent. Specific foods have been developed for several subcultures such as Vietnamese, Cuban, Puerto Rican, Navajo, Japanese, and Jewish.

When engaging in mutual goal setting with the client and a nutritionist to change harmful dietary practices, the team might need to consult culturally oriented magazines before prescribing particular food items. A number of popular magazines such as *Essence*, *Ebony*, and *Latina* have created healthier dishes from revised old family recipes for Hispanic and African American families. These dishes are tasty and resemble old traditions, yet they are nutritious. Although the foods may differ culturally, excesses often lead to similar risk factors. Box 7-3 identifies several questions that nurses should ask when conducting a nutritional assessment.

Many of clients' health lifestyle choices are associated with their nutritional practices. As a result, before nurses begin a dietary intervention, they should perform a nutritional assessment to determine food preferences, rituals, and taboos. For many cultures, eating is a social activity and people get together for celebration and to comfort each other. Table 7-2 depicts various food preferences that are present among some cultural groups in American society and the associated risk factors when there is excessive use. Efforts to understand dietary patterns of clients should go beyond relying on membership in a defined group. Knowing the client's nutritional practices makes it possible for nurses to develop treatment regimens that will not conflict with their cultural food practices.

## Religion

The expression of spiritually is a component of health and illness coping for most people. The Joint Commission requires that health professionals conduct a spiritual assessment on individuals. Prayer and religion play a dominant role in protecting health and supporting healing in many cultural traditions. Among all the ethnic groups in the United States, African Americans are most likely to report a formal religious affiliation (Pew Forum on Religion & Public Life, 2008). Among Hispanics, Roman Catholic and Pentecostal beliefs and practices are prevalent. Hispanics who practice Pentecostal beliefs may engage in prayer and believe in miraculous healing.

Muslims are the most racially diverse group and the second largest and fastest growing religion in the world. In the United States, the majority of Muslims are white (37%), African American (24%), Asian (20%), mixed race (15%), and Latino (4%). Muslims are considered either Sunni or Shia Muslim. Muslims face Mecca (which is northeast) when they pray, and when death is imminent they want their faces turned toward Mecca. Sunni Muslims pray five times a day and Shiite Muslims pray three times a day. Muslims gather for corporate worship on Fridays. Tradition says that Muslims pray on the floor, but during illness they may pray in bed. Exceptions from traditional Muslim practices can sometimes be permitted during

---

### BOX 7-3 Assessment of Dietary Practices and Food Consumption Patterns

1. Does the food have nutritional value based on *My Plate?*
2. What is the social significance of food in the family? Has the family adopted foods from other cultural groups?
3. What foods are most frequently purchased for family consumption? Who decides and from where is the food purchased?
4. What foods, if any, are prohibited for the family?
5. What variables play a significant role in food selection (cost, variability, family rituals, religion, family tradition, celebrations)?
6. How often does the family prepare food at home? Who prepares the food? How is it prepared?
7. How much food is eaten? When is it eaten and with whom?
8. Are fresh fruits and vegetables easily accessible for purchase in the community?
9. What spices do the family use in the preparation of the food? What are the family favorite recipes?
10. What are the characteristics of restaurants and other eating facilities that the family uses outside of the home?

---

### TABLE 7-2 Food Preferences and Associated Risk Factors in Selected Cultural Groups

| Cultural Group | Food Preferences | Nutritional Excess | Risk Factors |
|---|---|---|---|
| African Americans | Fried foods, greens, bread, pork, rice, foods with high sodium and starch content | Cholesterol, fat, sodium, carbohydrates, calories | Obesity, coronary heart disease, hypertension, cancer, diabetes, and HIV/AIDS |
| Asians | Soy sauce, rice, pickled dishes, raw fish, tea, balance between yin (cold) and yang (hot) concepts | Cholesterol, fat, sodium, carbohydrates, calories | Coronary heart disease, liver disease, cancer of the stomach, ulcers |
| Hispanics | Fried foods, beans and rice, chili, carbonated beverages, high-fat and high-sodium foods | Cholesterol, fat, sodium, carbohydrates, calories | Obesity, coronary heart disease, diabetes |
| American Indian/Alaskan Natives | Blue corn meal, beans, squash, game and fish | Carbohydrates, calories | Depression, suicide, diabetes, malnutrition, tuberculosis, infant and maternal mortality |

From Andrews MM, Boyle JS: *Transcultural Concepts in Nursing Care,* ed 6. Philadelphia, 2012, JB Lippincott; Giger JN: *Transcultural Nursing: Assessment and Intervention,* ed 6. St Louis, 2012, Mosby.

pregnancy, breast feeding, illness, or travel; but the nurse should always ask the client because some Muslims may observe the practices even though they may have received permission for an exception.

Some African Americans practice Muslim traditions although most belong to a Christian faith. Many African Americans find comfort and support in their spiritual beliefs, believe God is responsible for health, and view health professionals as God's instruments for healing. African Americans with Haitian background may practice voodoo in conjunction with a traditional religion.

Most Jews observe the holidays of Rosh Hashanah and Yom Kippur. Many Jews observe Sabbath, which extends from sundown on Friday until sundown on Saturday. Jews of European origin are called Ashkenazi Jews; Middle Easterners and non-European Jews are called Sephardic.

Chinese and other Asian people often practice Eastern religions such as Confucianism, Buddhism, and Taoism (Lai and Sunrood, 2009). Confucianism emphasizes respect for the elderly and people in authority. Practitioners believe that moral conduct and maintaining harmonious relationships are the keys to life. The five most important attributes are benevolence, righteousness, loyalty, filial piety, and virtue. The Buddhist principles embrace three attributes: mercy, thriftiness, and humility. Buddhists believe that people receive good fortune for doing the right thing and misfortune for doing the wrong thing. Taoism embraces selflessness and emotional calm. The most important thing to them is to be in harmony with nature. An important element of health is outdoor exercise for peace of mind and outside air. Part of achieving good health is to adjust the thinking and the body to fit in with the natural rhythm of the universe.

## Immigrants and Cultural Diversity

**Immigrants** to the United States are born in countries or territories external to the United States and migrate to the United States, contributing to its vast diversity. Place of origin for the immigrant is distinguished from nationality, which refers to the place where the individual has or had citizenship. For example, if individuals were born in the Dominican Republic, they may be naturalized citizens, but their ethnicity is likely to be Hispanic with a Dominican place of origin. It is estimated that the U.S. population consists of 39 million (foreign-born) immigrants accounting for 12% of the total population of which 11.7 million have illegal status (Congress of the United States, 2012). **Foreign-born** refers to all residents who were not a U.S citizen at birth, regardless of their current legal or citizen status or those whose parents were not U.S. citizens. More than two thirds of the foreign-born population lives in or around major metropolitan areas in four states: Nevada, Texas, California, and Arizona (Congress of the United States, 2012). Their employment tends to be associated with the region of the world from which they came. For example, persons from South America may be in construction- or agriculture-related occupations (21%), while persons from Asia tend to be associated with professional or technical occupations (39%). The foreign-born are likely to be poorer (23%) than the U.S.-born population

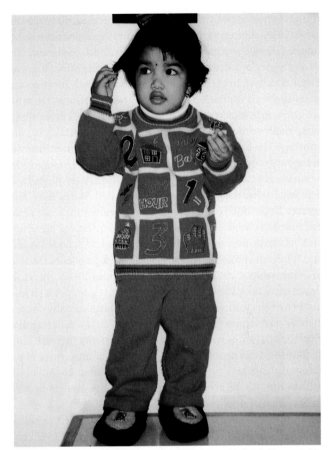

**FIG 7-4** A child from Nepal living in the United States. The child has a black dot on her forehead to protect her from the "evil eye."

(13.5%); 36% of immigrant-headed households use at least one major welfare program (primarily food assistance and Medicaid) compared to 23% of the U.S.-born population. They comprise 16% of the total adult workforce with more than 54% of the adults in the labor force having completed high school (Camarota, 2012). These immigrants bring with them unique cultural, health care, and religious backgrounds (Figure 7-4).

There are four categories of foreign-born. The first category is **legal immigrants**, also known as **lawful permanent residents**. This group constitutes about 85% of the immigrant population. They are not citizens but are legally allowed to live and work in the United States, usually because they fulfill labor demands or have family ties. Legal immigrants usually have a five-year waiting period living in the United States after receiving "qualified" immigration status before they are eligible to receive entitlements such as Medicaid and CHIP (Camarota, 2012). The second category of foreign-born consists of **refugees** and persons seeking asylum. The Refugee Act of 1980 provided a uniform procedure for refugees (based on the United Nations definition) to be admitted to the United States (U.S. Department of Health and Human Services, 2001). This included refugees from Cuba, Vietnam, Laos, Cambodia, and Russian Jewish refugees. These are people who seek protection in the United States because of fear of persecution (on the basis of race, religion, nationality, political view, or membership in a certain group) if they were to return to their homeland. Refugees are immediately eligible to receive Temporary Assistance for Needy Families, Supplemental Security Income, and Medicaid. The third category of foreign-born is the non-immigrants; these are people admitted to the United States for a limited duration and for a specified purpose. Non-immigrants include students, tourists, temporary workers, business executives, career diplomats, their spouses and children, artists, entertainers, and reporters. The fourth category of foreign-born is unauthorized immigrants, or undocumented or illegal aliens. These persons may have crossed a border into the United States illegally, or their legal permission to stay in the United States may have expired. Unauthorized immigrants are eligible to receive emergency medical services, immunizations, treatment for the symptoms of communicable diseases, and access to school lunches only. They are not eligible for federal public benefits through the Affordable Care Act. Between 2007 and 2012, increased apprehensions by the U.S. Border Patrol accounted for a smaller number of persons entering the United States illegally than in the previous decade (Pew Research Center, 2013). A description of the immigrant populations and what benefits they are eligible to receive can be found in *A Description of Immigrant Population: An Update* (Congress of the United States, 2012).

National debate about immigration policy has intensified, particularly about amnesty for illegal aliens, since the events of September 11, 2001. As a result, a variety of immigration laws have been enacted (*Changes in Immigration Law,* 2013). These changes reflect tightened and more restrictive visa procedures as well as greater scrutiny given to all visas and entry documents. The complex issues involved with the foreign-born population and health care accessibility restrict the opportunity for public health nurses to provide culturally competent care to this population.

Misperceptions abound about the economic value of allowing immigrants to enter, or to stay in, the United States. It is estimated that immigrants increase the gross domestic product by 37 billion dollars each year because of their presence in the labor force and contributions in skills, education and capital investments by adding workers to the pool (Immigration Policy Center, 2012), The dilemma for communities, however, is that immigrants typically pay federal taxes yet the services they receive are paid for by the states and localities. Although federal matching funds for Medicaid are not available to the states for immigrants, some states have found compelling public health reasons to use their own funds to cover even undocumented immigrant children, pregnant women with low incomes, disabled persons, and older adults (Camarota, 2012).

There are other health care issues in addition to financial constraints on providing health care for immigrants. Some of these are language barriers; differences in social, religious, and cultural backgrounds between the immigrant and the health care provider; and the use of traditional healing or folk health care practices that may be unfamiliar to U.S. health care providers. Providers may lack knowledge about high-risk diseases in the specific immigrant groups for whom they care. For example, some groups are more at risk for hepatitis B (with its attendant effects on the liver), tuberculosis, intestinal parasites, and visual,

hearing, and dental problems. Many of these conditions are either preventable or treatable if managed correctly. Nurses need to know the major health problems and risk factors that are specific to the immigrant populations for whom they provide care. Nurses need to understand the difficulty of the acculturation process for immigrant families and to treat individuals in the context of the culture from which they come. Often children and adolescents adjust to the new culture more easily than adults. This can lead to a shift in the balance of power between adults and children, contributing to family conflict and at times violence. Inability of elders to acculturate may play a large part in their lack of adherence to health care guidelines. When conducting a health history, nurses should be alert for warning signs of family stress and tension. Remember that older family members can help translate their culture, beliefs, religious practices, dietary habits, support systems, and risk factors for the health care provider. They can also assist with decision making and provide support to enable the person or group seeking care to change behaviors and increase their health promotion practices.

Similarly, understanding the role of the community in the care of immigrants is important. Communities can help clients (and thus providers) with communication, crisis intervention, housing, and emotional and other forms of support. Nurses need to carefully assess the community and learn what strengths, resources, and talents are available.

Nurses need knowledge about the traditional healing practices that immigrants use. Many of these practices have therapeutic value and can be blended with traditional Western medicine (Figure 7-5). The key is to know what practices are being used so the blending can be done knowledgeably. Community members are excellent sources of this information, and nurses working with immigrant populations should use the community assessment, group work, and family techniques described in other chapters to partner with immigrant clients.

Culturally appropriate nursing actions that can be implemented to increase authenticity, accuracy, and approachability when working with immigrant populations include the following:

1. Self-awareness: Recognize the values, beliefs, and practices that comprise your own culture. Nurses, like clients, are influenced by culture, values, and language.
2. Identify the client's preferred or native language. When nurses do not speak or understand the client's language, they must obtain assistance from an interpreter to ensure that full and effective communication occurs. Health care institutions must provide clients with an interpreter. The interpreter should have knowledge of the client's culture and medical terminology. Interpreters should be trained, qualified, and hired to ensure that they have met minimum standards to provide accurate and safe interpretation. Using family members, friends, and staff who are not trained as health/medical interpreters can create errors in understanding and communicating, pose grave risks for the client and liability to the health care institution. While both an interpreter and a translator interpret and translate information from one language to another, there are significant differences between the two. A translator is usually

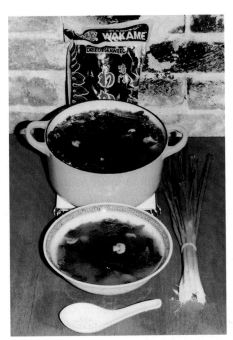

FIG 7-5 Mi-yuk kook (seaweed soup) is a Korean dish eaten by postpartum women to stop bleeding and to cleanse body fluids. It is also eaten every birthday.

associated with translating written documents such as medical records and legal documents; in contrast, the interpreter is associated with verbal communication that focuses on accurate expression of equivalent meanings rather than on word-to-word equivalence.

Many nurses cite linguistic barriers as the largest issue they encounter when trying to provide culturally competent care for linguistically different clients (Starr and Wallace, 2009). Experiences of success that nurses report when working with an interpreter include proper use of interpreters to assure that clients understand health care instructions; provision of linguistically appropriate educational material; ability to communicate in the client's language to provide health care instructions; and ensuring proper use of instructions. Experiences of difficulty include language barriers preventing appropriate communications; lack of available interpreters overall and for specific languages; and lack of appropriate translation by interpreter. Nurses can minimize some of these difficulties by learning basic words and sentences of the most commonly spoken languages in the community and observing client reactions when asking them questions. Also, nurses should provide written material in the client's primary language, so that family members can reinforce information when at home with the client. The How To Box provides guidelines for using an interpreter.

3. Learn the health-seeking behaviors of your client and their family members. In asking the client about family members, you might try using a simple genogram, which places family members on a diagram. Ask who the family members are, where they live, and who is missing or deceased. You might also ask them to talk about holiday celebrations: who comes, who is missing, what do they do?

4. Get to know the community where the immigrant client lives. Read about the culture of your clients. Take a course. Volunteer to participate in the acculturation process of the community (e.g., to give talks, hold forums with free-flowing and two-way communication), and learn who the formal and informal resources are.

5. Get to know some of the traditional practices and remedies used by families and communities. Coordinate health teaching seminars with traditional healing courses for the community so you can work with, not against them.

6. Learn how cultural subgroups explain common illnesses or events. In cultures where the body and mind are seen as one entity or in cultures in which there is a high degree of stigma associated with mental illness, people or individuals somaticize their feelings of psychological distress. In somatization, psychological distress is experienced as a physical illness.

7. Try to see things from the viewpoint of the client, family, and community and accommodate rather than squash the client's view.

8. Conduct a cultural assessment focusing on what is working, what is not working, and changes that need to be made to accommodate cultural norms and promote positive health behaviors.

---

**HOW TO** Guidelines for Selecting and Using an Interpreter

1. The interpreter must interpret everything that is said by all the people in the interaction and inform the public health nurse if the content might be perceived as insensitive or harmful to the dignity of the client.
2. The interpreter conveys the content, the spirit of what is said without omitting or adding.
3. The educational level and the socioeconomic status of the interpreter are important. The nurse should know that the interpreter understands the community's interpretation of the disease and the nurse should understand the community's health care practices around the disease.
4. The nurse needs to evaluate the interpreter's style, approach to clients, and ability to develop a relationship of trust and respect.
5. The gender and/or age of the interpreter may be of concern; in some cultures, women may prefer a female interpreter and men may prefer a male, and older clients may want a more mature interpreter. Avoid using children as interpreters, particularly when the client is an adult.
6. Identify the client's country of origin and language or dialect spoken before selecting the interpreter. For example, Chinese clients speak different dialects depending on the region in which they were born.
7. Observe the client for nonverbal messages such as facial expressions, gestures, and other forms of body language. If the client's responses do not fit with the question, the nurse should check to be sure that the interpreter understood the question.
8. Make phrase charts and picture cards available.
9. Increase accuracy in transmission of information by asking the interpreter to translate the client's own words, and ask the client to repeat the information that was communicated.
10. The interpreter must maintain confidentiality of all information and interactions. At the end of the interview, review the material with the client and the interpreter to ensure that nothing has been missed or misunderstood.

# CULTURAL DIVERSITY AND HEALTH DISPARITIES

## Disparities in Health

Disparities are used to describe incongruent elements. Health disparities are associated with inequity in social structures based on particular characteristics such as ethnicity, race, immigrant status, gender, age, and sexual orientation (Levine et al, 2011). Health disparities stem from characteristics historically linked to discrimination. They are also expressed in differences in morbidity and mortality rates among population groups linked to factors such as race or ethnicity, religion, socioeconomic status, gender, mental health, sexual orientation, place of origin, and residence. Health disparities are monitored annually by various departments within The U.S. Department of Health and Human Services as part of the national goal to achieve health equity for all within the United States (see the Healthy People 2020 box related to health disparities).

 **HEALTHY PEOPLE 2020**

### Goals and Objectives of Healthy People 2020 Related to Cultural Issues

**Goal:** Eliminate health disparities among different segments of the population as defined by gender, race or ethnicity, education, income, disability, living in rural areas, and sexual orientation.

**Selected Objectives**
- AHS-1: Increase the proportion of persons with health insurance.
- AHS-2: Increase the proportion of insured persons with clinical preventive services coverage.
- AHS-3: Increase the proportion of persons with a usual primary care provider.
- AHS-6: Increase the proportion of persons who have a specific source of ongoing care.
- AHS-7: Reduce the proportion of individuals who are unable to obtain or delay in obtaining necessary medical care, dental care, or prescription medicine.

## Social Determinants of Health

Social determinants of health are the circumstances in which people are born, grow up, live, work, age, and the systems put in place to deal with illness. These circumstances are in turn shaped by a wider set of forces such as economic stability (indicators such as poverty and unemployment), education (indicators such as reading levels, graduation rates, and enrollment in higher education), social and community context (indicators such as family structure and social cohesion), health and health care (indicators such as access to health services and access to primary care), and neighborhood (indicators such as quality of schools and housing, access to healthy foods, and incidences of crime and violence) (Healthy People 2020, 2013).

## Marginalization

Marginalization of vulnerable populations occurs when a segment of the population has been excluded from the mainstream in social, economic, cultural, or political life. Marginalization is brought about by policies, practices, and programs that have relegated these populations to the fringe of society and which prevents them from meaningfully participating in society. Examples of these vulnerable populations include but are not limited to groups excluded due to race/ethnicity, homelessness, immigrants with linguistic challenges, drug abuse, sexual orientation, economics, and gender, which are devalued and not granted certain privileges that are given to others. In some instances, vulnerable populations may be considered an equivalent term for marginalization.

## Health Equity

Health equity is concerned with providing social justice in health so that individuals are not disadvantaged from achieving the highest possible standard of health based on membership in a group that has historically been disadvantaged (Braveman, 2014). It is the principle underlying a commitment to reduce and ultimately eliminate disparities in health. Achieving health equity requires giving recognition to social barriers as well as barriers that have their origins in genetics, economics, and lifestyle factors that contribute to inequality of health. Health inequities are avoidable treatment between groups of people. They are reflected in differences in length of life, quality of life, rates of disease and disability, severity of disease, access to treatment among groups of people, and death.

## Social Justice

Social justice is concerned with values of impartiality and objectivity at a systems or governmental level and is founded on principles of fairness, equity, respect for self and human dignity, and tolerance. Practicing social justice is acting in accordance with fair treatment regardless of economic status, race, ethnicity, age, citizenship, disability, or sexual orientation.

## Health Literacy

The Centers for Disease Control and Prevention (CDC) define health literacy as the degree to which an individual has the capacity to obtain, communicate, process, and understand basic health information and services to make appropriate health care decisions. Low health literacy negatively influences understanding of medical information (such as illness condition, treatment plan), obtaining health care services, managing chronic conditions, and use of medication and avoidance of medication errors, and places individuals at a safety risk. Low literacy is more common among the elderly, minority populations, immigrants, individuals with lower socioeconomic status, and the medically underserved. Individuals with low health literacy are adversely affected by low educational skills, cultural barriers to health care, and by nurses who use language that the patient does not understand. Often these individuals may have a different perspective about their illness and what to do about it. The pattern in which they present their illness might be different from the pattern persons with high literacy skills would use to present their illness. When caring for persons with low literacy skills, nurses should ask the client to repeat instructions to assess the client's level of literacy, repeat information as needed, allow the client time to process the information, use face-to-face communication whenever possible, make the information personally relevant, give reasons for short-term benefits for taking the specific action, and provide sufficient follow-up for each person (CDC, 2009).

## Health Disparities and Socioeconomic Status

The relationship between health disparities and socioeconomic status is reflected in life expectancy, infant death rates, low birth rates, and many other health measures (Agency for Healthcare Research & Quality, 2013). Members of minority groups may be marginalized, preventing them from enjoying the same opportunities and resources for education, occupation, income earning, and property ownership that the dominant group has, thus relegating them to the fringe of society. Between 2007 and 2011 the poverty rate in the United States was 14.3% (Macartney et al, 2013), but there were differences in poverty rates associated with membership in various racial/ethnic groups. Table 7-3 indicates that there are more white families than minorities below the poverty level. However, the proportion of poor families in a minority group is greater. For example, 11.6% of white families are living in poverty, whereas 25.8% of African Americans, 23.2% of Hispanics, and 27% of American Indian/Alaskan Natives are doing so. Consequently, minority families are disproportionately represented on the lower tiers of the socioeconomic ladder. The mortality rate among individuals from lower socioeconomic status is significantly higher than among those from higher income levels (Cheng and Kindig, 2012).

Poor economic achievement is also a common characteristic found among populations at risk, such as single-parent head of households, the homeless, migrant workers, and refugees. Nurses should be able to distinguish between cultural and socioeconomic issues. Attributing behaviors stemming from socioeconomic deficits to behaviors embedded in cultural origins can result in misinterpretations of the client's motivation to adhere to treatment regimens. Data suggest that when nurses and clients come from the same social class, it is more likely that they operate from the same health belief model, and consequently there is less opportunity for misinterpretation and

communication problems. Nevertheless, research on health disparities has shown that individuals from minority racial and ethnic groups are disproportionately likely to develop severe health problems and to experience lower quality care and poor outcomes in relation to health problems even after controlling for socioeconomic status, insurance status, and age (Agency for Healthcare Research & Quality, 2014; 2013).

There is danger in believing that only individuals in the lower socioeconomic rung use cultural behaviors such as folk (natural and magico-religious) practices. More individuals in Western cultures, including health professionals, are integrating folk practices with the biomedical system to promote, protect, and restore their health. Acceptance of this is reflected in courses being offered in universities, the arrival of newer disciplines in health care such as homeopathic medicine, and more acceptance of traditional medicine (such as acupressure and acupuncture). Nurses can consult and seek guidance from non-Western practitioners to better understand how clients and families integrate cultural concepts with other aspects of client care to meet their clients' total health care needs.

## CULTURAL COMPETENT NURSING INTERVENTIONS

### Cultural Competence

Transcultural nursing recognizes and appreciates differences in health care values, beliefs, and customs. Transcultural theorists subscribe to the belief that nurses must acquire knowledge, skill, and attitudes in cultural competence and be committed to change to ensure positive outcomes, eliminate health disparities, and increase client satisfaction.

A number of governmental agencies such as the U.S. Department of Health and Human Services, state regulations, and private and quasi-governmental regulators such as The Joint Commission have attempted to address the need for cultural competence through various standards and legislation. For instance, standards of practice for culturally competent nursing care were developed by a task force of the expert panel for Global Nursing and Health of the American Academy of Nursing in concert with members of the Transcultural Nursing Society to help nurses apply these standards universally in the arenas of clinical practice, research, education, and administration (American Academy of Nursing Expert Panel, 2010). The 12 standards address core values inherent in professional nursing practice and include behaviors, attitudes, and skills requisite for cultural competence. These standards are described in Box 7-4.

Both of the accreditation bodies for nursing education, the Accreditation Commission for Education in Nursing (ACEN) and the Commission on Collegiate Nursing Education (CCNE), address the need for cultural competence as essential content in nursing education. State Boards of Nursing are requiring cultural competence education in nursing schools and recent legislation in many states includes requiring cultural competency training for health care providers to receive licensure or relicensure.

Cultural competence entails a combination of culturally congruent behaviors, practice attitudes, and policies that allow nurses to use interpersonal communication, relationship skills,

| TABLE 7-3 Poverty Rates by Ethnic Groups | | |
|---|---|---|
| Ethnic Groups | Percent of Total Populations | Percent of Poverty Rate |
| Non-Hispanic Whites | 42.4% | 11.6% |
| Blacks | 12.6% | 25.8% |
| Asians | 4.8% | 11.7% |
| Hispanics | 16.4% | 23.2% |
| American Indian/ Alaskan Natives | .09% | 27.0% |
| Native Hawaiians | 0.02% | 17.6% |

From U.S. Census Bureau: *Income, Poverty, and Health Insurance Coverage in the US: 2010* and Macartney S, Bishaw A, Fontenot K: *Poverty rates for selected detailed race and Hispanic groups by state and place: 2007–2011.*

### BOX 7-4 Standards of Practice for Culturally Competent Nursing Care

Standard 1. Social justice: Nurses use principles of social justice to guide them as they advocate for the patient, family, community, and other health care professionals.

Standard 2. Critical reflection: Nurses critically reflect on their own values, beliefs, and cultural heritage to determine the influence of these qualities and issues on providing culturally congruent nursing care.

Standard 3. Knowledge of cultures: Nurses understand the perspectives, traditions, values, practices, and family systems of culturally diverse individuals, families, communities, and populations for whom they care, as well as having knowledge of the complex variables that affect the achievement of health and well-being.

Standard 4. Culturally competent practice: Nurses use cross-cultural knowledge and culturally sensitive skills when implementing culturally congruent nursing care.

Standard 5. Cultural competence in health care systems and organizations: Health care organizations provide the structure and resources for nurses to evaluate and meet the cultural and language needs of their culturally diverse clientele.

Standard 6. Patient advocacy and empowerment: Nurses recognize the impact that health care policies, delivery systems, and resources have on their populations and advocate on the patients' behalf for inclusion of their cultural beliefs and practices in all dimensions of their health care.

Standard 7. Multicultural workforce: Nurses engage in activities to ensure multicultural workforce health care settings, such as those that strengthen recruitment and retention in hospitals and academic settings.

Standard 8. Education and training in culturally competent care: Nurses shall have knowledge and skills to ensure that the delivery of patient care is culturally congruent and includes global health care agendas that mandate formal education and clinical training as well as ongoing continuing education for all practicing nurses.

Standard 9. Cross-cultural communication: Nurses use culturally appropriate verbal and nonverbal communication skills to identify patient's values, beliefs, practices, perceptions, and unique health care needs.

Standard 10. Cross-cultural leadership: Nurses influence individuals, groups, and systems to achieve positive health outcomes of culturally competent care for diverse populations.

Standard 11. Policy development: Nurses have the knowledge and skills to work with public and private organizations, professional associations, and communities to develop policies and standards for comprehensive implementation and evaluation of culturally competent care.

Standard 12. Evidence-based practice and research: Nurses use tested interventions shown to be effective for the culturally diverse populations that they serve. The nurse also engages in research to test the effectiveness of interventions appropriate for specific culturally diverse clients.

Adapted from American Academy of Nursing Expert Panel: *Standards of practice for culturally competent nursing care*, 2010. Available at http://www.tcns.org/files/Standards_of_Practice_for_Culturally_Compt_Nsg_Care-Revised.pdf. Accessed February 25, 2014.

and behavioral flexibility to work effectively in cross-cultural situations. Cultural competence allows nurses to partner with the client to deliver health promotion, disease prevention, and health restoration (Campinha-Bacote, 2011; Leininger, 2002a). Culturally competent nurses respect individuals from different cultures, value diversity, and function effectively when caring for clients from other cultures. Cultural competence reflects a higher level of knowledge than cultural sensitivity, which was once thought to be all that was needed for nurses to effectively care for their client. In contrast, cultural sensitivity suggests that the nurse has basic knowledge of the client's culture but does not use the information to devise a plan of care that reflects the client's total cultural needs. Nurses should be aware of the social determinants of health in the environment that prevent individuals from achieving good health.

It is generally accepted that culturally competent nursing care is guided by the following principles (American Academy of Nursing Expert Panel, 2010):

1. Care must be client centered, that is, designed for the specific client, family, or community.
2. Care must be based on the uniqueness of the client's culture and incorporate the cultural norms and values of the client in the management of the care plan.
3. Self-empowerment strategies of the client are identified and viewed as strengths to facilitate client decision making and self-care management in health and illness situations.

Cultural competence is also one of the core attributes of public health nurses (Quad Council, 2011). Nurses work toward becoming culturally competent for a number of reasons. First, nurses who come from a culture different from that of the client may not be knowledgeable about the client's culture. Nurses come from a variety of cultural backgrounds and have their own cultural traditions. Each nurse has unique cultural experiences that give meaning and understanding to his or her behavior. Because of differences between the client's cultural system and the nurse's cultural system, when the client and the nurse interact they may have different understandings about the meaning of the health issue and different ideas about what to do to promote and protect health. In these circumstances, nurses who value and practice cultural competence use communication and relational strategies that respect clients' values, expectations, and goals without diminishing the nurses' own values, expectations, and goals. To illustrate, a recent Mexican immigrant who speaks little English goes to a community health center because of a urinary tract infection. The nurse understands that she must use strategies that would allow her to effectively communicate with the client. She also understands that the client has the right to receive effective care that is based upon culturally informed nursing science, to judge whether she has received the care she wanted, and to follow up with appropriate action if she did not receive the expected care. Nurses must be culturally competent to modify nursing interventions that are specific to the needs of cultural and ethnic groups.

Second, care that is not culturally competent may further increase the gap in racial and health disparities between minority and majority populations. Failure to effectively respond to the health care needs and preferences of culturally and linguistically diverse individuals may (1) increase barriers to equitable access to care, (2) inhibit effective communication between the client and the nurse, and (3) create obstacles in gathering assessment data, thus limiting the development and implementation of effective treatment plans.

Third, nurses use culturally competent practice to improve the quality, cost, and safety of care and health outcomes. The health care industry focuses on cost-effectiveness to balance cost and quality (Agency for Healthcare Research & Quality, 2012). **Quality of care** means that the client has access to health care and that the care is delivered by culturally competent nurses to help clients achieve positive health outcomes. Care that is not focused on the clients' values, expectations, and goals is likely to increase cost and diminish quality. For example, when clients are using both folk medicine and traditional Western medicine and nurses fail to assess and use this information in teaching, the clients may not get the full benefits of the treatment protocol. Positive outcomes, which are indicators of quality, may not be met. When quality is compromised, additional resources that typically increase costs may be needed to achieve the desired health care outcomes.

Fourth, legal regulations and accreditation mandates specify that culturally competent health care must be provided so that health disparities can be reduced and ultimately eliminated. For example, the specific *Healthy People 2020* objectives for persons of different cultures need to be met (USDHHS, 2010). To accomplish these objectives, the client's lifestyle and personal choices must be considered beyond the cursory ways that health care providers have interacted with clients in the past. Clients may present their symptoms vastly differently from the way they are presented in medical and nursing text books; they may present with different threshold for seeking care or expectations about their care. They may have beliefs about the origin and treatment of disease that affect their willingness to adhere to the treatment regimen, and they may have limited English proficiency and low health literacy.

For example, American health care professionals frequently view excessive drinking as a sign of disease and alcoholism as a mental illness. However, in the American Indian/Alaskan Native culture, these signify a disharmony between the individual and the spirit world, and biomedical interventions alone may not be adequate to reduce alcoholism within this culture. American Indians and Alaskan Natives have an alcohol-related death rate that is two times higher than it is in the general population. This is particularly devastating among American Indian males in the 35 to 49 age group, and contributes to a loss of 6.4 more years of potential life compared with those in the general population (CDC, 2008). The national goal is to reduce this disparity. However, many American Indian/Alaskan Natives view alcohol consumption as an acceptable way to participate in family celebrations and tribal ceremonies, and refusal to drink with family may be viewed as a sign of rejection. West (1993, p. 234) suggested that nurses understand the possible ramifications of not having culturally competent staff available to care for the American Indian/Alaskan Native population. She stated, "If the government sends Indians to a health clinic where personnel do not understand the holistic health practices of Indians and where young white people serve as caregivers and authority figures, failure is likely to result." To have successful outcomes, nurses who develop population-based programs to reduce alcohol-related deaths must be willing to respect the cultural uniqueness of Native Americans and to explore individuals' life experiences to find the underlying causes of their behaviors.

Fifth, to gain a competitive edge in the marketplace, the private sector is incorporating culturally competent policies

and care practices for its diverse populations and providers. Insurance companies, health maintenance organizations, and other private health entities have developed initiatives in cultural competence for their providers and engage in cultural competence strategies to improve patient satisfaction and patient care outcomes.

Sixth, in an effort to decrease the risk of liability from malpractice claims and to increase client satisfaction, health care providers and health care organizations are engaging in cultural negotiations. For example, a communication strategy focused on increasing productive health care services for clients was initiated. The strategy utilizes a nurse–client partnership and underscores openness, mutual respect, and flexibility when communicating.

## Developing Provider Cultural Competence

Cultural competence is an ongoing life process in which the nurse is challenged to break with the old and engage in new ways of thinking and performing.

Nurses develop cultural competence through the critical reflective use of self-awareness skills, communications skills, relationship-building skills, and intervention skills that promote mutual respect for differences in the use of participatory decision making. In developing cultural competence, nurses may be guided by two principles suggested by Leininger (2002a): (1) maintain a broad objective and open attitude toward individuals and their cultures, and (2) avoid seeing all individuals as alike. Because there are varying degrees of cultural competence, not all nurses will achieve the same level of development concurrently. For example, Starr and Wallace (2009) reported that public health nurses in a southeastern public health department rated themselves higher on cultural thoughts (cultural awareness and sensitivity) than on cultural competence behaviors. Over all, the nurses reported a moderate level of cultural competence that was increased through online and class room courses.

In an early model developed by Orlandi (1992), three stages to developing cultural competence were depicted (culturally incompetent, culturally sensitive, and culturally competent). Table 7-4 shows that each stage has three dimensions—cognitive

| TABLE 7-4 | The Cultural Competence Framework: Stages of Competence Development | | |
|---|---|---|---|
| | Culturally Incompetent | Culturally Sensitive | Culturally Competent |
| Cognitive | Oblivious | Aware | Knowledgeable |
| Affective | Apathetic | Sympathetic | Committed to change |
| Psychomotor (skills) | Unskilled | Lacking some skills | Highly skilled |
| Overall effect | Destructive | Neutral | Constructive |

From Orlandi MA: Defining cultural competence: an organizing framework. In Orlandi MA, editor: *Cultural Competence for Evaluators.* Washington, DC, 1992, U.S. Department of Health and Human Services.

(thinking), affective (feeling), and psychomotor (doing)—that have an overall effect on nursing outcomes. The most effective outcomes are knowledgeable, committed to change, and highly skilled. The most destructive outcomes are oblivious, apathetic, and unskilled.

A widely used model to explain the process of cultural competence was created by Campinha-Bacote (2011). The most recent model depicts five elements of cultural competence: (1) cultural awareness, (2) cultural knowledge, (3) cultural skill, (4) cultural encounter, and (5) cultural desire.

### Cultural Awareness

Cultural awareness refers to the self-examination and in-depth exploration of one's own biases, stereotypes, and prejudices as they influence behavior toward other cultural groups (Campinha-Bacote, 2011). Culturally aware nurses are conscious of culture as an influencing factor on differences between themselves and others, and are receptive to learning about the cultural dimensions of diverse clients. They understand the basis for their own behavior and how it helps or hinders the delivery of competent care to persons from cultures other than their own (American Academy of Nursing Expert Panel, 2010). Culturally aware nurses recognize that health is expressed differently across cultures and that culture influences an individual's responses to health, illness, disease, and death. Culturally competent care can be delivered in a variety of modes consistent with the client's health values. For example, at a community outreach program, a nurse was teaching a racially mixed group the screening protocol for breast and cervical cancer detection. An African American woman in the group refused to give the return demonstration for breast self-examination. When encouraged to do so, she said, "My breasts are much larger than those on the model. Besides, the models are not like me. They are all white." After hearing the client's comments, the nurse realized that she did not take into account the significance of breasts based on ethnicity and culture, the size of the breast, and had made no reference in her talk to the influence of culture or race on screening for breast and cervical cancer.

The nurse then talked with the client, asked for her recommendations, and encouraged her to return the demonstration. The nurse coached the client through the self-examination process while pointing out that regardless of breast size, shape, and color, the technique is the same for feeling the tissue and squeezing the nipple to make certain that there is no discharge. Because this nurse was culturally aware, she neither became angry with herself or the client nor imposed her own values on the client. Rather, she elicited a discussion with the client about her beliefs, attitudes, and feelings about screening for cancer that may have been influenced by her culture. The nurse understood that she had to tailor her teaching material to the needs of diverse client groups. Subsequently, she advocated for her agency to purchase a model of an African American woman's breast to be used in future health education programs with African American women.

If the nurse had not been culturally aware, she might have misunderstood the client's concerns and acted in a defensive manner. Such an interaction would have failed to identify client assets and barriers and appropriate intervention strategies. A confrontation might have ensued that would not have been helpful to the client or the nurse. Nurses should champion the cause for clients seeking health care to have health care professionals respect their cultural traditions.

### Cultural Knowledge

Cultural knowledge refers to the process of searching for and obtaining a sound educational understanding about culturally diverse groups (Campinha-Bacote, 2011). Emphasis is on learning about the clients' worldview from an emic (native) perspective as it pertains to health beliefs and practices, cultural values, and disease incidence and prevalence. For example, cultural knowledge indicates that Middle Eastern women might not attend prenatal classes without encouragement and support from the nurse (Meleis, 2005). Attendance at prenatal classes is about the future of the baby while the mother's main focus may be on the present and what is happening in the immediate environment. The nurse's understanding of the client's concept of time would decrease misinterpretation that the mother might undermine efforts to promote a healthy baby, and allows the nurse to select strategies to ensure the client's cooperation in providing the best care for the baby. In contrast, knowledge of Nigerian culture indicates that while women will start prenatal care as soon as pregnancy is confirmed, they view pregnancy and birth as natural events and may not continue to attend prenatal classes throughout the prenatal phase (Ogbu, 2005). Although the behavior of the women from these two countries may be the same, the rationale for their action is different. Leininger (2002a) points out that nurses who lack cultural knowledge may develop feelings of inadequacy and helplessness because they are often unable to effectively help their clients.

Although it is unrealistic to expect that nurses will have knowledge of all cultures, they should know how and where to obtain information that impacts the individual with whom they have frequent interaction. Missing or inadequate knowledge of the client's culture can contribute to negative situations such as client's inadequate use of health resources. Because cultural competence is a requirement in nursing education, students are now exposed to a variety of individuals who hold membership in cultures that are different from their own. Students therefore have an opportunity to assess gaps in their cultural knowledge about how to care for individuals, families, and communities from diverse groups. Students also learn that clients are a rich source of information about their own culture. The Evidence-Based Practice box provides an example of learning how to meet the needs of a cultural group that is different from that of the nurse.

### Cultural Skill

Cultural skill is the third element of developing cultural competence. Cultural skill refers to the ability of nurses to effectively integrate cultural awareness and cultural knowledge when conducting a cultural assessment as well as a culturally based physical assessment and to use the data to meet the specific client's needs (Campinha-Bacote, 2011). Culturally skillful nurses elicit

## EVIDENCE-BASED PRACTICE

The purpose of this descriptive correlation designed study was to assess the personal beliefs about the causes and meaning of having diabetes among members of the Lumbee Indian tribe living in rural southeastern North Carolina. The sample consisted of 40 adult men and women. A mixed method approach to consist of qualitative and quantitative data was used to conduct this study.

The participant responses indicated a moderate belief in the efficacy of diabetes treatment, a moderate belief in their ability to understand a coherent model of diabetes, and a low level of emotional distress related to having diabetes. Two major themes emerged from the open-ended questions about the causes of diabetes: (1) genetic predetermination and (2) lifestyle practices. Although participants believed that their prescribed diabetes medications were a necessary part of controlling their illness, several expressed fatigue and "felt worn out" with having to persist with their treatment expectations. Limitations were that the sample only included persons who were seeking health care treatment for diabetes and did not include those who were not scheduled for an appointment at the clinic during the data collection period, or included those who did not have access to health care.

### Nurse Use

Nurses should be aware that their Lumbee Indian clients may not always have a high degree of confidence in conventional treatment regimens nor understand the unpredictable course of diabetes. Nurses should work with these clients to provide culturally congruent education using appropriate communication to increase clients' knowledge about current treatment regimens. Nurses should incorporate culturally specific strategies that will empower clients to take a more active role in their illness management, dispel the attitude that a diagnosis of diabetes is genetically predetermined, link concrete behaviors to disease progression and outcomes, and demonstrate to clients how attainable decreases in blood sugar can reduce the risk of long-term consequences. Such strategies would help eliminate negative perceptions that may interfere with the health care delivery process. The researchers suggested that by using a broad systems approach, nurses will increase the availability of Native American health care providers who can serve as role models for the community as well as become activists for developing community infrastructure to support healthy lifestyles.

From Jacobs A, Kemppainen JK, Taylor JS, et al: Beliefs about diabetes and medication adherence among Lumbee Indians living in rural southeastern North Carolina. *J Transcult Nurs* 25:167–175, 2014.

from clients their perception of the health problem, discuss treatment protocol, negotiate acceptable options, select interventions that incorporate alternative treatment plans, and collaborate with all stakeholders. For example, culturally competent nurses use appropriate touch during conversation and modify the physical distance between themselves and others while meeting mutually agreed upon goals.

### Cultural Encounter

Cultural encounter is the fourth element essential to becoming culturally competent. Cultural encounter refers to the process that permits nurses to seek opportunities to directly engage in cross-cultural interactions with clients of diverse cultures to modify existing beliefs about a specific cultural group and possibly avoid stereotyping (Campinha-Bacote, 2011). Culture encounters, a key element in becoming culturally competent, have their roots in the nurse–client interpersonal relationship

that focuses on caring, compassion, presence, caring consciousness, and empathy. There are two types of cultural encounters: direct (face-to-face) and indirect. An example of a direct cultural encounter occurs when nurses learn directly from their Puerto Rican clients about spicy foods that they avoid during periods of breastfeeding. Indirect cultural encounters occur when nurses share these assessment findings with other nurses to help them develop their knowledge to effectively care for other Puerto Rican clients who are breastfeeding. The most important encounters are those in which nurses engage in effective communication, use appropriate language and literacy level, and learn about clients' life experiences and the significance of these experiences for health (Leininger, 2002a). In some communities, nurses may have few opportunities to work directly with persons of other cultures. Thus, when nurses come in contact with clients who are culturally different from the nurse, they should adapt general cultural concepts to the situation until they are able to learn directly from the clients about their culture. Developing cultural competence also comes from reading about, taking courses on, and discussing different cultures within multicultural settings. Successful cultural encounters embrace. Continuously interact with patients from diverse backgrounds to validate, refine, or modify existing values, beliefs and practices about a cultural group and to develop cultural desire, cultural awareness, cultural skill, and cultural knowledge (Figure 7-6).

### Cultural Desire

Cultural desire is the fifth element needed in the process of developing cultural competence. It refers to nurses' intrinsic motivation to want to engage in the previous four elements necessary to provide culturally competent care (Campinha-Bacote, 2012). It is based on the humanistic value of caring for the individual. Nurses who wish to become culturally competent do so because they want to, rather than because they are directed to do so. They demonstrate a sense of energy and enthusiasm about the possibility of providing culturally competent nursing interventions. Unlike the other elements, cultural desire cannot be directly taught in the classroom or in other educational or work settings. Nurses are more likely to demonstrate cultural desire when the environment at all levels of the organization reflects a philosophy that values cultural competence for all its clients.

Campinha-Bacote (2011) recommends that nurses who want to develop cultural competence should not fear making mistakes, but should internalize and incorporate into their own worldview selected beliefs, values, practices, life-ways, and problem-solving skills of other cultures with which they have the most frequent encounters. Several measures of the cultural competence construct have been reported in the nursing literature: the Interpersonal Process of Care survey (IPC-18, Chart Form: Stewart et al, 2007) and the Cultural Competent Assessment (CCA–25; Doorenbos et al, 2005). The IPC survey consists of two subscales that are used to determine disparities in interpersonal care, predict patient outcomes, and examine outcomes of quality improvement efforts to reduce health care disparities. The CCA consists of two subscales that

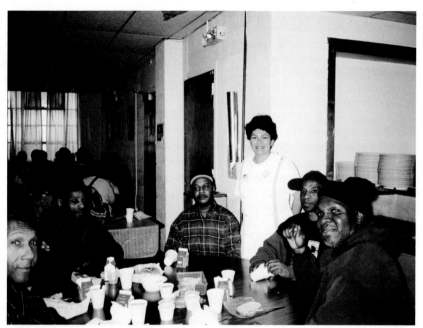

**FIG 7-6** A Hispanic nursing student interacting with African American men at a nutritional center. To interact in a culturally competent manner, the student needs to have awareness of and knowledge about the differences between her culture and the men's culture and the skill to portray this in her behavior toward them.

examine nurses' cultural diversity experience, cultural awareness and sensitivity, and performance of cultural competence behaviors.

## Barriers to Developing Cultural Competence

Nurses fail to provide culturally competent nursing care for a variety of reasons: they may have had minimal opportunity to learn about cross-cultural nursing; their supervisors may encourage them to increase productivity at the expense of quality; or they may be pressured by colleagues who are not knowledgeable about cultural concepts and are offended when others use the concepts. These and similar issues may result in nurses engaging in behaviors such as stereotyping, prejudice and racism, ethnocentrism, cultural imposition, cultural conflict, and culture shock.

### Stereotyping

Stereotyping is ascribing certain beliefs and behaviors about a given racial and ethnic group to an individual without assessing for individual differences. Stereotyping blocks the willingness of a person to be open and to learn about specific individuals or groups. When information is not immediately available, nurses may generalize about an individual's group behavioral pattern as a guide until they have had time to observe and assess the client's behavior. This can be a problem, and it may lead to a nurse's unwillingness to incorporate new and specific data about the client. New information may be distorted to fit with preconceived ideas. The generalizing that was a beginning point for understanding the individual becomes a final point. The individual is thus stereotyped on the basis of the group's ascribed behavior.

Stereotypes can be either positive or negative. For example, Asians are often positively stereotyped as the "model" minority

group, leading to an expectation that they will always behave in ways that reinforce the stereotypical notion. Other groups are stereotyped as "industrious and hard working," while some groups are stereotyped as negative and noncompliant. To illustrate, a nurse who believes that young African American women are sexually permissive may label a woman in this group who is complaining of abdominal pain as having symptoms of a sexually transmitted disease. Clients who perceive they are being stereotyped may respond with anger and hostility. This in turn perpetuates the stereotype and creates barriers to health-seeking behavior. To minimize the use of stereotypes, nurses should rely on their ability to conduct good health assessment and engage in culturally competent discussions.

### Prejudice

Prejudice is the emotional manifestation of deeply held beliefs (stereotypes) about a group. These beliefs are directed toward a person who is a member of that group, and who is presumed to have the qualities ascribed to the group. Prejudice is not based on reason or experience but rather on negative or favorable preconceived feelings. These feelings are often precursors for discriminatory acts based on prejudging, limited knowledge about, misinformation about, fear of, or limited contact with individuals from that group. Those who are prejudiced wish to deny the individuals, on the basis of race, skin color, ethnicity, or social standing, the opportunity to benefit fully from society's offerings of accessible health care, education, good jobs, and community activities.

### Racism

Racism is a form of prejudice that occurs through the exercise of power by individuals and institutions against people who are judged to be inferior on the basis of intelligence, morals, beauty, inheritance, and self-worth. Individuals are denied certain opportunities (e.g., jobs, housing, education, and health care) typically enjoyed by the larger group because of some characteristic over which they have no control. When racism is acted upon, it results in perceived or actual harm to the individual. Three types of racism exist: individual, institutional, and cultural. Individual racism refers to discriminatory behavior or acts directed toward individuals or groups because of identified characteristics, such as skin color, hair texture, and facial features. Institutional racism refers to discriminatory behavior or acts by an institution, as expressed in policies, priority setting, hiring, and resource allocation practices that are directed toward individuals and groups and restrict their access to opportunities or resources. Institutional racism provides the structure for racism at the individual level to be accepted and condoned. Cultural racism refers to discriminatory behavior or acts directed by the dominant group toward another cultural group. The cultural group is depicted in derogatory or stereotypical ways because of, for example, language or dress. All forms of racism can have individual, as well as community and population, effects.

The Tuskegee Syphilis Study is a well-known example of racism (Gamble, 1997). This study was conducted by the U.S. Public Health Service to observe the effects of syphilis on African American men over a period of 40 years, beginning in 1932. When African American men with syphilis were recruited for the study, they were told that they were being treated for "bad blood," and treatment for syphilis was withheld intentionally so that the study on the deleterious effect of syphilis could be completed. As a result, hundreds of men lost their lives because of discriminatory policies that promoted substandard health care. The consequence of such racism has contributed to the long-held beliefs by some African Americans that health research might be designed to harm them and that accessible health care for African Americans might be part of a research study, especially government-sponsored programs. In 2005, Dwayne, Isaac, and Laveist reported that a telephone survey revealed that no differences by race existed between African Americans and whites in knowledge about the Tuskegee study. There were significant race differences in medical care that the researchers attributed to broader historical and personal experiences of African Americans. Perceived racism by cultural groups can have physiological and psychological negative health outcomes that include high blood pressure, stroke, engaging in risky behaviors such as smoking and substance abuse, depression, and low self-esteem. Nurses too may be recipients of prejudicial or racist acts (Fielo and Degazon, 1997), but they do not have to accept such behavior from clients. Rather, they should set limits, discuss the behavior with other colleagues when appropriate, and avoid personalizing the behavior.

One way to depict the effects of prejudice and racism is to use a two-dimensional matrix: overt versus covert, and intentional versus unintentional. Locke and Hardaway (1992) depict four types of prejudice and racism that result from this matrix: overt intentional, covert intentional, overt unintentional, and covert unintentional. Overt intentional prejudice or racism means that the behavior is both apparent and purposeful. The nurse is aware of personal biases and beliefs and integrates them into a plan of action to negatively manage client problems. With overt unintentional, the behavior is apparent but not purposeful, and no harm is intended, although harm may result. Covert intentional means that the behavior is subtle and purposeful but the person tries to avoid being viewed as prejudicial or racist. Covert unintentional means that the person's behavior is neither apparent nor purposeful. The person is unaware of the behavior. Regardless of the type of prejudice or racism, the behavior is harmful to the client. Examples of each type of prejudice and racism are presented in Box 7-5.

### Ethnocentrism

Ethnocentrism, or cultural prejudice, is the belief that one's own cultural group determines the standards by which another group's behavior is judged. The implication is that one's own standards are better than and superior to the other person's standards. Ethnocentric nurses favor their own professional values and find unacceptable that which is different from their culture. Their inability to accept different worldviews often leads them to devalue the experiences of others, judge them to be inferior, and treat those who are different from themselves with suspicion or hostility (Andrews and Boyle, 2012).

Ethnoculturalism is in contrast to cultural blindness, in which there is an inability to recognize the differences between one's own cultural beliefs, values, and practices and those of another culture. The tendency is to believe that the recognition of racial, ethnic, religious, or gender difference is itself prejudicial and discriminatory. Hence, nurses who state that they treat all clients the same, regardless of cultural orientation, are demonstrating cultural blindness.

### Cultural Imposition

Cultural imposition is the belief in one's own superiority, or ethnocentrism, and is the act of imposing one's cultural beliefs, values, and practices on individuals from another culture. Nurses impose their values on clients when they forcefully promote biomedical traditions while ignoring the clients' valuing of non-Western treatments such as acupuncture, herbal therapy, or spiritualistic rituals. A goal for nurses is to develop an approach of cultural relativism, whereby they recognize that clients have different approaches to health, and that each culture should be judged on its own merit and not on the nurse's personal beliefs.

### Cultural Conflict

Cultural conflict is a perceived threat that may arise from a misunderstanding of expectations when nurses are unable to respond appropriately to another individual's cultural practice because of unfamiliarity with the practice (Andrews and Boyle, 2012). Although cultural conflicts are unavoidable, the nursing goal is to manage conflicts so that they do not affect the delivery of culturally competent nursing care. Knowing how conflict is managed in the particular culture can minimize the conflict. It is important, when resolving the conflict, that all persons involved in the conflict have a way to "save face."

## BOX 7-5   Types of Prejudice and Racist Behaviors

**Overt Intentional Prejudice/Racism**

Two homeless women, one African American and the other Irish, are clients at the oncology clinic at the free neighborhood health care center. Both of the women have a history of ovarian cancer and are experiencing financial difficulty from time to time due to the cost of medical care associated with the illness. Although the African American client has been homeless longer, both clients have health issues associated with diminished quality of life and functional status related to the length of the illness, the progression of the illness, and the seriousness of the illness. The nurse as case manager referred the Irish client to the social services department to inquire about available resources but did not refer the African American client. The nurse reasoned that minority clients have direct contact with some local and national government programs, know about available resources, and have experience negotiating the social system for themselves and their family. In contrast, the nurse reasoned that because the Irish woman had no prior experience negotiating government programs, she needed to advocate for her client. The nurse did not assess the health-seeking behaviors of either client before coming to these conclusions, stereotyped both women, and intentionally used her informational power to help one client while denying assistance to the other client.

**Overt Unintentional Prejudice/Racism**

The community health nurse was assigned to make an initial home visit to two clients recently discharged from the hospital with a diagnosis of hypertension. The nurse performed physical assessments on both clients. He developed an extensive culturally relevant teaching plan with the Filipino client that included information on sodium restriction and its effect on kidney functioning, ways to integrate cultural foods into the diet, and support in lifestyle changes. With the Puerto Rican client, the nurse performed a routine physical assessment and did not discuss the client's culturally special dietary requirements. The nurse reasoned that the Puerto Rican client was not capable of understanding such complex information and would most likely seek information from her *curandera* (a folk practitioner) to manage the hypertension. At the end of the visit, the nurse said to this client, "Take care of yourself. See you next time." This nurse did not realize that he had stereotyped the client and that his nursing interventions were

minimal. He believed that he had delivered patient-centered care and the difference in his assessment and implementation approach reflected his understanding of cultural competence theory.

**Covert Intentional Prejudice/Racism**

A Native American nurse works in a home health agency that serves an ethnically diverse community. The nurse has observed that her assigned clients are always among the poorest and live in the unsafe ZIP code areas of the community. Her nonminority nurse colleagues are not assigned to clients residing in those ZIP codes. In a recent staff meeting, the Native American nurse expressed discomfort about the assignment patterns that she had observed with her nursing supervisors. Upon hearing her observations, the supervisors looked at the nurse in a surprised and skeptical manner and asked her to give a specific example. This is an example of covert racism because the nursing supervisors were aware of the informal policy that they assign minority nurses to clients residing in designated minority neighborhoods. The nursing supervisors were aware of this long-standing practice to assign minority nurses to minority clients and Caucasian nurses to Caucasian clients but would never admit to it. The supervisors thought that the best way for minority clients to be the recipients of culturally competent care was to assign a minority nurse to care for their own.

**Covert Unintentional Prejudice/Racism**

Ashley is the seven-year-old daughter of a lesbian middle-class couple. The school nurse is frustrated that Ashley's parents refuse to disclose the father and insist on altering the demographic form to include the two mothers as parents. Ashley frequently shows up to the nurse's office with stomach upsets and the nurse attributes the upsets to the parents' sexual orientation. The school nurse has not conducted an in-depth assessment of the child's chief complaint. This is unusual behavior for the school nurse as she has been cited for her thorough assessments of children that have resulted in early diagnosis and treatment of disorders for this age group. This school nurse is unaware that her intolerance for the parents' sexual orientation and family's lifestyle has contributed to her decision to provide a cursory assessment for Ashley.

## Culture Shock

Culture shock is the feeling of helplessness, discomfort, and disorientation experienced by an individual attempting to understand or effectively adapt to a cultural group whose beliefs and values are radically different from the individual's culture. When nurses experience culture shock, it may be a normal reaction to a client's beliefs and practices that are not allowed or approved in the nurse's own culture (Andrews and Boyle, 2012). Culture shock is brought on by anxiety that results from losing familiar signs and symbols of social interaction. As nurses change their practice environments and leave the safety of the hospital for community settings, they may experience heightened discomfort and feelings of powerlessness to confront differences between themselves and clients. This is especially true when nurses have little knowledge or exposure to the culture from which the client comes. For example, nurses who are unfamiliar with "cupping" may experience culture shock when Cambodians use this practice to relieve headaches, to reduce stress and sinus tension, or to delay the onset of colds. Being aware of the clients' own cultural beliefs and having knowledge of other cultures may help nurses to be more accepting of cultural differences.

## Culturally Competent Nursing Interventions

In culturally competent nursing interventions nurses integrate their professional knowledge with the client's knowledge and practices to maintain, protect, and restore the client's health. Leininger (2002a) developed a nursing intervention framework to increase culturally competent care; this framework suggests three modes of action, based on negotiation between the client and nurse, which guide the nurse to deliver culturally competent care: cultural preservation, cultural accommodation, and cultural repatterning. When these decisions and actions are used with cultural brokering, the nurse is able to provide holistic care for culturally diverse clients (individual, family, or community).

### Cultural Preservation

Cultural preservation refers to assistive, supportive, facilitative, or enabling nurse actions and decisions that help the clients of a particular culture to retain and preserve traditional values, so they can maintain, promote, and restore health. For example, acupuncture, an ancient Chinese practice of inserting needles in specific points on the skin through which life energy flows, is used to relieve pain or cure diseases by restoring balance of yin and yang (Spector, 2012). This practice is being accepted by increasing numbers of Western practitioners as a legitimate treatment for many health problems. Thus, when Western practitioners integrate modalities such as acupuncture in the plan of care to maintain and protect the health of Asian clients who subscribe to the practice, they are providing care that is consistent with the clients' beliefs and values and helping to preserve their culture.

In another example, the nurse helps maintain cultural family values of Ms. Rodriquez, a 73-year-old Filipino woman who was discharged from hospital to home care after surgery for cancer of the large intestine. During the home visit, the nurse discussed with the client and her husband about making a referral to have a home health aide assist with physical care and light housekeeping chores. The family was gracious but seemed hesitant to accept the referral. The nurse knew that in the Filipino family the older daughter is expected to be the caregiver for her mother and father. She asked the couple if they would like to discuss the situation with their daughters. Both the client and her husband seemed pleased with the idea, and the nurse promised to get back to them the next day. When the nurse returned for her visit, Ms. Rodriquez's older daughter was present and told the nurse that she would manage without additional help. The three daughters had made a schedule to take turns caring for their parents. The nurse accepted and supported the family's decision and told them that if they decided at a later time to accept the services of a home health aide, they should call the agency. The nurse then gave the family the telephone number of the agency, and scheduled the next follow-up visit with them.

## Cultural Accommodation

Cultural accommodation refers to assistive, supportive, facilitative, or enabling nurse actions and decisions that help clients of a particular culture accept nursing strategies, or negotiate with nurses to achieve satisfying health care outcomes. Nurses may support and facilitate successful use of home burial of placenta alongside interventions from the biomedical health care system. For example, the delivery nurse was very helpful when Ms. Sanchez asked her not to discard a piece of the amniotic sac that was present on her grandbaby's face immediately after birth. Ms. Sanchez asked the nurse to give it to her instead. The grandmother believed that being born with a piece of the amniotic sac on the face was a visible sign that something special was going to happen in the person's life. The grandmother explained that after she dried the piece of the amniotic sac, she would keep it in a safe place. She would also spend extra time protecting the baby to prevent her from being harmed. Although the delivery room nurse was not knowledgeable about this practice, she was assistive and gave the grandmother the piece of the sac as she requested.

## Cultural Repatterning

Cultural repatterning refers to assistive, supportive, facilitative, or enabling nurse actions and decisions that help clients of a particular culture to change or modify a cultural practice for new or different health care patterns that are meaningful, satisfying, and beneficial. Successful repatterning is likely to occur when cultural values and beliefs are respected while at the same time there is a cocreation of interventions with the client to provide for a healthier pattern than before the changes were developed. For example, a culturally competent school nurse who works with Mexican Americans knows of the high incidence of obesity among women 20 years and older. Using this information, she developed a health education program for Mexican teenagers in the local high school. While respecting their cultural traditions, the nurse discussed weight management strategies with the teenagers. The nurse understood the teenagers' cultural issues pertaining to food and knew how to negotiate with them. She discouraged the use of fried foods (such as tortillas), sour cream, and regular cheese and encouraged and demonstrated the use of baked tortillas and salsa as dip and topping. In another example, a nurse discovered during her instructions on diabetes self-management that pregnant Haitian women were visiting an herbalist to obtain teas so they would not have to take insulin. The nurse asked for the names of the herbs in the teas that they were drinking and scheduled a conference with the pharmacist to discuss the specific ingredients in the herbs as well as ways that they might help clients meet their cultural needs. The nurse found out that one of the herbs contributed to high blood pressure, a problem that many of the women were experiencing. She negotiated with the women not to take the tea with the specific herb. The nurse understood the importance of supernatural causes of illness in the Haitian culture and sought cooperation from the herbalist. Another example of cultural repatterning occurs when nurses assist older Chinese clients to use low-sodium soy sauce, rather than soy sauce with high sodium, in their cooking as a means to more effectively manage their hypertension. Similarly, nurses should guide African Americans to eat more broiled and less fried foods.

## Culture Brokering

Culture brokering is advocating, mediating, negotiating, and intervening between the client's culture and the biomedical health care culture on behalf of clients. Nurses as culture brokers act as go-betweens or advocates between groups of persons or persons of different cultural backgrounds to reduce conflict or produce change to facilitate client access to health care. As client advocates, nurse brokers are positioned to understand both cultures (the client's culture and the culture of the health care system) and resolve or lessen problems that result when individuals in either culture do not understand the other person's values. To illustrate, migrant workers tend to have high occupational mobility; many are poor and have limited formal education. They may seek health care only when they are ill and cannot work. Nurses who staff mobile health care vans often come in contact with migrant workers and usually take the opportunity to teach these individuals about prevention, health maintenance, environmental sanitation, and nutrition because it may be the only opportunity they will ever have to care for that particular migrant worker. These public health nurses also advocate for the rights of the migrant worker to receive quality health care. In this instance mobile health care nurses who provide manpower for the health mobile care van clinic may contact the migrant health services for follow-up or referral care for the migrant workers who received health care from the mobile health care van.

---

>> **LINKING CONTENT TO PRACTICE**

As has been discussed throughout the chapter, culturally competent nursing care uses many of the standards, guidelines, and competencies from key nursing and public health documents. For example, the Council on Linkages (Council on Linkages, 2010) has a set of skills related to cultural competency and a set related to communication that are consistent with the information in this chapter. Likewise, the Quad Council further develops and applies the skills of the Council on Linkages related to both cultural competency and communication to public health nursing practice. As an example, the Council on Linkages states that a necessary skill in public health is to consider "the role of cultural, social, and behavioral factors in the accessibility, availability, acceptability and delivery of public health services." The Quad Council states that "public health nurses should consider the role of cultural, social, and behavioral factors in the accessibility, availability, acceptability and delivery of public health nursing services." Each of the competencies in the Council on Linkages core competencies is applied directly to public health nursing practice by the Quad Council (2011). Also, the American Academy Expert Panel on Global Nursing and Health (2010) identifies 12 standards that serve as a resource and guide for nurses in practice, administration, education, and research by underscoring cultural competence as a priority of care for the populations that they serve.

---

## Developing Organizational Cultural Competence

Cultural competence barriers extend beyond the individual health care provider. Institutions and agencies can facilitate cultural competence. For example, a number of organizations subscribe to the nine cultural competence strategies that Lie and colleagues (2010) targeted at the institutional level: (1) providing interpreter services, (2) establishing recruitment and retention policies to increase ethnic minority representation, (3) providing training in cultural competence and sensitivity, (4) coordinating with traditional healers in the community, (5) using community health workers, (6) carrying out culturally competent health promotion that incorporates cultural notions of health and well-being, (7) including families and community members in care and decision making, (8) facilitating provider immersion into another culture and administrative and organizational accommodation, such as providing a welcoming environment, and (9) ensuring linguistic appropriateness of materials and information. By incorporating culturally competent behaviors that are embedded in the culture of the organization into the cultural competence framework, institutions have expanded the reach of their resources into the community and are addressing social determinants of health care.

Tripp-Reimer et al (2001) described another organizational cultural competence intervention model. They described four levels of systems interventions: (1) being culturally neutral refers to the standard practice typically developed by whites for whites; (2) being culturally insensitive refers to addressing issues of accessibility of services by using bilingual and bicultural health informational material that incorporates surface-level cultural knowledge, such as dietary preferences into

practice; (3) being culturally innovative refers to the use of cultural symbols and notions of health and well-being to convey health promotion messages, working with established social institutions in the community; and (4) being cultural transformative refers to using principles of social activism and change to unearth power relationships and partnering with communities to alter aspects of the basic social structure. The assertion by these authors that social activism can and should be a part of social competence underscores the commitment that organized nursing has to address social justice issues rooted in larger systems problems of inequality and discrimination. Nurses, as providers, are expected to develop cultural competence to change the dynamic of the nurse–client relationship. As leaders, nurses are expected to use leadership skills to advocate for social justice by promoting community empowerment, liberation, and relief of suffering and human oppression.

Betancourt et al (2003) presented a three-tier cultural competence framework—clinical, organizational, and structural—through which culturally competent strategies can be implemented to reduce health disparities. According to Betancourt, the rationale for these three levels of focus is that all three levels contribute to disparate health outcomes; therefore they must all be addressed to level the playing field and equalize health outcomes. Social cultural barriers to culturally competent care in this model are clinical barriers (poor provider communication, provider stereotyping and discrimination, and misunderstanding of culture perspective on health issues), organizational barriers (the lack of minorities in institutional leadership and the health care workforce), and structural (lack of interpreter services, bureaucratic intake processes, and difficulties accessing specialty care for minorities). Interventions to overcome these barriers are suggested for each level. Structural interventions include improving access to processes within the delivery health care system that includes expanding interpreter services and health teaching; organizational interventions include increasing diversity within the workforce and the health care leadership; and clinical interventions include working to enhance provider knowledge of the relationship between sociocultural factors and health beliefs and behaviors, and equipping providers with tools and skills to manage these factors appropriately.

Institutional level interventions could include agency engagement with the broader community, increased access to care for socioeconomically disadvantaged groups, and selection of interventions that are culturally appropriate. This macro level model provides direction for agencies that want to adopt culturally competent practices as part of their operational procedures and to facilitate provider level culturally competent care. When describing these broad-base interventions, cultural competence becomes an umbrella term to address the many individual level skills, attitudes, and knowledge and organizational level structures, policies, and protocols that come together in a profession, organization, or community to provide effective care to culturally diverse populations.

How well do culturally competent interventions fare in improving positive health outcomes for culturally diverse clients? Many studies demonstrate a beneficial effect on

provider knowledge, provider attitudes, and provider skills. Favorable patient satisfaction measures and improvement in adherence to follow-up among client assignees to intervention group providers have also been reported. Interventions that focus on the avoidance of bias, gender concepts of culture, and client-centeredness demonstrate promise as lasting strategies to decrease health disparities. These strategies include availability and access to assessment of problems in their social and cultural context, selection of culturally and socially acceptable interventions, and increased accountability to recipients of services and their community. Institutional level interventions could include agency engagement with the broader community, increased access to care for socially disadvantaged groups, and selection of interventions that are culturally appropriate. These four macro level modes provide direction to agencies that want to adopt culturally competent practices as part of their operational procedure and to facilitate provider level culturally competent care. When describing these broad-based interventions, cultural competence becomes an umbrella term to address the many individual level competencies, skills, attitudes, and knowledge, and organizational level competencies, structures, policies, and protocols that come together in a profession, organization, or community to provide effective care to culturally diverse populations.

## Positive Health Outcomes Associated with Cultural Competence

Nurse clinicians and educators are beginning to understand how to provide critical learning environments and workplaces for students, faculty, and practitioners to apply the concepts of cultural competence in their practice in order to improve the effectiveness of their actions. The majority of nurses continue to believe that they are less confident and inadequately prepared to provide sustained culturally competent care to clients from diverse cultures (Esposito, 2014). It is important to disseminate cultural competence outcomes in nursing through public health and research conferences, staff development programs, continuing education programs, and the student nursing associations.

Sealey et al (2006) examined the cultural competence of nurse educators in Louisiana and found that very few of the nurse educators had formal preparation to teach transcultural nursing and that they felt uncomfortable attempting to do so. A study conducted on community-based nurses' perceptions of cultural competence offers some encouragement (Starr and Wallace, 2009). The study indicated that about 85% of clients participating in the study perceived that nursing care today contains key components of decision making, communication, and interpersonal styles that reflect cultural components, 57% indicated that their communication style was culturally competent, 61% rated their decision-making choices as reflective of cultural competence behaviors, and about 70% said their interpersonal style was indicative of cultural competence behaviors.

Evidence-based cultural competence practice in nursing connecting culturally competent health care goals with the professional values of nursing and patient care outcomes and satisfaction has been the subject of recent research activity in nursing. The majority of studies of the effectiveness of culturally competent nursing interventions are descriptive. Few studies have employed a randomized clinical trial design. Fisher et al (2007) identified 38 nursing interventions that used some form of culturally oriented interventions to target racial and ethnic disparities. Kulbok et al (2012) cited several examples from the evidence-based nursing literature of public health nursing using the technique of participatory practice, defined as the building of partnerships with community members to assess, plan, analyze data, and implement sustainable health promotion and prevention programs to reach marginalized populations in vulnerable communities. For instance, Andrews et al (2007) used participatory methods to assess an African American population living in an impoverished neighborhood. To gain in-depth insights about the community's assets and needs, the research team involved community advisory board members and community health workers to assist them in conducting a series of community forums and interpreting the data gathered at the forums. Anderson and her research team (2007) were able to identify multilevel factors related to smoking patterns of the community. Thomas et al (2009) worked with a tribal community council to attain culturally sensitive knowledge of the tradition, history, and strength of that community in projects to reduce substance abuse. McQuiston et al (2005) used ethnographic community participatory strategies to set up a nominal group process to obtain important cultural aspects of health when assessing health disparities in a Latino population. Zandee et al (2010) described how public health nursing students used cultural competence principles to better understand the cultural background of the communities in which they were placed. By partnering with community health workers, the students were able to improve their cultural competence.

## CULTURAL NURSING ASSESSMENT

A cultural nursing assessment is "a systematic identification and documentation of the culture care beliefs, meanings, values, symbols, and practices of individuals or groups within a holistic perspective, which includes the worldview, life experiences, environmental context, ethno history, language, and diverse social structure influences" (Leininger, 2002b, pp. 117-118). A cultural assessment is the basis for providing culturally competent health care and helps to ensure that nurses will understand and respect the client's beliefs, values, and health care practices and take these cultural data into consideration when creating a treatment plan for the client. A cultural assessment should focus on those aspects relevant to the presenting problem, necessary intervention, and participatory education. Nurses use the information gathered to help them identify and understand clients' beliefs and practices about health and illness. By adopting a relativistic approach, nurses avoid judging or evaluating the clients in terms of their own culture.

A nonjudgmental approach toward the client's culture is facilitated through having a skill set that includes understanding, eliciting, listening, explaining, acknowledging, recommending, and negotiating. It is vital that nurses listen to clients'

## QSEN FOCUS ON QUALITY AND SAFETY EDUCATION FOR NURSES

The six quality and safety competencies for nurses that were identified in the Quality and Safety Education for Nurses (QSEN) project are patient-centered care, teamwork and collaboration, evidence-based practice, quality improvement, safety, and informatics. While each of these is important and pertinent to the nursing actions taken with people from cultural groups other than that of the nurse, perhaps the most significant is that of patient-centered care. The chapter presents many guidelines and principles for aiding nurses in providing culturally competent care. One of the areas in which patient-centered care is lacking occurs when the nurse and the patient are not communicating effectively. The lack of communication may occur when they speak different languages, have different cultural practices and expectations that lead them to hear messages differently or when the persons being served simply do not understand what the nurse is saying and are reluctant to acknowledge this. Nurses must observe for both verbal and nonverbal cues that a message is either understood or not understood. When the latter occurs, the nurse should take action to clarify the message. This may include asking someone from that cultural group to assist or to enlist the aid of an interpreter. See: Issel LM, Bekemeier B: Safe practice of population-focused nursing care: Development of a public health nursing concept, *Nursing Outlook,* 58(5):226-232, 2010.

The following applies the QSEN competency of client-centered interventions that reflect cultural competence.

**Targeted Competency:** Client-Centered Intervention—Recognize the client or designee as the source of control and full partner in providing compassionate and coordinated interventions based on respect for the client's preferences, values, and needs.

Important aspects of client-centered intervention include:

* **Knowledge:** Describe strategies to empower clients or families in all aspects of the health care process
* **Skills:** Communicate client values, preferences, and expressed needs to other members of the health care team
* **Attitudes:** Willingly support client-centered care for individuals and groups whose values differ from your own.

### Client-Centered Care Question

Competence in providing client-centered interventions involves not only effective interviewing of individual clients, but developing an awareness of their context. As a community-based clinician, it is helpful to familiarize yourself with the cultural context of your clients. Learning about community resources can sometimes be helpful in learning about the cultural context. You have just been hired as a visiting nurse in a Hispanic community. What community resources could you explore to assist you in providing effective client-centered care?

### Answer

* You might explore community centers. Where are they? How well frequented are the community centers? Which programs are most popular? Which community center programs are health-oriented?
* Are community members very involved with one or more churches? You might familiarize yourself with elements of this faith tradition.
* Are there community elders who are publically recognized as leaders in the community? Can you meet with them to understand how the community has changed and evolved over time?

Prepared by Gail Armstrong, PhD(c), DNP, ACNS-BC, CNE, Associate Professor, University of Colorado Denver College of Nursing.

perceptions of their problem and, in turn, that nurses explain to clients their own perceptions of the problem. Nurses and clients should acknowledge and discuss similarities and differences between the two perceptions to develop recommendations and suggestions for management of problems. A variety of tools are available to assist nurses in conducting cultural assessments (Andrews and Boyle, 2012; Leininger, 2002b). The focus of such tools varies, and selection is determined by the dimensions of the culture to be assessed.

During an initial contact with clients, nurses should perform a general cultural assessment to obtain an overview of the clients' characteristics. Nurses ask clients about their ethnic background, language, education, religious affiliation, dietary practices, family relationships, hospital experiences, occupation and socioeconomic status, cultural beliefs, and language. Nurses also want to know about clients' distinctive features, perceptions of the health issue, causation, treatment, anticipated results, and the impact the issue might have on the client. Such basic data help nurses understand the clients from the clients' points of view and recognize their uniqueness, thus avoiding stereotyping. Data for an in-depth cultural assessment should be gathered over a period of time and not restricted to the first encounter with the client. This gives both the client and the nurse time to get to know each other, and it is especially beneficial for the client to see the nurse in a helping relationship. An in-depth cultural assessment should be conducted in two phases: a data collection phase and an organization phase.

The data collection phase consists of three steps:

1. The nurse collects self-identifying data similar to those collected in the brief assessment.
2. The nurse raises a variety of questions that seek information on the client's perception of what brings them to the health care system, the illness, and previous and anticipated treatments.
3. After the nursing diagnosis is made, the nurse identifies cultural factors that may influence the effectiveness of nursing care actions.

In the organization phase, data related to the client's and family's views on optimal treatment choices are routinely examined, and areas of difference between the client's cultural needs and the goals of Western medicine are identified. Nurses may use Leininger's (2002a) three actions (discussed previously in this chapter) to guide them in selecting and discussing culturally appropriate interventions with clients.

The key to a successful cultural assessment lies in nurses being aware of their own culture. The nurse should consider the following suggestions when eliciting cultural information:

* Be sensitive to the cues in the environment and be in tune with the verbal and nonverbal communications before taking action.
* Know about the resources in the community such as schools, churches, hospitals, tribal councils, restaurants, taverns, and bars.
* Know the specific areas to focus on before beginning the cultural assessment.
* Select a strategy for gathering cultural data. Possible strategies include in-depth interviews, informal conversations,

observations of the client's everyday activities or specific events, survey research, and a case method approach to study certain aspects of a client.

- Identify a confidante who will help "bridge the gap" between cultures. Be aware that in some cultures the woman's husband or a close male family friend may be the person from whom the nurse may need to obtain the cultural information.
- Know the appropriate questions to ask without offending the client.
- Interview other nurses or health care professionals who have worked with the specific individual, family, or community to get their input.

- Use a trained interpreter if the client has limited proficiency with English.
- Talk with formal and informal community leaders to gain a comprehensive understanding about significant aspects of community life.
- Be aware that all information has both subjective and objective aspects, and verify and cross-check the information that is collected before acting on it.
- Avoid the pitfalls that may occur when making premature generalizations.
- Be sincere, open, and honest with yourself and the client.

## PRACTICE APPLICATION

Mr. Nguyen, a 64-year-old man from rural Vietnam, entered the United States with his family 3 years ago through the refugee program. Mr. Nguyen was a farmer in his homeland, and since his arrival he has been unable to obtain a stable job that would allow him to adequately care for his family. His financial resources are limited, and he has no insurance. He speaks enough English to interact directly with people outside his family and community. His oldest daughter, Aeyoung, is enrolled in a 2-year program to become a registered nurse.

The Nguyen family attends the neighborhood church with other Vietnamese families. Mr. Nguyen has been attending the clinic at the hospital but refuses to discuss with his family, even with Aeyoung, the reason for these visits. Aeyoung became increasingly concerned as she observed her father to have insomnia, retarded motor activity, an inability to concentrate, and weight loss. However, Mr. Nguyen denied that he was not well. Aeyoung decided to discuss her concerns with a nurse, with whom she had developed an attachment, at the church. She invited the nurse to her home for lunch on a Saturday so she could meet her father and validate her impressions.

After several visits with the family, the nurse was able to establish a close enough relationship with Mr. Nguyen so that she could engage him in a discussion of his health. Because of her extensive work with other Vietnamese immigrants, the nurse was familiar with themes of loss and decided to focus her conversation with Mr. Nguyen on his adjustment to the new community living, gains and losses as a result of immigration, and coping strategies. After several discussions with

Mr. Nguyen, he confided in the nurse that he feared that he was dying because he had been diagnosed with cancer of the small intestine. He further revealed that he had not shared the diagnosis with the family because he did not want them to know of his "bad news." Mr. Nguyen had refused treatment because he knew that people never get better when they have cancer; they always die.

A. Which of the following actions best characterize the nurse's willingness to provide culturally competent care to Mr. Nguyen and his family?
  1. Discuss with the client his understanding of his diagnosis.
  2. Discuss with the client the prognosis for a person diagnosed with cancer of the small intestine in the United States.
  3. Discuss with the client the prognosis for a person diagnosed with cancer of the small intestine in Vietnam.
  4. Discuss the medical treatment and surgical intervention for cancer of the small intestine.
B. The way in which the nurse poses questions to Mr. Nguyen is very important and determines the kind of responses the client gives to the nurse. What types of questions should the nurse pose to Mr. Nguyen to get the best responses from him?
C. Which resources should a community health agency have available to assist Mr. Nguyen with his health care concerns?
**Answers can be found on the Evolve site.**

## KEY POINTS

- The U.S. population is becoming increasingly diverse, and nurses and health care organizations need to learn more about the culture of individuals to whom they provide care and the impact of culture on health care.
- Culture is a learned set of behaviors that are widely shared among a group of people and helps guide individuals in problem solving and decision making processes.
- Cultural differences exist among groups and they may be observed in areas such as biological variations, personal

space, perception of time, environmental control, family organization, communication, nutrition, and religion.
- There are individual differences among people within a cultural group.
- Changes in immigration laws and policies have increased migration, contributing to changes in community demographics and challenges for nurses to effectively communicate with their clients and help them understand the basic health information needed to make appropriate health

## KEY POINTS—cont'd

decisions. When nurses do not speak or understand the client's language, interpreters should be available to assist them in communicating with clients.

- In selecting an interpreter, nurses should not only consider the clients' cultural needs but also respect their right to privacy.

- Members of minority groups are over-represented on the lower tiers of the socioeconomic ladder. Poor economic achievement is also a common characteristic among populations at risk, such as the homeless, migrant workers, and refugees. Nurses should be able to distinguish between culture and socioeconomic class issues and not interpret behavior as having a cultural origin when in fact it is based on socioeconomic class.

- Clients who are excluded from full participation in the economic, social, and political life of the society may have more complex health issues and more difficulty accessing and receiving services from health care institutions.

- The social determinants of health are the circumstances in which people are born and grow up, live, work, and age, and the systems put in place to deal with illness. They are shaped by race, economics, education, the family structure, health, and access to health resources.

- Efforts to understand dietary practices should go beyond relying on the individual having membership in a specific group and include religious requirements.

- Culturally competent nursing care is designed for a specific client, reflects the nurse's knowledge and the individual's knowledge and practices, and is implemented with care and sensitivity. Such nursing care helps to improve health outcomes and reduce health care costs.

- Standards of practice have been developed to guide nurses around the world in the areas of clinical practice, research, education, and administration.

- Culturally competent nurses are empowered to provide equitable nursing care that is focused on meeting the physical, physiological, social, and cultural needs of the client.

- Culturally competent nurses are aware of their own cultures, use cultural knowledge, have cultural skill, and select culturally appropriate interventions to care for the client holistically. The most important aspect is cultural encounter with the client.

- Nurses must have the desire or intrinsic motivation to want to provide culturally competent nursing care.

- Barriers to providing culturally competent care include stereotyping, prejudice and racism, ethnocentrism, cultural imposition, cultural conflict, and culture shock.

- Culturally competent nurses may select from four modes of interventions when providing care: cultural preservation, cultural accommodation, cultural repatterning, and culture brokering.

- Organizations, institutions, and professional associations should have policies, procedures, and practices that support a climate in which nurses can deliver culturally competent care to clients whom they serve.

- Nurses should perform a cultural assessment on every client with whom they interact. Cultural assessments help nurses understand clients' perspectives of health and illness and thereby guide them to implement culturally competent interventions. The needs of clients vary with their age, education, religion, and socioeconomic status.

## CLINICAL DECISION-MAKING ACTIVITIES

1. Select a culture that you would like to study. Go to the appropriate websites and gather information about the cultural group. Identify the group's cultural beliefs and practices and health-seeking behaviors. Share what you have obtained from websites and ask the person to evaluate the information. Discuss this information with at least one member of that cultural group. Compare and contrast information obtained from the two sources. Describe how you would use this information in your clinical practice.

2. Discuss how you would interview older clients who are considering giving up their independence and living in a nursing home. Prepare them for the likelihood that their health care providers are likely to be culturally diverse and may not share the same race or ethnicity. How will they engage in communication with the care provider about their health needs, family of origin, and important routine behaviors? How will they share their daily routine, dietary practices, and memories of family and friends?

3. Identify an alternative health care practitioner in the community of your clinical placement where you have been

assigned. Prepare six questions and use them as a guide to interview the alternative healer about cultural health beliefs, healing practice, and alternative biomedical explanation of illness systems.

4. Select from one of the standards of practice for culturally competent care (Office of Minority Health, Expert Panel for Global Nursing and Health of the American Academy of Nursing and the Transculutral Nursing Society, the Quad Council, and the Joint Commission) and examine the extent to which the public health agency in your community is in compliance with cultural competence standards as identified by one of these organizations. Report your findings to a culturally competent leader in the organization.

5. On the basis of *Healthy People 2020* objectives, identify an at-risk aggregate in your community. Use the AHRQ website to access information for that year on the progress the community has made toward decreasing a specific health disparity. Work with the public health nurse to evaluate the effectiveness of the plan the community has developed to remedy the disparity.

# REFERENCES

Agency for Healthcare Research & Quality: National health care quality report, 2012. Available at http://www.ahqr.gov/news/newsletters/research. Accessed May 10, 2014.

Agency for Healthcare Research & Quality: Factors linked to racial or ethnic disparities in US fetal death rates differ among groups, 2013. Available at http://www.ahqr.gov/news/newsletters/research-activities /14mar/0314RA32htm. Accessed May 5, 2014.

Agency for Healthcare Research & Quality: Lack of insurance and poorer health creates double jeopardy for blacks and Hispanics, March 2014. Available at http://www.ahrq.gov/news/newsletters/research-activities/14mar/0314RA21.html. Accessed May 3, 2014.

American Academy of Nursing Expert Panel: 2010. Standards of practice for culturally competent nursing care. Available at http://www.tcns.org/files/Standards_of_Practice_for_Culturally_Compt_Nsg_Care-Revised.pdf. Accessed February 25, 2014.

American Association of Colleges of Nursing: Fact sheet: enhancing diversity in the nursing workforce, 2014. Available at http://www.aacn.nche.edu/media-relations/fact-sheets/enhancing-diversity. Accessed March 14, 2014.

Anderson NLR, Calvillo ER, Fongwa MN: Community-based approaches to strengthen cultural competency in nursing education and practice. J Transcult Nurs 18:49s–59s, 2007.

Anderson ET, McFarlane J: Community as Partner: Theory in Practice in Nursing, ed 6. Philadelphia, 2010, Lippincott Williams & Wilkins.

Andrews JO, Bentley G, Crawford S, et al: Using community-based participatory research to develop a culturally sensitive smoking cessation intervention with public housing neighborhoods. Ethnicity Dis 17:331–337, 2007.

Andrews MM, Boyle JS: Transcultural Concepts in Nursing Care, ed 6. Philadelphia, 2012, Lippincott Williams & Wilkins.

Beacham TD, Askew RW, William PR: Strategies to increase racial/ethnic student participation in the nursing profession. Assoc Black Nursing Faculty J 20:69–72, 2009.

Betancourt JR, Green AR, Carrillo JE, et al: Defining cultural competence: a practical framework for addressing racial/ethnic disparities in health and health care. Public Health Rep 1184:293–302, 2003.

Braveman P: What are health disparities and health equity? We need to be clear. Public Health Rep 129:5–8, 2014.

Camarota SA: Immigrants in the United States, 2010: a profile of America's foreign-born population. Center for Immigrant Studies, 2012. Available at http://cis.org/2012-profile-of-americas-foreign-born-population. Accessed April 1, 2014.

Campinha-Bacote J: Coming to know cultural competence: in evolutionary process. Internl J Human Caring 15:42–48, 2011.

Campinha-Bacote J: People of African heritage. In Purnell L, Paulanka BJ, editors: Transcultural Health Care: A Culturally Competent Approach, ed 4. Philadelphia, 2012, FA Davis, pp 91–114.

Centers for Disease Control and Prevention: Alcohol-attributable deaths and years of potential life lost among American Indians and Alaska Natives—United States, 2001-2005. MMWR 57:938–941, 2008.

Centers for Disease Control and Prevention: Improving health literacy for older adults: expert panel report, 2009. Available at http://www.cdc.gov/healthliteracy/pdf/olderadults.pdf. Accessed June 6, 2014.

Changes in immigration law, 2013. Available at http://www.lawcom.com/immigration/chngs.shtml. Accessed February 25, 2014.

Cheng ER, Kindig DA: Disparities in premature mortality between high- and low-income US Counties. Prev Chronic Dis 9:110120, 2012. Available at DOI: http://dx.doi.org/10.5888/pcd9.110120. Accessed May 16, 2014.

Congress of the United States: A Description of the Immigrant Population: An Update, Congressional Budget Office. Washington, DC, 2012, U.S. Government Printing Office.

Council on Linkages between Academic and Public Health Practice: Core Competencies for Public Health Professionals. Washington, DC, 2010, Public Health Foundation/Health Resources and Services Administration.

Degazon CE: A contrast in ethnic identification, social support, and coping strategies among subgroups of African elders. J Cult Div 1:79–85, 1994.

Doorenbos AZ, Schim SM, Benkert R, et al: Psychometric evaluation of the cultural competence assessment instrument among healthcare providers. Nurs Research 54:324–331, 2005.

Dwayne TB, Isaac LA, Laveist TA: The legacy of Tuskegee and trust in medical care: is Tuskegee responsible for race differences in

mistrust of medical care? J Natl Med Assoc 97:951–956, 2005.

Esposito CL: Provision of culturally competent health care: an interim status review and report. JNY State Nurses Assoc 43:4–11, 2014.

Fielo S, Degazon CE: When cultures collide: decision making in a multicultural environment. Nurs Health Care Perspect 18:238–243, 1997.

Fisher TL, Burnet DL, Huang ES, et al: Cultural leverage. Med Care Res and Rev 64(Suppl 5):243S–282S, 2007.

Gamble VN: Under the shadow of Tuskegee: African Americans and health care. Am J Public Health 87:1773–1778, 1997.

Giger JN: Transcultural Nursing: Assessment and Intervention, ed 6. St Louis, 2012, Mosby.

Healthy People 2020. Social determinants of health. 2013. Available at http://www.healthypeople.gov/2020/topicsobjectives2020/overview.aspx?topicid=39. Accessed April 11, 2014.

Immigration Policy Center: Strength in diversity, June 2012. Available at http://www.immigrationpolicy.org/sites/default/files/docs/Strength%20in%20Diversity%20updated%20061912.pdf. Accessed May 8, 2014.

Jacobs A, Kemppainen JK, Taylor JS, et al: Beliefs about diabetes and medication adherence among Lumbee Indians living in rural southeastern North Carolina. J Transcult Nurs 25:167–175, 2014.

Kulbok PA, Thatcher E, Park E, et al: Evolving public health nursing roles: focus on community participatory health promotion and prevention. Online J Issues Nurs 17:1, 2012.

Lai DWL, Sunrood S: Chinese health beliefs of older Chinese in Canada. J Aging and Health 21:38–62, 2009.

Leininger M: Essential transcultural nursing care concepts, principles, examples, and policy statements. In Leininger MM, McFarland M, editors: Transcultural Nursing: Concepts, Theories, Research, and Practices, ed 3. New York, 2002a, McGraw-Hill, pp 45–69.

Leininger M: Part 1: The theory of culture care and the ethnonursing research method. In Leininger MM, McFarland M, editors: Transcultural Nursing: Concepts, Theories, Research, and Practices, ed 3. New York, 2002b, McGraw-Hill, pp 71–98.

Levine DA, Neidecker MV, Kiefe CI, et al: Racial-ethnic disparities in access to physician care and medications among US stroke survivals. Neurology 76:53–61, 2011.

Lie D, Lee-Rey E, Gomez A, et al: Does cultural competency training of health professionals improve patient outcomes? a systematic review and proposed algorithm for future research. J of Gen Intern Med 2:317–325, 2010.

Locke DC, Hardaway YV: Moral perspectives in interracial settings. In Cochrane D, Manley-Casimir M, editors: Moral Education: Practical Approaches. New York, 1992, Praeger.

Macartney S, Bishaw A, Fontenot K: Poverty rates for selected detailed race and Hispanic groups by state and place: 2007-2011. 2013. Available at http://www.census.gov/prod/2013pubs/acsbr11-17.pdf. Accessed May 8, 2014.

McQuiston C, Parrado EA, Martinez AP, et al: Community-based participatory research with Latino community members: Horizonte Latino. J Professional Nurs 21:210–215, 2005.

Meleis AI: Arabs. In Lipson JG, Dibble SL, editors: Providing Culturally Appropriate Care in Culture and Clinical Care. San Francisco, 2005, UCSF Nursing Press, pp 42–57.

Morgan P, Barnett K, Perdue P, et al: African-American women with breast cancer and their spouses' perception of care received from physicians. ABNF 17:32–36, 2006.

Ogbu MA: Nigerians. In Lipson JG, Dibble SL, editors: Providing Culturally Appropriate Care in Culture and Clinical Care. San Francisco, 2005, UCSF Nursing Press, pp 243–259.

Orlandi MA: Cultural Competence for Evaluators. Washington, DC, 1992, U.S. Department of Health and Human Services.

Orque M: Orque's ethnic/cultural system: a framework for ethnic nursing care. In Orque MS, Bloch B, Monrroy LSA, editors: Ethnic Nursing Care. A Multicultural Approach. St. Louis, 1983, Mosby.

Pew Research Center: Pew Hispanic Center renamed Pew Research Center's Hispanic Trends Project 2013, Pew Hispanic Center. Available at http://www.pewresearch.org/2013/08/14/pew-hispanic-center-renamed-pew-research-centers-hispanic-trends-project/, Accessed February 18, 2014.

Phillips J, Malone B: Increasing racial/ethnic diversity in nursing to reduce health disparities and achieve health equity. Public Health Rep 129:45–50, 2014.

Purnell LD, Paulanka BJ: Transcultural Health Care: A Culturally Competent Approach, ed 4. Philadelphia, 2012, FA Davis.

Quad Council of Public Health Nursing Organizations: Quad Council PHN

*Competencies,* 2011, Quad Council Domains of Practice. Available at www.achne.org/files/Quad%20 Coouncil/QuadCouncilCompetences for Public Health Nurses.pdf. Accessed February 19, 2015.

Randall-David E: *Culturally Competent HIV Counseling and Education.* McLean, VA, 1994, Maternal and Child Health Clearinghouse.

Sealey LJ, Burnett M, Johnson G: Cultural competence of baccalaureate nursing faculty: are we up to the task? *J Cult Div* 13:131–140, 2006.

Smedley BD, Stith AY, Nelson AR, editors: *Unequal Treatment: Confronting Racial and Ethnic Disparities in Health Care.* Washington, DC, 2002, The National Academic Press.

Spector RE: *Cultural Diversity in Health and Illness,* ed 8. Norwalk, Conn, 2012, Appleton & Lange.

Starr S, Wallace DC: Self-reported cultural competence of public health nurses in a Southeastern U.S. public health department. *Public Health Nurs* 26:48–57, 2009.

Stewart AL, Napoles-Springer AM, Gregorich SE, et al: Interpersonal Processes of Care Survey: patient-reported measures for diverse groups. *Health Serv Res* 42:1235–1256, 2007.

The Pew Forum on Religion and Public Life 2008. US religious landscape survey: religious affiliation: diverse and dynamic. Available at http:// religions.pewforum.org/pdf/

report-religious-landscape-study-full.pdf, Accessed May 14, 2014.

Thomas LR, Donovan DM, Sigo RLW, et al: The community pulling together: a tribal community-university partnership project to reduce substance abuse and promote good health in a reservation tribal community. *J Ethn Substance Abuse* 8:1–13, 2009.

Tripp-Reimer T, Choi E, Kelley LS, et al: Cultural barriers to care: inverting the problem. *Diab Spect* 14:13–22, 2001.

U.S. Census Bureau: Income, poverty, and health insurance coverage in the United States: 2010. Available at http://www.census.gov/hhes/www/ poverty/data/threshld/index.html. Accessed April 24, 2014.

U.S. Department of Health and Human Services: *Mental Health: Culture, Race, and Ethnicity. Supplement to Mental Health: A Report of the Surgeon General.* Rockville, MD, 2001, U.S. Government Printing Office.

U.S. Department of Health and Human Services: *Healthy People 2020: Understanding and Improving Health.* Washington, DC, 2010, U.S. Government Printing Office.

West EA: The cultural bridge model. *Nurs Outlook* 41:229–234, 1993.

Zandee G, Bossenbroek D, Friesen M, et al: Effectiveness of community health worker/nursing student teams as a strategy for public health nursing education. *Public Health Nurs* 27:277–284, 2010.

# 8

# Public Health Policy

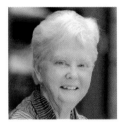

## *Marcia Stanhope, PhD, RN, FAAN*

Dr. Marcia Stanhope is currently an Associate of the Tufts and Associates Search Firm, Chicago, Ill. She is also a consultant for the nursing program at Berea College, Kentucky. She has practiced community and home health nursing, has served as an administrator and consultant in home health, and has been involved in the development of two nurse-managed centers. At one time in her career, she held a public policy fellowship and worked in the office of a U.S. senator. She has taught community health, public health, epidemiology, policy, primary care nursing, and administration courses. Dr. Stanhope formerly directed the Division of Community Health Nursing and Administration and served as Associate Dean of the College of Nursing at the University of Kentucky. She has been responsible for both undergraduate and graduate courses in population-centered nursing. She has also taught at the University of Virginia and the University of Alabama, Birmingham. During her career at the University of Kentucky she was appointed to the Good Samaritan Foundation Chair and Professorship in Community Health Nursing, and was honored with the University Provost's Public Scholar award. Her presentations and publications have been in the areas of home health, community health, and community-focused nursing practice, as well as primary care nursing.

## ADDITIONAL RESOURCES

**Evolve website http://evolve.elsevier.com/Stanhope**
- *Healthy People 2020*
- WebLinks
- Quiz

- Case Studies
- Glossary
- Answers to Practice Application

## OBJECTIVES

*After reading this chapter, the student should be able to do the following:*

1. Discuss the structure of the U.S. government and health care roles.
2. Identify the functions of key governmental and quasi-governmental agencies that affect public health systems and nursing, both around the world and in the United States.
3. Differentiate between the primary bodies of law that affect nursing and health care.
4. Define key terms related to policy and politics.
5. State the relationships between nursing practice, health policy, and politics.
6. Develop and implement a plan to communicate with policy makers on a chosen public health issue.

## KEY TERMS

advanced practice nurses, p. 182
Agency for Healthcare Research and Quality, p. 174
American Association of Colleges of Nursing, p. 184
American Nurses Association, p. 172
block grants, p. 169
boards of nursing, p. 177
categorical funding, p. 176
constitutional law, p. 176
devolution, p. 169
health policy, p. 168
judicial law, p. 177
law, p. 168
legislation, p. 177
legislative staff, p. 179

licensure, p. 179
National Institute of Nursing Research, p. 174
nurse practice act, p. 177
Occupational Safety and Health Administration, p. 173
Office of Homeland Security, p. 176
police power, p. 169
policy, p. 168
politics, p. 168
public policy, p. 168
regulations, p. 177
U.S. Department of Health and Human Services, p. 168
World Health Organization, p. 172
*—See Glossary for definitions*

*BRACHES OF GOV.* (handwritten)

*USDHHS* (handwritten)

Nurses are an important part of the health care system and are greatly affected by governmental and legal systems. Nurses who select the community as their area of practice must be especially aware of the impact of government, law, and health policy on nursing, health, and the communities in which they practice. Insight into how government, law, and political action have changed over time is necessary to understand how the health care system has been shaped by these factors. Also, understanding how these factors have influenced the current and future roles for nurses and the public health system is critical for better health policy for the nation.

Nurses have historically viewed themselves as advocates for the health of the population. It is this heritage that has moved the discipline into the policy and political arenas. To secure a more positive health care system, nurse professionals must develop a working knowledge of government, key governmental and quasi-governmental organizations and agencies, health care law, the policy process, and the political forces that are shaping the future of health care. This knowledge and the motivation to be an agent of change in the discipline and in the community are necessary ingredients for success as a population-centered nurse.

## DEFINITIONS

To understand the relationship between health policy, politics, and laws, one must first understand the definitions of the terms. Policy is a settled course of action to be followed by a government or institution to obtain a desired end (CDC, 2014). Public policy is described as all governmental activities, direct or indirect, that influence the lives of all citizens (Birkland, 2010). Health policy, in contrast, is a set course of action to obtain a desired health outcome for an individual, family, group, community, or society (WHO, 2014). Policies are made not only by governments, but also by such institutions as a health department or other health care agency, a family, a community, or a professional organization.

Politics plays a role in the development of such policies. Politics is found in families, professional and employing agencies, and governments. Politics determines who gets what and when and how they get it (Birkland, 2010). Politics is the art of influencing others to accept a specific course of action. Therefore, political activities are used to arrive at a course of action (the policy). Law is a system of privileges and processes by which people solve problems based on a set of established rules; it is intended to minimize the use of force (Yourdictionary, 2014). Laws govern the relationships of individuals and organizations to other individuals and to government. Through political action, a policy may become a law, a regulation, a judicial ruling, a decision, or an order.

After a law is established, regulations further define the course of action (policy) to be taken by organizations or individuals in reaching an outcome. Government is the ultimate authority in society and is designated to enforce the policy whether it is related to health, education, economics, social welfare, or any other society issue. The following discussion explains the role of government in health policy.

## GOVERNMENTAL ROLE IN U.S. HEALTH CARE

In the United States, the federal and most state and local governments are composed of three branches, each of which has separate and important functions (Truman, 2014). The *executive branch* is composed of the president (or state governor or local mayor) along with the staff and cabinet appointed by this executive, various administrative and regulatory departments, and agencies such as the U.S. Department of Health and Human Services (USDHHS). The *legislative branch* (i.e., Congress at the federal level) is made up of two bodies: the Senate and the House of Representatives, whose members are elected by the citizens of particular geographic areas. There is a federal Division of Nursing, a section within the Health Resources and Services Agency (HRSA) of the USDHHS, that refines criteria for nursing education programs as funded by Congress and affirmed by the President.

The *judicial branch* is composed of a system of federal, state, and local courts guided by the opinions of the Supreme Court. Each of these branches is established by the Constitution, and each plays an important role in the development and implementation of health law and public policy.

The executive branch suggests, administers, and regulates policy. The role of the legislative branch is to identify problems and to propose, debate, pass, and modify laws to address those problems. The judicial branch interprets laws and their meaning, as in its ongoing interpretation of states' rights to define access to reproductive health services to citizens of the states.

One of the first constitutional challenges to a federal law passed by Congress was in the area of health and welfare in 1937, after the 74th Congress had established unemployment compensation and old-age benefits for U.S. citizens (U.S. Law, 1937a). Although Congress had created other health programs previously, its legal basis for doing so had never been challenged. In *Stewart Machine Co. v. Davis* (U.S. Law, 1937b), the Supreme Court (judicial branch) reviewed this legislation and determined, through interpretation of the Constitution, that such federal governmental action was within the powers of Congress to promote the general welfare. It was obvious in 2008 and beyond that unemployment benefits are important to the economy and to individuals who lose jobs during a national economic crisis (BLS, 2010).

Most legal bases for the actions of Congress in health care are found in Article I, Section 8 of the U.S. Constitution, including the following:

1. Provide for the general welfare.
2. Regulate commerce among the states.
3. Raise funds to support the military.
4. Provide spending power.

Through a continuing number and variety of cases and controversies, these Section 8 provisions have been interpreted by the courts to appropriately include a wide variety of federal powers and activities. State power concerning health care is called police power (Legal Information Institute, 2014). This power allows states to act to protect the health, safety, and welfare of their citizens. Such police power must be used fairly, and the state must show that it has a compelling interest in taking actions, especially actions that might infringe on individual rights. Examples of a state using its police powers include requiring immunization of children before being admitted to school and requiring case finding, reporting, treating, and follow-up care of persons with tuberculosis. These activities protect the health, safety, and welfare of state citizens.

## Trends and Shifts in Governmental Roles

The government's role in health care at both the state and federal level began gradually. Wars, economic instability, and political differences between parties all shaped the government's role. The first major federal governmental action relating to health was the creation in 1798 of the Public Health Service (PHS). Then in 1890 federal laws were passed to promote the public health of merchant seamen and Native Americans. In 1934

Senator Wagner of New York initiated the first national health insurance bill. The Social Security Act of 1935 was passed to provide assistance to older adults and the unemployed, and it offered survivors' insurance for widows and children. It also provided for child welfare, health department grants, and maternal and child health projects. In 1948 Congress created the National Institutes of Health (NIH), and in 1965 it passed very important health legislation creating Medicare and Medicaid to provide health care service payments for older adults, the disabled, and the categorically poor. These legislative acts by Congress created programs that were implemented by the executive branch. In March 2010, the most recent legislation passed and signed by President Obama to improve the health of the nation and access to care was the health reform law, the Patient Protection and Affordable Care Act (US LAW, PL 111-148). See Chapter 3 for in-depth information (Kaiser Family Foundation, 2010a).

The U.S. Department of Health and Human Services (USDHHS) (known first as the Department of Health, Education, and Welfare [DHEW]) was created in 1953. The Health Care Financing Administration (HCFA) was created in 1977 as the key agency within the USDHHS to provide direction for Medicare and Medicaid. In 2002 HCFA was renamed the Center for Medicare and Medicaid Services (CMS). During the 1980s, a major effort of the Reagan administration was to shift federal government activities to the states, including federal programs for health care. The process of shifting the responsibility for planning, delivering, and financing programs from the federal level to the states is called **devolution**. Throughout the 1980s and 1990s, Congress has increasingly funded health programs by giving **block grants** to the states. Devolution processes including block granting should alert professional nurses that state and local policy has grown in importance to the health care arena. With the new health reform law, stimulus grants have been provided to state and local areas to improve health care access (HRSA, 2010).

The role of government in health care is shaped both by the needs and demands of its citizens and by the citizens' beliefs and values about personal responsibility and self-sufficiency. These beliefs and values often clash with society's sense of responsibility and need for equality for all citizens. A federal example of this ideological debate occurred in the 1990s over health care reform. The Democratic agenda called for a health care system that was universally accessible, with a focus on primary care and prevention. The Republican agenda supported more modest changes within the medical model of the delivery system. This agenda also supported reducing the federal government's role in health care delivery through cuts in Medicare and Medicaid benefits. The Democrats proposed the Health Security Act of 1993, which failed to gain Congress's approval. In an effort to make some incremental health care changes, both the Democrats and the Republicans in Congress passed two new laws. The Health Insurance Portability and Accountability Act (HIPAA) allows working persons to keep their employee group health insurance for up to 16 months after they leave a job (U.S. Law 107-105, 1996). The State Child Health Improvement Act (SCHIP) of 1997 provides insurance for children and families who cannot otherwise afford health insurance (U.S. Law, 1997).

With the latest health care reform, numerous debates occurred in the House of Representatives and the Senate until there was agreement that the Senate version of the bill would be passed. On March 30, 2010 President Obama signed into law the Health Care and Education Reconciliation Act of 2010, which made some changes to the comprehensive health reform law and included House amendments to the new law (Kaiser, 2010B). See Chapter 3 for further discussion.

This discussion has focused primarily on trends in and shifts between different levels of government. An additional aspect of governmental action is the relationship between government and individuals. Freedom of individuals must be balanced with governmental powers. After the terrorist attacks on the United States in September (World Trade Center attack) and October (anthrax outbreak) of 2001, much government activity was being conducted in the name of national security.

It is interesting to note that before September 11, 2001, the Congress and President, recognizing that the public health system infrastructure needed help, passed "The Public Health Threats and Emergencies Act" (PL 106-505) in 2000. This law "addresses emerging threats to the public's health and authorizes the Secretary of HHS to take appropriate response actions during a public health emergency, including investigations, treatment, and prevention" (Katz et al, 2014, p. 133). This legislation is said to have signaled the beginning of renewed interest in public health as the protector for entire communities. In June 2002 the Public Health Security and Bioterrorism Preparedness and Response Act was signed into law (US Law 2002, PL 107-188), with $3 billion appropriated by Congress, to implement the following antibioterrorism activities:

- Improving public health capacity
- Upgrading of health professionals' ability to recognize and treat diseases caused by bioterrorism
- Speeding the development of new vaccines and other countermeasures
- Improving water and food supply protection
- Tracking and regulating the use of dangerous pathogens within the United States (Katz et al, 2014)

Yet there is considerable debate on just how much governmental intervention is necessary and effective and how much will be tolerated by citizens. For example, in 2010 approximately 49% of citizens were against the new health care reform acts, and the Republicans were seen as being obstructionists. In 2014, 50% of citizens were for government intervention and 50% against (Debate.org, 2013).

## Government Health Care Functions

Federal, state, and local governments carry out five health care functions, which fall into the general categories of direct services, financing, information, policy setting, and public protection.

### Direct Services

Federal, state, and local governments provide direct health services to certain individuals and groups. For example, the federal government provides health care to members and dependents of the military, certain veterans, and federal prisoners. State and local governments employ nurses to deliver a variety of services to individuals and families, frequently on the basis of factors such as financial need or the need for a particular service, such as hypertension or tuberculosis screening, immunizations for children and older adults, and primary care for inmates in local jails or state prisons. The Evidence-Based Practice box presents a study that examined the use of a state health insurance program.

## EVIDENCE-BASED PRACTICE

The purpose of this study was to examine the changes in access to care, use of services, and quality of care among children enrolled in Child Health Plus (CHPlus), a state health insurance program for low-income children that became a model for the State Child Health Insurance Program (SCHIP). A before-and-after design was used to evaluate the health care experience of children the year before and the year after enrollment in the state health insurance program. The study consisted of 2126 children from New York State, ranging from birth to 12.99 years of age. Results indicated that the state health insurance program for low-income children was associated with improved access, use, and quality of care. The development and implementation of SCHIP was an outcome of the soaring costs of health care and the fact that there were 11 million uninsured children in the United States at the time of the study. It was the largest public investment in child health in 30 years.

### Nurse Use

This study supports the value of health policy and the need to evaluate the effectiveness of policy in accomplishing the purposes of the policy.

From U.S. Department of Health and Human Services: Healthy People 2010: understanding and improving health, ed 2, Washington, DC, 2000, U.S. Government Printing Office.

### Financing

Governments pay for some health care services; the 2011 percentage of the bill paid by the government was about 46.3%, and this is projected to increase to 47.6% by the year 2015. The government also pays for training some health personnel and for biomedical and health care research (NCHS, 2014). Support in these areas has greatly affected both consumers and health care providers. Federal governments finance the direct care of clients through the Medicare, Medicaid, Social Security, and SCHIP programs. State governments contribute to the costs of Medicaid and SCHIP programs. Many nurses have been educated with government funds through grants and loans, and schools of nursing in the past have been built and equipped using federal funds. Governments also have financially supported other health care providers, such as physicians, most significantly through the program of Graduate Medical Education funds.

The federal government invests in research and new program demonstration projects, with NIH receiving a large portion of the monies. The National Institute of Nursing Research (NINR) is a part of the NIH and, as such, provides a substantial sum of money to the discipline of nursing for the purpose of developing the knowledge base of nursing and promoting nursing services in health care (NINR, 2014).

### Information

All branches and levels of government collect, analyze, and disseminate data about health care and health status of the citizens.

## TABLE 8-1  International and National Sources of Data on the Health Status of the U.S. Population

| Organization | Data Sources |
|---|---|
| **International** | |
| United Nations | http://www.un.org/ |
| | *Demographic Yearbook* |
| World Health Organization | http://www.who.int/en/ |
| | *World Health Statistics Annual* |
| **Federal** | |
| Department of Health and Human Services | http://www.hhs.gov |
| | National Vital Statistics System |
| | National Survey of Family Growth |
| | National Health Interview Survey |
| | National Health Examination Survey |
| | National Health and Nutrition Examination Survey |
| | National Master Facility Inventory |
| | National Hospital Discharge Survey |
| | National Nursing Home Survey |
| | National Ambulatory Medical Care Survey |
| | National Morbidity Reporting System |
| | U.S. Immunization Survey |
| | Surveys of Mental Health Facilities |
| | Estimates of National Health Expenditures |
| | AIDS Surveillance |
| | Nurse Supply Estimates |
| Department of Commerce | http://www.commerce.gov |
| | U.S. Census of Population |
| | Current Population Survey |
| | Population Estimates and Projections |
| Department of Labor | http://www.dol.gov |
| | Consumer Price Index |
| | Employment and Earnings |

An example is the annual report *Health: United States, 2013,* compiled each year by the USDHHS (NCHS, 2014). Collecting vital statistics, including mortality and morbidity data, gathering of census data, and conducting health care status surveys are all government activities. Table 8-1 lists examples of available federal and international data sources on the health status of populations in the United States and around the world. These sources are available on the Internet and in the governmental documents' section of most large libraries. This information is especially important because it can help nurses understand the major health problems in the United States and those in their own states and local communities.

### Policy Setting

Policy setting is a chief governmental function. Governments at all levels and within all branches make policy decisions about health care. These health policy decisions have broad implications for financial expenses, resource use, delivery system change, and innovation in the health care field. One law that has played a very important role in the development of public health policy, public health nursing, and social welfare policy in the United States is the Sheppard-Towner Act of 1921 (USDHHS, HRSA, 2010).

The Sheppard-Towner Act made nurses available to provide health services for women and children, including well-child and child-development services; provided adequate hospital services and facilities for women and children; and provided grants-in-aid for establishing maternal–child welfare programs. The act helped set precedents and patterns for the growth of modern-day public health policy. It defined the role of the federal government in creating standards to be followed by states in conducting categorical programs such as the Women, Infants, and Children (WIC) and Early Periodic Screening and Developmental Testing (EPSDT) programs. The act also defined the position of the consumer in influencing, formulating, and shaping public policy; the government's role in research; a system for collecting national health statistics; and the integrating of health and social services. This act established the importance of prenatal care, anticipatory guidance, client education, and nurse–client conferences, all of which are viewed today as essential nursing responsibilities.

### Public Protection

The U.S. Constitution gives the federal government the authority to provide for the protection of the public's health. This function is carried out in numerous venues, such as by regulating air and water quality and protecting the borders from the influx of diseases by controlling food, drugs, and animal transportation, to name a few. The Supreme Court interprets and makes decisions related to public health, such as affirming a woman's rights to reproductive privacy *(Roe v. Wade),* requiring vaccinations, and setting conditions for states to receive public funds for highway construction/repair by requiring a minimum drinking age.

## *HEALTHY PEOPLE 2020:* AN EXAMPLE OF NATIONAL HEALTH POLICY GUIDANCE

In 1979 the surgeon general issued a report that began a 30-year focus on promoting health and preventing disease for all Americans (DHEW, 1979). In 1989, *Healthy People 2000* became a national effort with many stakeholders representing the perspectives of government, state, and local agencies; advocacy groups; academia; and health organizations (USDHHS, 1991).

Throughout the 1990s states used *Healthy People 2000* objectives to identify emerging public health issues. The success of this national program was accomplished and measured through state and local efforts. The *Healthy People 2010* document focused on a vision of healthy people living in healthy communities. *Healthy People 2020* has four overarching goals, which can be found in the Healthy People 2020 box; this box compares the goals of *Healthy People* documents from 2000 to 2020.

## ORGANIZATIONS AND AGENCIES THAT INFLUENCE HEALTH

### International Organizations

In June 1945, following World War II, many national governments joined together to create the United Nations (UN). By charter, the aims and goals of the UN deal with human rights,

**HEALTHY PEOPLE 2020**

### A Comparison of the Goals of Healthy People 2000, Healthy People 2010, and Healthy People 2020

| Healthy People 2000 | Healthy People 2010 | Healthy People 2020 |
|---|---|---|
| Increase the years of healthy life for Americans | Increase quality and years of healthy life | Attaining high quality, longer lives free of preventable disease, disability, injury, and premature death |
| Reduce health disparities among Americans | Eliminate health disparities | Achieving health equity, eliminating disparities, and improving the health of all groups |
| Achieve access to preventive services for all Americans | | Creating social and physical environments that promote good health for all |
| | | Promoting quality of life, healthy development, and healthy behaviors across all life stages |

From U.S. Department of Health and Human Services: Leading indicators.In Healthy People 2000, 2010, & 2020, Washington, DC, 1989,1999, 2010, U.S. Government Printing Office.

world peace, international security, and the promotion of economic and social advancement of all the world's peoples. The UN, headquartered in New York City, is made up of six principal divisions, several subgroups, and many specialized agencies and autonomous organizations. With the approval and support of the UN Commission on the Status of Women, five world conferences on women have been held. At these conferences, the health of women and children and their rights to personal, educational, and economic security as well as initiatives to achieve these goals at the country level were debated and explored, and policies were formulated (United Nations, 1975, 1980, 1985, 1995, 2000). The work of the UN and the world conferences continues with agendas to include the development of human beings, eradication of poverty, protection of human rights, investment in health, education, training, trade, economic growth, and a continued emphasis on women (United Nations, 2014).

One of the special autonomous organizations growing out of the UN is the World Health Organization (WHO). Established in 1946, WHO relates to the UN through the Economic and Social Council to achieve its goal to attain the highest possible level of health for all persons. "Health for All" is the creed of the WHO. Headquartered in Geneva, Switzerland, the WHO has six regional offices. The office for the Americas is located in Washington, DC, and is known as the Pan American Health Organization (PAHO).

The WHO provides services worldwide to promote health, it cooperates with member countries in promoting their health efforts, and it coordinates the collaborating efforts between countries and the disseminating of biomedical research. Its services, which benefit all countries, include a day-to-day information service on the occurrence of internationally important diseases; the publishing of the international list of causes of disease, injury, and death; monitoring of adverse reactions to

drugs; and establishing of world standards for antibiotics and vaccines. Assistance available to individual countries includes support for national programs to fight disease, to train health workers, and to strengthen the delivery of health services. The World Health Assembly (WHA) is the WHO's policy-making body, and it meets annually. The WHA's health policy work provides policy options for many countries of the world in their development of in-country initiatives and priorities; however, although WHA policy statements are important everywhere, they are guides and not law. The WHA's most recent policy statement on nursing and midwifery was released in 2013, and the current worldwide shortage of professional nurses is now on the WHO agenda and is being addressed by country (WHA, 2011; WHO, 2010; WHO, 2013).

The World Health Report, first published in 1995, is WHO's leading publication. Each year the report combines an expert assessment of global health, including statistics relating to all countries, with a focus on a specific subject. The main purpose of the report is to provide countries, donor agencies, international organizations, and others with the information they need to help them make policy and funding decisions. In the 2010 report, the WHO mapped out what countries can do to modify their financing systems so they can move more quickly toward this goal—universal coverage—and sustain the gains that have been achieved. The report builds on new research and lessons learned from country experience. It provides an action agenda for countries at all stages of development and proposes ways that the international community can better support efforts in low-income countries to achieve universal coverage and improve health outcomes (WHO, 2010).

The presence of nursing in international health is increasing. Besides offering direct health services in every country in the world, nurses serve as consultants, educators, and program planners and evaluators. Nurses focus their work on a variety of public health issues, including the health care workforce and education, environment, sanitation, infectious diseases, wellness promotion, maternal and child health, and primary care. Dr. Naeema Al-Gasseer of Bahrain has served as the scientist for nursing and midwifery at the WHO; Marla Salmon, former dean of nursing at The University of Washington, chaired a Global Advisory Group on Nursing and Midwifery; and Linda Tarr Whelan served as the U.S. Ambassador to the UN Commission on the Status of Women. Virginia Trotter Betts, past president of the American Nurses Association (ANA), served as a U.S. delegate to both the WHA and the Fourth World Conference on Women in Beijing in 1995, where she participated on the negotiating team of the conference to develop a platform on the health of women across the life span. Many U.S. nurse leaders, such as Dr. Carolyn Williams, current author in this book, have been WHO consultants.

## Federal Health Agencies

Laws passed by Congress may be assigned to any administrative agency within the executive branch of government for implementing, supervising, regulating, and enforcing. Congress decides which agency will monitor specific laws. For example, most health care legislation is delegated to the USDHHS. However, legislation concerning the environment would most

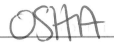

likely be implemented and monitored by the Environmental Protection Agency (EPA), and that concerning occupational health by the Occupational Safety and Health Administration (OSHA) in the U.S. Department of Labor.

## U.S. Department of Health and Human Services

The USDHHS is the agency most heavily involved with the health and welfare of U.S. citizens. It touches more lives than any other federal agency. The following agencies have been selected for their relevance to this chapter.

*Health Resources and Services Administration.* The Health Resources and Services Administration (HRSA) has been a long-standing contributor to the improved health status of Americans through the programs of services and health professions education that it funds. The HRSA contains the Bureau of Health Professions (BHPr), which includes the Division of Nursing as well as the Divisions of Medicine, Dentistry, and Allied Health Professions. The Division of Nursing is the key federal focus for nursing education and practice, and it provides national leadership to ensure an adequate supply and distribution of qualified nursing personnel to meet the health needs of the nation.

At the 122nd meeting of the Division of Nursing's National Advisory Council for Nursing Education and Practice (NACNEP), the participants discussed the role of public health nurses in participating in primary care in their communities. The speaker indicated several factors that need to be in place to support the public health nurse role:

- Baccalaureate standard for entry into practice
- Ongoing stable funding for health departments
- Competitive salaries commensurate with responsibilities
- Interventions grounded in and responsive to community needs
- Consideration of health determinants
- Experience in health promotion and prevention
- Long-term trusting relationships in the community (i.e., with clients)
- Established network of community partners
- Commitment to social justice and eliminating health disparities

In the council's twelfth report to Congress (USDHHS, 2013a) the council recommended further investment by the government in public health nursing, arguing the need based on system changes and the Affordable Care Act implementation, greater need to connect public health and care delivery with front-line public health nurses, plus the economic benefits of supporting this investment. Through the input of the NACNEP, the Division of Nursing sets policy for nursing nationally.

*Centers for Disease Control and Prevention.* The Centers for Disease Control and Prevention (CDC) serve as the national focus for developing and applying disease prevention and control, environmental health, and health promotion and education activities designed to improve the health of the people of the United States. The mission of the CDC is to protect America from health, safety and security threats, both foreign and in the United States. Whether diseases start at home or abroad, are chronic or acute, curable or preventable, human error or deliberate attack, CDC fights disease and supports communities and citizens to do the same. As such CDC increases

the health security of our nation (CDC, 2014A) The CDC seeks to accomplish its mission by working with partners throughout the nation and the world in the following ways:

- To provide health security
- To detect and investigate health threats
- To tackle the biggest health problems causing death and disability
- To conduct research that will enhance prevention
- To promote healthy and safe behaviors, communities, and environments
- To develop leaders and train the public health workforce, including disease detectives
- To develop and advocate sound public health policies
- To implement prevention strategies
- To promote healthy behaviors
- To foster safe and healthful environments
- To provide leadership and training

The outbreak of summer 2014 is an example of how the CDC fulfills its mission. The Shiga toxin-producing *Escherichia coli* outbreak linked to raw clover sprouts affected six states and 19 people, and 44% were hospitalized. Idaho was the state that was most likely the source of the outbreak. The CDC regularly collects data about foodborne illnesses through the National Notifiable Disease Surveillance System on a weekly basis through the CDC MMWR weekly report from states. Because of the recognized increase in cases, states were asked to report aggregate numbers of cases twice a week along with foodborne-related hospitalizations and complications. The CDC implemented an investigation to track the cases and worked with state and local health departments to perform the following:

- Detect the possible outbreak
- Define and find cases
- Generate hypotheses about the likely source
- Test the hypothesis
- Find the point of contamination
- Control the outbreak from further spread
- Decide when the outbreak is over.

By August 2014, there had been about 19 cases beginning in June 2014. In 3 months there were cases in 6 states. Figure 8-1 presents a CDC map indicating cases per state (CDC, MMWR Dispatch, 2014b). The six states involved were California (1), Idaho (3), Michigan (1), Montana (2), Utah (1), and Washington (11). By August 2014 CDC determined the outbreak to be over. Although few people were involved in this outbreak, the outcome could have been deadly to the persons who ate the sprouts. While the Ebola virus of West Africa continues to spread, the CDC is monitoring the effects of the virus as part of their global monitoring system. CDC has information and training materials ready for those who may need to use the materials (CDC, 2014c). The CDC has taken an active role in the recent outbreak of measles as a result of exposure to the virus at Disneyland in California. This outbreak resulted in 140 people from seven states being infected. On 1/23/2015, the CDC issued a health advisory to all public health and health care facilities nationwide (Zipprich et al, 2015).

*National Institutes of Health.* Founded in 1887, NIH today is one of the world's foremost biomedical research centers, and the federal focus point for biomedical research in the United States.

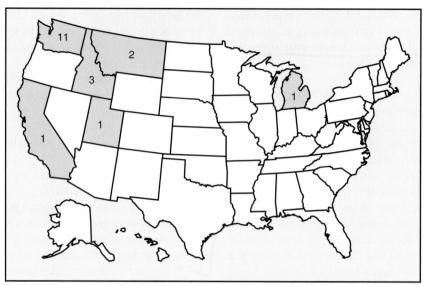

**FIG 8-1** The number of reported *Escherichia coli* cases linked to multistate outbreak, by state—United States, May to August, 2014 (From Centers for Disease Control and Prevention: *Epidemiology of* Escherichia coli *outbreak, United States,* Atlanta, 2014 USDHHS.)

The NIH is composed of 27 separate institutes and centers. The goal of NIH research is to acquire new knowledge to help prevent, detect, diagnose, and treat disease and disability, from the rarest genetic disorder to the common cold. The NIH mission is to uncover new knowledge that will lead to better health for everyone. The NIH works toward that mission by conducting research in its own laboratories; supporting the research of nonfederal scientists in universities, medical schools, hospitals, and research institutions throughout the country and abroad; helping in the training of research investigators; and fostering communication of medical and health sciences' information (NIH, 2010a).

In late 1985 Congress overrode a presidential veto, allowing the creation of the National Center for Nursing Research within the NIH. In 1993 the Center became one of the divisions of the NIH and was renamed the **National Institute of Nursing Research** (NINR). The research and research-related training activities previously supported by the Division of Nursing were transferred to the new Institute. The NINR is the focal point of the nation's nursing research activities. It promotes the growth and quality of research in nursing and client care, provides important leadership, expands the pool of experienced nurse researchers, and serves as a point of interaction with other bases of health care research. The mission of NINR is to promote and improve the health of individuals, families, communities, and populations.

NINR supports and conducts clinical and basic research and research training on health and illness across the life span. The research focus encompasses health promotion and disease prevention, quality of life, health disparities, and end of life. NINR seeks to extend nursing science by integrating the biological and behavioral sciences, using new technologies to research questions, improving research methods, and developing the scientists of the future (NINR, 2011).

*Agency for Healthcare Research and Quality.* The **Agency for Healthcare Research and Quality** (AHRQ) is the lead federal agency charged with improving the quality, safety, efficiency, and effectiveness of health care for all Americans. As one of 12 agencies within the USDHHS, AHRQ supports health services research that will improve the quality of health care and promote evidence-based decision making. AHRQ is committed to improving care safety and quality by developing successful partnerships and generating the knowledge and tools required for long-term improvement. The goal of AHRQ research is to promote measurable improvements in health care in America. The outcomes are gauged in terms of improved quality of life and client outcomes, lives saved, and value gained for what we spend (AHRQ, 2014a).

By examining what works and what does not work in health care, the AHRQ fulfills its missions of translating research findings into better client care and providing consumers, policy makers, and other health care leaders with information needed to make critical health care decisions. In 1999, Congress, through legislation, specifically directed AHRQ to focus on measuring and improving health care quality; promoting client safety and reducing medical errors; advancing the use of information technology for coordinating client care and conducting quality and outcomes research; and seeking to eliminate disparities in health care delivery for the priority populations of low-income groups, minorities, women, children, older adults, and individuals with special health care needs.

The AHRQ published protocols for care of clients with a variety of health problems. These protocols became the standards of health care delivery. The agency continues to maintain a clinical practice guidelines clearinghouse for use by clinicians and others. In addition, the AHRQ had a project called "Put Prevention into Practice" to promote the use of standardized protocols for primary care delivery for clients across the age span (see Schedule of Clinical Preventive Services in AHRQ, 2014b). Today there is a program titled The Practice-Based Research Network that rapidly develops and assesses methods and tools to ensure that new scientific evidence is incorporated into real-world practice settings (AHRQ, 2014c).

*Centers for Medicare and Medicaid Services.* One of the most powerful agencies within the USDHHS is the CMS, which administers Medicare and Medicaid accounts and guided payment policy and delivery rules for services for 100 million people in 2014 (CMS, 2014). In addition to providing health insurance, CMS also performs a number of quality-focused health care or health-related activities, including regulating of laboratory testing, developing coverage policies, and improving quality of care. CMS maintains oversight of the surveying and certifying of nursing homes and continuing care providers (including home health agencies, intermediate care facilities for the developmentally disabled, and hospitals). It makes available to beneficiaries, providers, researchers, and state surveyors information about these activities and nursing home quality.

## Federal Non-Health Agencies

Although the USDHHS has primary responsibility for federal health functions, several other departments of the executive branch carry out important health functions for the nation. Among these are the Defense, Labor, Agriculture, and Justice Departments.

## Department of Defense

The Department of Defense delivers health care to members of the military, to their dependents and survivors, to National Guard and reserve members, and to retired members and their families. The assistant secretary of defense for health affairs administers a variety of health care plans for service personnel: TriCare Prime (a managed care arrangement) and an option for fee-for-service plans called TriCare Standard as well as TriCare Extra with many other options available. In each branch of the uniformed services, nurses of high military rank are part of the administration of these health services (U.S. Department of Defense, 2014).

## Department of Labor

The Department of Labor houses OSHA, which imposes workplace requirements on industries. These requirements shape the functions of nurses and the types of health services provided to workers in the workplace. A record-keeping system required by OSHA greatly affects health records in the workplace. Each state has an agency similar to OSHA that also monitors and inspects industries, as well as the health services delivered to them by nurses.

Needlestick injuries and other sharps-related injuries that result in occupational bloodborne pathogen exposure continue to be an important public health concern, especially to health care workers. In response to this serious situation, Congress passed the Needle Stick Safety and Prevention Act, which became law on November 6, 2000. To meet the requirements of this act, OSHA revised its Bloodborne Pathogen Standard to become effective on April 18, 2002. This act clarified the responsibility of employers to select safer needle devices as they become available and to involve employees in identifying and choosing the devices. The updated standard also required employers to maintain a log of injuries from contaminated sharps (OSHA, 2008; 2011; OSHA, 2013).

## Department of Agriculture

The Department of Agriculture houses the Food and Nutrition Service, which oversees a variety of food assistance activities. This service collaborates with state and local government welfare agencies to provide food stamps to needy persons to increase their food purchasing power. Other programs include school breakfast and lunch programs, WIC, and grants to states for nutrition education and training. In 2013, WIC provided support for 53% of all infants born in the United States. Although these programs have been successful, the increasing use of the process of giving federal block grants to states (rather than implementing national programs) may threaten the effectiveness of these programs because of differences in how decisions are made at the state level on how to spend money on nutrition (USDA, 2013).

## Department of Justice

Health services to federal prisoners are administered within the Department of Justice. The Federal Bureau of Prisons is responsible for the custody and care of approximately 214,000 federal offenders (Bureau of Federal Prisons, 2014). The Medical and Services Division of the Bureau of Prisons includes medical, psychiatric, dental, and health support services with community standards in a correctional environment. Health promotion is emphasized through counseling during examinations, education about effects of medications, infectious disease prevention and education, and chronic care clinics for conditions such as cardiovascular disease, diabetes, and hypertension. The Bureau also provides forensic services to the courts, including a range of evaluative mental health studies outlined in federal statutes. Health care for prisoners is highly regulated because of a series of court decisions on inmates' rights.

## State and Local Health Departments

Depending on funding, public commitment and interest, and access to other resources, programs offered by state and local health departments vary greatly. Many state and local health officials report that employees in public health agencies lack skills in the core sciences of public health, and that this has hindered their effectiveness. The lack of specialized education and skill is a significant barrier to population-based preventive care and the delivery of quality health care to the public. Public health workforce specialists report that the number of retirees expected in this decade will result in a major shortage of public health workers, including nurses. More often than at other levels of government, nurses at the local level provide direct services. Some nurses deliver special or selected services, such as follow-up of contacts in cases of tuberculosis or venereal disease or providing child immunization clinics. Other nurses have a more generalized practice, delivering services to families in certain geographic areas (PHF, 2010; University of Michigan Center of Excellence in Public Health Workforce Studies, 2013).

At the local and state levels, coordinating health efforts between health departments and other county or city departments is essential. Gaps in community coordination are showing up in glaring ways as states and communities scramble to address bioterrorism preparedness since September 11, 2001, and since such natural disasters as Hurricane Katrina. The United States had 220,000 people lose their homes in 2013 due to extreme storms and tornadoes in Oklahoma and another 100,000 from flooding in Colorado. Health departments are on the front line in such occurrences (see Chapter 46).

## IMPACT OF GOVERNMENT HEALTH FUNCTIONS AND STRUCTURES ON NURSING

The variety and range of functions of governmental agencies have had a major impact on the practice of nursing. Funding, in particular, has shaped roles and tasks of population-centered nurses. The designation of money for specific needs, or **categorical funding,** has led to special and more narrowly focused nursing roles. Examples are in emergency preparedness, school nursing, and family planning. Funds assigned to antibioterrorism cannot be used to support unrelated communicable disease programs or family planning.

The events of September 11, 2001, have had the public and the profession of nursing concerned about the ability of the present public health system and its workforce to deal with bioterrorism, especially outbreaks of deadly and serious communicable diseases. For example, smallpox vaccinations were stopped in 1972, but immunity lasts for only 10 years; although there have been no reported cases since the early 1970s, almost no one in the United States retains their immunity. Thus, the population is vulnerable to a smallpox outbreak, and smallpox could be used as a weapon of bioterrorism. Two laboratories in the world retain a small amount of the smallpox virus. Because of these potential threats, the U.S. government has begun to increase production of the vaccine (NIH, 2010b). Few public health professionals are knowledgeable of the symptoms, treatment, or mode of transmission of this disease. Most health professionals, including registered nurses (RNs), who currently work in the United States, have never seen a case of anthrax, smallpox, or plague—the three major biological weapons of concern in the world today. A few have now seen the effects of the Ebola virus. The USDHHS and the federal **Office of Homeland Security** have provided funds to address this serious threat to the people of the United States.

One of the first things being done is the rebuilding of the crumbling public health infrastructures of each state to provide surveillance, intervention, and communication in the face of future bioterrorism events and natural disasters. On December 19, 2006, President George W. Bush signed the Pandemic and All-Hazards Preparedness Act (PAHPA), which was intended to improve the organization, direction, and utility of preparedness efforts. PAHPA centralizes federal responsibilities, requires state-based accountability, proposes new national surveillance methods, addresses surge capacity, and facilitates the development of vaccines and other scarce resources (Morhard and Franco, 2013). On March 13, 2013, President Barrack Obama signed the Pandemic and All-Hazards Preparedness Reauthorization Act into law. The 2013 law reauthorizes funding for public health and medical preparedness programs that enable communities to build systems to support people in need during and after disasters (USDHHS, 2013B).

## THE LAW AND HEALTH CARE

The United States is a nation of laws, which are subject to the U.S. Constitution. The law is a system of privileges and processes by which people solve problems on the basis of a set of established rules. It is intended to minimize the use of force. Laws govern the relationships of individuals and organizations to other individuals and to government. After a law is established, regulations further define the course of actions to be taken by the government, organizations, or individuals in reaching an agreed-on outcome. Government and its laws are the ultimate authority in society and are designed to enforce official policy whether it is related to health, education, economics, social welfare, or any other society issue. The number and types of laws influencing health care are ever increasing. Definitions of law (Catholic University of America, 2010) include the following:

- A rule established by authority, society, or custom
- The body of rules governing the affairs of people, communities, states, corporations, and nations
- A set of rules or customs governing a discrete field or activity (e.g., criminal law, contract law)

These definitions reflect the close relationship of law to the community and to society's customs and beliefs.

The law has had a major impact on nursing practice. Although nursing emerged from individual voluntary activities, society passed laws to give formality to public health and, through legal mandates (i.e., laws), positions and functions for nurses in community settings were created. These functions in many instances carry the force of law. For example, if the nurse discovers a person with smallpox, the law directs the nurse and others in the public health community to take specific actions. In another example, in a mumps outbreak, a nurse and other health professionals are required to report mumps cases. This reporting requirement helps with locating and treating cases so cases can be treated or isolated as they occur to prevent further spreading of disease. Three types of laws in the United States have particular importance.

### Constitutional Law

**Constitutional law** derives from federal and state constitutions. It provides overall guidance for selected practice situations. For example, on what basis can the state *require* quarantine or isolation of individuals with tuberculosis? The U.S. Constitution specifies the explicit and limited functions of the federal government. All other powers and functions are left to the individual states. The major constitutional power of the states relating to population-centered nursing practice is the state's right to intervene in a reasonable manner to protect the health, safety, and welfare of its citizens. The state has *police power* to act through its public health system, but it has limits. First, it must be a "reasonable" exercise of power. Second, if the power interferes or infringes on individual rights, the state must demonstrate that there is a "compelling state interest" in exercising its power. Isolating an individual or separating someone from a community because that person has a communicable disease has been deemed an appropriate exercise of state powers. The state can isolate an individual even though it infringes on individual rights (such as freedom and autonomy), under the following conditions (Lee et al, 2012):

- There is a compelling state interest in preventing an epidemic.
- The isolation is necessary to protect the health, safety, and welfare of individuals in the community or the public as a whole.
- The isolation is done in a reasonable manner.

The legal and medical communities along with AIDS (acquired immunodeficiency syndrome) activists rejected (and made the case) that the social quarantine of individuals with AIDS was unnecessary. Thus, individual freedom and autonomy of the individual come before "compelling state interest" unless science warrants another conclusion (Swendiman and Elsea, 2010).

## Legislation and Regulation

Legislation is law that comes from the legislative branches of federal, state, or local government. This is referred to as Statute Law because it becomes coded in the statutes of a government (Birkland, 2010). Much legislation has an effect on nursing. Regulations are specific statements of law related to defining or implanting individual pieces of legislation or statute law. For example, state legislatures enact laws (statutes) establishing boards of nursing and defining terms such as registered nurse and nursing practice. Every state has a board of nursing. The board may be found either in the department of licensing boards of the health department or in an administrative agency of the governor's office. Created by legislation known as a state nurse practice act, the board of nursing is made up of nurses and consumers. The functions of this board are described in the nurse practice act of each state and generally include licensing and examination of RNs and licensed practical nurses; licensing and/or certification of advanced practice nurses; approval of schools of nursing in the state; revocation, suspension, or denying of licenses; and writing of regulations about nursing practice and education.

The state boards of nursing operationalize, implement, and enforce the statutory law by writing explicit statements (rules) on what it means to be an RN, and on the nurse's rights and responsibilities in delegating work to others and in meeting continuing education requirements.

All nurses employed in community settings are subject to legislation and regulations. For example, home health care nurses employed by private agencies must deliver care according to federal Medicare or state Medicaid legislation and regulations, so the agency can be reimbursed for those services. Private and public health care services rendered by nurses are subject to many governmental regulations for quality of care, standards of documentation, and confidentiality of client records and communications. All state health departments have a public health practice reference that governs the practice of nurses and others, and state public health laws that define the essential public health services that must be offered in the state as well as the optional services that may also be offered.

## Judicial and Common Law

Both judicial law and common law have great impact on nursing. Judicial law is based on court or jury decisions. The opinions of the courts are referred to as *case law* (Birkland, 2010). The court uses other types of laws to make its decisions, including previous court decisions or cases. Precedent is one principle of common law. This means that judges are bound by previous decisions unless they are convinced that the older law is no longer relevant or valid. This process is called *distinguishing*, and it usually involves a demonstration of how the current situation in dispute differs from the previously decided situation. Other principles of common law such as justice, fairness, respect for individual's autonomy, and self-determination are part of a court's rationale and the basis upon which to make a decision.

## LAWS SPECIFIC TO NURSING PRACTICE

Despite the broad nature and varied roles of nurses in practice, two legal arenas are most applicable to nurse practice situations. The first is the statutory authority for the profession and its scope of practice, and the second is professional negligence or malpractice.

### Scope of Practice

The issue of scope of practice involves defining nursing, setting its credentials, and then distinguishing between the practices of nurses, physicians, and other health care providers. The issue is especially important to nurses in community settings, who have traditionally practiced with much autonomy.

Health care practitioners are subject to the laws of the state in which they practice, and they can practice only with a license. The states' nurse practice acts differ somewhat, but they are the most important statutory laws affecting nurses. The nurse practice act of each state accomplishes at least four functions: defining the practice of professional nursing, identifying the scope of nursing practice, setting educational qualifications and other requirements for licensure, and determining the legal titles nurses may use to identify themselves. The usual and customary practice of nursing can be determined through a variety of sources, including the following:

- Content of nursing educational programs, both general and special
- Experience of other practicing nurses (peers)
- Statements and standards of nursing professional organizations
- Policies and procedures of agencies employing nurses
- Needs and interests of the community
- Updated literature, including research, books, texts, and journals
- Internet sites if it can be determined that the site is a professional source of information

All of these sources can describe, determine, and refine the scope of practice of a professional nurse. Every nurse should know and follow closely any proposed changes in the practice acts of nursing, medicine, pharmacy, and other related professions. The nurse should always examine all legislation, rules, and regulations related to nursing practice. For example, a review of the pharmacy act will let the nurse know whether to question the right to dispense medications in a family planning clinic in a local health department. Defining the scope of practice forces one to clarify independent, interdependent, and dependent nursing functions.

Just as practice acts vary by state, so do the evolving issues and tensions of scopes of practice among the health professions. In past years, several state legislatures (working closely with the National Council of State Boards of Nursing) embarked on a legislative effort to develop the Interstate Nurse Licensure Compact. The compact allows mutual recognition of generalist nursing licensure across state lines in the compact states. By 2014, 24 states had adopted the compact (NCSBN, 2014).

## Professional Negligence

*Professional negligence*, or *malpractice*, is defined as an act (or a failure to act) that leads to injury of a client. To recover money damages in a malpractice action, the client must prove all of the following:

1. That the nurse owed a duty to the client or was responsible for the client's care
2. That the duty to act the way a reasonable, prudent nurse would act in the same circumstances was not fulfilled
3. That the failure to act reasonably under the circumstances led to the alleged injuries
4. That the injuries provided the basis for a monetary claim from the nurse as compensation for the injury

Reported cases involving negligence and population-centered nurses are rare. However, the following is an example:

> ### Home Nurse Fails to Properly Supervise Bottle Feeding of Child With Tracheal Tube for Oxygen—Death—$4.5 Million Verdict
>
> *The plaintiff, a child, age sixteen months, suffered insufficiency of her lungs and required a continuous supply of oxygen via a tracheal tube. She required constant supervision by a home health nurse.*
>
> *In January 2008, during the day a bottle of formula was given by the nurse. The formula entered the tracheal tube and lungs. After several minutes the nurse observed that the child had stopped breathing and began cardiopulmonary resuscitation. The child did not survive. It was determined that the child had suffered asphyxiation due to ingestion of vomited material.*
>
> *The plaintiff claimed that the child had choked and gagged throughout the nurse's resuscitation attempts and that CPR was not the correct method of resuscitating the child. The plaintiff claimed that the tracheal tube should have been cleared or changed.*
>
> *The case was initially brought against the defendant nurse's employer, the home care agency, and the hospital which had provided the tracheal tube. The claims against the hospital were discontinued and the matter proceeded to trial against the home care agency. The defendant did not contest liability.*
>
> *According to a published account a $4.5 million verdict was returned for the child's pain and suffering. A defense motion to set aside the verdict was pending.*
>
> **With permission from**
> **Medical Malpractice Verdicts,**
> **Settlements & Experts; Lewis Laska, Editor,**
> **901 Church St., Nashville,**
> **TN 37203-3411, 2013 1-800-298-6288.**

An integral part of all negligence actions is the question of who should be sued. When a nurse is employed and functioning within the scope of employment, the employer is responsible for the nurse's negligent actions. This is referred to as the doctrine of *respondeat superior*. By directing a nurse to carry out a particular function, the employer becomes responsible for negligence, along with the individual nurse. Because employers are usually better able to pay for the injuries suffered by clients, they are sued more often than the nurses themselves, although an increasing number of judgments include the professional nurse by name as a co-defendant. In some instances, if the agency is found liable, the agency may in turn sue the nurse for negligence. At least, the nurse often loses the job.

Thus, it is imperative that all nurses engaged in clinical practice carry their own professional liability insurance. Nurses may have personal immunity for particular practice areas, such as giving immunizations. In some states, the legislature has granted personal immunity to nurses employed by public agencies to cover all aspects of their practice under the legal theory of *sovereign immunity* (Cherry and Jacobs, 2013).

Nursing students need to be aware that the same laws and rules that govern the professional nurse govern them. Students are expected to meet the same standard of care as that met by any licensed nurse practicing under the same or similar circumstances. Students are expected to be able to perform all tasks and make clinical decisions on the basis of the knowledge they have gained or been offered, according to their progress in their educational programs and along with adequate educational supervision.

## LEGAL ISSUES AFFECTING HEALTH CARE PRACTICES

Specific legal issues of nursing vary depending on the setting where care is delivered, the clinical arena, and the nurse's functional role. The law, including legislation and judicial opinions, significantly affects each of the following areas of nursing practice. Nurses responsible for setting and implementing program priorities need to identify and monitor laws related to each special area of practice.

### School and Family Health

Nurses employed by health departments or boards of education may deliver school and family health nursing. School health legislation establishes a minimum of services that must be provided to children in public and private schools. For example, most states require that children be immunized against certain communicable diseases before entering school. Children must have had a physical examination by that time, and most states require at least one physical at a later time in their schooling. Legislation also specifies when and what type of health screening will be conducted in schools (e.g., vision and hearing testing). These requirements are found in statutory laws of states. Some states are now requiring a simple dental examination in schools for the purpose of referring children to a dental health professional if needed.

Statutes addressing child abuse and neglect make a large impact on nursing practice within schools and families. Most states require nurses to notify police and/or a social service agency of any situation in which they suspect a child is being abused or neglected. This is one instance in which the law mandates that a health professional breach client confidentiality to protect someone who may be in a helpless or vulnerable position. There is *civil immunity* for such reporting, and the nurse may be called as a witness in a court hearing of the case.

Occupational health is another special area of practice that has specific legal requirements as a result of state and federal statutes. Of special concern are the state workers' compensation statutes, which provide the legal foundation for claims of workers injured on the job. Access to records, confidentiality, and the use of standing orders are legal issues that have great practice significance to nurses employed in industries.

## Home Care and Hospice

Home care and hospice services rendered by nurses are shaped through state statutes and have specific nursing requirements for licensure and certification. Compliance with these laws is directly linked to the method of payment for the services. For example, a service must be licensed and certified to obtain payment for services through Medicare. Federal regulations implementing Medicare/Medicaid have an enormous effect on much of nursing practice, including how nurses record details of their visits, record time spent in care activities, and document client care and the client's status and progress.

In addition, many states have passed laws requiring nurses to report elder abuse to the proper authorities, as is done with children and youth. Laws affecting home care and hospice services have focused on such issues as the right to death with dignity, rights of residents of long-term facilities and home health clients, definitions of death, and the use of living wills and advance directives. The legal and ethical dimensions of nursing practice are particularly important. Individual rights, such as the right to refuse treatment, and nursing responsibilities, such as the legal duty to render reasonable and prudent care, may appear to be in conflict in delivering home and hospice services. Much case discussion (sometimes including outside ethics consultation) may be needed to resolve such conflicts.

## Correctional Health

Correctional health nursing practice is significantly shaped by federal and state laws and regulations and by recent Supreme Court decisions. The laws and decisions primarily relate to the type and amount of services that must be provided for incarcerated individuals. For example, physical examinations are required for all prisoners after they are sentenced. Regulations specify basic levels of care that must be provided for prisoners, and access to care during illness is a particular focus. Court decisions requiring adequate health services are based on constitutional law. If minimal services are not provided, it is a violation of a prisoner's right to freedom from cruel and unusual punishment. Such decisions provide a framework that strongly influences the setting of nursing priorities. For example, providing care to the sick would take priority over wellness or health education classes.

## THE NURSE'S ROLE IN THE POLICY PROCESS

The number and types of laws influencing health care are increasing. Because of this, nurses need to be involved in the policy process and understand the importance of involvement of nursing to the clients they serve.

For nurses to effectively care for their client populations and their communities in the complex U.S. health care system, professional advocacy for logical health policy that considers equality is essential. Professional nurses working in the community know all too well about the health care problems they and their clients encounter daily, and it is through policy and political activism that both big-picture and long-term solutions can be developed.

Although the term *policy* may sound rather lofty, health policy is quite simply the process of turning health problems into workable action solutions. Health policy is developed on the three-legged stool of *access, cost,* and *quality.* The policy process, which is very familiar to professional nurses, includes the following:
- Statement of a health care problem
- Statement of policy options to address the health problem
- Adoption of a particular policy option
- Implementation of the policy product (e.g., a service)
- Evaluation of the policy's intended and unintended consequences in solving the original health problem

Thus the policy process is very similar to the nursing process, but the focus is on the level of the larger society and the adoption strategies require political action. For most professional nurses, action in the policy arena comes most easily and naturally through participation in nursing organizations such as the ANA at the state level or the Association of Community Health Nursing Educators (ACHNE) or the Association of State and Territorial Directors of Nursing (ASTDN) at the national or state level, and in certain specialty organizations like the American Association of Specialty Nursing Organizations.

## Legislative Action

It is often helpful to review the legislative and political processes that may have been a part of high school education. It becomes important material to remember as a professional career is embarked upon.

The people within geographic jurisdictions elect their legislative representatives and senators. An important part of the legislative process is the work of the legislative staff. These individuals do the legwork, research, paperwork, and other activities that move policy ideas into bills and then into law. In addition to the individual legislator's office, the congressional committee staffs are also important. They are usually experts in the content of the work of a committee, such as a health and welfare committee. Frequently, developing a working relationship with key legislative staffers can be as important to achieving a policy objective as the relationship with the policy maker (i.e., the legislator).

The legislative process begins with ideas (policy options) that are developed into bills. After a bill is drafted, it is introduced to the legislature, given a number, read, and assigned to a committee. Hearings, testimony, lobbying, education, research, and informal discussions follow. If the bill is passed from the legislative committee, the entire House of Representatives hears the bill, amends it as necessary, and votes on it. A majority vote moves the bill to Senate where it is read and amended, and then a vote is taken. Figure 8-2 shows the necessary formal process of the legislative pathway.

Nurses can be involved in the legislative process at any point. Many professional nursing associations have legislative committees made up of volunteers, governmental relations staff professionals, and sometimes political action committees (PACs), all engaged in efforts to monitor, analyze, and shape health policy.

Common methods of influencing health policy outcomes include face-to-face encounters, personal letters, mailgrams, electronic mail, telephone calls, testimony, petitions, reports, position papers, fact sheets, letters to the editor, news releases, speeches, coalition building, demonstrations, and lawsuits. Depending on the issue, any of these can be effective. Although most business, including politics and the policy agendas, are dependent upon the Internet today for instant communication and quick response, all of these methods continue to be of great importance in influencing policy agendas. For example, if a face-to-face encounter is used with a legislator or a staffer, these persons can put a "face on the policy" agenda, and the reality that the policy affects real persons is an important consideration when the legislator or staff pushes the policy agenda forward. Guidelines on communication are provided in the How To box. Tips on communication and visiting legislators and their staffs, as well as general tips on political action, are presented in Boxes 8-1, 8-2, and 8-3. Political activities in which nurses can and should be involved include a wide variety of activities such as being informed voters (a must!), participating in a political party, registering others to vote, getting out the vote, fundraising for candidates, building networks or communication links for issues (e.g., a phone tree or Internet distribution list), and participating in organizations to ensure their effective involvement in health policy and politics.

## BOX 8-1    Tips for Visits with Legislators

- Face-to-face visits are viewed as the most effective.
- Call ahead and ask how much time the staff or legislator is able to give you.
- When you arrive, ask if the appointment time is the same or if a scheduled vote on the House/Senate floor is going to need the legislator's attention.
- Engage in small talk at the beginning of the conversation only if the staff or legislator has time.
- Structure time so that the issue can be briefly presented. The visit will probably be 15 minutes or less.
- Allow an opportunity for the staff or Congress member to seek clarity or ask questions.
- Offer to provide additional information or find answers to questions asked.

- Do not assume that the legislator or the legislator's staff is well informed on the issue.
- Leave a one- or two-page fact sheet on the issue.
- Numbers count. If the views you express are shared by a local nurses' organization or by nurses employed at a health care facility, let the legislator know.
- Invite Congress members and their staffs to conferences or meetings of nurses' organizations, or to tour nursing facilities to meet others interested in the same policy issues.
- If appropriate, invite the media and let the legislator know.
- Follow up with a letter of thanks to both the legislator and the staffer.

Modified from Mason D et al: Policy and politics in government, ed 5, St Louis, 2007, Elsevier.

## BOX 8-2    Tips for Written Communication with Legislators

- Communicate in writing to express opinions.
- Identify yourself as a nurse.
- Acknowledge the Congress member's work as positive or negative, but be courteous.
- Follow up on meetings or phone calls with a letter or e-mail.
- Share knowledge about a particular problem.
- Recommend policy solutions so the legislator or staff will know why you are writing.
- The letter should be typed, a maximum of two pages, and focused on one or two issues at most.
- The purpose of the letter should be stated at the beginning.
- Present clear and compelling rationales for your concern or position on an issue.
- If the purpose of the letter is to express disappointment regarding a stance on an issue or a vote that has been cast, the letter should be as positive as possible.

- Write letters thanking a Congress member for taking a particular position on an issue.
- A letter to the editor of the local newspaper or a nursing newsletter praising a legislator's position (with a copy forwarded to the legislator) is welcome publicity, especially during an election year.
- If you visited with the legislator or a staffer, review the major points covered in person and answer any questions that were raised during conversation.
- Have personal business cards and include them with letters.
- Address written correspondence as follows (the same general format applies to state and local officials):

| U.S. Senator | U.S. Representative |
|---|---|
| Honorable Jane Doe | Honorable Jane Doe |
| United States Senate | House of Representatives |
| Washington, DC 20510 | Washington, DC 20515 |
| Dear Senator Doe: | Dear Representative Doe: |

Modified from Mason D et al: Policy and politics in government, ed 5, St Louis, 2007, Elsevier.

**The Federal Level**

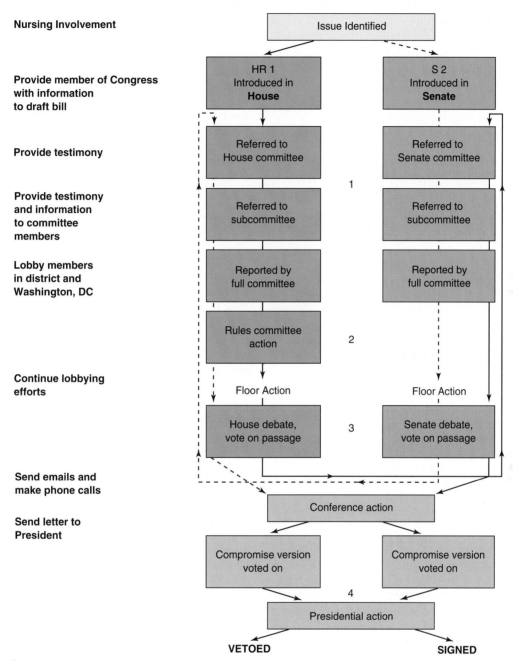

Nursing Involvement

Provide member of Congress with information to draft bill

Provide testimony

Provide testimony and information to committee members

Lobby members in district and Washington, DC

Continue lobbying efforts

Send emails and make phone calls

Send letter to President

Issue Identified

HR 1 Introduced in **House**

S 2 Introduced in **Senate**

Referred to House committee

Referred to Senate committee

Referred to subcommittee

Referred to subcommittee

Reported by full committee

Reported by full committee

Rules committee action

Floor Action

Floor Action

House debate, vote on passage

Senate debate, vote on passage

Conference action

Compromise version voted on

Compromise version voted on

Presidential action

**VETOED**   **SIGNED**

1

2

3

4

1 A bill goes to full committee first, then to special subcommittees for hearings, debate, revisions, and approval. The same process occurs when it goes to full committee.  It either dies in committee or proceeds to the next step.
2 Only the House has a Rules Committee to set the "rule" for floor action and conditions for debate and amendments. In the Senate, the leadership schedules action.
3 The bill is debated, amended, and passed or defeated.  If passed, it goes to the other chamber and  follows the same path.
If each chamber passes a similar bill, both versions go to conference.
4 The President may sign the bill into law, allow it to become law without his signature, or veto it and return it to Congress. To override the veto, both houses must approve the bill by a two-thirds majority vote.

**FIG 8-2**  How a bill becomes a law. (From Mason DJ, Leavitt JK, Chaffee MW: *Policy and politics in nursing and health care,* ed 6, St Louis, 2011, Elsevier.)

---

### BOX 8-3  Tips for Action

- Become informed.
- Become acquainted with elected officials.
- Become involved in the state nurses' association.
- Build communication and leadership skills.
- Increase your knowledge about a range of professional issues.
- Expand and strengthen your professional network.
- Build relationships within the profession and with representatives of public and private sector organizations with an interest in health care.
- Be aware of what is taking place in health care beyond the environment and the practice in which you work.
- Communicate with legislators regularly and share expertise and perspective on issues related to health care and nursing.
- Offer your expertise to assist in developing new legislation, modifying existing legislation or regulations.

- Identify yourself as a nurse with associated education and expertise.
- Let people know that nurses are capable of functioning in many different roles and making substantial contributions.
- Be confident.
- Do not burn bridges.
- Be friendly.
- Lend a hand to other nurses. It benefits all of us.
- Find an experienced mentor to work with you if you are new to the policy arena.
- Volunteer, seek appointments, or participate in elections in campaigns.
- Explore opportunities for involvement through internships, fellowships, and volunteer work at all levels (local, state, and national).

Modified from Mason D, Keavitt JK, Chaffee MW: Policy and politics ingovernment, ed 5, St Louis, 2007, Elsevier.

---

### HOW TO  Be an Effective Communicator

- *Use simple communications that will be readily understood.*
- *Choose language that clearly conveys information to individuals of diverse cultures, different ages, and different educational backgrounds.*
- *Target oral or written communication to the issue and omit jargon unique to medicine and nursing.*
- *State your expertise on the issue first.*
- *Briefly describe your education and experience.*
- *Identify the relevance of the issue beyond nursing.*
- *Provide information regarding the impact of the issue on the legislator's constituents.*
- *Present accurate, credible data.*
- *Do not oversell or give inaccurate information about the problem.*
- *Present information in an organized, thorough, concise form that is based on factual data (when available).*
- *Give examples.*

The direct reimbursement of advanced practice nurses (APNs) in the Medicare program is one example of how nurses can use their influence. The inclusion of amendments to Medicare that authorized APN reimbursement regardless of specialty or client location in the Balanced Budget Act of 1997 required the sustained efforts of the ANA and other national nursing organizations over a long period (Nursing World, 2000; USDHHS, CMS, 2011. During that time, individual nurses provided testimony to Congress and to MEDPAC (the physicians' political action committee) on the importance of direct reimbursement to APNs. Many APNs worked closely and vigorously with their congressional representatives to lobby for this Medicare amendment. Even more wrote letters and provided position papers and fact sheets to help legislators understand the value of APNs. Although the process took more than 10 years to achieve fully, APN reimbursement in Medicare became a reality. Both the nursing profession and Medicare beneficiaries will benefit from the enhanced access of Medicare clients to APNs.

The ANA was likewise a strong supporter for the Patient Safety Act of 1997 (ANA, 1997). This law requires health care agencies to make public some information on nurse staff levels, staff mix, and outcomes, and it requires the USDHHS to review and approve all health care acquisitions and mergers. All of these requirements are to determine any long-term effect on the health and safety of clients, communities, and staff.

On the state legislative level, all 50 states have passed title protection for APNs; this was achieved by individual nurses, state nurses associations, and various nursing specialty groups participating in the legislative process with the 50 state legislators. Title protection means that only certain nurses who meet state criteria can call themselves *advanced practice nurses.*

### Regulatory Action

The regulatory process, although it may not be as visible a process as legislation, can also be used to shape laws and dramatically affect health policy. This process should be on the radar screen of professional nurses who wish to successfully participate in policy activity.

At each level of government, the executive branch can and, in most cases, must prepare regulations for implementing policy for new laws and new programs. These regulations are detailed, and they establish, fix, and control standards and criteria for carrying out certain laws. Figure 8-3 shows the steps in the typical process of writing regulations. When the legislature passes a law and delegates its oversight to an agency, it gives that agency the power to make regulations. Because regulations flow from legislation, they have the force of law.

### The Process of Regulation

After a law is passed, the appropriate executive department begins the process of regulation by studying the topic or issue. Advisory groups or special task forces are sometimes formed to provide the content for the regulations. Nurses can influence these regulations by writing letters to the regulatory agency in charge or by speaking at open public hearings. Many letters are now accepted by Internet.

After rewriting, the proposed regulations are put into final draft form and printed in the legally required publication (e.g., at the federal level, the *Federal Register*). Similar registers exist in most states, where regulations from state executive

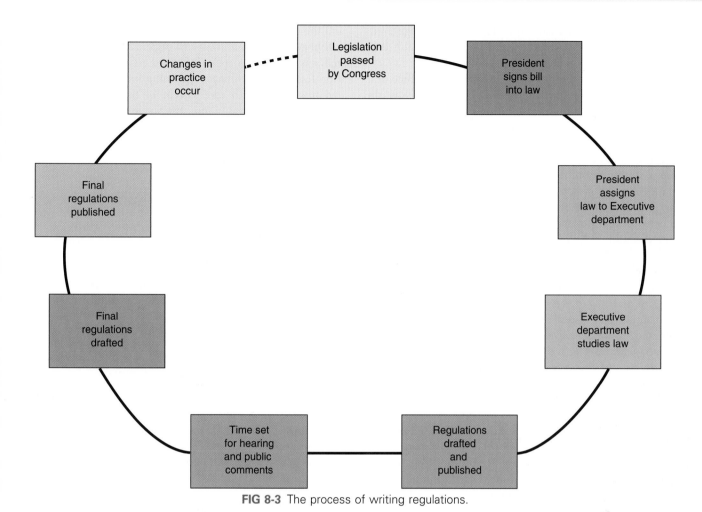

**FIG 8-3** The process of writing regulations.

departments, including state health departments, are published. Public comment is called for in written form or oral presentation within a given period.

Revisions made to proposed regulations are based on public comment and public hearing. Depending on the amount and content of the public reaction, final regulations are prepared or more study of the area and issues is conducted. Final published regulations carry the force of law. When regulations become effective, health care practice is changed to conform to the new regulations. Monitoring administrative regulations is essential for the professional nurse, who can influence regulations by attending the hearings, providing comments, testifying, and engaging in lobbying aimed at individuals involved in the writing of the regulations. Concrete written suggestions for revision submitted to these individuals are frequently persuasive and must be acknowledged by government in publishing the final rules. An excellent example of how nurses must continue to influence health policy outcomes, even after positive legislation has passed, occurred after the passage of the Balanced Budget Act of 1997 (PL 105-33, 1997). The HCFA began to implement the BBA '97 through the publication of draft regulations seeking to define APN practice and Medicare reimbursement. The nursing community responded vigorously with negative opinions about the initial restrictive definitions and requirement. Their reactions were effective and reshaped the final regulations to recognize the state definitions for APN practice autonomy.

Final regulations, published in a *Code of Regulations* (both federal and state), usually lead to changes in practice. For example, Medicare regulations setting standards for nursing homes and home health are incorporated into these agencies' manuals. In the case of APN reimbursement, some Medicare fiscal intermediaries have had difficulty in recognizing APNs as appropriate providers, but professional nursing organization advocates have forcefully addressed these implementation barriers.

## Nursing Advocacy

Advocacy begins with the art of influencing others (politics) to adopt a specific course of action (policy) to solve a societal problem. This is accomplished by building relationships with the appropriate policy makers—the individuals or groups that determine a specific course of action to be followed by a government or institution to achieve a desired end (policy outcome). Relationships for effective advocacy can be built in a number of ways.

In January 2006, Medicare Part D—the prescription drug benefits policy—became effective. Public health professionals need to continue to assist many vulnerable persons to understand the value of enrolling in Part D, to educate them on how to use the benefits, and to ensure that the populations who are "dually" enrolled in both Medicare and Medicaid are registered. Coordinating efforts between civic, religious, and health care agencies to provide health education is a necessity.

A letter or visit to the district, state, or national office of a legislator to discuss a particular policy or health care issue can be interesting, educational, and effective. Contributions of money, labor, expertise, or influence may also be welcomed by the policy makers involved in setting a course of action to obtain a desired health outcome for an individual, a family, a group, a community, or society (health policy). In addition, one may develop a grassroots network of community and professional friends with a mutual interest in health policy advocacy. The network may be able to promote health policy initiatives for the community. During the Obama presidential campaign, many advocacy networks were established via the Internet and monies were solicited using this process.

Many special-interest groups in health care have the potential, desire, and resources to influence the health policy process. A tremendous advantage that nursing has in advocating for issues and in influencing policy makers is the force of its numbers, since nursing is the largest of the health professions. However, nursing must organize its numbers in such a way that each nurse joins with others to speak with one voice. The greatest effect will be had when all nurses make similar demands for policy outcomes.

During 2002, the nursing profession spoke clearly, distinctly, and together on a serious problem for the health arena and for the profession: the nursing shortage. Health care facilities and employers were having ever-increasing difficulty finding experienced nurses to employ. In addition, the need for RNs was predicted to balloon in the next 20 years because of the aging of the U.S. population, technological advances, and economic factors. Demand for RNs was anticipated to increase by 22% by the year 2008. This increased demand for professional nurses, coupled with the expected retirement of a rapidly aging nursing workforce, placed a tremendous stress on the health care system.

The workforce shortage resulted from a complex set of factors such as fewer young people entering the profession, declining nursing school enrollment, the aging of the current nurse workforce, and uncomfortable working conditions in which nurses felt pressured to "do more with less." On December 4, 2009, the BLS (2009) reported that the health care sector of the economy was continuing to grow, despite significant job losses in nearly all major industries. During the same time period a shortage of registered nurses was projected to spread across the country between 2009 and 2030 (AJMQ, 2012).

The American Association of Colleges of Nursing (AACN) remained concerned about the shortage of RNs and worked with schools, policy makers, other organizations, and the media to bring attention to this health care crisis. AACN worked to enact legislation, identify strategies, and form collaborations to address the nursing shortage (AACN, 2010). However, in June 2011 it was reported that employers and staffing agencies posted more than 121,000 new job ads for Registered Nurses in May, up 46% from May 2010 (AACN, 2014).

Advocacy by expert and committed health professionals can bring about positive change for the profession, the community, and the clients that nurses serve. Keeping up to date on issues within government, professional organizations, law, and public policy is vitally important. Informed activism directed toward a professional role, image, and value for professional nurses, and toward a health care system in the United States that provides high quality and affordable universal access to health care, should be a life-long commitment for all professional nurses.

---

## ⏩ LINKING CONTENT TO PRACTICE

An example of how the policy process works follows, involving a nursing organization and individual members. Whether you are a member of a group as described below, or working on your own to influence health policy, the steps described here apply.

Over a 15-month time frame, the American Nurses Association was involved in advocating for health care reform. During the presidential campaign, candidates were educated about the nursing profession and ANA's *Agenda for Health System Reform*. ANA and its members participated in national media interviews and local media events. The message was that the association and its members believed that health care is a basic right. ANA collaborated with the nursing community to outline the profession's priorities as proposals were developed in Congress. Testimony was given before three key congressional committees. ANA representatives met with White House and congressional health care reform staff, and took part in two presidential press conferences at the White House.

As reported by ANA, thousands of nurses joined ANA's health care reform team, sending letters to representatives of Congress, sharing their stories, and meeting with members of Congress. They also participated in rallies and events.

For more information on ANA's health care reform work, visit http://www.rnaction.org/toolkit.

---

## QSEN FOCUS ON QUALITY AND SAFETY EDUCATION FOR NURSES

- **Targeted competency:** Quality improvement
- **Knowledge:** Describe strategies for learning about the outcomes of care in the public setting
- **Skills:** Seek information about outcomes of care for populations served in care settings
- **Attitudes:** Appreciate that continuous quality improvement is an essential part of the daily work of all professionals

**QI Question**

The Quad Council competency of policy development and program planning skills indicates that the beginning PHN collects information that will inform policy decisions. Also the PHN describes the legislative policy development process and identifies outcomes of current health policy relevant to PHN practice. The 2014 outbreak of the Ebola virus in the United States brought quick recognition that there was a need for improvement in policies related to infectious disease control. What were the indicators that the infection control policies in place were not sufficient to prevent the spread of disease? Describe the CQI data collection processes that determined the need for policy change. What role did nurses and organized nursing play in improving the infection control policy and guidelines nationally? What has been the outcome of the new policy and how were populations affected both locally and nationally?

## PRACTICE APPLICATION

Larry was in his final rotation in the Bachelor of Science in nursing program at State University. He was anxious to complete his final nursing course, because upon graduation he would begin a position as a staff nurse specializing in school health at the local health department. His wife was expecting their first child, and she had been receiving prenatal care at the health department.

Larry was aware that a few years ago the federal government had, by law, provided block grants to states for primary care, maternal–child health programs, and other health care needs of states. He had read the *Federal Register* and knew that the regulations for these grants had been written through USDHHS departments. He was aware that these regulations did not require states to fund specific programs.

Larry read in the local newspaper that the health department was closing its prenatal clinic at the end of the month. When his state had received its block grant, it decided to spend the money for programs other than prenatal care. Larry found that a 3-year study in his own state showed improved pregnancy outcomes as a result of prenatal care. The results were further improved when the care was delivered by population-centered nurses. After Larry's daughter was born, he read in the *Federal Register* that states could apply for federal stimulus funds and receive a grant for home visiting services to support mothers and new babies.

Larry was concerned that, as a student, he would have little influence on how such grant dollars would be spent. However, he decided to call his classmates together to plan a course of action.

What would such an action plan include?

Answers can be found on the Evolve site.

## KEY POINTS

- The legal basis for most congressional action in health care can be found in Article I, Section 8, of the U.S. Constitution.
- The five major health care functions of the federal government are direct service, financing, information, policy setting, and public protection.
- The goal of the World Health Organization is the attainment by all people of the highest possible level of health.
- Many federal agencies are involved in government health care functions. The agency most directly involved with the health and welfare of Americans is the U.S. Department of Health and Human Services (USDHHS).
- Most state and local governments have activities that affect nursing practice.
- The variety and range of functions of governmental agencies have had a major impact on nursing. Funding, in particular, has shaped the role and tasks of nurses.
- The private sector (of which nurses are a part) can influence legislation in many ways, especially through the process of writing regulations.
- The number and types of laws influencing health care are increasing. Because of this, involvement in the political process is important to nurses.
- Professional negligence and the scope of practice are two legal aspects particularly relevant to nursing practice.
- Nurses must consider the legal implications of their own practice in each clinical encounter.
- The federal and most state governments are composed of three branches: the executive, the legislative, and the judicial.

- Each branch of government plays a significant role in health policy.
- The U.S. Public Health Service was created in 1798.
- The first national health insurance legislation was challenged in the Supreme Court in 1937.
- *Health: United States* (NCHS, 2013) is an important source of data about the nation's health care problems.
- In 1921 the Sheppard-Towner Act was passed, and it had an important influence on child health programs and population-centered nursing practice.
- The Division of Nursing, the National Institute of Nursing Research, and the Agency for Healthcare Policy and Research are governmental agencies important to nursing.
- Nurses, through state and local health departments, function as consultants, policy advocates, population level and direct care providers, researchers, teachers, supervisors, and program managers.
- The state governments are responsible for regulating nursing practice within the state.
- Federal and state social welfare programs have been developed to provide monetary benefits to the poor, older adults, the disabled, and the unemployed.
- Social welfare programs affect nursing practice. These programs improve the quality of life for special populations, thus making the nurse's job easier in assisting the client with health needs.
- The nurse's scope of practice is defined by legislation and by standards of practice within a specialty.

## CLINICAL DECISION—MAKING ACTIVITIES

1. Conduct an interview with a local health officer. Ask for information from a 10-year period. Try to see trends in population size, health needs and corresponding roles, and activities of government that were implemented to meet these changes. What were some of the problems you identified?

2. Examine a current health department budget and compare it with a budget from previous years. Has there been any impact on health care because of changes in government spending (especially before and after the passing of the Patient Protection and Affordable Care Act)? Give an example.

3. Locate your state register or other documents, such as newspapers, that publish proposed regulations. Select one set of proposed regulations and critique them. Submit your opinion in writing as public comment, or attend the hearing and testify on the regulations. Be sure to submit something in writing. Evaluate your participation by stating what you learned and whether the proposed regulations were changed in your favor.

4. Find and review your state nurse practice act and define your scope of practice. Give examples of your practice boundaries.

5. Contact your local public health agency to discuss the state's official powers in regulating epidemics, such as the measles outbreak in Orange County, California, (HCA, 2014) and anthrax exposures related to bioterrorism.

6. Explore the state's right to protect the health, safety, and welfare of its citizens.

7. Ask about the conflict between the state's rights and individual rights and how such issues are resolved.

8. Ask about the standards of care that apply to this issue and how it is decided which services offered to clients should be mandatory and which should be voluntary.

9. Explore how the role of public health differs in these epidemics compared with the past epidemics of smallpox and tuberculosis. Be specific.

## REFERENCES

Agency for Healthcare Research and Quality: *At a Glance*. Bethesda, MD, 2014a, USDHHS. Accessed at: www.AHRQ.gov. on 8/15/2012.

Agency for Healthcare Research and Quality: *Clinical Practice Guidelines*. Bethesda, MD, 2014b, USDHHS. Accessed at: www.AHRQ.gov. on 9/15/2014.

Agency for Healthcare Research and Quality: *Practice Based Research Network*. Bethesda, MD, 2014c, USDHHS. Accessed at: www.AHRQ.gov. on 9/15/2014.

American Association of Colleges of Nursing: *Fact Sheet on the Nursing Shortage*. Washington, DC, May 2010, AACN.

American Association of Colleges of Nursing: *About AACN: Mission and Strategic Plan*. Washington, DC, May 2014, AACN.

American Journal of Medical Quality: United States Registered Nurse Workforce Report Card and Shortage Forecast. January 2012.

American Nurses Association: *Press Release, ANA Applauds Introduction of Patient Safety Act of 1997*. March 1997. Available at: http://www.nursingworld.org. Accessed December 10, 2010.

Birkland T: *An Introduction to the Policy Process*, ed 3. Armonk, NY, 2010, M.E. Sharpe.

Bureau of Federal Prisons: Weekly population report. 2014. Available at: http://www.bop.gov. Accessed 9/15/2014.

Catholic University of America: Definitions of law. 2010. Available at: http://www.faculty.cua.edu. Accessed August 2010.

Centers for Disease Control and Prevention: *Public Health Policy, United States*. Atlanta, 2014a, USDHHS. Accessed at: www.cdc.gov. on 9/16/2014.

Centers for Disease Control and Prevention: *Epidemiology of Escherichia Coli and Multistate Outbreak, United States*. Atlanta, 2014b, USDHHS. Accessed at: www.cdc.gov. on 9/16/2014.

Centers for Disease Control and Prevention: *Ebola Outbreak*. Atlanta, 2014c. Accessed at: www.cdc.gov. on 9/16/2014.

Centers for Medicare and Medicaid Services. Washington, DC, 2014. Accessed at: www.CMS.gov. on 9/15/2014.

Cherry B, Jacobs SR: *Contemporary Nursing Issues, Trends and Management*, ed 6. St Louis, 2013, Elsevier.

Debate.Org: Is government intervention ruining health care in America. 2013. Accessed at: www.debate.org. on 9/15/2014.

Department of Health, Education and Welfare: Improving Health. *Healthy People: The Surgeon General's Report on Health Promotion and Disease Prevention, DHEW Publication No. 79-55-71*. Washington, DC, 1979, U.S. Government Printing Office. http://www.census.gov/statab/. Accessed July 2002.

HCA: Measles Outbreak Orange County California. May 2014. Accessed at: OC.gov. on 9/16/2014.

Health Resources and Services Administration: *Open

*Opportunities*. Rockville, MD, 2010, USDHHS. www.hrsa.gov. Accessed December 11, 2010.

Kaiser Family Foundation: *Fastfacts*. Menlo Park, CA, 2010A, Kaiser.

Kaiser Family Foundation: *Summary of New Health Reform Law*, PowerPoint "New Insurance Market Rules. Menlo Park, CA, June 2010B, Kaiser. www.healthreform.kff.org.

Katz R, Macintyre A, Barbera J: Emergency public health. In Pines JM, Abualenain J, Scott J, et al, editors: *Emergency Care and the Public's Health*. Hoboken, NJ, 2014, John Wiley and Sons, Ltd.

Lee LM, Heilig CM, White A: Ethical justification for conducting public health surveillance without patient consent. *Am J Public Health* 102(1):38–44, 2012.

Legal Information Institute: Police power of governments. Ithaca, NY, Cornell University. Accessed at: www.law.cornell.edu. on 9/15/2014.

Mason DJ, Leavitt JK, Chaffee MW: *Policy and Politics in Nursing and Health Care*, ed 6. St Louis, 2011, Elsevier.

Morhard R, Franco C: The Pandemic and All-Hazards Preparedness Act: Its contributions and new potential to increase public health preparedness. *Biosecur Bioterror* 11(2):145–152, 2013. Available at: http://online.liebertpub.com/doi/pdf/10.1089/bsp.2013.0042. Accessed May 7, 2014.

National Center for Health Statistics: *Health: United States, 2013*.

Hyattsville, MD, 2014, U.S. Government Printing Office.

National Council of State Boards of Nursing: Map of NLC states. 2014. https://www.ncsbn.org. Accessed on 9/15/2014.

National Institutes of Health: *Structure and Goals*. Bethesda, MD, 2010a, USDHHS.

National Institutes of Health: *Smallpox Vaccines*. Bethesda, MD, July 2, 2010b, USDHHS.

National Institute of Nursing Research: *National Institutes of Health: Mission and Strategic Plan*. Bethesda, MD, 2011, USDHHS.

National Institute of Nursing Research: *National Institutes of Health: Funding Opportunities*. Bethesda, MD, 2014, USDHHS.

Nursing World, Legislative Branch: State government relations: advanced practice recognition with Medicaid reimbursement. 2000. Available at: http://www.nursingworld.org. Accessed December 10, 2010.

Occupational Safety and Health Administration: *Clarification of the Use and Selection of Blood Bourne Pathogen Safety Devices*. Washington, DC, May 5, 2008, U.S. Department of Labor.

Occupational Safety and Health Administration: *OSHA fact sheet*: OSHA's bloodborne pathogen standard. 2011. Available at: https://www.osha.gov/OshDoc/data_BloodborneFacts/bbfact01.pdf. Accessed May 7, 2014.

Occupational Safety and Health Administration: Bloodborne pathogens 2013 Update. 2013.

Available at: https://www.uawgmjas.org/j/index.php?option=com_docman&task=doc_view&gid=15. Accessed May 7, 2014.

Public Health Foundation: *Improving Public Health Infrastructure and Performance through Innovative Solutions and Measurable Results.* Washington, DC, 2010, The Foundation.

Swendiman K, Elsea J: *Federal and State Quarantine and Isolation Authority: CRS Report to Congress.* Washington, DC, August 2010, Legislative Attorneys American Law Division.

Truman Library: Branches of Government, Independence Missouri. Accessed at: www.trumanlibrary@wara.gov. on 9/15/2014.

United Nations: *Report of the World Conference of the International Women's Year, Mexico City, June 19 to July 2, Chapter I, Section A.2, Publication No. E.76.IV.1.* New York, 1975, UN.

United Nations: *Report of the World Conference of the United Nations Decade for Women: Equality, Development and Peace, Copenhagen, July 24-30, Chapter I, Section A, Publication No. E.80. IV.3.* New York, 1980, UN.

United Nations: *Report of the World Conference to Review and Appraise Achievements of the United Nations Decade for Women: Equality, Development and Peace, Nairobi, July 15-26.* New York, 1985, UN.

United Nations: *Report of the Fourth World Conference on Women, Beijing, September 4-15, Chapter I, Resolution 1, Annex I, Publication No. E.96.IV.13.* New York, 1995, UN.

United Nations: *Women 2000: Gender Equality, Development and Peace for the 21st Century, Beijing, 23rd session of the United Nations General Assembly.* New York, 2000, UN.

United Nations: *Report of Future World Conferences.* New York, 2014, UN.

U.S. Bureau of Labor Statistics (BLS): *Employment Summary.* Washington, DC, December 4, 2009, U.S. Department of Labor.

U.S. Bureau of Labor Statistics (BLS): *The Importance of Unemployment Benefits.* Washington, DC, August 2010, The U.S. Department of Labor.

U.S. Department of Agriculture: *Food and Nutrition Services: 40 Years 1979-2009.* Washington, DC, 2013, USDA.

U.S. Department of Defense: *TRICARE Management Activity, the Military Health System.* Falls Church, VA, 2014, DOD. www.tricare.com. Accessed on 9/15/2014.

U.S. Department of Health and Human Services: *Healthy People 2000: National Health Promotion and Disease Prevention Objectives.* Washington, DC, 1991, U.S. Government Printing Office. http://www.health.gov/healthypeople.

U.S. Department of Health and Human Services: Leading indicators. In *Healthy People 2010: Understanding and Improving Health*, ed 2. Washington, DC, 2000, U.S. Government Printing Office.

U.S. Department of Health and Human Services: *Healthy People 2020. Proposed Healthy People 2020 Objectives.* Washington, DC, 2010. Available at: http://www.healthypeople.gov/hp2020/

default.asp. Accessed December 10, 2010.

U.S. Department of Health and Human Services: Health Resources and Services Administration (HRSA): *America's Children in Brief: Key National Indicators of Well-Being.* Washington, DC, 2010, Maternal and Child Health Bureau.

U.S. Department of Health and Human Services: *The Division of Nursing's National Advisory Committee on Nursing Education and Practice.* Rockville, MD, 2013a, Division of Nursing.

U.S. Department of Health and Human Services: *Assistant Secretary Nicole Lurie statement on the Pandemic and All Hazards Preparedness Reauthorization Act.* March 13, 2013b, HHS Press Office. Available at: http://www.hhs.gov/news/press/2013pres/03/20130313a.html. Accessed May 7, 2014.

U.S. Department of Health and Human Services, Centers for Medicare and Medicaid Services: Medicare information for advanced practice registered nurses, anesthesiologist assistants, and physician assistants. 2011. ICN 901623. Available at: http://www.cms.gov/Outreach-and-Education/Medicare-Learning-Network-MLN/MLNProducts/downloads/Medicare_Information_for_APNs_and_PAs_Booklet_ICN901623.pdf. Accessed May 8, 2014.

U.S. Law: 49 Stat 622, Title II. 1937a.

U.S. Law: 42 SC 301, *Stewart Machine Co. v. Davis.* 1937b.

U.S. Law (Public Law 107-105): Health Insurance Portability and Accountability Act (HIPAA). 1996.

U.S. Law: 105-33, Title XXL of the Social Security Act, BBA. 1997.

U.S. Law (Title XXI of the Social Security Act, BBA '97): State Child Health Improvement Act (SCHIP). 1997.

U.S. Law: 107-188: Public Health Security and Bioterrorism and Response Act. 2002.

U.S. Law (Public Law 111-148): Patient Protection and Affordable Care Act (PPACA). 2010.

University of Michigan Center of Excellence in Public Health Workforce Studies: *Enumeration and Characteristics of the Public Health Nurse Workforce: Findings of the 2012 Public Health Nurse Workforce Surveys.* Ann Arbor, MI, 2013, University of Michigan.

World Health Assembly: Strengthening nursing and midwifery, 64th session WHA. May 24, 2011. Available at: http://apps.who.int/gb/ebwha/pdf_files/WHA64/A64_R7-en.pdf. Accessed May 6, 2014.

World Health Organization: Health systems financing: the path to universal coverage. The World Health Report. 2010. Available at: http://www.who.org:Accessed. December 10, 2010.

World Health Organization: Health policy defined. Accessed at: www.WHO.org. 9/15, 2014.

World Health Organization: WHO nursing and midwifery progress report: 2008-2012. 2013. Available at: http://www.who.int/hrh/nursing_midwifery/progress_report/en/. Accessed May 6, 2014.

Your Dictionary: Law 2014. Accessed at: www.yourdictionary.com/law. on 9/15/2014.

# PART 3

# Conceptual and Scientific Frameworks Applied to Population-Centered Nursing Practice

In recent years many foundations, organizations and associations have developed important documents that discuss the importance of public health nursing and that define the essential competencies for public health nursing practice. Because of the emerging public health threats in the United States and many other countries it has been important to focus on the essential role of public health nursing in dealing effectively with these threats. Specifically, there has been a reemergence of communicable diseases, and other diseases previously limited in scope have now become more virulent. At the same time, there has been an increased incidence of drug-resistant organisms. Also, environmental hazards that affect the water, land, air, and food that animals and people eat and drink and the locations where people live have increased. As will be discussed in other sections of the book, chronic diseases consume an increasing portion of health care expenditures, and many of these diseases are associated with lifestyle choices.

Many factors influence behavior and subsequently health. Edberg (2015) says that "ecological models integrate the various influences on health behavior, including interpersonal, organizational, community and public policy factors, to name a few" (p.12). Public health nursing incorporates an ecological approach as it responds to the needs of families, communities, and populations. Public health nurses are in an ideal position to identify risk factors as well as protective factors for the populations they serve.

Documents that can guide and assist public health nurses in developing strategies to serve their populations include the "Scope and Standards of Public Health Nursing" revised in 2013 by the American Nurses Association. This document provides a framework for the practice of public health nursing that builds on the current information about the influences on practice and the issues facing public health nurses. Similarly, in 2013, the American Association of Colleges of Nursing developed a supplement to the "Essentials of Baccalaureate Education for Professional Nursing Practice" entitled "Public Health: Recommended Baccalaureate Competencies and Curricular Guidelines for Public Health Nursing." Another useful document that is cited in many chapters in the text is "Core Competences for Public Health Professionals" which was developed by the Council on Linkages Between Academia and Public Health Practice and revised in 2014. In 2011 the Quad Council of Public Health Nursing developed a companion document for the Core Competences for Public Health Professionals that aligns the work of the Council on Linkages directly with public health nursing. Also, the Institute

Edberg M: *Essentials of Health Behavior*, ed 2, Burlington MA, Jones & Bartlett Learning, 2015.

of Medicine developed "For the Public's Health: Investing in a Healthier Future" in 2012 which provides considerable information about population-based prevention efforts designed to improve the health of Americans.

The chapters in Part Three support the tenants of these documents and provide information about how to use conceptual models, epidemiology, genomics, environmental health, infectious and communicable diseases, principles of education, and how evidence helps to organize population-centered nursing practice to meet the core functions of public health. Each chapter provides readers with tools that can be used to influence population-centered nursing practice.

# 9

# Population-Based Public Health Nursing Practice: The Intervention Wheel

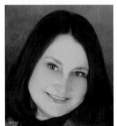

*Linda Olson Keller, DNP, CPH, APHN-BC, RN, FAAN*

Linda Olson Keller is a Clinical Associate Professor at the University of Minnesota School of Nursing. Her research focuses on evidence-based public health nursing practice and the infrastructure of the public health nursing workforce. She spent 20 years of her career in the Office of Public Health Practice at the Minnesota Department of Health. Dr. Olson Keller is certified in Public Health, board certified as an Advanced Public Health Nurse, and is a Fellow of the American Academy of Nursing. She is a frequent national speaker and consultant on public health leadership and practice.

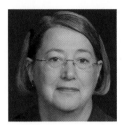

*Sue Strohschein, MS, RN/PHN, APRN, BC*

Sue Strohschein's public health nursing career spans more than 40 years and includes practice in both local and state health departments in Minnesota. She was a generalized public health nurse consultant for the Minnesota Department of Health for 25 years. Since 2008 she has been with the University of Minnesota School of Nursing as a senior research fellow.

## ADDITIONAL RESOURCES

Ⓔ **Evolve Website http://evolve.elsevier.com/Stanhope**
- *Healthy People 2020*
- WebLinks
- Quiz
- Case Studies
- Glossary
- Answers to Practice Application

## OBJECTIVES

*After reading this chapter, the student should be able to do the following:*
1. Identify the components of the Intervention Wheel.
2. Describe the assumptions underlying the Intervention Wheel.
3. Define the wedges and interventions of the Intervention Wheel.
4. Differentiate among three levels of practice (community, systems, and individual/family).
5. Apply the nursing process at three levels of practice.

## KEY TERMS

In these times of change, the public health system is constantly challenged to keep focused on the health of populations. The Intervention Wheel is a conceptual framework that has proved to be a useful model in defining population-based practice and explaining how it contributes to improving population health.

The Intervention Wheel provides a graphic illustration of population-based public health practice (Keller et al, 1998, 2004a,b). It was previously introduced as the Public Health Intervention Model and was known nationally as the "Minnesota Model"; it is now often simply referred to as the "Wheel." The Wheel depicts how public health improves population

health through interventions with communities, the individuals and families that comprise communities, and the systems that impact the health of communities (Figure 9-1). The Wheel was derived from the practice of public health nurses (PHNs) and intended to support their work. It gives PHNs a means to describe the full scope and breadth of their practice.

This chapter applies the Intervention Wheel framework to public health nursing practice. However, it is important to note that other public health members of the interprofessional team such as nutritionists, health educators, planners, physicians, and epidemiologists also use these interventions.

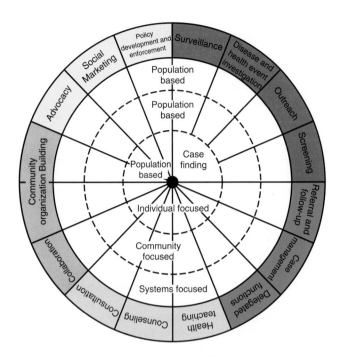

The Intervention Wheel is composed of three distinct elements of equal importance:

- First, the model is population based.

- Second, the model encompasses three levels of practice (community, systems, individual/family).

- Third, the model identifies and defines 17 public health interventions.

Each intervention and level of practice contributes to improving population health.

**FIG 9-1** The Intervention Wheel components. (Used with permission from Keller LO, Strohschein S, Lia-Hoagberg B, et al: Population-based public health interventions: practice-based and evidence-supported, part I. *Public Health Nurs* 21:453–468, 2004.)

## THE INTERVENTION WHEEL ORIGINS AND EVOLUTION

The original version of the Wheel resulted from a grounded theory process carried out by PHN consultants at the Minnesota Department of Health in the mid-1990s. This was a period of relentless change and considerable uncertainty for Minnesota's public health nursing community. Debates about health care reform and its impact on the role of local public health departments created confusion about the contributions of public health nursing to population-level health improvement. In response to the uncertainty, the consultant group presented a series of workshops across the state highlighting the core functions of public health nursing practice (see Chapter 1 for a description of these core functions). A workshop activity required participants to describe the actions they undertook to

carry out their work. The consultant group analyzed 200 practice scenarios developed at the workshops that ranged from home care and school health to home visiting and correctional health. In the final analysis, 17 actions common to the work of PHNs regardless of their practice setting were identified. The analysis also demonstrated that most of these interventions were implemented at three levels: (1) with individuals, either singly or in groups, and with families; (2) with communities as a whole; and (3) with systems that impact the health of communities. A wheel-shaped graphic was developed to illustrate the set of interventions and the levels of practice (see Figure 9-1).

The interventions were subjected to an extensive review of supporting evidence in the literature through a grant from the federal Division of Nursing awarded to the Minnesota Department of Health in the 1990s. In 1999 the PHN consultant group at the Minnesota Department of Health designed and implemented a systematic process identifying more than 600 items from supporting evidence in the literature. These items were rated for their quality and relevancy by a group of graduate nursing students. The resulting subset of 221 items was further analyzed by two expert panels. One panel was composed of public health nursing educators and expert practitioners from five states (Iowa, Minnesota, North Dakota, South Dakota, and Wisconsin). The other panel was a similarly composed national panel. The result was a slightly modified set of 17 interventions. Figure 9-2 graphically illustrates the systematic critique. Each intervention was defined at multiple levels of practice; each was accompanied by a set of basic steps for applying the framework and recommendations for best practices.

Adoption of the model was rapid and worldwide. Since its first publication in 1998, the Intervention Wheel has been incorporated into the public/community health coursework of numerous undergraduate and graduate curricula. The Wheel serves as a model for practice in many state and local health departments and has been presented in Mexico, Norway, Poland, Hungary, Namibia, Kazakhstan, and Japan. It has served as an organizing framework for inquiry for topics ranging from honors theses examining residents' perceptions regarding environmental hazards in their community (Kariuki, 2012) to nursing curriculum reviews (Schoneman et al, 2014) to building breast cancer screening coalitions (Depke and Onitilo, 2011). The Wheel's strength comes from the common language it affords PHNs to discuss their work (Keller et al, 1998).

## ASSUMPTIONS UNDERLYING THE INTERVENTION WHEEL

As with all conceptual frameworks and models, assumptions are made that help to explain the model or framework. The Intervention Wheel framework is based on 10 assumptions.

### Assumption 1: Defining Public Health Nursing Practice

Public health nursing is defined as "the practice of promoting and protecting the health of populations using knowledge from nursing, social, and public health sciences" (APHA, 2013, p. 2).

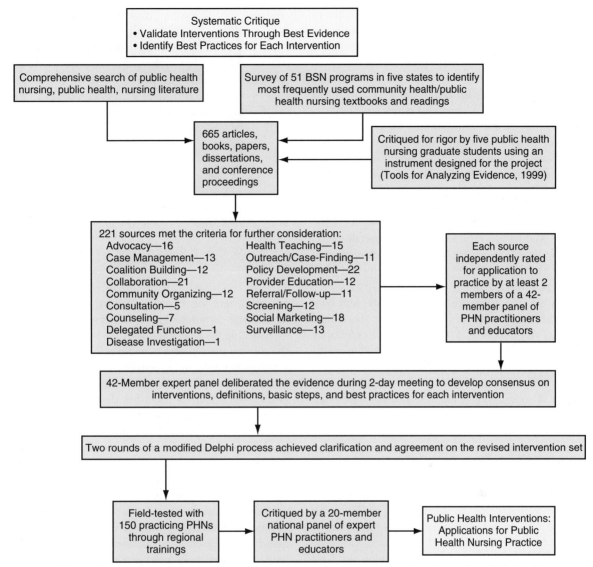

FIG 9-2 Development of a conceptual framework using an evidence-based process. (Used with permission from Keller LO, Strohschein S, Lia-Hoagberg B, et al: Population-based public health interventions: practice-based and evidence-supported, part I. *Public Health Nurs* 21:459, 2004.)

The title "public health nurse" designates a registered nurse with educational preparation in both public health and nursing. The primary focus of **public health nursing** is to promote health and prevent disease for entire population groups. This is done by working with individuals, families, communities, and/or systems.

## Assumption 2: Public Health Nursing Practice Focuses on Populations

The focus on populations as opposed to individuals is a key characteristic that differentiates public health nursing from other areas of nursing practice. A **population** is a collection of individuals who have one or more personal or environmental characteristics in common (Williams and Highriter, 1978). Populations may be understood as two categories. A **population at risk** is a population with a common identified risk factor or risk exposure that poses a threat to health. For example, all

adults who are overweight and hypertensive constitute a population at risk for cardiovascular disease. All under-immunized or un-immunized children are a population at risk for contracting vaccine-preventable diseases. A **population of interest** is a population that is essentially healthy but that could improve factors that promote or protect health. For instance, healthy adolescents are a population of interest that could benefit from social competency training. All first-time parents of newborns are a population of interest that could benefit from a public health nursing home visit. Populations are not limited to only individuals who seek services or individuals who are poor or otherwise vulnerable.

## Assumption 3: Public Health Nursing Practice Considers the Determinants of Health

Health inequities are defined as health status inequalities that society deems to be avoidable or unnecessary (Bleich, Jarlenski,

Bell, and LaVeist, 2012). Significant health disparities related to race, gender, age, and socioeconomic status exist within the United States. The CDC's (2013) *Health Disparities and Inequalities Report—United States, 2013* provides the following examples:

- In 2008, the U.S. rate of infant deaths per 1000 live births was 6.61 for all races; across races and ethnicities the rates varied. For infants born to white women the rate was 5.52; for black and African American women, 12.67; for Asian or Pacific Islander women, 4.51; for American Indian or Alaskan Native women, 8.42, for Hispanic women, 5.59 (Table 1, pp 172).
- Infant mortality rates also differed based on the geographic location of the mother. The rates were generally higher in the Southern and Midwestern regions. The infant mortality rates were highest in DC (11.97 per 1000 live birth) and Mississippi (10.16 per live birth) and lowest in Massachusetts and Utah (both at 4.94 per 1000 live births) (Table 2, pp 173).
- Disparities in life expectancy exist between gender and race. In 2008, the life expectancy at birth for men in the United States was 75.6 years; yet for U.S. women, the life expectancy at birth was 80.6 (Table 1, p. 89). Furthermore, the life expectancy at birth for black populations in the U.S. was 74.0 years, compared to 78.5 years for white populations (Table 1, p. 89).

What are the factors driving these differences? Factors that influence health status across the life cycle are known as the determinants of health. They include income, education, employment, social support, biology and genetics, physical environment, housing, transportation, and personal health practices.

Resolving health inequities and addressing the determinants of health are key distinguishing characteristics of public health nursing. For example, historically, Lillian Wald's Henry Street Settlement House offered numerous social programs, including drama and theater productions, vocational training for boys and girls, three kindergartens, summer camps for children, two large scholarship funds, study rooms staffed with people to help children with their homework, playgrounds for children, a neighborhood library, and classes in carpentry, sewing, art, diction, music, and dance. The following photo shows the settlement house's backyard playground.

In a recent interpretive qualitative study of PHNs' practice in Nova Scotia, researchers found that PHNs routinely implemented "ecosocial surveillance functions" that focused on monitoring changes in social determinants of health. The researchers observed that PHNs "…monitored both bottom-up changes in individual, family, and community determinants of health, and top-down vertical changes or policy directives in the larger system" (Meagher-Stewart et al, 2009, p 557).

## Assumption 4: Public Health Nursing Practice Is Guided by Priorities Identified Through an Assessment of Community Health

In the context of the Intervention Wheel, a community is defined as "a group of people who share common culture, values and/or interests, based on social identity and/or territory,

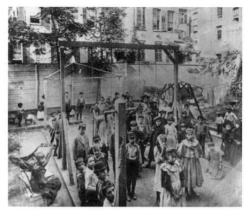

From Jewish Women's Archive: This day in history, March 10, 1893, Resource information for backyard of a Henry Street branch. Available at http://www.jwa.org/archive/jsp/gresInfo.jsp?resID=297. Accessed December 11, 2010.

and who have some means of recognizing, and (inter)acting upon, these commonalities" (Gregory et al, 2009, p. 103).

Assessing the health status of the populations that comprise the community requires ongoing collection and analysis of relevant quantitative and qualitative data. Community assessment includes a comprehensive assessment of the determinants of health. Data analysis identifies deviations from expected or acceptable rates of disease, injury, death, or disability as well as risk and protective factors. Community assessment generally results in a lengthy list of community problems and issues. However, communities rarely possess sufficient resources to address the entire list. This gap between needs and resources necessitates a systematic priority-setting process. Although data analysis provides direction for priority setting, the community's beliefs, attitudes, and opinions as well as the community's readiness for change must be assessed (Keller et al, 2002). PHNs, with their extensive knowledge about the communities in which they work, provide important information and insights during the priority-setting process.

## Assumption 5: Public Health Nursing Practice Emphasizes Prevention

Prevention is "anticipatory action taken to prevent the occurrence of an event or to minimize its effect after it has occurred" (Turnock, 2011). Prevention is customarily described as a continuum moving from primary to tertiary prevention (Leavell and Clark, 1965; Shi and Johnson, 2013; Turnock, 2011). The Levels of Prevention box provides definitions and examples of the levels of prevention.

A hallmark of public health nursing practice is a focus on health promotion and disease prevention, emphasizing primary prevention whenever possible. Although not every event is preventable, every event has a preventable component.

## Assumption 6: Public Health Nurses Intervene at All Levels of Practice

To improve population health, the work of PHNs is often carried out sequentially and/or simultaneously at three levels of prevention (see Figure 9-2).

## LEVELS OF PREVENTION

### Examples of Interventions Applied to Definition of Prevention

#### Primary Prevention

Primary prevention promotes health and protects against threats to health. It keeps problems from occurring in the first place. It promotes resiliency and protective factors or reduces susceptibility and exposure to risk factors. Primary prevention is implemented before a problem develops. It targets essentially well populations. Immunizing against a vaccine-preventable disease is an example of reducing susceptibility; building developmental assets in young persons to promote health is an example of promoting resiliency and protective factors.

#### Secondary Prevention

Secondary prevention detects and treats problems in their early stages. It keeps problems from causing serious or long-term effects or from affecting others. It identifies risk or hazards and modifies, removes, or treats them before a problem becomes more serious. Secondary prevention is implemented after a problem has begun, but before signs and symptoms appear. It targets populations that have risk factors in common. Programs that screen populations for hypertension, obesity, hyperglycemia, hypercholesterolemia, and other chronic disease risk factors are examples of secondary prevention.

#### Tertiary Prevention

Tertiary prevention limits further negative effects from a problem. It keeps existing problems from getting worse. It alleviates the effects of disease and injury and restores individuals to their optimal level of functioning. Tertiary prevention is implemented after a disease or injury has occurred. It targets populations who have experienced disease or injury. Provision of directly observed therapy (DOT) to clients with active tuberculosis to ensure compliance with a medication regimen is an example of tertiary prevention.

Data from Keller LO, Strohschein S, Lia-Hoagberg B, et al: Population-based *public health nursing* interventions: a model from practice. *Public Health Nurs* 15(3):207-15, 1998.

**Community-level practice** changes community norms, community attitudes, community awareness, community practices, and community behaviors. It is directed toward entire populations within the community or occasionally toward populations at risk or populations of interest. An example of community-level practice is a social marketing campaign to promote a community norm that serving alcohol to under-aged youth at high school graduation parties is unacceptable. This is a community-level primary prevention strategy.

**Systems-level practice** changes organizations, policies, laws, and power structures within communities. The focus is on the systems that impact health, not directly on individuals and communities. Conducting compliance checks to ensure that bars and liquor stores do not serve minors or sell to individuals who supply alcohol to minors is an example of a systems-level **secondary prevention** strategy practice.

**Individual-level practice** changes knowledge, attitudes, beliefs, practices, and behaviors of individuals. This practice level is directed at individuals, alone or as part of a family, class, or group. Even though families, classes, and groups are comprised of more than one individual, the focus is still on

individual change. Teaching effective refusal skills to groups of adolescents is an example of individual secondary prevention strategy level of practice.

## Assumption 7: Public Health Nursing Practice Uses the Nursing Process at All Levels of Practice

Although the components of the nursing process (assessment, diagnosis, planning, implementation, and evaluation) are integral to all nursing practice, PHNs must customize the process to the three levels of practice. Table 9-1 outlines the nursing process at the community, systems, and individual/family levels of practice.

## Assumption 8: Public Health Nursing Practice Uses a Common Set of Interventions Regardless of Practice Setting

**Interventions** are "actions taken on behalf of communities, systems, individuals, and families to improve or protect health status" (ANA, 2010). The Intervention Wheel encompasses 17 interventions: surveillance, disease and other health investigation, outreach, screening, case finding, referral and follow-up, case management, delegated functions, health teaching, consultation, counseling, collaboration, coalition building, community organizing, advocacy, social marketing, and policy development and enforcement.

The interventions are grouped with related interventions; these **wedges** are color coordinated to make them more recognizable (Figure 9-3, *A*). For instance, the five interventions in the *red wedge* are frequently implemented in conjunction with one another. Surveillance is often paired with disease and health event investigation, even though either can be implemented independently. Screening frequently follows either surveillance or disease and health event investigation and is often preceded by outreach activities in order to maximize the number of those at risk who actually get screened. Most often, screening leads to case finding, but this intervention can also be carried out independently.

The green wedge consists of referral and follow-up, case management, and delegated functions—three interventions that, in practice, are often implemented together (Figure 9-3, *B*).

Similarly, health teaching, counseling, and consultation—the blue wedge—are more similar than they are different; health teaching and counseling are especially often paired (Figure 9-3, *C*).

The interventions in the orange wedge—collaboration, coalition building, and community organizing—although distinct, are grouped together because they are all types of collective action and are most often carried out at systems or community levels of practice (Figure 9-3, *D*).

Similarly, advocacy, social marketing, and policy development and enforcement—the yellow wedge—are often interrelated when implemented (Figure 9-3, *E*). In fact, advocacy is often viewed as a precursor to policy development; social marketing is seen by some as a method of carrying out advocacy.

The interventions on the right side of the Wheel (i.e., the red, green, and blue wedges) are most commonly used by PHNs who focus their work more on individuals, families, classes, and

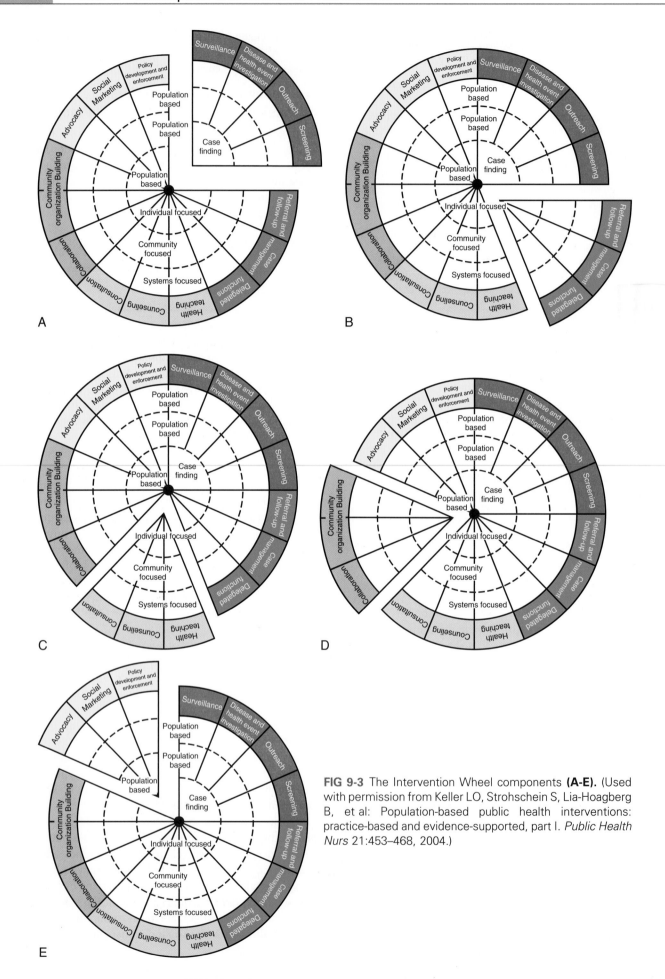

**FIG 9-3** The Intervention Wheel components **(A-E).** (Used with permission from Keller LO, Strohschein S, Lia-Hoagberg B, et al: Population-based public health interventions: practice-based and evidence-supported, part I. *Public Health Nurs* 21:453–468, 2004.)

## TABLE 9-1    Public Health Nursing Process

| Public Health Nursing Process | Systems Level | Community Level | Individual/Family Level |
|---|---|---|---|
| Recruit additional partners. | Recruit additional partners (local, regional, state, national) from systems that are key to impacting and/or who have an interest in the health issue/problem. | Recruit community organizations, services, and citizens who are part of the community intervention that have an interest in this health issue/problem. | |
| Identify population of interest. | Identify those systems for which change is desired. | Identify the population of interest at risk for the problem. | Identify new and current clients in caseload who are at risk for the priority problem. |
| Establish relationship. | Begin/continue establishing relationship with system partners. | Begin/continue establishing relationship with community partners and population of interest. | Begin/continue establishing relationship with the family. |
| Assess priority. | Assess the impact and interrelationships of the various systems on the development and extent of the health issue/problem. | Assess the health issue/problem (demographics, health determinants, past and current efforts). Identify the particular strengths, health risks, and health influences of the population of interest | Identify the particular strengths, health risks, social supports, and other factors influencing the health of the family and each family member. |
| Elicit perceptions. | Develop a common consensus among system partners of the health issue/problem and the desired changes. | Elicit the population of interest's perception of their strengths, problems, and health influences. | Elicit family's perception of their strengths, problems, and other factors influencing their health. |
| Set goals. | In conjunction with system partners, develop system goals to be achieved. | In conjunction with the population of interest, negotiate and come to agreement on community-focused goals. | In conjunction with the family, negotiate and come to agreement on meaningful, achievable, measurable goals. |
| Select health status indicators. | Based on systems goals, select meaningful, measurable health status indicators that will be used to measure success. | Based on the refined community goal/problem, select meaningful, measurable health status indicators that will be used to measure success. | Select meaningful, measurable health status indicators that will be used to measure success. |
| Select interventions. | Select system-level interventions considering evidence of effectiveness, political support, acceptability to community, cost-effectiveness, legality, ethics, greatest potential for successful outcome, nonduplicative, levels of prevention. | Select community-level interventions considering evidence of effectiveness, acceptability to community, cost-effectiveness, legality, ethics, nonduplicative, greatest potential for successful outcome. | Select interventions considering evidence of effectiveness, acceptability to family, cost-effectiveness, legality, ethics, greatest potential for successful outcome. |
| Select intermediate outcome indicators. | Determine measurable, meaningful intermediate outcome indicators. | Determine measurable and meaningful intermediate outcome indicators. | Determine measurable, meaningful intermediate outcome indicators. |
| Determine strategy frequency and intensity. | Using best practices, determine intensity, sequencing, frequency of interventions considering urgency, political will, resources. | Using best practices, determine intensity, sequencing, frequency of interventions. | Using best practices, determine intensity, sequencing, frequency of interventions. |
| Determine evaluation methods. | Determine evaluation methods for measuring process, intermediate, and outcome indicators. | Determine evaluation methods for measuring process, intermediate, and outcome indicators. | Determine evaluation methods for measuring process, intermediate, and outcome indicators. |
| Implement the interventions. | Implement the interventions. | Implement the interventions. | Implement the interventions. |
| Regularly reassess interventions. | Regularly reassess the system's response to the interventions and modify plan as indicated. | Reassess the population of interest's response to the interventions on an ongoing basis and modify plan as indicated. | Reassess and modify plan at each contact as necessary. |
| Adjust interventions. | Adjust the frequency and intensity of the interventions according to the needs and resources of the community. | Adjust the frequency and intensity of the interventions accordingly. | Adjust the frequency and intensity of the interventions according to the needs and resources of the family. |
| Provide feedback. | Provide feedback to system's representatives. | Provide feedback to the population of interest and informal and formal organizational representatives. | Provide regular feedback to family on progress (or lack thereof) of client goals. |
| Collect evaluation. | Regularly and systematically collect evaluation information. | Regularly and systematically collect evaluation information. | Regularly and systematically collect evaluation information. |
| Compare results to plan. | Compare actual results with planned indicators. | Compare actual results with planned indicators. | Compare actual results with planned indicators. |

*Continued*

| TABLE 9-1 | Public Health Nursing Process—cont'd | | |
|---|---|---|---|
| **Public Health Nursing Process** | **Systems Level** | **Community Level** | **Individual/Family Level** |
| Identify differences. | Identify and analyze differences in those systems that achieved outcomes compared with those that did not. | Identify and analyze differences in those in the population of interest who achieved outcomes compared with those who did not. | Identify and analyze differences in services received by families who achieved outcomes compared with those who did not. |
| Apply results to practice. | Apply results to identify needed systems changes. Depending on readiness of the system to accept the results, present results to decision makers and the general population. | Apply results to modify community interventions. Present results to community for policy considerations as appropriate. | Report results to supervisor and other service providers as appropriate. Apply results to personal practice and agency for policy considerations as appropriate. |

groups and to a lesser extent on work with systems and communities. The orange and yellow wedges, on the other hand, are more commonly used by PHNs who focus their work on effecting systems and communities. However, a PHN may use any or all of the interventions. No single PHN is expected to perform every intervention at all three levels of practice. From a management perspective, however, it is useful to ensure that a public health workforce has the capacity to implement all 17 interventions at all three practice levels.

## Assumption 9: Public Health Nursing Practice Contributes to the Achievement of the 10 Essential Services

Implementing the interventions ultimately contributes to the achievement of the 10 essential public health services (see Chapter 1). The 10 essential public health services describe *what* the public health system does to protect and promote the health of the public. Interventions are the means through which public health practitioners implement the 10 essential services. Interventions are the *how* of public health practice (Public Health Functions Steering Committee, 1995).

## Assumption 10: Public Health Nursing Practice Is Grounded in a Set of Values and Beliefs

The Cornerstones of Public Health Nursing (Box 9-1) were developed as a companion document to the Intervention Wheel. The Wheel defines the "what and how" of public health nursing practice; the Cornerstones define the "why." The Cornerstones synthesize foundational values and beliefs from both public health and nursing. They inspire, guide, direct, and challenge public health nursing practice (Keller, Strohschein, and Schaffer, 2010).

## USING THE INTERVENTION WHEEL IN PUBLIC HEALTH NURSING PRACTICE

The Wheel is a conceptual model. It was conceived as a common language or catalog of general actions used by PHNs across all practice settings. When those actions are placed within the context of a set of associated assumptions or relations among

---

### BOX 9-1   Cornerstones of Public Health Nursing

**Public Health Nursing Practice**
- Focuses on the health of entire populations
- Reflects community priorities and needs
- Establishes caring relationships with the communities, families, individuals, and systems that comprise the populations PHNs serve
- Is grounded in social justice, compassion, sensitivity to diversity, and respect for the worth of all people, especially the vulnerable
- Encompasses the mental, physical, emotional, social, spiritual, and environmental aspects of health
- Promotes health through strategies driven by epidemiologic evidence
- Collaborates with community resources to achieve those strategies, but can and will work alone if necessary
- Derives its authority for independent action from the Nurse Practice Act

| Cornerstones from Public Health | Cornerstones from Nursing |
|---|---|
| Population-based/focused | Relationship-based |
| Grounded in social justice | Grounded in an ethic of caring |
| Focus on greater good | Sensitivity to diversity |
| Focus on health promotion and disease prevention | Holistic focus |
| Does what others cannot or will not | Respect for the worth of all |
| Driven by the science of epidemiology | Independent practice |
| Organizes community resources | Long-term commitment to the community |

---

concepts, the Intervention Wheel serves as a conceptual model for public health nursing practice (Fawcett and DeSanto-Madeya, 2013). It creates a structure for identifying and documenting interventions performed by PHNs and captures the nature of their work. The Intervention Wheel provides a framework, a way of thinking about public health nursing practice. The *Public Health Nursing: Scope and Standards of Practice* includes the Intervention Wheel as one of several public health nursing frameworks used in practice today (ANA, 2013).

## COMPONENTS OF THE MODEL

As depicted in Figure 9-1, the model has three components: a population basis, three levels of practice, and 17 interventions.

## Component 1: The Model Is Population Based

The upper portion of the Intervention Wheel clearly illustrates that all levels of practice (community, systems, and individual/family) are population based. Public health nursing practice is population focused. It identifies populations of interest or populations at risk through an assessment of community health status and an assignment of priorities. Services to individuals and families are population based only if they meet the following criteria: (1) Individuals receive services because they are members of an identified population, and (2) services to individuals clearly contribute to improving the overall health status of the identified population.

The population of Sherburne County (Minnesota) increased almost 175% in 25 years (Minnesota Departments of Education, Health, Human Services, and Public Safety, 2013). The numerous new housing developments characterized urban sprawl, which has been implicated in the current obesity epidemic in both children and adults (Ferdinand et al, 2012; Renalds, Smith, and Hale, 2010). The local health department staff was concerned about the prevalence of obesity in its population. Data from the U.S. Department of Agriculture's Food Environment Atlas website showed that 25.7% of the population's adults were considered obese in 2012 (USDA, 2014).

A 2013 state student health survey documented that 16% of ninth-grade girls and 26% of ninth-grade boys in the county were overweight or obese. In this same age group, 26% of girls and 21% of boys reported they had been active less than 60 minutes daily for two days or less of the previous seven days. It was clear that Sherburne County had an obesity problem (Minnesota Departments of Education, Health, Human Services, and Public Safety, 2013).

Reversing this trend required reducing barriers to exercise. Health department staff recognized the impact of urban sprawl on their built environment (Renalds, Smith, and Hale, 2010), or the "collective availability of sidewalks, parks, trails, recreational facilities, traffic safety, and other neighborhood characteristics that promote recreational physical activity as well as active transport to work, school, or errands" (Ferdinand et al, 2012).

One of the first factors they considered was the walkability of their communities, or the extent to which planned transportation networks and public spaces accommodate walking and other forms of physical exercise. Walkability includes: (1) continuous and well-maintained sidewalks, (2) easy access, path directness, and street network connectivity, (3) crossing safety, (4) absence of heavy and high-speed traffic, (5) pedestrian buffering from traffic, (6) land-use density and diversity, (7) street trees and landscaping, (8) visual interest and sense of place, and (9) security (Lo, 2009; Walkability Checklist).

With these data, the public health staff engaged community members to determine the next steps to improve their community walkability. The department asked undergraduate nursing students who were in their public health nursing clinical program to design, implement, and evaluate a walkability project. The students walked over 100 miles and rated the walkability of three different Sherburne County communities. The students analyzed the results and presented recommendations for improvements to the city councils of the three communities. The findings were used by two of the three communities to secure funding for improvements to their community's walkability (Zoller, 2010).

## Component 2: The Model Encompasses Three Levels of Practice

Public health nursing practice intervenes with communities, the individuals and families that comprise communities, and the systems that impact the health of communities. Interventions at each level of practice contribute to the overall goal of improving population health. The work of PHNs is accomplished at all levels. No one level of practice is more important than another; in fact, many public health priorities are addressed simultaneously at all three levels.

One public health priority that almost every PHN will encounter is the potential for the occurrence of vaccine-preventable disease because of delayed or missing immunizations. A recent task analysis of 60 PHNs from 29 states revealed that 93% of all PHNs participated in immunization activities (Keller, 2008). This held true regardless of the PHN's work setting (e.g., home, clinic, school, correctional facility, childcare center) or the population focus (e.g., maternal–child health, elderly chronic disease management, refugee health, disease prevention and control).

Vaccine-preventable diseases, or diseases that may be prevented through recommended immunizations, include diphtheria, pertussis, tetanus, polio, mumps, measles, rubella, hepatitis A, hepatitis B, varicella, meningitis, *Haemophilus influenzae* type b (Hib), pneumococcal pneumonia, rotavirus, human papillomavirus (HPV), herpes zoster, and seasonal influenza (CDC, 2012).

This section illustrates strategies for reducing the occurrence of vaccine-preventable diseases at all three levels of practice. These are only selected examples of strategies to improve immunization rates; it is not an inclusive list.

### Community Level of Practice

The goal of community-level practice is to increase the knowledge and attitude of the entire community about the importance of immunization and the consequences of not being immunized. These strategies will lead to an increase in the percentage of people who obtain recommended immunizations for themselves and their children.

At the community level, PHNs work with health educators on public awareness campaigns. They perform outreach at schools, senior centers, county fairs, community festivals, and neighborhood laundromats.

PHNs conduct or coordinate audits of immunization records of all children in schools and childcare centers to identify children who are under-immunized. The PHNs refer them to their medical providers or administer the immunizations through health department clinics.

When a confirmed case of a vaccine-preventable disease occurs, PHNs work with epidemiologists to identify and locate everyone exposed to the index case. PHNs assess the immunization status of people who were exposed and ensure appropriate treatment.

In the event of an outbreak in the community, all PHNs have a role and ethical responsibility to take part in mass dispensing clinics. Mass dispensing clinics disperse immunizations or medications to specific populations at risk. For example, clinics may be held in response to an epidemic of mumps, a case of hepatitis A attributable to a foodborne exposure in a restaurant, or an influenza pandemic in the general population.

### Systems Level of Practice

The goal of systems-level practice is to change the laws, policies, and practices that influence immunization rates, such as promoting population-based immunization registries and improving clinic and provider practices.

PHNs work with schools, clinics, health plans, and parents to develop population-based immunization registries. Registries, known officially by the Centers for Disease Control and Prevention (CDC) as "Immunization Information Systems," combine immunization information from different sources into a single electronic record. A registry provides official immunization records for schools, daycare centers, health departments, and clinics. Registries track immunizations and remind families when an immunization is due or has been missed.

PHNs conduct audits of records in clinics that participate in the federal vaccine program. PHNs ascertain if a clinic is following recommended immunization standards for vaccine handling and storage, documentation, and adherence to best practices. PHNs also provide feedback and guidance to clinicians and office staff for quality improvement.

PHNs also work with health care providers in the community to ensure that providers accurately report vaccine-preventable diseases as legally required by state statute.

### Individual/Family Level of Practice

The goal of individual/family-level strategies is to identify individuals who are not appropriately immunized, identify the barriers to immunization, and ensure that the individual's immunizations are brought up to date.

At the individual level of practice, PHNs conduct health department immunization clinics. Unlike mass dispensing clinics, immunization clinics are generally available to anyone who needs an immunization and do not target a specific population. These clinics often provide an important service to individuals without access to affordable health care.

PHNs use the registry to identify children with delayed or missing immunizations. They contact families by phone or through a home visit. The PHNs assess for barriers and consult with the family to develop a plan to obtain immunizations either through a medical clinic or from a health department clinic. The PHN follows up at a later date to ensure that the child was actually immunized.

PHNs routinely assess the immunization status for clients in all public health programs, such as well-child clinics, family planning clinics, maternal–child health home visits, or case management of elderly and disabled populations, and they ensure that immunizations are up to date.

---

**BOX 9-2** **Screening**

A school nurse was approached by the school's health and physical education staff who expressed interest in implementing a BMI screening program for children in 4th through 8th grades. Their plan was to do height, weight, and BMI measurements during gym class and requested that the school nurse do the follow-up with the parents of children found to be overweight or obese and encourage that these children be seen by their family health care provider. Although aware that prevalence of obesity in that age group was growing, she was also aware that most local health care providers believed that "chunkiness" in the middle years was a natural occurrence for children. She was also aware that a cardinal rule of screening is that it is unethical to screen if effective treatment and other resources for follow-up do not exist.

In 2008 the U.S. Task Force on Community Preventive Services found insufficient evidence to recommend school-based programs to prevent or reduce obesity. In addition, the American Academy of Pediatrics expressed caution to schools when considering implementing such a program (AAP, 2010). Based on this knowledge, the school nurse suggested to the health and physical education staff that together they find other means of addressing the issue.

---

## Component 3: The Model Identifies and Defines 17 Public Health Interventions

The Intervention Wheel encompasses 17 interventions: surveillance, disease and other health investigation, outreach, screening, case finding, referral and follow-up, case management, delegated functions, health teaching, consultation, counseling, collaboration, coalition building, community organizing, advocacy, social marketing, and policy development and enforcement.

All interventions, except case finding, coalition building, and community organizing, are applicable at all three levels of practice. Community organizing and coalition building cannot occur at the individual level. Case finding is the individual level of surveillance, disease and other health event investigation, outreach, and screening. Altogether, a PHN selects from among 43 different intervention-level actions.

Table 9-2 provides examples of the intervention at the three levels of practice for each of the 17 interventions.

- **Surveillance** describes and monitors health events through ongoing and systematic collection, analysis, and interpretation of health data for the purpose of planning, implementing, and evaluating public health interventions, and disseminating this data to those who need to know to prevent and control outbreaks (adapted from *Morbidity and Mortality Weekly Review*, 2012).
- **Disease and other health event investigation** systematically gathers and analyzes data regarding threats to the health of populations, ascertains the source of the threat, identifies cases and others at risk, and determines control measures.
- **Outreach** locates populations of interest or populations at risk and provides information about the nature of the concern, what can be done about it, and how services can be obtained.
- **Screening** identifies individuals with unrecognized health risk factors or asymptomatic disease conditions in populations (Box 9-2).

*Text continued on p. 206*

## TABLE 9-2 Examples of 17 Interventions at Three Levels of Practice

| Interventions | Systems | Community | Individual |
|---|---|---|---|
| Surveillance | PHNs participated in dead bird reporting (i.e., making "dead bird calls"). People were asked to report the sighting of dead birds to a health department as part of surveillance activities for the West Nile virus. PHNs collected dead birds found in atypical places, such as the middle of a backyard or on a hiking trail. Birds were tested until a positive was found in the county. | PHNs implemented a program that tracked the growth and development of all newborns in the county. Parents were mailed questionnaires at regular intervals that they completed and returned to the public health office. PHNs screened the questionnaires for potential problems or delays and contacted the families by phone or home visits to determine if further action was indicated. | Surveillance at the Individual Level is CASE FINDING (see Case Finding Intervention). |
| Disease and other health event investigation | During a flood, the PHNs spent part of the day doing "rounds" among the rows of people living in a large emergency shelter set up in a gymnasium. The PHNs were concerned about the stresses that this population experienced, so they assessed for withdrawal, depression, and inability to cope. The PHNs observed that the children were not coping well. They questioned parents and heard stories about night terrors and atypical behavior. In response, the PHNs requested child mental health counselors from the Emergency Response Team. They also worked with parents in the shelter to set up a "toddler corner" where children could play and act like children. Parents took turns staffing the corner. | A PHN worked with a Catholic church that served a parish with a rapidly growing Hispanic population to connect mothers and children with community resources. The priest mentioned that he was seeing an unusual number of stillbirths among his parishioners. His comment led the PHN into a series of questions and investigation. The PHN discovered that the church allowed its kitchen facilities to store foods brought from Mexico. Suspecting a possible foodborne contaminant, the PHN took samples to the health department lab for testing. A supply of queso blanco fresco obtained from the church's refrigerator was found to be contaminated with *Listeria*. After an outreach and education campaign within the parish and the community, the rate of stillbirths decreased. | Disease and other health event investigation at the Individual Level is CASE FINDING (see Case Finding Intervention). |
| Outreach | Prior to launching a universally offered home visiting program for newborns, focus group interviews revealed the best strategies to encourage participation were as follows:<br>• Send letters or postcards announcing the program to pregnant women<br>• Make hospital visits to moms after delivery<br>• Include photos of visitors on business cards and brochures<br>• Be recommended by trusted individuals, such as physicians, nurses, and other new mothers<br>• Have program staff visit Lamaze and other childbirth education programs, and early childhood development classes | PHNs were part of a coalition that received a grant to do community education on depression to an elderly Hmong population. Many Hmong elders were isolated but did not view depression as a disease. The PHNs tailored an outreach event to the Hmong population during a community market. Even though the program targeted persons over 50, people were allowed to determine their own eligibility. That is, if they "felt old," they qualified. Second, since it was considered unlikely that the elders would come to the booth, the coalition members talked with elders in more casual settings, approaching elders sitting under shade trees or at their market booth. All the interviews were conducted in the Hmong language. | Outreach at the Individual Level is CASE FINDING (see Case Finding intervention). |

Continued

## TABLE 9-2    Examples of 17 Interventions at Three Levels of Practice—cont'd

| Interventions | Systems | Community | Individual |
|---|---|---|---|
| Screening | Vision screening is a core PHN activity with the school-aged population. PHNs worked with a community group to determine why school children who failed vision screening and were referred did not receive the recommended follow-up. Issues included the expense of eye-care services and glasses, lack of convenient appointment times with eye-care specialists, and whether parents valued eye care. The PHNs participated in a task force that facilitated an agreement among eye-care providers to schedule evening and weekend appointments, arranged support from the Lions International Service Club toward the purchase of eyewear, and communicated the need for follow-up to parents at parent-teacher conferences. | PHNs collaborated with a high school on a prevention program to address physical inactivity and unhealthy dietary behaviors. The PHNs conducted health screenings that gave each student a "snapshot" of his or her health (height, weight, BMI, blood pressure, total cholesterol, HDL). Students received a report of their nutritional and physical activity levels with information about how to begin building lifestyle changes. One hundred ninety-two students from five schools were screened and 71 were referred (37% referral rate). Upon completion of the educational components, students who were rescreened had a total cholesterol decrease of 219 points. | Screening at the Individual Level is CASE FINDING (see Case Finding Intervention). |
| Case finding | Does not apply at this practice level | Does not apply at this practice level | A state's newborn blood screening program detected an infant with a possible case of congenital hypothyroidism. The information was sent to the infant's medical provider, who was expected to contact the family. The mother of the infant was a single Hispanic woman who did not speak English and did not respond to the clinic's numerous calls. The provider referred the situation to a PHN for assistance in locating the mother. After talking with contacts in the Hispanic community, the PHN located friends of the young mother who confirmed she had returned to Mexico with the infant. They did not know how to contact her but agreed to alert those within the Hispanic community of the seriousness of the baby's problem. About 2 months later the mother did return, sought the PHN's assistance, and received care for the baby. |
| Referral and follow-up | PHNs providing health services to inmates in a county jail noticed that individuals with mental health issues, chronic health concerns, chemical dependency issues, or homelessness frequently returned to jail. Few of these issues were typically addressed prior the inmates' release. The PHNs initiated RAPP (Release Advance Planning Program), a voluntary "discharge planning" process through which referrals and other arrangements with community resources could be made prior to the inmates returning to the community. Recidivism rates decreased by 57% by the third year of the program's operation. | PHNs often serve as community resource directories. PHNs are known by community members for their extensive knowledge of whom or where to call for a variety of problems or issues. For example, PHNs in a rural health department responded to calls ranging from rats to cockroaches to bedbugs, from septic tank failures to peeling paint, and from air quality to blue-green algae. The PHNs often followed up with community members to ensure that their issues were resolved. | A PHN received a referral on a mentally ill young man from a small town. He needed regular injections to prevent rehospitalization. When the PHN was unable to locate this client at home, she found him at his regular "hangout"—the local bar—where he drank only soda pop. While creatively maintaining confidentiality, the PHN worked with the bartender in this establishment to set up regular appointment times for the client. |

| | | | |
|---|---|---|---|
| **Case management** | Public health nurses representing 10 county health departments, medical clinics, a large health plan company, and the state health department worked together to provide coordinated prenatal care to improve birth outcomes. The group created an integrated prenatal care system that promoted early prenatal care, improved nutrition, and linked women to services in the communities. | | A local physician reported a highly contagious active infectious tuberculosis (TB) case that was determined to be multidrug resistant. The client did not speak English. The PHN coordinated his care with the physician, the CDC, and a home health department's TB unit, the CDC, and a home health agency. Neither the hospital outpatient department nor any home health agency would agree to treat this client in their facility or make home visits. *(Continued under delegated functions below.)* |
| **Delegated functions** | In a county of 120,000 residents, PHNs from the local health department led a coalition of hospitals, clinics, schools, and emergency managers in designing and implementing a community-wide mass immunization plan to administer influenza vaccine. The design included the establishment of administration protocols approved by the health department's medical advisor. The health department also served as the central distribution point for all vaccines available within the county. | PHNs administered immunizations at "drive-thru" flu clinics held in a county highway garage. Residents received their assessment and flu shots in their vehicles. This unique access increased the numbers of immunizations received by elderly and disabled residents, particularly those with limited mobility. The drive-thru clinic also reduced the exposure potential to infectious diseases that was inherent in regular clinic waiting rooms. | *(See above case management.)* In addition to doing daily direct observed therapy (DOT), the PHN was the only health care provider who would do weekly lab draws, daily IV therapy, and biweekly dressing changes for the first 7 months of treatment. Without PHN involvement, this client would have likely succumbed to TB. The client completed a full 18 months of therapy and recovered. |
| **Health teaching** | PHNs worked with the epidemiologist in their health department to develop "best practice" guidelines for pediculosis (lice) treatment from the perspectives of the scientific literature and the practice community. Recommendations included both suffocating and chemical agents. Clinics, schools, and pharmacists used the new guidelines. The public health department created an internal standardized pediculosis response procedure, and the county's social services department developed a new policy for school truancy issues related to pediculosis. | Several rural counties launched a program to help youth incorporate a healthy diet and exercise into their lives. A health fair was held in conjunction with parent–teacher conferences. Committees composed of youth and adults planned activities such as "Dance 'n' Dips," a dance followed by a dip at the city pool. Members of a church began offering evening exercise classes. A small town sponsored the "Run, Walk 'n Roll" that was open to runners, walkers, strollers, and wheelchairs. The "Toilet Paper" document, a monthly nutrition and health tip sheet designed to resemble toilet paper, was displayed in 152 bathrooms, next to the toilet paper dispensers. The tips were popular; PHNs reported that people came up to them on the street to discuss the tips. PHNs reported seeing changes in community attitudes. | A PHN works with pregnant and parenting teens at an alternative high school program that provides educational options for teens whose lives did not fit the traditional school day. The program included teens from a variety of cultures and backgrounds. The program had an onsite childcare center; students were able to visit their child during the school day. The PHNs taught weekly prenatal classes in conjunction with life skills and child development classes. PHNs also worked with each student to look at family planning options. Their "Pregnancy Free Club" provided each student private time with a PHN to look at barriers that prevented the student from effectively using birth control. The program had a repeat adolescent pregnancy rate significantly lower than the national average, declining from a baseline of 25% to a mean of 4.7% over 9 years of the program. |
| **Counseling** | PHNs partnered with a community family center to promote prenatal attachment for families who were isolated, who had experienced previous pregnancy loss, or who had other attachment issues. The project promoted attachment to the baby through the use of doulas, guided videotaping, nutrition counseling, and relaxation through music and imagery. | In response to multiple deaths within an American Indian community, PHNs in a tribal health department worked with the community to design and implement a culturally appropriate grief and loss program. Interventions included drumming activities for youth, traditional healers, and peer counselors. | A PHN led monthly support groups for family members and volunteers providing in-home care to individuals with Alzheimer's disease. The PHN provided one-to-one caregiver coaching to those needing additional support. |

*Continued*

## TABLE 9-2  Examples of 17 Interventions at Three Levels of Practice—cont'd

| Interventions | Systems | Community | Individual |
|---|---|---|---|
| Consultation | After hearing about the risk for serious infectious disease for children in daycare, PHN daycare consultants from eight local health departments developed a curriculum on handwashing for children. They obtained a grant to develop a video in several languages and widely distributed the handwashing materials. | PHNs providing postpartum home visits to new mothers noted that women employed by a certain large company often gave up breastfeeding upon returning to work. Reasons included lack of private space to express milk and nonsupportive supervisors. The PHNs approached the company's human resources director and presented a business case for breastfeeding. After several meetings the company agreed to revamp its policies on breastfeeding in the workplace and requested PHNs' assistance in providing training. | The older sister of an elderly bachelor farmer died. The sister had kept house and cooked for her brother for their entire adult lives. Upon her death, he was unable to live independently. Neighbors concerned for his well-being convinced him to talk with a PHN/social worker team to explore his preferences and determine the best options for a living situation that respected his need for self-determination. He eventually moved into an assisted living facility that met his needs. |
| Collaboration | PHNs changed the way they had traditionally related to the 26 medical clinics in their community. They visited each clinic quarterly to provide information about change in vaccine policy and improving the reporting of notifiable diseases as required by law. They also answered questions, promoted disease prevention programs, and resolved problems together, such as vaccine shortages. This relationship benefited the public health department and the medical clinics. | Everyone is a bully, is being bullied, or is a bystander. School nurses worked with a community action team to develop community assets—caring, encouraging environment for youth and valuing of youth by adults. Through strategies such as a mentoring program for at-risk elementary school students and a revitalized orientation program for ninth graders entering high school, the incidence of bullying behavior was reduced. | Over a period of years, a PHN was able to establish a trusting relationship with a Haitian client with HIV. Through her transactions with this client, the PHN came to understand her own values differently and honored the client's spiritual values and practices. |
| Coalition building | PHNs were part of a coalition that formed to address the exploding bedbug issue in the community. The coalition was a response to requests from local housing providers for assistance. Coalition members included PHNs along with property owners and managers, commercial pest management operators, university entomologists, and the local housing authority. They provided education about the eradication and prevention of bedbug infestations, cost implications, and potential litigation issues to local apartment managers, fraternity house operators, and housing officials. | A student health survey revealed a greater than expected number of overweight or obese children in a school district. A coalition of school nurses, educators, and health care providers concerned about childhood obesity developed a school-based program for elementary students. As a result of the work of this coalition, parents received a report card about their child's BMI. Parents also received educational materials that offered tips for healthy living and a directory of physical activity options. A follow-up evaluation revealed that parents who received a report card were more likely to have initiated dietary changes or a physical activity plan than parents who had not. | Coalition building is not implemented at the individual level of practice. |
| Community organizing | A local newspaper reported that a statewide student health survey revealed their school district had one of the highest teen alcohol-use rates in the state. Numerous letters to the editors questioned why the community was not doing anything about the problem and demanded community action. In response, a PHN from the public health department partnered with other community groups and organizations to develop a plan to address alcohol use in the community. The plan included enforcing existing laws, such as enforcing "not a drop" laws with minors and developing social media messages for adolescents that emphasized "Not everyone drinks…" | In response to a public safety meeting where 750 angry residents showed up to complain about what they saw as the deterioration of their community, a city health department dispersed a team of PHNs to develop "social capital." The PHNs facilitated the development of social connections, relationships, and trust in a community that had experienced an influx of mainly poor, minority renters. Their goal was to ensure that neighbors know and care about each other enough to run next door to borrow a cup of sugar or offer to help the elderly woman down the block. PHNs helped organize exercise classes, a farmer's market, community gardens, and neighborhood dinners, which were free with the only requirement that diners eat next to somebody they did not know. | Community organizing is not implemented at the individual level of practice. |

| | | | |
|---|---|---|---|
| **Advocacy** | A worker at a large meat packing plant that employed over 1000 people speaking 12 languages was diagnosed with active infectious tuberculosis (TB). Initially the plant managers were more concerned about losing production than being exposed. The PHNs worked with the managers to convince them that exposure to TB was a serious problem and that they could cooperate with public health without decreasing production. Although the managers would not mandate testing, they did allow PHNs to offer free Mantoux tests during work time on all three shifts to any employee who wanted to be tested. Over 700 employees were tested, with over 70 positives. Many of the employees with positive Mantoux tests lacked access to health care. The PHNs negotiated reduced clinic fees and secured community grant funds to pay for x-rays and prescribed treatment for infected persons who were uninsured and without resources. (See individual advocacy example.) | A visiting nurse agency (VNA) served many families with small children living at or below poverty level. Many were homeless, experiencing mental health issues, alcohol or drug abuse, or domestic violence. Club 100 was a voluntary organization of community women and men associated with the VNA. It is a program that reaches out into the community to ask people of means to help care for people who have very little. It paired men and women with VNA nurses and their at-risk family clientele. The volunteers of Club 100 were divided into teams that worked with a PHN. The PHN selected clients who would benefit from the program and presented the client's case to the team on a quarterly basis. The club provided "gifts" such as high chairs, strollers, diapers, books, toys, and tools to support family self-sufficiency and improved the lives of these men, women and children. | A PHN received a referral on a 9-month-old boy with a recent diagnosis of meningitis resulting from active TB. The child's parents were a young Hispanic couple who did not speak English. The child's mother was pregnant and stayed at home with her two small children. The family had no telephone and neither parent had a driver's license. The entire family reacted positively to the Mantoux tests that the PHN administered. At this point, the PHN arranged an appointment at the local clinic for the entire family, complete with transportation and interpreters. The father was found to have active infectious TB. He was ordered not to return to his job at the meat packing plant and consequently lost his health insurance. The PHN assisted the family in applying for medical assistance and other services for which they were eligible. *(The fact that a meat packing plant employee had infectious TB required this PHN to intervene at the systems level——see systems advocacy example.)* |
| **Social marketing** | A partnership of health departments, managed care organizations, pharmaceutical companies, health care insurers, and others sought to decrease unnecessary antimicrobial use and reduce the spread of antimicrobial resistance. "Moxie Cillin" and "Annie Biotic" were mascots that appeared on pamphlets, posters, stickers, and in person. They urged discontinuation of inappropriate requesting of antibiotics by parents and unnecessary prescribing of antibiotics by health care providers. | A PHN working in a small rural county was assigned to work on a Fetal Alcohol Syndrome prevention grant in partnership with the local hospital. The PHN coordinated the grant activities, which included mass media efforts such as billboards, radio spots read by local celebrities, and newspaper articles. Multiple posters were placed in every bar in the community, and local bartenders were engaged as partners in the effort to reduce alcohol use among pregnant women. After 2 years, the project documented an increase in community awareness, which is the first step in changing the community norm regarding alcohol use among pregnant women. | PHNs routinely conducted home safety checks with pregnant and parenting families to prevent childhood injuries. As incentives, they distributed safety kits that included items to child-proof a home, such as cupboard safety locks, outlet covers, door knob safety covers, and drawer latches. While having a PHN checking contents in cupboards and water temperatures may have felt intrusive to some families, the kits increased the number of families who were receptive to home safety checks. |
| **Policy development and enforcement** | Local health department PHNs and health educators partnered with law enforcement to establish ordinances prohibiting the sale of tobacco to under-age youth. Part of the initiative included recruiting and training youth to conduct compliance checks, in which under-age youth attempted to purchase cigarettes in retail stores. PHNs also created an electronic compliance tracking system that was eventually used by the entire state. | A PHN investigated a public health complaint about a fly problem originating from the manure pit of a farm that housed millions of chickens. Garbed in protective equipment, the intrepid PHN crawled under the chicken cages that dumped into the manure pits and found masses of maggots. After determining that the situation constituted a public health nuisance, the PHN successfully worked with the business owners to find a solution that involved the drying of manure to prevent the maggots from surviving. | A PHN received a referral regarding the safety of an 80-year-old woman living alone on a littered farm site. The woman lived with 18 cats in a house without heat that was ankle-deep with cans, clothes, and cat feces. The PHN initiated a vulnerable adult evaluation that resulted in a "not sufficiently vulnerable" finding under state statute. Through repeated contacts, the PHN was able to establish a trusting relationship; the women accepted a referral for care to a physician. However, she was not successful in changing the woman's living situation. |

---

**BOX 9-3   Health Teaching**

- Health teaching communicates facts, ideas, and skills that change knowledge, attitudes, values, beliefs, behaviors, practices, and skills of individuals, families, systems, and/or communities.
- Knowledge is familiarity, awareness, or understanding gained through experience or study.
- Attitude is a relatively constant feeling, predisposition, or set of beliefs directed toward an object, person, or situation, usually in judgment of something as good or bad, positive or negative.
- Value is a core guide to action.
- Belief is a statement or sense, declared or implied, intellectually and/or emotionally accepted as true by a person or group.
- Behavior is an action that has a specific frequency, duration, and purpose, whether conscious or unconscious.
- Practice is the act or process of doing something or the habitual or customary performance of an action.
- Skill is proficiency, facility, or dexterity that is acquired or developed through training or experience.

---

**QSEN  FOCUS ON QUALITY AND SAFETY EDUCATION FOR NURSES**

**Targeted competency:** Client-centered care
**Knowledge:** Integrate understanding of multiple dimensions of client-centered care including communication, information, and education.
**Skills:** Communicate values, preferences, and expressed needs to all members of the team
**Attitudes:** Values seeing health care situation through the client's health
**Question:** The Quad Council competency, community dimensions of practice, supports the application of the Intervention Wheel's PHN intervention of community organizing. The Quad Council suggests beginning PHN's participate effectively in activities that facilitate community involvement.

A statewide behavioral risk survey was conducted by the state health department. The survey shows that in your community there is still a high rate of smoking among the population. What types of activities could be planned to identify common goals among the population and the health care system? How could you participate? What might your role be in resource mobilization and development of strategies to be implemented for reaching goals?

---

- **Case finding** locates individuals and families with identified risk factors and connects them with resources.
- **Referral and follow-up** assists individuals, families, groups, organizations, and/or communities to identify and access necessary resources in order to prevent or resolve problems or concerns.
- **Case management** optimizes self-care capabilities of individuals and families and the capacity of systems and communities to coordinate and provide services.
- **Delegated functions** are direct care tasks a registered professional nurse carries out under the authority of a health care practitioner as allowed by law. Delegated functions also include any direct care tasks a registered professional nurse entrusts to other appropriate personnel to perform.
- **Health teaching** communicates facts, ideas, and skills that change knowledge, attitudes, values, beliefs, behaviors, and practices of individuals, families, systems, and/or communities (Box 9-3).
- **Counseling** establishes an interpersonal relationship with a community, system, family, or individual intended to increase or enhance their capacity for self-care and coping. Counseling engages the community, system, family, or individual at an emotional level.
- **Consultation** seeks information and generates optional solutions to perceived problems or issues through interactive problem solving with a community, system, family, or individual. The community, system, family, or individual selects and acts on the option best meeting the circumstances.
- **Collaboration** commits two or more persons or organizations to achieve a common goal through enhancing the capacity of one or more of the members to promote and protect health (Freshman et al, 2010; Henneman et al, 1995).
- **Coalition building** promotes and develops alliances among organizations or constituencies for a common purpose. It builds linkages, solves problems, and/or enhances local leadership to address health concerns.

- **Community organizing** helps community groups to identify common problems or goals, mobilize resources, and develop and implement strategies for reaching the goals they collectively have set (Bezboruah, 2013; Minkler, 2012).
- **Advocacy** pleads someone's cause or acts on someone's behalf, with a focus on developing the capacity of the community, system, individual, or family to plead their own cause or act on their own behalf.
- **Social marketing** uses commercial marketing principles and technologies for programs designed to influence the knowledge, attitudes, values, beliefs, behaviors, and practices of the population of interest.
- **Policy development** places health issues on decision makers' agendas, acquires a plan of resolution, and determines needed resources. Policy development results in laws, rules, regulations, ordinances, and policies.
- **Policy enforcement** compels others to comply with the laws, rules, regulations, ordinances, and policies created in conjunction with policy development.

In addition to the definition and examples, each intervention has basic steps for implementation at each of the three levels (i.e., community, systems, and individual/family) as well as a listing of best practices for each intervention. The basic steps are intended as a guide for the novice public health nurse or the experienced public health nurse wishing to review his/her effectiveness. Box 9-4 describes the basic steps of the counseling intervention.

The best practices are provided as a resource for PHNs seeking excellence in implementing the interventions. They were constructed by a panel of expert public health nursing educators and practitioners after a thorough analysis of the literature. Many practices of public health nursing are either not researched or, if they are researched, not published. The process used to develop this model considered this limitation and met the challenge with the use of expert practitioners

## BOX 9-4   Basic Steps for the Intervention of Counseling*

Working alone or with others, PHNs:
1. Meet the "client"—the individual, family, system, or community.
2. Establish rapport by listening and attending to what the client is saying and how it is said.[†]
3. Explore the issues.
4. Gain the client's perception of the nature and cause of the identified problem or issue and what needs to change.[‡]
5. Identify priorities.
6. Gain the client's perspective on the urgency or importance of the issues; negotiate the order in which they will be addressed.
7. Establish the emotional context.
8. Explore, with the client, emotional responses to the problem or issue.
9. Identify alternative solutions.
10. Establish, with the client, different ways to achieve the desired outcomes and anticipate what would have to change in order for this to happen.
11. Agree on a contract.
12. Negotiate, with the client, a plan for the nature, frequency, timing, and end point of the interactions.
13. Support the individual, family, system, or community through the change.
14. Provide reinforcement and continuing motivation to complete the change process.
15. Bring closure when the PHN and client mutually agree that the desired outcomes are achieved.

*Complete version available at http://www.health.state.mn.us/divs/cfh/ophp/resources/docs/phinterventionsmanual2001.pdf.
[†]Modified from Burnard P: Counseling: a guide to practice in nursing, Oxford, England, 1992, Butterworth-Heineman.
[‡]Understanding the client's cultural or ethnic context is important to perception. For further information, please see Sue DW: Counseling the Culturally Diverse: Theory and Practice, ed. 6, New Jersey, 2013, Wiley.

## BOX 9-5   Best Practices for the Intervention of Referral and Follow-up

**Best Practice**
Successful implementation is increased when the:
- PHN respects the client's right to refuse a referral.
- PHN develops referrals that are timely, merited, practical, tailored to the client, client controlled, and coordinated.
- Client is an active participant in the process and the PHN involves family members as appropriate.
- PHN establishes a relationship based on trust, respect, caring, and listening.
- PHN allows for client dependency in the client–PHN relationship until the client's self-care capacity sufficiently develops.
- PHN develops comprehensive, seamless, client-sensitive resources that routinely monitor their own systems for barriers.

**Evidence**
McGuire, Eigsti Gerber, Clemen-Stone, 1996 (expert opinion)
Stanhope and Lancaster, 1984 (text)
Will, 1977 (expert opinion)
Wolff, 1962 (expert opinion)

**Expert Panel Recommendation**
McGuire, Eigsti Gerber, Clemen-Stone, 1996 (expert opinion)
Stanhope and Lancaster, 1984 (text)
Will, 1977 (expert opinion)
Wolff, 1962 (expert opinion)

McGuire S, Eigsti Gerber D, Clemen-Stone S: Meeting the diverse needs of clients in the community: effective use of the referral process. *Nursing Outlook* 44(5):218–222, 1996; Stanhope M, Lancaster J: *Community health nursing: process and practice for promoting health.* St Louis, 1984, Mosby, p 357; Will M: Referral: a process, not a form. *Nursing* 77:44–55, 1977; Wolff I: Referral—a process and a skill. *Nurs Outlook* 10(4):253–262, 1962.

and educators. The best practices are a combination of research and other evidence from the literature and/or the collective wisdom of experts. Box 9-5 outlines an example of a set of best practices for the intervention of referral and follow-up, some supported by evidence and others supported by practice expertise.

## ADOPTION OF THE INTERVENTION WHEEL IN PRACTICE, EDUCATION, AND MANAGEMENT

The speed at which the Intervention Wheel was adopted may be attributed to the balance between its practice base and its evidence-based support. The Intervention Wheel has led to numerous innovations in practice and education since it was first published in 1998 (Keller et al, 2004a). Further dissemination of the model has occurred through the hundreds of graduate and undergraduate schools of nursing that use the Intervention Wheel as a framework for teaching public health nursing.

The Intervention Wheel has been widely adopted as a framework for public health nursing practice:
- In 2007, the American Nurses Association officially recognized the Intervention Wheel as a framework in the Public Health Nursing Scope and Standards of Practice (ANA, 2007, 2012).
- The Los Angeles County Department of Health Services used the Intervention Wheel in their initiative to reinvigorate public health nursing practice—orientation, practice standards, documentation, recruitment, and retention—for their 500 public health nurse generalists and specialists (LACDHS, 2002; Avilla and Smith, 2003; Smith and Bazini-Barakat, 2003).
- The Massachusetts Association of Public Health Nurses used the Intervention Wheel as the framework for their state "Leadership Guide and Resource Manual" (Massachusetts Association of Public Health Nurses, 2009).
- PHNs in the Shiprock Service Unit of the Indian Health Service use the Wheel in their practice and adapted it to reflect the Navajo culture. The Navajo Intervention Wheel (Figure 9-4) is presented as a Navajo basket and uses the traditional colors of the Navajo nation.
- From 2001 to 2005, the Intervention Wheel served as the framework for a Division of Nursing grant that successfully brought together education and practice communities to collaboratively redesign the public health nursing student's clinical experience. Several of these collaboratives remain viable and active.

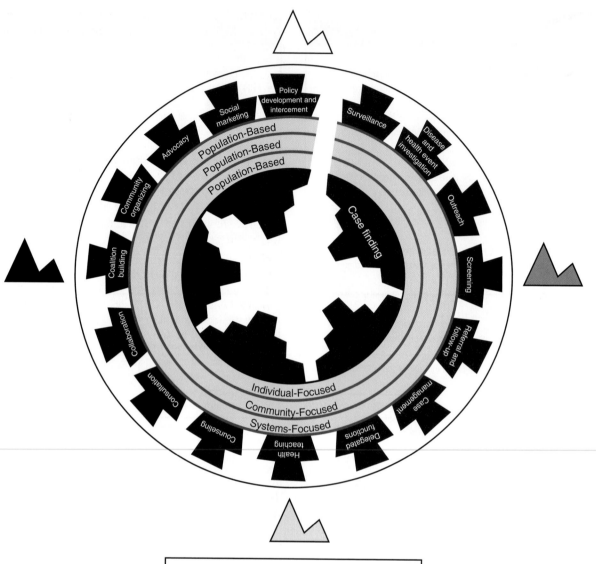

The Navajo basket represents mother earth (the tan area), the black design represents the four sacred mountains that surround the Navajo Nation, and the red area represents the rainbow, which symbolizes harmony. In Navajo philosophy, one should not enclose oneself without an opening. Therefore, the basket has an opening, or doorway, to receive all that is good/positive, and allow all the bad/negative to exit.

Neva Kayaani

**FIG 9-4** Navajo Wheel. (Courtesy Shiprock Service Unit, Shiprock, NM, Indian Health Service.)

- PHN consultants at the Wisconsin Department of Health used the Intervention Wheel to differentiate levels of nursing practice in local health departments related to educational preparation and to outline the role of the associate degree and diploma nurse in public health. (Although the baccalaureate degree is the accepted standard for entry to public health nursing practice, shortages of baccalaureate prepared nurses sometimes result in health departments employing associate degree and diploma nurses.)

- PHNs at the St. Paul-Ramsey County (MN) Department of Health used the Intervention Wheel to illustrate the activities of their refugee health program. Their display (Figure 9-5) identified the most common interventions implemented with the refugee population and illustrated each intervention with a photograph.

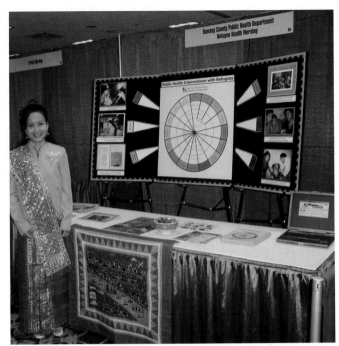

FIG 9-5 St. Paul-Ramsey County Public Health Family Health International Team. (Courtesy Sophia Emang, Public Health Nurse, St. Paul-Ramsey.)

## EVIDENCE-BASED PRACTICE BOX

Nursing informatics is relatively new for many public health departments in the United States. Community health nurses typically use the Omaha System to document their practice; however, this system is used by various disciplines working in public health. The Omaha System taxonomy is the conceptual framework for the Automated Community Health Information System (ACHIS), which is the longstanding electronic data system used to document nursing practice in community nursing centers. However, researchers identified a gap in the Omaha System and ACHIS in that both were better at capturing individual-level interventions than community- and system-level interventions. Therefore, researchers in this study incorporated interventions from the Intervention Wheel into the existing electronic record system in hopes that community- and system-level activities could be documented better. Nine Wheel interventions were added to the ACHIS: "Policy Development," "Social Marketing," "Advocacy," "Community Organizing," "Coalition Building," "Collaboration," "Consultation," "Screening," and "Outreach." The newly expanded system was piloted by two community/public health nurses and the data indicated the system was successful in capturing a broad scope of the nurses' practice. The researchers documented their methodology so that other administrators in public health may replicate the adaptation of the electronic health record for community nursing practice.

### Nurse Use

By having a systematic data collection method, better evaluation of processes and outcomes of public health nursing and other public health professionals would be possible. Such data would also aid in providing evidence-based decision support for public health practice that could be used for quality improvement, funding proposals, and policy decisions.

Baisch MJ: A systematic method to document population-level nursing interventions in an electronic health system. *Public Health Nursing* 29(4):352–360, 2012.

The Wheel provides a meaningful frame of reference and common language for staff to communicate about the nature of their work and is used in orientation programs in several states.

- The Alaskan Public Health Nurse Leadership Academy uses the Intervention Wheel to familiarize new staff with population-based practice (http://www.hss.state.ak.us/dph/nursing/PFDs/Troshynski-Academy.pdf).
- Several universities have developed online applications of the Intervention Wheel, including the Virginia Commonwealth University (http://www.people.vcu.edu/~elmiles/interventions/) and the University of Minnesota School of Public Health (http://www.sph.umn.edu/ce/tools/wheel.asp).

The concepts of the model have also been used internationally. The Intervention Wheel was used in public health nursing projects in New Zealand and Ireland. The Institute of Primary Health & Ambulatory Care in the Townsville Health Service District, Queensland Health in Australia used the Intervention Wheel to develop a set of competencies (http://www.health.qld.gov.au/townsville/Clinicians/default.asp).

The significance of the contributions of the Intervention Wheel has been recognized by the nursing community. The authors of the Intervention Wheel received Sigma Theta Tau International and National Pinnacle Awards for Research Dissemination and a Creative Achievement Award from the American Public Health Association, Section of Public Health Nursing.

## HEALTHY PEOPLE 2020

The objectives chosen to be highlighted in this chapter show how many of the interventions from the Wheel are applied in the *Healthy People 2020* document. It further indicates how appropriate these interventions are to improving the health of individuals, populations, and communities, thus improving the health of the nation.

## APPLYING THE NURSING PROCESS IN PUBLIC HEALTH NURSING PRACTICE

PHNs use the nursing process at all levels of practice. PHNs must customize the components of the nursing process (assessment, diagnosis, planning, implementation, evaluation) to the three levels of practice. See Table 9-2 for an outline of the nursing process at the community, systems, and individual/family levels of practice.

## APPLYING THE PROCESS AT THE INDIVIDUAL/FAMILY LEVEL

### Community Assessment

During a health department's community assessment process, information on the health status of children was obtained from the following:

- Staff public health nurses who worked with families in clinics, schools, and homes
- Community partners who worked with families, including health care providers, mental health workers, social workers, and school personnel

**HEALTHY PEOPLE 2020**

*Healthy People 2020* identifies action steps for 38 health priorities that the United States must take to achieve better population health by the year 2020. The 500 recommended objectives offer numerous opportunities for public health nurses to contribute through implementing interventions at any or all of the levels. Here are a few examples:

- AH-8: Adolescent Health Objective: *Increase the proportion of adolescents who have had a wellness check-up in the past 12 months.* PHNs who provide well-child screening services in school settings or local health departments will need well-designed outreach interventions to convince teens that even healthy kids can benefit from check-ups. This will require consulting with parents and groups of teens themselves to identify what "benefits" would attract them and incorporating them into the outreach design. PHNs will also need to collaborate with other health care providers in the community to ensure that diagnostic and treatment services are available for teens who require additional services.

- DH-7: Disability and Secondary Conditions Objective: *Reduce the proportion of older adults with disabilities who use inappropriate medications.* The case management that PHNs provide to elderly or disabled populations in their communities includes an assessment of clients' medications to ensure compliance with the regimen prescribed by health care providers under delegated functions.

- ECBP-10: Education and Community-Based Programs Objective: *Increase the number of community-based organizations providing population-based primary prevention services in the following areas: injury, violence, mental illness, tobacco use, substance abuse, unintended pregnancy, chronic disease programs, nutrition, and physical activity.* PHNs may convene coalitions to address an issue or serve as facilitators or participants of coalitions already organized. For instance, PHNs with expertise in substance use prevention might offer health teaching and consultation to a coalition organized to find ways to reduce substance use during pregnancy. It could also mean the establishment of a new screening and referral system among providers to identify early pregnant women and their partners struggling with drug or alcohol use and link with resources for treatment.

- EH-8.1: Environmental Health Objective: *Eliminate elevated blood lead levels in children.* PHNs providing services to families with young children assess (surveillance) the living conditions for lead. Housing constructed prior to 1978, the year lead-based paint for residential use was banned, is particularly suspect. Depending on the community's housing and lead-abatement codes, PHNs may provide health teaching and counseling to the families regarding the dangers of lead exposure to small children or provide advocacy on their behalf with housing authorities.

- MICH-18: Maternal Infant and Child Health Objective: *Decrease postpartum relapse of smoking among women who quit smoking during pregnancy.* A recent systematic review of the literature on effective strategies to prevent postpartum smoking relapse concluded that PHNs would more likely be effective in assisting new mothers to resist returning to smoking and exposing their child to second-hand smoke if they: (1) consistently used the U.S. Preventive Services Task Forces "5 A's" when counseling with smokers, (2) tailored health teaching regarding the dangers of second-hand smoke to the client's specific situation, (3) empowered the mother and family members to adopt a smoke-free home smoking policy, and (4) advocated for the importance of partners also quitting (Ashford et al, 2009).

From Ashford K, Hahn E, Hall L, et al: Postpartum smoking relapse and secondhand smoke, Public Health Rep 124:515-526, 2009.

- Preschool screening program data on the number of young children with developmental delays and problems for the past 5 years
- Data from the county social services department on the number of substantiated child maltreatment and neglect cases for the past 5 years

PHNs participated in the community meeting that prioritized the long list of issues identified in the community assessment. One of the top community priorities that emerged was the following: *Decreasing numbers of children at risk for delayed development, injury, and disease because of inadequate parenting by parents experiencing mental health problems.*

The community health plan developed a goal to decrease the number of children with delayed development, injury, and disease attributable to inadequate parenting. The local health department, with the support of community partners, decided they would address this priority through a home visiting strategy. Home visiting enhances a child's environment and increases the capacity of parents to behave appropriately. Although parental mental health problems are a major source of stress for children, this vulnerability can be tempered through support from others and a caring environment.

Home visiting to families is an example of practice at the individual level because the interventions are delivered to families with the goal of changing parental knowledge, attitudes, practices, and behaviors.

## Public Health Nursing Process: Assessment of a Family

A PHN received a referral on Tyler, age 3. He was the only child of Ashley, a 19-year-old single mother with severe depression. Ashley lived in an old rented house in the small town where she grew up. She had a boyfriend who was not Tyler's biological father. Ashley survived on limited public assistance and occasional help from her mom.

The PHN assessed the resilience, assets, and protective factors as well as the problems, deficits, and health risks of this family. The PHN also tried to elicit Ashley's perception of her situation, which was difficult because of her depressed state. This step is important because often a client's perception of their problems or strengths may not align with the PHN's professional assessment.

All public health nursing practice is relationship based, regardless of level of practice. An established trust relationship increases the likelihood of a successful outcome. One of the PHN's main priorities was to establish a trusting relationship with Ashley. This was difficult because Ashley was seldom out of bed when the PHN arrived, but the PHN persisted and eventually developed the relationship.

## Public Health Nursing Process: Diagnosis

- *Diagnosis:* Increased risk for delayed development, injury, and disease because of inadequate parenting by a primary parent experiencing depression

- *Population at risk:* Young children who are being parented by a primary parent who is experiencing mental health problems
- *Prevention level:* Secondary prevention, because the families have an identified risk

## Public Health Nursing Process: Planning (Including Selection of Interventions)

Based on the assessment of this family, the PHN negotiated with Ashley to establish meaningful, measurable, achievable inter-mediate goals. In families experiencing mental illness (actually, in most families), behavior change occurs in very small steps. For this family, client goals included the following outcomes:

- Ashley will get out of bed at least 3 days in the week.
- Tyler will be dressed when the PHN arrives.
- Tyler will get to the bus on time 3 days in a row.
- The clutter will be cleaned off the steps.
- Ashley will call to make a doctor's appointment for Tyler's well-child check.
- Ashley will use "time outs" instead of spanking.
- Ashley will read a story to Tyler twice a week. (Intermediate indicators at the individual level of practice are changes in an individual's knowledge, attitudes, motivation, beliefs, values, skills, practices, and behavior that lead to desired changes in health status.)

The PHN also selected meaningful, measurable outcome health status indicators to measure the impact of the interventions on population health. Examples include no signs or reports of child maltreatment; child regularly attends preschool; child receives well-child examinations according to recommended schedule; child's immunizations are up to date; the family seeks medical care for acute illness as needed and does not seek medical care inappropriately; and child falls within normal limits on developmental tests.

The PHN selected the interventions, which included collaboration, case management, health teaching, delegated functions, and referral and follow-up. In selecting these interventions, the PHN considered evidence of effectiveness, political support, acceptability to the family, cost-effectiveness, legality, ethics, greatest potential for successful outcome, and level of prevention.

## Public Health Nursing Process: Implementation

The PHN determined the sequence and frequency of her home visits based on her assessment of each family. Some families received home visits once a week, some twice a week, and others twice a month. The PHN visited this family weekly in the beginning and then spaced the home visits farther apart. She used the following interventions.

### Collaboration

The PHN identified and involved as many alternative caregivers in Tyler's care as possible, including Tyler's biological father, aunt and uncle, and grandparents as well as Ashley's boyfriend.

### Case Management

The PHN arranged childcare services and coordinated transportation for Tyler to spend significant portions of his day outside of the home.

### Health Teaching

The PHN provided information on child growth and development, nutrition, immunizations, safety, medical and dental care, and discipline to Ashley and the alternative caregivers.

### Delegated Functions (Public Health Nurse to Paraprofessional)

The PHN placed a family health aide in the home to provide role modeling for Ashley. As part of this intervention, the PHN monitored and supervised the aide.

### Referral and Follow-up

Based on the assessment, the PHN referred Ashley to community resources and services that included early childhood services, legal aid, food stamps, mental health counselors, and transportation.

## Public Health Nursing Process: Evaluation

The PHN reassessed and modified her plan at each home visit. She provided regular feedback to Ashley and the other caregivers on their progress. The PHN documented her results and compared them with the selected indicators. After 6 months of home visits, Ashley got out of bed most days of the week but rarely got dressed. Ashley was more successful in getting Tyler to the bus and to preschool. The family health aide helped Ashley clean the clutter off the steps. Ashley scheduled a doctor's appointment for Tyler's well-child visit but failed to get him to the appointment. Ashley was successful in learning to substitute "time outs" for spanking, with the help of the family aide. Tyler exhibited no signs of child maltreatment. He attended preschool regularly. Tyler was still behind on his immunizations because of the missed appointment. All of Tyler's developmental tests were within normal limits.

The PHN reported her results to her supervisor during their regular supervisory meetings. The PHN also talked with other PHNs who worked with similar families about common issues and best practices, and applied what she had learned to her practice.

## APPLYING THE PUBLIC HEALTH NURSING PROCESS AT THE COMMUNITY LEVEL OF PRACTICE SCENARIO

*Note:* At the community level of practice, the community assessment, program planning, and evaluation process is the public health nursing process.

### Community Assessment (Public Health Nursing Process: Assessment)

Childhood obesity is a rapidly growing community problem. An increasing number of children ages 2 to 11 are considered overweight, as defined by a body mass index (BMI) at or above the 95th percentile (based on CDC Growth Charts; Ogden et al, 2010). The 2011-2012 National Health and Nutrition Examination Survey data estimated that 9.5% of boys and 7.2% of girls aged 2 to 5 were obese in the United

States. Among children aged 6 to 11 years, the percentages were 16.4% for boys and 19.1% for girls (CDC, 2014). Childhood obesity and hyperplasia of adipose cells are linked to obesity later in life.

A health department recognized the well-established association between overweight and obesity in childhood and the development of both continuing overweight/obesity as adults and a host of chronic diseases (CDC, 2010). In response, the public health nursing director of a health department convened a childhood obesity prevention summit. Over 80 participants representing area health care providers, schools, child care, and governmental and community-based health organizations met for an entire day to discuss the problem and frame solutions.

### Community Diagnosis (Public Health Nursing Process: Diagnosis)

The percentage of children aged 2 to 11 who are overweight or obese is unacceptable and threatens the future health status of the community.

- *Population of interest:* Children aged 2 to 11
- *Level of prevention:* Primary prevention

### Community Action Plan (Public Health Nursing Process: Planning, Including Selection of Interventions)

At the conclusion of the summit, each organization represented committed to promoting healthy eating and physical activity habits for all residents, with an emphasis on parents of young children. The health department recognized that a substantial portion of a child's caloric intake occurs at child care.

Based on its assessment of the community, the health department initiated a 24-week evidence-based program that promotes the consumption of fruits and vegetables by young children through intervention with licensed home childcare providers. "LANA the Iguana" (Learning About Nutrition Through Activities) encourages eating eight targeted fruits and vegetables: broccoli, sweet red pepper, cherry tomatoes, apricots, sugar snap peas, kiwi, sweet potatoes, and strawberries (Figure 9-6). These fruits and vegetables were featured in activities throughout the program related to menu changes, classroom activities, and family involvement.

### Menu Changes

Home childcare providers increased opportunities for children to eat more fruits and vegetables by serving the targeted fruits and vegetables on the menu, alternating four for one week and four the next. Fruits and vegetables were served as the morning and afternoon snack every day.

### Classroom Activities

Home childcare providers increased children's preference for and knowledge of fruits and vegetables by featuring one of the targeted fruits and vegetables each week throughout the program. During that week, the featured fruit or vegetable was

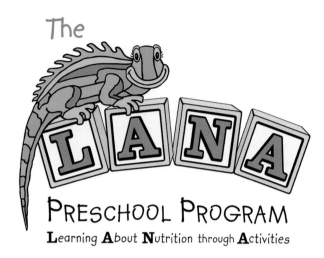

FIG 9-6 LANA the Iguana. (Used with permission from Minnesota Department of Health, Center for Health Promotion.)

the focus of tasting and cooking activities as well as the topic of stories and games.

### Family Involvement

Home childcare providers gave families information about the program and activities to do at home. These included quick and easy kid-tested recipes and take-home fruit/vegetable tasting kits.

The PHNs selected their interventions, which included consultation, health teaching, social marketing, collaboration, and surveillance. In selecting these interventions, the PHNs considered evidence of effectiveness, acceptability to community, cost-effectiveness, legality, ethics, and greatest potential for successful outcome.

### Community Implementation Plan (Public Health Nursing Process: Implementation)

1. *Social marketing:* LANA the Iguana was a social marketing program. It incorporated a range of age-appropriate social marketing techniques including iguana puppets and storybooks, recipe cards, and activities. The PHNs promoted retention by providing home childcare providers with incentives, including two grocery store gift cards and plastic fruit/vegetable toys for the children. They worked with librarians to place LANA the Iguana kits (comprised of iguana puppets, activities, and storybooks) in the local library for parents to check out. PHNs also donned the LANA the Iguana costume to implement the curriculum directly to children as well as train the home childcare providers and parents.
2. *Health teaching:* The PHNs trained the home childcare providers on the LANA curriculum to ensure fidelity to the program.
3. *Consultation:* The public health nurses consulted with home childcare providers about the program on a regular and ongoing basis.
4. *Collaboration:* PHNs collaborated with health educators to develop and distribute LANA materials, including a curricu-

lum guide, recipe books, storybooks, parent newsletters, and LANA the Iguana puppets. They also collaborated with public health nursing students to collect program evaluation data.

5. *Surveillance:* The PHNs collected data on the consumption of fruits and vegetables in the home childcare setting.

## Community Evaluation (Public Health Nursing Process: Evaluation)

Follow-up surveys with the county's 75 licensed home childcare providers, who served about 500 children, found that 67% of children were more or much more likely to eat fruits and 78% were more likely to eat vegetables; 92% of children were more likely to try new foods; and 76% of providers offered fruits and vegetables more often at snack time (Dakota County, 2010). Establishing healthy eating habits among young children will lead to reduced levels of obesity.

## APPLYING THE PUBLIC HEALTH NURSING PROCESS TO A SYSTEMS LEVEL OF PRACTICE SCENARIO

Health departments conduct assessments of community health status, a core function of public health, on an ongoing basis. The identification of some community problems emerges out of practice, rather than through a formal community assessment. This scenario is such an example.

## Public Health Nursing Process: Assessment

For several years, PHNs had been very concerned about the poor living conditions in an apartment complex in which many of their clients lived. The walls were moldy, the carpet was unclean and deteriorated, and closet doors had fallen off their runners and struck children living in the apartment. The PHNs were suspect of the required cash payments that the manager required for repairs, extra security deposits, and increased rent after the birth of a baby.

Many of the tenants were undocumented Latinos and tried not to create problems. Most could not speak or read English well, and often signed lease agreements without taking note of damage or existing problems in the apartment and were therefore blamed for them. In addition, the manager blamed the tenants for the mold on the walls, implying that their cooking created too much humidity. Citing these "problems," the manager often gave bad references for the tenants, which made it difficult for them to move.

Over the years, the PHNs had diligently worked with their clients to correct these problems, but with little success. When the PHNs met with the manager to discuss the issues, he became angry. As a result, the manager had the PHNs' cars towed whenever he saw them in the parking lot. The PHNs also had sought help from city officials, but the officials had no legal recourse to remedy the situation.

Finally, several events occurred that spurred the PHNs to action. One of the PHNs found a nonfunctioning smoke detector in an apartment during a home safety check. The family reported that the apartment manager had dismantled the smoke detector and left it that way. At the same time, another PHN was working with a family that was trying to move to a new, safer, cleaner apartment. The family had found a new apartment but could not move because the manager gave them a bad (although false) reference. The family no longer had a lease, but the manager said they could not move. The PHNs realized that there were many complex legal issues related to the living conditions of their clients.

## Public Health Nursing Process: Diagnosis

- *Diagnosis:* Families at risk of illness and injury because of hazardous housing and abuse of legal rights
- *Population at risk:* Families living in hazardous housing in an apartment complex
- *Prevention level:* Secondary, because families are at risk for injury and illness

## Public Health Nursing Process: Planning (Including Selection of Interventions)

At the systems level of practice, the goal is to change policies, laws, and structures. The PHNs' goals were to enforce the tenants' legal rights and improve the living conditions in the apartment complex. Their plan was to seek advice from a housing advocate service and connect their clients with legal counsel. Before they could pursue this plan, the PHNs consulted with their supervisor. Their supervisor supported their decision but also had to clear the plan with the health department director and the city manager.

The PHNs selected their interventions, which included consultation, referral and follow-up, advocacy, policy development, and surveillance. In selecting these interventions, the PHNs considered evidence of effectiveness, political support, acceptability to the family, cost-effectiveness, legality, ethics, greatest potential for a successful outcome, non-duplication, and level of prevention.

## Public Health Nursing Process: Implementation

The PHNs worked with the tenants and the housing advocacy service to implement the following interventions.

### Consultation

The PHNs consulted with attorneys at a housing advocate service.

### Referral and Follow-up

The attorneys informed the PHNs that they needed to hear directly from the tenants in order to proceed. The PHNs set up a meeting time between the tenants and the attorneys from the housing advocate service.

### Advocacy

The PHNs arranged for their public health interpreter to go door to door with an advocate from the housing service to invite tenants to the meeting. They also arranged for the interpreter to attend the meeting to interpret each family's concerns. The PHNs strongly encouraged all of the tenants to attend.

## Policy Development

The public health nurses worked with the attorneys from the housing advocate service to develop the meeting agenda.

## Surveillance

The PHNs continued to conduct ongoing monitoring of living conditions in the apartment complex.

## Public Health Nursing Process: Evaluation

Many of the tenants attended the meeting. As a result of the meeting, the attorney chose to have the rent paid to the court and put in escrow until a legal determination could be made. During this process the apartment owner became aware of these issues and dismissed the manager, who was discovered to have been acting fraudulently. A new manager was employed who worked to improve the living conditions of the apartments.

### ▶▶ LINKING CONTENT TO PRACTICE

The discussions of the application of the nursing process to a variety of clients beginning on page 209 and Tables 9-1 and 9-2 provide numerous examples of how the content in this chapter is applied in practice. Please review these for examples of how you may apply this model in your practice.

## ▌ PRACTICE APPLICATION

Outreach locates populations of interest or populations at risk and provides information about the nature of the concern, what can be done about it, and how services can be obtained. Outreach activities may be directed at whole communities, at targeted populations within those communities, and/or at systems that impact the community's health. Outreach success is determined by the proportion of those considered at risk that receive the information and act on it.

The chance of a 20-year-old woman developing breast cancer within the next 10 years is 1 in 1681. At age 30, a woman's chance of developing breast cancer within the next 10 years is 1 in 232; at age 40, it is 1 in 69; at age 50, it is 1 in 42; at age 60, it is 1 in 29; and at age 70, it is 1 in 27 (Susan G. Komen Foundation, 2013).

A health system decided to offer free mammograms in recognition of National Breast Cancer Month. They sponsored a mobile mammography van at a large shopping mall every Saturday in October. The van offered mammograms to everyone, regardless of age. The health system advertised the service by placing windshield flyers on all the cars in the shopping mall parking lot. The van provided 180 mammograms, mostly to women in their 30s who had health insurance that covered preventive services.

1. What is the population most at risk of breast cancer?
2. Did the mammograms in the parking lot reach this population?
3. What types of outreach would public health nurses conduct to reach the population at risk?
   **Answers can be found on the Evolve site.**

## ▌ KEY POINTS

- In these times of change, the public health system is constantly challenged to keep focused on the health of populations.
- The Intervention Wheel is a conceptual framework that has proved to be a useful model in defining population-based practice and explaining how it contributes to improving population health.
- The Wheel depicts how public health improves population health through interventions with communities, the individuals and families that comprise communities, and the systems that impact the health of communities.
- The Wheel serves as a model for practice in many state and local health departments.
- The Wheel is based on 10 assumptions.
- The Intervention Wheel encompasses 17 interventions.
- Other public health members of the interprofessional team such as nutritionists, health educators, planners, physicians, and epidemiologists also use these interventions.
- Implementing the interventions ultimately contributes to the achievement of the 10 essential public health services.
- The *Cornerstones of Public Health Nursing* was developed as a companion document to the Intervention Wheel.
- The original version of the Wheel resulted from a grounded theory process carried out by public health nurse consultants at the Minnesota Department of Health in the mid-1990s.
- The interventions were subjected to an extensive review of supporting evidence in the literature.
- The Wheel is a conceptual model. It was conceived as a common language or catalog of general actions used by public health nurses across all practice settings.
- The Intervention Wheel serves as a conceptual model for public health nursing practice and creates a structure for identifying and documenting interventions performed by public health nurses and captures the nature of their work.
- The Wheel has three main components: a population basis, three levels of practice, and 17 interventions.

## KEY POINTS—cont'd

- The Wheel has led to numerous innovations in practice and education since the original Intervention Wheel was first published in 1998.
- Public health nurses in the Shiprock Service Unit of the Indian Health Service adapted the Intervention Wheel to reflect the Navajo culture.

- Numerous graduate and undergraduate schools of nursing throughout the United States have adopted the Intervention Wheel as a framework for teaching public health nursing practice.

## CLINICAL DECISION-MAKING ACTIVITIES

1. Describe the three components of the Intervention Wheel. How do the components relate to each other? Explain how you can apply them to your clinical practice.
2. Go to Chapter 1 and reread the definitions of the core functions of public health practice and look at the 10 essential services. How does the Wheel address the core functions? How does it relate to the 10 essential services?

3. Go to the Wheel website: www.health.state.mn.us/divs/cfh/ophp/resources/docs/wheel.pdf. Choose one of the 17 interventions to explore. Read about the recommended strategies to use when intervening with a client. Explain the level of practice and how you can apply the intervention. Give a concrete example.

## REFERENCES

American Academy of Pediatrics: Active healthy living: prevention of childhood obesity through increased physical activity. *Pediatrics* 117(5):1834–1842, 2010. This policy is a revision of the policy posted on May 1, 2000.

American Nurses Association: *Public health nursing: scope and standards of practice.* Silver Spring, MD, 2007, ANA. http://www.nursesbooks.org.

American Nurses Association: *Public health nursing: scope and standards of practice,* ed 2. Silver Spring, MD, 2013, ANA. http://www.nursesbooks.org.

American Nurses Association Task Force: *Nursing social policy statement: the essence of the profession,* ed 2010. Washington, DC, 2010, American Nurses Publishing.

American Public Health Association, Public Health Nursing Section: *Definition and role of public health nursing.* Washington, DC, 2013, APHA. Available at: http://www.apha.org/NR/rdonlyres/284CE437-6AF3-4B23-88BA-52F2A0E329E6/0/PHNdefinitionNov2013_final125142.pdf. Accessed July 9, 2014.

Avilla M, Smith K: The reinvigoration of public health nursing: methods and innovations. *J Public Health Manag Pract* 9:16–24, 2003.

Bezboruah KC: Community organizing for health care: an analysis of the process. *J Community Practice* 21(1/2):9–27, 2013.

Bleich SN, Jarlenski MP, Bell CN, et al: Health inequalities—trends, progress, and policy. *Annu Rev Public Health* 33:7–40, 2012.

doi: 10.1146/annurev-publhealth-031811-124658.

Burnard P: *Counseling: a guide to practice in nursing.* Oxford, England, 1992, Butterworth-Heineman.

Centers for Disease Control and Prevention: *Obesity: halting the epidemic by making health easier,* 2010. Available at: http://www.cdc.gov/chronicdisease/resources/publications/aag/pdf/2010/AAG_Obesity_2010_Web_508.pdf. Accessed July 10, 2014.

Centers for Disease Control and Prevention: *Vaccines and preventable diseases,* 2012. Available at: http://www.cdc.gov/vaccines/vpd-vac/default.htm. Accessed July 10, 2014.

Centers for Disease Control and Prevention: CDC health disparities and inequalities report—United States, 2013. *MMWR* 62(Supp3):89, 172–173, 2013. Available: http://www.cdc.gov/mmwr/pdf/other/su6203.pdf. Accessed July 9, 2014.

Centers for Disease Control and Prevention: *NCHS Obesity Data.* May 2014, National Center for Health Statistics. Available: http://www.cdc.gov/nchs/data/factsheets/factsheet_obesity.pdf. Accessed July 10, 2014.

Dakota County (MN) Public Health: Factsheet: tackling childhood obesity with Lana the Iguana. 2010. Available at: http://www.co.dakota.mn.us.

Depke JL, Onitilo AA: Coalition building and the Intervention Wheel to address breast cancer screening in Hmong women. *Clin Med Res* 9(1):1–6, 2011.

Fawcett J, DeSanto-Madeya S: *Contemporary Nursing Knowledge: Analysis and Evaluation of Nursing Models and Theories,* ed 3. Philadelphia, 2013, FA Davis.

Ferdinand AO, Sen B, Rahurkar S, et al: The relationship between built environments and physical activity: a systematic review. *Am J Pub Health* 102(10):e7–e13, 2012. doi: 10.2105/AJPH.2012.300740.

Freshman B, Rubino L, Chassiakos YR: *Collaboration Across the Disciplines in Health Care.* Sudbury, MA, 2010, Jones and Bartlett.

Gregory D, Johnston R, Pratt G, et al, editors: *The Dictionary of Human Geography,* ed 5. Oxford, England, 2009, Blackwell, pp 103–104.

Henneman EA, Lee J, Cohn JI: Collaboration: a concept analysis. *J Adv Nurs* 21:103–109, 1995.

Jewish Women's Archive: *Resource information for Backyard of a Henry Street Branch,* 2010. Available at: http://jwa.org/archive/jsp/gresInfo.jsp?resID=297. Accessed December 11, 2010.

Kariuki JC: *What Community Residents Perceive Can Be Done to Address Concerns Regarding Litter and Brownfields in Weinland Park,* Honors thesis. 2012, Ohio State University College of Nursing. Available at: http://kb.osu.edu/dspace/bitstream/handle/1811/51986/HONORS_RESEARCH_PROPOSAL_3.pdf?sequence=1. Accessed July 10, 2014.

Keller LO: *Report on a Public Health Nurse to Population Ratio.* 2008, Association of State and Territorial Directors of Nursing. Available at: http://

www.astdn.org/downloadablefiles/draft-PHN-to-Population-Ratio.pdf. Accessed December 11, 2010.

Keller LO, Strohschein S, Lia-Hoagberg B, et al: Population-based public health nursing interventions: a model from practice. *Public Health Nurs* 15:311–320, 1998.

Keller LO, Strohschein S, Lia-Hoagberg B, et al: Assessment, program planning, and evaluation in population-based public health practice. *J Public Health Manag Pract* 8:30–43, 2002.

Keller LO, Strohschein S, Lia-Hoagberg B, et al: Population-based public health interventions: practice-based and evidence-supported, part I. *Public Health Nurs* 21:453–468, 2004a.

Keller LO, Strohschein S, Schaffer M, et al: Population-based public health interventions: innovations in practice, teaching, and management, part II. *Public Health Nurs* 21:469–487, 2004b.

Keller LO, Strohschein S, Schaffer M: Cornerstones of public health nursing. *Public Health Nurs* 28(3):249–260, 2010.

Leavell HR, Clark EG: *Preventive Medicine for the Doctor in His Community,* ed 3. New York, 1965, McGraw-Hill.

Lo R: Walkability: what is it? *J Urbanism* 2(2):145–166, 2009.

Los Angeles County Department of Health Services: Public Health Nursing Administration: *Public health nursing administration model,* 2002. Available at: http://lapublichealth.org/phn/whatphn.htm, narrative available at: http://lapublichealth.org/phn/docs/

Narrative2002.PDF. Accessed December 11, 2010.

Massachusetts Association of Public Health Nurses: Leadership guide and resource manual, 2009. Available at: www.maphn.org. Accessed January 20, 2011.

McGuire S, Eigsti Gerber D, Clemen-Stone S: Meeting the diverse needs of clients in the community: effective use of the referral process. *Nurs Outlook* 44:218–222, 1996.

Meagher-Stewart D, Edwards N, Aston M, et al: Population health surveillance practice public health nurses. *Public Health Nurs* 26(6):553–560, 2009.

Minkler M, editor: *Community Organizing and Community Building for Health*, ed 3. New Brunswick, NJ, 2012, Rutgers University Press.

Minnesota Departments of Education, Health, Human Services, and Public Safety: *2013 Minnesota Student Survey County Tables, Fall*, 2013, Available at: http://

www.health.state.mn.us/divs/chs/mss/countytables/sherburne13.pdf. Accessed July 9, 2014.

Morbidity and Mortality Weekly Review: CDC's Vision for Public Health Surveillance in the 21st Century report. 61(Suppl: July 27, 2012):10–14, 2012.

Ogden CL, Carroll MD, Curtin LR, et al: Prevalence of high body mass index in U.S. children and adolescents, 2007–2008. *JAMA* 303(3):242–249, 2010.

Public Health Functions Steering Committee: *Public health in America*, 1995. Available at: www.health.gov/phfunctions/public.htm. Accessed December 11, 2010.

Renalds A, Smith T, Hale P: A systematic review of built environment and health. *Fam Community Health* 33(1):68–78, 2010.

Schoneman D, Simandl G, Hansen JM, et al: Competency-based project to review community/public health

curricula. *Public Health Nurs* 31(4):373–383, 2014.

Shi L, Johnson JA: *Novick & Morrow's Public Health Administration: Principles for Population-Based Management*, ed 3. Gaithersburg, MD, 2013, Aspen.

Smith K, Bazini-Barakat N: A public health nursing practice model: melding public health principles with the nursing process. *Public Health Nurs* 20:42–48, 2003.

Stanhope M, Lancaster J: *Community Health Nursing: Process and Practice for Promoting Health*. St Louis, 1984, Mosby, p 357.

Sue DW, Sue D: *Counseling the Culturally Different: Theory and Practice*. New York, 1999, Wiley.

Susan G, Komen Foundation: *Breast cancer risk factors factsheet*, 2013. Available at: http://ww5.komen.org/uploadedfiles/Content_Binaries/

806-372a.pdf. Accessed July 10, 2014.

Turnock BJ: *Public Health: What It Is and How It Works*, ed 5. Gaithersburg, MD, 2011, Aspen Publishers.

U.S. Department of Agriculture: *Food Environment Atlas for Sherburne, MN, Health and Physical Activity, 2012*. Available at: http://www.ers.usda.gov/data-products/food-environment-atlas/go-to-the-atlas.aspx#.U76q7JRdVLN. Accessed July 10, 2014.

Walkability Checklist: (no date). Partnership for a Walkable America. Retrieved from: http://www.walkableamerica.org/checklist-walkability.pdf.

Williams CA, Highriter ME: Community health nursing: population focus and evaluation. *Public Health Rev* 7:197–221, 1978.

Zoller, Kara, personal communication, August 16, 2010.

# 10

# Environmental Health

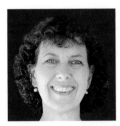

## Barbara Sattler, RN, DrPH, FAAN

Dr. Barbara Sattler has a diploma in nursing from Pilgrim State Psychiatric Center School of Nursing, a BS in political science from the University of Baltimore, and the MPH and DrPH from the Johns Hopkins University. She is a Professor at the University of San Francisco. She is a founding member of the Alliance of Nurses for Healthy Environments (www.enviRN.org), a national network of nurses who are addressing the integration of environmental health into our nursing education, practice, research, and policy/advocacy efforts. She has been working in the area of environmental health and nursing for three decades and has been involved in issues associated with air, water, food, and products, as well as climate change and energy policies as they relate to human health.

## ADDITIONAL RESOURCES

**Evolve Website http://evolve.elsevier.com/Stanhope**
- Healthy People 2020
- WebLinks—Of special note see the link for these sites:
  - Envirotools
  - www.enviRN.org: Alliance of Nurses for Healthy Environments
  - National Library of Medicine online toxicology tutorial

- Case Studies
- Glossary
- Answers to Practice Application

**Appendix**
- Appendix F.3: Comprehensive Occupational and Environmental Health History

## OBJECTIVES

*After reading this chapter, the student should be able to do the following:*

1. Explain the relationship between the environment and human health and disease.
2. Understand the key disciplines that inform nurses' work in environmental health.
3. Apply the nursing process to the practice of environmental health.
4. Describe legislative and regulatory policies that have influenced the impact of the environment on health and disease patterns in communities.
5. Explain and compare the environmental health roles and skills for nurses practicing in public health, as well as those practicing in practice settings.
6. Incorporate environmental principles into practice.

## KEY TERMS

agent, p. 222
bioaccumulated, p. 236
biomonitoring, p. 221
climate change, p. 223
compliance, p. 236
consumer confidence reports, p. 228
environment, p. 222
environmental justice, p. 236
environmental standards, p. 236
epidemiologic triangle, p. 222
epidemiology, p. 222
epigenetics, p. 221
geographic information systems, p. 222
host, p. 222
indoor air quality, p. 227
Industrial Hygiene Hierarchy of Controls, p. 232
methylmercury, p. 236

monitoring, p. 236
non–point sources, p. 226
permit, p. 236
permitting, p. 234
persistent bioaccumulative toxins, p. 236
persistent organic pollutants, p. 236
point sources, p. 226
precautionary principle, p. 231
right to know, p. 228
risk assessment, p. 228
risk communication, p. 233
risk management, p. 232
route of exposure, p. 233
toxicants, p. 229
toxicology, p. 221
*—See Glossary for definitions*

# CHAPTER OUTLINE

"Environmental health *comprises those aspects of human health, including quality of life, that are determined by physical, chemical, biological, social, and psychosocial factors in the environment. It also refers to the theory and practice of assessing, correcting, controlling, and preventing those factors in the environment that can potentially affect adversely the health of present and future generations.*"

**United Nations University, 1993 (UNU)**

An estimated 24% of the global burden of disease and 23% of all deaths can be attributed to environmental factors (WHO, 2015). As nurses there are a number of ways in which we can define our environment. Our homes, schools, workplaces, and communities are the environments in which most of us can be found at any given time. Each location holds potential health risks. As nurses, who are among the most trusted conveyors of information to the public, it is our responsibility to understand as much as possible about these risks—how to assess them, how to eliminate or reduce them, how to communicate and educate about them, and how to advocate for policies that support healthy environments.

We can also divide and examine the environment from the perspective of the media in which environmental degradation takes place: air, water, soil, and food. And a third approach would be to divide environmental exposures into categories: biological, chemical, and radiological. In this chapter we will look at the environment as comprehensively as possible and consider the roles that nurses can have in assessing and addressing environmental health.

Environmental exposures are rarely limited to one location or to one source. For example, the broad category of pesticides includes the insecticides we may use in our homes, the herbicides we may use in our gardens, the pesticide residues on fruits and vegetables, and our antimicrobial soaps. Each of these

forms of pesticides comes with a potential health risk. If you have children and regularly use pesticides in your home, you increase their risk of contracting leukemia. The more you use insecticides, the greater the risk of leukemia (Metayer et al, 2013; Wigle et al, 2009; Turner et al, 2010; Brown, 2004). The childhood risk for leukemia increases if the mother was exposed to pesticides, including occupational exposures (Bailey et al, 2014). Many playing fields where children compete in sports are regularly sprayed with pesticides (Gilden et al, 2012).

In May 2010, the President's Cancer Panel proclaimed that the contribution environmental carcinogens have made to the burden of cancer in the United States has been grossly underestimated. In addition to the main focus on chemical carcinogens, the panel noted the importance of radiation sources—ionizing and nonionizing. In a letter to President Obama, they wrote: "The Panel urges you most strongly to use the power of your office to remove the carcinogens and other toxins from our food, water, and air that needlessly increase our health care costs, cripple our Nation's productivity and devastate American lives" (President's Cancer Panel, 2010). With this call came a range of recommendations for reducing the risk of cancer, both through individual choices and through national policy. The recommendations for individuals are found in Resource 10.A on the Evolve resources website.

Cancer is not the only health endpoint of environmental exposures. An estimated 52 million homes in the United States contain some lead-based paint that is associated with risks for premature births, learning disabilities in children, hypertension in adults, and many other health problems. Lead poisoning is a completely preventable disease (Figure 10-1). Of the top 20 environmental pollutants that were reported to the Environmental Protection Agency (EPA), nearly three fourths were known or suspected neurotoxins. Thirty million Americans drink water that exceeds one or more of the EPA's safe drinking

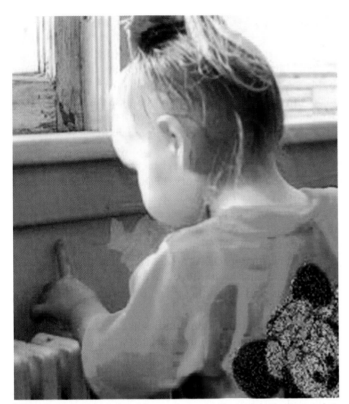

FIG 10-1 Although lead is no longer allowed in house paint, over 34 million homes in the United States have lead-based paint U.S. Department of Housing and Urban Development (US DHUD, 2011). Pregnant women and parents who live in homes built before 1978 should be encouraged to have their homes tested for lead-based paint dust. (From State of Hawaii Department of Public Health. Available at http://hawaii.gov/health/environmental/noise/asbestoslead/images2/child.jpg. Accessed December 15, 2010.)

water standards, and 50% of Americans live in an area that exceeds current national ambient air quality standards. When these standards are exceeded, there is an increased risk to the public for a wide range of health effects.

Although food labeling includes nutrition information, there is no requirement to label whether pesticides are used in the food production; whether nontherapeutic antibiotics were given to the livestock, poultry, or farmed fish; the presence of genetically modified organisms (GMOs) in a product; or whether recombinant bovine growth hormone (rBGH) was given to the dairy cows. Nurses have declared that the "right to know" about potentially hazardous exposures is one of the basic principles of environmental health (see Box 10-1). Nurses have a range of potential public health responsibilities in protecting the public from exposures and environmental health risks (ANA 2007).

A range of influences including genetics, socioeconomic status, and environmental exposures impact environmental health. In evaluating environmental exposures in a home, nurses' assessments can begin with a set of questions: What exposures can you identify in your own home? Do you use pesticides? Does your home have lead-based paint? (The age of a home is a good proxy for identifying the presence of

## BOX 10-1  American Nurses Association's Principles of Environmental Health for Nursing Practice

The ANA calls for all nurses to understand basic environmental health concepts, invokes the Precautionary Principle, recognizes the multidisciplinary nature of environmental health, and promotes and supports nurses' roles in developing and maintaining environmentally healthy workplaces for themselves and their patients. Principles include knowledge about environmental health and its effect on nursing practice, the Precautionary Principle, nurses' rights to work in a safe workplace and use materials, products, technology, and practices that reflect an evidence-based approach. Other principles relate to quality assessment of the environment, interdisciplinary work in environmental health, involvement in research, and support of nurses who advocate for a safe environment (ANA, 2007).

From American Nurses Association. Principles of environmental health for nursing practice, Silver Spring, MD, 2007.

lead-based paint because it is most likely found in homes built before 1978, when the use of lead was banned in household paint.) Is the paint chipping or peeling? Are any of your appliances or heat sources producing unhealthy levels of carbon monoxide? Have you checked your home for radon, the second largest cause of lung cancer in the United States? How about your workplace? Do you eat fish on a regular basis? (Some fish can have unhealthy levels of mercury.) A more comprehensive home assessment tool can be found in the Resources.

## ⟩⟩ LINKING CONTENT TO PRACTICE

The Council on Linkages Between Academic and Public Health Practice, 2010 a key document that guides practice in both nursing and public health. Specifically, the core competencies of the Council on Linkages includes, within the domain of public health science skills, a competency that says practitioners will apply "the basic public health sciences (including, but not limited to, environmental health sciences, health services administration, and social and behavioral health sciences) to public health policies and programs." The Quad Council of Public Health Nursing Organizations (2011) further applies this competency specifically to public health nursing practice by adding that these skills are applied to public health nursing practice, policies, and programs. In 2007, the ANA adopted 10 principles of environmental health. Although all 10 are essential, three are highlighted here. Nurses should know about environmental health concepts, participate in assessing the quality of the environment in which they practice, and live and use the Precautionary Principle (which is discussed later in the chapter) to guide their work. A third principle points out that healthy environments are sustained through multidisciplinary collaboration, which is a key concept discussed throughout the chapter.

In 2010, the American Nurses Association (ANA) established an environmental health standard within the Scope and Standards of Professional Practice that define the profession of nursing. This means that all nurses are now expected to have knowledge of and skills associated with environmental health.

Underpinning many of these organizational decisions to include environmental health in nursing were the recommendations made in the report *Nursing, Health and Environment* (Pope, Snyder, and Mood, 1995) from the Institute of Medicine (IOM) of the National Academy of Science, which recommended that all nurses have a basic understanding of environmental health principles and integrate these principles into our practice, education, advocacy, policies, and research. In this chapter, we will explore the basic competencies recommended by the IOM. Box 10-2 presents the competencies.

## BOX 10-2    General Environmental Health Competencies for Nurses Recommended by the Institute of Medicine in *Nursing, Health and the Environment*

### Basic Knowledge and Concepts

All nurses should understand the scientific principles and underpinnings of the relationship between individuals or populations and the environment (including the work environment). This understanding includes the basic mechanism and pathways of exposure to environmental health hazards, basic prevention and control strategies, the interprofessional nature of effective interventions, and the role of research.

### Assessment and Referral

All nurses should be able to successfully complete an environmental health history, recognize potential environmental hazards and sentinel illnesses, and make appropriate referrals for conditions with probable environmental causes. An essential component is the ability to access and provide information to clients and communities and to locate referral sources.

### Advocacy, Ethics, and Risk Communication

All nurses should be able to demonstrate knowledge of the role of advocacy (case and class), ethics, and risk communication in client care and community intervention with respect to the potential adverse effects of the environment on health.

### Legislation and Regulation

All nurses should understand the policy framework and major pieces of legislation and regulations related to environmental health.

From Pope AM, Snyder MA, Mood LH, editors: Nursing, health, and environment, Washington, DC, 1995, Institute of Medicine, National Academy Press.

## *HEALTHY PEOPLE 2020* OBJECTIVES FOR ENVIRONMENTAL HEALTH

Environmental health is one of the priority areas of the *Healthy People 2020* objectives. The federal government has long recognized the importance of the relationship between environmental risks and the underlying factors contributing to diseases. Selected examples of the *Healthy People 2020* environmental health objectives are outlined in the following Healthy People 2020 box (U.S. Department of Health and Human Services, Healthy People 2020, 2010).

 **HEALTHY PEOPLE 2020**

### *Examples of Objectives Related to Environmental Health*

- EH-8.1: Eliminate elevated blood lead levels in children.
- EH-9: Minimize the risks to human health and the environment posed by hazardous sites.
- EH-10: Reduce pesticide exposures that result in visits to the health care facility.
- EH-11: Reduce the amount of toxic pollutants released into the environment.
- EH-13: Reduce indoor allergen levels.
- EH-18: Decrease the number of U.S. homes that are found to have lead-based paint or related hazards.

From U.S. Department of Health and Human Services: Healthy People 2020. Available at http://www.healthypeople.gov/2020topicsobjectives 2020/default.aspx. Accessed January 1, 2011.

## HISTORICAL CONTEXT

Historically, nurses and physicians have been taught little about the environment and environmental threats to health. In the IOM report mentioned previously, quotes from Florence Nightingale are used extensively, not only because she is a recognized symbol of nursing (i.e., the lady with the lamp), but also because of the central focus of environment in her practice and writings. She promoted the use of clean water and safe sanitary conditions and connected these elements to disease prevention. Early in the twentieth century, Lillian Wald, who coined the name "public health nurses," spent her life improving the environment of the Henry Street neighborhood and encouraging her broad network of influential contacts to make changes in the physical environment, as well as social conditions that had direct health impacts. As modern day nurses are rediscovering environmental health, they are reintegrating many of the observations and skills that were practiced by early nurse pioneers.

There are still many communities like the ones that Lillian Wald served. Poverty is highly associated with health disparities and is also associated with disproportionately higher environmental exposure, which compounds the health disparities. Poverty is linked to living in substandard housing, living closer to hazardous waste sites, working in more hazardous jobs, having poorer nutrition, and having less access to quality health care (particularly preventative services). The term *environmental justice* refers to the disproportionate environmental exposures that poor people and people of color experience in the United States and elsewhere, including lead paint dust exposure, the presence of pests (resulting in increased use of pesticides), and the use of supplemental heating sources that may cause dangerous carbon monoxide exposure. These combined circumstances multiply the risk for health disparities.

It is important to note how we began to understand the relationship between environmental chemical exposures and their potential for harm. There are several ways in which we have historically made such discoveries:

- When humans present with signs and symptoms that can be connected to a specific chemical exposure. This may occur with acute pesticide poisoning or carbon monoxide poisoning. It often occurs when workers are occupationally exposed. In such instances, the temporal and geographic relationships to the exposures and health effects help to identify health hazards in the environment (e.g., the diagnosis of mesothelioma from asbestos exposure).
- When large accidental releases of chemicals occur in a community that contaminate air, water, soil, or food, resulting in health effects. Such events show us how toxic chemicals are to humans and animals. For example, in the Love Canal incident outside of Buffalo, NY, an entire community was affected by hazardous chemicals that were dumped on the land where a housing development was built.
- In rare instances, when human environmental (and occupational) epidemiologic studies have been performed. Through such studies, we have learned about the toxic effects of chemicals.

However, the most common way in which the relationships between chemical exposures and health risks are identified is when toxicologists study the effects of chemicals on animals and then use models to estimate what the effects might be on humans. This estimation process is called *extrapolation*. More than 84,000 man-made (synthetic) chemical compounds have been developed and introduced to our environment since World War II, and we are most often reliant on the data that are created in animal studies to warn us about their potential toxicity to humans. For many of these chemicals, no toxicity data are available. Surprisingly, there is no current requirement for original toxicological research to be completed when a product or process is being brought to market.

We live in a radically different environment compared to a century ago. In addition to man-made pollutants contaminating our air, water, and food, many of the same pollutants are now also found in our bodies (including breast milk). In 2001, the Centers for Disease Control and Prevention began biomonitoring—the testing of human fluids and tissues for the presence of potentially toxic chemicals, as part of its National Health and Nutrition Exam Study. For instance, most Americans carry pesticides, solvents, heavy metals and other potentially toxic chemicals in their bodies. In 2005, an Environmental Working Group tested the umbilical cord blood of newborn babies and found that they also contained a similar range of potentially harmful chemicals (EWG, 2005). Each of these potentially hazardous substances creates a health risk. Nurses need to understand the environmental exposures and the health effects that may be associated with chemicals in order to develop assessment tools, implement hazard reduction programs, and advocate for safe and healthy chemical policies. For example, when a woman is pregnant for the first time, this is an ideal time for a nurse to help her assess and reduce or eliminate preventable environmental health risks in her home and workplace. A good environmental health history can help uncover a number of exposures from the products she may use, the ways in which she addresses pests in her home and garden, to the way in which she may set up a new nursery room.

In the Resource Section under chemical policies, there are a number of links to organizations that track federal and state legislation on chemical issues.

## ENVIRONMENTAL HEALTH SCIENCES
### Toxicology

Toxicology is the basic science that contributes to our understanding of health effects associated with chemical exposures. Historically, it was referred to as the "study of poisons." Its corollary in health care is pharmacology, which studies the human health effects, both desirable and undesirable, associated with drugs. In toxicology, only the negative effects of chemical exposures are studied. However, the key principles of pharmacology and toxicology are the same. Just as the dose of a drug makes the difference in its efficacy and its toxicity, the quantity of an air or water pollutant to which we may be exposed can determine whether or not (and the extent to which) we experience a risk of a health effect. In addition, the timing

of the exposure—over the human life span—can make a difference. For example, during embryonic and fetal development, exposure to toxic chemicals can create immediate harm or create a critical pathway for future disease. Very young children, whose systems are still immature, are also more vulnerable to exposures. *In Harm's Way*, an online report by Physicians for Social Responsibility (with associated training materials) describes the neurological damage that several common chemicals can cause to developing children (Schettler et al, 2000). Just as is true of medications, the same dose that one would give an adult will have a much greater effect on a child and certainly on a fetus. As we age our liver and renal functions slow, thereby creating opportunities for toxic chemicals to accumulate, and thus creating higher risks for harm.

Both drugs and pollutants can enter the body from a variety of routes. Most drugs are given orally and absorbed by the gastrointestinal (GI) tract. Water- and food-associated pollutants, including pesticides and heavy metals, enter the body via the digestive tract. Some drugs are administered as inhalants, and some pollutants in the air (including indoor air) enter the body via the lungs. Some drugs are applied topically. In work settings, employees can receive dermal exposures from toxic chemicals when they immerse their unprotected hands in chemical solutions, especially solvents. Pollution can enter our bodies via the lungs (inhalation), GI tract (ingestion), skin, and even the mucous membranes (dermal absorption). Most chemicals cross the placental barrier and can affect the fetus, just as most chemicals cross the blood–brain barrier. In addition to direct damage to cells, tissues, organs and organ systems, there can be changes to the DNA from chemical exposures that can change gene expression, which in turn can predict disease. This latter effect is the focus of a relatively new field of biological study: epigenetics. Scientists now understand that there are many variables that predict disease outcomes, including environmental exposures.

In the same way that we consider age, weight, other drugs taken, and underlying health status of a client when we administer drugs, we must consider that these same factors can affect an individual's response to environmental exposures. For example, children are much more vulnerable to virtually all pollutants. People who are immunosuppressed (people with HIV/AIDS or those on immunosuppressant drugs like steroids or anti-cancer medications) are especially at risk for foodborne and waterborne pathogens. Because our communities are comprised of people of different ages and different health statuses, their vulnerabilities to the effects of pollution will also vary. When assessing a community's environmental health status, be sure to review the general health status of the community and to identify members who may have higher risk factors.

Chemicals that are similar are often grouped into categories or "families" so that it is possible to understand the actions and risks associated with those groupings. Examples are metals and metallic compounds (e.g., arsenic, cadmium, chromium, lead, mercury), hydrocarbons (e.g., benzene, toluene, ketones, formaldehyde, trichloroethylene), irritant gases (e.g., ammonia, hydrochloric acid, sulfur dioxide, chlorine), chemical asphyxiants (e.g., carbon monoxide, hydrogen sulfide, cyanides), and pesticides (e.g., organophosphates, carbamates, chlorinated hydrocarbons). Although some common health risks exist within these families of chemicals, the possible health risks for each chemical should be evaluated individually when a potential human exposure exists. The best source of peer-reviewed information for this is the National Library of Medicine (NLM). The NLM has a set of databases that are focused on toxicology and environmental health called TOXNET. You will find the link to several of these helpful informational programs and databases in the Referral Resources.

## Epidemiology

Whereas toxicology is the science that studies the poisonous effects of chemicals, **epidemiology** is the science that helps us understand the strength of the association between exposures and health effects. Epidemiology is often used for occupationally related illnesses but has been used less often to study environmentally related diseases. It is difficult to characterize and/or distinguish among the many exposures that we all experience, and it can be challenging to find control groups when the environmental exposure of concern is in the air, water, or food.

Epidemiologic studies have helped us to understand the association between learning disabilities and exposure to lead-based paint dust, asthma exacerbation and air pollution (Smargiassi et al, 2014; Habre et al, 2014), and GI disease and waterborne *Cryptosporidia* (Yoder et al, 2012). Environmental surveillance, such as childhood lead registries, provides data with which to track and analyze incidence and prevalence of health outcomes. The results of such analyses can help to target scarce public health resources. Scientists are now approaching epidemiology at the molecular level, looking at gene/environment interactions.

As described in Chapter 12, three major concepts—agent, host, and environment—form the classic **epidemiologic triangle**. (See Figure 12-2, *A* in Chapter 12.) This simple model belies the often-complex relationships between **agent**, which may include chemical mixtures (i.e., more than one agent); **host**, which may refer to a community with people of multiple ages, genders, ethnicities, cultures, and disease states; and **environment**, which may include dynamic factors such as air, water, soil, and food, as well as temperature, humidity, and wind. Limitations of environmental epidemiologic data include reliance on occupational health studies to characterize certain toxic exposures. The occupational health studies were performed on healthy adult workers whose biological systems were different from those of neonates, pregnant women, children, people who are immunosuppressed, and the elderly. Nevertheless, nurses can review epidemiologic studies regarding exposures of concern to their communities and use epidemiologic techniques to assess environmental risks in communities.

## Geographic Information Systems

Another research tool for environmental health studies is **geographic information systems** (GIS), a methodology that requires the coding of data so that it is related spatially to a place on Earth. By layering geographically related data, maps can be created to note where the data may be related. For instance, by taking a data set that geographically notes where children under 10 years of age live and overlaying another data set that notes geographical areas designated by the age of housing stock, a public health nurse could see where there are the largest number of children who live in areas with older housing stock. With this information, the nurse could target a lead surveillance and educational program. Nurse researcher Mona Choi used GIS to study the relationship between air pollution and emergency visits for cardiovascular and pulmonary diagnosis. Community-based maps that are created using GIS technologies are helpful in educating community members and local policy makers. The maps can provide useful graphic depictions of public health problems.

Environmental health requires a combination of tried and tested nursing tools mixed with new tools, such as GIS, and the recognition that many disciplines may be involved in the identification and the resolution of environmental health issues.

Nurse scientists Wade Hill and Patricia Butterfield (2006) developed a model for environmental risk interventions, which can be provided by public health nurses, that improves children's health by addressing home-related sources such as lead paint, contaminated drinking water, and environmental tobacco smoke, among others. These risks can cause health effects ranging from minor learning deficiencies to serious and life-threatening diseases such as cancer. Many of the environmental risks children encountered were prevented or reduced by taking practical and affordable steps. Butterfield developed an environmental justice framework by which to consider environmental exposures in rural areas (Butterfield & Postma, 2009).

## Multidisciplinary Approaches

In addition to toxicology and epidemiology, there are a number of earth sciences to help us understand how pollutants travel in air, water, and soil. Geologists, meteorologists, physicists, and chemists all contribute information to help explain how and when humans may be exposed to hazardous chemicals, radiation (e.g., radon), and biological contaminants. Key public health professionals include food safety specialists, sanitarians, radiation specialists, and industrial hygienists.

The nature of environmental health demands a multidisciplinary approach to assess and reduce/eliminate environmental health risks. For instance, to assess and address a lead-based paint poisoning case we might include a housing inspector with expertise in lead-based paint or a sanitarian to assess the lead-associated health risks in the home; clinical specialists to manage the client's health needs; laboratories to assess the blood lead levels, as well as lead levels in the paint and house dust and drinking water; and then lead-based paint remediation specialists to reduce the lead-based paint risk in the home.

We might also add a health educator and outreach worker to educate the family and encourage compliance with environmental health behaviors and clinical treatments. And finally, we may need to work with public health lawyers to address noncompliant landlords. Such combined approaches could potentially involve the local health department, the state department of environmental protection, the housing department, a primary and tertiary care setting, public or private sector labs, and the legal system. The nurse's responsibility is to understand the roles of each respective agency and organization, know the public health laws (particularly as they pertain to lead-based paint poisoning in their communities), and work with the community to coordinate services to meet their needs. The nurse also might set up a blood lead screening program through the local health department, educate local health providers to encourage them to systematically test children for lead poisoning, and/or work with advocacy organizations to improve the condition of local housing stock. Note that although lead-based paint is no longer in use in the United States, it is still widely used in developing countries.

---

### QSEN FOCUS ON QUALITY AND SAFETY EDUCATION FOR NURSES

**Targeted Competency:** Function effectively within nursing and interprofessional teams, fostering open communication, mutual respect, and shared decision making to achieve quality client care.

**Knowledge:** Describe scopes of practice and roles of health care team members.

**Skills:** Assume the role of team member or leader based on the situation.

**Attitudes:** Value the perspectives and expertise of all health team members.

**Safety Question:** One of the objectives of *Healthy People 2020* related to environmental health is "Reduce pesticide exposures that result in visits to a health care facility" (ED 8-10). The public health nurse, who is working on a project to help mothers learn parenting skills, visits a new mother who lives and works on a large farm. When the nurse drives into the farm on her way to the housing where workers live, she sees that the fields are being sprayed with pesticides from a truck and that two young children are riding in the back of the truck. What action should she take?

**Answer:** At the individual level, she should talk with the owner or manager of the farm and remind him or her of the toxicity of pesticides and the danger to those who are in the vicinity of the spraying. She should recommend that he or she not allow anyone to ride in the open portion of the vehicle and that the driver should leave the window closed and wear a mask to protect his or her nose and mouth.

**Systems level:** She should identify areas where the workers on the farms congregate, such as churches, social halls, and so forth. Then she should ask if she could provide an educational program on the dangers of coming into contact with pesticides. She could distribute pamphlets about this hazard in local venues where both farm managers and workers will be able to access them. What else might the nurse do?

---

## CLIMATE CHANGE

According to the World Health Organization, "climate change is a significant and emerging threat to public health, and changes the way we must look at protecting vulnerable populations" (WHO, 2014b). The 2014 report of the Intergovernmental Program on Climate Change, a WHO-related group of scientists, concludes that "climate change will act mainly, at least until the middle of this century, by exacerbating health problems that already exist, and the largest risks will apply in populations that are currently most affected by climate-related diseases" (IPCC, 2014). In the United States we are already seeing some of the earlier climate change predictions materialize: long-term warming trends, extreme weather conditions, as well as

disruption in water supplies, agriculture, ecosystems, and coastal communities.

There are two concurrent categories of roles for nurses: mitigation and response. There is still much we can do to mitigate the steep upward slope that we are now observing for temperatures, $CO_2$ levels, desertification, and sea water levels. Working at the individual, community, institutional (school, hospital, etc.), and governmental levels, there is much work to be done to ensure energy-conserving policies and practices, rational transportation practices, and changes in our consumption patterns.

Regarding response preparation, public health nurses must lead the development of contingencies for long-term, high-heat weather conditions, as well as increased storm activities (that include more severe storm patterns), more extensive fires in areas prone to fires, and the associated disaster preparedness. For more on disaster preparedness, see Chapter 23 on nurses' roles in disaster management. Nurses should also be prepared for threats to food security from shifting weather patterns that may deter/eliminate food production and for acute shifts of populations as they migrate away from low-lying, coastal regions or other areas acutely affected by storm or fire damage. These shifts are likely to create climate change–related refugee migrations.

The oil spill in the Gulf of Mexico was the largest in history and caused devastating damage. It is expected that its effects on birds, fish, and other sea animals, as well as the environment, will continue for many more years. Since fish populations were affected, many fishermen lost their jobs and the livelihood that they knew (Gulf Oil Spill, n.d.). This type of ecosystem destruction and economic disruption will be typical if we do not address climate change and our associated need to reduce/eliminate our reliance on fossil fuels (gas, oil, coal). It is important to explore the science underpinning climate change, consider the human and ecological health threats, and reflect on nurses emerging roles as climate change unfold.

## ENVIRONMENTAL HEALTH ASSESSMENTS

There are a number of ways to assess environmental health risks in a community. For example, risks can be assessed by medium: air, water, soil, or food. Or exposures could be listed according to urban, rural, or suburban settings, with many exposures being common to all three settings. Nurses may also divide the environment into functional locations such as home, school, workplace, and community. Each of these locations will have unique environmental exposures, as well as overlapping exposures. For instance, ethylene oxide, the toxic gas that is used in the sterilizing equipment in hospitals, is typically found only in a workplace. However, pesticides might be found in any of the four areas. When assessing environments, be sure to determine if an exposure is in the air, water, soil, and/or food and whether it is a chemical, biological, or radiological exposure.

### Information Sources

The NLM has developed some of the most useful, comprehensive, and reliable sources of environmental health information.

The NLM's website for ToxTown (http://toxtown.nlm.nih.gov/) is one of the best places to start when developing environmental assessment skills. Within ToxTown, there is a Household Products page where nurses can research common products such as those for personal care, cleaning, pet care, lawn care, and others to see the potential health risks that may be associated with them. Also, chemicals can be researched by brand or chemical name or by Chemical Abstract System number. (The NLM website can be accessed at www.nlm.nih.gov; at the website, search for the environmental assessment section.)

Also within ToxTown, you can search for general environmental health risks in the "city," "town," and "farm," or even go to a "US–Mexico Border Community." While in the virtual "city" you can visit a hair salon, hospital, or funeral home to see what kinds of environmental health risks are posed in such places. ToxTown brings together governmental and well-vetted nongovernmental sources for a rich web resource in which to learn about environmental health.

Another database that is specific to personal care products, which includes over 68,000 products that can be searched by brand name and specific product descriptors, is the Skin Deep database (http://www.ewg.org/skindeep/). The Safe Cosmetics website, which links to the Skin Deep database, additionally provides information on better protecting your health by selecting products that have simpler ingredients and fewer synthetic chemicals. For example, the site points out that even top-selling brands of natural and organic products may have some toxic components. Specifically, they say that some top-selling herbal shampoos contain 1,4-dioxane, a synthetic chemical carcinogen. They also comment on the number of lipsticks that they found to contain lead. Note that in both the NLM and the Safe Cosmetics databases, the information is predicated on what the manufacturers place on the label as ingredients (Figure 10-2). If the manufacturer claims that a component is a "trade secret," it will not appear on the label. Rarely are the chemicals that make up a "fragrance" listed on the label; instead, it is likely to only read "fragrance" on the label. And finally (and this is especially true with pesticides), the label may merely say "inerts"

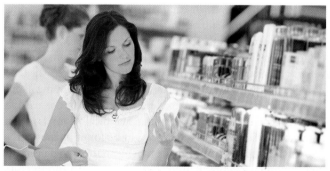

**FIG 10-2** Some of the chemicals in our personal care products can be hazardous to our health. You can look up the chemicals in your products and learn about the potential health risks by going to the SkinDeep database: http://www.ewg.org/skindeep/. (Photo from the U.S. Food and Drug Administration. Available at http://www.fda.gov/Cosmetics/default.htm?wvsessionid=1724ec6bbda343c6b7d0e092db6c2f30.)

without any further information about their chemical identity. Thus, it is sometimes impossible to make a true assessment about the health risks based on the information provided by the manufacturer.

One of the ANA Environmental Health Principles is the tenet of the "Right to Know," which recommends the need for access to all information necessary to make informed decisions and protect our health. There are still a number of ways in which full disclosure of chemical exposure is lacking in terms of air and water pollution, food contents, and product ingredients. Nurses, both individually and through their professional organizations, can advocate for increasing access to information through "right to know," labeling, and other legislative and regulatory efforts.

## APPLYING THE NURSING PROCESS TO ENVIRONMENTAL HEALTH

If you suspect that a client's health problem is being influenced by environmental factors, follow the nursing process and note the environmental aspects of the problem in every step of the process:

1. *Assessment.* Use your observational skills (e.g., windshield surveys); interview community members; ask your individual clients; and ask the families of your clients. Review web-based data on existing exposures, such as air and water pollution monitoring data, drinking water testing, and contaminated soil. Relate the disease and the environmental factors in the diagnosis.
2. *Planning.* Look at community policy and laws as methods to facilitate the care needs for the client; include environmental health personnel in planning.
3. *Intervention.* Coordinate medical, nursing, and public health actions to meet the client's needs. Ensure that the affected person or family is referred for appropriate clinical care.
4. *Evaluation.* Examine criteria that include the immediate and long-term responses of the client as well as the recidivism of the problem for the client.

### Individual Environmental Exposure History

When working with individuals, it is important to include environmental health risks as part of a client's history. Ask certain questions to assess exposures that may occur in all of the settings in which they spend time. A helpful mnemonic was developed to assist health professionals in remembering the areas of concern when taking an environmental history: "I PREPARE." The mnemonic (see Box 10-3) can be used when interviewing an individual client or when assessing a family or it can be adapted for use with a group of community members.

### Community-wide Environmental Health Assessment Tools

Nurses have developed several exposure assessment tools, including forms for pregnant women, home and school assessments, community-wide assessments, and assessment tools for hospital-related exposures. The web links on the Evolve site for this book include several examples of environmental assessment tools.

substandard housing (with attendant risks of chipping and peeling paint, pests, and unsafe neighborhoods), live closer to pollution sources, are employed in more dangerous occupations, and have less access to healthy food options. In addition, vulnerability is variable through the human life cycle. The embryo and fetus are the most vulnerable to chemical exposures because of the rapid growth of cells and the development of tissues, organs, and organ systems. Following is a section on children's special vulnerabilities. The very young and the very old also are vulnerable because their body systems are either still developing or are less efficient, respectively. For more information about the special vulnerabilities of the elderly, see the EPA's dedicated information site on older Americans (www.epa.gov/aging/) and look at their report "Growing Smarter/Living Healthier: A Guide to Smart Growth and Active Aging (http://www.epa.gov/aging/docs/growing-smarter-living-healthier.pdf). For more information on the effects of perinatal exposures, the University of California San Francisco has a Program on Reproduction and Environment that provides informational webinars, factsheets, the latest research and policy/advocacy information available at http://www.prhe.ucsf.edu.

## Children's Environmental Health

Consider some of the current childhood health statistics with which environmental factors are associated: approximately 9% of American children suffer from asthma, with higher rates in black children (CDC, 2012). About 20% of the world's children and adolescents suffer from a mental health problem (WHO, n.d.), and this statistic is mirrored in the United States (DHHS, 2005). The CDC monitoring system for autism spectrum disorders reports that the prevalence of autism among 8-year-olds in the United States is 1 in every 68 children (CDC, 2014a). The global prevalence of autism has increased twentyfold to thirtyfold since the earliest epidemiologic studies were conducted in the late 1960s and early 1970s. And millions of homes in the United States continue to have chipping and peeling lead-based paint.

Developmental disorders and attention deficit hyperactivity disorder (ADHD) collectively are estimated to affect 17% of school-age children (AHRQ, 2002; Anney et al, 2006). Child obesity has doubled and adolescent obesity has more than quadrupled in the last 30 years (CDC, 2014b). From 1975 to 2010 the incidence rates for 4 cancer types, acute lymphocytic leukemia, non-Hodgkin lymphoma, acute myeloid leukemia, and testicular germ cell tumors, increased in children (ACS, 2014). The most common cancers among children ages 0 through 14 are acute lymphocytic leukemia, brain and CNS, neuroblastoma, and non-Hodgkin lymphoma (ACS, 2014, p. 25). "All cancers involve the malfunction of genes that control cell growth and division. Only a small proportion of cancers are strongly hereditary..." (ACS, 2014, p. 1). According to the American Cancer Society (ACS), about 5% of all cancers are strongly associated with heredity (ACS, 2010). The rest occur from environmental exposures, lifestyle choices (diet, smoking, etc.), and other factors during our lifetimes.

Over the past 25 years there has been great improvement in the 5-year survival rate of major childhood cancers. The 5-year survival rate for children for all cancer sites improved from 58% for those diagnosed between 1975 and 1977 to 81% for children diagnosed between 1999 and 2007 (Jemal et al, 2010). The list of possible causes of children's cancers includes the following: genetic abnormalities, ultraviolet and ionizing radiation, electromagnetic fields, viral infections, certain medications, food additives, tobacco, alcohol, and industrial and agricultural chemicals (Ross and Olshan, 2004; Bassil et al, 2007). Clearly, the environment is playing an important role.

### EVIDENCE-BASED PRACTICE

Gilden et al examined the use of pesticides on athletic fields where children play sports. This cross-sectional descriptive study used a survey to assess playing field maintenance practices related to the use of pesticides on the field. The authors gave the survey to 33 field managers in order to assess maintenance practices. Their data were analyzed using descriptive statistics and generalized estimating equations.

They found that 65.3% of the managers said they applied pesticides, primarily herbicides, to the fields. They also found that managers of urban and suburban fields were less likely to apply pesticides than were managers of rural fields. The use of pesticides presents many health hazards, and the results of this study demonstrated that children who engage in sports activities on athletic fields are exposed to health hazards.

- Nurse Use: Nurses can inform people such as school officials, coaches, and field managers of the dangers of using pesticides on athletic fields.

Gilden R, Friedmann E, Sattler B, et al: Potential health effects related to pesticide use on athletic fields. *Public Health Nursing* 29(3):198-207, May/June 2012.

Children are not just little adults. They are different in many ways, particularly with regard to their exposures and responses to the environment. As nurses, we know that infants and young children breathe more rapidly than adults, and this increase in respiratory rate translates to a proportionately greater exposure to air pollutants. While infants' lungs are developing they are particularly susceptible to environmental toxicants. Although full function of the lungs is attained at approximately age 6, changes continue to occur in the lungs through adolescence (Dietert et al, 2000). Children are short and, as such, their breathing zones are lower than adults, causing them to have closer contact to the chemical and biological agents that accumulate on floors and carpeting. Children of color and poor children in America are disproportionately affected by a range of environmental health threats, including lead, air pollution, pesticides, incinerator emissions, and exposures from hazardous waste sites (Suk and Davis, 2008; Landrigan et al, 2010).

In clinical settings, there is little that can be done to address a child's body burden of toxic chemicals; however, the nursing community as a profession has a weighty obligation to understand the science and risks associated with environmental pollutants and to engage in the political and economic decisions regulating the environment that have a profound effect on human health, especially the health of our children. This engagement occurs in policy-making arenas including legislative, regulatory, and international treaties. Nurses have increasingly become involved in the policy arena. The Alliance of Nurses for Healthy Environments is actively engaging nurses in state and federal chemical policies and energy policies (including fracking) as they relate to health, and policies related to sustainable foods.

Children's bodies also operate differently. Some of the protective mechanisms that are well developed in adults, like the blood–brain barrier, are immature in young children, thereby increasing their vulnerability to the effects of toxic chemicals. And finally, the kidneys of young children are less effective at filtering out undesirable toxic chemicals, and these chemicals then continue to circulate and accumulate.

Infants and young children drink more fluids per body weight than adults, thus increasing the dose of contaminants found in their drinking water, milk (hormones and antibiotics), and juices (particularly pesticides). If an adult were to drink a proportionate amount of water to an infant, the adult would have to drink about 50 glasses of water a day. Children also eat more per body weight, eat different proportions of food, and absorb food differently than adults (EPA, 2013). How many adults could eat the same amount of raisins pound-for-pound as the average 2-year-old? Children consume much greater quantities of fruits and fruit juices than adults, once again adding exposure to doses of pesticide residues. The average 1-year-old drinks 21 times more apple juice, 11 times more grape juice, and nearly 5 times more orange juice per unit of body weight than the average adult (Rawn et al, 2004). The Food Quality Protection Act (FQPA) was passed to specifically address the consumption patterns and special vulnerabilities of children (Box 10-5).

---

**BOX 10-5    Provisions Under the Food Quality Protection Act Regarding Pesticide Exposure to Children from Multiple Sources**

New provisions under the Food Quality Protection Act of 1996 related to protection of infants and children:

*Health-based standard:* A new standard of a reasonable certainty of "no harm" that prohibits taking into account economic considerations when children are at risk.

*Additional margin of safety:* Requires that the EPA use an additional 10-fold margin of safety when there are adequate data to assess prenatal and postnatal development risks.

*Account for children's diet:* Requires the use of age-appropriate estimates of dietary consumption in establishing allowable levels of pesticides on food to account for children's unique dietary patterns.

*Account for all exposures:* In establishing acceptable levels of a pesticide on food, the EPA must account for exposures that may occur through other routes, such as drinking water and residential application of the pesticide.

*Cumulative impact:* The EPA must consider the cumulative impact of all pesticides that may share a common mechanism of action.

*Tolerance reassessments:* All existing pesticide food standards must be reassessed over a 10-year period to ensure that they meet the new standards to protect children.

*Endocrine disruption testing:* The EPA must screen and test all pesticides and pesticide ingredients for estrogen effects and other endocrine disruptor activity.

*Registration renewal:* Establishes a 15-year renewal process for all pesticides to ensure that they have up-to-date science evaluations over time.

From Environmental Protection Agency: Food Quality Protection Act of 1996. Available at http://www.epa.gov/pesticides/regulation/laws/fgpa/. Accessed December 15, 2010.

---

Toxic chemicals can have different effects depending on the timing of exposure. During fetal development, there are periods of exquisite sensitivity to the effects of toxic chemicals. During such times, even extraordinarily small exposures can prevent or change a process that may permanently affect normal development. The brain undergoes rapid structural and functional changes during late pregnancy and in the neonatal period. Therefore, it is extremely important to safeguard women's environments when they are pregnant (Table 10-1).

Alarmingly, 27 states have issued mercury contamination advisories for fish in *every* lake and river within their state's borders (EPA, 2009). According to the EPA, more than 1 million women in the United States of childbearing age eat sufficient amounts of mercury-contaminated fish to risk damaging brain development of their children. Nurses in all settings need to understand the implications that the fish advisories have for their clients and communities, and the contribution that the health sector has in creating this health risk, while at the same time counseling on the positive contribution of fish to a nutritionally balanced diet.

About 84,000 chemicals are used in commerce in the United States (EPA, 2014). Almost all are man-made; 15,000 of them are produced annually in quantities greater than 10,000 lb and 2800 of them are produced in quantities greater than 1 million pounds per year (Goldman and Koduru, 2000). Of the 2,800, only 7% have been tested for developmental effects and only 43% have been tested for any human health effects.

Companies are not required to divulge the results of their private testing. A full battery of neurotoxicity tests is not required even for pesticides that may be sprayed in nurseries and labor and delivery areas, not to mention in homes. To make things even more complicated, risks from multiple chemical exposures are rarely considered when regulations are drafted. Such an omission ignores the reality that both children and adults are exposed to many toxic chemicals, often concurrently. The only exception to this rule is in the case of regulations regarding pesticides that are used on food (Figure 10-4). This exception was created by the 1996 FQPA, in which Congress acknowledged that children eat foods that may be contaminated by more than one pesticide residue. See Box 10-5 for the provisions under the FQPA.

## PRECAUTIONARY PRINCIPLE

With thousands of chemical compounds now creating a chemical soup in our air and water (and in our bodies, in our breast milk), it is increasingly difficult to prove specific hypotheses regarding the relationship of exposure to a singular chemical and disease outcome in humans. It has been suggested that we adopt a precautionary approach when research and other indicators demonstrate a possible toxic relationship between a chemical and health. Box 10-6 presents the *Wingspread Statement on the Precautionary Principle*. This precautionary approach calls for action to reduce potentially toxic exposure to humans in light of data or other indicators, rather than delaying until more "conclusive" studies are performed. We will never have the perfect studies. Nurses, who are trained in disease

## TABLE 10-1    Workplace Hazards to Women of Reproductive Age*

| Agent | Observed Effects | Potentially Exposed Workers |
|---|---|---|
| Cancer treatment drugs (e.g., methotrexate) | Infertility, miscarriage, birth defects, low birth weight | Health care workers, pharmacists |
| Organic solvents (e.g., toluene, xylene, formaldehyde) | Miscarriage | Health care workers, laboratory workers, print shop and manufacturing employees |
| Lead | Infertility, miscarriage, low birth weight, developmental disorders | Battery makers, solderers, welders, bridge repainters, firing range workers, home remodelers |
| Strenuous physical tabor (e.g., prolonged standing, shift/night work) | Miscarriage, preterm delivery | Many types of workers |
| Cytomegalovirus | Birth defects, low birth weight, developmental disorders | Health care workers, workers who have contact with infants and children |
| Parvovirus B19 | Miscarriage | Health care workers, workers who have contact with infants and children |
| Rubella | Birth defects, low birth weight | Health care workers, workers in who have contact with infants and children |
| Toxoplasmosis | Miscarriage, birth defects, developmental disorders | Animal care workers, veterinarians |
| Varicella zoster | Birth defects, low birth weight | Health care workers, workers who have contact with infants and children |

*This list is not complete. Information about these hazards is constantly being revised. Readers should not assume that a substance is safe if it is missing from this list.
Source: National Institute for Occupational Safety and Health (www.cdc.gov/niosh/99-104.html)

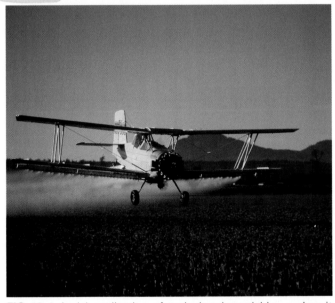

FIG 10-4 Aerial application of agricultural pesticides makes it very difficult to control exposures. The chemicals get tracked into homes in farming communities. (Copyright © 2011 Photos. com, a division of Getty Images. All rights reserved. Photo #87531230.)

prevention, appreciate and should advocate for a precautionary approach when it may prevent injuries or illnesses. The ANA has adopted the precautionary principle as the basic tenet on which to guide its environmental advocacy work.

The bottom line is that life depends on the environment, and what humans do collectively can affect this vital resource for present and future generations. A central concept in Native American cultures is that humans are stewards, not proprietors, of the environment. Native Americans make the "Rule of Seven" central to all environmental decisions: What will be the effect on the seventh generation? A quote (Myths-Dreams-Symbols, 2006) attributed to Chief Seattle, a nineteenth-century Native American, illustrates the need to think more holistically when we consider environmental impacts: "Whatever befalls the earth befalls the sons of the earth. Man did not weave the web of life; he is merely a strand in it. Whatever he does to the web, he does to himself." McDonough suggests that, as we make policies, plans, and designs, we ask ourselves how these decision are evidence that "we love all the children of all the species for all times" (Huff interview with McDonough, 2013).

Mary O'Brien, in her book *Making Better Environmental Decisions: An Alternative to Risk Assessments*, notes that we are repeatedly given a very short list of risk reduction choices, and that the public is not effectively engaged in the decision-making process. She suggests that a broader range of options would allow us to see the possibilities for further reducing (or even eliminating) risks and that the process should be much more democratic in nature. O'Brien suggests the best approach to making effective environmental decisions is to use information, emotion, and a sense of relationship to others concurrently. By "others" she means other species, cultures, and generations (O'Brien, 2000). Her method is consistent with a nursing approach. Using her approach will require that nurses more actively engage in environmental health—assessing environmental health risks, developing risk reduction strategies, and supporting policies that embrace the precautionary principle and care for all of the children of all of the species for all times.

## ENVIRONMENTAL HEALTH RISK REDUCTION

Prevention is a core goal in every public health intervention. Preventing problems is less costly whether the cost is measured in resources consumed or in human health effects. Policies, as well as practices, can promote primary prevention. After we have assessed the environmental risks in our communities, we

### BOX 10-6    Wingspread Statement on the Precautionary Principle

In 1998 an international group of health and public health professionals, scientists, government officials, lawyers, grassroots activists, and labor activists met at a conference center called "Wingspread" in Wisconsin to define the "precautionary principle." The group issued the following consensus statement:

The release and use of toxic substances, the exploitation of resources, and physical alterations of the environment have had substantial unintended consequences affecting human health and the environment. Some of these concerns are high rates of learning deficiencies, asthma, cancer, birth defects and species extinctions, along with global climate change, stratospheric ozone depletion and worldwide contamination with toxic substances and nuclear materials.

We believe existing environmental regulations and other decisions, particularly those based on risk assessment, have failed to protect adequately human health and the environment the larger system of which humans are but a part.

We believe there is compelling evidence that damage to humans and the worldwide environment is of such magnitude and seriousness that new principles for conducting human activities are necessary.

While we realize that human activities may involve hazards, people must proceed more carefully than has been the case in recent history. Corporations, government entities, organizations, communities, scientists and other individuals must adopt a precautionary approach to all human endeavors.

Therefore, it is necessary to implement the Precautionary Principle: When an activity raises threats of harm to human health or the environment, precautionary measures should be taken even if some cause and effect relationships are not fully established scientifically. In this context the proponent of an activity, rather than the public, should bear the burden of proof.

The process of applying the Precautionary Principle must be open, informed and democratic and must include potentially affected parties. It must also involve an examination of the full range of alternatives, including no action.

Wingspread Statement on the Precautionary Principle, Racine WI, 1998. Available at http://www.gdrc.org/u-gov/precaution-3.html. Retrieved March 12, 2015.

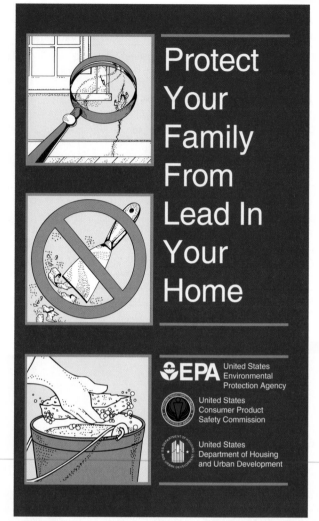

**FIG 10-5** Lead can be found in many places in a home. Nurses should help families learn about these sources and take actions to remove any lead-based paint using certified professionals. Good hygiene is key to reducing lead dust exposure, especially given that urban soot will often have lead from the legacy of lead used in gasoline for many decades. (From U.S. Environmental Protection Agency. Available at http://www.epa.gov/lead/pubs/leadpdfe.pdf. Accessed December 29, 2010.)

can apply the basic principles of disease prevention when planning intervention strategies. For lead exposure, remediating a home with lead-based paint to make it lead safe applies the primary prevention strategy of removing the exposure (at least from that specific source of lead) (Figure 10-5). Even good lead poisoning surveillance will not prevent lead exposure, but may help with early detection of rising blood lead levels. Such surveillance is a secondary prevention strategy. Finally, when a symptomatic child is seen, it is important to have a health care system readily available in which specialists familiar with lead poisoning will provide swift medical interventions to reduce blood lead levels, thus reducing the risk of further harm. This is a tertiary prevention response. Box 10-7 presents examples of risk reduction strategies for nurses in the health care setting.

### Industrial Hygiene Hierarchy of Controls

For workplace exposures, industrial hygienists have developed a "hierarchy of control" for avoiding or minimizing employee exposures to potentially hazardous chemicals. Industrial hygienists are public health professionals who specialize in workplace exposures to hazards—physical, chemical, and biological—that create the conditions for health risks (Box 10-8 presents the industrial hygiene hierarchy of controls). Once it is established that a human health threat exists, develop a plan of action—a way of eliminating or managing (reducing) the risk. Risk management should be informed by the risk assessment process and involves the selection and implementation of a strategy to eliminate or reduce risks.

Box 10-9 lists the 3 Rs for reducing environmental pollution.

Nursing interventions to reduce environmental health risks can take many forms. Education is one example of a nursing intervention. By working with a wide array of community

## BOX 10-7 Risk Reduction: Every Nurse's Role

In the health care setting (hospital, clinic, home health), we have many opportunities to make environmentally friendly and healthy choices:

- Shift to electronic records, thus avoiding the use of paper. When paper is a must, use products that are made from recycled ingredients
- Recycle: paper, glass, cans, plastic, small batteries, blue wrap, electronic equipment
- Work with suppliers to get products with minimum packaging and the safest ingredients possible: "environmentally preferable purchasing"
- Promote the use of green cleaners
- Go fragrance free by using fragrance-free products in the hospital and creating a policy that requires employees to use fragrance-free personal care products (shampoos, creams, etc.)
- Turn off lights AND computers AND patient monitoring equipment when rooms are not being used
- Report leaky sinks, toilets, and other plumbing sources
- Promote the purchase of local, sustainably grown foods (with a preference for organic, no use of GMOs, no use of unnecessary antibiotics, and no pesticides)
- Start a hospital/clinic/health department garden
- Start a Green Team, or join the existing one in your institution
- Create community while doing these activities and build relationships—it makes the whole process more meaningful and fun!

## BOX 10-8 Industrial Hygiene Hierarchy of Controls*

**Eliminate** unnecessary toxic chemicals.
**Substitute** less hazardous or nonhazardous substances (e.g., using water-based vs. solvent-based products).
**Isolate** the hazardous chemicals from human exposure (e.g., use closed systems).
**Apply engineering controls** (e.g., ventilation systems, including exhaust hoods).
Reduce the exposures through **administrative controls** (e.g., rotating employees in areas with high exposures).
Use **personal protective equipment** (e.g., gloves, respirators, protective clothing).

*In addition, education is a critical tool in the hierarchy of controls. Modified from Levy B, Wegman D: Occupational health: recognizing and preventing work-related disease and injury, ed 4, Philadelphia, 2000, Lippincott Williams & Wilkins.

## BOX 10-9 The 3 Rs for Reducing Environmental Pollution

The "3 Rs" adage of the environmentalist community—*reduce, reuse,* and *recycle*—helps us consider ways to decrease our personal impact on the environment, and thereby decrease environmental health risks. These concepts can apply to our health care settings, as well as our homes. By recycling, we prevent the need to extract more resources from the earth to manufacture products. By recycling, we also prevent products from unnecessary landfilling or incineration. Choosing reusable products, versus single-use devices and products, similarly prevents the need for manufacturing more products and decreases the waste stream. Reducing our waste stream can also be accomplished generally by a reduction in consumption (buying less "stuff," as well as by reducing unnecessary packaging and other nonessential goods). The "Story of Stuff" (www.thestoryofstuff.org) provides an excellent overview of the "cradle to grave" travels of products and the full range of their human and ecological impacts.

members, nurses can help a community understand the relationship between harmful environmental exposures and human health and guide the community toward risk reduction on the basis of both individual behavior changes, as well as community-wide approaches. In communities in which radon is likely to be a naturally occurring exposure, nurses can educate the community about the health risks, methods to measure radon levels in a home, and how to address unhealthy radon levels.

Nurses work with individuals, families, and communities in all three levels of prevention. For example, in Planned Parenthood Clinics in the United States, as a form of primary prevention, clinicians ask clients about possible environmental health risks in their everyday lives and then direct them to safer products and healthier behaviors to decrease potentially toxic exposures. Secondary prevention takes place when pediatric clinics include lead screening as part of their protocols. By doing so they are apt to find children with elevated blood lead levels, which then allow them to act to decrease the child's environmental lead exposures. This form of secondary prevention does not actually prevent the exposure but calls for action based on evidence of exposure. If a child has a seriously high blood lead level, the child would be admitted to the hospital for chelation therapy which is a process used to decrease the body's burden of lead.

## LEVELS OF PREVENTION

### Example Applied to Lead-Based Paint Exposure

**Primary Prevention**
Eliminate lead-based paint and lead-based paint dust from the home.

**Secondary Prevention**
Provide blood lead testing of children in communities with older housing stock.

**Tertiary Prevention**
When a child presents with extremely elevated blood lead levels, make sure the child is being cared for by a health professional who is familiar with clinical interventions to reduce blood lead levels using clinical (chelating medications) interventions, **while concurrently assuring that the child returns to a lead-safe place.**

The clinical intervention is tertiary prevention. It neither prevents the exposure, nor focuses on decreasing the exposure, but rather focuses on decreasing the potential health sequela associated with elevated lead levels.

## Risk Communication

Risk communication is both an area of practice and a skill that is a composite of two separate words: "risk" and "communication." *Risk* is a familiar term in nursing practice. It is understood in the health context when we counsel patients about the risks of pregnancy, communicable disease (especially sexually transmitted disease), unintentional injury, and risk associated with personal choices (e.g., smoking, alcohol consumption, and diet). Risk assessment in environmental health focuses on characterizing the hazard (the "source"), its physical and chemical properties, its toxicity, and the potential exposure pathways—mode of transmission, route of exposure, receptor population, and dose. In their seminal work on risk communication,

---

### BOX 10-10    Definitions of Risk

Risk has traditionally been defined by the following equation:

$$Risk = magnitude \times probability$$

There is a growing body of literature from practitioners and researchers who have studied the human reaction to risk—real and perceived. Sandman et al (1991) were the first to examine the "outrage" factor that can influence the way in which we perceive risk, particularly to environmental risks.

$$Risk = hazard + outrage$$

Addressing only the hazard is doing only half of the necessary work; addressing the response (outrage) is equally important.

From Sandman PM, Chess C, Hane BJ: Improving dialogue with communities, New Brunswick, NJ, 1991, Rutgers University.

---

### BOX 10-11    Outrage Factors: Characteristics of Risk That Contribute to the Public's Feeling of Outrage

| Safer = Less Outrage | Less Safe = More Outrage |
|---|---|
| **12 Principal Outrage Components** | |
| Voluntary | Involuntary (coerced) |
| Natural | Industrial (artificial) |
| Familiar | Exotic |
| Not memorable | Memorable |
| Not dreaded | Dreaded |
| Chronic | Catastrophic |
| Knowable (detectable) | Unknowable (undetectable) |
| Individually controlled | Controlled by others |
| Fair | Unfair |
| Morally irrelevant | Morally relevant |
| Trustworthy sources | Untrustworthy sources |
| Responsive process | Unresponsive process |

---

Sandman, Chess, and Hane (1991) noted that risk has traditionally been formulated as magnitude (the size, severity, extent of area, or population affected) multiplied by the probability (how likely exposure or damage is to occur) (Box 10-10). For example, an environmental risk assessment of a contaminated site would involve a calculation of the dose that might be received through all routes of exposure, the toxicity of the chemical, the size and vulnerability (age, health) of the population potentially exposed (resident, future resident, transient), and the likelihood of exposure. Sandman et al (1991) also noted that the reaction to things that scare people and the things that kill people are often not related to the actual hazard. They have gone further to probe what is behind those differences and identified a list of "outrage factors" to explain people's responses to risk (Box 10-11). They maintain that the outrage is just as predictable and open to intervention as the science of addressing the hazard.

"Communication" of risk involves understanding the outrage factors relevant to the risk being addressed so they can be incorporated in the message—the information—either to create action to ensure safety or prevent harm or to reduce unnecessary fear. An example of raising outrage to produce action can be seen in the shift from emphasis on smokers (voluntary) to victims of passive smoking (involuntary) to stimulate public policy that limits or bans smoking in public places. When the emphasis on risk went from a voluntary choice of smokers to an involuntary exposure of nonsmokers, the outrage level of the nonsmoking public became high enough to result in legislation guaranteeing smoke-free public spaces (e.g., public buildings, airplanes, and restaurants).

On the other hand, outrage decreases when people receive information on the situation from a trusted source, and physicians and nurses are often cited in surveys as trusted sources of information on environmental risks (Kaiser Foundation, 2013). The public trust is a compelling incentive to match professional knowledge and skills to a community's expectations. The outrage factor can also be a driving force in building credibility and trustworthiness in every person whose work involves interacting with the public.

Risk communication includes all the principles of good communication in general. It is a combination of the following:
- *The right information:* Accurate, relevant, in a language that audiences can understand. A good risk assessment is essential information for shaping the message.
- *To the right people:* Those affected and those who are worried but may not be affected. Information on the community is essential: geographic boundaries, who lives there (i.e., demographics), how they obtain information (e.g., flyers or newspapers, radio, television, word of mouth), where they congregate (e.g., school, church, community center), and who within the community can help plan the communication.
- *At the right time:* For timely action or to allay fear.

## GOVERNMENTAL ENVIRONMENTAL PROTECTION

The government has a variety of tools to address environmental exposures. In addition to passing legislation, creating and enforcing standards and regulations, deciding how land should be used, providing permits, and supporting research, the government is actively engaged in educating the public. Many federal agencies are involved in environmental health regulation, such as the EPA, the FDA, and the Department of Agriculture. The Department of Health and Human Services (DHHS) has two major research institutes, the National Institute of Environmental Health Science (NIEHS) and the National Institute of Occupational Safety and Health (NIOSH). Within DHHS is the CDC (which includes the National Center for Environmental Health [NCEH] that is responsible for tracking environmental health trends, recommending clinical and public health practices, and also engaging in research). Every state has an agency responsible for environmental quality. At the city or county level, the local health department most often manages environmental health issues. However, environmental protection issues are typically directed by the state using both federal and state laws. Box 10-12 lists key environmental protection laws.

Potentially harmful pollution that cannot be prevented must be controlled. An important step in the process of controlling pollution is permitting, a process by which the government

## BOX 10-12   Environmental Laws

### National Environmental Policy Act (NEPA)
The NEPA established the Environmental Protection Agency (EPA) and a national policy for the environment and provides for the establishment of a Council on Environmental Policy. All policies, regulations, and public laws shall be interpreted and administered in accordance with the policies set forth in this act.

### Federal Insecticide, Fungicide, and Rodenticide Act (FIFRA)
FIFRA provides federal control of pesticide distribution, sale, and use. The EPA was given the authority to study the consequences of pesticide usage and requires users such as farmers and utility companies to register when using pesticides. Later amendments to the law required applicators to take certification examinations, registration of all pesticides used in the United States, and proper labeling of pesticides that, if in accordance with specifications, will cause no harm to the environment (summary from FIFRA, 1972).

### Clean Water Act (CWA)
The CWA sets basic structure for regulating pollutants to U.S. waters. The law gave the EPA the authority to set effluent standards on an industry basis and continued the requirements to set water quality standards for all contaminants in surface water. The 1977 amendments focused on toxic pollutants. In 1987 the CWA was reauthorized, and again focused on toxic pollutants, authorized citizen suit provisions, and funded sewage treatment plants.

### Clean Air Act (CAA)
The Clean Air Act regulates air emissions from aerial, stationary, and mobile sources. The EPA was authorized to establish National Ambient Air Quality Standards (NAAQS) to protect public health and the environment. The goal was to set and achieve the NAAQS by 1975. The law was amended in 1977 when many areas of the country failed to meet the standards. The 1990 amendments to the Clean Air Act intended to meet unaddressed or insufficiently addressed problems such as acid rain, ground level ozone, stratospheric ozone depletion, and air toxics. Also in the 1990 reauthorization was a mandate for Chemical Risk Management Plans. This mandate requires industry to identify "worst case scenarios" regarding the hazardous chemicals that they transport, use, or discard (summary from Clean Air Act, 1970).

### Occupational Safety and Health Act (OSHA)
The OSHA was passed to ensure worker and workplace safety. The goal was to make sure employers provide an employment place free of hazards to health and safety such as chemicals, excessive noise, mechanical dangers, heat or cold extremes, or unsanitary conditions. To establish standards for the workplace, the Act also created NIOSH (National Institute for Occupational Safety and Health) as the research institution for OSHA.

### Safe Drinking Water Act (SDWA)
The SDWA was established to protect the quality of drinking water in the United States. The Act authorized the EPA to establish safe standards of purity and required all owners or operators of public water systems to comply with primary (health-related) standards.

### Resource Conservation and Recovery Act (RCRA)
The RCRA gave the EPA the authority to control the generation, transportation, treatment, storage, and disposal of hazardous waste. The RCRA also proposed a framework to manage nonhazardous waste. The 1984 Federal Hazardous and Solid Waste Amendments to this Act required phasing out land disposal of hazardous waste. The 1986 amendments enabled the EPA to address problems from underground tanks storing petroleum and other hazardous substances.

### Toxic Substances Control Act (TSCA)
The TSCA gives the EPA the ability to track the 75,000 industrial chemicals currently produced in or imported into the United States. The EPA can require reporting or testing of chemicals that may pose environmental health risks and can ban the manufacture and import of those chemicals that pose an unreasonable risk. TSCA supplements the Clean Air Act and the Toxic Release Inventory.

### Comprehensive Environmental Response, Compensation, and Liability Act (CERCLA or Superfund)
This law created a tax on the chemical and petroleum industries and provided broad federal authority to respond directly to releases or threatened releases of hazardous substances that may endanger public health or the environment.

### Superfund Amendments and Reauthorization Act (SARA)
SARA amended the Comprehensive Environmental Response, Compensation, and Liability Act with several changes and additions. These changes included increased size of the trust fund; encouragement of greater citizen participation in decision making on how sites should be cleaned up; increased state involvement in every phase of the Superfund program; increased focus on human health problems related to hazardous waste sites; new enforcement authorities and settlement tools; emphasis on the importance of permanent remedies and innovative treatment technologies in clean-up of hazardous waste sites; and Superfund actions to consider standards in other federal and state regulations. (Under Superfund legislation, the Federal Agency for Toxic Substances and Disease Registry was established.)

### Emergency Planning and Community Right to Know Act (EPCRA)
The EPCRA, also known as Title III of SARA, was enacted to help local communities protect public health safety and the environment from chemical hazards. Each state was required to appoint a State Emergency Response Commission that was required to divide their state into Emergency Planning Districts and establish a Local Emergency Planning Committee (LEPC) for each district.

### National Environmental Education Act
The National Environmental Education Act created a new and better coordinated environmental education emphasis at the EPA. It created the National Environmental Education and Training Foundation.

### Pollution Prevention Act (PPA)
The PPA focused industry, government, and public attention on reduction of the amount of pollution through cost-effective changes in production, operation, and use of raw materials. Pollution prevention also includes other practices that increase efficient use of energy, water, and other water resources, such as recycling, source reduction, and sustainable agriculture.

### Food Quality Protection Act (FQPA)
The FQPA amended the Federal Insecticide, Fungicide, and Rodenticide Act and the Federal Food, Drug, and Cosmetic Act. The Act changed the way the EPA regulates pesticides. The requirements included a new safety standard of reasonable certainty of no harm to be applied to all pesticides used on foods.

### Chemical Safety Information, Site Security, and Fuels Regulatory Act (Amendment to Section 112 of Clean Air Act)
This act removed from coverage by the Risk Management Plan (RMP) any flammable fuel when used as fuel or held for sale as fuel by a retail facility (flammable fuels used as a feedstock or held for sale as a fuel at a wholesale facility are still covered). This Act required certain facilities to have in place a risk management program and submit a summary of that program, called a Risk Management Plan (RMP) to the EPA. The law has two distinct parts that pertain to: flammable fuels and public access to Off-Site Consequence Analysis (OCA) data. OCA is "worst-case scenario" data.

places limits on the amount of pollution emitted into the air or water. A permit is a legally binding document.

Environmental standards may describe a permitted level of emissions, a maximum contaminant level (MCL), an action level for environmental clean-up, or a risk-based calculation; environmental standards are required to address health risks. It is the responsibility of potential polluters to operate within the regulations and standards. Compliance and enforcement are the next building blocks in controlling pollution. Compliance refers to the processes for ensuring that permit/standard/regulatory requirements are met. Clean-up or remediation of environmental damage is another control step. Public information and involvement processes, such as citizen advisory panels or community forums, are integral to the development of standards, on-going monitoring, and remediation.

## POLICY AND ADVOCACY

There are almost 3 million nurses in the United States today—approximately 1 in every 100 Americans is a registered nurse! Nurses can and should be a strong voice for a healthy environment. As informed citizens, nurses can take a variety of actions to protect the environmental health of families, clients, and communities. Nurses are perceived as trusted messengers and as reliable sources of environmental health information and as such, have a responsibility to be informed and take action in the best interest of public health. Often, legislators are called to vote on environmental legislation without a sound understanding of how the legislation may affect public health. Nurses can serve as a resource for state and federal legislators and their staff. Although every nurse may not be an expert in all aspects of environmental health, every nurse does have a basic education in human health and has a sufficient understanding of who may be most vulnerable to environmental insult. Nurses' thoughts about the potential impacts of new laws on the health of individuals and communities are valuable to legislators and other policy makers, as well as the public.

Grounded in science and using sound risk communication skills, nurses become the most credible sources of information at community gatherings, formal governmental hearings, and professional nursing forums. Nurses work as advocates for environmental justice so that all members of the community have a right to live and work in an environment that is healthy and safe (Mood, 2002). Public health nurses also volunteer to serve on state, local, or federal commissions, and they know about zoning and permit laws that regulate the impact of industry and land use on the community. Many nurse legislators began their careers by advocating for the rights of others. Nurses must read, listen, and ask questions. Then, as informed citizens, they will be leaders, fostering community action to address environmental health threats.

In 2008 the Alliance of Nurses for Healthy Environments was created to coalesce individual nurses and nursing organizations around issues associated with the environmental exposures and human health. This organization addresses the integration of environmental health into nursing education, practice (including greening the health care sector), research, and advocacy.

## Environmental Justice and Environmental Health Disparities

Some diseases differentially affect different populations. Certain environmental health risks disproportionately affect poor people and people of color in the United States. If you are a poor person of color, you are more likely to live near a hazardous waste site or an incinerator, and more likely to have children who are lead poisoned. You are also more likely to have children with asthma, which has a strong association with environmental exposures. Campaigns to improve the unequal burden of environmental risks in communities of color and in poor communities are striving to achieve environmental justice or environmental equity.

In 1993 the Environmental Justice Act was passed, and in 1994 Executive Order 12898, "Federal Actions to Address Environmental Justice in Minority Populations," was signed. This Act and the subsequent actions created policies to more comprehensively reduce the incidence of environmental *injustice* by mandating that every federal agency act in a manner to address and prevent illnesses and injuries. Nursing interventions and involvement in environmental health policies can have a significant effect on the health disparities experienced by our most challenged communities.

## Environmental Health Threats from the Health Care Industry: New Opportunities for Advocacy

Many choices in the health care setting affect environmental health. Nurses often lead in reducing the use of mercury-containing products in hospitals. The use of mercury-containing thermometers and sphygmomanometers leads to a risk of breakage, which releases a highly toxic substance into the workplace. Further, when a hospital uses incineration to dispose of their waste, the mercury-containing products will create significant releases of mercury into the air, thus contaminating communities. This airborne mercury will be present in raindrops; when the airborne mercury lands on water bodies (e.g., lakes, rivers, or oceans), it is converted by the microorganisms in the water to methylmercury, which is highly toxic to humans. The methylmercury is then bioaccumulated in the fish: as larger fish eat smaller fish, the body burden of methylmercury increases significantly.

Many synthetic chemicals that contaminate the environment are referred to as persistent bioaccumulative toxins (PBTs) or persistent organic pollutants (POPs). These are chemicals that do not break down in air, water, or soil, or in the plant, animal, and human bodies to which they may be passed. Ultimately, since humans are at the top of the food chain, these chemicals may come to reside in our bodies. For instance, lead, which should not be found in the human body, can be found in the long bones of almost any human in the world because of its ubiquitous use and presence in our environment.

Dioxin, another pollutant that contaminates our communities, is created, in part, by the health care industry. Dioxins are created when we manufacture or burn (incinerate) products that contain chlorine, such as bleached white paper or polyvinyl chloride (PVC) plastics. When dioxins are released into the environment, they are consumed by agricultural animals (e.g., beef and dairy cows, hogs, and poultry) and fish, where they are stored in fat cells as they work their way up the food chain. This phenomenon has resulted in dioxin deposition in breast tissue and been found in both cow and human milk. Virtually all women now have dioxin in their breast tissue. Dioxin, an endocrine-disrupting chemical and a strong carcinogen, is associated with several neurodevelopmental problems including learning disabilities and is now in every human's body. The solution to this problem is to stop releasing dioxins into the environment. In the health care setting, one way to eliminate the creation and release of dioxins is to stop using products like PVC plastics and selecting safer alternatives by employing environmentally preferable purchasing policies and practices.

An international campaign called Health Care Without Harm is working to reduce and eliminate mercury and PVC plastic in the health care industry, as well as the elimination of incineration of medical waste. The ANA was a founding member of the Health Care Without Harm campaign, and nurses have taken many leadership roles in the activities in the United States and around the world. The Health Care Without Harm website (http://www.noharm.org) provides outstanding information on greening hospitals and resources about pollution prevention in the health care sector.

## REFERRAL RESOURCES

There is no one source of information about environmental health nor is there a single resource to which a public health nurse can refer an individual or community should an environmentally related problem be suspected. As mentioned earlier, the NLM's ToxTown is a great starting place, and it allows the interested browser to dig deeply into environmental health content. TOXNET has an amalgamation of important databases and environmental health literature and additional peer-reviewed environmental health literature. The EPA is another rich source of information (www.epa.gov). Use of the Internet

makes information widely accessible, but finding an actual person to assist you or the communities you serve may not be as easy. One starting point may be the environmental epidemiology unit or toxicology unit of the state health department or department of environmental quality. The Association of Occupational and Environmental Clinics (AOEC) (http://www.aoec.org) is a national network of specialty clinics and individual practitioners available for consultation and sometimes for provision of educational programs for health professionals. Through AOEC, you can also find the Pediatric Environmental Health Specialty Units; there are 10 throughout the country. These specialty units were specifically established to provide consultation on environmental health issues. Another local or state resource may be environmental health experts in nursing or medical schools or schools of public health.

Local resources include local health and environmental protection agencies; poison control centers; agricultural extension offices; and occupational and environmental departments in schools of medicine, nursing, and public health. Some local and state agencies have developed topical directories to assist in accessing the appropriate staff for specific questions. Many of the resources have websites that allow ready access through the Internet and can be located by using any of the popular search methods. Box 10-13 presents an extensive list of environmental health agency resources.

The most active advocates for environmental health policies are grassroots organizations, the big environmentalist organizations, and environmental justice organizations. To learn more about who these organizations are, see the Resource Section under nongovernmental organizations.

## ROLES FOR NURSES IN ENVIRONMENTAL HEALTH

Nurses can be involved in many environmental health roles, in full-time work, as an adjunct to existing roles, and as informed citizens. Nurses who are passionate about this issue can develop

---

### BOX 10-13 Information and Guidance Sources for Referrals

The websites for each of these agencies can be accessed directly through the WebLinks feature on the book's website at http://evolve.elsevier.com/Stanhope.

**Federal Agencies**
Agency for Toxic Substances and Disease Registry
Centers for Disease Control and Prevention
Consumer Product Safety Commission
Environmental Protection Agency
Office of Children's Environmental Health
Food and Drug Administration
National Institute for Occupational Safety and Health
National Institute of Environmental Health Sciences
National Institutes of Health
National Cancer Institute
National Institute of Nursing Research
Occupational Safety and Health Administration
National Library of Medicine—TOXNET

**State Agencies**
State Health Departments
State Environmental Protection Agencies

**Associations and Organizations**
American Association of Poison Control Centers
American Association of Occupational Health Nurses
Association of Occupational and Environmental Clinics
Beyond Pesticides
Center for Health and Environmental Justice
Children's Environmental Health Network
Environmental Defense
Environmental Working Group
Health Care Without Harm
National Environmental Education Foundation
Natural Resources Defense Council
Pediatric Environmental Health Specialty Units
Society for Occupational and Environmental Health

research expertise, sit on commissions, write articles, and take national leadership roles. All nurses can include environmental exposures in their history taking; consider the environmental impacts of the products they select for their clinics, hospitals, schools, and other settings; promote recycling and reuse of products; and promote environmentally preferable purchasing. Each type and level of engagement is important. The following are some ways in which nurses can get involved both professionally and as informed citizens:

- *Community involvement/public participation.* Organizing, facilitating, and moderating; making public notices effective and public forums accessible; welcoming input. Making information exchange understandable and problem solving acceptable to culturally diverse communities are valuable assets a nurse contributes. Skills in community organizing and mobilizing can be essential for a community to have a meaningful voice in decisions that affect them.
- *Individual and population risk assessment.* Using nursing assessment skills to detect potential and actual exposure pathways and outcomes for clients cared for in the acute, chronic, and healthy communities of practice.
- *Risk communication.* Interpreting, applying principles to practice. Nurses may serve as skilled risk communicators

within agencies, working for industries or working as independent practitioners. Amendments to the Clean Air Act require major industrial sources of air emissions to have risk management plans and to inform their neighbors of specifics of the risks and plans (Clean Air Act, 1996).

- *Epidemiologic investigations.* Nurses need to have the skills to respond in scientifically sound and humanely sensitive ways to community concerns about cancer, birth defects, and stillbirths when citizens fear environmental causation.
- *Policy development.* Proposing, informing, and monitoring action from agencies, communities, and organization perspectives.

The assimilation of the concepts of environmental health into a nurse's daily practice gives new life to traditional public health values of prevention, community building, and social justice. Box 10-14 presents the work of three nurses currently working in environmental health.

As nurses learn more about the environment, opportunities for integration into their practice, education programs, research, advocacy, and policy work will become evident and will evolve. Opportunities abound for those pioneering spirits within the nursing profession who are dedicated to creating healthier environments for their clients and communities.

---

### BOX 10-14    Examples of Three Modern-Day Environmental Health Nursing Pioneers

In Baltimore, MD, **Dr. Claudia Smith** (a nurse who is on the faculty at the University of Maryland) directed a project in which nurses worked with community members to address a variety of health problems associated with poor housing conditions. For this project, which was funded by the U.S. Department of Housing and Urban Development, Dr. Smith hired and trained community members to assess and reduce unhealthy conditions caused by lead-based paint, high levels of carbon monoxide, and asthma triggers (e.g., dust mites, pet dander, and pests); she taught community members about safer choices for pest control using the least toxic approach to pest management by using an integrated pest management approach.

After **Denise Choiniere**, a graduate student in community health who was working in the cardiac care unit (CCU) at the University of Maryland Medical Center, learned about the health effects associated with heavy metals, she was very uncomfortable with simply throwing away the batteries that were used in the many small devices, such as Holter monitors. Instead, she developed a battery recycling program for the CCU and the telemetry unit. She then discovered that her hospital purchased 97,000 small batteries every year. Each of these small batteries contains a heavy metal—mercury, lithium, cadmium, or lead. She was the driving force in developing a hospital-wide, small battery recycling program. This activity created a whole new career trajectory for Ms. Choiniere, who was recently appointed to the executive position of Sustainability Coordinator for the whole hospital. She has since addressed green cleaning products, promoted the recycling of "blue wrap" used in the operating rooms, and organized a farmers' market that meets weekly in front of the hospital, thus bringing locally grown and sustainably farmed products to hospital employees and the surrounding community. She then was given oversight for all of the 650-bed hospital's purchases.

**Dr. Robyn Gilden** is a nursing faculty member who worked for 5 years with communities that knew or suspected that they were living near a hazardous waste site. She learned about the many laws and agencies involved in hazardous waste site assessments and clean-ups. Hazardous wastes can affect soil, water,

and air. Sources of contamination may come from old, unlined landfills; uncontrolled dump sites; spills or discharges from industry; leaking underground storage tanks (like gasoline tanks); or runoff from fields. The Agency for Toxic Substances and Disease Registry (ATSDR), a federal agency responsible for documenting the health hazards associated with environmental exposures, maintains a listing of the most problematic contaminants found at polluted sites. They include a wide range of highly toxic chemicals including arsenic, lead, mercury, vinyl chloride, benzene, polychlorinated biphenyls (PCBs), and cadmium. These toxic chemicals top the list because they are the most commonly found contaminants and pose a significant threat to human health based on routes of exposure and level of toxicity. Dr. Gilden learned about the resources that are available for the best and most current toxicological information. The National Library of Medicine's TOXNET and ATSDR's websites, including their ToxFAQs, are some of the best sources of navigable information.

In working with communities, Dr. Gilden met with government officials, including mayors of small towns, as well as concerned parents, people from local governments, health departments, educational institutions, businesses, developers, bankers, realtors, and other community members. She has also learned about the many statutes that cover hazardous waste sites, such as the Superfund legislation (which covers the most polluted waste sites) and Brownfields legislation (which covers contaminated sites where economic development is involved). Both these pieces of legislation mandate community involvement, which is where Dr. Gilden's community health and risk communication skills are used. Regardless of who is responsible for or in charge of a contaminated site, the nurse understands that the community must be an active and equal participant. It is the community members who will be impacted by decisions and have to live with the results of clean-up and redevelopment. As is true of most nurses, Dr. Gilden quickly became a trusted person to the community members.

When she discovered the "Pesticide Warning" signs on the playing fields where her children played sports, this launched Dr. Gilden into a new area of research and advocacy regarding children's exposures.

## PRACTICE APPLICATION

Following are two case scenarios related to exposure pathways. The first involves lead poisoning and the second, fracking-related concerns.

At the county health department, a 3-year-old boy named Billy presents with gastric upset and behavioral changes. These symptoms have persisted for several weeks. During your history taking, you discover that Billy's parents have been renovating their old home. A parent in Billy's daycare center suggested that Billy's symptoms might be associated with lead, so Billy's parents have brought him in to the clinic.

You relay this information to the primary care practitioner who, in turn, orders a blood lead level, which comes back at 45 mcg/dL. This is a very high value.

You research lead poisoning and discover that there are many potential health effects of lead exposure and that children are at greatest risk because their bodies, especially their nervous systems, are still developing. You also find that chronic lead poisoning may lead to long-term effects, such as developmental delays and impaired learning ability.

You let the health professional know about the lead poisoning specialists in the nearby children's hospital. On further investigation, you find that Billy's home was built before 1950 and is still under renovation. Billy should not return to the home. At this point, the sanitarian from the local health department tests the dust in the home and finds high lead levels. Because of Billy's age and associated behaviors, such as hand-to-mouth activities, you determine that the lead dust in the home is the probable exposure. However, you must also consider multiple sources of exposure.

1. What other sources of exposure might exist?
2. What would you include in an assessment of this situation?
3. What prevention strategies would you use to resolve this issue? At the individual level? At the population level?

Mrs. Bell calls the local health department to report that her drinking water, from their private well, is discolored and that her son has been experiencing headaches and nose bleeds. You talk with Dan, the health department's environmental health professional (sanitarian) who tells you that there is new "fracking" activity on the east side of your rural county, where Mrs. Bell and her family live, and that this may be the reason for the water discoloration and the child's symptoms. You look up "fracking" and discover that the word is shorthand for hydraulic fracturing, a new technique for extracting natural gas that is fraught with community and health concerns. (For more information on fracking, see the Resource Section.) Dan and you agree to make a site visit to the Bell's farm.

1. What will you be looking for on your visit?
2. How can you help the Bells, if any of their issues seem to be associated with the nearby fracking site?
3. What other experts are available to you and the Bells?

**Answers can be found on the Evolve site.**

## KEY POINTS

- Nurses need to be informed professionals and advocates for citizens in their community regarding environmental health issues.
- Models describing the determinants of health acknowledge the role of the environment in health and disease.
- Climate change is creating profound risks to human health globally and in the United States.
- For most chemicals in our homes, work, schools, and communities, no research has been completed to determine whether or not they will cause health effects.
- Prevention activities include education, reduction/elimination of exposures, waste minimization, energy policies, and land use planning.
- Pollution control activities include use of technologies; environmental permitting; environmental standards, monitoring, compliance, and enforcement; and clean-up and remediation.
- Each nursing assessment should include questions and observations concerning potential and existing environmental exposures.

- Useful environmental exposure data are difficult to acquire. Those data that exist can be used to aid in the assessment, diagnosis, intervention, and evaluation of environmentally related health problems.
- Both case advocacy and class advocacy are important skills for nurses in environmental health practice.
- Risk communication is a critical skill and must acknowledge the outrage factor experienced by communities with environmental hazards.
- Federal, state, and local laws and regulations, as well as international treaties, exist to protect the health of people from environmental hazards.
- Environmental health practice engages multiple disciplines, and nurses are important members of the environmental health team.
- Environmental health practice includes principles of health promotion, disease prevention, and health protection.
- *Healthy People 2020* objectives address both targets for the reduction of risk factors and diseases related to environmental causes.

## CLINICAL DECISION-MAKING ACTIVITIES

1. Explain why the source of drinking water is important to investigate in the assessment of an unusually high number of infertility cases in a community; in increased lead levels in children from a certain school; and in an outbreak of a gastrointestinal epidemic in an agricultural community.

2. Discuss the use of the epidemiologic triangle in explaining the determinants of health.

3. Discover if your jurisdiction has a law or regulation for the disclosure of lead-based paint or radon levels for personal property as part of the act of sale for real estate. If your community does not, investigate with the government officials of the community the reasons for the lack of a disclosure requirement.

## REFERENCES

Agency for Healthcare Research and Quality: *Focus on Research: Children with Chronic Illness and Disabilities, AHRQ Publication No. 02-M025.* Rockville, MD, 2002, U.S. Department of Health and Human Services, AHRQ Publications Clearing House.

American Cancer Society: *Cancer Facts and Figures,* 2010. Available at: http://www.cancer.org. Accessed June 19, 2014.

American Cancer Society: *Cancer Facts & Figures, 2014.* Atlanta GA, 2014, ACS.

American Nurses Association: *ANA's Principles of Environmental Health in Nursing Practice with Implementation Strategies.* Silver Spring MD, 2007, Author.

Anney R, Hawi Z, Sheehan K, et al: Epigenetic effects in ADHD: parent-of-origin effects in image sample. *Am J Med Genet B Neuropsychiatr Genet* 141(7):736–737, 2006.

Bassil KL, Vakil C, Sanborn M, et al: Cancer health effects of pesticides: systematic review. *Can Fam Physician* 53(10):1704–1711, 2007.

Bailey HD, Fritschi L, Infante-Rivard C, et al: (2014) Parental occupational pesticide exposure and the risk of childhood leukemia in the offspring: findings from the childhood leukemia international consortium. *Int J Cancer* 2014. doi: 10.1002/ijc.28854.

Brown RC: Windows of exposure to pesticides and childhood leukemia: an analysis of the current literature. *Birth Defects Res A Clin Mol Teratol* 70(5):301, 2004.

Butterfield P, Postma J: ERRNIE research team: The TERRA framework: conceptualizing rural environmental health inequities through an environmental justice lens. *ANS Adv Nurs Sci* 32(2):107–117, 2009.

Centers for Disease Control (CDC): Asthma: data and surveillance, 2012. Available at: http://www.cdc.gov/asthma/asthmadata.htm. Accessed March 16, 2014.

Centers for Disease Control (CDC): Prevalence of autism spectrum disorder among children aged 8 years—Autism and Developmental Disabilities Monitoring Network, 11 sites, United States, 2010. *MMWR Surveill Summ* 63(SS02):1–21, 2014a.

Centers for Disease Control (CDC): Adolescent and school health: childhood obesity, 2014b. facts. http://www.cdc.gov/healthyyouth/obesity/facts.htm. Accessed March 16, 2014.

Clean Air Act: Risk management programs, Section 112(7). *Federal Register,* Part III EPA, 40 CFR, Part 68, 2014a.

Clean Air Act 1970. http://www.epa.gov/air/caa/. Accessed June 29, 2014.

Council on Linkages Between Academic and Public Health Practice: *Core Competencies for Public Health Professionals.* Washington DC, 2010, Public Health Foundation/Health Resources and Services Administration.

Department of Health and Human Services (DHHS): SAMHSA: fast facts about children and mental health, 2005. http://www.dbhds.virginia.gov/documents%5CCFS%5CFact%20Sheet-About-Children-and-Mental-Health-16.pdf. Accessed March 16, 2014.

Dietert RR, Etzel RA, Chen D, et al: Workshop to identify critical windows exposure for children's health: immune and respiratory systems work group summary. *Environ Health Perspect* 108(Suppl 3):483–490, 2000.

Environmental Protection Agency (EPA): America's children and the environment, 3 ed (ACE3) 2013—Frequently asked questions, 2013. http://www.epa.gov/envirohealth/children/basics/background.html#4. Accessed March 16, 2014.

Environmental Protection Agency: 2009. Available at: http://www.epa.gov/waterscience/fish/advisories/fs2008.html. Accessed December 15, 2010.

Environmental Protection Agency: Chemicals in commerce: TSCA Chemical Substance Inventory, 2014 (Last updated 3/13/14). http://www.epa.gov/oppt/existingchemicals/pubs/tscainventory/basic.html. Accessed March 16, 2014.

Environmental Working Group: *Body Burden—The Pollution in Newborns: A Benchmark Investigation of Industrial Chemicals, Pollutants and Pesticides in Umbilical Cord Blood,* July 14, 2005.

Federal Insecticide, Fungicide, and Rodenticide Act: 1972. http://www.epa.gov/oecaagct/lfra.html. Accessed June 29, 2012.

Gilden R, Friedmann E, Sattler B, et al: Potential health effects related to pesticide use on athletic fields. *Pub Health Nurs* 29(3):198–207, 2012.

Goldman LR, Koduru SH: Chemicals in the environment and developmental toxicity in children: a public health and policy perspective. *Environ Health Perspect* 108:S443–S448, 2000.

Gulf Oil Spill: BP ruined the Gulf, N.d. http://www.fulf-oil-spill.us/. Accessed December 29, 2010.

Habre R, Moshier E, Castro W, et al: The effects of PM 2.5 and its components from indoor and outdoor sources on cough and wheeze symptoms in asthmatic children. *J Expo Sci Environ Epidemiol* 2014. doi: 10.1038/jes.2014.21.

Hill WG, Butterfield PG: Environmental risk reduction for rural children. In Lee HJ, Winters CA, editors: *Rural Nursing: Concepts, Theory, and Practice,* ed 2. New York, 2006, Springer.

Huff M: Ensia Magazine Interview by Mary Huff with William McDonough, 2013. http://ensia.com/interviews/william-mcdonough-remaking-the-way-we-make-things/. Accessed March 16, 2014.

Intergovernmental Program on Climate Change: Climate Change 2014: impacts, adaptation, and vulnerability, IPCC Working Group II Contribution to the 5th assessment report, 2014. http://www.who.int/globalchange/environment/climatechange-2014-report/en/. Retrieved June 10, 2014.

Jemal A, Siegel R, Xu J, et al: Cancer statistics 2010. *CA Cancer J Clin* 60(5):277–300, 2010.

Kaiser Foundation: Nurses trusted source—Kaiser health tracking poll, 2013. http://kff.org/health-reform/poll-finding/kaiser-health-tracking-poll-august-2013/. Accessed March 16, 2014.

Landrigan PJ, Rauh VA, Galvez MP: Environmental justice and the health of children. *Mt Sinai J Med* 77(2):178–187, 2010. doi: 10.1002/msj.20173.

Louv R: *No Child Left Inside: Saving Our Children from Nature-Deficit Disorder.* Chapel Hill, NC, 2005, Algonquin Books.

Metayer C, Colt JS, Buffler PA, et al: Exposure to herbicides in house dust and risk of childhood acute lymphoblastic leukemia. *J Expo Sci Environ Epidemiol* 23(4):363–370, 2013. doi: 10.1038/jes.2012.115.

Mood LH: Environmental health policy: environmental justice. In Mason DJ, Leavitt JK, editors: *Policy and Politics in Nursing and Health Care,* ed 4. Philadelphia, 2002, Saunders.

Myths-Dreams-Symbols: 2006. Available at: http://www.mythsdreamssymbols.com/seattle.html. Accessed December 15, 2010.

O'Brien M: *Making Better Environmental Decisions: An Alternative to Risk Assessment.* Cambridge, MA, 2000, MIT Press.

Pope AM, Snyder MA, Mood LH, editors: *Nursing, Health and Environment.* Washington, DC, 1995, Institute of Medicine, National Academy Press.

President's Cancer Panel: *Reducing Environmental Cancer Risk: What Can We Do Now?* NOTE: the actual quote comes from the letter transmitting the report to the President, April 2010. Annual report 2008-2009. Released 2010. http://deainfo.nci.nih.gov/advisory/pcp/annualReports/pcp08-09rpt/PCP_Report_08_09_509.pdf. Retrieved June 10, 2014.

Public Health, Environment and Social Determinants of Health (PHE): 2015. http://www.who.int/phe/about_us/en/. Accessed February 17, 2015.

Quad Council of Public Health Nursing Organizations: *Competencies for*

*Public Health Nursing Practice.* Washington DC, 2011, ASTDN.

Rawn DF, Roscoe V, Krakalovich T, et al: *N*-methyl carbamate concentrations and dietary intake estimates for apple and grape juices available on the retail market in Canada. *Food Addit Contam* 21(6):555–563, 2004.

Ross JA, Olshan AF: Pediatric cancer in the United States: the Children's Oncology Group Epidemiology Research Program. *Cancer Epidemiol Biomarkers Prev* 13:1552–1554, 2004.

Sandman PM, Chess C, Hane BJ: *Improving Dialogue with Communities.* New Brunswick, NJ, 1991, Rutgers University.

Schettler T, Stein J, Reich F, et al: *In Harm's Way: Toxic Threats to Development, a Report by Greater Boston Physicians for Social Responsibility, Prepared for a Joint Project with Clean Water.* Cambridge, MA, 2000, PSR. Available at: http://www.psr.org/chapters/boston/resources/in-harms-way-materials-download.html. Accessed June 29, 2014.

Smargiassi A, Goldberg MS, Wheeler AJ, et al: Associations between personal exposure to air pollutants and lung function tests and cardiovascular indices among children with asthma living near an industrial complex and petroleum refineries. *Environ Res* 132C:38–45, 2014. doi: 10.1016/j.envres.2014.03.030.

Suk WA, Davis EA: Strategies for addressing global environmental health concerns. *Ann N Y Acad Sci* 1140:40–44, 2008.

Turner MC, Wigle DT, Krewski D: Residential pesticides and childhood leukemia: a systematic review and meta-analysis. *Environ Health Perspect* 118(1):33–41, 2010.

U.S. Department of Health and Human Services: *Healthy People 2020*, 2010. Available at: http://www.healthypeople.gov/2020topicsobjectives/default.aspx. Accessed June 10, 2014.

U.S. Department of Housing and Urban Development: American Healthy Homes Survey, lead and arsenic findings. April 2011, Office of Healthy Homes and Lead Hazard Control.

Wigle DT, Turner MC, Krewski D: A systematic review and meta-analysis of childhood leukemia and parental occupational pesticide exposure. *Environ Health Perspect* 117(10):1505–1513, 2009.

United Nations University: WHO quote found from 1993 document, 1993. http://unu.edu/publications/articles/environmental-health-governance-for-sustainable-development.html. Retrieved June 7, 2014.

*Wingspread Statement on the Precautionary Principle.* Racine, WI, 1998. Available at: http://www.gdrc.org/u-gov/precaution-3.html. Retrieved to March 12, 2015.

U.S. Department of Housing and Urban Development: American Healthy Homes Survey, lead and arsenic findings, April 2011, Office of Healthy Homes and Lead Hazard Control. http://portal.hud.gov/hudportal/documents/huddoc?id=AHHS_REPORT.pdf. Accessed February 17, 2015.

World Health Organization: Public Health and the Environment. , Public Health, Environment, and Social Determinants of Health (PHE). http://www.who.int/phe/about_us/en/. Accessed February 17, 2015.

World Health Organization: Climate Change and Human Health, 2014. http://www.who.int/globalchange/en/. Accessed March 16, 2014b.

World Health Organization: Fact File: 10 facts on mental health, N.d. http://www.who.int/features/factfiles/mental_health/mental_health_facts/en/. Accessed March 16, 2014.

Yoder JS, Wallace RM, Collier SA, et al: Cryptosporidiosis surveillance—United States, 2009-2010. Centers for Disease Control and Prevention (CDC). *MMWR Surveill Summ* 61(5):1–12, 2012. http://www.cdc.gov/mmwr/preview/mmwrhtml/ss6105a1.htm. Accessed June 29, 2014.

learn about this area of science in order to respond effectively to the challenges of this new knowledge.

An example of this challenge is that of genetic testing for mutations associated with hereditary disease. The best way to identify whether there is a mutation in a family where a hereditary disease is suspected is to test the person who displays the most evidence of being a mutation carrier. This is usually a relative who has had a cancer that occurs typically as part of the hereditary cancer syndrome (e.g., breast or ovarian) that is suspected in the family.

The previous example could present a difficulty because family members who have had cancer may not agree to being tested for genetic mutations. This refusal presents challenges to the person who desires information that might affect decision making and his or her health. An additional ethical challenge encountered involves individuals without an insurance carrier that reimburses for genetic testing, or who may have a high deductible in the insurance policy. Some individuals also think that testing will decrease the quality of their life and make them anxious about the future if they were to discover they have a mutation. Other people fear a positive test result may lead to feelings of guilt about passing along a disease to children and grandchildren.

## Case Example 1

K.N. is a 42-year-old mother with three daughters, ages 16, 18, and 22. She has an extensive family history of ovarian cancer. Because of her family history, K.N. is regularly screened per current treatment guidelines. K.N.'s mother, who was diagnosed with ovarian cancer at age 55, underwent genetic testing and was discovered to be a carrier of the *BRCA2* gene mutation predisposing to breast and ovarian cancer. Despite undergoing frequent screening, several of K.N.'s aunts have died of ovarian cancer at an early age. K.N.'s husband wants her to be tested for the *BRCA2* gene and, if positive, has encouraged her to undergo a prophylactic salpingo-oophorectomy. K.N. is concerned that a positive genetic test may result in loss of insurance coverage. She is also concerned that this will have a negative psychological impact on her children.

Joan Akins is a public health nurse at the county health department serving the area where K.N. resides. Ms. Akins has recently conducted a cancer awareness campaign that included public health education on hereditary cancer syndromes. K.N. contacts Ms. Akins to request advice on whether to undergo genetic testing. Ms. Akins actively listens to K.N.'s concerns and provides general information on genetic testing and the implications of the test results for K.N. and for her children. She also discusses the newly enacted Genetic Information Nondiscrimination Act (GINA) legislation that protects the public from genetic discrimination by employers and insurers. Ms. Akins encourages K.N. to talk with her gynecologist about her concerns and to make an appointment for genetic counseling, providing names and contact information for local genetic counselors who specialize in cancer genetics.

As mentioned, genetic testing decisions are personal and complex and can be controversial, leading to dissonance in families. It is important for public health nurses to respect individuals' and family members' decision-making processes. They must, at the same time, be well informed about genetic testing to provide accurate education to members of the public in order to support appropriate decision making.

Also, current methods of testing do not detect all of the mutations that can occur in some diseases, including hereditary cancer syndrome–related genes. If a mutation is detected during DNA testing, this would not confirm an absolute risk for cancer, but rather would indicate that a person is at increased risk to develop the cancers that are part of the particular hereditary cancer syndrome and may need high-risk management. Such a finding has implications for family members who might have inherited the same mutation, enabling them to undergo DNA testing specific to the identified mutation. Such focused testing is more accurate and cost-effective than testing for multiple potential mutations (NCI, 2014). In contrast, if DNA testing in a cancer-affected relative is negative, this does not indicate family members are not at risk. There might be a mutation in a different hereditary cancer syndrome gene than those tested. It is important to remember that many mutations associated with cancer susceptibility and familial syndromes have yet to be identified.

For these reasons, family history must also be considered. However, caution is needed in interpreting family history for several reasons: an inherited syndrome may not be evident for someone with a small family; not everyone is informed of their family's history of disease; death of a family member may be unrelated to cancer, such as early accidental death; or members may have been adopted and this may not be known to others in the family. Finally, because most cancers are not hereditary, family history should be accompanied by assessment of shared familial environments.

## Case Example 2

Sickle cell anemia is an autosomal recessive disease in which a gene mutation results in the production of structurally abnormal hemoglobin called hemoglobin S. Gene carriers have one normal form of the hemoglobin gene and one mutation, a condition called sickle cell trait. The highest rates of disease are among African Americans, with sickle cell anemia affecting approximately 1 in 500 African Americans and 8% of the population being carriers (anemia, sickle, National Center for Biotechnology Information [n.d.]; see http://www.ncbi.nlm.nih.gov/books/NBK22238).

Marge Covington is a public health nurse employed by a nonprofit, community-based organization that provides health care education and outreach services to members of the African American community in a large metropolitan area. The rate of sickle cell anemia among members of the community is higher than the national average. In response, Ms. Covington has implemented a program with the projected outcome to reduce disease rates among African Americans in the community. The program objectives are to (1) increase awareness of the disease in the community and (2) increase rates of carrier testing to support informed decision making regarding childbearing. To meet these objectives, Ms. Covington has initiated monthly educational sessions on sickle cell anemia and sickle cell trait at community centers throughout the area. She has also collaborated with a local hospital system to provide free biannual genetic counseling sessions with optional carrier screening at community health clinics.

Continuing education is important for public health nurses during this time of rapid integration of new genetic tests into health care practice. Only through ongoing education will public health nurses have the basis from which to appropriately educate the public regarding genetic testing. In addition, recognition of the role of gene–environment interactions in susceptibility to cancer and many other diseases underscores the importance of assessing risk from an environmental perspective. Public health nurses offer this perspective as part of the larger interprofessional team needed to address the complex issues involved in genetic testing.

## CURRENT ISSUES IN GENOMICS AND GENETICS

*"Translating the knowledge we are gaining from gene discoveries into practical clinical and public health applications will be critical for realizing the potential of personalized health care and improving the health of the nation."*

**Muin J. Khoury, MD, PhD, Director,
CDC Office of Public Health Genomics**

Many issues are involved in the growing field of genetics/genomics. Selected issues are discussed in this section. Individuals are learning the importance of having a family medical history. Some health care providers are unclear about how to accurately interpret the family history of a client who has had the initiative to collect it. Moreover, many clients are reluctant to disclose this family history for fear that it will affect their health insurance status or eligibility despite current laws in place designed to protect these clients.

Helping patients and families navigate through the disclosure process and uncovering their personal and family health history and understanding specific genetic tests is an important role for public health nurses. In addition, if patients are willing to make lifestyle changes or health decisions, the appropriate psychosocial support and education can be provided to clients and their families. Nurses play an important role in answering questions and assisting in challenges these clients and families face with making decisions when there is any suspicion of increased risk for genetically based diseases. To make things more confusing, companies market their tests and advertise directly to the public. This type of marketing has implications for nurses and other health care providers who need to provide the appropriate counseling about the implications and indications for such testing. For example, marketing on the Internet complicates client decision making since it can provide consumers with easy access to genetic tests without involving a health care professional in the testing process. Even the clinically available genetic tests, which may provide legitimate test results, are difficult to interpret without genetic counseling. Currently, the Centers for Disease Control and Prevention (CDC), the Centers for Medicare Services (CMS), and the

Federal Drug Administration (FDA) have oversight of genetic tests and products, whereas the Federal Trade Commission (FTC) has oversight of the advertising of these tests and products. The National Institutes of Health (NIH), Health Resources and Services Administration (HRSA), and Agency for Healthcare Research and Quality (AHRQ) support research related to genetic tests and products (CDC, 2014).

Keeping current with the changes in this scientific field with many complex systems in place is a challenging task. The National Human Genome Research Institute of the National Institutes of Health (NIH) provides reliable, up-to date genetics and genomics information related to patient management, curricular resources, new National Institutes of Health and NHGRI research activities, and ethical, legal and social issues. Additionally, the Centers for Disease Control and Prevention (CDC) provides a "Genomics & Health Impact Update" periodically on their website for public use (NIH, 2014; CDC 2014).

Helping patients and families understand genetic predisposition to disease versus normal population risk and the impact of lifestyle and environment on health is another role for public health nurses. According to the CDC (2014), genomics plays a role in nine of the ten leading causes of death in the United Sates, most notably chronic diseases such as cancer and heart disease. There are multifactorial influences acting together to influence disease risk, physiological and mental health conditions, pathogenic DNA, and the therapies used to treat disease (Perry, 2011). For example, "common congenital malformations, such as cleft lip and palate and neural tube defects, result from multifactorial inheritance, a combination of genetic and environmental factors" (Perry, 2011, p. 147). Box 11-1 presents examples of multifactorial diseases, or those caused by gene and environment interaction.

The issue of multifactorial interactions that lead to disease is becomingly increasingly recognized in occupational health. According to the CDC, advances in technology in the last few decades have increased our knowledge of the role that genetics plays in occupational diseases. In occupational health, one of the key issues relates to genetic changes that are acquired during a lifetime as a result of exposures and the interaction between genes and environmental factors. However, the use of genetic information in occupational safety and health research and

---

**BOX 11-1  Examples of Multifactorial Disorders**

| | |
|---|---|
| Autism (strong genetic basis) | Multiple sclerosis |
| Neural tube disorders | Asthma |
| Cleft lip, palette | Allergies |
| Congenital heart disease | Autoimmune disorders |
| Coronary artery disease | Bipolar disorder |
| Type I diabetes | Schizophrenia |
| Type II diabetes | Kidney stones |
| Breast cancer | Gallstones |
| Colon cancer | Obesity |
| Lung cancer | Peptic ulcer disease |
| Rheumatic heart disease | Gout |
| Alcoholism | |

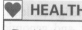

## PRACTICE APPLICATION

T.S., a 4-year-old with hemophilia B, is attending his Head Start program this fall. His mother brought all of his medical supplies and needles so that staff could start an emergency IV infusion if the need arose. The possibility of needing to start an IV concerned the staff who were teachers, not health care workers. The mother was also anxious about her son being away from home and attending preschool for the first time. As the public health nurse who is responsible for providing health care for Head Start programs in your community, how do you manage the health care for this child while also ensuring safety and making sure that adequate plans are in place for this facility?

A. Let T.S.'s mother know that she needs a note from T.S.'s physician before he can bring any medications to the facility.

B. Notify all of the student's parents/guardians of T.S.'s condition in order to set the guidelines and prevent possible bleeds. The children at the center should be aware of the condition, and the parents also need to educate their children to ensure extra precaution around T.S.

C. Organize a meeting between staff, educators, and parents of T.S. to educate about hemophilia. The aim is to educate key people to ensure T.S.'s safety while at Head Start.
**Answers can be found on the Evolve site.**

## KEY POINTS

- Genetics is the study of the function and effect of single genes that are inherited by children from their parents. Genomics is the study of individual genes in order to understand the interplay of genetic, environmental, cultural, and psychosocial factors in disease.
- DNA is a nucleic acid that contains genetic information called genes.
- Genetic mutations can be caused by the environment or can be spontaneous and arise naturally during the process of DNA replication.
- Human disease comes from the collision between genetic variations and environmental factors.
- Genetic testing decisions are personal and complex and can be controversial, leading to challenging situations in families.
- The Genetic Information Nondiscrimination Act (GINA) of 2008 was designed to prohibit the improper use of genetic information in health insurance and employment.
- The use of genomics and how it relates to drug treatment will enable personalized health care and medicine to be tailored to each person's needs; health, therefore, can be predictive and preventive in nature.
- According to the International Society of Nurses in Genetics (ISONG), the genetic nurse carries out the responsibility for identifying genetic risk factors, providing nursing interventions, making referrals, and providing health promotion education. The advanced practice nurse can provide genetic counseling or refer to a genetic counselor and act as case manager for a person with or at risk for a disease that arises from a genetic susceptibility.
- Nurses can promote assurance for access to care, including genetic screening, the privacy of health information, and certainty that no discrimination will be allowed in treatment or screening for disease.
- The field of genetics/genomics is growing rapidly and will require nurses to continue to learn and to be aware of advances in research in this area.
- Genomics affects individuals, families, and communities.
- Epigenetics is the study of heritable changes in gene activity that are *not* caused by changes in the DNA sequence; it also can be used to describe the study of stable, long-term alterations in the transcriptional potential of a cell that are not necessarily heritable. Unlike simple genetics based on changes to the DNA sequence (the genotype), the changes in gene expression or cellular phenotype of epigenetics have other causes.

## CLINICAL DECISION-MAKING ACTIVITIES

1. Choose a disorder that has a genetic basis. Look at three sites on the Internet to see what information is available for clients, families, and health professionals. Then evaluate the sites according to the following criteria:
   - Who wrote the information on the site? Is it written by a health professional? Is it sponsored by a government organization that is a reliable source of health information such as the CDC? Is it peer reviewed?
   - Is the information written at the literacy level that a client could understand?
   - How would you improve the usefulness of these three sites based on the clients, families, and communities with whom you work?

2. Since public health nurses often identify groups within a community who are considered high risk for illness and then provide care to them as individuals, or to their families or in groups, choose a group in your community. Then develop a plan of care including appropriate referrals to other agencies and a comprehensive plan for follow-up.

3. Identify parent support groups in your community and inquire about attending a meeting.

# REFERENCES

American Academy of Nursing: Nurses transforming health care using genetics and genomics, revisions submitted to American Academy of Nursing Board of Directors, January 22, 2009. Available at: http://www.aannet.org/files/public/Genetic_White_Paper_1-22-09.pdf. Accessed June 12, 2014.

American Cancer Society: Breast cancer facts & figures 2013-2014. Atlanta, American Cancer Society, Inc. Available at: http://www.cancer.org/acs/groups/content/@research/documents/document/acspc-042725.pdf. Accessed June 20, 2014.

American Nurses Association: Code of Ethics for Nurses with Interpretive Statements. Kansas City, MO, 2001, ANA. Available at: http://www.nursingworld.org/MainMenuCategories/EthicsStandards/CodeofEthicsforNurses/Code-of-Ethics.pdf.

Calzone KA, Cashion A, Feetham S, et al: Nurses transforming health care using genetics and genomics. Nurs Outlook 58(1):26–35, 2010. Available at: http://www.nursingoutlook.org/article/S0029-6554(09)00073-6/fulltext. Accessed on June 20, 2014.

Centers for Disease Control and Prevention: Genomics Translation: Genomic Workforce Competencies, 2001. Available at: http://www.cdc.gov/genomics/translation/competencies/. Accessed on June 20, 2014.

Centers for Disease Control and Prevention: Genetics in the workplace, 2010. http://www.cdc.gov/niosh/topics/genetics/. Accessed on June, 20, 2014.

Centers for Disease Control and Prevention: Genomic testing, 2013. Retrieved from: http://www.cdc.gov/genomics/gtesting/. Accessed on June 20, 2014.

Centers for Disease Control and Prevention: Genomics and health, 2014. Retrieved from: http://www.cdc.gov/genomics/public/. Accessed on June 20, 2014.

Clark A, Adamian M, Taylor J: An overview of epigenetics in nursing. Nursing Clin N Am 48(4):649–659, 2013. Retrieved from: http://

www.sciencedirect.com/science/article/pii/S0029646513000856. Accessed on June 20, 2014.

Collins FS, Green E, Guttmacher AE, et al: A vision for the future of genomic research. Nature 422:835–847, 2003. Available at: http://www.nature.com/nature/journal/v422/n6934/full/nature01626.html. Accessed on June 20, 2014.

Collins FS: An overview of the human genome project, 2006. Available at doi: 10.1111/j.1749-6632.1999.tb08532.x. Accessed June 20, 2014.

Consensus Panel on Genetic/Genomic Nursing Competencies: Essentials of Genetic and Genomic Nursing: Competencies, Curricula Guidelines, and Outcome Indicators, ed 2. Silver Spring, MD, 2009, ANA. Available at: http://www.nursingworld.org/MainMenuCategories/EthicsStandards/Genetics-1/EssentialNursingCompetenciesandCurriculaGuidelinesforGeneticsandGenomics.pdf. Accessed on June 20, 2014.

European Society of Human Genetics: Quotes from DNA-Day 2012. Quote from L. Haven Figari. Retrieved from: http://www.dnaday.eu/quotes.htm. on June 20, 2014.

Evaluation of Genomic Applications in Practice and Prevention; EGAPP Working Group Recommendation, 2013. Retrieved from: http://www.egappreviews.org/recommendations/lynch.htm. Accessed on June 20, 2014.

Genetics in Primary Care: Genetic red flags, 2014. Available at: http://www.geneticsinprimarycare.org/YourPractice/family-Health-History/Pages/Genetic%20Red%20Flags.aspx. Accessed June 23, 2014.

International Council of Nurses: The ICN Code of Ethics for Nurses. Geneva, Switzerland, 2012, ICN.

International Society of Nurses in Genetics: Statement on Scope and Standards of Genetics Clinical Nursing Practice. Washington DC, 1998, ANA.

Jenkins J, Calzone KA: Establishing the essential nursing competencies for genetics and genomics.

J Nurs Scholarsh 39(1):10–16, 2007. Available at: http://www.ncbi.nlm.nih.gov/pmc/articles/PMC3099038/. Accessed on June 20, 2014.

Jirtle RL, Skinner MK: Environmental epigenomics and disease susceptibility. Nat Rev Genet 8:253–262, 2007. Retrieved from: http://www.nature.com/nrg/journal/v8/n4/full/nrg2045.html.

Jorde LB, Carey JC, Bamshad MJ, editors: Medical Genetics, ed 4. Philadelphia, 2010, Elsevier.

Karns L, Genetics Counselor UVA Health System (2010). Interview by E. J. Zschaebitz (phone interview). Accessed May 5, 2010.

Lumey LH, Stein AD, Susser A: Prenatal famine and adult health. Ann Rev Pub Health 32:237–262, 2011. Available at: http://www.annualreviews.org/doi/pdf/10.1146/annurev-publhealth-031210-101230. Accessed on December 17, 2014.

McKusick VA: History of medical genetics. In Rimoin DL, Connor JM, Pyertiz RE, et al, editors: Emery and Rimoin's Principles and Practice of Medical Genetics, vol 1, ed 5. London, 2007, Churchill Livingstone, pp 3–32.

National Cancer Institute: Genetics of breast and ovarian cancer, 2014. Available at: http://www.cancer.gov/cancertopics/pdq/genetics/breast-and-ovarian/HealthProfessional/page2. Accessed June 20, 2014.

National Center for Biotechnology Information: Anemia, sickle cell, n.d. Available at: http://www.ncbi.nlm.nih.gov/books/NBK22238. Accessed June 20, 2014.

National Coalition of Health Professional Education in Genetics: Core competencies for all health professionals, September 2009. Available at: www.nchpeg.org. Accessed June 12, 2014.

National Coalition of Health Professional Education in Genetics: Core principles in genetics, ed 3. September 2007. www.nchpeg.org. Accessed June 12, 2014.

National Institutes of Health: All about the Human Genome Project (HGP). From the National Human

Genome Research Institute, 2014. Retrieved from: http://www.genome.gov/10001772. Accessed June 20, 2014.

National Society of Genetic Counselors: Your genetic health:patient information, 2014. Accessed at: http://nsgc.org/p/cm/ld/fid=143. Accessed on June 20, 2014.

Perry SE: Genetics, conception and fetal development. In Lowdermilk DL, Perry SE, editors: Maternity Nursing, ed 8. St Louis, 2011, Mosby, pp 135–167.

Quad Council of Public Health Nursing Organizations: Public health nursing competencies. Wheat Ridge, CO, 2011, QCPHNO.

Szoka B: FDA Oversteps on genetic testing: opposing view. USA Today December 16, 2013. Retrieved from http://www.usatoday.com/story/opinion/2013/12/16/genetic-tests-23andme-editorials-debates/4045823/?AID=10709313&PID=4003003&SID=m50q5aac4nvt.

U. S. Department of Health and Human Services: Personalized health care, 2007. Available at: http://www.hhs.gov/myhealthcare/. Accessed June 23, 2014.

U.S. Department of Health and Human Services: Guidance on the Genetic Information Nondiscrimination Act: implications for investigators and institutional review boards, 2009. Available at: http://www.hhs.gov/ohrp/policy/gina.pdf. Accessed June 12, 2014.

U.S. Department of Health and Human Services: Healthy People 2020. Washington, DC, 2010. Accessed at: http://www.healthypeople.gov/2020/topicsobjectives2020/overview.aspx?topicid=15U.S. on June 20, 2014.

Wellcome Trust & the Sanger Institute: The first draft of the Book of Humankind has been read, 2012. Quoting Michael Dexter. Retrieved from: http://www.sanger.ac.uk/about/press/2000/draft2000/mainrelease.html. on June 20, 2014.

Williams JK: Education for genetics and nursing practice. AACN Clin Issues 13(4):492–500, 2002.

# Epidemiology

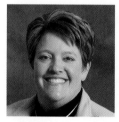

### Swann Arp Adams, MS, PhD

Dr. Swann Arp Adams has over 17 years of experience in clinical epidemiology. She holds a PhD in epidemiology and an MS in biomedical sciences. Dr. Adams has previous experience in a variety of research fields including physical activity, bone marrow transplantation, diabetes, breast cancer, and cancer disparities. She is the Associate Director of the Cancer Prevention and Control Program and is an associate professor with a joint appointment in the College of Nursing and the Department of Epidemiology and Biostatistics at the University of South Carolina. Her current research work focuses on reducing the burden of cancer disparities experienced by African Americans. Past honors include the Doctoral Achievement Award (2004) and the Gerry Sue Arnold Alumni Award (2008) from the Arnold School of Public Health of the University of South Carolina.

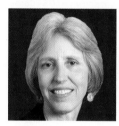

### DeAnne K. Hilfinger Messias, PhD, RN, FAAN

Dr. DeAnne K. Hilfinger Messias is an international community health nurse, educator, and researcher. She spent more than two decades in Brazil, where she directed a primary health care project on the lower Amazon, taught women's health and community health nursing, and organized women's health initiatives among poor urban populations. Her research and scholarship focuses on women's work and health, immigrant women's health, language access, and community empowerment. She is currently involved in a community-based intervention trial of a promotora-delivered physical activity intervention among low-income Latinas. Dr. Messias was a fellow with the International Center for Health Leadership Development at the School of Public Health, University of Illinois at Chicago (2002–2004) and a Fulbright Senior Scholar in Global/Public Health at the Federal University of Goiás, Brazil (2005). She is a professor and director of the PhD Program in the University of South Carolina College of Nursing, with a joint appointment in the Women's and Gender Studies Program.

## ADDITIONAL RESOURCES

**ⓔ Evolve Website http://evolve.elsevier.com/Stanhope**
- Healthy People 2020
- WebLinks
- Quiz

- Case Studies
- Glossary
- Answers to Practice Application

## OBJECTIVES

*After reading this chapter, the student should be able to do the following:*

1. Define epidemiology and describe its essential elements and approach.
2. Describe current and historical contexts of the development of the field of epidemiology.
3. Identify key elements of the epidemiologic triangle and the ecological model and describe the interactions among these elements in both models.
4. Explain the relationship of the natural history of disease to the three levels of prevention and to the design and implementation of community interventions.
5. Interpret basic epidemiologic measures of morbidity (disease) and mortality (death).
6. Discuss descriptive epidemiologic parameters of person, place, and time.
7. Describe the key features of common epidemiologic study designs.
8. Describe essential characteristics and methods of evaluating a screening program.
9. Identify the most common sources of bias in epidemiologic studies.
10. Evaluate epidemiologic research and apply findings to nursing practice.
11. Discuss the role of the nurse in epidemiologic surveillance and primary, secondary, and tertiary prevention.

The authors would like to acknowledge the contribution of Robert E. McKeown, PhD, FACE, who contributed to this chapter for previous editions.

## KEY TERMS

## CHAPTER OUTLINE

Epidemiology is considered the basic science of public health. Like public health nursing, epidemiology is a complex and continually evolving field with a common focus: the optimal health for all members of all communities, local and global. Nurses use epidemiologic frameworks, methods, and data to better understand factors that contribute to health and disease; to develop health promotion and disease prevention interventions and measures; to identify the presence of infectious agents in individuals and groups; to design, implement, and evaluate community health programs; and to develop and evaluate public health policies. Since nurses care for individuals and families, it is important that they consider the broader context in which these individuals live and the complex interplay of social and environmental factors that affect individual and collective

DEF. OB HUTH.

well-being. Basic knowledge of epidemiology is essential to the practice of nursing across all settings and populations.

## DEFINITIONS OF HEALTH AND PUBLIC HEALTH

Health is the core concept in nursing and epidemiology. In 1978 the World Health Organization (WHO) affirmed that "health, which is a state of complete physical, mental and social well-being, and not merely the absence of disease or infirmity, is a fundamental human right and the attainment of the highest possible level of health is a most important world-wide social goal" (WHO, 1978, p. 1). As defined by the American Nurses Association (ANA), "Nursing is the protection, promotion, and optimization of health and abilities, prevention of illness and injury, alleviation of suffering through the diagnosis and treatment of human response, and advocacy in the care of individuals, families, communities, and populations" (ANA, 2012). This definition reflects the WHO goal and coincides with epidemiologic principles. A holistic approach to health, including the incorporation of epidemiologic principles, is particularly appropriate for nurses. Nurses incorporate concepts of health into their nursing practice on a daily basis.

Public health has been described as a system and social enterprise; a profession; a collection of methods, knowledge, and techniques; governmental health services, especially medical care for the poor and underserved; and the health status of the public (Turnock, 2011). In the early twentieth century, C.E.A. Winslow defined public health as "the science and art of preventing disease, prolonging life and promoting physical health and efficiency through organized community effort." The Institute of Medicine (IOM) report The Future of Public Health drew upon Winslow's definition in stating the mission of public health is to fulfill "society's interest in assuring conditions in which people can be healthy" (IOM, 1988, p. 40). This mission statement clearly indicates a societal interest in the health of all its members. More specifically, the mission of the public health enterprise is to *ensure conditions* that promote health and well-being. From both public health and nursing perspectives, *health* encompasses much more than the presence or absence of a physical disease or disability; it involves optimal functioning across a broad range of systems—physiological, somatic, psychological, social, and environmental. The authors of the 1988 IOM report caution that this broad view of health and the role of public health professionals and agencies forces "practitioners to make difficult choices about where to focus their energies and raises the possibility that public health could be so broadly defined so as to lose distinctive meaning" (IOM, 1988, p. 40). Nurses are especially well suited to address this concern because of their holistic view of health and broad, interprofessional approach to intervention.

The practice of public health nursing is based on definitions of health and public health that go beyond a narrow biomedical model of individual health. Ensuring the public's health includes delivery of specific services to individuals, but also includes the establishment and implementation of public policies and programs. Public health and public health nursing activities focus on community prevention, disease control, and personal and community health services. The IOM report The Future of the Public's Health in the 21st Century (IOM, 2002) highlights the importance of intersectoral collaborations to accomplish the mission of public health. There is further emphasis on an ecological approach to research and practice (discussed later). Interprofessional collaboration between nurses and other health professionals, including epidemiologists, is critical to efforts to create and sustain the conditions necessary for health promotion, health maintenance, and overall improvements in public health (Baldwin, 2007).

 **HEALTHY PEOPLE 2020**

### Examples of New Epidemiologic Objectives Included in Healthy People 2020

- AH-2: Increase the percentage of adolescents who participate in extracurricular and out-of-school activities.
- AOCBC-4: Reduce the proportion of adults with doctor-diagnosed arthritis who find it "very difficult" to perform specific joint-related activities.
- C-9: Reduce invasive colorectal cancer.
- D-16: Increase prevention behaviors in persons at high risk for diabetes with prediabetes.
- FS-5: Increase the proportion of consumers who follow key food safety practices.
- HAI-2: Reduce invasive methicillin-resistant *Staphylococcus aureus* (MRSA) infections.

From U.S. Department of Health and Human Services. Healthy People 2020. Available at www.healthypeople2020. Accessed January 14, 2011.

## DEFINITIONS AND DESCRIPTIONS OF EPIDEMIOLOGY

Epidemiology has been defined as "the study of the occurrence and distribution of health-related states or events in specified populations, including the study of the determinants influencing such states, and the application of this knowledge to control the health problems" (Porta, 2008, p. 81). The word *epidemiology* comes from the Greek words *epi* (upon), *demos* (people), and *logos* (thought), and it originally referred to the spread of diseases of infectious origin. In the past century the definition and scope of epidemiology have broadened and now include the examination of the occurrence of chronic diseases, such as cancer and cardiovascular disease; mental health and health-related events, such as accidents, injuries, and violence; occupational and environmental exposures and their effects; and positive health states.

Epidemiologists investigate the distribution or patterns of health events in populations to characterize health outcomes in terms of *what, who, where, when, how,* and *why*: What is the outcome? Who is affected? Where are they? When do events occur? This focus is called descriptive epidemiology, because it seeks to describe the occurrence of a disease in terms of person, place, and time (Koepsell and Weiss, 2003). The *how* and *why*, or determinants of health events, are those factors, exposures, characteristics, behaviors, and contexts that determine (or influence) the patterns: How does it occur? Why are some affected more than others? Determinants may be individual, relational or social, communal, or environmental. This focus on investigation of causes and associations is called ana-lytic epidemiology, in reference to the goal of understanding the etiology (or origins and causal factors) of disease; the broad consideration of many levels of potential determinants is called the *ecological approach* (IOM, 2002). The results of these investigations are used to guide or evaluate policies and programs that improve the health of the community. The differentiation between *descriptive* and *analytic* epidemiologic studies is not clear-cut: analytic studies rely on descriptive comparisons, and descriptive comparisons shed light on determinants.

> ## ≫ LINKING CONTENT TO PRACTICE
>
> It is important that nurses understand the relationship between population health concepts and clinical practice. Within the field of epidemiology, the definition of *population* is not necessarily confined to large groups of people, such as the population of the United States. Population health concepts also apply to other types of groups, such as the collective group of clients at one clinical practice site. In this case, the clinical epidemiologic application of population health concepts is evident in questions such as: What are the factors that contribute to the health and illness issues among clients I see in my clinic? Why do some of my clients fare better than others with the same disease conditions? Are there alternative clinical practices that might positively impact the health of my clients? All of these very clinical questions incorporate epidemiologic concepts of describing the *burden of disease* in a population, identifying and understanding *determinants of health,* and examining possible *root causes* of health outcomes. Two important nursing documents recently highlighted ways in which epidemiologic knowledge and skills are essential to nursing practice. The Council on Linkages Between Academia and Public Health Practice (2014) outlined essential analytic/assessment and public health science skills, and The Quad Council of Public Health Nursing Competencies (Swider et al, 2013) provided details and examples of ways to implement these skill sets in nursing practice.

The first step in the epidemiologic process is to answer the "what" question by defining a health outcome. The case definition usually refers to cases of disease, but also may include instances of injuries, accidents, or even wellness (Koepsell and Weiss, 2003). Epidemiology has played an important role in the refinement of the case definition for acquired immunodeficiency syndrome (AIDS) and other emerging infectious diseases and in the development of more precise diagnostic criteria for psychiatric disorders. Epidemiologic methods are used to quantify the frequency of occurrence and characterize both the case group and the population from which they come. The aim is to describe the distribution (i.e., determine who has the disease and where and when the disease occurs) and to search for factors that explain the pattern or risk of occurrence (i.e., answer the questions of why and how the disease occurs).

An **epidemic** occurs when the rate of disease, injury, or other condition exceeds the usual (endemic) level of that condition. There is no specific threshold of incidence that indicates the existence of an epidemic. Because of the virtual eradication of smallpox globally, any occurrence of smallpox could be considered an epidemic. In contrast, given the high rates of ischemic heart disease in the United States, an increase of many cases would be needed before an epidemic was noted; some would

argue the current high rates compared with earlier periods already indicate an epidemic. The rising rates of obesity in the United States have led the Centers for Disease Control and Prevention (CDC) to consider adult obesity as an epidemic (CDC, 2012). Recent epidemiologic data show that 35.7% of U.S. adults 20 years of age and older—more than 78 million people—are obese. Approximately 19% of the population ages 6 to 12 and 17% of those 12 to 19 years old are considered overweight (Ogden et al, 2012). Obesity contributes to increased risk for heart disease, hypertension, diabetes, arthritis-related disabilities, and certain cancers.

Epidemiology builds on and draws from other disciplines and methods, including clinical medicine and laboratory sciences, social sciences, quantitative methods (especially biostatistics), and public health policy, among others. Epidemiology differs from clinical medicine, which focuses on the diagnosis and treatment of disease in individuals. Epidemiology is the study of populations in order to (1) monitor the health of the population, (2) understand the determinants of health and disease in communities, and (3) investigate and evaluate interventions to prevent disease and maintain health. Effective nursing practice bridges the disciplines of clinical medicine and epidemiology, incorporating a focus on both individual and collective strategies. Nurses working in the community provide clinical services to individuals as they also tend to the broader context in which these individuals live and the complex interplay of social and environmental factors that affect their well-being. Nurses apply epidemiologic methods in their daily practice, as they note trends in specific illnesses (e.g., sexually transmitted infections) or conditions (e.g., accidents) and in designing, implementing, and evaluating community health programs. The AIDS epidemic was first identified because clinicians, using basic epidemiology methods, realized that much higher numbers of *Pneumocystis jiroveci (carinii pneumonia)* were being diagnosed than had ever been seen previously.

## HISTORICAL PERSPECTIVES

The roots of epidemiology have been traced to ancient Greece (Merrill and Timmreck, 2006). In the fourth century BC, Hippocrates maintained that to understand health and disease in a community, one should look to geographic and climatic factors, the seasons of the year, the food and water consumed, and the habits and behaviors of the people. Yet modern epidemiology did not emerge until the nineteenth century and it was only in the twentieth century that the field developed as a discipline with a distinctive identity (Susser, 1985).

Two refinements in research methods in the eighteenth and nineteenth centuries were critical for the formation of epidemiologic methods: (1) use of a comparison group, and (2) the development of quantitative techniques (numerical measurements, or counts). One of the most famous studies using a comparison group is the pivotal mid-nineteenth-century investigation of cholera by John Snow, who is often credited with being the "father of epidemiology" (Merrill and Timmreck, 2006). By mapping cases that clustered around a single public water pump in one London cholera outbreak, Snow demonstrated a connection between water supply and cholera. He later observed that cholera rates were higher among households supplied by water companies whose water intakes were downstream from the city than among households whose water came from further upstream, where it was subject to less contamination (Table 12-1). Snow realized that his investigation was an example of what epidemiologists call a *natural experiment* and his findings added credibility to his argument that foul water was the vehicle for transmission of the agent that caused cholera (Gordis, 2013; Koepsell and Weiss, 2003).

 Development and application of epidemiologic methods in the twentieth century were stimulated by dramatic changes in society and population dynamics (the combined effects of birth rates, death rates, life expectancy, and patterns of illness and causes of death) (McKeown, 2009). Contributing factors included improved nutrition, new vaccines, better sanitation, the advent of antibiotics and chemotherapies, and declining infant and child mortality and birth rates. Societal changes also

resulted from large-scale events including the Great Depression and World War II, followed by a rising standard of living for many but continued deep poverty for others. These changes led to increasing longevity and significant shifts in the age distribution of the population, resulting in increases in age-related diseases, such as coronary heart disease (CHD), stroke, cancer, and senile dementia (Susser, 1985; IOM, 2002). However, disparities remain among population subgroups in life expectancy and risk of many acute and chronic diseases. Figure 12-1 shows the 10 leading causes of death in the United States in 1900, 1950, and 2010, with the percentage of all deaths attributed to each cause. The top three causes of death have not changed since 1950, whereas the composition of the remaining seven leading causes *has* changed.

With the increase in chronic disease, epidemiologists realized the necessity of looking beyond single agents (e.g., the infectious agent that causes cholera) toward a multifactorial etiology (i.e., many factors or combinations and levels of factors contributing to disease, such as the complex set of factors that cause cardiovascular disease), referred to as an ecologic model (IOM, 2002). Researchers and practitioners also recognized the contribution of behavioral and environmental causes to some chronic conditions formerly considered to be degenerative diseases of aging. This understanding prompted new thinking about the possibility of preventing or delaying the onset of certain chronic diseases (Susser, 1985). In addition, the development of genetic and molecular techniques (such as genetic markers for increased risk of breast cancer and sophisticated tests for antibodies to infectious agents or for other biological markers of exposures to environmental toxins, such as lead or pesticides) has increased the ability to identify and classify persons in terms of exposures or inherent susceptibility to disease.

### TABLE 12-1   Household Cholera Death Rates by Source of Water Supply in John Snow's 1853 Investigation

| Company | No. of Houses | Deaths from Cholera | Deaths Per 10,000 Households |
|---|---|---|---|
| Southwark and Vauxhall | 40,046 | 1263 | 315 |
| Lambeth | 26,107 | 98 | 37 |
| Rest of London | 256,423 | 1422 | 59 |

From Snow J: On the mode of communication of cholera. In *Snow on Cholera.* New York, 1855, The Commonwealth Fund.

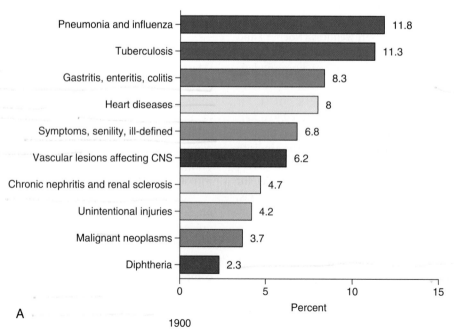

FIG 12-1 Ten leading causes of death as a percentage of all deaths, United States. **A,** 1900.

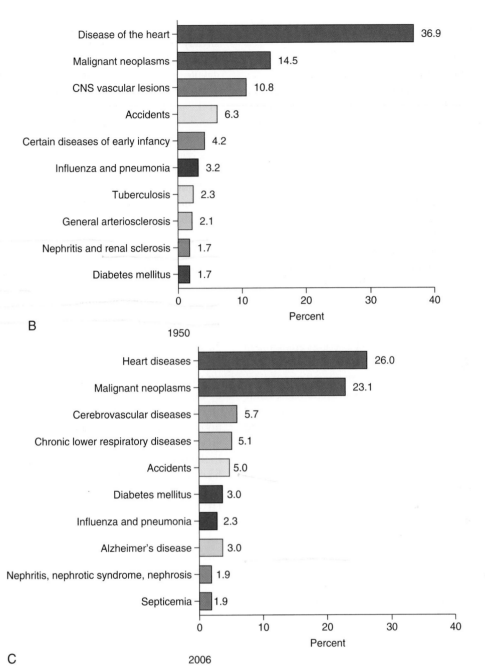

FIG 12-1, cont'd **B,** 1950. **C,** 2006. (**B,** Data from Anderson RN: Deaths: leading causes for 2000. *Natl Vital Stat Rep* 50:16, 2002; Brownson RC, Remington PL, Davis JR: *Chronic Disease Epidemiology and Control,* ed 2. Washington, DC, 1998, APHA; U.S. Department of Health, Education, and Welfare: *Vital Statistics of the United States: 1950,* vol 1, Washington, DC, 1954, USDHEW, Public Health Service.) **C,** Heron M. Deaths: Leading causes for 2010. *National Vital Statistics Reports* 62(6). Hyattsville, MD: National Center for Health Statistics, 2013; Martin JA, Hamilton BE, Sutton PD, et al: Births, final data for 2006. *Natl Vital Stat Rep* 57:7, 2009.)

# BASIC CONCEPTS IN EPIDEMIOLOGY

## Measures of Morbidity and Mortality

### Proportions, Rates, and Risk

The distribution of health states and events is an important focus of epidemiology. Because people differ in their probability or risk of disease, a primary concern is the identification of how they differ. Today, epidemiologists use tools such as geographic information systems (GISs) to study health-related events to identify disease distribution patterns, similar to John Snow's mapping of cholera cases in London in the nineteenth century. However, mapping cases is limited in what it can reveal. A higher number of cases may simply be the result of a larger population with more people who are potential cases, or of a longer period of observation. Any description of disease patterns should take into account the size of the population at risk for the disease. That is, we should look not only at the numerator (the number of cases), but also at the denominator (the number of people in the population at risk) and at the length of time the population was observed. For example, 50 cases of influenza in a month might be viewed as a serious epidemic in a population of 250 but would indicate a low rate in a population of 250,000. On the other hand, even in a small population, one might observe 50 cases over a period of several years. Using rates and proportions instead of simple counts of cases takes the size of the population at risk into account (Koepsell and Weiss, 2003). How time is considered differs according to the measure being used.

Epidemiologic studies rely on proportions and rates. A proportion is a type of ratio in which the denominator includes the numerator. For example, in 2006 there were 2,426,264 deaths recorded in the United States, of which 631,636 were reported as caused by heart disease; so the proportion of deaths attributable to heart disease in 2006 was 631,636/2,426,264 = 0.260, or 26.0%. Because the numerator must be included in the denominator, proportions can range from 0 to 1. Proportions are often multiplied by 100 and expressed as a percent, literally meaning per 100. In public health statistics, however, if the proportion is very small, we use a larger multiplier to avoid small fractions; thus the proportion may be expressed as a number per 1000 or per 100,000.

A rate is a measure of the frequency of a health event in "a defined population, usually in a specified period of time" (Porta, 2008, p. 207). A rate is a ratio, but it is not a proportion because the denominator is a function of both the population size and the dimension of time, whereas the numerator is the number of events (Rothman, 2012; Koepsell and Weiss, 2003; Gordis, 2013). Furthermore, depending on the units of time and the frequency of events, a rate may exceed 1. As its name suggests, a rate is a measure of how rapidly something is happening: how rapidly a disease is developing in a population or how rapidly people are dying. Conceptually, a rate is the instantaneous change in a continuous process. Notice the use of the words *event* and *happening*. Rates deal with change over time, as individuals move from one state of being to another (e.g., from well to ill, alive to dead, or ill to cured). In observing a population over time to observe such changes in status, we typically exclude from the population being followed those persons who have already experienced the event.

Using the same health event of death from heart disease detailed previously, we can also compute a rate. To calculate the death rate, the denominator will be the number of individuals in the population *during the year in which the deaths occurred*, rather than total number of deaths. For example, in 2006, the U.S. population estimate was 299,398,484. Since rates are commonly expressed per 100,000 or per 1000, we will divide this total population figure by 100,000, to get 2993.98484. The resulting calculation of the rate of death from heart disease in the United States in 2006 would be 631,636/2993.98484 = 211 per 100,000.

Risk refers to the probability that an event will occur within a specified time period. A population at risk is the population of persons for whom there is some finite probability (even if small) of that event. For example, although the risk of breast cancer in men is small, a few men do develop breast cancer and therefore could be considered part of the population at risk. There are some outcomes for which certain people would never be at risk (e.g., men cannot be at risk of ovarian cancer, nor can women be at risk of testicular cancer). A high-risk population, on the other hand, would include those persons who, because of exposure, lifestyle, family history, social or environmental context, or other factors, are at greater risk for disease than the population at large. Although anyone may be susceptible to HIV infection, the degree of susceptibility does vary. Everyone in the population is at risk for HIV and AIDS, but persons who have multiple sexual partners without adequate protection or who use intravenous drugs are in the high-risk population for HIV infection. However, others who do not fit these categories may unknowingly be at high risk. An example is women who consider themselves to be in monogamous relationships but are unaware that their partners have sexual relations with other women or men. As proportions, risk estimates have no dimensions, but they are a function of the length of time of observation. Given a continuous rate, increasing time will mean that a larger proportion of the population will eventually become ill.

Epidemiologists and other health professionals are interested in measures of morbidity, especially incidence proportions, incidence rates, and prevalence proportions (Gordis, 2013). These measures provide information about the risk of disease, the rate of disease development, and the levels of existing disease in a population, respectively.

---

| **HOW TO**  **Quantify a Health Problem in the Community** |
| --- |

*Planning for resources and personnel often requires quantifying the level of a problem in a community. For example, to know how different districts compare in the rates of very-low-birth-weight (VLBW) infants, one would calculate the prevalence of VLBW births in each district:*

1. *Determine the number of live births in each district from birth certificate data obtained from the vital records division of the health department.*
2. *Use the birth weight information from the birth certificate data to determine the number of infants born weighing less than 1500 g in each district.*

3. *Calculate the prevalence of VLBW births by district as the number of infants weighing less than 1500 g at birth divided by the total number of live births.*
4. *If the number of VLBW births in each district is small, use several recent years of data to obtain a more stable estimate.*

## Measures of Incidence

Measures of incidence reflect the number of *new* cases or events in a population at risk during a specified time. An incidence rate quantifies the rate of development of new cases in a population at risk, whereas an incidence proportion indicates the proportion of the population at risk who experience the event over some period of time, for example, the proportion of the population who develop influenza during a given year (Rothman, 2012). The population at risk is considered to be persons without the event or outcome of interest but who are at risk of experiencing it. Note that existing (or prevalent) cases are excluded from the population at risk for this definition, since they already have the condition and are no longer at risk of developing it. The incidence proportion is also referred to as the **cumulative incidence rate** (and erroneously simply as the incidence rate) because it reflects the cumulative effect of the incidence rate over the time period, whether it is a month, a year, or several years. A constant incidence rate operating over a period of time results in an increasing proportion of the population who are affected, that is, the incidence rate may stay constant while the cumulative incidence rate increases with time because the pool of people who have the disease is becoming larger. An incidence proportion can be interpreted as an estimate of risk of disease in that population over that period. An example of this might be the incidence proportion for cancer. Using statistics published for a 5-year period of time, one could calculate that 20 of 200 individuals were newly diagnosed with cancer (hypothetical example). The incidence proportion would then be $20/200 = 0.10$ or 10%. This could be interpreted that over a 5-year period of time, the risk of cancer in the population was 10%. The risk of disease is a function of both the rate of new disease development and the length of time the population is at risk. The interpretation can be for an individual (i.e., the probability that the person will become ill) or for a population (i.e., the proportion of a population expected to become ill over the specified period). For further examples of these calculations as it relates to mortality, see Table 12-2.

Another common risk measure used by both the science and general community is relative risk. Essentially, the relative risk compares the incidence of disease in an "exposed" population to the incidence of disease in an "unexposed" population. In this way, the relative risk is based on the calculations that are performed for the cumulative incidence rate. As an example, one could conceptualize the exposure as "taking hormone replacement therapy" and the outcome as breast cancer. In this case, we would identify a group of women who would be of an age to take hormone replacement therapy. Next, we would categorize these women into two groups—those women not taking hormone replacement therapy and those who are taking hormone replacement. Within these two groups, then we would

calculate the *cumulative incidence rate for each group*. The *relative risk* would then be expressed as the cumulative incidence rate of breast cancer among women taking hormone replacement therapy divided by the cumulative incidence rate of breast cancer among those *not* taking hormone replacement therapy.

Because the relative risk is based upon a ratio, the actual value can range anywhere from >0 to infinity (theoretically). When the cumulative incidence rates are exactly equal, the relative risk is 1.00. This is often termed the "null value," indicating that the exposure of interest has no effect on the outcome of interest. This is the statistic most often cited in media releases about scientific studies. Using the hormone replacement therapy and breast cancer example, a research study that indicated a relative risk of 1.75 can be interpreted to indicate that the risk of developing breast cancer among those women taking hormone replacement therapy is 75% times the risk of developing breast cancer among women not taking hormone replacement therapy. This is also the statistic that the nurses can use to estimate the probability of disease among their patients. This concept will be discussed in more detail later in this chapter in the section on cohort studies.

---

**HOW TO Use Epidemiologic Concepts in Nursing**
*Epidemiologic concepts and data are used in ongoing assessments of both community and individual health problems. An initial component of a community health assessment is the collection of incidence, morbidity, and mortality rates for specific diseases. Health service data, such as immunization rates, causes of hospitalization, and emergency department visits, are also obtained. Additional areas for community assessment are outlined in the How To box on page 264. Individual health problems should incorporate evaluations of health risk based on lifestyle patterns along with the standard history and clinical examinations.*

---

## Prevalence Proportion

The prevalence proportion is a measure of existing disease in a population at a particular time (i.e., the number of existing cases divided by the current population). We can also calculate the prevalence of a specific risk factor or exposure. When used alone, the term *prevalence* typically refers to the *prevalence proportion*, although the term is sometimes used to refer to the count of existing cases (i.e., the numerator of the prevalence proportion). For example, consider the following data from a breast cancer screening program that had reached 8000. Among these 8000 women, if 35 had previously been diagnosed with breast cancer and an additional 20 cases of breast cancer were identified as a result of the screening program, the prevalence proportion of current and past breast cancer events in this population would be 55 out of 8000, expressed as a rate of 687.5 per 100,000.

It is important to note that a prevalence proportion is not an estimate of the risk of developing disease. The prevalence proportion is a function of both the rate at which new cases of the disease develop and how long these cases remain in the population. To illustrate this point, consider the prevalence of

## TABLE 12-2   Common Mortality Rates

| Rate/Ratio | Definition and Example |
|---|---|
| Crude mortality rate | Usually an annual rate that represents the proportion of a population who die from any cause during the period, using the midyear population as the denominator<br>Example: In 2006 there were 2,426,264 deaths in a total population of 299,398,484, or 810.4 per 100,000:<br>$$\frac{2,426,264}{299,398,484} = 810.4 \text{ per } 100,000$$ |
| Age-specific rate | Number of deaths among persons of given age group per midyear population of that age group<br>Example: 2006 age-specific mortality rate for 20- to 24-year-olds:<br>$$\frac{21,148}{21,111,240} = 100.2 \text{ per } 100,000$$ |
| Cause-specific rate | Number of deaths from a specific cause per midyear population<br>Example: 2006 cause-specific rate for accidents:<br>$$\frac{121,599 \text{ deaths from accidents}}{299,398,484 \text{ midyear population}} = 40.6 \text{ per } 100,000$$ |
| Case-fatality rate | Number of deaths from a specific disease in a given period divided by number of persons diagnosed with that disease<br>Example: If 87 of every 100 persons diagnosed with lung cancer die within 5 years, the 5-year case fatality rate is 87%. The 5-year survival rate is 13%. |
| Proportionate mortality ratio | Number of deaths from a specific disease per total number of deaths in the same period<br>Example: In 2006 there were 631,636 deaths from diseases of the heart, and 2,426,264 deaths from all causes:<br>$$\frac{631,636}{2,426,264} = 0.26 \text{ or } 26 \text{ of all deaths in 2006 were attributable to heart disease}$$ |
| Infant mortality rate | Number of infant deaths before 1 year of age in a year per number of live births in the same year<br>Example: In 2006 there were 28,527 infant deaths and 4,265,555 live births:<br>$$\frac{28,527}{4,265,555} = 668.79 \text{ per } 100,000 \text{ live births or } 6.69 \text{ per } 1000 \text{ live births}$$ |
| Neonatal mortality rate | Number of infant deaths under 28 days of age in a year per number of live births in the same year<br>Example: In 2006 there were 18,989 neonatal deaths and 4,265,555 live births:<br>$$\frac{18,989}{4,265,555} = 445.17 \text{ per } 100,000 \text{ or } 4.45 \text{ per } 1000 \text{ live births}$$ |
| Postneonatal mortality rate | Number of infant deaths from 28 days to 1 year in a year per number of live births in the same year<br>Example: In 2006 there were 9538 postneonatal deaths and 4,265,555 live births:<br>$$\frac{9538}{4,265,555} = 223.61 \text{ per } 100,000 \text{ or } 2.24 \text{ per } 1000 \text{ live births}$$ |

From Heron M. Deaths: Leading causes for 2010. *Natl Vital Stat Rep* 62(6), Hyattsville, MD, 2013, National Center for Health Statistics; Martin JA, Hamilton BE, Sutton PD, et al: Births: Final data for 2006. *Natl Vital Stat Rep* 57(7), Hyattsville, MD, 2009, National Center for Health Statistics.

prostate cancer. The number of people with prostate cancer at any given time reflects both the number of new cases diagnosed at that specific point in time and the number of previously diagnosed men currently living with the diagnosis of prostate cancer. The duration of a specific disease is affected by both case fatality and cure. For example, a disease with a short duration (e.g., an intestinal virus) may not have a high prevalence proportion, even if the rate of new cases is high, because cases do not accumulate (see Point Epidemic later in this chapter). A disease with a long course (e.g., Crohn's disease) will have a higher prevalence proportion than a rapidly fatal disease that has the same rate of new cases.

### Comparing Prevalence and Incidence

The prevalence proportion measures existing cases of disease and is affected by factors that influence risk (incidence) and by factors that influence survival or recovery (duration). Prevalence proportions are useful in planning health care services because they indicate the level of disease existing in the population and therefore the size of the population in need of services. However, prevalence measures are less useful when we are looking for factors related to disease etiology. Because prevalence proportions reflect duration in addition to the risk of getting the disease, it is difficult to sort out what factors are related to risk and what factors are related to survival or recovery.

For example, the 5-year survival rate for breast cancer is about 85%, but the 5-year survival rate for lung cancer in women is only about 15%. Even if the incidence rates of breast and lung cancer were the same in women (and they are not), the prevalence proportions would differ because, on average, women live longer after a diagnosis of breast cancer than do women diagnosed with lung cancer. In other words, the duration of breast cancer is longer.

The measures of choice in studying disease etiology are incidence rates and incidence proportions, because incidence is affected only by factors related to the risk of developing disease and not to survival or cure. At the level of a local health department, epidemiologists and nurses would rely on both incidence and prevalence data in planning services focused on the prevention and control of tuberculosis (TB). They would examine the existing level of TB within the community (prevalence) to plan services and direct prevention and control measures, and they would take into consideration the rate of new TB cases (incidence) to study risk factors and evaluate the effectiveness of prevention and control programs.

---

**HOW TO**   **Assess Health Problems in a Community**

1. Examine local epidemiologic data (e.g., incidence, morbidity, and mortality rates) to identify major health problems.
2. Examine local health services data to identify major causes of hospitalizations and emergency department visits. Consult with key community leaders (e.g., political, religious, business, educational, health, and cultural leaders) about their perceptions of identified community health problems.
3. Mobilize community groups to elicit discussions and identify perceived health priorities within the community (e.g., focus groups, neighborhood forums, or community-wide forums).
4. Analyze community environmental health hazards and pollutants (e.g., water, sewage, air, toxic waste).
5. Examine indicators of community knowledge and practices of preventive health behaviors (e.g., use of infant car seats, safe playgrounds, lighted streets, seat belt use, designated driver programs).
6. Identify cultural priorities and beliefs about health among different social, cultural, racial, or national origin groups.
7. Assess community members' interpretations of and degrees of trust in federal, state, and local assistance programs.
8. Engage community members in conducting surveys to assess specific health problems.

---

\*\*For Further Note: This process is very similar to the intake/assessment process that all nurses are familiar with such as obtaining medical and family history (analogous to #1 and #2 above), identifying health concerns of the patient (analogous to #3 and #5 above), perform clinical exam (analogous to #4 above), and evaluate patient knowledge, beliefs, and personal risk (analogous to #5-#8).

## Attack Rate   — EX: Food poisoning

Another measure of morbidity, often used in infectious disease investigations, is the attack rate. This form of incidence proportion is defined as the proportion of persons who are exposed to an agent and develop the disease. Attack rates are often specific to an exposure; food-specific attack rates, for example, are the proportion of persons becoming ill after eating a specific food item.

## Mortality Rates

Mortality rates are key epidemiologic indicators of interest to nurses (Table 12-2). Although measures of mortality reflect serious health problems and changing patterns of disease, they are limited in their usefulness. Mortality rates are informative only for fatal diseases and do not provide direct information about either the level of existing disease in the population or the risk of contracting any particular disease. Also, it is not uncommon for a person who has one disease (e.g., prostate cancer) to die from a different cause (e.g., stroke).

Note that many commonly used mortality rates in Table 12-2 are in fact proportions, not true rates (Rothman, 2012; Gordis, 2013). Because the population changes during the course of a year, we typically take an estimate of the population at midyear as the denominator for annual rates, because the midyear population approximates the amount of person-time contributed by the population during a given year. Using the approximation noted previously for small rates when the period of observation is a single unit of time, the annual mortality rate is an estimate of the risk of death in a given population for that year. These rates are multiplied by a scaling factor (usually 100,000) to avoid small fractions. The result is then expressed as the number of deaths per 100,000 persons. Although a crude mortality rate is calculated easily and represents the actual death rate for the total population, it has certain limitations. It does not reveal specific causes of death, which change in relative importance over time (see Figure 12-1). Also, it is affected by the age distribution of the population because older people are at much greater risk of death than younger people. For example, in 2005 the U.S. crude mortality rate for African Americans was 749.4 per 100,000, compared with a rate of 873.7 per 100,000 for white Americans, even though the mortality rate was higher for African Americans than for whites in every age group up to age 85 (Heron, 2010).

Mortality rates are also calculated for specific groups (e.g., age-, sex-, or race-specific rates). In these instances, the number of deaths occurring in the specified group is divided by the population at risk, now restricted to the number of persons in that group. This rate may be interpreted as the risk of death for persons in the specified group during the period of observation.

The cause-specific mortality rate is an estimate of the risk of death from some specific disease in a population. It is the number of deaths from a specific cause divided by the total population at risk, usually multiplied by 100,000. Two related measures should be distinguished from the cause-specific mortality rate. The case fatality rate (CFR) is usually a proportion: the proportion of persons diagnosed with a particular disorder (i.e., cases) that die within a specified period of time. The CFR may be interpreted as an estimate of the risk of death within that period for a person newly diagnosed with the disease (e.g., the proportion of persons with breast cancer who die within 5 years). Because the CFR is the proportion of diagnosed persons who die within the period, 1 minus the CFR yields the survival rate. For example, if the 5-year CFR for lung cancer is 86%, then the 5-year survival rate is only 14% (Remington et al, 2010). Persons diagnosed with a particular disease often want to know the probability of survival. These rates provide an estimate of that probability.

The second measure to be distinguished from the cause-specific mortality rate is the proportionate mortality ratio (PMR)—the proportion of all deaths that are attributable to a specific cause. The denominator is not the population at risk of death but the total number of deaths in the population; therefore, the PMR is not a rate nor does it estimate the risk of death. The magnitude of the PMR is a function of both the number of deaths from the cause of interest and the number of deaths from other causes. If deaths from certain causes decline over time, the PMR for deaths from other causes that remain fairly constant (in absolute numbers) may increase. For example, motor vehicle accidents accounted for 3.3 deaths per 100,000 persons 5 to 14 years of age in the United States in 2006, which is 21.8% of all deaths in this age group (the PMR). By comparison, motor vehicle accidents caused 22.3 deaths per 100,000 persons 75 to 84 years of age in 2006, which was less than 0.5% of all deaths in this older age group (Heron, 2010). This demonstrates that, although the risk of death from a motor vehicle accident was almost 6.8 times greater in the older group (based on the rates), such accidents accounted for a far greater proportion of all deaths in the younger group (based on the PMR). The reason is that there is a much greater risk of death from other causes in the older group.

Measures of infant mortality are used around the world as an indicator of overall health and availability of health care services. The most common measure, the infant mortality rate (IMR), is the number of deaths to infants in the first year of life divided by the total number of live births. Because the risk of death declines rather dramatically during the first year of life, neonatal and postneonatal mortality rates are also of interest (see Table 12-2). To effectively plan and evaluate community health interventions, nurses need to be able to understand and interpret these key epidemiologic indicators. One of the benefits of epidemiologic studies is that the results may demonstrate which disease prevention and control interventions are more useful and effective.

## Epidemiologic Triangle, Web of Causality, and the Ecologic Model

Epidemiologists understand that disease results from complex relationships among causal agents, susceptible persons, and environmental factors. These three elements—**agent**, **host**, and **environment**—are traditionally referred to as the **epidemiologic triangle** (Figure 12-2, *A*). This model was originally developed as a way of identifying causative factors, transmission, and risk related to infectious diseases. Changes in one of the elements of the triangle can influence the occurrence of disease by increasing or decreasing a person's risk for disease. As illustrated in Figure 12-2, *B*, specific characteristics of agent and host, as well as the interactions between agent and host, are influenced by the environmental context in which they exist, and may in turn influence the environment. Examples of these three components are listed in Box 12-1.

Although the interactions of host, environment, and agent are clearly key elements in disease causation, causal relationships are often more complex than implied by the concept of the epidemiologic triangle. The concept of a web of causality reflects the more complex interrelationships among the numerous factors interacting, sometimes in subtle ways, to increase (or decrease) risk of disease. Furthermore, associations are sometimes mutual, with lines of causality going in both directions. More recently, some epidemiologic researchers have advocated a new paradigm that goes beyond the two-dimensional causal web to consider multiple levels of factors that affect health and disease (Krieger, 1994; Macintyre and Ellaway, 2000).

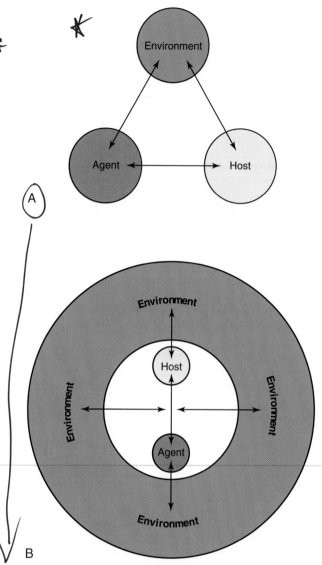

**FIG 12-2** Two models of the agent-host-environment interaction (the epidemiologic triangle).

### BOX 12-1   Examples of Agent, Host, and Environmental Factors in the Epidemiologic Triangle

**Agent**
Infectious agents (e.g., bacteria, viruses, fungi, parasites)
Chemical agents (e.g., heavy metals, toxic chemicals, pesticides)
Physical agents (e.g., radiation, heat, cold, machinery)

**Host**
Genetic susceptibility
Immutable characteristics (e.g., age, sex)
Acquired characteristics (e.g., immunological status)
Lifestyle factors (e.g., diet and exercise)

**Environment**
Climate (e.g., temperature, rainfall)
Plant and animal life (e.g., agents or reservoirs or habitats for agents)
Human population distribution (e.g., crowding, social support)
Socioeconomic factors (e.g., education, resources, access to care)
Working conditions (e.g., levels of stress, noise, satisfaction)

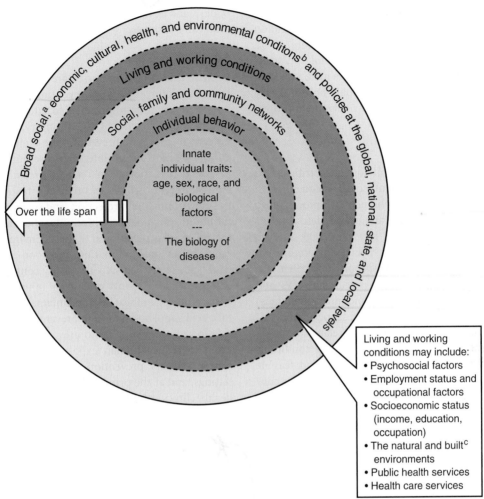

Living and working conditions may include:
• Psychosocial factors
• Employment status and occupational factors
• Socioeconomic status (income, education, occupation)
• The natural and built[c] environments
• Public health services
• Health care services

**FIG 12-3** Determinants of population health. This is a guide to thinking about the determinants of population health. (Reprinted with permission from *The Future of the Public's Health in the 21st Century*, Copyright 2002 by the National Academy of Sciences, courtesy of the National Academies Press, Washington, DC). [a] Social conditions include, but are not limited to: economic inequality, urbanization, mobility, cultural values, attitudes and policies related to discrimination and intolerance on the basis of race, gender, and other differences. [b] Other conditions at the national level might include major sociopolitical shifts, such as recession, war, major environmental disasters, and governmental collapse. [c] The built environment includes transportation, water and sanitation, housing, and other dimensions of urban planning.

Krieger (1994) has suggested that in addition to research on the relationships within the web, we need to look for "the spider"—that is, focus on those larger factors and contexts that influence or create the causal web itself.

With this shift in the scientific thinking, practitioners and researchers are thinking more broadly about the multiple underlying determinants of health. There is increasing recognition of the widespread and profound influence of external factors on the health of individuals, communities, and populations. This is consistent with the ecologic model for population health illustrated in Figure 12-3. This approach expands epidemiologic studies both upward to broader contexts (such as neighborhood characteristics and social context) and downward to the genetic and molecular level. Of course the relative impact of the various factors depicted in this figure is not fixed, and would vary across different populations, contexts, and

settings. However, the model does provide a useful guide for considering the potential relative impact for intervention across various sectors.

Like the web of causality model, the ecologic model recognizes multiple determinants of health and treats them as interrelated and acting synergistically (or antagonistically), rather than as a list of discrete factors. The ecologic model spans a broader spectrum of systems and etiological factors than the more traditional web of causality model and it encompasses determinants at many levels: biological, mental, behavioral, social, and environmental factors, including policy, culture, and economic environments. Another way of thinking of this is that the ecologic model moves from a two-dimensional perspective to a multidimensional perspective. Nurses have a significant role in shaping the health of the population and need to be mindful of the many environmental factors that may contribute to health behaviors and health outcomes. In addressing health behavior change, nurses often focus on patient education (within the domain of "health behaviors" in Figure 12-3). However, lack of attention to other environmental and social issues (i.e., lack of transportation, lack of adequate childcare arrangements, financial constraints, inadequate housing) may mean that the patient is unable to access or respond appropriately to the health education efforts.

## Social Epidemiology

A renewed interest in social epidemiology is attributed in part to the recognition of persistent social inequalities in health. Social epidemiology is the branch of epidemiology that studies the social distribution and social determinants of health and disease (Berkman and Kawachi, 2000; Krieger, 2000; Kawachi and Berkman, 2003). Social epidemiologists focus on the roles and mechanisms of specific social phenomena (e.g., socioeconomic stratification, social networks and support, discrimination, work and employment demands) in the production of health and disease states. Social epidemiologists examine social inequalities and data related to neighborhoods, communities, employment, and family conditions to analyze health issues and design appropriate and feasible public health interventions. Public health professionals are concerned with relationships between social conditions and patterns of health and disease in individuals, families, groups, and populations.

The complex factors that influence or lead to social inequalities in health are being increasingly examined or "rediscovered" through the lens of epidemiology. Berkman and Kawachi (2000) identified several key concepts within the subfield of social epidemiology. These include a population perspective (IOM, 2002), the social context of behavior, contextual and multilevel analysis (Sampson et al, 1997; Diez-Roux, 2002), a developmental and life-course perspective, and general susceptibility to disease. The aim of social epidemiology is to identify ways in which the structure of society influences the public's health, through the interactions of social context, environmental factors, biological mechanisms, and the timing and accumulation of risk, as represented by the ecologic model and the lifespan perspective. Social epidemiologists have called for further research to examine the impact of extra-individual factors (institutions, communities, macroeconomic conditions, and economic and social policy) on exposure to resources (Lynch and Kaplan, 2000).

## Levels of Preventive Interventions

The goal of epidemiology is to identify and understand the causal factors and mechanisms of disease, disability, and injuries so that effective interventions can be implemented to prevent the occurrence of these adverse processes before they begin or before they progress. The natural history of disease is the course of the disease process from onset to resolution (Porta, 2008). The three levels of prevention provide a framework commonly used in public health practice (see the Levels of Prevention box later in the chapter). As practicing epidemiologists, nurses working in the community are involved in primary, secondary, and tertiary prevention of communicable and noncommunicable diseases.

## Primary Prevention

In their daily practice, nurses are often involved in activities related to all three levels of prevention (see Levels of Prevention box). Primary prevention refers to interventions aimed at preventing the occurrence of disease, injury, or disability. Interventions at this level of prevention are aimed at individuals and groups who are susceptible to disease but have no discernible pathology (i.e., they are in a state of prepathogenesis). This first level of prevention includes broad efforts such as health promotion, environmental protection, and specific protection. Health promotion includes nutrition education and counseling and the promotion of physical activity. Environmental protection ranges from basic sanitation and food safety, to home and workplace safety plans, to air quality control. Examples of specific protection against disease or injury include immunizations, proper use of seat belts and infants' car seats, preconception folic acid supplementation to prevent neural tube defects, fluoridation of water supplies to prevent dental caries, and actions taken to reduce human exposure to agents that may cause cancer. Primary prevention occurs in homes, in community settings, and at the primary level of health care (e.g., in public health clinics, physicians' offices, community health centers, and rural health clinics).

### LEVELS OF PREVENTION

#### Examples Related to Cardiovascular Disease

**Primary Prevention**
Counsel clients about low-fat diet and regular physical exercise.

**Secondary Prevention**
Implement blood pressure and cholesterol screening; give treadmill stress test.

**Tertiary Prevention**
Provide cardiac rehabilitation, medication, surgery.

Examples of nurses' involvement in primary prevention include health education and promotion programs, such as nutrition education and counseling, sex education, and family planning services. Primary prevention efforts focus on both the general population and on specific vulnerable groups (e.g., the homeless, HIV-positive persons, certain immigrant groups) to improve the general health status and to reduce the incidence of specific diseases such as TB. An example of a primary prevention intervention is the provision of health education and training for daycare workers regarding health and hygiene issues, such as proper hand hygiene, diapering, and food preparation and storage. Immunizations are another example of primary prevention. In terms of environmental protection, nurses work proactively to develop and advocate for policies and legislation that lead to prevention of environmental hazards. They can also provide consultation to industries, local governments, and groups of concerned citizens as well as public education for a wide range of preventable environmental health problems.

## Secondary Prevention

Secondary prevention encompasses interventions designed to increase the probability that a person with a disease will have that condition diagnosed at a stage when treatment is likely to result in cure. Health screenings are the mainstay of secondary prevention. Early and periodic screenings are critical for diseases for which there are few specific primary prevention strategies, such as breast cancer. (Screening programs are discussed in more detail later in the chapter.) As noted above, primary prevention is a major focus of health education. However, nurses often use health education interventions when caring for individuals with a diagnosed health problem with the aim of preventing further complications or exacerbations. For example, at the individual and family level, teaching the asthmatic child to recognize and avoid exposure to potential asthma triggers and helping the family implement specific protection strategies, such as replacing carpets, keeping air systems clean and free of mold, and avoiding contact with household pets and second-hand smoke could be considered secondary prevention.

Interventions at the secondary level of prevention may occur in community settings as well as within primary and secondary levels of health care services. Oral rehydration therapy (ORT) for infant diarrheal disease is an excellent example of secondary prevention in the community. Particularly in developing countries, when safe water can be made available, ORT is a low-cost and effective way to treat infant diarrheal disease. When mothers identify the early signs of infant dehydration and administer a homemade ORT solution of water, sugar, and salt, they are putting secondary prevention into practice. When taking a health history with clients, nurses can integrate secondary prevention into practice by asking about family history of cancer, heart disease, diabetes, and mental illness, and then providing follow-up education about appropriate screening procedures.

Other examples of secondary prevention interventions include screening tests to detect breast cancer (i.e., mammography), cervical cancer (i.e., Pap tests), colon cancer (i.e., colonoscopy), prenatal screening of pregnant women to detect gestational diabetes, routine tuberculin testing of specific groups (e.g., health care providers, childcare workers), and identification and screening of persons who have had contact with an individual known to have TB. In all these examples, the aim of secondary prevention is to identify the presence of a disease or condition at an early stage and begin necessary treatment early to increase the likelihood of cure or to prevent further complications.

## Tertiary Prevention

Tertiary prevention includes interventions aimed at disability limitation and rehabilitation from disease, injury, or disability. Tertiary prevention interventions occur most often at secondary and tertiary levels of care (e.g., specialized clinics, hospitals, rehabilitation centers) but may also occur in community and primary care settings. Medical treatment, physical and occupational therapy, and rehabilitation are interventions characterized as tertiary prevention. With the emergence of new drug-resistant strains of TB, nurses now face the challenge of designing and implementing programs to increase long-term compliance and provide aftercare for clients in a variety of community settings. An example of tertiary prevention is a public health nurse providing directly observed therapy (DOT) to individuals diagnosed with active TB.

## An Intervention Spectrum

The standard classification of preventive measures in public health is composed of the primary, secondary, and tertiary levels of prevention. However, this standard classification has been revised and refined for application to diverse settings and health issues. In the field of cancer, this potential for intervention has been conceptualized across the entire continuum of care (Figure 12-4). As cancer is a disease which, for most anatomical sites,

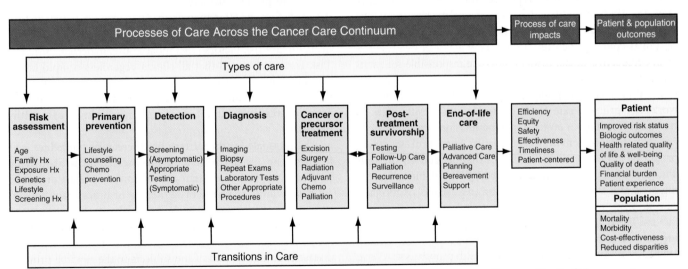

**FIG 12-4** Multilevel interventions in health care across the cancer care continuum. (Taplin SH, Price RA, Edwards HM, et al: Introduction: Understanding and Influencing Multilevel Factors Across the Cancer Care Continuum. *J Natl Cancer Inst Monogr* (44): 2–10, 2012. Oxford University Press.)

has a relatively long period of development, this creates a longer timeline for potential intervention by the researcher or health practitioner. For example, family history of breast cancer is known to be a strong risk factor among specific subgroups of women. Knowing this, the nurse can advocate for genetic testing (first intervention) and also (regardless of the test result) promote healthy lifestyle choices when counseling patients (second intervention). In patients diagnosed with hormone positive breast cancer, the nurse can counsel and facilitate treatment adherence for the woman to her hormonal therapy (third intervention point). Other interventions would include facilitating communication with patients and their families in order to expedite the treatment trajectory from the point of diagnosis to the scheduled surgery (fourth intervention point). Clearly, nurses have critical roles in prevention at all points across the intervention spectrum.

## SCREENING

Screening, a key component of many secondary prevention interventions, involves the testing of groups of individuals who are at risk for a certain condition but are as yet asymptomatic. The purpose is to classify these individuals with respect to the likelihood of having the disease. From a clinical perspective, the aim of screening is early detection and treatment when these result in a more favorable prognosis. From a public health perspective, the objective is to sort out efficiently and effectively those who probably have the disease from those who probably do not, again to detect early cases for treatment or begin public health prevention and control programs. A screening test is *not* a diagnostic test. Effective screening programs must have built-in referral mechanisms for subsequent diagnostic evaluation for those who screen positive, to determine if they actually have the disease and need treatment, and there must be effective protocols in place for referral to accessible and appropriate follow-up care and treatment. If there is no effective treatment, or if the individuals or groups targeted for screening experience considerable barriers in accessing appropriate treatment, the justification of the screening program must be assessed ethically as well as epidemiologically (Childress et al, 2002).

As public health advocates, nurses are responsible for planning and implementing screening and prevention programs targeted to the at-risk populations. Nurses working in schools, worksites, primary care facilities, and public health agencies may work together to target at-risk populations on the basis of occupational and environmental risks. Successful screening programs have several characteristics that depend on the tests and on the population screened (Box 12-2). In planning screening programs for a specific population (e.g., school, workplace, community), nurses need to take into consideration various factors. These include the characteristics of the health problem, the screening tests available, and the population (Harkness, 1995). Screening is recommended for health problems that have a high prevalence, are relatively serious, can be detected in early states, and for which effective treatment is available. The population should be easily identifiable and assessable, amenable to screening, and willing and able to seek treatment or follow-up

procedures. Criteria for evaluating the suitability of screening tests include cost-effectiveness, ease and safety of administration, availability of treatment, ethics of administration or widespread implementation, sensitivity, specificity, validity, and reliability (Gordis, 2013; McKeown and Learner, 2009).

Screening procedures exist for a wide range of health conditions, including cancer (e.g., breast, cervical, testicular, colon, rectal, and skin), diabetes, hypertension, TB, lead poisoning, hearing loss, and sexually transmitted diseases (e.g., gonorrhea, chlamydia, syphilis). Nurses must keep abreast of recommended screening guidelines, which are regularly reviewed and revised on the basis of epidemiologic research results. For example, the latest U.S. Preventive Services Task Force guidelines (USPSTF, 2008) strongly recommend routine screening for lipid disorders in men 35 years and older and women 45 years and older. Screening for younger adults (men ages 20 to 35 and women ages 20 to 45) is recommended when any of the following risk factors are present: diabetes, family history of cardiovascular disease before age 50 in men or age 60 in women, family history suggestive of familial hyperlipidemia, or multiple coronary heart disease risk factors (e.g., tobacco use, hypertension). The Task Force also noted that all clients, regardless of lipid levels, should be offered counseling about the benefits of a diet low in saturated fat and high in fruits and vegetables, regular physical activity, avoidance of tobacco, and maintenance of healthy weight.

The rationale for the current lipid screening guidelines is as follows. The clearest benefit of lipid screening is identifying individuals whose near-term risk of coronary heart disease is sufficiently high to justify drug therapy or other intensive lifestyle interventions to lower cholesterol levels. Screening men older than age 35 years and women older than age 45 years will identify nearly all individuals whose risk of coronary heart disease is as high as that of the subjects in the existing primary prevention trials. Younger people typically have a substantially lower risk, unless they have other important risk factors for coronary heart disease or familial hyperlipidemia. The primary goal of screening younger people is to promote lifestyle

---

**BOX 12-2    Characteristics of a Successful Screening Program**

1. *Valid (accurate):* A high probability of correct classification of persons tested
2. *Reliable (precise):* Results consistent from place to place, time to time, and person to person
3. *Capable of large group administration:*
   a. Fast in both the administration of the test and the procurement of results
   b. Inexpensive in both personnel required and materials and procedures used
4. *Innocuous:* Few, if any, side effects; minimally invasive test
5. *High yield:* Able to detect enough new cases to warrant the effort and expense (*yield* defined as the amount of previously unrecognized disease that is diagnosed and treated as a result of screening)
6. *Ethical and effective:* Meets the desired public health goal with health benefits that outweigh any moral or ethical infringements.

changes, which may provide long-term benefits later in life. The average effect of diet interventions is small, and screening is not needed to advise young adults about the benefits of a healthy diet and regular exercise because this advice is considered useful for all age groups. Although universal screening may detect some clients with familial hyperlipidemia earlier than selective screening, it has yet to be determined if universal screening would lead to significant reductions in coronary events (USPSTF, 2008).

## Reliability and Validity

### Reliability

The precision, or reliability, of the measure (i.e., its consistency or repeatability) and its validity or accuracy (i.e., whether it really measures what we think it is measuring, and how exact the measurement is) are important considerations for any measurement. For example, suppose you are planning to conduct a blood pressure screening in a community setting. You will probably be taking blood pressure measurements on a large number of people and then following up with repeated measures for individuals identified as having higher levels of blood pressure. If the sphygmomanometer used for the blood pressure screening varies in its measurement so that it does not record a similar reading for the same person twice in a row, it lacks precision (or reliability). The instrument would be unreliable even if the overall mean of repeated measurements was close to the true overall mean for the persons measured. The problem would be that the readings would not be reliable for any individual, which is what a screening program requires. On the other hand, suppose the readings are reliably reproducible, but, unknown to you, they tend to be about 10 mm Hg too high. This instrument is producing precise readings, but the uncorrected (or uncalibrated) instrument lacks accuracy (or validity). In short, a measure can be *consistent* without producing *valid* results.

Three major sources of error can affect the reliability of measurement:

- Variation inherent in the trait being measured (e.g., blood pressure changes with time of day, activity, level of stress, and other factors)
- Observer variation, which can be divided into intra-observer reliability (the level of consistency by the same observer) and inter-observer reliability (the level of consistency from one observer to another)
- Inconsistency in the instrument, which includes the internal consistency of the instrument (e.g., whether all items in a questionnaire measure the same thing) and the stability (or test-retest reliability) of the instrument over time

### Validity: Sensitivity and Specificity

Validity in a screening test is measured by sensitivity and specificity. Sensitivity quantifies how accurately the test identifies those *with* the condition or trait. In other words, sensitivity represents the proportion of persons with the disease whom the test correctly identifies as positive (true positives). High sensitivity is needed when early treatment is important and when identification of every case is important.

Specificity indicates how accurately the test identifies those *without* the condition or trait—in other words, the proportion of persons whom the test correctly identifies as negative for the disease (true negatives). High specificity is needed when rescreening is impractical and when reduction of false positives is important. The sensitivity and specificity of a test are determined by comparing the results from the screening test with results from a definitive diagnostic procedure (sometimes called the gold standard). For example, the Pap smear is used frequently to screen for cervical dysplasia and carcinoma. The definitive diagnosis of cervical cancer requires a biopsy with histologic confirmation of malignant cells.

The ideal for a screening test is 100% sensitivity and 100% specificity. That is, the test is positive for 100% of those who actually have the disease, and it is negative for all those who do not have the disease. In practice, sensitivity and specificity are often inversely related. That is, if the test results are such that one can choose some point beyond which a person is considered positive (a "cutpoint"), as in a blood pressure reading to screen for hypertension or a serum glucose reading to screen for diabetes, then moving that critical point to improve the sensitivity of the test will result in a decrease in specificity. In other words, an improvement in specificity can be made only at the expense of sensitivity. Table 12-3 shows how to calculate sensitivity and specificity. Some authors refer to a false-positive rate, which is 1 minus the specificity, and a false-negative rate, or 1 minus the sensitivity. These "rates" are simply the proportions of subjects incorrectly labeled as *nondiseased* and *diseased*, respectively.

A third measure associated with sensitivity and specificity is the predictive value of the test. The positive predictive value (also called predictive value positive) is the proportion of persons with a positive test who actually have the disease, interpreted as the probability that an individual with a positive test has the disease. The negative predictive value (or predictive value negative) is the proportion of persons with a negative test who are actually disease free. Although sensitivity and specificity are relatively independent of the prevalence of disease, predictive values are affected by the level of disease in the screened population and by the sensitivity and specificity of the test. When the prevalence is very low, the positive predictive value will be low, even with tests that are sensitive and specific. In

**TABLE 12-3 Classification of Subjects According to True Disease State and Screening Test Results for Calculation of Indices of Validity**

| Result of Screening Test | Disease | No Disease |
|---|---|---|
| Positive | True positive (TP) | False positive (FP) |
| Negative | False negative (FN) | True negative (TN) |

Sensitivity = TP/(TP + FN); specificity = TN/(TN + FP); false-negative "rate" = 1 − sensitivity = FN/(FN + TP); false-positive "rate" = 1 − specificity = FP/(TN + FP); positive predictive value = TP/(TP + FP); often multiplied by 100 and expressed as a percentage.

addition, lower specificity produces lower positive predictive values because of the increase in the proportion of false-positive results.

In setting cut points, it is necessary to consider the potential human and economic costs of missing true cases by lowering the sensitivity versus the cost of falsely classifying noncases by lowering the specificity. In making such decisions, factors to be considered include the importance of capturing all cases, the likelihood that the population will be rescreened, the interval between screenings relative to the rate of disease development, and the prevalence of the disease. A low prevalence typically requires a test with high specificity; otherwise, the screening will produce too many false positives in the largely nondiseased population. On the other hand, a disease with a high prevalence usually requires high sensitivity; otherwise, too many of the real cases will be missed by the screening (false negatives).

Two or more tests can be combined, in series or in parallel, to enhance sensitivity or specificity. In series testing, the final result is considered positive only if all tests in the series were positive, and it is considered negative if any test was negative. For example, if a blood sample were screened for HIV, a positive enzyme-linked immunosorbent assay (ELISA) might be followed up with a Western blot, and the sample would be considered positive only if both tests were positive. Series testing enhances specificity, producing fewer false positives, but sensitivity will be lower. In series testing, sequence is important; a very sensitive test is often used first to pick up all cases including false positives, and then a second, very specific test is used to eliminate the false positives. In parallel testing, the final result is considered positive if *any* test was positive and negative only if all tests were negative. To return to the example of a blood sample being tested for HIV, a blood bank might consider a sample positive if a positive result was found on either the ELISA or the Western blot. Parallel testing enhances sensitivity, leaving fewer false negatives, but specificity will be lower.

## SURVEILLANCE

Surveillance involves the systematic collection, analysis, and interpretation of data related to the occurrence of disease and the health status of a given population. Surveillance systems are often classified as either active or passive (Teutsch and Churchill, 2010). Passive surveillance is the more common form used by most local and state health departments. Health care providers in the community report cases of notifiable diseases to public health authorities through the use of standardized reports. Passive surveillance is relatively inexpensive but is limited by variability and incompleteness in provider reporting practices. Active surveillance is the purposeful, ongoing search for new cases of disease by public health personnel, through personal or telephone contacts or the review of laboratory reports or hospital or clinic records. Because active surveillance is costly, its use is often limited to brief periods for specific purposes as in the emergence of a newly identified disease, a particularly severe disease, or the reemergence of a previously eradicated disease. In situations that do not require ongoing active surveillance, or

where it may not be feasible to maintain a surveillance system across larger geographic areas, sentinel surveillance systems may be instituted. Representative populations may be selected and sentinel providers identified to provide information on specific diseases or conditions. Nurses engage in surveillance activities as they monitor the health status of individuals, families, and groups in their care. They use surveillance data to assess and prioritize the health needs of populations, design public health and clinical services to address those needs, and evaluate the effectiveness of public health programs.

## BASIC METHODS IN EPIDEMIOLOGY

### Sources of Data

One of the first issues to address in any epidemiologic study is how to obtain the data (Koepsell and Weiss, 2003; Gordis, 2013). Three major categories of data sources are commonly used in epidemiologic investigations:

1. Routinely collected data, such as census data, vital records (birth and death certificates), and surveillance data as carried out by the CDC.
2. Data collected for other purposes but useful for epidemiologic research, such as medical, health department, and insurance records.
3. Original data collected for specific epidemiologic studies.

The first two types of data are often referred to as *secondary data*, and the third type is commonly considered *primary data*.

### Routinely Collected Data

Vital records are the primary source of birth and mortality statistics. Although registration of births and deaths is mandated in most countries, thus providing one of the most complete sources of health-related data, the quality of specific information varies. For example, on birth certificates, sex and date of birth are fairly reliable, whereas gestational age, level of prenatal care, and smoking habits of the mother during pregnancy are less reliable. On death certificates, the quality of the cause of death information varies over time and from place to place, depending on diagnostic capabilities and custom. Vital records, readily available in most areas, are inexpensive and convenient and allow study of long-term trends. Mortality data, however, are informative only for fatal diseases or events.

Since 1790, the U.S. Census has been conducted every 10 years. The U.S. Census provides population data, including demographic distribution (e.g., age, race, sex), geographic distribution, and additional information about economic status, housing, and education. Census data are used as denominators for various rates. The American Community Survey is an ongoing survey also conducted by the U.S. Census Bureau. Data from these surveys provide important information on the status of the population and for public health planning and evaluation activities.

### Data Collected for Other Purposes

Hospital, physician, health department, laboratory, and insurance records provide information on morbidity, as do surveillance systems, such as cancer registries and health department reporting systems, which solicit reports of all cases of a particular disease within a geographic region. Other information, such as occupational exposures, may be available from employer records. School and employment attendance and absenteeism records are another potential source of data that may be used in epidemiologic investigations.

## Epidemiologic Data

The National Center for Health Statistics sponsors periodic health surveys and examinations in carefully drawn samples of the U.S. population. Examples are the National Health and Nutrition Examination Survey (NHANES), the National Health Interview Survey (NHIS), and several National Health Care Surveys including the National Hospital Discharge Survey (NHDS), the National Ambulatory Medical Care Survey (NAMCS), and the National Nursing Home Survey (NNHS). The CDC also conducts or contracts for surveys such as the Youth Risk Behavior Survey (YRBS), the Pregnancy Risk Assessment Monitoring System (PRAMS), and the Behavioral Risk Factor Surveillance System (BRFSS). These surveys provide information on the health status and behaviors of the population. For many studies, however, the only way to obtain the needed information is to collect the required data in a study specifically designed to investigate a particular question. The design of such studies is discussed later.

With the technological advances available through GIS, the use of cartographic data for epidemiologic studies is becoming more widespread. For example, GIS systems are now an integral component of malaria vector control in Mexico and Central America (Najera-Aguilar et al, 2005). Local health professionals and authorities who survey their communities to identify mosquito breeding sites now use global positioning system (GPS) and GIS technology to display and analyze their data. The resulting GIS maps are graphic illustrations of their communities, including buildings, streets, rivers, mosquito breeding sites, and dwellings where individuals with malaria live. These maps allow the calculation of preventive treatments for dwellings located inside various radiuses, from 50 to 250 meters, around the houses with malaria cases. The standardization and integration of cartographic data collection in countries with endemic malaria are part of coordinated international efforts to strengthen malaria control. GIS technology has been used to examine other health issues, such as access to prenatal care. McLafferty and Grady (2005) compared levels of geographic access to prenatal clinics among immigrant groups in Brooklyn, New York. They used kernel estimation—a technique to depict the density of points (in this case, prenatal clinics) as a spatially continuous variable that can be represented as a smooth contour map. Then, using birth record data for the year 2000, which included the mother's country of birth, they compared clinic density levels among different immigrant groups. The authors noted the usefulness of these methods for public health departments in exploring demographic transitions and developing health service networks that are responsive to immigrant populations. GIS technology can be applied in a variety of situations, such as mapping the distribution of health exposures or outcomes, linking data with geo-coded addresses of individuals to

sources of potentially toxic exposures, and mapping water quality measures in sensitive ecosystems.

## Rate Adjustment

Rates, which are of central importance in epidemiologic studies, can be misleading when compared across different populations. For example, the risk of death increases rather dramatically after 40 years of age; therefore, a higher crude death rate is expected in a population of older people compared with a population of younger people (Rothman, 2012; Koepsell and Weiss, 2003; Gordis, 2013). Because the direct comparison of the overall mortality rate in an area with a large population of older adults to the mortality rate in an area with a much younger population would be misleading, there are methods that adjust for such differences in populations. Age adjustment is based on the assumption that a population's overall mortality rate is a function of the age distribution of the population and the age-specific mortality rates. Rates for any outcome can be adjusted by the methods described here, but we focus our discussion on age adjustment of death rates because it is most common. As noted previously: as the population ages, the risk of death increases.

Age adjustment can be performed by direct or indirect methods. Both methods require a *standard population,* which can be an external population, such as the U.S. population for a given year; a combined population of the groups under study; or some other standard chosen for relevance or convenience. A direct age-adjusted rate applies the age-specific death rates from the study population to the age distribution of the standard population. The result is the (hypothetical) death rate of the study population if it had the same age distribution as the standard population.

The indirect method, as the name suggests, is more complicated. The age-specific death rates of the standard population applied to the study population's age distribution produce an index rate that is used with the crude rates of both the study and standard populations to produce the final indirect adjusted rate, which is also hypothetical. The indirect method may be required when the age-specific death rates for the study population are unknown or unstable (e.g., based on relatively small numbers). Often, instead of an indirect adjusted rate, a standardized mortality ratio (SMR) is calculated. This is the number of observed deaths in the study population divided by the number of deaths expected on the basis of the age-specific rates in the standard population and the age distribution of the study population (Szklo and Nieto, 2012; Gordis, 2013).

Although this discussion has focused on age adjustment, the process can be used to adjust for any factor that might vary from one population to another. For example, to compare infant mortality rates across populations with different birth weight distributions, these methods may be used to produce birth weight–adjusted infant mortality rates. Note that all adjusted rates are fictitious rates. They may resemble crude rates if the distribution of the study sample is similar to the distribution of the standard population. The magnitude of adjusted rates depends on the standard population used. The choice of a different standard would produce a different adjusted rate. The change from the 1940 U.S. population to the 2000 U.S. population as the standard for age-adjusted rates from the NCHS demonstrates the difference a change in standard population can make (Anderson and Rosenberg, 1998; Sorlie et al, 1999).

## Comparison Groups

The use of comparison groups is at the heart of the epidemiologic approach. Incidence or prevalence measures in groups that differ in some important characteristic must be compared to gain clues about which factors influence the distribution of disease (i.e., disease determinants or risk factors). Observing the rate of disease only among persons exposed to a suspected risk factor will not show clearly that the exposure is associated with increased risk until the rate observed in the exposed group is compared with the rate in a group of comparable unexposed persons. To illustrate, one might investigate the effect of smoking during pregnancy on the rate of birth of low-birth-weight infants by calculating the rate of low-birth-weight infants born to women who smoked during their pregnancy. However, the hypothesis that smoking during pregnancy is a risk factor for low birth weight is supported only when the low-birth-weight rate among smoking women is compared with the (lower) rate of low-birth-weight infants born to nonsmoking women.

The ideal approach would be to compare one group of people who all have a certain characteristic, exposure, or behavior, with a group of people *exactly* like them except that they all *lack* that characteristic, exposure, or behavior. In the absence of that ideal, researchers either randomize people to exposure or treatment groups in experimental studies, or they select comparison groups that are comparable in observational studies. Advances in statistical techniques now make it possible to control for differences between groups, but these advanced techniques are effective only in reducing the bias that results from confounding by variables we have measured.

## DESCRIPTIVE EPIDEMIOLOGY

Descriptive epidemiology describes the distribution of disease, death, and other health outcomes in the population according to person, place, and time, providing a picture of how things are or have been—the who, where, and when of disease patterns. Analytic epidemiology, on the other hand, searches for the determinants of the patterns observed—the how and why. That is, epidemiologic concepts and methods are used to identify what factors, characteristics, exposures, or behaviors might account for differences in the observed patterns of disease occurrence. Descriptive and analytic studies are observational, meaning the investigator observes events as they are or have been and does not intervene to change anything or introduce a new factor. Experimental or intervention studies, however, include interventions to test preventive or treatment measures, techniques, materials, policies, or drugs.

### Person

Personal characteristics of interest in epidemiology include race, ethnicity, sex, age, education, occupation, income (and related socioeconomic status), and marital status. As noted previously, the most important predictor of overall mortality is age. The mortality curve by age drops sharply during and after the first year of life to a low point in childhood, then it begins to increase through adolescence and young adulthood, and after that it increases sharply (exponentially) through middle and older ages (Gordis, 2013).

There are also substantial differences in mortality and morbidity rates by sex. Female infants have a lower mortality rate than comparable male infants, and the survival advantage continues throughout life (Xu, Kochanek, and Tejada-Vera, 2009). However, patterns for specific diseases vary. For example, women have lower rates of CHD until menopause, after which the gap narrows. For rheumatoid arthritis, the prevalence among women is greater than among men (Remington, Brownson, and Wegner, 2010).

Although the concept of race as a variable for public health research has come under scrutiny (CDC, 1993; Fullilove, 1998), there are clear differences in morbidity and mortality rates by race in the United States (USDHHS, 2000; NCHS, 2009). According to the Office of Minority Health (OMH, 1999), racial and ethnic minority groups are among the fastest-growing populations in the United States, yet they have poorer health and remain chronically underserved by the health care system. Data in the OMH report *Elimination of Racial and Ethnic Disparities in Health* highlighted some of the significant health disparities within the leading categories of death in the United States. For example, in 2007 the overall infant mortality rate (IMR) was 6.8 deaths per 1000 live births, but the IMR among African Americans was 12.9 per 1000 live births (Xu, Kochanek, and Tejada-Vera, 2009), and the gap has been widening in recent years. Racial and ethnic health disparities have been observed in a wide range of diseases and health behaviors, from infant mortality to diabetes, heart disease, cancer, and HIV. Although there has been some progress toward meeting the goal of eliminating racial/ethnic disparities, with improvement in rates for most health status indicators across all racial/ethnic groups, the improvements have not been uniform across groups and "substantial differences among racial/ethnic groups persist" (Keppel, Pearcy, and Wagener, 2002). Among Native Americans and Native Alaskans, several health indicators actually worsened from 1990 to 1998. The IMR declined in all groups, but it remains 2.3 times higher for infants born to non-Hispanic African American mothers than for those born to white non-Hispanic mothers. Similarly, the overall age-adjusted mortality rate was 22% higher in the African American population than in the white population in 2006, and it was higher for 10 of the 15 leading causes of death (Heron, 2010). Although individual characteristics such as race, gender, and immigration status are of interest to epidemiologists, there has been increasing focus on social, economic, and cultural contexts and processes underlying racial and ethnic inequalities in health, such as discrimination (Krieger, 2000; Fuller et al, 2005).

### Place

When considering the distribution of a disease, geographic patterns come to mind: Does the rate of disease differ from place to place (e.g., with local environment)? If geography had no effect on disease occurrence, random geographic patterns might be seen, but that is often not the case. For example, at high altitudes there is lower oxygen surface tension, which might result in smaller babies. Other diseases reflect distinctive geographic patterns. For example, Lyme disease is transmitted from animal reservoirs to humans by a tick vector. Thus, the disease is more likely to be found in areas where there are animals carrying the disease, a large tick population for transmission to humans, and contact between the human population and the tick vectors (Heymann, 2014).

The influence of place on disease may certainly be related to geographic variations in the chemical, physical, or biological environment. However, variations by place also may result from differences in population densities, or in customary patterns of behavior and lifestyle, or in other personal characteristics. For example, geographic variations might occur because of high concentrations of a religious, cultural, or ethnic group who practice certain health-related behaviors. The high rates of stroke found in the southeastern United States are likely to be the result of a number of social, economic, cultural, and personal factors that have little to do with geographic features per se. Recent epidemiologic research has also focused on neighborhood-level variables, such as unemployment and crime rate, social cohesion, educational levels, racial segregation, and access to important services (Cohen et al, 2000; Caughy, O'Campo, and Patterson, 2001; Bradman et al, 2005; Fuller et al, 2005; McLafferty and Grady, 2005). For example, recent research on adolescent injection drug users (IDUs) found that African American IDUs from neighborhoods with large percentages of minority residents and low adult educational levels were more likely to initiate injection use during adolescence than white IDUs from neighborhoods with low percentages of minority residents and high adult education levels. Nurses need to pay attention to this wide range of community-level variables as they assess the health of communities.

## Time

Time is the third component of descriptive epidemiology. In relation to time, epidemiologists ask these questions: Is there an increase or decrease in the frequency of the disease over time? Are other temporal (and spatial) patterns evident? Temporal patterns of interest to epidemiologists include secular trends, point epidemic, cyclical patterns, and event-related clusters.

## Secular Trends

Long-term patterns of morbidity or mortality rates (i.e., over years or decades) are called secular trends. Secular trends may reflect changes in social behavior or health practices. For example, the increased lung cancer mortality rates among men and women in recent years reflect a delayed effect of increased smoking in prior years. Similarly, the decline in cervical cancer deaths is primarily attributable to widespread screening with the Pap test (Remington, Brownson, and Wegner, 2010). Some secular trends may result from increased diagnostic capability or changes in survival (or case fatality) rather than in incidence. For example, case fatality from breast cancer has decreased

in recent years although the incidence of breast cancer has increased. Some, although not all, of the increased incidence is a result of improved diagnostic capability. These two trends result in a breast cancer mortality curve that is flatter than the incidence curve (Remington et al, 2010). Mortality data alone do not accurately reflect the true situation. For example, changes in case definition or revisions in the coding of a disease according to the International Classification of Diseases (ICD) can produce an artificial change in mortality rates.

## Point Epidemic

One temporal and spatial pattern of disease distribution is the point epidemic. This time-and-space–related pattern is important in infectious disease investigations and is a significant indicator for toxic exposures in environmental epidemiology. A point epidemic is most clearly seen when the frequency of cases is plotted against time. The sharp peak characteristic of such graphs indicates a concentration of cases in some short interval of time. The peak often indicates the response of the population to a common source of infection or contamination to which they were all simultaneously exposed. Knowledge of the incubation or latency period (the time between exposure and development of signs and symptoms) for the specific disease entity can help to determine the probable time of exposure. A common example of a point epidemic is an outbreak of gastrointestinal illness from a foodborne pathogen. Nurses who are alert to a sudden increase in the number of cases of a disease can chart the outbreak, determine the probable time of exposure, and, by careful investigation, isolate the probable source of the agent.

## Cyclical Patterns

In addition to secular trends and point epidemics, there are also cyclical time patterns of disease. One common type of cyclical variation is the seasonal fluctuation seen in a number of infectious illnesses. Seasonal changes may be influenced by changes in the agent itself, changes in population densities or behaviors of animal reservoirs or vectors, or changes in human behavior that result in changing exposures (e.g., being outdoors in warmer weather and indoors in colder months). There may also be artificial seasons created by calendar events (e.g., holidays and tax-filing deadlines) that may be associated with patterns of stress-related illness. Patterns of accidents and injuries may also be seasonal, reflecting differing employment and recreational patterns. Some disease cycles, such as influenza, have patterns of smaller epidemics every few years, depending on strain, with major pandemics occurring at longer intervals (Heymann, 2014). Workers in public health can prepare to meet increased demands on resources by paying careful attention to these cyclical patterns.

## Event-Related Clusters

A fourth type of temporal pattern is nonsimultaneous event-related clusters. These are patterns in which time is not measured from fixed dates on the calendar but from the point of some exposure or event, presumably experienced in common by affected persons, although not occurring at the same time.

## KEY POINTS—cont'd

- A key concept in epidemiology is that of the levels of prevention, based on the stages in the natural history of disease.
- Primary prevention involves interventions to reduce the incidence of disease by promoting health and preventing disease processes from developing.
- Secondary prevention includes programs (such as screening) designed to detect disease in the early stages, before signs and symptoms are clinically evident, to intervene with early diagnosis and treatment.
- Tertiary prevention provides treatments and other interventions directed toward persons with clinically apparent disease, with the aim of lessening the course of disease, reducing disability, or rehabilitating.
- Epidemiologic methods are also used in the planning and design of community health promotion (primary prevention) strategies and screening (secondary prevention) activities, and in the evaluation of the effectiveness of these interventions.
- Basic epidemiologic methods include the use of existing data sources to study health outcomes and related factors and the use of comparison groups to assess the association between exposures or characteristics and health outcomes.
- Epidemiologists rely on rates and proportions to quantify levels of morbidity and mortality. Prevalence proportions provide a picture of the level of existing cases in a population at a given time. Incidence rates and proportions measure the rate of new case development in a population and provide an estimate of the risk of disease.
- Descriptive epidemiologic studies provide information on the distribution of disease and health states according to personal characteristics, geographic region, and time. This knowledge enables practitioners to target programs and allocate resources more effectively and provides a basis for further study.
- Analytic epidemiologic studies investigate associations between exposures or characteristics and health or disease outcomes, with a goal of understanding the etiology of disease. Analytic studies provide the foundation for understanding disease causality and for developing effective intervention strategies aimed at primary, secondary, and tertiary prevention.

## CLINICAL DECISION-MAKING ACTIVITIES

1. Interview a local public health nurse or other public health professional from the local health department.
   A. Ask about the current public health priorities and how those priorities were determined.
   B. Describe the type of epidemiologic data used in determining local public health priorities.
2. Identify a current health issue in your local community (e.g., childhood lead poisoning, diabetes, HIV/AIDS).
   A. Describe primary, secondary, and tertiary prevention interventions related to this health issue.
   B. How could nurses improve the effectiveness of their prevention activities related to this health issue?
3. Look at a recent issue of the *Final Mortality Statistics* from the National Center for Health Statistics, or the most recent issue of *Health: United States.* Examine the trends in cause-specific mortality and choose one or two of the leading causes of death.
   A. On the basis of current epidemiologic evidence, explain the factors that have contributed to the following: the observed trend in mortality rates for this disease; the changes in survival; the changes in incidence.
   B. Are the changes the result of better (or worse) primary, secondary, or tertiary prevention? Are there modifiable factors, such as health behaviors, that lend themselves to better prevention efforts? What would they be?
4. Identify existing inequalities among the counties in your state, using infant mortality data.
   A. Describe the distribution of infant mortality in your state (by county), using rate ratio and population attributable risk data.
   B. Compare the infant mortality rates in your state with national and international data.
   C. Compare the characteristics of the counties (e.g., urban, rural, racial/ethnic distribution, economic indicators, distribution of health care facilities) with the highest and lowest infant mortality rates.
   D. Identify local, state, and national initiatives that are addressing infant mortality.
5. Examine the leading causes of infant death in the United States.
   A. What differences in intervention approaches are suggested by the various causes of death?
   B. How would you design an epidemiologic study to examine risk factors for specific causes of neonatal and postneonatal death? What types of epidemiologic measures would be useful? What study design(s) would be appropriate?
   C. How would you use the information from your study to develop an intervention program and to define the target population for your intervention?
6. Find a report of an epidemiologic study in one of the major public health, nursing, or epidemiology journals. How do the findings of this study, if valid, affect your nursing practice? How do you incorporate the results of epidemiologic research into your nursing practice?

# REFERENCES

American Nurses Association: *The Essential Guide to Nursing Practice: Applying ANA's Scope and Standards of Practice and Education.* Washington, DC, 2012, ANA.

Anderson RN: Deaths: leading causes for 2000. *Natl Vital Stat Rep* 50:1–85, 2002.

Anderson RN, Rosenberg HM: Age standardization of death rates: implementation of the year 2000 standard. *Natl Vital Stat Rep* 47:1–16, 1998.

Baldwin DC: Some historical notes on interdisciplinary and interprofessional education and practice in health care in the USA. *J Interprofess Care* 21:23–37, 2007.

Bell RA, Hillers VN, Thomas TA: The Abuela project: safe cheese workshops to reduce the incidence of Salmonella typimurium from consumption of raw-milk cheese. *Am J Public Health* 89:1421–1424, 1999.

Berkman LF, Kawachi I: A historical framework for social epidemiology. In Berkman LF, Kawachi I, editors: *Social Epidemiology.* New York, 2000, Oxford University Press.

Bradman A, Chevier J, Tager I, et al: Association of housing disrepair indicators with cockroach and rodent infestations in a cohort of pregnant Latina women and their children. *Environ Health Perspect* 113:1795–1801, 2005.

Brown P, Ferguson FIT: "Making a big stink": women's work, women's relationships, and toxic waste activism. *Gender Society* 9:145–172, 1995.

Brown P, Masterson-Allen S: Citizen action on toxic waste contamination: a new type of social movement. *Soc Natural Res* 7:269–286, 1994.

Brownson RC, Petitti DB, editors: *Applied Epidemiology: Theory to Practice,* ed 2. New York, 2006, Oxford University Press.

Caughy MO, O'Campo PJ, Patterson J: A brief observational measure for urban neighborhoods. *Health Place* 7:225–236, 2001.

Centers for Disease Control and Prevention: Use of race and ethnicity in public health surveillance: summary of the CDC/ATSDR workshop. *MMWR Morb Mortal Wkly Rep* 42(RR–10):1993.

Centers for Disease Control and Prevention: *Overweight and Obesity,* 2012. Accessed at: http://www.cdc.gov/obesity/data/adult.html. on 6/26/14.

Childress JF, Faden RR, Gaare RD, et al: Public health ethics: mapping the terrain. *J Law Med Ethics* 30:169–177, 2002.

Cohen D, Spear S, Scribner R, et al: "Broken windows" and the risk of gonorrhea. *Am J Public Health* 90:230–236, 2000.

Council on Linkages Between Academic and Public Health Practice: *Core Competencies for Public Health Professionals.* Washington DC, 2014, Public Health Foundation/Health Resources and Services Administration.

DiChiro G: Local actions, global visions: remaking environmental expertise. *Frontiers (Boulder)* 18:203, 1997.

Diez-Roux AV: A glossary for multilevel analysis. *J Epidemiol Community Health* 56:588–594, 2002.

Fuller CM, Borrell LN, Latkin CA, et al: Effects of race, neighborhood, and social network on age at initiation of injection drug use. *Am J Public Health* 95:689–695, 2005.

Fullilove MT: Comment: abandoning "race" as a variable in public health research: an idea whose time has come. *Am J Public Health* 88:1297, 1998.

Gebbie KM, Hwang I: Preparing currently employed public health nurses for changes in the health system. *Am J Public Health* 20:716–721, 2000.

Gordis L: *Epidemiology,* ed 5. Philadelphia, 2013, Saunders.

Harkness GA: *Epidemiology in Nursing Practice.* St Louis, 1995, Mosby.

Heron M: *Deaths: Leading Causes for 2010.* Natl Vital Stat Rep 62:6, 2013. Hyattsville, MD, 2013, National Center for Health Statistics.

Heymann DL, editor: *Control of Communicable Diseases Manual,* ed 20. Washington, DC, 2014, American Public Health Association.

Institute of Medicine: *The Future of Public Health.* Washington, DC, 1988, National Academy Press.

Institute of Medicine: *The Future of the Public's Health in the 21st Century.* Washington, DC, 2002, NAP. Available at: http://www.iom.edu/Reports/2002/The-Future-of-the-Publics-Health-in-the-21st-Century.aspx. Accessed December 23, 2010.

Kawachi I, Berkman LF: *Neighborhoods and Health.* New York, 2003, Oxford University Press.

Keppel KG, Pearcy JN, Wagener DK: *Trends in Racial and Ethnic-specific Rates for The Health Status Indicators: United States, 1990-98, Healthy People Statistical Notes.* Hyattsville, MD, 2002, NCHS. No. 23.

Koepsell TD, Weiss NS: *Epidemiologic Methods: Studying the Occurrence of Illness.* New York, 2003, Oxford University Press.

Krieger N: Epidemiology and the web of causation: has anyone seen the spider? *Soc Sci Med* 39:887, 1994.

Krieger N: Discrimination and health. In Berkman LF, Kawachi I, editors: *Social Epidemiology.* Oxford, 2000, Oxford University Press, pp 36–75.

Lynch J, Kaplan G: Socioeconomic position. In Berkman LF, Kawachi I, editors: *Social Epidemiology.* New York, 2000, Oxford University Press, pp 13–35.

Lynch JW, Kaplan GA, Pamuk ER, et al: Income inequality and mortality in metropolitan areas of the United States. *Am J Public Health* 88:1074, 1998.

Macintyre S, Ellaway A: Ecological approaches: rediscovering the role of the physical and social environment. In Berkman LF, Kawachi I, editors: *Social Epidemiology.* New York, 2000, Oxford University Press, pp 332–348.

Martin JA, Hamilton BE, Sutton PD, et al: Births, final data for 2006. *Natl Vital Stat Rep* 57:7, 2009.

McKeown RE: The epidemiologic transition: changing patterns of mortality and population dynamics. *Am J Lifestyle Med* 3(S1):19S–26S, 2009.

McKeown RE, Learner RM: Ethics in public health practice. In Coughlin S, Beauchamp T, Weed D, editors: *Ethics and Epidemiology,* ed 2. New York, 2009, Oxford University Press, pp 147–181.

McLafferty S, Grady S: Immigration and geographic access to prenatal clinics in Brooklyn, NY: a geographic information systems analysis. *Am J Public Health* 95:638–640, 2005.

Merrill RM, Timmreck TC: *Introduction to Epidemiology,* ed 4. Sudbury, MA, 2006, Jones & Bartlett.

Mood L: Toxic waste: deep in the roots of nursing comes a search for harmful sources. *Reflect Nurs Leadership* 26:21–25, 2000.

Najera-Aguilar P, Martinez-Piedra R, Vidaurre-Arenas M: From sketch to digital maps: a geographic information system (GIS) model and application for malaria control without the use of pesticides. *Pan Am Health Org Epidemiol Bull* 26:11, 2005.

National Center for Health Statistics: *Health, United States: with Chartbook.* Hyattsville, MD, 2009, National Center for Health Statistics, p 2008.

Ogden CL, Carroll MD, Kit BK, et al: *Prevalence of Obesity in the United States, 2009-2010.* Hyattsville, MC, 2012, National Center for Health Statistics Data Brief, p 82.

Office of Minority Health, U.S. Department of Health and Human Services: *Elimination of Racial and Ethnic Disparities in Health: Report to Congress.* Washington, DC, 1999, OMH.

Porta M: *A Dictionary of Epidemiology,* ed 5. New York, 2008, Oxford University Press.

Remington PL, Brownson RC, Wegner MV: *Chronic Disease Epidemiology and Control,* ed 3. Washington, DC, 2010, American Public Health Association.

Rothman KJ: *Epidemiology: an Introduction,* ed 2. New York, 2012, Oxford University Press.

Sampson RJ, Raudenbush SW, Earls F: Neighborhoods and violent crime: a multilevel study of collective efficacy. *Science* 277:918, 1997.

Schlesselman JJ: *Case-control Studies: Design, Conduct, Analysis.* New York, 1982, Oxford University Press.

Snow J: On the mode of communication of cholera. In *Snow on Cholera.* New York, 1855, The Commonwealth Fund.

Sorlie PD, Thom TJ, Manolio T, et al: Age-adjusted death rates: consequences of the year 2000 standard. *Ann Epidemiol* 9:93–100, 1999.

Susser M: *Causal Thinking in the Health Sciences.* New York, 1973, Oxford University Press.

Susser M: Epidemiology in the United States after World War II: the evolution of technique. *Epidemiol Rev* 7:147, 1985.

Swider SM, Krothe J, Reyes D, et al: The Quad Council Practice Competencies for Public Health Nursing. *Publ Health Nurs* 30:519–536, 2013.

Szklo M, Nieto FJ: *Epidemiology: Beyond the Basics,* ed 3. Boston, 2012, Jones & Bartlett.

Teutsch SM, Churchill RE: *Principles and Practice of Public Health Surveillance,* ed 3. New York, 2010, Oxford.

Turnock BJ: *Public Health: What it is and How it Works,* ed 5. Gaithersburg, MD, 2011, Aspen.

U.S. Department of Health, Education, and Welfare: *Vital Statistics of the United States: 1950,* vol 1. Washington, DC, 1954, USDHEW, Public Health Service.

U.S. Department of Health and Human Services: *Healthy People 2010: Understanding and Improving Health,* ed 2. Washington, DC, 2000, U.S. Government Printing Office.

U.S. Preventive Services Task Force: *Screening for Lipid Disorders in Adults: U.S. Preventive Services Task Force Recommendation Statement.* Rockville, MD, 2008, Agency for Healthcare Research and Quality.

Victoria CG, Habicht J-P, Bryce J: Evidence-based public health: moving beyond randomized trials. *Am J Public Health* 94(3):400–405, 2004.

World Health Organization: *Declaration of Alma-Ata: International Conference on Primary Health Care.* Geneva, Switzerland, 1978, WHO, p 1.

Xu J, Kochanek KD, Tejada-Vera B: *Deaths: Preliminary Data for 2007,* Natl Vital Stat Rep 58:1. Hyattsville, MD, 2009, National Center for Health Statistics.

# Infectious Disease Prevention and Control

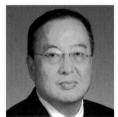

## Francisco S. Sy, MD, PhD

Dr. Francisco S. Sy is the Director of the Division of Extramural Activities and Scientific Programs at the National Center on Minority Health and Health Disparities (NCMHD) at the National Institutes of Health (NIH) in Bethesda, MD. Before joining NIH, he served as a Senior Health Scientist in the Division of HIV/AIDS Prevention (DHAP), National Center for HIV, STD and TB Prevention (NCHSTP), at the Centers for Disease Control and Prevention (CDC) in Atlanta, GA. Dr. Sy was a tenured professor at the University of South Carolina (USC) School of Public Health in Columbia, SC, where he taught infectious disease epidemiology for 15 years. Dr. Sy has written several book chapters and scientific articles on various infectious and tropical diseases, HIV disease epidemiology, prevention, and program evaluation. He is the editor of the *AIDS Education and Prevention: An Interprofessional Journal* since its inception in 1988. Dr. Sy earned his Doctor of Public Health (DrPH) degree in Immunology and Infectious Diseases from Johns Hopkins University in 1984, Master of Science in Tropical Public Health from Harvard University in 1981 and Doctor of Medicine degree from the University of the Philippines in 1975.

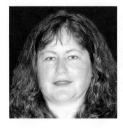

## Susan C. Long-Marin, DVM, MPH

Susan C. Long-Marin developed an interest in infectious disease and public health while serving as a Peace Corps Volunteer in the Philippines in the 1970s. Training in veterinary medicine further increased her respect for the ingeniousness of microbes and the importance of primary prevention. Today she manages the epidemiology program of a county health department in Charlotte, NC, which serves a growing and rapidly changing population from a variety of racial, ethnic, and national backgrounds. Dr. Long-Marin earned her Doctor of Veterinary Medicine degree from Virginia Tech and her Master of Public Health in Epidemiology degree from the University of South Carolina.

## ADDITIONAL RESOURCES

**Evolve website http://evolve.elsevier.com/Stanhope**
- Healthy People 2020
- WebLinks—Of special note, see the links for these sites:
  - Centers for Disease Control and Prevention
  - *Emerging Infectious Diseases,* Centers for Disease Control and Prevention
  - *MMWR Morbidity and Mortality Weekly Report,* Centers for Disease Control and Prevention
- World Health Organization
- *WER/Weekly Epidemiological Record,* World Health Organization
- Quiz
- Case Studies
- Glossary
- Answers to Practice Application

## OBJECTIVES

*After reading this chapter, the student should be able to do the following:*
1. Discuss the current impact and threats of infectious diseases on society.
2. Explain how the elements of the epidemiologic triangle interact to cause infectious diseases.
3. Provide examples of infectious disease control interventions at the three levels of public health prevention.
4. Explain the multisystem approach to control of communicable diseases.
5. Discuss the factors contributing to newly emerging or re-emerging infectious diseases.
6. Define the bloodborne pathogen reduction strategy and universal precautions.

## KEY TERMS

The topic of infectious diseases includes the discussion of a wide and complex variety of organisms; the pathology they may cause; and their diagnosis, treatment, prevention, and control. This chapter presents an overview of the communicable diseases that nurses encounter most often. Diseases are grouped according to descriptive category (by mode of transmission or means of prevention) rather than by individual organism (e.g., *Escherichia coli*) or taxonomic group (e.g., viral, parasitic). Detailed discussion of sexually transmitted diseases, human immunodeficiency virus (HIV), acquired immunodeficiency syndrome (AIDS/HIV stage III), viral hepatitis, and

tuberculosis (TB) is provided in Chapter 14. Although not all infectious diseases are directly communicable from person to person, the terms *infectious disease* and *communicable disease* are used interchangeably throughout this chapter.

## HISTORICAL AND CURRENT PERSPECTIVES

In the United States at the beginning of the twentieth century, infectious diseases were the leading cause of death. By 2000 improvements in nutrition and sanitation, the discovery of antibiotics, and the development of vaccines had put an end to infectious disease epidemics like diphtheria and typhoid fever that once ravaged entire populations. In 1900 respiratory and diarrheal diseases were major killers. For example, tuberculosis (TB) led to over 11% of all deaths in the United States and was the second leading cause of death; in 2010, 536 deaths or 0.02% were attributed to this once frequently fatal disease (CDC, 2012a). As individuals live longer, chronic diseases—heart disease, cancer, and stroke—have replaced infectious diseases as the leading causes of death.

Infectious diseases, however, have not vanished, and they remain a continuing cause for concern. They remain the leading cause of death for children and adolescents worldwide and the second-leading cause overall, killing an estimated 8 million people a year (WHO, 2013). In the United States, the downward trend in mortality from infectious diseases seen since 1900—with the exception of the 1918 influenza pandemic—reversed itself in the 1980s, with the emergence of new entities such as HIV disease and the increasing development of antibiotic resistance. Respiratory diseases in the form of pneumonias and influenza remain among the 10 leading causes of death, and new strains such as novel influenza A H1N1 and avian influenza A H5N1 test our disease control abilities and consume resources. Previously unknown causal connections between infectious organisms and chronic diseases have been recognized, such as *Helicobacter pylori* and peptic ulcer disease, and human papillomaviruses (HPVs) and cervical cancer. Also, in the twenty-first century, infectious diseases have become a means of terrorism, as illustrated by the anthrax letters of 2001.

New killers emerge and old familiar diseases take on different, more virulent characteristics. Consider the following developments from the past 30 years. HIV disease reminds us of plagues from the past and challenges our ability to control and contain infection like no other disease in recent history. Because drugs have been developed to slow the progression but there is still neither vaccine nor cure, this initially infectious disease is now a chronic condition as well. Legionnaires' disease and toxic shock syndrome, unknown at mid-twentieth century, have become part of the common vocabulary. The identification of infectious agents causing Lyme disease and ehrlichiosis provided two new tickborne diseases to worry about. And, in the summer of 1993 in the southwestern United States, healthy young adults were stricken with a mysterious and unknown but often fatal respiratory disease that is now known as hantavirus pulmonary syndrome. The summer of 1994 brought public attention to a severe, invasive strain of *Streptococcus pyogenes* group A, referred to by the press as the "flesh-eating" bacteria.

In the 1990s the transmission of infectious disease through the food supply became a newsworthy concern when the consumption of improperly cooked hamburgers and unpasteurized apple juice contaminated with a highly toxic strain of *E. coli* (*E. coli* 0157:H7) caused illness and death in children across the country. In 1996 multiple states reported outbreaks of diarrheal disease traced to imported fresh berries; the implicated organism in these outbreaks, *Cyclosporacayetanensis* (a coccidian parasite), was first diagnosed in humans in 1977. Also in 1996, the fear that "mad cow disease" (bovine spongiform encephalopathy [BSE]) could be transferred to humans through beef

consumption led to the slaughter of thousands of British cattle and a ban on the international sale of British beef. Initially seen only in Europe and Japan as well as Great Britain, the first case of BSE was diagnosed in the United States in 2003. Variant Creutzfeldt-Jakob disease (vCJD), which attacks the brain with fatal results, is the human disease hypothesized but not yet proven to result from eating beef infected with the transmissible agent causing BSE; only three acquired cases of vCJD have been seen in the United States, but these individuals were born outside of and resided in the country for only a short period (CDC, 2013a).

In 1997 vancomycin-resistant *Staphylococcus aureus* (VRSA) was first reported; previously, vancomycin had been considered the only effective antibiotic against methicillin-resistant *S. aureus* (MRSA). Although MRSA is still largely a health care–associated infection, community-associated disease is becoming more common with outbreaks frequently associated with school athletic programs and prison populations. Also in 1997, the first reported outbreak of avian flu affecting humans occurred in Hong Kong. Lack of subsequent reports suggested an isolated incident, but in 2004 avian influenza A H5N1 again emerged in Southeast Asia with resulting human cases. This virus has now infected avian populations in Asia, Europe, the Near East, and North Africa, and it continues to cause sporadic human cases, especially in Southeast Asia and Egypt. Human cases are determined to spread largely through direct contact with infected poultry or infected surfaces, with human to human transmission largely ineffective and only a few rare cases thought to have occurred. In 1999 the first Western Hemisphere activity of West Nile virus (WNV), a mosquito-transmitted illness that can affect livestock, birds, and humans, occurred in New York City. By 2002 WNV, thought to be carried by infected birds and possibly mosquitoes in cargo containers, had spread across the United States as far west as California and was reported in Canada and Central America as well.

The viral hemorrhagic fevers (HF) Ebola and Marburg, unknown to most people 30 years ago, have become the premise of movies and novels, and recently the cause of widespread international concern. While earlier reported Ebola virus outbreaks largely occurred in Central Africa and were limited and quickly contained, an outbreak of Ebola virus that began in the spring of 2014 in Guinea, West Africa resisted containment and in spite of international assistance, spread rapidly through neighboring Liberia and Sierra Leone. A small number of cases also occurred in several other West African countries but were contained. An air traveler brought a case to the United States resulting in the infection of two nurses who cared for him. Health care workers returning from work in West Africa were diagnosed, one in the United States and one in Great Britain, and a nurse in Spain was also infected caring for a patient who had been transported from the Ebola-infected region of Africa. By January 2015, this on going epidemic had resulted in over 21,700 reported cases in nine countries (the majority in Guinea, Liberia and Sierra Leone) and almost 8,650 reported deaths. In response to the imported and health care-transmitted cases, infectious disease policies and procedures within hospitals were modified, and screening and surveillance tactics were introduced at airports around the world for passengers arriving from West Africa (CDC, 2015a).

Although caused by different viruses within the *Filoviridae* family, Ebola and Marburg hemorrhagic fevers (HF) have similar clinical presentations. The reservoir host of Ebola viruses remains unknown but there is an association with non-human primates, and evidence is also beginning to point toward a bat reservoir (CDC, 2014a). Marburg HF virus had been reported only five times since its recognition in 1967 before a major outbreak in Angola occurred during 2004 and 2005, affecting more than 350 people with a fatality rate of close to 90%. Since then, a much smaller outbreak occurred in Uganda in 2007 among gold miners and another in Uganda in 2012 affecting 15 people. The reservoir host of Marburg virus is the African fruit bat, *Rousettusa egyptiacus* (CDC, 2014b).

Severe acute respiratory syndrome (SARS) was first recognized in China in February 2003 and, as if in a bestselling thriller, this newly emerging infectious disease quickly achieved pandemic proportions. By the summer of 2003, major outbreaks had occurred in Hong Kong, Taiwan, Vietnam, Singapore, and Canada. Three months after the first official news of SARS, over 8000 cases with more than 700 deaths had been reported to the World Health Organization (WHO) from 28 countries. Played out on television in pictures of people wearing facemasks for protection, the rapid spread of a previously unknown disease with an initially unknown cause and no definitive treatment contributed to the creation of a perception of risk of infection far greater than actually existed. Frightened Americans canceled trips to China and Hong Kong and avoided people who had recently returned from Asia. Then, as suddenly as it began, the pandemic subsided. SARS was found to be caused by a new strain of coronavirus, but since 2003, only a few cases, largely associated with laboratory workers, have been reported. A large number of individuals infected by SARS could be traced back to unrecognized cases in hospitals, suggesting that prompt identification and isolation of symptomatic people is the key to interrupting transmission. No new cases of SARS have been reported since 2004. Global efforts continue to clarify the epidemiology of this disease as well as develop a reliable diagnostic test and vaccine. In 2012, SARS coronavirus was officially declared a select agent—a bacterium, virus, or toxin that has the potential to pose a severe threat to public health and safety. Additional information on SARS can be obtained at the CDC SARS website (http://www.cdc.gov/sars/).

In the first decade of the twenty-first century, foodborne infections again have made headlines as *E. coli*–infected spinach sickened and killed individuals across the United States. In 2008, tomatoes were blamed for a nationwide outbreak of salmonellosis but were ruled innocent when the green chilies that accompanied them in salsa were found to be the actual culprit. Salmonella made the news as contaminated peanut butter forced recalls across the United States, sickened hundreds, and resulted in several deaths, and again in 2012 when contaminated cantaloupes resulted in 261 reported illnesses and 3 deaths across 24 states. Even chocolate chip cookie dough was not safe; a national recall in 2009 followed the discovery that people had been sickened after eating raw dough contaminated by *E. coli*.

Perhaps the most publicized infectious disease event of 2009 was the advent of a new strain of flu, novel influenza A H1N1. First reported from Mexico and rapidly acquired by travelers to that country, H1N1 spread quickly across the world, causing the WHO to declare a pandemic and stimulate the race for a vaccine. While H1N1 did not become the major killer it was feared to, it did disproportionately result in hospitalizations and deaths in younger and middle-aged adults. H1N1 did not disappear and has been included in the seasonal vaccine since 2009. During the 2013-2014 flu season in the United States, H1N1 once more became the predominant circulating strain, and once more hit hardest the young and middle-aged.

The year 2012 brought the first reports of another novel coronavirus that, like SARS, results in acute respiratory distress with a high mortality rate. Middle Eastern Respiratory Syndrome Coronavirus or MERS-CoV has only been seen in individuals living in or who have traveled to countries in the Arabian Peninsula. It seems to spread by close contact and many of the cases have been in health care workers. The reservoir is unknown but there appears to be an association with camels. The first cases of MERS-CoV in the United States were reported in 2014 in individuals who had traveled from Saudi Arabia. Read more about MERS at http://www.cdc.gov/coronavirus/mers/index.html.

Worldwide, infectious diseases are the leading killer of children and young adults and are responsible for almost half of all deaths in developing countries. Of these infectious disease deaths, 90% result from six causes: acute respiratory infections, diarrheal diseases, malaria, and measles among children; and TB and HIV infection among adults. TB alone is estimated to kill a million people a year and malaria another 625,000 (WHO, 2013). The CDC in its *Ounce of Prevention* campaign notes that in the United States as many as 160,000 people die per year with infectious diseases as an underlying cause. The economic burden of infectious diseases is staggering. Foodborne illnesses alone are estimated to cost $77.7 billion annually in the United States (Scharff, 2012). The CDC estimates the costs to the U.S. health care system of almost 19 million new STD infections each year to be as much as $15.9 billion annually (USDHHS, 2014). In 2013, the annual cost for five of the most significant health care–associated infections was estimated at $9.8 billion (Zimlichman et al, 2013).

Because of the morbidity, mortality, and associated cost of infectious diseases, the national health promotion and disease prevention goals outlined in *Healthy People 2020* list a number of objectives for reducing the incidence of these illnesses in a variety of the sections, including Immunization & Infectious disease. Objectives for reducing salmonellosis and other foodborne infections are found in the section on Food Safety, an objective for reducing malaria cases reported in the United States may be seen under Global Health, there is a section on sexually transmitted diseases, and there are objectives related to health care–associated infections (see the Healthy People 2020 box for examples). Although infectious diseases are not currently the leading causes of death in the United States, they continue to present varied, multiple, and complex challenges to all health care providers. Nurses must know about these diseases to effectively participate in diagnosis, treatment, prevention, and control.

## HEALTHY PEOPLE 2020

### *Selected Objectives Related to Infectious Diseases*

- IID-1: Reduce, eliminate, or maintain elimination of cases of vaccine-preventable diseases.
- IID-12: Increase the percentage of children and adults who are vaccinated against seasonal influenza.
- FS-1: Reduce infections caused by key pathogens transmitted commonly through food.
- HAI-2 Reduce invasive health care–associated methicillin-resistant *Staphylococcal aureus* (MRSA) infections.

From U.S. Department of Health and Human Services: *Healthy People 2020: The Road Ahead.* 2009, USDHHS. Available at http://www.healthypeople.gov/HP2020/. Accessed January 26, 2010.

## TRANSMISSION OF COMMUNICABLE DISEASES

### Agent, Host, and Environment

The transmission of communicable diseases depends on the successful interaction of the infectious agent, the host, and the environment. These three factors make up the epidemiologic triangle (Figure 13-1), as discussed in Chapter 12. Changes in the characteristics of any of the factors may result in disease transmission. Consider the following examples. Antibiotic therapy not only may eliminate a specific pathologic agent, but also alter the balance of normally occurring organisms in the body. As a result, one of these agents overruns another and disease, such as a yeast infection, occurs. HIV performs its deadly work not by directly poisoning the host but by destroying the host's immune reaction to other disease-producing agents. Individuals living in the temperate climate of the United States do not normally contract malaria at home, but they may become infected if they change their environment by traveling to a climate where malaria-carrying mosquitoes thrive. As these examples illustrate, the balance among agent, host, and environment is often precarious and may be unintentionally disrupted. At present, the potential results of such disturbance require attention as advances in science and technology, destruction of natural habitats, explosive population growth, political instability, and a worldwide transportation network combine to alter the balance among the environment, people, and the agents that produce disease.

### Agent Factor

Four major categories of agents cause most infections and infectious disease: bacteria (e.g., *Salmonella* and *E. coli*), fungi (e.g., *Aspergillus* spp. and *Candida* spp.), parasites (e.g., helminthes and protozoa), and viruses (e.g., hepatitis A and B and HIV). Less commonly seen is the prion, a transmissible agent that causes abnormal folding of normal cellular prion proteins in the brain, resulting in a family of rare progressive neurodegenerative disorders that affect both humans and animals. Variant Creutzfeldt-Jakob disease and kuru are examples of prion diseases. The individual agent may be described by its ability to cause disease and by the nature and the severity of the disease. *Infectivity, pathogenicity, virulence, toxicity, invasiveness,* and *antigenicity,* terms commonly used to characterize infectious agents, are defined in Box 13-1.

### Host Factor

A human or animal host can harbor an infectious agent. The characteristics of the host that may influence the spread of disease are host resistance, immunity, herd immunity, and infectiousness of the host. Resistance is the ability of the host to withstand infection, and it may involve natural or acquired immunity.

Natural immunity refers to species-determined, innate resistance to an infectious agent. For example, opossums rarely contract rabies. Acquired immunity is the resistance acquired by a host as a result of previous natural exposure to an infectious agent. Having measles once protects against future infection. Acquired immunity may be induced by active or passive immunization. Active immunization refers to the immunization of an individual by administration of an antigen (infectious agent or vaccine) and is usually characterized by the presence of an antibody produced by the individual host.

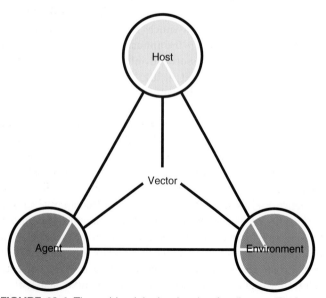

**FIGURE 13-1** The epidemiologic triangle of a disease (Redrawn from Gordis L: *Epidemiology*, ed 5, Philadelphia, 2005, Saunders.)

### BOX 13-1   Six Characteristics of an Infectious Agent

- *Infectivity:* The ability to enter and multiply in the host
- *Pathogenicity:* The ability to produce a specific clinical reaction after infection occurs
- *Virulence:* The ability to produce a severe pathological reaction
- *Toxicity:* The ability to produce a poisonous reaction
- *Invasiveness:* The ability to penetrate and spread throughout a tissue
- *Antigenicity:* The ability to stimulate an immunological response

Vaccinating children against childhood diseases is an example of inducing active immunity. <u>Passive immunization</u> refers to immunization through the transfer of a specific antibody from an immunized individual to a nonimmunized individual, such as the transfer of antibody from mother to infant or by administration of an antibody-containing preparation (immunoglobulin or antiserum). Passive immunity from immunoglobulin is almost immediate but short lived. It is often induced as a stopgap measure until active immunity has time to develop after vaccination. Examples of commonly used immunoglobulins include those for hepatitis A, rabies, and tetanus.

<u>Herd immunity</u> refers to the immunity of a group or community. It is the resistance of a group of people to invasion and spread of an infectious agent. Herd immunity is based on the resistance of a high proportion of individual members of a group to infection. It is the basis for increasing immunization coverage for vaccine-preventable diseases. Through studies, experts determine what percent coverage (e.g., >90%) of a specified group of people (e.g., children entering school) by a specified vaccine (e.g., one dose of measles vaccine) is necessary to ensure adequate protection for the entire community against a given disease and target immunization campaigns and initiatives to meet that goal. The higher the immunization coverage, the greater the herd immunity.

**Infectiousness** is a measure of the potential ability of an infected host to transmit the infection to other hosts. It reflects the relative ease with which the infectious agent is transmitted to others. Individuals with measles are extremely infectious; the virus spreads readily on airborne droplets. A person with Lyme disease cannot spread the disease to other people (although the infected tick can).

## Environment Factor

The environment refers to everything that is external to the human host, including physical, biological, social, and cultural factors. These environmental factors facilitate the transmission of an infectious agent from an infected host to other susceptible hosts. Reduction in communicable disease risk can be achieved by altering these environmental factors. Using mosquito nets and repellants to avoid bug bites, installing sewage systems to prevent fecal contamination of water supplies, and washing utensils after contact with raw meat to reduce bacterial contamination are all examples of altering the environment to prevent disease.

## Modes of Transmission

Infectious diseases can be transmitted horizontally or vertically. <u>Vertical transmission</u> is the passing of the infection from parent to offspring via sperm, placenta, milk, or contact in the vaginal canal at birth. Examples of vertical transmission are transplacental transmission of <u>HIV and syphilis</u>. Horizontal transmission is the <u>person-to-person</u> spread of infection through one or more of the following <u>four routes: direct/indirect contact, common vehicle, airborne, or vector borne.</u> Most sexually transmitted infections are spread by direct sexual contact. Enterobiasis, or pinworm infection, can be acquired through direct contact or indirect contact with contaminated

objects such as toys, clothing, and bedding. <u>Common vehicle</u> refers to transportation of the infectious agent from an infected host to a susceptible host via food, water, milk, blood, serum, saliva, or plasma. Hepatitis A can be transmitted through contaminated food and water, and hepatitis B through contaminated blood. Legionellosis and TB are both spread via contaminated droplets in the air. <u>Vectors</u> are arthropods such as ticks and mosquitoes or other invertebrates such as snails that transmit the infectious agent by biting or depositing the infective material near the host. Vectors may be necessary to the life cycle of the organism (e.g., mosquitoes and malaria) or may act as mechanical transmitters (e.g., flies and food).

## Disease Development

<u>Exposure to an infectious agent does not always lead to an infection. Similarly, infection does not always lead to disease.</u> Infection depends on the infective dose, the infectivity of the infectious agent and the immunocompetence of the host. It is important to differentiate infection and disease, as clearly illustrated by the HIV disease epidemic. <u>Infection</u> refers to the entry, development, and multiplication of the infectious agent in the susceptible host. <u>Disease</u> is one of the possible outcomes of infection and it may indicate a physiological dysfunction or pathologic reaction. An individual who tests positive for HIV is infected, but if that person shows no clinical signs, the individual is not diseased. Similarly, if an individual tests positive for HIV and also exhibits clinical signs consistent with AIDS (HIV stage III), that individual is both infected and diseased.

Incubation period and communicable period are not synonymous. The <u>incubation period</u> is the time interval between invasion by an infectious agent and the first appearance of signs and symptoms of the disease. The incubation periods of infectious diseases vary from between 2 and 4 hours for staphylococcal food poisoning to between 10 and 15 years for AIDS (HIV stage III). The <u>communicable period</u> is the interval during which an infectious agent may be transferred directly or indirectly from an infected person to another person. The period of communicability for influenza is 3 to 5 days after the clinical onset of symptoms. Hepatitis B–infected persons are infectious many weeks before the onset of the first symptoms and remain infective during the acute phase and chronic carrier state, which may persist for life.

## Disease Spectrum

*Exposure & infect. not automatic.*

Persons with infectious diseases may exhibit a <u>broad spectrum of disease that ranges from subclinical infection to severe and fatal disease.</u> Those with subclinical or inapparent infections are important from the public health point of view because they are a source of infection but may not be receiving care like those with clinical disease. They should be targeted for early diagnosis and treatment. Those with clinical disease may exhibit localized or systemic symptoms and mild to severe illness. The final outcome of a disease may be recovery, death, or something in between, including a carrier state, complications requiring extended hospital stay, or disability requiring rehabilitation.

<u>At the community level</u>, the disease may occur in endemic, epidemic, or pandemic proportion. <u>Endemic</u> refers to the

constant presence of a disease within a geographic area or a population. Pertussis is endemic in the United States. Epidemic refers to the occurrence of disease in a community or region in excess of normal expectancy. Although people tend to associate large numbers with epidemics, even one case can be termed epidemic if the disease is considered previously eliminated from that area. For example, one case of polio, a disease considered eliminated from the United States, would be considered epidemic. Pandemic refers to an epidemic occurring worldwide and affecting large populations. HIV disease is both epidemic and pandemic, as the number of cases continues to grow across various regions of the world as well as in the United States. SARS and novel influenza A H1N1 are both emerging infectious diseases and responsible for recent pandemics.

## SURVEILLANCE OF COMMUNICABLE DISEASES

During the first half of the twentieth century, the weekly publication of national morbidity statistics by the U.S. Surgeon General's Office was accompanied by the statement, "No health department, state or local, can effectively prevent or control disease without knowledge of when, where, and under what conditions cases are occurring" (CDC, 1996). Surveillance gathers the "who, when, where, and what"; these elements are then used to answer "why." A good surveillance system systematically collects, organizes, and analyzes current, accurate, and complete data for a defined disease condition. The resulting information is promptly released to those who need it for effective planning, implementation, and evaluation of disease prevention and control programs.

### Elements of Surveillance

Infectious disease surveillance incorporates and analyzes data from a variety of sources. Box 13-2 lists 10 commonly used data elements.

### Surveillance for Agents of Bioterrorism

Since September 11, 2001, increased emphasis has been placed on surveillance for any disease that might be associated with the intentional release of a biological agent. The concern is that, because of the interval between exposure and disease, a covert release may go unrecognized and without response for some time if the resulting outbreak closely resembles a naturally

occurring one. Health care providers are asked to be alert to (1) temporal or geographic clustering of illnesses (people who attended the same public gathering or visited the same location), especially those with clinical signs that resemble an infectious disease outbreak—previously healthy people with unexplained fever accompanied by sepsis, pneumonia, rash, or flaccid paralysis, and (2) an unusual age distribution for a common disease (e.g., chickenpox-like disease in adults without a child source case).

Because of the heightened concern about possible bioterrorist attacks, various sorts of syndromic surveillance systems have been developed by public health agencies across the country. These systems incorporate factors such as the previously mentioned temporal and geographic clustering and unusual age distributions with groups of disease symptoms or syndromes (e.g., flaccid paralysis, respiratory signs, skin rashes, gastrointestinal symptoms) with the goal of detecting early signs of diseases that could result from a bioterrorism-related attack. Syndromic surveillance systems may include tracking emergency department visits sorted by syndrome symptoms as well as other indicators of illness including school absenteeism and sales of selected over-the-counter medications. Early on, CDC developed EARS (Early Aberration Reporting System), a surveillance tool available at no charge and used by various public health officials across the country and abroad. Work continues to enhance and strengthen these tools. Although more active infectious disease surveillance is being encouraged because of the potential for bioterrorism, the positive benefit is increased surveillance for other communicable diseases as well. Such heightened surveillance can just as easily warn of a community salmonellosis or influenza outbreak. Although the benefit of syndromic surveillance as a warning system has not been proved, it has been valuable in tracking disease outbreaks such as the 2009 H1N1 pandemic. (For additional information on preparedness surveillance, see the CDC website at http://www.bt.cdc.gov/episurv/.)

Nurses are frequently involved at different levels of the surveillance system. They play important roles in collecting data, making diagnoses, investigating and reporting cases, and providing information to the general public. Examples of possible activities include investigating sources and contacts in outbreaks of pertussis in school settings or shigellosis in daycare; performing TB testing and contact tracing; collecting and reporting information pertaining to notifiable communicable diseases; performing infection control in hospitals; and providing morbidity and mortality statistics to those who request them, including the media, the public, service planners, and grant writers.

### List of Reportable Diseases

"A notifiable disease is one for which regular, frequent, and timely information regarding individual cases is considered necessary for the prevention and control of the disease" (CDC, 2013b). Requirements for disease reporting in the United States are mandated by state rather than federal law and, as such, vary slightly from state to state. State health departments, on a voluntary basis, report cases of selected diseases to the CDC through the National Notifiable Diseases Surveillance System (NNDSS). State public health officials collaborate with the CDC

---

**BOX 13-2    Ten Basic Data Elements of Surveillance**

1. Mortality registration
2. Morbidity reporting
3. Epidemic reporting
4. Epidemic field investigation
5. Laboratory reporting
6. Individual case investigation
7. Surveys
8. Utilization of biological agents and drugs
9. Distribution of animal reservoirs and vectors
10. Demographic and environmental data

X

## BOX 13-3   Nationally Notifiable Infectious Conditions—United States 2014

1. Anthrax
2. Arboviral diseases, neuroinvasive and non-neuroinvasive
3. Babesiosis
4. Botulism
5. Brucellosis
6. Chancroid
7. *Chlamydia trachomatis* infection
8. Cholera
9. Coccidioidomycosis
10. Congenital syphilis
11. Cryptosporidiosis
12. Cyclosporiasis
13. Dengue virus infections
14. Diphtheria
15. Ehrlichiosis and anaplasmosis
16. Giardiasis
17. Gonorrhea
18. *Haemophilus influenzae*, invasive disease
19. Hansen's disease
20. Hantavirus pulmonary syndrome
21. Hemolytic uremic syndrome, post-diarrheal
22. Hepatitis A, acute
23. Hepatitis B, acute
24. Hepatitis B, chronic
25. Hepatitis B, perinatal infection
26. Hepatitis C, acute
27. Hepatitis C, past or present
28. HIV infection (AIDS has been reclassified as HIV Stage III)
29. Influenza-associated pediatric mortality
30. Invasive pneumococcal disease
31. Legionellosis
32. Leptospirosis
33. Listeriosis
34. Lyme disease
35. Malaria

36. Measles
37. Meningococcal disease
38. Mumps
39. Novel influenza A virus infections
40. Pertussis
41. Plague
42. Poliomyelitis, paralytic
43. Poliovirus infection, nonparalytic
44. Psittacosis
45. Q fever
46. Rabies, animal
47. Rabies, human
48. Rubella
49. Rubella, congenital syndrome
50. Salmonellosis
51. Severe acute respiratory syndrome–associated coronavirus disease
52. Shiga toxin–producing *Escherichia coli*
53. Shigellosis
54. Smallpox
55. Spotted fever rickettsiosis
56. Streptococcal toxic-shock syndrome
57. Syphilis
58. Tetanus
59. Toxic shock syndrome (other than Streptococcal)
60. Trichinellosis
61. Tuberculosis
62. Tularemia
63. Typhoid fever
64. Vancomycin-intermediate *Staphylococcus aureus* and Vancomycin-resistant *Staphylococcus aureus*
65. Varicella
66. Varicella deaths
67. Vibriosis
68. Viral hemorrhagic fever
69. Yellow fever

From Centers for Disease Control and Prevention: *Nationally Notifible Infectious Conditions United States 2010.* 2010, CDC. Available at http://www.cdc.gov/ncphi/disss/nndss/phs/infdis2010.htm. Accessed March 25, 2010.
*AIDS has been reclassified as HIV stage III.

to determine which diseases should be nationally notifiable. The list of nationally notifiable diseases may be revised as new diseases emerge or disease incidence declines. The 69 diseases designated as notifiable at the national level and reported in 2014 are listed in Box 13-3. The NNDSS data are collated and published weekly in the *Morbidity and Mortality Weekly Report* (MMWR). Final reports are published annually in the *Summary of Notifiable Diseases.* (Learn more about the NNDSS at the CDC website at http://wwwn.cdc.gov/nndss/default.aspx. A brief history of the reporting of nationally notifiable infectious diseases in the United States is available at http://wwwn.cdc.gov/nndss/script/history.aspx.)

## EMERGING INFECTIOUS DISEASES

### Emergence Factors   *

Emerging infectious diseases are those in which the incidence has actually increased in the past several decades or has the potential to increase in the near future. These emerging diseases

may include new or known infectious diseases. Consider the following selected examples. Identified only in 1976 when sporadic outbreaks occurred in Sudan and Zaire, Ebola virus is a mysterious killer with a frightening mortality rate that sometimes reaches 90%, has no known treatment, and has no recognized reservoir in nature. It appears to be transmitted through direct contact with bodily secretions and as such can be contained once cases are identified. Why outbreaks occur is not understood, although index cases have been associated with the handling of wild primates and evidence is increasing for a bat reservoir. Ebola and its fellow virus Marburg are examples of new viruses that may appear as civilization intrudes farther and farther into previously uninhabited natural environments, changing the landscape and disturbing ecological balances that may have existed unaltered for hundreds of years. (Read more about the viral hemorrhagic viruses Ebola and Marburg at the CDC's viral special pathogens website: http://www.cdc.gov/ncezid/dhcpp/vspb/index.html.) See also World Health Organization, 2014a.

Hantavirus pulmonary syndrome was first detected in 1993 in the Four Corners area of Arizona and New Mexico, when young, previously healthy Native Americans fell ill with a mysterious and deadly respiratory disease. The illness was soon discovered to be a variant of, but to exhibit different pathology from, a rodent-borne virus previously known only in Europe and Asia. Transmission is thought to occur through aerosolization of rodent excrement. One explanation for the outbreak in the Southwest is that an unseasonably mild winter led to an unusual increase in the rodent population; more people than usual were exposed to a virus that had until that point gone unrecognized in this country. Infection in Native Americans first brought attention to hantavirus pulmonary syndrome because of a cluster of cases in a small geographic area, but no evidence suggests that any ethnic group is particularly susceptible to this disease. Hantavirus pulmonary syndrome has now been diagnosed in sites across the United States. The best protection against this virus seems to be avoiding rodent-infested environments.

Not only is HIV disease relatively new but the resultant immunocompromise gave rise to previously rare opportunistic infections such as cryptosporidiosis, toxoplasmosis, and *Pneumocystis* pneumonia (PCP). HIV may have existed in isolated parts of sub-Saharan Africa for years and emerged, only recently, into the rest of the world as the result of a combination of factors, including new roads, increased commerce, and prostitution.

*Esherichia coli* 0157:H7 and other shiga toxin–producing *E. coli* show a more virulent nature than strains of the past. TB is another familiar face turned newly aggressive. After years of decline, it has resurged as a result of infection resulting from HIV disease and the development of multidrug resistance. New influenza viruses like A H1N1 and A H5N1 challenge scientists to rapidly develop vaccines to protect a world population with little or no immunity.

West Nile Virus (WNV), a mosquito-borne seasonal disease, was first identified in Uganda in 1937 and first detected in the United States in 1999. How WNV arrived in the United States may never be known, but the answer most likely involves infected birds or mosquitoes. Because the virus was new in this country and the outbreak of 2002 caused numerous deaths, WNV garnered a great deal of media attention. However, for the majority of people, infection with WNV results in no clinical signs (about 80%) or only mild flu-like symptoms. In a small percentage of individuals, approximately 1 of 150 cases, a more severe, potentially fatal neuroinvasive form may develop, which may leave permanent neurologic deficits for those who survive. The incidence of neuroinvasive disease increases with age, with the highest rates in those 70 years and older. After first appearing in New York City in 1999, the virus spent several years quietly spreading up and down the East Coast without remarkable morbidity or mortality. This situation changed abruptly in the summer of 2002 when it began moving across the country, accompanied by significant avian, equine, and human mortality. WNV has now been reported in every state except Hawaii and Alaska and is the most common arbovirus (virus carried by arthropods) disease in the country. The CDC estimates that

during its introduction into the United States, between 1999 and 2008, WNV led to almost 30,000 confirmed and probable cases and over 1000 deaths. The number of reported cases varies widely per year. These periodic outbreaks appear to result from a complex interaction of multiple factors, including weather: hot, dry summers followed by rain, which influences mosquito breeding sites and population growth. Because the ecology of WNV is not fully understood, the future pattern and nature of the virus in the United States is uncertain. Until a human vaccine is developed (a vaccine for horses does exist), preventing human infection is dependent on mosquito control and preventing mosquito bites. Rarely, WNV has been transmitted through blood transfusions, in utero exposure, and possibly breastfeeding (CDC, 2010a). (Learn more about WNV and view maps of recent activity at the CDC website: http://www.cdc.gov/ncidod/dvbid/westnile/index.html.)

Other examples of emerging pathogens newly recognized in the past 30 years include viruses (Australian bat lyssavirus and Hendra or equine morbilli virus); bacteria (*Bartonella henselae, Ehrlichiae,* and *Borrelia burgdorferi*); and parasites (*Babesia microti* and *Acanthameoba*). *B. henselae* causes cat scratch fever. *Ehrlichiae, B. burgdorferi* (causes Lyme disease), and *B. microti* are all transmitted by ticks.

As shown in Table 13-1 several factors, operating singly or in combination, can influence the emergence of these diseases (Table 13-1) (CDC, 1994). Except for microbial adaptation and changes made by the infectious agent, such as those likely in the emergence of *E. coli* 0157:H7, most of the emergence factors are consequences of activities and behavior of the human hosts, and of environmental changes such as deforestation,

## TABLE 13-1    Factors that Can Influence the Emergence of New Infectious Diseases

| Categories | Specific Examples |
|---|---|
| Societal events | Economic impoverishment, war or civil conflict, population growth and migration, urban decay |
| Health care | New medical devices, organ or tissue transplantation, drugs causing immunosuppression, widespread use of antibiotics |
| Food production | Globalization of food supplies, changes in food processing and packaging |
| Human behavior | Sexual behavior, drug use, travel, diet, outdoor recreation, use of childcare facilities |
| Environmental | Deforestation/reforestation, changes in water ecosystems, flood/drought, famine, global changes (e.g., warming) |
| Public health | Curtailment or reduction in prevention programs, inadequate communicable disease infrastructure surveillance, lack of trained personnel (epidemiologists, laboratory scientists, vector and rodent control specialists) |
| Microbial adaptation | Changes in virulence and toxin production, development of drug resistance, microbes as co-factors in chronic diseases |

From Centers for Disease Control and Prevention: *Addressing emerging infectious disease threats: a prevention strategy for the U.S.,* Atlanta, 1994, CDC.

*Emerging Diseases*

urbanization, and industrialization. The rise in households with two working parents has increased the number of children in daycare and with this shift has come an increase in diarrheal diseases such as shigellosis. Changing sexual behavior and illegal drug use influence the spread of HIV disease as well as other sexually transmitted infections. Before the use of large air-conditioning systems with cooling towers, legionellosis was virtually unknown. Modern transportation systems closely and quickly connect regions of the world that for centuries had little contact. Insects and animals as well as humans may carry disease between continents on ships and planes. Immigrants, both legal and undocumented, as well as travelers, bring with them a variety of known and potentially unknown diseases.

## Examples of Emerging Infectious Diseases

Selected emerging infectious diseases, including a brief description of the diseases and symptoms they cause, their modes of transmission, and causes of emergence, are listed in Table 13-2. Progress in addressing emerging infectious disease as well as current findings and topics can be found in the CDC journal *Emerging Infectious Diseases*. (The journal is published monthly and is available online at http://www.cdc.gov/ncidod/EID/about/about.html)(Figure 13-2).

## PREVENTION AND CONTROL OF INFECTIOUS DISEASES

### Planning to Address Infectious Disease

In 2011, the CDC published *A CDC Framework for Preventing Infectious Disease: Sustaining the Essentials and Innovating for the Future*, a plan for preventing and controlling infectious threats through a "strengthened, adaptable, and multi-purpose U.S. public health system." Reflecting technological advances of the past decade, the plan places a heavy emphasis on the role of technology in surveillance, detection, and control. Three elements for action are identified: (1) Strengthen public health fundamentals, including infectious disease surveillance, laboratory detection, and epidemiologic investigation; (2) Identify and implement high-impact public health interventions to reduce infectious diseases; and (3) Develop and advance policies to prevent, detect, and control infectious diseases. It also discusses linkages between infectious and chronic disease; lists a timeline of disease threats, emerging pathogens, and unusual health events worldwide from 2000-2011; and identifies infectious disease issues of special concern: (1) antimicrobial resistance, (2) chronic viral hepatitis, (3) food safety, (4) health care–associated infections, (5) HIV/AIDS,

## TABLE 13-2 Examples of Emerging Infectious Diseases

| Infectious Agent | Diseases/Symptoms | Mode of Transmission | Causes of Emergence |
|---|---|---|---|
| *Borrelia burgdorferi* | Lyme disease: rash, fever, arthritis, neurologic and cardiac abnormalities | Bite of infective Ixodes tick | Increase in deer and human populations in wooded areas |
| *Cryptosporidium* | Cryptosporidiosis; infection of epithelial cells in gastrointestinal and respiratory tracts | Fecal–oral, person-to-person, waterborne | Development near watershed areas; immunosuppression |
| Ebola-Marburg viruses | Fulminant, high mortality, hemorrhagic fever | Direct contact with infected blood, organs, secretions, and semen | Unknown, likely human invasion of virus ecological niche |
| *Escherichia coli* 0157:H7 | Hemorrhagic colitis; thrombocytopenia; hemolytic uremic syndrome | Ingestion of contaminated food, especially undercooked beef and raw milk | Likely caused by a new pathogen |
| Hantavirus | Hemorrhagic fever with renal syndrome; pulmonary syndrome | Inhalation of aerosolized rodent urine and feces | Human invasion of virus ecological niche |
| Human immunodeficiency virus (HIV-1) | HIV infection; AIDS (HIV stage III); severe immune dysfunction, opportunistic infections | Sexual contact with or exposure to blood or tissues of infected persons; perinatal | Urbanization; lifestyle changes; drug use; international travel; transfusions; transplant |
| Human papillomavirus (HPV) | Skin and mucous membrane lesions (warts); strongly linked to cancer of the cervix and penis | Direct sexual contact, contact with contaminated surfaces | Newly recognized; changes in sexual lifestyle |
| Influenza A H1N1 virus (novel, pandemic) | Influenza: fever, cough, headache, myalgia, prostration, possibly GI signs | Person-to-person, airborne (droplet), and contact (direct and indirect) | Antigenic shift |
| Influenza A H5N1 virus (novel, avian) | Influenza: fever, cough, headache, myalgia, prostration | Direct contact with infected poultry or birds; limited person-to-person transmission | Antigenic shift |
| *Legionella pneumophila* | Legionnaires' disease: malaise, myalgia, fever, headache, respiratory illness | Air cooling systems, water supplies | Recognition in an epidemic situation |
| *Pneumocystis jiroveci* | Acute pneumonia | Unknown; possibly airborne or reactivation of latent infection | Immunosuppression |
| SARS | Severe and acute pneumonia | Person-to-person, airborne (droplet) and direct and indirect contact with respiratory secretions and other bodily fluid | Unknown; newly recognized coronavirus; possible animal transmission into Chinese population |
| West Nile virus | No clinical signs to mild flu-like symptoms to fatal neuroinvasive disease | Bite of infected mosquitoes; infected birds serve as reservoirs | International travel and commerce |

Based on information from Heymann DL, editor: *Control of communicable diseases manual*, ed 20, Washington, DC, 2014, American Public Health Association; Fauci AS, Touchette NA, Folkers GK: Emerging infectious diseases: a 10-year perspective from the National Institute of Allergy and Infectious Diseases, *Emerg Infect Dis* 11(4):519-525, 2005.

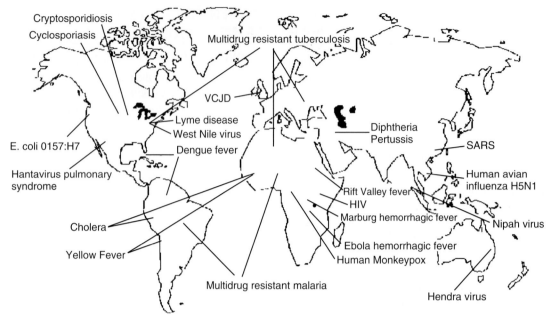

**FIGURE 13-2** Examples of recent emerging and reemerging infectious diseases. (Based on Institute of Medicine: *Microbial threats to health: emergence, detection, and response.* Washington, DC, 2003, National Academy Press.)

(6) respiratory infections, (7) safe water, and (8) zoonotic and vectorborne diseases (CDC, 2011a). (This plan may be viewed at http://www.cdc.gov/oid/docs/ID-Framework.pdf .)

### Prevention and Control Programs

Infectious disease can be prevented and controlled. The goal of prevention and control programs is to reduce the prevalence of a disease to a level at which it no longer poses a major public health problem. In some cases, diseases may even be eliminated or eradicated. The goal of elimination is to remove a disease from a large geographic area such as a country or region of the world. Eradication is removing a disease worldwide by ending all transmission of infection through the complete extermination of the infectious agent. WHO officially declared the global eradication of smallpox on May 8, 1980 (Evans, 1985). After the successful eradication of smallpox, the eradication of other communicable diseases became a realistic challenge, and in 1987 WHO adopted resolutions for eradication of paralytic poliomyelitis and dracunculiasis (Guinea worm infection) from the world by the year 2000.

These eradication goals were not reached in 2000, but substantial progress has been made. When the resolution was made in 1987 for the eradication of Guinea worm disease, there were an estimated 3.5 million cases a year in 20 countries in Asia and Africa and 120 million people were at risk for the disease. In 2013, only 148 cases were reported worldwide, making the goal of global eradication appear within reach (CDC, 2013c). Read more about Guinea worm disease eradication at http://www.cdc.gov/parasites/guineaworm/.

With the Global Polio Eradication Initiative, the World Health Organization (WHO) partnered with national governments, Rotary International, the CDC, and UNICEF in what has been called the world's largest public health initiative. Since 1988, over 2 billion children around the world have been immunized against polio through the cooperation of more than 200 countries and 20 million volunteers, supported by an international investment of over $3 billion. At the end of 2008, WHO reviewed the progress of the initiative with two independent outside agencies and concluded that the remaining technical and operational challenges to eradication could be overcome in each of the polio-endemic countries by ensuring the political commitment of all polio-affected countries to attain the highest possible coverage and enhancing routine vaccination and surveillance (CDC, 2009a).

As a result of the Global Polio Eradication Initiative launch in 1988, the number of polio-endemic countries has decreased from 125 to 3 (Afghanistan, Nigeria, and Pakistan); 4 of the 6 regions of the World Health Organization (WHO) are certified polio free—the Americas, Europe, South East Asia, and the Western Pacific; and the number of worldwide polio cases has fallen from an estimated 350,000 to 407 in 2013, a decrease of more than 99% in reported cases. However, importation of cases resulting from the ease of worldwide travel or breakdowns in coverage in a neighboring country continues to lead to outbreaks in nonendemic countries. Between January and May of 2014, 77 cases of wild polio were reported from 8 countries: Afghanistan, Cameroon, Equatorial Guinea, Ethiopia, Iraq, Nigeria, Pakistan, and Syria. Such outbreaks point to the necessity of maintaining mass vaccination campaigns in polio-free countries to protect against cases imported from endemic areas. Challenges to maintaining coverage include political instability and sporadic violence, cultural beliefs about immunization, religious fears, and distrust of immunization. With the potential for eradication so close, in May of 2014, the WHO declared the recent international spread of wild poliovirus a public health emergency of international concern and issued Temporary

Recommendations under the International Health Regulations (2005) to prevent further spread of the disease (CDC, 2014c). (Read more about global polio eradication efforts at http://www.polioeradication.org/.)

## Primary, Secondary, and Tertiary Prevention

There are three levels of prevention in public health: primary, secondary, and tertiary. In prevention and control of infectious disease, primary prevention seeks to reduce the incidence of disease by preventing occurrence, and this effort is often assisted by the government. Many interventions at the primary level, such as federally supplied vaccines and "no shots, no school" immunization laws, are population based because of public health mandates. Nurses deliver childhood immunizations in public and community health settings, check immunization records in daycare facilities, and monitor immunization records in schools.

The goal of secondary prevention is to prevent the spread of infection and/or disease once it occurs. Activities center on rapid identification of potential contacts to a reported case. Contacts may be (1) identified as new cases and treated, or (2) determined to be possibly exposed but not diseased and appropriately treated with prophylaxis. Public health disease control laws also assist in secondary prevention because they require investigation and prevention measures for individuals affected by a communicable disease report or outbreak. These laws can extend to the entire community if the exposure potential is deemed great enough, as could happen with an outbreak of smallpox or epidemic influenza. Nurses perform much of the communicable disease surveillance and control work in this country.

Although many infections are acute, with either recovery or death occurring in the short term, some exhibit chronic courses (AIDS/HIV stage III) or disabling sequelae (leprosy/Hansen's disease). Tertiary prevention works to reduce complications and disabilities through treatment and rehabilitation. The Levels of Prevention box has examples of communicable disease prevention and control interventions at the three levels of prevention.

## Role of Nurses in Prevention

Prevention is at the center of public health, and nurses perform much of this work. Examples include immunizations for vaccine-preventable disease, especially childhood immunization and the monitoring of immunization status in clinic, daycare, school, and home settings. Nurses work in communicable disease surveillance and control, teach and monitor bloodborne pathogen control, and advise on prevention of vector borne diseases. They teach methods for responsible sexual behavior, screen for sexually transmitted infection, and provide HIV disease counseling and testing. They screen for TB, identify TB contacts, and deliver directly observed TB treatment in the community.

## Multisystem Approach to Control

Communicable diseases represent an imbalance in the harmonious relationship between the human host and the

### LEVELS OF PREVENTION
*Examples of Infectious Disease Interventions*

**Primary Prevention**
To prevent the occurrence of disease:
- Responsible sexual behavior
- Malaria chemoprophylaxis
- Tetanus boosters, flu shots
- Rabies pre-exposure immunization
- Safe food-handling practices in the home
- Repellants for preventing vector borne disease
- Following childhood immunizations recommendations, and "no shots, no school" laws
- Regulated and inspected municipal water supplies
- Bloodborne pathogen regulations
- Restaurant inspections
- Federal regulations protecting American cattle from exposure to bovine spongiform encephalopathy (BSE)

**Secondary Prevention**
To prevent the spread of disease:
- Immunoglobulin after hepatitis A exposure
- Immunization and chemoprophylaxis as appropriate in meningococcal outbreak
- Rabies postexposure immunization
- Tuberculosis screening for health care workers
- Sexually transmitted disease (STD) partner notification
- Human immunodeficiency virus (HIV) testing and treatment
- Quarantine

**Tertiary Prevention**
To reduce complications and disabilities through treatment and rehabilitation:
- *Pneumocystis* pneumonia (PCP) chemoprophylaxis for people with AIDS/HIV stage III
- Regular inspection of hands and feet as well as protective footwear and gloves to avoid trauma and infection for leprosy clients who have lost sensation in those areas

environment. This state of imbalance provides the infectious agent an opportunity to cause illness and death in the human population. Given the many factors that can disrupt the agent-host-environment relationship, a multisystem approach to control of communicable diseases as shown in Table 13-3 must be developed (Wenzel, 1998).

## AGENTS OF BIOTERRORISM

September 11, 2001, made real the specter of terrorism on American soil. The anthrax attacks that followed further highlighted the possibilities for the intentional release of a biological agent, or bioterrorism. The CDC suggests that the agents most likely to be used in a bioterrorist attack are those having the potential for both high mortality and easy dissemination—factors most likely to result in major public panic and social disruption. Six infectious agents are considered of highest concern: anthrax (*Bacillus anthracis*), plague (*Yersinia pestis*), smallpox (variola major), botulism (*Clostridium botulinum*), tularemia (*Francisella tularensis*), and selected hemorrhagic viruses (filoviruses such as Ebola and Marburg; arenaviruses

**TABLE 13-3    A Multisystem Approach to Communicable Disease Control**

| Goal | Example |
|------|---------|
| Improve host resistance to infectious agents and other environmental hazards | Hygiene, nutrition, and physical fitness; increased immunization coverage; provision of drugs for prevention and treatment; stress control and improved mental health |
| Improve safety of the environment | Sanitation, clean water and air; proper cooking and storage of food; control of vectors and animal reservoir hosts |
| Improve public health systems | Increased access to health care; appropriate health education; improved surveillance systems |
| Facilitate social and political change to ensure better health for all people | Individual, organizational, and community action; legislation |

Modified from Wenzel RP: Control of communicable diseases: overview. In Wallace RB, editor: *Public health and preventive medicine,* ed. 15, 2008, New York.

such as Lassa fever, Junin virus, and related viruses). The CDC urges health care providers to be familiar with the epidemiology of these diseases as well as illness patterns possibly indicating an unusual infectious disease outbreak associated with the intentional release of a biological agent. (More information on recognition of illness associated with the intentional release of a biological agent as well as possible agents may be found at the CDC Emergency Preparedness and Response website: http://www.bt.cdc.gov.)

## Anthrax

Until the fall of 2001, anthrax was more commonly a concern of veterinarians and military strategists than the general public. After September 11th, the news of deaths caused by letters deliberately contaminated with anthrax and transmitted through the postal service profoundly changed our view of this infectious disease. Anthrax is an acute disease caused by the spore-forming bacterium *B. anthracis.* It is thought that anthrax may have caused the biblical fifth and sixth plagues of Exodus as well as the Black Bane of Europe in the 1600s. In 1881 anthrax became the first bacterial disease for which immunization was available. More commonly seen in cattle, sheep, and goats, anthrax in modern times has rarely and sporadically affected humans, usually through the handling or consumption of infected animal products (Cieslak and Eitzen, 1999).

Anthrax is a clever organism that perpetuates itself by forming spores. When animals dying from anthrax suffer terminal hemorrhage and infected blood comes into contact with the air, the bacillus organism sporulates. These spores are highly resistant to disinfection and environmental destruction and may remain in contaminated soil for many years. In the United States, anthrax zones are said to follow the cattle drive trails of the 1800s. Sometimes referred to as wool handler's disease, anthrax has commonly posed the greatest risk to people who work directly with dying animals, such as veterinarians, or those

who handle infected animal products such as hair, wool, and bone or bone meal or products made from these materials such as rugs and drums. Products made from infected materials may transmit this disease around the world. Person-to-person transmission is rare (Heymann, 2014).

Anthrax disease may manifest in one of three syndromes: cutaneous, gastrointestinal, and respiratory or inhalational. Cutaneous anthrax, the form most commonly seen, occurs when spores come in contact with abraded skin surfaces. Itching is followed in 2 to 6 days by the development of a characteristic black eschar, usually surrounded by some degree of edema and possibly secondary infection. The lesion itself is usually not painful. If untreated, infection may spread to the regional lymph nodes and bloodstream, resulting in septicemia and death. The fatality rate for untreated cutaneous anthrax is between 5% and 20%, but if appropriately treated, death seldom occurs. Before 2001 the last cutaneous case in the United States was reported in 1992. Gastrointestinal anthrax is considered rare and occurs from eating undercooked, contaminated meat. Inhalational anthrax is also considered rare, typically seen in occupations with exposure to hide tanning or bone processing. Before 2001 the last case reported in the United States was in 1976. Initially, symptoms are mild and nonspecific and may include fever, malaise, mild cough, or chest pain. These symptoms are followed 3 to 5 days later, often after an apparent improvement, by fever and shock, rapid deterioration, and death. Untreated cases of inhalational anthrax are fatal; treated cases may show as high as a 95% fatality rate if treatment is initiated after 48 hours from the onset of symptoms.

Because of factors such as the ability for aerosolization, the resistance to environmental degradation and a high fatality rate, inhalational anthrax has long been considered to have an extremely high potential for being the single greatest biological warfare threat (Cieslak and Eitzen, 1999). An accidental release from a biological research institute in Sverdlovsk, Russia, in 1979 resulted in the documented death of 66 individuals and demonstrated the capacity of this organism as a weapon. Manufacture and delivery of the spores have been considered a challenge because of a tendency for the spores to clump. During 1998 in the United States, more than two dozen anthrax threats (letters purporting to be carrying anthrax) were made. None of them were real. The events of the fall of 2001, when 11 people were sickened and 5 died from deliberate exposure, have shown that the threat of anthrax as a weapon of bioterror is all too real.

Any threat of anthrax should be reported to the Federal Bureau of Investigation and to local and state health departments. Anthrax is sensitive to a variety of antibiotics including the penicillins, chloramphenicol, doxycycline, and the fluoroquinolones. In cases of possible bioterrorism activity, individuals with a credible threat of exposure, with confirmed exposure, or at high risk of exposure are immediately started on antibiotic prophylaxis, preferably fluoroquinolones. Immunization is recommended as well. People who have been exposed are not contagious, so quarantine is not appropriate (Heymann, 2014).

In recent years, although no more deliberate acts of bioterrorism have been reported, England and the United States have seen rare cases of cutaneous, inhalational, and gastrointestinal anthrax associated with drumming circles using drums covered with imported animal hides. Since December 2009, in the United Kingdom there has been an ongoing outbreak of anthrax among injecting drug users, in some cases resulting in death. The infection is believed to be caused by contaminated heroin. With no new cases after the summer, Scotland declared the outbreak over in December 2010 but concluded the possibility of an ongoing risk of anthrax in heroin users supported by sporadic cases occurring in England. In 2012, 13 cases were reported from Germany, Denmark, France, and the United Kingdom. Ongoing European investigation continues (Grunow et al, 2013).

## Smallpox ✳

Formerly a disease found worldwide, smallpox has been considered eradicated since 1979. The last known natural case in the United States was in 1949. The last known case of smallpox worldwide occurred in Somalia in 1977. The United States stopped routinely immunizing for smallpox in 1982. The only documented existing virus sources are located in freezers at the CDC in Atlanta and at a research institute in Novosibirsk, Russia. Controversy exists over the destruction of these viral stocks, and despite an earlier call by WHO for destruction in 2002, the date was postponed to allow for additional research needed should clandestine supplies fall into terrorist hands. The World Health Assembly expected to debate this issue in 2014.

Smallpox has been identified as one of the leading candidate agents for bioterrorism. Susceptibility is 100% in the unvaccinated (those vaccinated before 1982 are not considered protected, although they may have some immunity) and the fatality rate is estimated at 20% to 40% or higher. Immunization with a vaccinia vaccine, the immunizing agent for smallpox, can be protective even after exposure. In 2007 the U.S. Food and Drug Administration (FDA) licensed a new smallpox vaccine, derived from the only other smallpox vaccine licensed by the FDA: Dryvax, approved in 1931 and now in limited supply because it is no longer manufactured. The WHO does not recommend vaccination of the general public because currently the risk of death (1 per 1 million doses) or serious side effects is greater than that of the disease. Those who routinely are exposed to smallpox virus such as laboratory workers should be vaccinated. Because of the potential for bioterrorism and the fact that many health care providers have never seen this disease, it is important to become familiar with the clinical and epidemiologic features of smallpox and how it is differentiated from chickenpox (see the How To box). Should a nonvaricella, smallpox-like disease be detected, immediate contact with local and national health authorities is obligatory (Heymann, 2014).

---

**HOW TO  Distinguish Chickenpox from Smallpox**

*Despite the availability of a vaccine, chickenpox is still a common disease of childhood and may be seen in susceptible adults as well. Although many health care providers are familiar with chickenpox, most have never seen a case of smallpox. Because of the potential for smallpox to be used as a bioweapon, the CDC suggests that nurses and other practitioners familiarize themselves with the differences in presentation between the two diseases. The rash*

*pattern for each disease is distinctive, but in the first 2 to 3 days of development, the two may be indistinguishable. Infectious disease texts and posters provide a pictorial description. If a smallpox infection is suspected, the local health department should be notified immediately.*

| Chickenpox (Varicella) | Smallpox (Historical Variola Major) |
|---|---|
| *Sudden onset with slight fever and mild constitutional symptoms (both may be more severe in adults)* | *Sudden onset of fever, prostration, severe body aches, and occasional abdominal pain and vomiting, as in influenza* |
| *Rash is present at onset* | *Clear-cut prodromal illness, rash follows 2-4 days after fever begins decreasing* |
| *Rash progression is maculopapular for a few hours, vesicular for 3-4 days, followed by granular scabs* | *Progression is macular, papular, vesicular, and pustular, followed by crusted scabs that fall off after 3-4 weeks if client survives* |
| *Rash is "centrifugal" with lesions most abundant on the trunk or areas of the body usually covered by clothing* | *Rash is "centripetal" with lesions most abundant on the face and extremities* |
| *Lesions appear in "crops" and can be at various stages in the same area of the body* | *Lesions are all at same stage in all areas* |
| *Vesicles are superficial and collapse on puncture; mild scarring may occur* | *Vesicles are deep-seated and do not collapse on puncture; pitting and scarring are common* |

---

From Heymann DL, editor: *Control of communicable diseases manual*, ed 19. Washington, DC, 2008, American Public Health Association; Henderson DA: Smallpox: clinical and epidemiologic features. *Emerg Infect Dis* 5:537–539, 1999.

## Plague ✳

Plague is a vector borne disease transmitted by rodent fleas carrying the bacterium *Y. pestis*. Portrayed vividly in the Bible and events throughout history, plague is believed responsible for the epidemic of Black Death that killed over a quarter of the population of Europe during the Middle Ages. The disease is endemic in much of South Asia, parts of South America, and the western United States, but the majority of outbreaks and cases today are reported from Africa, especially from the Democratic Republic of the Congo. Plague arrived in the United States as a consequence of a pandemic that began in China during the late 1800s and spread to the West Coast via shipboard rats. Although resulting plague in cities was largely controlled, the disease spread to and became enzootic in wild rodents. The current primary vertebrate reservoirs in the United States are usually ground squirrels rather than rats, rabbits, wild carnivores, and in some cases cats. Human plague in the western United States occurs infrequently and sporadically with fewer than 20 cases reported a year since 1970. Veterinarians have contracted the disease from infected cats. People with regular outdoor exposure such as hunters, trappers, and those living in rural areas as well as cat owners are at highest risk for natural transmission (Heymann, 2014).

Initial signs and symptoms of plague are nonspecific and include myalgia, malaise, fever, chills, sore throat, and headache. As the disease progresses, lymphadenitis commonly develops in the lymph nodes, draining the area nearest the bite. This swollen node, or bubo, most frequently seen in the inguinal area, gives rise to the name bubonic plague. Whether lymphadenitis is present or not, bubonic plague may progress to septicemic plague and secondary pneumonic plague. Secondary pneumonic plague can spread through respiratory droplets, resulting in primary pneumonic plague and human-to-human outbreaks. No such transmission has been reported in the United States since 1924, but several cases of primary pneumonic plague have developed from exposure to infected cats.

Untreated cases of primary septicemic and pneumonic plague are most often fatal; the case fatality rate for untreated bubonic plague is 50% to 60%. Streptomycin is the treatment of choice; gentamicin, tetracyclines, and chloramphenicol are alternatives. Immunization may confer some protection against bubonic plague but not pneumonic. Commercial plague vaccine is no longer available in the United States. Naturally acquired plague is usually bubonic. Plague used as a means of a terrorist attack would most likely be aerosolized, resulting in pneumonic disease and human-to-human transmission (Heymann, 2014). Read more about plague at the CDC website: http://www.cdc .gov/plague/.

## Tularemia

Sometimes referred to as "rabbit fever" or "deer fly fever," tularemia is a zoonotic disease caused by the bacterial agent *F. tularensis* which is carried commonly by wild animals, especially rabbits, as well as muskrats, voles, beavers, some domestic animals, and some ticks, mosquitoes, and flies. Tularemia may be transmitted by the bite of an infected arthropod; contact of eyes, skin, or mucous membranes with infected tissues, blood, or water; ingestion of inadequately cooked infected meat or contaminated water; inhalation of contaminated dust; and handling of contaminated pelts and paws. Hunters handling rabbit and rodent carcasses, lawn care workers, and those working outside in rural areas may be at higher risk. Tularemia has also occurred from running over an infected rabbit with a lawn mower and by handling sick pets including dogs, cats, hamsters, and prairie dogs. Tularemia is not transmitted from person to person (Heymann, 2014).

How tularemia presents varies depending on how the infection was acquired and the virulence of the infecting agent. There are two subspecies of *F. tularensis*—one causing few deaths even without treatment and one resulting in a 5% to 15% fatality rate without treatment, primarily from respiratory disease. Commonly the onset of tularemia is sudden and may resemble influenza with high fever, myalgia, headache, nausea, and chills. Frequently an ulcerative lesion appears at the point of inoculation accompanied by swelling of associated lymph nodes. However, lymphadenitis can occur without a primary lesion. In either case, the presence of these buboes can cause

confusion with plague. Inoculation, or introduction of the organism, into the eye results in a purulent conjunctivitis accompanied by regional lymphadenitis. Ingestion of infected tissue or contaminated water produces a sore throat, abdominal pain, diarrhea, and vomiting. Infection by inhalation may cause respiratory involvement and possible sepsis. Pneumonia is a potential complication with all forms and requires prompt treatment to prevent potentially fatal complications. Aminoglycosides or ciprofloxacin are the treatment drugs of choice. There is no vaccination for tularemia currently in widespread use in the United States, although live attenuated vaccine applied intradermally by scarification is available to high-risk workers (Heymann, 2014).

Tularemia has been reported from every state except Hawaii but is not a particularly common disease, with an average of 130 cases per year reported from 2003 through 2012. The only two reported outbreaks of pneumonic tularemia in the United States have come from Martha's Vineyard, where the disease is endemic and cases are frequently reported in lawn care workers (Feldman et al, 2003). Because of the low incidence of naturally occurring disease, tularemia was removed from the nationally notifiable disease list in 1994 but reinstated in 2000 with the growing concern over bioterrorism. Aerosolized tularemia with resulting pneumonic disease is considered the most likely scenario for use as an agent of bioterrorism (CDC, 2009b). (Read more about tularemia at the CDC website: http://www.cdc.gov/ tularemia/index.html.)

## VACCINE-PREVENTABLE DISEASES

Vaccines are one of the most effective methods of preventing and controlling communicable diseases. The smallpox vaccine, which left distinctive scars on so many shoulders, is no longer in general use because the smallpox virus has been declared eradicated from the world's population. Despite threats of bioterrorism, there are no plans to reintroduce universal smallpox immunization because of potential side effects. Diseases such as polio, diphtheria, pertussis, and measles, which previously occurred in epidemic proportions, are now controlled by routine childhood immunization. They have not, however, been eradicated, so children need to be immunized against them. In the United States, "no shots, no school" legislation has resulted in the immunization of most children by the time they enter school. However, many infants and toddlers, the group most vulnerable to these potentially severe diseases, do not receive scheduled immunizations despite the availability of free vaccines. And infants less than six months of age who are not yet fully immunized may be susceptible to infections in unimmunized individuals around them (see the Evidence-Based Practice box). Surveys show inner-city children from minority and ethnic groups are particularly at risk for incomplete immunization, and children from religious communities whose beliefs prohibit immunization and children with parents who have philosophical objections to immunization may receive no protection at all. Studies also show low levels of vaccination against pneumonia in senior citizens and lower levels of influenza coverage in adults from minority and ethnic groups. *Healthy People*

*2020* includes several objectives about obtaining and maintaining appropriate levels of immunization in all age groups. (Additional information on vaccine-preventable diseases may be found at the CDC website: http://www.cdc.gov/vaccines/.)

---

## EVIDENCE-BASED PRACTICE

Because they are too young to be fully immunized, infants under six months of age are at greatest risk for complications and death from pertussis. New mothers, fathers, caretakers, and close contacts to the infant are frequently the source of infection, leading to the concept of cocooning the infant against pertussis through immunizing individuals who have close contact with the baby. In examining ways to increase Tdap (tetanus, reduced diphtheria, acellular pertussis) uptake in new mothers, researchers looked at two hospitals with zero postpartum Tdap immunization rates. One followed standard procedures and the other instituted a standing order for new mothers to receive Tdap before discharge. Implementing the standing orders raised the zero starting rate to 69%. At the hospital that followed standard procedures, the rate for postpartum Tdap immunization remained at zero. Since this study, the Advisory Committee on Immunization Practices has updated its recommendation to say women should receive Tdap, if they have not already, toward the end of their second trimester or during their third trimester of pregnancy. However, even with this new recommendation, studies find only a small percentage of unimmunized pregnant women receive a Tdap vaccination (LABioMed, 2014).

### Nurse Use

The adult public has been slow to embrace Tdap. One reason may be lack of awareness of the availability of the vaccine and/or of the importance it plays in keeping infants safe. There are a variety of ways to approach this issue, starting with consumer awareness and provider education and advocacy. This study shows how a change in standard practice within an institution had a dramatic effect on Tdap immunization in postpartum mothers. Whether Tdap or other issues that require attention, nurses manage clinics and take leadership roles in hospitals, physicians' offices, health departments, and safety-net health services, which puts them in a position to both assess where there are opportunities for intervention and to change practice to address important public health concerns.

---

Because many children receive their immunizations at public health departments, nurses play a major role in increasing immunization coverage of infants and toddlers. Nurses track children known to be at risk for underimmunization and call or send reminders to their parents. They help avoid missed immunization opportunities by checking the immunization status of every young child encountered, whether or not the clinic or home visit is related to immunization. In addition, they organize immunization outreach activities in the community; provide answers to parents' questions and concerns about immunization; and educate parents about why immunizations are needed, inappropriate contraindications to immunization, and the importance of completing the immunization schedule on time.

### Routine Childhood Immunization Schedule

The 2014 recommended immunization schedule for children and adolescents in the United States includes routine immunization against the following 16 diseases: hepatitis B, diphtheria, pertussis, tetanus, measles, mumps, rubella, polio, *Haemophilus influenzae* type B meningitis, *Varicella* (chickenpox*)*, *Streptococcus pneumoniae*–related illnesses, rotavirus, hepatitis A, influenza, HPV, and meningococcal disease (CDC, 2014d). The vaccine schedule is a rather complex and frequently changing document that makes continuing adjustments for the latest research and recommendations and is issued annually by the Advisory Committee on Immunization Practices (ACIP). More recent additions to the schedule include hepatitis A, rotavirus, seasonal influenza for all children ages 6 months through 18 years, and Tdap (the tetanus, reduced-strength diphtheria, and acellular pertussis vaccine licensed for older children, adolescents, and adults). Because many of these vaccines require three to four doses, the schedule begins at birth with succeeding staggered vaccinations designed to achieve recommended immunization levels by 2 years of age. Additional doses may be required before a child enters school and at adolescence or on entering college. The ACIP, the American Academy of Pediatrics and the American Academy of Family Physicians regularly update recommended immunization schedules. The ACIP also issues a recommended adult immunization schedule for those over 18 years old, by age group and immune status. The 2014 schedule includes, as appropriate, HPV, varicella, measles, mumps and rubella, pneumococcus, zoster to prevent shingles, and tetanus every 10 years with one dose given as Tdap. Other immunizations available in special circumstances include, but are not limited to, rabies, yellow fever, typhoid, smallpox, and anthrax. (Recommended vaccine schedules may be viewed at http://www.cdc.gov/vaccines/schedules/index.html.)

### Measles

Measles is an acute, highly contagious disease that, although considered a childhood illness, may be seen in the United States in adolescents and young adults. Symptoms include fever, sneezing and coughing, conjunctivitis, small white spots on the inside of the cheek (Koplik's spots), and a red, blotchy rash beginning several days after the respiratory signs. Measles is caused by the rubeola virus and is transmitted by inhalation of infected aerosol droplets or by direct contact with infected nasal or throat secretions or with articles freshly contaminated with the same nasal or throat secretions. A very contagious nature, combined with the fact that people are most contagious before they are aware they are infected, makes measles a disease that can spread rapidly through the population. Infection with measles confers lifelong immunity (Heymann, 2014).

Measles and malnutrition form a deadly combination for many children in the developing world. Despite the introduction in 1963 of a live attenuated measles vaccine that is safe, effective, and widely available, measles is still endemic in many countries. The WHO estimates 20 million people are affected each year with over 100,000 deaths—mostly children under the age of five. Much of this mortality is preventable by immunizing all infants. The good news is that with the launch of the Measles and Rubella Initiative in 2001, global measles deaths have decreased by 78 percent worldwide in recent years—from 562,400 deaths in 2000 to 122,000 in 2012 (WHO, 2014b).

Immunization has dramatically decreased measles cases in the United States to the point that, in March 2000, a panel of experts declared measles no longer endemic in the United States. Before introduction of the vaccine in 1963, 200,000 to 500,000 cases of measles were reported yearly, but by 1983 reported cases had fallen to an all-time low of less than 1500. In the late 1980s, the incidence of measles began to climb again, with more than 55,000 cases reported between 1989 and 1991. This increase resulted from low immunization rates among preschool children and was countered with efforts to increase immunization rates and the routine use of two doses of measles vaccine for all children. Except for outbreaks in 1994 that occurred predominantly among high school and college-age persons, many of whom had not received two doses of measles vaccine, reported measles cases dropped continuously from 1991 to 2004 when only 37 confirmed cases were reported to the CDC—the lowest number since measles became a nationally reportable disease in 1912.

Since measles elimination was documented in the United States in 2000, annual reported cases have ranged from the low of 37 in 2004 to a high of 644 in 2014. Years with high numbers of reports are driven by outbreaks. In 2008, 140 cases were reported with 3 outbreaks. This increase was attributed to spread in communities with groups of unvaccinated people. The 220 cases in 2011 largely resulted from cases imported from a large outbreak in France. The United States experienced 11 outbreaks in 2013, three of which had more than 20 cases and in 2014 saw 23 outbreaks and 644 cases, many of which were associated with a large, ongoing measles outbreak in the Philippines. The first three weeks of January 2015 saw 68 cases from 11 states, most of which were linked with a large outbreak in a California amusement park (CDC, 2015b).

These recent outbreaks in the United States highlight the ongoing risk of measles importation from other countries by people who travel. With first-dose vaccine coverage of preschool children at greater than 90% and schools in 49 states requiring two doses of vaccine, the pattern of infection has shifted from under immunization of infants and school-age children to disease acquired from other countries. Because imported cases had not previously resulted in large outbreaks, it appeared that vaccination efforts had been successful in increasing herd immunity against measles, but groups who remain at greatest risk for infection are those who do not routinely accept immunization, such as people with religious or philosophical objections, students in schools that do not require two doses of vaccine, and infants in areas where immunization coverage is low. The exposure of these groups to an imported case can result in a major outbreak and, indeed, beginning with the 2008 outbreaks, most increases have not been the result of a greater number of imported cases but of greater viral transmission after importation into the United States, leading to a larger number of importation-associated cases. These importation-associated cases largely occur among the unvaccinated, frequently among school-aged children who are eligible for vaccination but whose parents choose not to have them vaccinated and infants who are too young for vaccination. States vary in the ease of obtaining philosophical exemptions from immunization and requirements for vaccination of home-schooled children. The increase in importation-associated cases may result in an increase in measles morbidity, especially in communities with many unvaccinated residents (CDC, 2015b; CDC, 2014e).

*Healthy People 2020* calls for the reduction, elimination or maintained elimination of vaccine-preventable diseases including the reduction of indigenous measles cases. Efforts to meet this goal will require (1) rapid detection of cases and implementation of appropriate outbreak control measures, (2) achievement and maintenance of high levels of vaccination coverage among preschool-age children in all geographic regions, (3) continued implementation and enforcement of the two-dose schedule among young adults, (4) the determination of the source of all outbreaks and sporadic infections, and (5) cooperation among countries in measles control efforts. Nurses receive reports of cases, investigate them, and initiate control measures for outbreaks. They use every opportunity to immunize adolescents and young adults who lack documentation of two doses of measles vaccine. Nurses who work in regions where undocumented residents are common, where groups obtain exemption from immunization on religious grounds or who choose not to vaccinate for philosophical reasons, where preschool coverage is low and/or where international visitors are frequent need to be especially alert for measles cases and the necessity of prompt outbreak control among particularly susceptible populations.

## Rubella

The rubella (German measles) virus causes a mild febrile disease with enlarged lymph nodes and a fine, pink rash that is often difficult to distinguish from measles or scarlet fever. In contrast to measles, rubella is only a moderately contagious illness. Transmission is through inhalation of or direct contact with infected droplets from the respiratory secretions of infected persons. Children may show few or no constitutional symptoms, whereas adults usually experience several days of low-grade fever, headache, malaise, runny nose, and conjunctivitis before the rash appears. Many infections occur without a rash (Heymann, 2014).

For many years, because it caused only a mild illness, rubella was considered to be of minor importance. Then, in 1941 the link between maternal rubella and poor pregnancy outcomes was recognized and the disease suddenly assumed major public health significance. Rubella infection, in addition to causing intrauterine death and spontaneous abortion, may result in anomalies referred to as congenital rubella syndrome (CRS), affecting single or multiple organ systems. Defects include cataracts, congenital glaucoma, deafness, microcephaly, mental retardation, cardiac abnormalities, and diabetes mellitus. CRS occurs in up to 90% of infants born to women who are infected with rubella during the first trimester of pregnancy (Heymann, 2014). During the 1962 to 1965 rubella pandemic, an estimated 12.5 million cases of rubella occurred in the United States, resulting in 2000 cases of encephalitis, 11,250 fetal deaths, 2100 neonatal deaths, and 20,000 infants born with CRS. The economic impact of this epidemic was estimated at $1.5 billion (CDC, 2005).

The United States has established and achieved the goal of eliminating indigenous rubella transmission and CRS. Rubella elimination is defined as the absence of continuous endemic transmission lasting ≥12 months. With the introduction of a vaccine in 1969, cases of rubella in the United States fell precipitously from 57,686 to less than 10 cases per year 2003 and 2004 with a large percentage of the cases imported or import linked. By the beginning of 2005, at the 39th National Immunization Conference, the director of the CDC announced that rubella was no longer endemic in the United States. From 2005 through 2011, 67 rubella cases were reported as well as two rubella outbreaks involving three cases and four cases of CRS. Of these 67 cases, 28 cases (42%) were known importations. Elimination of endemic rubella was once again documented and verified in the United States in December 2011 (CDC, 2013d).

Rubella remains endemic in parts of the world, however, and because of international travel and countries without routine rubella vaccination, imported cases of rubella and CRS cases are possible. In 2012, WHO estimated 110,000 cases of CRS worldwide, many of them in Asia and Africa where vaccination coverage is lowest. WHO also reports that intensive and widespread rubella vaccination efforts have largely eliminated rubella and CRS in many developed and in some developing countries. The WHO Region of the Americas has had no endemic (naturally transmitted) cases of rubella infection since 2009.

Unimmunized immigrants do not necessarily import disease, but their unimmunized status may leave them vulnerable to infection once they arrive. In addition to a focus on identifying and vaccinating foreign-born adults, the continued elimination of rubella and CRS in the United States will require (1) maintaining high immunization rates among children, (2) ensuring vaccination among women of child-bearing age, especially those who are foreign-born, (3) continuing aggressive surveillance, and (4) responding rapidly to any outbreak.

## Pertussis

Pertussis (whooping cough) begins as a mild upper respiratory tract infection progressing to an irritating cough that within 1 to 2 weeks may become paroxysmal (a series of repeated violent coughs). The repeated coughs occur without intervening breaths and can be followed by a characteristic inspiratory "whoop." Pertussis is caused by the bacterium *Bordetella pertussis* and is transmitted via an airborne route through contact with infected droplets. It is highly contagious and considered endemic in the United States. Vaccination against pertussis, delivered in combination with diphtheria and tetanus, is a part of the routine childhood immunization schedule. Treatment of infected individuals with antibiotics such as erythromycin may shorten the period of communicability but does not relieve symptoms unless given early in the course of the infection. Prophylactic treatment with antibiotics is recommended for family members and close contacts of infected individuals, regardless of immunization status and age, if there is a child in the house under the age of 1 year or a woman in the last 3 weeks of pregnancy or to prevent ongoing transmission within the family. Infection with pertussis does not offer permanent immunity (Heymann, 2014).

Before the development of a whole-cell vaccine—DTP (diphtheria, tetanus, pertussis)—in the 1940s, pertussis led to hundreds of thousands of cases and thousands of deaths per year, the majority in children younger than 5 years. After vaccine licensure and the introduction of universal vaccination, reported cases in the United States steadily declined, hitting a record low of just over 1000 in 1976. However, beginning in the early 1980s, pertussis cases began to show cyclical increases peaking every 3 to 5 years with the peaks getting higher and reported cases going up. In 2012, over 48,000 cases were reported, the highest number since 1955 (CDC, 2014f).

In the mid 2000s the epidemiology of pertussis appears to have changed. While infants less than 6 months were still the most likely to be infected as they are not old enough to be fully vaccinated, incidence began increasing in children 7 to 10 years old, many of whom had been fully vaccinated, suggesting that the acellular vaccine DTaP, introduced in 1997 for the entire childhood series in response to concerns over serious side effects in some children after DTP, may not offer the duration of protection seen with the whole-cell vaccine. Tdap (tetanus, reduced strength diphtheria, acellular pertussis) was licensed in 2005 as a booster for adults in place of their next tetanus vaccination and adolescents, with routine recommendation for immunization at 11 to 12 years. The reduction in rates in preteens 11 to 12 years old demonstrates immediate protection from Tdap, but increasing incidence in 13- to 14-year-olds suggests waning immunity with no durable protection. But while waning immunity may not be completely protective, evidence suggests that when infected, people who have been boostered will experience milder disease. While positive for those thus protected, this lack of symptoms may have the unintended consequence of making them excellent inapparent carriers. Nonetheless, vaccination with DTaP and Tdap continues to be recommended as the single most effective strategy in reducing illness and death from pertussis. Pregnant women and close contacts to their babies are especially encouraged to be vaccinated in an effort to prevent disease in infants, the group most likely to experience severe complications and death. In addition to maintaining high rates of immunization, prevention efforts also included publicizing Tdap, increasing awareness of pertussis in adolescents and adults among providers, and promptly implementing treatment and control in the face of outbreaks (CDC, 2012b).

Because pertussis does have a cyclical pattern (there are periodic outbreaks such as those seen in California in 2010 and in Washington state as well as numerous other states across the country in 2012), it is important for nurses to work with the community to maintain the highest possible levels of immunization coverage to minimize these occurrences. Because of the contagious nature of pertussis, nurses play a major role in limiting transmission during outbreaks by ensuring appropriate treatment of family members and close contacts. The Quality and Safety in Nursing Education box describes safety factors related to pertussis.

## Influenza

Influenza is a viral respiratory tract infection often indistinguishable from the common cold or other respiratory diseases.

Transmission is airborne and through direct contact with infected droplets. Unlike many viruses that do not survive long in the environment, the flu virus is thought to exist for many hours in dried mucus. Outbreaks are common in the winter and early spring in areas where people gather indoors such as in schools and nursing homes. Gastrointestinal and respiratory symptoms are common. Because symptoms do not always follow a characteristic pattern, many viral diseases that are not influenza are often called flu. The most important factors to note about influenza are its epidemic nature and the mortality that may result from pulmonary complications, especially in older adults and children less than 2 years of age (Heymann, 2014).

There are three types of influenza viruses: A, B, and C. Type A is usually responsible for large epidemics, whereas outbreaks from type B are more regionalized; type C epidemics are sporadic, less common, and usually result in only mild illness. Influenza viruses often change in the nature of their surface appearance or their antigenic makeup. Types B and C are fairly stable viruses, but type A changes constantly. Minor antigenic changes are referred to as antigenic drift, and they result in yearly epidemics and regional outbreaks. Major changes such as the emergence of new subtypes are called antigenic shift; these occur only with type A viruses. Antigenic shift and drift lead to epidemic outbreaks every few years and pandemic outbreaks every 10 to 40 years as seen with novel influenza A H1N1 in 2009. Mortality rates associated with epidemics may or may not be higher than those in nonepidemic situations.

The preparation of influenza vaccine each year is based on the best possible prediction of what type and variant of virus will be most prevalent that year. Because of the changing nature of the virus, yearly immunization is necessary and in the United States is given in early fall before the flu season begins. In recent history, if vaccine were available, immunization for seasonal flu was particularly recommended for children ages 6 months up to 19 years, pregnant women, people 50 years of age and older, people of any age with certain chronic medical conditions, people who live in nursing homes and other long-term care facilities, and people who live with or care for those at risk for complications from flu. During the 2009-2010 influenza season, pandemic novel influenza A H1N1 replaced other seasonal flu viruses as the predominantly circulating virus, and the recommended priority groups shifted from seniors to the young; high school students and pregnant women seemed particularly hard hit, whereas those over 65 appeared to perhaps have some degree of protection. For the 2010-2011 flu season, novel influenza A H1N1 was included in the vaccine and the ACIP recommended universal coverage for everyone ages 6 months and older (CDC, 2010b).

Flu immunizations, when matched appropriately with circulating virus strains, are estimated to provide 70% to 90% protection against infection in healthy young adults; although they do not always prevent infection, they do result in milder disease symptoms. There are now a variety of vaccines available including one that is not grown in eggs for those with egg sensitivity and one that is administered nasally as a mist. Although influenza is often self-limiting in the healthy population, serious complications, particularly viral and bacterial pneumonias, can be deadly to older adults, children under 2 years of age, and those debilitated by chronic disease. When appropriate, it is important to couple influenza immunization of this population with immunization against pneumococcal pneumonia.

The use of influenza antiviral drugs should be considered in the nonimmunized or groups at high risk for complications. New evidence also suggests that antivirals can decrease the number of deaths in hospitalized influenza patients. The neuraminidase inhibitors (oseltamivir, zanamivir) have activity against influenza A and B viruses, whereas the adamantanes (amantadine, rimantadine) have activity only against influenza A viruses. Since January 2006, the neuraminidase inhibitors have been the only recommended influenza antiviral drugs because of widespread resistance to the adamantanes among influenza A (H3N2) virus strains. There have been incidences, worldwide and in the United States, of H1N1 virus resistance to oseltamivir. Current guidelines indicate antiviral treatment should be guided by surveillance data on circulating viruses and confirmatory testing of viral subgroups. CDC annually publishes Recommendations for Influenza Antiviral Medications (CDC, 2014g). (Read more about influenza at http://www.cdc.gov/flu/index.html.)

*Healthy People 2020* targets increasing the proportion of the population vaccinated annually against influenza and pneumococcal disease. Nurses often spearhead influenza immunization campaigns that target older adults. Examples include conducting flu clinics at polling places during elections or at community centers and churches during "senior vaccination Sundays." Inhabitants of residences and nursing homes for older adults are at risk, since influenza can spread rapidly with severe consequences through such living arrangements. As with children, nurses should check immunization history and encourage immunization for every older adult encountered in a clinic or home visit.

But while children, the elderly, and those with health conditions that put them at high risk for complications have traditionally been targets for immunizations, new strains of influenza such as H1N1 have more seriously affected young adults, leading to the recommendation that everyone over 6 months of age receive flu immunization. Nurses not only can promote this message, they can provide an example by choosing immunization as well. The CDC estimates that in the early flu season of 2013, 64% of health care providers were immunized against flu, and while this is higher than the general population (who were at closer to 40%), it is far from the *Healthy People 2020* goal of 90%. When nurses get immunized against influenza, they are protecting not only themselves but their patients (CDC, 2014h).

## Pandemic Novel Influenza A (H1N1)

Novel influenza A H1N1, a new flu virus that quickly reached pandemic proportions, was first recognized in Mexico and the United States in the spring of 2009. Originally called swine flu, the virus is of swine origins but does not spread from swine to people. Instead, it is transmitted rapidly and easily from person to person and in some cases is suspected to have spread from humans to swine as well as other animals such as dogs, cats, and ferrets. Because the virus was new, the population lacked immunity and visitors to Mexico quickly became infected and carried it to people around the globe. By June of 2009 more than 70 countries had reported cases of novel H1N1 infection, and ongoing community-level outbreaks of novel H1N1 occurred in multiple parts of the world, prompting the WHO to declare a global pandemic. This action was a reflection of the spread of the new H1N1 virus, not the severity of illness caused by the virus.

Although novel H1N1 appeared to spread in the same manner as seasonal influenza viruses, the groups most affected were children, young adults (especially those with underlying chronic disease), and pregnant women, as opposed to seniors who are the usual targets of seasonal flu but were thought in this case to perhaps have some degree of immunity. Initial reports made it appear that the virus inflicted a high case fatality rate, but as surveillance strengthened and expanded, this did not prove to be the case; however, by the end of the year, pediatric deaths were higher than in previous years and pediatric hospitalizations higher than other age groups. The majority of 2009 novel H1N1 deaths occurred in people between the ages of 50 and 64 years of age, 80% of whom have had an underlying health condition (CDC, 2010c).

With the identification of the virus, the scramble was on for a vaccine, which became available in the fall of 2009 in limited doses and was initially targeted to priority groups, including those 6 months to 24 years of age, caretakers, infants less than 6 months of age, pregnant women, adults 25 to 64 years of age with chronic conditions, health care providers, and first responders. Initial demand for vaccine was high, but since the

virus did not appear to prove overall any more frightening than seasonal flu and more vaccine came on the market, the available supply was more than enough for anyone who wished to be immunized. The delivery of the vaccine, in addition to seasonal flu vaccine, proved a planning and logistical challenge to the public health system, demanded considerable resources, and provided a valuable exercise in implementation of preparedness strategies. Nurses were at the forefront of this expansive operation by planning for, scheduling, and immunizing—in a variety of community settings, schools, and clinics—a large portion of the population, including two doses to children. During the summer of 2009, novel H1N1 outbreaks extended the normal flu season far beyond the usual period and dominated reported circulating flu viruses from the Southern Hemisphere as well. Activity peaked at the end of October in the United States, but novel H1N1 continued into 2010 as the dominant circulating strain. Resistance to antiviral neuraminidase inhibitors was reported but remained low, and the vast majority of 2009 H1N1 viruses tested did not appear to change significantly, remaining related to the A/California/7/2009 H1N1 reference virus selected by WHO as the 2009 H1N1 vaccine virus. An H1N1 component was included in the 2010 seasonal vaccine (CDC, 2010c). H1N1 returned as the predominant strain seen during the 2013-2014 flu season.

## Avian Influenza A (H5N1)

In 1997 in Hong Kong, the first known cases of human illness associated with an avian influenza type A virus H5N1 were reported. Referred to in the press as Hong Kong bird flu, this virus appeared to have been transmitted to people through contact with infected poultry. As a result of this association, Hong Kong officials ordered the slaughter of all chickens in and around Hong Kong with a resulting halt in the spread of disease. No cases were reported outside Hong Kong and, despite recurring outbreaks of avian flu in poultry, no further H5N1 virus activity in humans was reported (CDC, 1998). This situation changed dramatically in late 2003 and early 2004 when H5N1 outbreaks occurred among poultry, people, and, in some cases, other animals in nine Asian countries. And unlike the earlier situation in Hong Kong, these outbreaks have not disappeared but only subsided to again reappear. As of the beginning of 2014, human infections with H5N1 have been reported from 16 different countries with some fatality rates as high as 70%. The largest numbers have been reported from Indonesia (195), Egypt (173), and Vietnam (125). Canada has reported one case. To date, there have not been any reports of highly pathogenic avian influenza H5N1 virus infections among wild birds, poultry, or other animals or humans in the United States.

An unanswered question is whether there are actually many more human cases than are identified because symptoms are not severe enough to recognize. Most of the reported cases have resulted from contact with infected poultry, but it is believed that a few cases of human-to-human transmission have occurred. So far, the documented spread from human to human has been rare and not sustained, but because influenza viruses have the ability to change, concern exists among scientists that

H5N1 may modify to the point where people could easily infect each other; also, because H5N1 does not usually infect humans, they would have little immune protection. Such a change could give rise to pandemic influenza with a virus that appears to exact a high toll in human lives. Given this possibility, surveillance becomes of utmost importance and close attention is paid to H5N1 virus activity among poultry and humans in Asia, Europe, and North Africa. Vaccine development efforts are underway and, although licensed in some countries, are not yet generally available (CDC, 2014i).

# FOODBORNE AND WATERBORNE DISEASES

In recent years attention has focused on stories related to foodborne illness associated with peanut butter, cookie dough, spinach, lettuce, tomatoes, chili peppers, strawberries, raspberries, oysters, uncooked eggs, poultry and hamburger, raw milk, unpasteurized apple cider, and so forth. Cans of beef stew suspected to be contaminated with botulism have been pulled off grocery store shelves and the term *mad cow disease* has entered the popular vocabulary. Recalls of food products have become a common occurrence. Highly centralized food production and processing systems that use food produced in far-reaching areas and distribute it through widespread distribution networks increase the potential for any contamination to result in large-scale, multistate outbreaks. One incident of contamination may affect hundreds of people across the country and result in numerous deaths. Anyone can acquire foodborne illness, regardless of socioeconomic status, race, sex, age, occupation, education or area of residence, but the very young, old, and debilitated are most susceptible and bear the highest burden of morbidity and mortality.

In 2010, the CDC developed new lower than previously estimated but more precise estimates for foodborne illness suggesting that in the United States, as many as 1 in 6 Americans (or 48 million people) gets sick, 128,000 are hospitalized, and 3,000 die from foodborne illnesses each year, most the result of unidentified agents (CDC, 2010d). Known pathogens cause an estimated 9.4 million foodborne illnesses annually in the United States (Scallan et al, 2011). Because their presentations are often not clinically distinctive and frequently self-limiting, single cases of foodborne illness may be difficult to identify. Affected individuals in single cases or in outbreak situations may not see a physician or are treated presumptively and not tested. In either case, the illness goes unreported, resulting in statistics that underestimate the true magnitude of the problem.

FoodNet is a CDC sentinel surveillance system targeting 10 sites across the country and collecting information from laboratories on disease caused by enteric pathogens transmitted commonly through food. It is a collaborative effort among CDC, the U.S. Department of Agriculture (USDA), and the FDA. In 2011 FoodNet reported 18,964 laboratory-diagnosed cases of infection, the majority caused by *Salmonella, Campylobacter,* and *Shigella* (CDC, 2012c).

Confirmed foodborne outbreaks are reported by states to the CDC through the Foodborne Disease Outbreak Surveillance System. During 2009-2010, a total of 1,527 foodborne disease outbreaks were reported from all 50 states, Puerto Rico, and the District of Columbia. These outbreaks resulted in 29,444 cases of illness, 1,184 hospitalizations, and 23 deaths. Among the 790 outbreaks with a single laboratory-confirmed etiologic agent, norovirus was the most commonly reported, accounting for 42% of outbreaks, and *Salmonella* was second, accounting for 30% of outbreaks. Of the 653 outbreaks where a food source was identified, 299 were determined to originate from only one ingredient with the most outbreaks attributed to beef, fish, dairy, and poultry. The most illnesses were associated with eggs, followed by beef and poultry. Of organisms paired with food sources, the most outbreaks were from *Campylobacter* in unpasteurized dairy, *Salmonella* in eggs, STEC O157 in beef, ciguatoxin in fish, and scombroid toxin (histamine fish poisoning) in fish, and the most outbreak-related illnesses by far resulted from *Salmonella* in eggs (2,231 illnesses) followed by *Salmonella* in sprouts (493) and *Salmonella* in vine-stalk vegetables such as tomatoes (422). The combinations responsible for the most hospitalizations were *Salmonella* in vine-stalk vegetables, STEC O157 in beef, and *Salmonella* in sprouts; those that caused the most deaths were STEC O157 in beef (three deaths), *Salmonella* in pork, and *Listeria* in dairy (two each). Thirty-eight multistate outbreaks were reported; twenty-one were caused by *Salmonella* (CDC, 2013e). (Learn more about the Foodborne Disease Outbreak Surveillance System at http://www.cdc.gov/foodborne burden/surveillance-systems.html.)

The ability to identify multistate outbreaks has been greatly enhanced through technology now routinely used in public health laboratories (serotyping and pulsed-field gel electrophoresis) and the rapid sharing of this information among public health officials through PulseNet, the national molecular subtyping network for foodborne disease surveillance. Since 1996, this DNA fingerprinting has allowed the detection of thousands of individual and multistate outbreaks including people sickened from eating *Salmonella* contaminated peanut butter, tomatoes and cantaloupes, *E. coli* in leafy vegetables, and *Vibrio parahaemolyticus* in oysters. (Learn more about PulseNet at http://www.cdc.gov/pulsenet/index.html.)

The CDC recommends three goals in achieving food safety: (1) control or eliminate pathogens in domestic and imported food, (2) reduce or prevent contamination during growing, harvesting, and processing, and (3) continue the education of restaurant workers and consumers about risks and prevention measures. Also noted is the need for continued efforts to understand how contamination of fresh produce and processed foods occurs and to develop and implement measures that reduce it.

Foodborne illness, or "food poisoning," as it is erroneously but commonly called, is often categorized as either food infection or food intoxication. Food infection results from bacterial, viral, or parasitic infection of food by pathogens such as *Salmonella, Campylobacter,* hepatitis A, *Toxoplasma,* and *Trichinella.* Food intoxication is caused by toxins produced by bacterial growth, chemical contaminants (heavy metals), and a variety of disease-producing substances found naturally in certain foods such as mushrooms and some seafood. Examples of food intoxications are botulism, mercury poisoning, and paralytic

## TABLE 13-4 Commonly Encountered Food Intoxications

| Causal Agent | Incubation Period | Duration | Clinical Presentation | Associated Food |
|---|---|---|---|---|
| Staphylococcus aureus | 30 min to 7 hr | 1-2 days | Sudden onset of nausea, cramps, vomiting, and prostration, often accompanied by diarrhea; rarely fatal | All foods, especially those likely to come into contact with food-handlers' hands that may be contaminated from infections of the eyes and skin |
| Clostridium perfringens (strain A) | 6-24 hr | 1 day or less | Sudden onset of colic and diarrhea, maybe nausea; vomiting and fever unusual; rarely fatal | Inadequately heated meats or stews; food contaminated by soil or feces becomes infective when improper storage or reheating allows multiplication of organism |
| Vibrio parahaemolyticus | 4-96 hr | 1-7 days | Watery diarrhea and abdominal cramps; sometimes nausea, vomiting, fever, headache; rarely fatal | Raw or inadequately cooked seafood; period of time at room temperature usually required for multiplication of organism |
| Clostridium botulinum | 12-36 hr, sometimes days | Slow recovery, maybe months | Central nervous system signs; blurred vision, difficulty in swallowing and dry mouth, followed by descending symmetrical flaccid paralysis in an alert person; "floppy baby" in infant; fatality <15% with antitoxin and respiratory support | Home-canned fruits and vegetables that have not been preserved with adequate heating; infants have become infected from ingesting honey |

Based on information from Heymann DL, editor: *Control of communicable diseases manual,* ed 20, Washington, DC, 2014, American Public Health Association.

shellfish poisoning. Table 13-4 presents some of the most common agents of food intoxication and their incubation period, source, symptoms, and pathology. Although it is not a hard-and-fast rule, food infections are associated with incubation periods of 12 hours to several days after ingestion of the infected food, whereas intoxications become obvious within minutes to hours after ingestion. Botulism is a clear exception to this rule, with an incubation period up to several days or more in adults. Possessing a potent preformed toxin, capable of producing severe intoxication resulting in flaccid paralysis and death if not identified and treated early, *C. botulinum* is one of the organisms considered a strong candidate for a weapon of bioterrorism (Heymann, 2014).

### The Role of Safe Food Preparation

Protecting the nation's food supply from contamination by virulent microbes is a multifaceted issue that is and will continue to be incredibly costly, controversial, and time-consuming to address. The specter of terrorist threats to the food supply adds an additional layer of complexity. However, much foodborne illness, regardless of causal organism, can easily be prevented through simple changes in food preparation, handling, and storage. Common errors include (1) cross-contamination of food during preparation, (2) insufficient cooking or reheating temperatures, (3) holding cooked food or storing food at temperatures that promote growth of pathogens and/or formation of toxins, and (4) poor personal hygiene. Because these measures are so important in preventing foodborne disease, *Healthy People 2020* has continued to include an objective directed toward them. WHO estimates that 2.2 million people, 1.9 million of them children, die annually from foodborne and waterborne diarrheal diseases in less-developed countries. In 2001 WHO released a new campaign entitled *Five Keys to Safer Food,* which reduces the former *Ten Golden Rules for Food*

### BOX 13-4   WHO Five Keys to Safer Food

1. Keep food clean.
2. Separate raw and cooked food.
3. Cook thoroughly.
4. Keep food at safe temperatures.
5. Use safe water and raw materials.

From the World Health Organization: *Five Keys to Safer Food campaign.* 2009b, WHO. Available at http://www.who.int/foodsafety/consumer/5keys/en. Accessed March 25, 2010; Heymann DL, editor: *Control of communicable diseases manual,* ed 19. Washington, DC, 2008, American Public Health Association.

*Preparation* developed in the early 1990s to five even simpler and easier to remember principles (presented in Box 13-4). A poster explaining the *Five Keys* is available in 25 languages and is accompanied by a training manual titled *Bring Food Safety Home* (Heymann, 2014). (Read more about the Five Keys at the WHO website: http://www.who.int/foodsafety/consumer/5keys/en/index.html.)

### Salmonellosis

Salmonellosis is a bacterial disease characterized by sudden onset of headache, abdominal pain, diarrhea, nausea, sometimes vomiting, and almost always fever. Onset is typically within 48 hours of ingestion, but the clinical signs are impossible to distinguish from other causes of gastrointestinal distress. Diarrhea and lack of appetite may persist for several days, and dehydration may be severe. Although morbidity can be significant, death is uncommon except among infants, older adults, and the debilitated. The rate of infection is highest among infants and small children. It is estimated that only a small proportion of cases are recognized clinically and that only 1% of clinical cases are reported. The number of

*Salmonella* infections yearly may actually be in the millions (Heymann, 2014).

Outbreaks occur commonly in restaurants, hospitals, nursing homes, and institutions for children. The transmission route is eating food derived from an infected animal or contaminated by feces of an infected animal or person. Unchlorinated municipal water supplies have also been implicated in *Salmonella* outbreaks. Raw or undercooked meat and meat products, raw or undercooked poultry, uncooked eggs, unpasteurized milk and dairy products, and contaminated produce are the foods most often associated with salmonellosis. Recent large outbreaks have been linked with eating tomatoes, jalapeño peppers, and peanut butter. Meat and poultry may be contaminated during preparation or cross-contaminate food being prepared with them. Improper food preparation temperatures (cooking and holding) and cross-contamination appear to be the biggest risk factors for food-associated outbreaks. Animals are the common reservoir for the various *Salmonella* serotypes, although infected humans may also fill this role. Animals are more likely to be chronic carriers. Reptiles such as iguanas have been implicated as *Salmonella* carriers along with pet turtles, poultry, cattle, swine, rodents, dogs, and cats. People have also been infected by handling *Salmonella*-contaminated dry dog food and treats. Person-to-person transmission is an important consideration in daycare and institutional settings (Heymann, 2014).

### Enterohemorrhagic *Escherichia coli* (EHEC or *E. coli* 0157:H7)

*Escherichia coli* 0157:H7 belongs to the enterohemorrhagic category of *E. coli* serotypes producing a strong cytotoxin called a Shiga toxin and are collectively known as Shiga toxin–producing *E. coli* (STEC). *E. coli* serotypes in this group can cause a potentially fatal hemorrhagic colitis. This pathogen was first widely described in humans in 1992 following the investigation of two outbreaks of illness associated with consumption of hamburger from a fast-food restaurant chain. Transmission is through ingestion of food contaminated by infected feces. Ruminants, particularly cattle, are the most important reservoir, although humans may also serve as a source for person-to-person transmission. Undercooked hamburger has been implicated in several outbreaks, as have roast beef, alfalfa sprouts, melons, lettuce, uncooked spinach, unpasteurized milk and apple cider, municipal water, and person-to-person transmission in daycare centers, homes, and institutions. Recent large outbreaks have been associated with uncooked spinach and petting zoos. Infection with *E. coli* 0157:H7 causes bloody diarrhea, abdominal cramps, and, infrequently, fever. Children and older adults are at highest risk for clinical disease and complications. Hemolytic uremic syndrome (HUS) is seen in approximately 15% of cases among children and a smaller number of adults and may result in acute renal failure. The case fatality rate for infection that results in HUS can be as great as 5% (Heymann, 2014).

Hamburger often appears to be involved in outbreaks because the grinding process exposes pathogens on the surface of the whole meat to the interior of the ground meat, effectively mixing the once-exterior bacteria thoroughly throughout the hamburger so that searing the surface no longer suffices to kill

all bacteria. Tracking the contamination is complicated by the fact that hamburger is often made of meat ground from several sources. The best protection against this pathogen, as with most foodborne agents, is to thoroughly cook food before eating it.

### WATERBORNE DISEASE OUTBREAKS AND PATHOGENS

Waterborne pathogens usually enter water supplies through animal or human fecal contamination and frequently cause enteric disease. They include viruses, bacteria, and protozoans. Hepatitis A virus is probably the most publicized waterborne viral agent, although other viruses may also be transmitted by this route (enteroviruses, rotaviruses, and paramyxoviruses). The most important waterborne bacterial diseases are cholera, typhoid fever, and bacillary dysentery. However, other *Salmonella* spp. as well as *Shigella, Vibrio,* and *Campylobacter* species and various coliform bacteria including *E. coli* 0157:H7 may be transmitted in the same manner. Recently, since added to surveillance in 2001, *Legionella* spp. have frequently been implicated in waterborne disease outbreaks (WBDOs) in the United States. In the past, the most important waterborne protozoans have been *Entamoeba histolytica* (amebic dysentery) and *Giardia lamblia,* but major outbreaks of cryptosporidiosis in municipal water, as seen in the diarrheal outbreak that crippled the city of Milwaukee in 1993, have pushed *Cryptosporidium* into the debate over how to best safeguard municipal water supplies. Protozoans do not respond to traditional chlorine treatment as do enteric and coliform bacteria, and their small size requires special filtration.

The CDC defines a WBDO as an incident in which two or more persons experience similar illness after consuming water that epidemiologic evidence implicates as the source of that illness. Recreational water and other water not intended for drinking as well as drinking water may be involved in waterborne outbreaks. Facilities with inadequate chlorination and pools allowing diapered children pose particular risk for infection, as does drinking water without adequate disinfection while hiking and camping in the backcountry.

Since 1971, the CDC, the U.S. Environmental Protection Agency (EPA), and the Council of State and Territorial Epidemiologists have maintained a collaborative Waterborne Disease and Outbreaks Surveillance System for collecting and reporting data related to occurrences and causes of waterborne disease and outbreaks. This surveillance system is the primary source of data concerning the scope and effects of WBDOs in the United States. The CDC and the EPA, to improve timeliness and completeness of reporting, are collaborating with public health jurisdictions to implement electronic reporting through the National Outbreak Reporting System (NORS) (CDC, 2013f).

### VECTORBORNE DISEASES

Vectorborne diseases refer to illnesses for which the infectious agent is transmitted by a carrier, or vector, which is usually an arthropod (mosquito, tick, fly), either biologically or mechanically. With biological transmission, the vector is necessary for the developmental stage of the infectious agent. Examples include the mosquitoes that carry WNV and the fleas that transmit plague. Mechanical transmission occurs when an insect simply contacts the infectious agent with its legs or mouth parts and carries it to the host. For example, flies and cockroaches may contaminate food or cooking utensils. Most vector borne diseases involve zoonotic cycles requiring some sort of animal host or reservoir.

Vectorborne diseases commonly encountered in the United States are those associated with ticks, such as Lyme disease (*Borrelia burgdorferi*), Rocky Mountain spotted fever (*Rickettsia rickettsii*), ehrlichiosis (*Ehrlichiae*), and anaplasmosis (*Anaplasma phagocytophilum*), formerly known as human granulocytic ehrlichiosis. Nurses who work with large immigrant populations or with international travelers may encounter malaria and dengue fever, both carried by mosquitoes. More recently in the news, WNV is an example of endemic mosquito-borne viruses that include St. Louis, LaCrosse, and western and eastern equine encephalitis. Plague (*Y. pestis*) is carried by fleas of wild rodents. Other more rarely seen tick-associated diseases include babesiosis (*Babesia microti*), tularemia (*F. tularensis*), and Q fever (*Coxiella burnetii*). Southern tick-associated rash illness (STARI) is a newly described illness for which the causative organism has not been determined. STARI resembles Lyme disease in appearance but does not result in the neurologic, arthritic, and other chronic conditions seen with Lyme disease. It is mainly found in the southeast and is associated with the bite of the Lonestar tick (*Amblyomma americanum*) (CDC, 2011b) and ticks (CDC, 2014j).

## Lyme Disease

Parents in Lyme, CT, concerned about the unusual incidence of juvenile rheumatoid arthritis in their children, were the first to bring attention to this tick borne infection that now bears their town's name. First described in 1975, Lyme disease became a nationally notifiable disease in 1991 and is now the most common vector borne disease in the United States, with over 30,000 confirmed cases and probable cases reported to CDC in 2012. However, new studies suggest that the actual number of diagnosed cases may be as many as 10 times that number, making Lyme disease a major public health problem and with an urgent need for improved prevention (Kuehn, 2013). The causative agent, the spirochete *B. burgdorferi,* was identified in 1982. Lyme disease is transmitted by ixodid ticks that are associated with white-tailed deer (*Odocoileus virginianus*) and the white-footed mouse (*Peromyscus leucopus*). Lyme disease usually occurs in summer during tick season and it has been reported throughout the United States, with 95% of cases concentrated in rural and suburban areas of the northeast, mid-Atlantic and north-central states, particularly Wisconsin and Minnesota.

The clinical spectrum of Lyme disease can be divided into three stages. Stage I is characterized by erythema chronicum-migrans, a distinctive skin lesion often called a bull's-eye lesion because it begins as a red area at the site of the tick attachment that spreads outward in a ring-like fashion as the center clears. About 50% to 70% of infected persons develop this lesion 3 to 30 days after a tick bite. The skin lesion may be accompanied

or preceded by fever, fatigue, malaise, headache, muscle pains, and a stiff neck, as well as tender and enlarged lymph nodes and migratory joint pain. Most clients diagnosed in this early stage respond well to 10 to 14 days of oral tetracycline or penicillin.

If not treated during this first stage, Lyme disease can progress to stage II, which may include additional skin lesions, headache, and neurologic and cardiac abnormalities. Clients who progress to stage III have recurrent attacks of arthritis and arthralgia, especially in the knees, which may begin months to years after the initial lesion. The clinical diagnosis of classic Lyme disease with the distinctive skin lesion is straightforward. Illness without the lesion is more difficult to diagnose, because serologic tests are more accurate in stages II and III than in stage I (Heymann, 2014).

## Rocky Mountain Spotted Fever

Contrary to its name, Rocky Mountain spotted fever (RMSF) is seldom seen in the Rocky Mountains and most commonly occurs in the southeast, Oklahoma, Kansas, and Missouri. The infectious agent is *R. rickettsii.* The tick vector varies according to geographic region. The dog tick, *Dermacentor variabilis,* is the vector in the eastern and southern United States. RMSF is not transmitted from person to person. It is thought that one attack confers lifelong immunity.

Clinical signs include sudden onset of moderate to high fever, severe headache, chills, deep muscle pain, and malaise. About 50% of cases experience a rash on the extremities that spreads to most of the body. Many cases of what has been referred to as "spotless" RMSF may actually be caused by recently identified forms of human ehrlichiosis, another tick-borne infection. RMSF responds readily to treatment with tetracycline. Definitive diagnosis can be made with paired serum titers. Because early treatment is important in decreasing morbidity and mortality, treatment should be started in response to clinical and epidemiologic considerations rather than waiting for laboratory confirmation (Heymann, 2014).

## Prevention and Control of Tickborne Diseases

In *Healthy People 2020,* the *HP2010* objective for reducing Lyme disease has been archived because of lack of proven interventions to prevent transmission. A vaccine for Lyme disease, recommended for use by persons living in high-risk areas, was licensed in 1998; however, in 2002 the manufacturer withdrew it from the commercial market because of low demand and sales. Measures for preventing exposure to ticks include reducing tick populations, avoiding tick-infested areas, wearing protective clothing when outdoors (long sleeves and long pants tucked into socks), using repellants, and immediately inspecting for and removing ticks when returning indoors. The CDC reports that landscaping modifications such as removing brush and leaf litter or creating a buffer zone of wood chips or gravel between yard and forest may reduce exposure to ticks as well as appropriate pesticide application to lawns. Ticks require a prolonged period of attachment (6 to 48 hours) before they start blood-feeding on the host; prompt tick discovery and removal can help prevent transmission of disease. Ticks should be removed with steady, gentle traction on tweezers applied to the head parts of the tick. The tick's body should not be squeezed during the removal process to avoid infection that could be transmitted from resultant tick feces and tissue juices (Heymann, 2014). When outdoors, permethrin sprayed on clothing and tick repellents on bare skin containing 20% to 30% diethyltoluamide (DEET) can offer effective protection; use of DEET should be avoided on children less than 2 years of age because of reports of significant toxicity, including skin irritation, anaphylaxis, and seizures. Read more about tick-associated diseases at the CDC website (http://www.cdc.gov/ticks/index.html) and the prevention of tick-associated diseases on the Lyme Disease Resources CDC website, which includes handouts that can be ordered and the Handbook on Tick Management produced by the state of Connecticut (http://www.cdc.gov/ncidod/dvbid/Lyme/ld_resources.htm) (CDC, 2014j).

## DISEASES OF TRAVELERS

Individuals traveling outside the United States need to be aware of and take precautions against potential diseases to which they may be exposed. Which diseases and what precautions to take depend on the individual's health status, the destination, the reason for travel, and the length of travel. Persons who plan to travel in remote regions for an extended period may need to consider rare diseases and take special precautions that would not apply to the average traveler. Consultation with public health officials can provide specific health information and recommendations for a given situation. Nurses often staff public health travel clinics and provide this information based on CDC recommendations. The CDC offers information for both medical professionals and travelers at their Travelers' Health webpage including the Yellow Book, *CDC Health Information for International Travel,* which in addition to being available online, can be ordered in hardcopy or accessed from mobile devices. (To read more about Travelers' Health and the Yellow Book, see http://wwwnc.cdc.gov/travel/page/yellowbook-home -2014.)

On return from visiting exotic places, travelers may bring back with them an unplanned souvenir in the form of disease. Therefore, in a presenting client, it is important to ask about a history of travel. Even the apparently healthy returned traveler, especially one who was in a tropical country for some time, should undergo routine screening to rule out acquired infections. Likewise, refugees and immigrants may arrive with infectious disease problems ranging from helminthic infections to diseases of major public health significance, such as TB, malaria, cholera, HIV disease, and hepatitis. Nurses may find themselves dealing with these diseases, since refugees and immigrants, especially the undocumented, are often treated through the public health system.

### Malaria

Caused by the bloodborne parasite *Plasmodium,* malaria is a potentially fatal disease characterized by regular cycles of fever and chills. Transmission is through the bite of an infected *Anopheles* mosquito. The word *malaria* is based on an association between the illness and the "bad air" of the marshes where

the mosquitoes breed. Malaria is an old disease that appears in recorded history in 2700 BC China. Although no longer endemic in most temperate countries, malaria is the most prevalent vector borne disease worldwide, occurring in over 100 countries and territories. Half of the world's population is considered at risk; 90% of cases occur in Africa. Malaria is the fifth-leading cause of infectious disease death worldwide and the second-leading cause of infectious disease death (after HIV disease) in Africa. There is no vaccine available to protect against this disease, which in 2012 resulted in an estimated 207 million cases and 627,000 deaths, most in the Africa Region. The WHO reports malaria mortality rates have fallen by 42% globally since 2000, and by 49% in the WHO African Region. This move in a positive direction is attributed to international funding for bed net campaigns and increased access to treatment (WHO, 2014c).

Malaria prevention depends on protection against mosquitoes and appropriate chemoprophylaxis. Drug resistance is an increasing problem in combating malaria. Of the four *Plasmodium* species causing human malaria, *P. ovale* and *P. vivax* result in disease that can progress to relapsing malaria and *P. vivax* is increasingly drug resistant. *P. falciparum* causes the most serious malarial infection and is highly drug resistant. Thus decisions about antimalarial drugs must be tailored individually on the basis of the type of malaria in the specific area of the country to be visited, the purpose of the trip, and the length of the visit. The CDC and the WHO publish guides on the status of malaria and recommendations for prophylaxis on a country-by-country basis. At this time, there is no one drug or drug combination known to be safe and efficacious in preventing all types of malaria. Antimalarials are generally started a week to several weeks before leaving the country and are continued for 4 to 6 weeks after returning.

Despite appropriate prophylaxis, malaria may still be contracted. Travelers should be advised of this fact and urged to seek immediate medical care if they exhibit symptoms of cyclical fever and chills up to 1 year after returning home. Immigrants and visitors from areas where malaria is endemic may become clinically ill after entering the United States. Approximately 1500 cases of malaria in travelers and immigrants are reported in the United States every year. Also, although malaria is eliminated from the United States, the mosquito vectors are not, so local cases still can occur if these vector mosquitoes bite people infected outside the country. From 1957 to 2011, 63 outbreaks of locally transmitted mosquito-borne malaria have been reported in the United States. In these outbreaks, local mosquitoes become infected by biting persons carrying malaria parasites (acquired in endemic areas) and then transmit malaria to local residents. From 1963 to 2011, 97 individuals have acquired malaria through blood transfusions (CDC, 2014k). (For more information about malaria in the United States as well as worldwide, visit the malaria homepage at the CDC website: http://www.cdc.gov/malaria/.)

### Foodborne and Waterborne Diseases

As in the United States, much foodborne disease abroad can be avoided if the traveler eats thoroughly cooked foods prepared with reasonable hygiene; eating foods from street vendors may not be a good idea. Trichinosis, tapeworms, and fluke infections, as well as bacterial infections, result from eating raw or under-cooked meats. Raw vegetables may act as a source of bacterial, viral, helminthic, or protozoal infection if they have been grown with or washed in contaminated water. Fruits that can be peeled immediately before eating, such as bananas, are less likely to be a source of infection. Dairy products should be pasteurized and appropriately refrigerated.

Water in many areas of the world is not potable (safe to drink), and drinking this water can lead to infection with a variety of protozoal, viral, and bacterial agents including amoebae, *Giardia, Cryptosporidium,* hepatitis, cholera, and various coliform bacteria. Unless traveling in an area where the piped water is known to be safe, only boiled water (boiled for 1 minute), bottled water, or water purified with iodine or chlorine compounds should be consumed (CDC, 2013g). Ice should be avoided because freezing does not inactivate these agents. If the water is questionable, choose coffee or tea made with boiled water, carbonated beverages without ice, beer, wine, or canned fruit juices.

## Diarrheal Diseases

Travelers often suffer from diarrhea, so much so that colorful names, such as Montezuma's revenge, turista, and Colorado quickstep, exist in our vocabulary to describe these bouts of intestinal upset. Some of these diarrheas do not have infectious causes; they result from stress, fatigue, schedule changes, and eating unfamiliar foods. Acute infectious diarrheas are usually of viral or bacterial origin. *E. coli* probably causes more cases of traveler's diarrhea than all other infective agents combined. Protozoan-induced diarrheas such as those resulting from *Entamoeba* and *Giardia* are less likely to be acute, and they more commonly present once the traveler returns home. Travelers need to pay special attention to what they eat and drink. (Read more about travelers' health at the CDC website: http://www.cdc.gov/travel/.)

## ZOONOSES

A zoonosis is an infection transmitted from a vertebrate animal to a human under natural conditions. The agents that cause zoonoses do not need humans to maintain their life cycles; infected humans have simply managed somehow to get in their way. Means of transmission include animal bites (bats and rabies), inhalation (rodent excrement and hantavirus), ingestion (milk and listeriosis), direct contact (rabbit carcasses and tularemia), and arthropod intermediates. This last transmission route means that many vector borne diseases are also zoonoses. For example, white-tailed deer harbor ticks that can carry Lyme disease, and rats and ground squirrels may be infested with fleas capable of transmitting plague. Other than vector borne diseases, some of the more common zoonoses in the United States include toxoplasmosis (*Toxoplasma gondii*), cat-scratch disease (*Bartonella henselae*), brucellosis (*Brucella* species), leptospirosis (*Leptospira interrogans*), listeriosis (*Listeria monocytogenes*), salmonellosis (*Salmonella* serotypes), and

rabies (family Rhabdoviridae, genus *Lyssavirus*). Many of the emerging infectious diseases such as avian influenza A H5N1, WNV, monkey pox, hantavirus pulmonary syndrome, and variant Creutzfeldt-Jakob disease are examples of zoonoses. Also, among the diseases considered best candidates for weapons of bioterrorism, anthrax, plague, tularemia, and some of the hemorrhagic fever viruses (e.g., Lassa) are all zoonoses. The CDC estimates that 75% of recently emerging infectious diseases affecting humans are diseases of animal origin and that approximately 60% of all human pathogens are zoonotic.

## Rabies (Hydrophobia)

One of the most feared of human diseases, rabies has the highest case fatality rate of any known human infection, essentially 100%. Despite the availability of intensive medical care, only six individuals have been known to recover after the onset of rabies, three in the United States, and only one survivor who did not receive pre-exposure or postexposure prophylaxis (PEP) has been reported (CDC, 2012d). A significant public health problem worldwide with as many as 50,000 deaths a year, mostly in developing countries, rabies in humans in the United States is a rare event because of the widespread vaccination of dogs begun in the 1950s. Today, the major carriers of rabies in the United States are not dogs but wild animals—raccoons, skunks, foxes, coyotes, and bats. Small rodents, rabbits and hares, and opossums rarely carry rabies. Epidemiologic information should be consulted for information on the potential carriers for a given geographic region. When the virus spreads from wild to domestic animals, cats are often involved. Of the 31 human cases of rabies reported in the United States from 2003 through June 2013, 36% were acquired outside the continental United States. Domestically acquired cases were largely associated with insectivorous bats (85%) and raccoons (15%). However, five of these domestic cases occurred not through direct contact but as the result of organ transplant. Cases contracted outside the United States most commonly resulted from the bites of infected dogs (82%), with one fox and one bat exposure (Dyer et al, 2013). Rabies is transmitted to humans by introducing virus-carrying saliva into the body, usually via an animal bite or scratch. Transmission may also occur if infected saliva comes into contact with a fresh cut or intact mucous membranes. Rabies is found in neural tissue and is not transmitted via blood, urine, or feces. Airborne transmission has been documented in caves with infected bat colonies. Transmission from human to human is theoretically possible but has not been documented except through transplant organs harvested from individuals who died of undiagnosed rabies. Guidelines for organ donation exist to minimize this possibility (Heymann, 2014).

The best protection against rabies remains vaccinating domestic animals—dogs, cats, cattle, and horses. If a person is bitten, the bite wound should be thoroughly cleaned with soap and water and a physician consulted immediately. Be suspicious of bites from a wild animal or an unprovoked attack from a domestic animal. Even when there is no suspicion of rabies, contact a physician because tetanus or antibiotic prophylaxis may be needed. An estimated 23,000 people per year require

PEP after being in contact with potentially rabid animals (Christian et al, 2009).

No successful treatment exists for rabies once symptoms appear, but if given promptly and as directed, PEP with human rabies immunoglobulin (RIG) and rabies vaccine can prevent the development of the disease. Three products are licensed for use as rabies vaccine in the United States: human diploid cell vaccine (HDCV), purified chick embryo cell culture vaccine (PCECV), and rabies vaccine adsorbed (RVA); only HDCV and PCECV are available for use in the United States (CDC, 2008a). In 2010, the previously recommended series of five 1-mL doses of vaccine injected into the deltoid muscle was changed to four (CDC, 2010e). Reactions to the vaccine are fewer and less serious than with previously used vaccines. Individuals who deal frequently with animals, such as zookeepers, laboratory workers, and veterinarians, may choose to receive the vaccine as pre-exposure prophylaxis. The decision to administer the vaccine to a bite victim depends on the circumstances of the bite and is made on an individual basis.

The Compendium of Animal Rabies Prevention and Control compiled by the National Association of State Public Health Veterinarians, Inc. gives recommendations for prevention of and vaccination for rabies in animals. Recommendations for administering PEP are provided by the Advisory Committee for Recommendations on Immunization Practices and are available through local public health officials or the CDC. In general, cats and dogs that have bitten someone and have verified rabies vaccinations are confined for 10 days for observation. Treatment is initiated only if signs of rabies are observed during this period. If the animal is known or suspected to be rabid, treatment begins immediately. If the animal is unknown to the victim and escapes, public health officials should be consulted for help in deciding whether treatment is indicated. With wild animal bites, treatment is begun immediately. With bites from livestock, rodents, and rabbits, treatment is considered on an individual basis. Decisions to treat become more complicated for possible nonbite exposure to saliva from known infected animals, and again public health officials are helpful in making these treatment decisions (CDC, 2011c).

## PARASITIC DISEASES

Parasites are organisms that depend on a host to survive. Endoparasites, those that live within the body, are classified into four major groups: nematodes (roundworms), cestodes (tapeworms), trematodes (flukes), and protozoa (single-celled animals). Nematodes, cestodes, and trematodes are all referred to as helminths along with acanthocephalins or thorny-headed worms, which are not as commonly involved in human infections. Table 13-5 presents examples of relatively common diseases caused by parasites from these groups. Parasites that remain on the surface of a host's body to feed rather than within it such as ticks, fleas, lice, and mites that attach or burrow into the skin are called *ectoparasites*. Many parasitic infections are vector borne and/or zoonotic.

Parasitic diseases are more prevalent in rural areas of low-income countries than in the United States. Contributing

**TABLE 13-5    Examples of Diseases Resulting from Endoparasitic Infection by Category**

| Category | Parasite | Disease |
|---|---|---|
| Cestodes | *Taeniasaginata, Taeniasolium* | Beef tapeworm, pork tapeworm |
| Nematodes | *Ancylostoma, Necator* | Ancylostomiasis, necatoriasis (hookworm) |
| Intestinal | *Ascaris, Toxocara* | Ascariasis, toxocariasis (roundworm) |
|  | *Enterobius vermicularis* | Enterobiasis (pinworm) |
|  | *Trichuris trichiura* | Trichuriasis (whipworm) |
| Blood/Tissue | *Drancunculiasis medinensis* | Guinea worm |
|  | *Onchocerca volvulus* | Onchoserciasis (river blindness) |
|  | *Wuchereria bancrofti* | Lymphatic filariasis (elephantiasis) |
| Trematodes | *Schistosoma* sp. | Schistosomiasis (snail fever) |
| Protozoans | *Entamoeba histolytica* | Amebiasis |
|  | *Giardia lamblia* | Giardiasis |
|  | *Leishmania* spp. | Leishmaniasis |
|  | *Plasmodium* spp. | Malaria |
|  | *Toxoplasma gondii* | Toxoplasmosis |
|  | *Trichomonas vaginalis* | Trichomoniasis |
|  | *Trypanosoma* spp. | African sleeping sickness, Chagas' disease |

Based on information from Heymann DL, editor: *Control of communicable diseases manual,* ed 20, Washington, DC, 2014, American Public Health Association.

factors are tropical climate and inadequate prevention and control measures. Poor sanitation, a lack of cheap and effective drugs, and a scarcity of funding lead to high reinfection rates even when control programs are attempted. Parasitic organisms result in a wide spectrum of diseases including leading causes of death and disability in Africa, Asia, Central America, and South America. Examples include malaria, guinea worm disease, river blindness (onchocerciasis), leishmaniasis, amoebiasis, African sleeping sickness, Chagas' disease, schistosomiasis, and lymphatic filariasis. These parasitic diseases not only cause major mortality in endemic regions but also tremendous morbidity. Debilitation from infection may result in an inability to attend school or work as well as growth retardation, developmental disabilities, and cognitive impairment in young children, all of which contribute to significant economic burden for the countries affected.

Parasitic infections also affect persons living in developed countries. In the United States parasitic organisms frequently cause foodborne and waterborne diarrheal illness (*Giardia, Entamoeba, Cryptosporidia*) and sexually transmitted infections (*Trichomonas*), and they pose a particular problem for immunodeficient individuals (*Cryptosporidia, Toxoplasma, Cyclospora*). Trichomoniasis is a common, easily treated with antibiotics, sexually transmitted disease caused by the protozoan parasite *Trichomonas vaginalis*. An estimated 3.7 million people are estimated to be infected but only 30% may show symptoms (CDC, 2012e). *Giardiasis* is a diarrheal illness caused by the parasite *Giardia intestinalis*. It is the most common intestinal parasitic infection in the United States and results in 19,000 to 20,000 reported cases annually (CDC, 2012f). Cryptosporidiosis is also a diarrheal disease caused by the microscopic parasite *Cryptosporidium*. Because *Cryptosporidium* possesses an outer shell that allows it to survive outside the body for extended periods of time and tolerate low levels of chlorine disinfection, it is a frequent cause of water-related disease outbreaks in swimming pools and splash parks. In the United States "crypto" is a common cause of both foodborne and waterborne disease resulting in an estimated 740,000 cases each year (Scallan et al, 2011).

New technology for recognizing protozoan parasites, the ease of international travel, immigration from developing countries, and diseases that affect the immune system such as HIV disease (thus leaving individuals susceptible to secondary parasitic infections) all contribute to rising reports of and a greater attention to parasitic diseases in the United States. The CDC speaks about the major neglected diseases of poverty in the United States, which it defines as diseases that disproportionately affect people in poverty, infect a significant number of people, and receive limited attention in tracking, prevention, and treatment. Five of the six are parasitic: Chagas' disease, cysticercosis, toxocariasis, toxoplasmosis, and trichomoniasis. To ensure an accurate diagnosis, nurses and other health professionals need to familiarize themselves with the clinical presentations and risk factors associated with these parasitic diseases.

## Intestinal Parasitic Infections

Although intestinal parasites are major contributors to morbidity and mortality in developing countries, climate, improved sanitary conditions, and effective drug therapy have served to greatly reduce widespread indigenous transmission in the United States, so much so that surveillance for many of these organisms is not widely practiced. A study using 1988-1994 NHANES III data reported that 14% of Americans have antibodies to *Toxocara*, a roundworm carried by dogs and cats that can be passed to humans. While this suggests that tens of millions of Americans have been exposed, it does show how many are actually infected (Won et al, 2008). Although most people show no signs of infection, this parasite can cause systemic illness and blindness. Technological advances have allowed for improved recognition of protozoans, leading to increased reporting of some organisms like *Cryptosporidium*. Cryptosporidiosis became a nationally notifiable disease in 1995 and giardiasis in 2002. However, many other parasitic infections such as toxocariasis and toxoplasmosis are not reportable.

Enterobiasis (pinworm) is the most common helminthic infection in the United States. Pinworm infection is seen most often among school-aged children and is most prevalent in crowded and institutional settings. Transmission is via consumption of infected eggs found in soil contaminated by human feces. Pinworms resemble small pieces of white thread and can be seen with the naked eye. Diagnosis is usually accomplished by pressing cellophane tape to the perianal region early in the morning. Treatment with oral vermicides and concurrent disinfection is highly effective (CDC, 2013h).

## Parasitic Opportunistic Infections

Opportunistic infections (OIs) are infections that occur more frequently or more severely in individuals immunocompromised by HIV infection. Before the introduction of routine prophylactic treatment and potent-combination, highly active antiretroviral therapies (ARTs) in the 1990s, OIs were the leading cause of illness and death in this group. Some of the protozoan parasitic OIs seen in clients with HIV disease and others who are immunocompromised include PCP; cryptosporidiosis, microsporidiosis and isosporiasis, all producing diarrheal disease and transmitted by fecal–oral contact; and toxoplasmosis. With the advent of ARTs, the incidence of OIs in American HIV disease clients has dropped dramatically. Isosporiasis was always rare, but the rates for cryptosporidiosis and microsporidiosis have also declined markedly. Although no longer seen with the frequency of the past, toxoplasmosis and PCP have not disappeared. OIs are more likely to appear in individuals unaware of their HIV disease or without good access to health care. Guidelines for prevention and treatment of OIs are now regularly updated by the Panel on Opportunistic Infections in HIV-Infected Adults and Adolescents representing opinion from the Centers for Disease Control and Prevention, the National Institutes of Health, and the HIV Medicine Association of the Infectious Diseases Society of America. Because of rapid evolution in HIV management, the Panel makes the most recent information readily available on the AIDS information website (http://aidsinfo.nih.gov).

*Toxoplasma gondii* is a coccidial organism harbored by cats infected by eating other infected animals. While rodents, ruminants, swine, poultry, and other birds may have infective organisms in their muscle tissue, only cats carry this parasite in their intestinal tract, allowing the excretion of infected eggs. People contract the disease through contact with infected cat feces or eating improperly cooked meat. In most healthy people, toxoplasmosis produces a mild to inapparent infection, but in immunodeficient individuals, the disease may, in addition to rash and skeletal muscle involvement, result in cerebritis, pneumonia, chorioretinitis, myocarditis, and/or death. Infection early in pregnancy may cause fetal death or deformity. CNS infection is common with HIV disease. Because toxoplasmosis is not a nationally reportable disease, reliable case numbers are not readily available. On their website, CDC estimates there are over a million new *Toxoplasma* infections and 400 to 4000 cases of congenital toxoplasmosis in the United States each year; an estimated 4,800 people experience ocular involvement as part of infection; and toxoplasmosis is a leading cause of foodborne illnesses deaths, resulting in an estimated 327 deaths and 4,428 hospitalizations per year (CDC, 2014l).

## Control and Prevention of Parasitic Infections

Correct diagnosis by nurses and other health care workers allows the provision of early and appropriate treatment and client education for preventing and controlling parasitic infections. Diagnosis of parasitic diseases is based on history, including travel, characteristic clinical signs and symptoms, and the use of appropriate laboratory tests to confirm the clinical diagnosis. Knowing what specimens to collect, how and when to collect, and what laboratory techniques to use are all important in establishing a correct diagnosis. Effective drug treatment is available for most parasitic diseases. The high cost of the drugs, drug resistance, and toxicity are some of the common therapeutic problems. Measures for prevention and control of parasitic diseases include early diagnosis and treatment, improved personal hygiene, safer sex practices, community health education, vector control, and improvements in sanitary control of food, water, and waste disposal.

## HEALTH CARE–ASSOCIATED INFECTIONS

Previously referred to as nosocomial infections and hospital-acquired infections, health care–associated infections (HAIs) are, as the name implies, those transmitted during hospitalization or developed within a hospital or other health care setting. They may involve clients, health care workers, visitors, or anyone who has contact with a hospital or doctor's office. Invasive diagnostic and surgical procedures, broad-spectrum antibiotics, and immunosuppressive drugs, along with the original underlying illness, leave hospitalized clients particularly vulnerable to exposure to virulent infectious agents from other clients and indigenous hospital flora from health care staff. In this setting, the simple act of performing hand hygiene before approaching every client becomes critical. A CDC prevalence survey of U.S. acute care hospitals in 2011 estimated 722,000 HAIs annually, suggesting that on any given day, 1 in 25 hospital patients has at least one health care–associated infection. An estimated 75,000 hospital patients with HAIs died during their hospitalizations. More than half of all HAIs occurred outside of the intensive care unit (Magill et al, 2014). Another recent report estimates total annual costs for five major health care–associated infections (HAIs) at $9.8 billion, with surgical site infections contributing the most to overall costs (Zimlichman et al, 2013). In addition, HAIs have a high likelihood of involving and contributing to antibiotic resistance.

The CDC maintains the National Healthcare Safety Network (NHSN), a voluntary, Internet-based surveillance system that provides national data on the epidemiology of HAIs in the United Sates. (Read more about preventing health care–associated infections and antibiotic resistance at the CDC HAI website: http://www.cdc.gov/ncidod/dhqp/hai.html.)

Infection control practitioners play a key role in hospital infection surveillance and control programs. Without a qualified and well-trained person in this position, the infection control program is ineffective. A great majority of infection control practitioners are nurses. Their common job titles are infection control nurse, infection control coordinator, and nurse epidemiologist.

## Universal Precautions

In 1985, in response to concerns regarding the transmission of HIV infection during health care procedures, the CDC recommended a universal precautions policy for all health care settings. This strategy requires that blood and body fluids from *all clients* be handled as if infected with HIV or other bloodborne pathogens. When in a situation where potential contact with blood or other body fluids exists, health care workers must always perform hand hygiene and wear gloves, masks, protective clothing, and other indicated personal protective barriers. Needles and sharp instruments must be used and disposed of properly (CDC, 1989). The CDC also made recommendations for preventing transmission of HIV and hepatitis B during medical, surgical, and dental procedures (CDC, 1991). Updated guidelines and recommendations for preventing HAIs including universal precautions were published in 2007 (Siegel et al, 2009). Today the Healthcare Infection Control Practices and Advisory Committee is charged with providing guidance on hospital infection control and developing strategies for surveillance, prevention and control of HAIs. The most recent guidance may be found on the Guidelines and Recommendations page of the CDC's Healthcare Associated Infection web pages at http://www.cdc.gov/hai/prevent/prevent_pubs.html. The following Linking Content to Practice box applies the three public health core functions to infectious diseases.

---

## ⟫ LINKING CONTENT TO PRACTICE

Public health involves the prevention of disease, promotion of health, and protection against hazards that threaten the health of the community as reflected in the public health logo and summed up in the mission "assuring conditions in which people can be healthy." The three core functions of public health in achieving this mission as defined in 1988 by the Institute of Medicine in Recommendations for the Future of Public Health are *Assessment, Policy Development,* and *Assurance.* These three have been further divided into the "Ten Essential Services of Public Health" as a means of evaluating the effectiveness of public health efforts.

This chapter presents communicable diseases that commonly challenge the health of a community as well as prevention and control roles for public health nurses. Examples of some of the "Essential Services" under which these roles fall are presented by core function.

**Assessment:** (1) Monitor health/identify problems and (2) Diagnose and investigate health problems. Examples include surveillance, investigation, and identification of reportable communicable disease cases. **Policy Development:** (3) Inform, educate, and empower and (4) Mobilize community partnerships. Examples include evaluating immunization status, explaining the reason for immunizations and how to comply with the immunization schedule, organizing community partners to provide immunizations and documentation through a registry, and mounting a community campaign to inform the community of the importance of age-appropriate immunization. **Assurance:** (5) Enforce laws and regulations and (6) Link to services and provide care. Examples include assuring compliance with communicable disease control laws through treatment or prophylaxis for exposure to reportable diseases; excluding diseased students from daycare or school; linking individuals without insurance to follow-up care for communicable disease treatment or exposure.

## PRACTICE APPLICATION

The rising numbers of foreign-born residents in communities that did not previously have large immigrant populations provides a challenge to those involved with communicable disease control, especially in outbreak situations. Language barriers, specific cultural practices, and undocumented status all contribute to opportunities for infection as well as presenting obstacles to prevention and control. Diseases such as TB, brucellosis, measles, hepatitis B, and parasitic infections often originate in other countries and are diagnosed only after the individual arrives in the United States. People coming from countries without, with newly established, or with poorly enforced vaccination programs may be unimmunized. These people are particularly susceptible to infection in outbreak situations. For example, many people coming from Latin America have not been immunized against rubella. Differences in cultural practices can lead to outbreaks of foodborne illness. Listeriosis outbreaks have been traced to the use of unpasteurized milk in cottage industry cheese production.

In the face of a single infectious disease report or an outbreak situation, when working with communities whose members speak limited English, it is vital (1) to have a means of communication, (2) to be able to provide a culturally appropriate message, and (3) to have an established level of trust. Ideally, these requirements are addressed before an outbreak occurs, allowing a prompt and efficient response when immediate action is needed.

A. What would be a useful first step in building trust with a largely non–English-speaking immigrant community?
1. Hold a health fair in the community.
2. Provide incentives to use health department services.
3. Identify trusted community leaders such as religious leaders and ask their help in developing a plan.
4. Distribute a brochure in the target community language.

B. What might best encourage undocumented residents to respond to a request to be immunized during an outbreak situation?
1. Using an already established public health program to provide interpreter services, making it clear that proof of immigration status is not required for services
2. Printing a request in the newspaper in the language of the targeted individuals
3. Involving trusted community leaders in making the request
4. Emphasizing to the individuals the severity of the consequences if immunization does not occur

C. What means of communication would work best when targeting largely non–English-speaking communities of recent immigrants?
1. Newspaper articles in target language
2. Radio announcements in target language
3. Fliers in target language posted in the community
4. Announcements from trusted community leaders

D. How would public health officials best undertake the development of information to effectively reach a largely non–English-speaking community of recent immigrants?
1. Use the services of the local university communications department.
2. Ask community leaders to work with translators and prevention specialists to develop messages using their own words.
3. Hire a professional to translate an existing well-developed English-language brochure.
4. Use brochures provided by the state health department.
**Answers can be found on the Evolve site.**

## KEY POINTS

- The burden of infectious diseases is high in both human and economic terms. Preventing these diseases must be given high priority in our present health care system.
- The successful interaction of the infectious agent, host, and environment is necessary for disease transmission. Knowledge of the characteristics of each of these three factors is important in understanding the transmission, prevention, and control of these diseases.
- Effective intervention measures at the individual and community levels must be aimed at breaking the chain linking the agent, host, and environment. An integrated approach focused on all three factors simultaneously is an ideal goal to strive for but may not be feasible for all diseases.
- Health care professionals must constantly be aware of vulnerability to threats posed by emerging infectious diseases. Most of the factors causing the emergence of these diseases are influenced by human activities and behavior.

- Communicable diseases are preventable. Avoiding infection through primary prevention activities is the most cost-effective public health strategy.
- Health care professionals must always apply infection control principles and procedures in the work environment. They should strictly adhere to universal blood and body fluid precautions to prevent transmission of HIV and other blood-borne pathogens.
- Effective control of communicable diseases requires the use of a multisystem approach focusing on enhancing host resistance, improving safety of the environment, improving public health systems, and facilitating social and political changes to ensure health for all people.
- Communicable disease prevention and control programs must move beyond providing drug treatment and vaccines. Health promotion and education aimed at changing individual and community behavior must be emphasized.

## KEY POINTS—cont'd

- Nurses play a key role in all aspects of prevention and control of communicable diseases. Close cooperation with other members of the interprofessional health care team must be maintained. Mobilizing community participation is essential to successful implementation of programs.

- The successful global eradication of smallpox proved the feasibility of eradication of selected communicable diseases. As professionals and concerned citizens of the global village, health care workers must support the current global eradication campaigns against poliomyelitis and dracunculiasis.

## CLINICAL DECISION-MAKING ACTIVITIES

1. Accompany a nurse who makes home visits. Discuss living situations and other risk factors that may contribute to the development of infectious diseases, as well as possible points at which the nurse may intervene to help prevent these diseases, such as checking the immunization status of all individuals in the household. What are realistic interventions and how much responsibility should a nurse take in attempting to affect the living situation?

2. To become familiar with the reportable diseases that are a problem in your community, look at how many cases have been reported during the past month, 6 months, and year. Contrast these numbers with national and state statistics. How is your county or city different from or similar to these larger jurisdictions? If different, what environmental, political, or demographic features may contribute to this difference?

3. Spend time with the persons who are responsible for reporting and investigating communicable disease in your community. Discuss types of surveillance conducted and outbreak procedures that may accompany the reporting of some of these diseases. If possible, attend an outbreak investigation. Would the existing surveillance systems and outbreak control policies be sufficient in the case of a bioterrorism event?

4. Review the demographic profile of your community including trends from the past 10 years and projections for the next decade. Pay special attention to growth patterns of particular populations such as racial and ethnic groups or specific age groups (e.g., children under 18, adults 65 and older).

How do changes in these populations affect the delivery of interventions for infectious disease control such as immunization?

5. Visit a clinic that serves a refugee, immigrant, or migrant labor population to observe the infectious diseases commonly seen in these groups. Compare and contrast this visit with a visit to a clinic that serves an inner-city population and a visit to a clinic that serves a rural population. How are the infectious disease control issues different and/or similar for these varied populations?

6. Sit in a clinic waiting room for immunization services and talk with parents about their concerns and the barriers they may perceive in obtaining immunizations for their children. How can this information be used to better facilitate immunization services?

7. Spend time with a school nurse to see what infectious diseases are routinely encountered in the educational setting. Discuss risk factors for disease in school-age youths and the strategies used to prevent infectious diseases in this age group. Do school policies support the strategies needed for the prevention of infectious diseases in students?

8. Visit a daycare center. Observe potential situations for the communication of infectious diseases and discuss with the director the steps taken to prevent and control infection, including immunization requirements and procedures for hand hygiene and food preparation. Does the center have specific infection control policies and procedures, and does the staff appear to be following them?

## REFERENCES

Centers for Disease Control and Prevention: Guidelines for prevention of transmission of HIV and hepatitis B virus to health care and public safety workers. *MMWR Morb Mortal Wkly Rep* 37(S–6):1, 1989.

Centers for Disease Control and Prevention: Recommendations for preventing transmission of HIV and hepatitis B virus to patients during exposure-prone invasive procedures. *MMWR Morb Mortal Wkly Rep* 40(RR–8):1, 1991.

Centers for Disease Control and Prevention: Addressing emerging infectious disease threats: a prevention strategy for the U.S,

1994. *MMWR Morb Mortal Wkly Rep* 43(RR–5):1–18, 1994.

Centers for Disease Control and Prevention: Notifiable disease surveillance and notifiable disease statistics—United States, June 1946 and June 1996. *MMWR Morb Mortal Wkly Rep* 45:530, 1996.

Centers for Disease Control and Prevention: Update: isolation of avian influenza A (H5N1) viruses from humans—Hong Kong, 1997-1998. *MMWR Morb Mortal Wkly Rep* 46:1245, 1998.

Centers for Disease Control and Prevention: Achievements in public health: elimination of rubella and congenital rubella

syndrome—United States, 1969-2004. *MMWR Morb Mortal Wkly Rep* 4(11):279–282, 2005.

Centers for Disease Control and Prevention: Human rabies prevention—United States, 2008 recommendations of the Advisory Committee on Immunization Practices. *MMWR Morb Mortal Wkly Rep* 57(RR03):1–26, 2008a.

Centers for Disease Control and Prevention: Progress toward interruption of wild poliovirus transmission—worldwide, 2008. *MMWR Morb Mortal Wkly Rep* 58(12):308–312, 2009a.

Centers for Disease Control and Prevention: Tularemia—Missouri, 2000-2007. *MMWR Morb Mortal*

*Wkly Rep* 58(27):744–748, 2009b.

Centers for Disease Control and Prevention: Surveillance for human West Nile virus disease—United States, 1999-2008. *MMWR Morb Mortal Wkly Rep* 59(2):1–17, 2010a.

Centers for Disease Control and Prevention: Update: influenza activity—United States, August 30, 2009-January 9, 2010. *MMWR Morbid Mortal Wkly Rep* 59(02):38–43, 2010b.

Centers for Disease Control and Prevention: *CDC's Advisory Committee on Immunization Practices (ACIP) Recommends Universal Annual Influenza*

Vaccination, Media Advisory. 2010c, CDC. Available at: http://www.cdc.gov/media/pressrel/2010/r100224.htm. Accessed May 16, 2014.

Centers for Disease Control and Prevention: *CDC Media Telebriefing on the Burden of Foodborne Disease, Media Advisory*. 2010d, CDC. Available at: http://www.cdc.gov/media/pressrel/2010/a101215.html. Accessed May 16, 2014.

Centers for Disease Control and Prevention: Use of a reduced (4-dose) vaccine schedule for postexposure prophylaxis to prevent human rabies, recommendations of the Advisory Committee on Immunization Practices. *MMWR Morb Mortal Wkly Rep Recomm Rep* 59(02):1–9, 2010e.

Centers for Disease Control and Prevention: A CDC framework for preventing infectious diseases: sustaining the essential and innovating for the future. 2011a. Available at: http://www.cdc.gov/oid/docs/ID-Framework.pdf. Accessed May 16, 2014.

Centers for Disease Control and Prevention: *Southern Tick-Associated Rash Illness Webpage*. 2011b, CDC. Available at: http://www.cdc.gov/stari/. Accessed May 16, 2014.

Centers for Disease Control and Prevention: Compendium of animal rabies prevention and control, 2011. *MMWR Morb Mortal Wkly Rep Recomm* 60(6):1–12, 2011c.

Centers for Disease Control and Prevention: Deaths: preliminary data for 2011. *Natl Vital Stats Rep* 61(6):16, 2012a.

Centers for Disease Control and Prevention: MMWR pertussis epidemic—Washington, 2012. *MMWR Morb Mortal Wkly Rep* 61(28):517–522, 2012b.

Centers for Disease Control: *Foodborne Diseases Active Surveillance Network (FoodNet): FoodNet Surveillance Report for 2011 (Final Report)*. 2012c, CDC.

Centers for Disease Control and Prevention: Recovery of a patient from clinical rabies—California, 2011. *MMWR Morb Mortal Wkly Rep* 61(04):61–65, 2012d.

Centers for Disease Control: *Trichomoniasis—CDC Fact Sheet, Last Updated August 3, 2012*. 2012e, CDC. Available at: http://www.cdc.gov/std/trichomonas/STDFact-Trichomoniasis.htm. Accessed May 16, 2014.

Centers for Disease Control and Prevention: Giardiasis surveillance—United States, 2009-2010. *MMWR Morb Mortal Wkly Rep* 61(SS05):13–23, 2012f.

Centers for Disease Control and Prevention: Fact sheet: variant Creutzfeldt-Jakob disease. 2013a. Available at: http://www.cdc.gov/ncidod/dvrd/vcjd/factsheet_nvcjd.htm#surveillance. Accessed May 16, 2014.

Centers for Disease Control and Prevention: Summary of notifiable diseases—United States 2011. *MMWR Morb Mortal Wkly Rep* 60(53):3, 2013b.

Centers for Disease Control and Prevention: Progress toward global eradication of dracunculiasis, January 2012-June 2013. *MMWR Morbid Mortal Wkly Rep* 62(42):829–833, 2013c.

Centers for Disease Control and Prevention: Prevention of measles, rubella, congenital rubella syndrome, and mumps, 2013: summary recommendations of the Advisory Committee on Immunization Practices (ACIP). *MMWR Morbid Mortal Wkly RepRecomm Rep* 62(RR04):1–34, 2013d.

Centers for Disease Control: Surveillance for foodborne disease outbreaks—United States, 2009-2010. *MMWR Morbid Mortal Wkly Rep* 62(03):41–47, 2013e.

Centers for Disease Control: Surveillance for waterborne disease outbreaks associated with drinking water and other nonrecreational water—United States, 2009-2010. *MMWR Morbid Mortal Wkly Rep* 6(35):714–720, 2013f.

Centers for Disease Control and Prevention: Water treatment methods. 2013g. Available at: http://wwwnc.cdc.gov/travel/content/water-treatment.aspx. Accessed May 16, 2014.

Centers for Disease Control and Prevention: Parasites—enterobious, epidemiology and risk factors. 2013h. Available at: http://www.cdc.gov/parasites/pinworm/epi.html. Accessed May 16, 2014.

Centers for Disease Control and Prevention: Ebola hemorrhagic fever. 2014a. Available at: http://www.cdc.gov/vhf/ebola/. Accessed May 16, 2014.

Centers for Disease Control and Prevention: Marburg hemorrhagic fever. 2014b. Available at: http://www.cdc.gov/vhf/marburg/. Accessed May 16, 2014.

Centers for Disease Control and Prevention: Global health—polio. 2014c. Available at: http://www.cdc.gov/polio/updates/. Accessed May 16, 2014.

Centers for Disease Control and Prevention: Recommended immunization schedules for persons aged 0 through 18 years—United States, 2014. *MMWR Morb Mortal Wkly Rep* 63(05):108–109, 2014d.

Centers for Disease Control and Prevention: Measles cases and outbreaks. 2014e. Available at: http://www.cdc.gov/measles/cases-outbreaks.html. Accessed May 16, 2014.

Centers for Disease Control and Prevention: Pertussis—surveillance and reporting. 2014f. Available at: http://www.cdc.gov/pertussis/surv-reporting.html. Accessed May 16, 2014.

Centers for Disease Control and Prevention: CDC recommendations for influenza antiviral medications remain unchanged. 2014g. Available at: http://www.cdc.gov/media/haveyouheard/stories/Influenza_antiviral2.html. Accessed May 16, 2014.

Centers for Disease Control and Prevention: 2013-14 Flu season FluVaxView information and coverage, seasonal influenza. 2014h. Available at: http://www.cdc.gov/flu/fluvaxview/1314season.htm. Accessed May 16, 2014.

Centers for Disease Control and Prevention: Highly pathogenic avian influenza A (H5N1) in people, seasonal flu. 2014i. Available at: http://www.cdc.gov/flu/avianflu/h5n1-people.htm. Accessed May 16, 2014.

Centers for Disease Control and Prevention: Ticks. 2014j. Available at: http://www.cdc.gov/ticks/. Accessed May 16, 2014.

Centers for Disease Control and Prevention: Malaria facts. 2014k. Available at: http://www.cdc.gov/malaria/about/facts.html. Accessed May 16, 2014.

Centers for Disease Control and Prevention: Neglected parasitic infections in the United States—toxoplasmosis. 2014l. Available at: http://www.cdc.gov/parasites/resources/pdf/npi_toxoplasmosis.pdf. Accessed May 16, 2014.

Centers for Disease Control and Prevention: Ebola virus disease. 2015a. Available at: http://www.cdc.gov/vhf/ebola/. Accessed January 25, 2015.

Centers for Disease Control and Prevention: Measles cases and outbreaks. 2015b. Available at: http://www.cdc.gov/measles/cases-outbreaks.html. Accessed January 25, 2015.

Christian KA, Blanton JD, Auslander M, et al: Epidemiology of rabies post-exposure prophylaxis—United States of America 2006-2008. *Vaccine* 27(51):7156–7161, 2009.

Cieslak TJ, Eitzen EM Jr: Clinical and epidemiologic principles of anthrax. *Emerg Infect Dis* 5:552–555, 1999.

Dyer JL, Wallace RW, Orciari L, et al: Rabies surveillance in the United States during 2012. *JAVMA* 243(6):811–812, 2013.

Evans AS: The eradication of communicable diseases: myth or reality? *Am J Epidemiol* 122:199, 1985.

Fauci AS, Touchette NA, Folkers GK: Emerging infectious diseases: a 10-year perspective from the National Institute of Allergy and Infectious Diseases. *Emerg Infect Dis* 2005. Available at: http://www.cdc.gov/ncidod/EID/vol11no04/04-167.htm. Accessed May 16, 2014.

Feldman KA, Stiles-Enos D, Julian K, et al: Tularemia on Martha's Vineyard: seroprevalence and occupational risk. *Emerg Infect Dis* 2003. Available at: http://www.cdc.gov/ncidod/EID/vol9no3/02-0462.htm. Accessed May 16, 2014.

Grunow R, Klee SR, Beyer W, et al: Anthrax among heroin users in Europe possibly caused by same bacillus anthracis strain since 2000. *Eurosurveillance* 18(13):1–9, 2013. Available at: http://www.eurosurveillance.org/ViewArticle.aspx?ArticleId=20437. Accessed May 16, 2014.

Heymann DL, editor: *Control of Communicable Diseases Manual*, ed 20. Washington, DC, 2014, American Public Health Association.

Kuehn BM: CDC estimates 300,000 US cases of Lyme disease annually. *JAMA* 310(11):1110, 2013.

Los Angeles Biomedical Research Institute at Harbor-UCLA Medical Center (LA BioMed): Changes in hospital orders increase pertussis immunization rates. *Science Daily* 2014. Available at: www.sciencedaily.com/releases/2014/03/140305110923.htm. Accessed May 16, 2014.

Magill SS, Edwards JR, Bamberg W, et al: Multistate point-prevalence survey of health care–associated infections. *N Engl J Med* 370:1198–1208, 2014.

Scallan E, Hoekstra RM, Angulo FJ, et al: Foodborne illness acquired in the United States—major pathogens. *Emerg Infect Dis* 17(1):2011. Available at: http://dx.doi.org/10.3201/eid1701.P11101 http://wwwnc.cdc.gov/eid/article/17/1/p1-1101_article.htm. Accessed May 16, 2014.

Scharff RL: Economic burden from health losses due to foodborne illness in the United States. *J Food Prot* 75(1):123–131, 2012.

Siegel JD, Rhinehart E, Jackson M, et al: *Guidelines for Isolation Precautions: Preventing Transmission of Infectious Agents in Healthcare Settings*. 2009, CDC. Available at: http://www.cdc.gov/hicpac/2007IP/2007isolationPrecautions.html. Accessed May 16, 2014.

Knowledge about the risk of communicable diseases has changed dramatically in recent years. For example, in the decades following the development of antibiotics in the 1940s, sexually transmitted diseases (STDs) were considered to be a problem of the past. The recent emergence of new viral STDs and antibiotic-resistant strains of bacterial STDs has posed new challenges. Left unchecked, STDs can cause poor pregnancy outcomes, infertility, and cervical cancers. There is also the problem of co-infection, with one STD increasing the susceptibility to other STDs, such as human immunodeficiency virus (HIV). STDs are also called sexually transmitted infections (STIs) because many times, the infections are asymptomatic. In this chapter, the term STDs will be used.

This concern about infectious diseases has prompted the development of standards for STDs, HIV and acquired immunodeficiency syndrome (AIDS), hepatitis, and tuberculosis (TB) in the *Healthy People 2020* report. The Healthy People 2020 box shows some objectives used to evaluate progress toward decreasing communicable diseases by the year 2020.

### ♥ HEALTHY PEOPLE 2020

The following selected objectives pertain to the communicable diseases discussed in this chapter:
• HIV-3: Reduce the rate of HIV transmission among adults and adolescents.
• STD-8: Reduce congenital syphilis.
• IID-26: Reduce new hepatitis C infections.
• STD-1: Reduce the proportion of adolescents and young adults with *Chlamydia trachomatis* infections.

From U.S. Department of Health and Human Services: *Healthy People 2020 Objectives*, Washington, DC, 2010, Office of Disease Prevention and Health Promotion, USDHHS.

Several communicable diseases and all STDs are acquired through behaviors that can be avoided or changed, and thus intervention efforts by nurses have focused on disease prevention. Prevention can take the form of vaccine administration (as with hepatitis A and hepatitis B), early detection (of infections like TB, for example), or instruction of clients about abstinence or safer sex. Individuals who live with chronic infections can transmit them to others.

This chapter describes selected communicable diseases and their nursing management. It concludes with implications for nursing care in primary, secondary, and tertiary prevention.

## HUMAN IMMUNODEFICIENCY VIRUS INFECTION

Human immunodeficiency virus (HIV) infection has had an enormous political and social impact on society. Controversies have arisen over many aspects of HIV. Fears about HIV may lead to attitudes of blaming clients for their infections and to discrimination. These beliefs are magnified by the fact that this disease has commonly afflicted two groups who have been largely scorned by society: homosexuals and injection drug users (Fair and Ginsberg, 2010). Debates have arisen over how to control disease transmission and how to pay for related health services. An ongoing debate involves whether clean needles should be distributed to injection drug users to prevent the spread of HIV.

Economic costs of HIV/AIDS result from premature treatment and disability. The fact that nearly 55% of HIV infections occur in persons between the ages of 20 and 39 years may result in disrupted families and lost creative and economic productivity at a period of life when vitality is the norm (CDC, 2013l). In 2009, 39% of new HIV infections occurred in the 13- to 29-year-old age group (CDC, 2013i). Medicaid and Medicare primarily support the health care delivery costs of those infected. Many people with HIV qualify for Medicaid or Medicare because they are indigent or fall into poverty when paying for health care over the course of the illness. The lifetime cost of HIV care for one client is $379,668 (CDC, 2013j). The Ryan White HIV/AIDS Program, through the Ryan White HIV/AIDS Treatment Extension Act of 2009, provides care for persons with HIV infection (USDHHS, 2014a). This program provides funds for health care in the geographic areas with the largest number of AIDS cases. Health services that are covered include emergency services, services for early intervention and care (sometimes including coverage of health insurance), and drug reimbursement programs for HIV-infected individuals. The AIDS Drug Assistance Programs (ADAPs) are awards that pay for medications on the basis of the estimated number of persons living with AIDS in the individual state (USDHHS, 2014b).

## Natural History of HIV

The natural history of HIV includes three stages: the primary infection (within about 1 month of contracting the virus), followed by a period when the body shows no symptoms (clinical latency), and then a final stage of symptomatic disease (Buttaro et al, 2013).

When HIV enters the body, a person may experience a mononucleosis-like syndrome, referred to as a primary infection, which lasts for a few weeks. This may go unrecognized. The body's CD4 white blood cell count drops for a brief time when the virus is most plentiful in the body. The immune system increases antibody production in response to this initial infection, which is a self-limiting illness. Symptoms include lymphadenopathy, myalgias, sore throat, lethargy, rash, and fever (CDC, 2013g). Even if the client seeks medical care at this time, the antibody test at this stage is usually negative, so it is often not recognized as HIV.

After a variable period of time, commonly from 6 weeks to 3 months, HIV antibodies appear in the blood. Although most antibodies serve a protective role, HIV antibodies do not. However, their presence helps in the detection of HIV infection because screening tests show their presence in the bloodstream.

HIV-infected persons live several years before developing symptomatic disease. During this prolonged incubation period, clients have a gradual deterioration of the immune system and can transmit the virus to others. The use of highly active antiretroviral therapy (HAART) has greatly increased the survival time of persons with HIV/AIDS.

Acquired immunodeficiency syndrome (AIDS, a.k.a. HIV Stage 3) is the last stage in the long continuum of HIV infection and may result from damage caused by HIV, secondary cancers, or opportunistic organisms. AIDS is defined as a disabling or life-threatening illness caused by HIV; it is diagnosed in a person with a CD4 T-lymphocyte count of less than 200/mL with documented HIV infection (CDC, 2008).

Many of the AIDS-related opportunistic infections are caused by microorganisms that are commonly present in healthy individuals but do not cause disease in persons with an intact immune system. These microorganisms proliferate in persons with HIV/AIDS because of a weakened immune system. Opportunistic infections may be caused by bacteria, fungi, viruses, or protozoa. The most common opportunistic diseases are *Pneumocystis jiroveci (carinii)* pneumonia and oral candidiasis, but also include pulmonary TB, invasive cervical cancer, or recurrent pneumonia.

In 2008 the case definition for HIV infection was revised to include the HIV classification/staging system based on the number of CD4+ T-lymphocytes. Criteria for defining HIV infection include a positive result from the antibody screening test or a positive result from a nucleic acid test (DNA or RNA). In situations where the mother of a newborn is HIV infected, the HIV nucleic acid test (DNA or RNA) is used to identify HIV/AIDS in infants (CDC, 2008).

TB, an infection that is becoming more prevalent because of HIV infection, can spread rapidly among immunosuppressed individuals. Thus, HIV-infected individuals who live in close proximity to one another, such as in long-term care facilities, prisons, drug treatment facilities, or other settings, must be carefully screened and in some instances deemed noninfectious before admission to such settings. TB is covered in more depth later in this chapter. See the following QSEN box for suggestions about implementing quality and safety in the care of patients with HIV and other communicable and infectious diseases.

---

### QSEN FOCUS ON QUALITY AND SAFETY EDUCATION FOR NURSES

#### Sexually Transmitted Diseases

**Targeted Competency**
Evidence-based practice (EBP): Integrate best current evidence with clinical expertise and client/family preferences and values for delivery of optimal care.
**Knowledge:** Explain the role of evidence in determining best clinical practice.
**Skills:** Locate evidence reports related to clinical practice topics and guidelines
**Attitudes:** Value the concept of EBP as integral to determining best clinical practice.

*Client-centered Care Question*
Evidence supports the fact that some medications previously effective in treating STDs no longer are effective. If you learned that a colleague was planning to use a treatment that is no longer considered effective to treat a specific STD, what would you do to assure that the care the client receives is based on current evidence?

Answer: With your colleague collect current treatment guidelines information about that specific STD. The first place that you might look would be the Centers for Disease Control and Prevention guidelines for that disease. For example, you might look at "HIV treatment guidelines for adults and adolescents updated" at the following website to find out what is the most effective antiretroviral therapy (ART) for the treatment of HIV infection. See http://aids.info.nih.gov/guidelines.

## Transmission

HIV is transmitted through exposure to blood, semen, transplanted organs, vaginal secretions, and breast milk (Heymann, 2014). Persons who had blood exposure or sexual or needle-sharing contact with an HIV-infected person are at risk for contracting the virus. The virus is not transmitted through casual contact such as touching or hugging someone who has HIV infection or through mosquitoes or other insects. Although HIV has been found in saliva and tears in some instances, there are no reports of transmission through contact with these body fluids (Heymann, 2014). The modes of transmission are listed in Box 14-1, and the exposure categories of HIV are shown in Figure 14-1.

Potential donors of blood and tissues are screened through interviews to assess for a history of high-risk activities and screened with the HIV antibody test. Blood or tissue is not used from individuals with a history of high-risk behavior or who are HIV infected. In addition to being screened, coagulation

---

**BOX 14-1  Modes of Transmission of Human Immunodeficiency Virus (HIV)**

HIV can be transmitted in the following ways:
- Sexual contact, involving the exchange of body fluids, with an infected person
- Sharing or reusing needles, syringes, or other equipment used to prepare injectable drugs
- Perinatal transmission from an infected mother to her fetus during pregnancy or delivery, or to an infant when breastfeeding
- Transfusions or other exposure to HIV-contaminated blood or blood products, organs, or semen

From Heymann D: *Control of Communicable Diseases Manual,* Washington, DC, 2008, APHA.

---

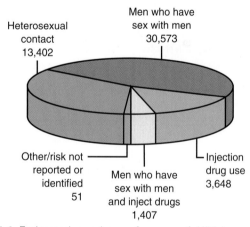

FIG 14-1 Estimated numbers of cases of HIV by exposure category in 2011, United States. Note that the "other" category includes hemophilia, blood transfusion, perinatal exposure, and risk factors not reported or not identified. (Data from Centers for Disease Control and Prevention: *HIV Surveillance Report*, vol. 23, Diagnoses of HIV infection in the United States and Dependent Areas, 2011. Published February 2013. Available at http://www.cdc.gov/hiv/library/reports/surveillance/2011/surveillance_Report_vol_23.html. Accessed March 9, 2014.)

---

factors used to treat hemophilia and other blood disorders are made safe through heat treatments to inactivate the virus. Screening has significantly reduced the risk of transmission of HIV by blood products and organ donations.

When a person has an STD infection such as chlamydia or gonorrhea, the risk of HIV infection increases and HIV may also increase the risk for other STDs. This may result from any of the following: open lesions providing a portal of entry for pathogens; STDs decreasing the host's immune status, resulting in a rapid progression of HIV infection; and HIV changing the natural history of STDs or the effectiveness of medications used in treating STDs (Heymann, 2014).

The nurse serves both as an educator about the modes of transmission and as a role model for how to behave toward and provide supportive care for those with HIV infection. An understanding of how transmission does and does not occur will help family and community members feel more comfortable in relating to and caring for persons with HIV (see Box 14-1).

## Epidemiology of HIV/AIDS

Worldwide 35.3 million persons live with HIV infection. Sub-Saharan Africa accounts for more than 70% of all HIV infections (UNAIDS, 2013). The epidemic is also growing in Eastern Europe, the Middle East, and central Asia (UNAIDS, 2012). Women are at highest risk for infection because of unprotected sex with infected partners. However, there is some evidence that HIV prevention programs may be changing risk behavior in southern Africa. Worldwide, the treatment of HIV infection has been given higher priority, and the use of highly active antiretroviral therapy has increased to 61% for those who need it under the 2010 WHO Guidelines, and 34% of those eligible under the 2013 guidelines (UNAIDS, 2013).

Nurses must identify the trends of HIV infection in the populations they serve, so that they can screen clients who may be at risk and can adequately plan prevention programs and illness care resources. For example, knowing that AIDS disproportionately affects minorities helps nurses set priorities and plan services for these groups. Factors such as geographic location, age, and ethnic distribution are tracked to more effectively target programs. It is important to identify persons infected with HIV before symptomatic AIDS develops, so that treatment can begin as early as needed. It is estimated that about 1.1 million people in the United States are infected with HIV, but 15.8% (180,900 people) are not aware of their infection (CDC, 2013k).

Since the first cases of AIDS were identified in 1981, the total reported number of persons living with AIDS in the United States grew to 487,692 by the end of 2010 (CDC, 2013l). Note that this number reflects only those who are living; it does not include those who have died. The prevalence of AIDS has increased from 2004 to 2007, reflecting increased life expectancy from the use of antiretroviral therapy (CDC, 2013l).

Figure 14-1 shows the exposure categories for persons with HIV in 2011. Men who have sex with men (MSM) make up the largest group with HIV in the United States, and the number of persons contracting HIV through heterosexual transmission is the second largest. Heterosexual transmission has surpassed injection drug use (IDU) as the primary mode of HIV transmission in women (CDC, 2013l).

The distribution of pediatric HIV infection has fallen dramatically as a result of prenatal care that includes HIV testing, antiretroviral therapy for the mother, and cesarean delivery. Perinatal HIV transmission has declined, and two thirds of pediatric HIV infection results from perinatal exposure (CDC, 2013l).

As seen in Table 14-1, HIV has disproportionately affected minority groups. African Americans have the largest HIV disease burden of any racial/ethnic group in the United States; African American rates of new HIV infection are 8 times higher than in whites, the highest prevalence of those living with HIV is in the African American community, and the highest proportions of people diagnosed with HIV Stage 3 (AIDS) are African American (CDC, 2014h). This overrepresentation is associated with poverty, since African Americans have a higher poverty rate than other groups do. This reflects decreased access to prevention and treatment, and lack of awareness of HIV infection. Stigma, fear, and homophobia play a role as well (CDC, 2014h). Transgender people are also at high risk, particularly transgender women. Because of data collection limitations, it is difficult to estimate HIV prevalence in transgender communities. However, data from countries that collect data for transgender women separately from men who have sex with men indicate that HIV prevalence is nearly 50 times higher than for other adults of reproductive age (CDC, 2013h).

As seen in Figure 14-2, the geographic distribution of HIV infection is clustered in urban areas. Regionally, the southern

United States and the U.S. territories of the Virgin Islands and Puerto Rico report the highest rates (CDC, 2013l). States with AIDS prevalence greater than 12.5 per 100,000 population in 2011 were Delaware (13.8), Florida (21.2), Georgia (27.9), Louisiana (22.4), Maryland (24.0), Mississippi (16.4), New

## TABLE 14-1 Estimated Numbers of New HIV Infections and Stage 3 (AIDS) Infections in Adults and Adolescents, 2011 (50 States, the District of Columbia, and 6 U.S. Dependent Areas)

| Race/Ethnicity | HIV Infection | Rate Per 100,000 | Rate, Males | Rate, Females | Stage 3 (AIDS) |
|---|---|---|---|---|---|
| Black, African American | 23,168 | 60.4 | 112.8 | 40.0 | 15,966 |
| White | 13,846 | 7.0 | 14.5 | 2.0 | 8,304 |
| Hispanic/Latino | 10,159 | 19.5 | 43.4 | 7.9 | 6,849 |
| Asian | 982 | 6.5 | 13.8 | 2.3 | 492 |
| American Indian/Alaska Native | 212 | 9.3 | 18.0 | 5.5 | 146 |
| Native Hawaiian/Pacific Islander | 78 | 15.3 | 34.2 | 3.9 | 51 |
| Multiple races | 827 | 14.2 | 38.5 | 7.5 | 753 |
| Total | 49,272 | 15.8 | 30.8 | 7.7 | 32,561 |

Centers for Disease Control and Prevention: *HIV Surveillance Report: Diagnoses of HIV Infection and AIDS in the United States and Dependent Areas*, 2011; vol. 23. Accessed at http://www.cdc.gov/hiv/topics/surveillance/resources/reports/. Published, February 2013. Accessed February 22. 2014.

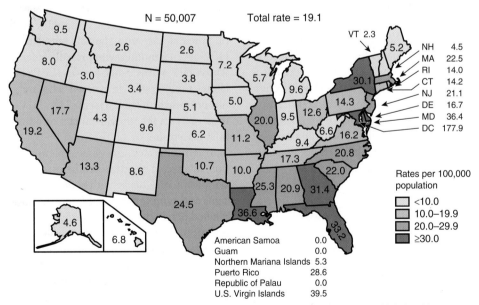

*Note.* Data include persons with a diagnosis of HIV infection regardless of stage of disease at diagnosis. All displayed data have been statistically adjusted to account for reporting delays, but not for incomplete reporting

**FIG 14-2** Map of rates of diagnosis of HIV infection among adults and adolescents, 2011, in the United States and 6 dependent areas. (Data from Centers for Disease Control and Prevention: *HIV Surveillance Report*, vol. 23, Diagnoses of HIV infection in the United States and Dependent Areas, 2011. Published February 2013. Available at http://www.cdc.gov/hiv/library/reports/surveillance/2011/surveillance_Report_vol_23.html. Accessed March 9, 2014.)

**TABLE 14-2  Estimated Numbers of New HIV Infections and Stage 3 (AIDS) Infections in Adults and Adolescents, 2011 (50 States, the District of Columbia, And 6 U.S. Dependent Areas) By Age**

| Age | HIV Infection | Rate per 100,000 | Stage 3 (AIDS) | Rate per 100,000 |
|---|---|---|---|---|
| <13 | 193 | 0.4 | 15 | 0 |
| 13-14 | 53 | 0.6 | 49 | 0.6 |
| 15-19 | 2263 | 10.3 | 510 | 2.4 |
| 20-24 | 8140 | 36.3 | 2429 | 10.9 |
| 25-29 | 7608 | 35.3 | 3433 | 16.1 |
| 30-34 | 6318 | 30.4 | 4001 | 19.5 |
| 35-39 | 5384 | 27.1 | 4071 | 20.8 |
| 40-44 | 5883 | 27.6 | 4783 | 22.7 |
| 45-49 | 5706 | 25.4 | 4994 | 22.5 |
| 50-54 | 4051 | 17.7 | 3567 | 15.8 |
| 55-59 | 2369 | 11.6 | 2198 | 10.9 |
| 60-64 | 1258 | 7.0 | 1107 | 6.2 |
| ≥65 | 974 | 2.3 | 899 | 2.2 |

Centers for Disease Control and Prevention: *HIV Surveillance Report: Diagnoses of HIV Infection and AIDS in the United States and Dependent Areas*, 2011; vol. 23. Accessed at http://www.cdc.gov/hiv/topics/surveillance/resources/reports/. Published, February 2013. Accessed February 22. 2014.

Jersey (13.0), New York (21.7), South Carolina (16.4), Texas (16.5), and the District of Columbia (94.2) (CDC, 2013l). As shown in Table 14-2, both HIV and HIV Stage 3 (AIDS) affect people across the life span, with peak HIV rates occurring for those in the 25- to 29-year-old age group. Peak HIV Stage 3 (AIDS) rates occur in individuals age 40 to 44.

## HIV Surveillance

A study of diagnosed cases of AIDS does not reveal current HIV infection patterns because of the interval between infection with HIV and the onset of clinical disease. Moreover, the effectiveness of antiretroviral drugs given early in the HIV infection before symptoms start provides impetus for early identification of infection. Thus in 2008 confidential laboratory reporting of HIV-positive status by name was required in all 50 states and the District of Columbia (CDC, 2013l), although not all states require viral load and CD4 counts (CDC, 2013o).

## HIV Testing

The HIV antibody test is the most commonly used screening test for determining infection. This test does just as its name implies: it does not reveal whether an individual has symptomatic AIDS, nor does it isolate the virus. It does indicate the presence of the antibody to HIV. The most commonly used form of this test is the enzyme-linked immunosorbent assay (EIA). The EIA effectively screens blood and other donor products. To minimize false-positive results, a confirmatory test, the Western blot, is used to verify the results. False-negative results may also occur after infection and before antibodies are produced. Sometimes referred to as the window period, this can last from 6 weeks to 3 months.

Rapid HIV antibody testing using oral fluid samples (e.g., OraQuick, Home Access HIV-1 Test System) is 99.5% accurate and provides results within 20 minutes, allowing immediate results to be given (CDC, 2013q; USPSTF 2013). In addition to the rapid results, this test may appeal to persons who fear having their blood drawn. If the test is positive, it requires a second specific confirmatory test.

Routine voluntary HIV testing is recommended for all adults ages 15 to 65 (USPSTF, 2013). Voluntary screening programs for HIV may be either confidential or anonymous; the process for each is unique. Confidential testing involves reporting by identifying the person's name and other identifying information; this information is considered protected by confidentiality. With anonymous testing, the client is given an identification code number that is attached to all records of the test results and is not linked to the person's name and address (CDC, 2013q). Demographic data such as the person's sex, age, and race may be collected, but there is no record of the client's name and associated identifying information. An advantage of anonymous testing may be that it increases the number of people who are willing to be tested, because many of those at risk are engaged in illegal activities. The anonymity eliminates their concern about the possibility of arrest or discrimination. However, anonymous testing does not allow for follow-up if the test is positive because the client's name and address are not available.

## Perinatal and Pediatric HIV Infection

Perinatal transmission accounts for nearly all HIV infection in children and can occur during pregnancy, labor and delivery, or breastfeeding. The effectiveness of antiretroviral therapy in pregnant women and newborns in preventing transmission from mother to fetus or infant has made pediatric HIV rates decline sharply. On the basis of the effectiveness of antiviral therapy, it is recommended that HIV testing be a routine part of prenatal care and that all pregnant women be tested for HIV—even a mother who presents in labor who is untested and whose HIV status is not known (USPSTF, 2013). Rapid testing allows rapid results in women who are giving birth, but have not been previously tested for HIV. HIV prevention in women must remain the primary focus of efforts to reduce pediatric HIV infection.

If left untreated, the clinical picture of pediatric HIV infection involves a shorter incubation period than in adults, and symptoms may occur within the first year of life. The physical signs and symptoms in children include failure to thrive, unexplained persistent diarrhea, developmental delays, and bacterial infections such as TB and severe pneumonia (WHO, 2010b).

Detection of HIV infection in infants of infected mothers is made through different tests from those used in children over 18 months. Virologic assays that directly detect HIV (e.g., nucleic acid amplification tests [NAT] such as HIV DNA, RNA polymerase chain reaction [PCR] assays, and related RNA qualitative or quantitative assays) must be used (Panel on Antiretroviral Therapy and Medical Management of HIV-Infected Children, 2014). The EIA test is not valid because it tests for antibodies, which in the infant reflect passively acquired maternal antibodies.

Despite having an HIV-infected mother, many children do not acquire HIV. However, one or both parents may die from HIV infection. The families of many children with AIDS are impoverished, with limited financial, emotional, social, and health care resources. The added strain of this illness makes many individuals and families unable to provide for the emotional, physical, and developmental needs of affected children.

## HIV Stage 3 (AIDS) in the Community

AIDS is a chronic disease, so individuals continue to live and work in the community. Persons with AIDS have bouts of illness interspersed with periods of wellness when they are able to return to school or work. When ill, much of their care is provided in the home. The nurse teaches families and significant others about personal care and hygiene, medication administration, standard precautions to ensure infection control, and healthy lifestyle behaviors such as adequate rest, balanced nutrition, and exercise.

Adherence to HAART is critical for clients because administration must be consistent to be effective (CDC, HRSA, NIH, et al., 2014). It is important for nurses to educate clients about accurate medication administration. Peer advocates and persons living with HIV infection who are trained to work with infected persons play a vital role in advocacy and teaching self-care management.

The Americans with Disabilities Act of 1990 and other laws protect persons with asymptomatic HIV infection and AIDS against discrimination in housing, at work, and in other public situations (USDJ, 2012). Policies regarding school and worksite attendance have been developed by most states and localities on the basis of these laws. These policies provide direction for the community's response when a person develops HIV infection. The nurse can identify resources such as social and financial support services and interpret school and work policies.

Mental health issues such as depression, substance abuse, and bipolar disorder are often present in someone newly diagnosed with HIV. These conditions must be addressed prior to or simultaneously with HIV treatment to be effective. It is vitally important that a variety of health and social services be available to support persons with HIV (CDC, HRSA, NIH, et al, 2014).

Nurses can assist employers by educating managers about how to deal with ill or infected workers to reduce the risk of breaching confidentiality or wrongful actions such as termination. Disclosing a worker's infection to other workers, terminating employment, and isolating an infected worker are examples of situations that have led to litigation between employees and employers. The CDC supports workplace issues through programs offered by its Business and Labor Resource Service. (See resources on the Evolve website at http://evolve.elsevier.com/Stanhope.)

HIV-infected children should attend school because the benefit of attendance far outweighs the risk of transmitting or acquiring infections. None of the cases of HIV infection in the United States have been transmitted in a school setting. An interprofessional team that includes the child's physician, the nurse, and the child's parent or guardian about educational and care needs.

Because of impaired immunity, chi are more likely to get childhood di sequellae. Therefore, DPT (diphther (inactivated polio virus), and MMR (measles, vaccines should be given at regularly scheduled times for dren infected with HIV. HiB (*Haemophilus influenzae* type B), hepatitis B, pneumococcus, and influenza vaccines may be recommended after medical evaluation (CDC, 2009a). Additionally the Panel on Opportunistic Infections in HIV-Exposed and HIV–Infected Children guidelines (2013) recommends meningococcal disease vaccination, as well as hepatitis A and varicella vaccination, provided that the infant or child is not severely immunocompromised.

Individual decisions about risk to the infected child or others should be based on the behavior, neurological development, and physical condition of the child. Attendance may be inadvisable in the presence of cases of childhood infections, such as chickenpox or measles, within the school, because the immunosuppressed child is at greater risk of suffering complications. Alternative arrangements, such as homebound instruction, might be instituted if a child is unable to control body secretions or displays biting behavior.

### Resources

As the number of individuals with HIV/AIDS has increased, services to meet these needs have grown. Voluntary and faith-based service organizations, such as community-based organizations or AIDS support organizations, have developed in many localities to address these needs. These services may include counseling, support groups, legal aid, personal care services, housing programs, and community education programs. Nurses collaborate with workers from community-based organizations in the client's home and may advise these groups in their supportive work. The federal government and many organizations have established toll-free numbers and websites to provide information, as noted on the Evolve website at http://evolve.elsevier.com/Stanhope.

## SEXUALLY TRANSMITTED DISEASES

The number of new cases (the **incidence**) of STDs such as gonorrhea, herpes simplex virus, human papillomavirus (HPV), and chlamydia continues to increase. Chlamydia is the most commonly reported infectious disease; gonorrhea is the second most common. Because of the impact of STDs on long-term health and the emergence of eight new STDs since 1980, continued attention to their prevention and treatment is vital.

The common STDs listed in Table 14-3 are categorized by cause, either viral or bacterial. The bacterial infections include gonorrhea, syphilis, and chlamydia. Most of these are curable with antibiotics, with the exception of the newly emerging antibiotic-resistant strains of gonorrhea.

STDs caused by viruses cannot be cured. These are chronic diseases resulting in a lifetime of symptom management and infection control. The viral infections include herpes simplex

## TABLE 14-3    Summary of Sexually Transmitted Diseases

| Disease/ Pathogen | Incubation | Signs and Symptoms | Diagnosis | Treatment | Nursing Implications |
|---|---|---|---|---|---|
| **Bacterial** | | | | | |
| Chlamydia: *Chlamydia trachomatis* | 3-21 days | *Man:* None or non-gonococcal urethritis (NGU); painful urination and urethral discharge; epididymitis<br>*Woman:* None or mucopurulent cervicitis (MPC), vaginal discharge; if untreated, progresses to symptoms of PID: diffuse abdominal pain, fever, chills | Nucleic acid amplification test (NAAT) of male urine and female endocervix | One of following treatments:<br>Doxycycline 100 mg PO bid × 7 days<br>Azithromycin 1 g PO × 1<br>Alternative regimens:<br>Erythromycin base 500 mg PO qid × 7 days<br>Erythromycin ethylsuccinate 800 mg PO qid × 7 days<br>Levofloxacin 500 mg PO, daily × 7 days<br>Ofloxacin 300 mg PO bid × 7 days<br>Doxycycline, effective and cheap<br>Azithromycin, good because single dose is sufficient | Refer partners of past 60 days; counsel client to use condoms and to avoid sex for 7 days after start of therapy and until symptoms are gone in both client and partners; medication teaching<br>Annual screening recommended for all sexually active women under 25, and women over 25 with new or multiple sexual partners |
| Gonorrhea: *Neisseria gonorrhoeae* | 3-21 days | *Man:* Urethritis, purulent discharge, painful urination, urinary frequency; epididymitis<br>*Woman:* None, or symptoms of PID | Nucleic acid amplification test (NAAT) | For uncomplicated gonorrhea:<br>Ceftriaxone 250 mg. IM PLUS EITHER<br>Azithromycin 1 gm PO × 1<br>OR<br>Doxycycline 100 mg PO qd × 7 days<br>If ceftriaxone not readily available, PO cefixime may be used in combination with doxycycline or azithromycin, but patient should return at one week for a test-of-cure at the site of infection | Refer partners of past 60 days; return for evaluation if symptoms persist; counsel client to use therapy until complete and symptoms are gone in both client and partners; medication teaching |
| Syphilis: *Treponema pallidum* | 10-90 days 6 weeks to 6 months<br>Within 1 year of infection<br>After 1 year from date of infection<br>*Late active:*<br>2-40 years<br>20-30 years<br>10-30 years | *Primary:* usually single, painless chancre; if untreated, heals in few weeks<br>*Secondary:* low-grade fever, malaise, sore throat, headache, adenopathy, and rash<br>*Early latency:* Asymptomatic, infectious lesions may recur<br>*Late latency:* Asymptomatic, noninfectious except to fetus of pregnant women<br>Gummas of skin, bone, mucous membranes, heart, liver<br>*CNS involvement:* Paresis, optic atrophy<br>*Cardiovascular involvement:* Aortic aneurysm, aortic value insufficiency | Visualization of pathogen on dark field microscopic examination; single painless ulcer (chancre); FTA-ABS or MHA-TP, VDRL (reactive 14 days after appearance of chancre)<br>Clinical signs of secondary syphilis<br>*VDRL:* FTA-ABS or MHA-TP<br>Lumbar puncture, CSF cell count, protein level determination and VDRL | Penicillin G 2.4 million units, IM once<br>If penicillin allergy:<br>Doxycycline 100 mg PO bid × 14 days (p.30)<br>Tetracycline 500 mg four times daily × 14 days<br>Tetracycline should not be administered to pregnant women or those with neurosyphilis or congenital syphilis<br>*Early syphilis:*<br>Ceftriaxone (1 g daily either IM or IV for 10-14 days)<br>Azythromomycin 2-g PO once<br>*Early latent:*<br>Benzathine penicillin G 2.4 million units IM in a single dose<br>*Late latent or latent:*<br>Benzathine penicillin G 7.2 million units total in three doses of 2.4 million units IM at 1-week intervals<br>*Tertiary:*<br>Benzthine penicillin G 7.2 million units total, in three doses of 2.4 million units IM each at 1-week intervals<br>In general, penicillins are prescribed in varying doses depending on diagnosis | Counsel to be tested for HIV; screen all partners of past 3 months; re-examine client at 3 and 6 months |

## TABLE 14-3   Summary of Sexually Transmitted Diseases—cont'd

| Disease/ Pathogen | Incubation | Signs and Symptoms | Diagnosis | Treatment | Nursing Implications |
|---|---|---|---|---|---|
| **Viral** | | | | | |
| Human immunodeficiency virus (HIV) | 4-6 weeks *Seroconversion:* 6 weeks to 3 months *AIDS:* month to years (average, 11 years) | *Possible:* Acute mononucleosis-like illness (lymphadenopathy, fever, rash, joint and muscle pain, sore throat) Appearance of HIV antibody *Opportunistic diseases:* Most commonly *Pneumocystis jiroveci* pneumonia, oral candidiasis, Kaposi's sarcoma | *HIV antibody test:* EIA or Western blot test; OraSure (SmithKline Beecham) is an oral HIV-1 antibody testing system, test results in about 3 days CD4+ T-lymphocyte count of less than 200/μl with documented HIV infection, or diagnosis with clinical manifestation of AIDS as defined by CDC | Prophylactic administration of zidovudine (ZDV) immediately after exposure may prevent seroconversion Post-exposure prophylaxis (PEP) should begin as soon as possible. Choice of antiviral drug therapy is made based on toxicity and drug resistance. Combinations of drugs are considered such as zidovudine (ZDV) and 3TC. Drug selection is complicated and evolving. Pre-exposure prophylaxis (PrEP) was approved in 2012, consisting of daily tenofovir disoproxil fumarate plus emtricitabine (TDF/FTC), for use among sexually active, at-risk adults. | HIV education and counseling; partner referral for evaluation; medication education; assessment and referral Men who have sex with men should be tested annually for HIV, chlamydia, syphilis, and gonorrhea |
| Genital warts: human papillomavirus (HPV) | 4-6 weeks most common; up to 9 months | Often subclinical infection; painless lesions near vaginal openings, anus, shaft of penis, vagina, cervix; lesions are textured, cauliflower appearance; may remain unchanged over time | Visual inspection for lesions; Pap smear; hybrid capture 2 HPV DNA test; colposcopy | Prevention: Gardasil vaccine No cure; one third of lesions will disappear without topical treatment Client-applied: topical podofilix 0.5% bid × 3 days, 4 days of no therapy; or imiquimod 5% cream daily at bedtime for up to 16 weeks Provider-administered: podophyllum resin 10%-25% or trichloroacetic acid 80%-90%; repeat weekly if needed; cryotherapy with liquid nitrogen, laser, or surgical removal | Education about HPV vaccine Warts and surrounding tissues contain HPV, so removal of warts does not completely eradicate virus; examination of partners not necessary, since treatment is only symptomatic; condom use may reduce transmission; medication application |
| Genital herpes simplex virus (HSV) | 2-20 days; average, 6 days | Vesicles, painful ulceration of penis, vagina, labia, perineum, or anus; lesions last 5-6 weeks and recurrence is common; may be asymptomatic | Presence of vesicles; viral culture (obtained only when lesions present and before they have scabbed over) | No cure; treatment may be episodic or suppressive for frequent recurrence *Episodic treatment:* acyclovir 400 mg PO tid × 7-10 days; OR Acyclovir 200 mg PO five times a day × 7-10 days; OR famciclovir 250 mg PO tid 7-10 days; or valacyclovir 1 g PO bid × 7-10 days | Refer partners for evaluation; teach client about likelihood of recurrent episodes and ability to transmit to others even if asymptomatic; condom use; annual Pap smear |

**From:** Centers for Disease Control and Prevention: Sexually Transmitted Diseases Treatment Guidelines, 2010. *MMWR Morb Mortal Wkly Rep* 59(RR-12), 2010.
Centers for Disease Control and Prevention: Update to CDC's Sexually Transmitted Diseases Treatment Guidelines 2010: Oral Cephalosporins no longer a recommended treatment for Gonococcal infections. *MMWR Morb Mortal Wkly Rep* 61(31), 2012.
Centers for Disease Control and Prevention: *Pre-exposure prophylaxis* (2013m). Available at: http://www.cdc.gov/hiv/prevention/research/prep/. Accessed March 12, 2014.
Centers for Disease Control and Prevention: Recommendations for the laboratory-based detection of *Chlamydia trachomatis* and *Neisseria gonorrhoeae. MMWR Morb Mortal Wkly Rep* 63(RR-2), 2014.

virus and human papillomavirus (HPV), also referred to as genital warts. The hepatitis A, B, and C viruses, which may also be transmitted via sexual activity, are discussed later in this chapter.

## Gonorrhea

*Neisseria gonorrhoeae* is a gram-negative intracellular diplococcal bacterium that infects the mucous membranes of the genitourinary tract, rectum, and pharynx. It is transmitted through genital–genital contact, oral–genital contact, and anal–genital contact.

Gonorrhea is identified as either uncomplicated or complicated. Uncomplicated gonorrhea refers to limited cervical or urethral infection. Complicated gonorrhea includes salpingitis, epididymitis, systemic gonococcal infection, and gonococcal meningitis. The signs and symptoms of infection in males are purulent and copious urethral discharge and dysuria. Symptoms in males are usually sufficient to seek treatment. Gonococcal infection in women however, is commonly asymptomatic, and treatment may not be sought. The disease will continue to be spread to others through sexual activity and may not be recognized until pelvic inflammatory disease (PID) occurs (CDC, 2010b).

Some individuals may continue to be sexually active and infect others while symptomatic. Co-infection with gonorrhea and chlamydia is common; therefore treatment containing ceftriaxone combined with either doxycycline or azithromycin is recommended (CDC, 2012g).

Reported gonorrhea rates are on the rise again after a long period of decline, particularly in the Northeast, Midwest, and West, although overall rates are still highest in the South (CDC, 2014b). The reported number of cases in the United States in 2012 was 334,826. The difference between the actual cases and reported cases occurs because gonorrhea may be unreported by health care providers, and because clients who are asymptomatic do not seek treatment and are therefore not identified. Groups with the highest incidence of gonorrhea are African Americans, persons living in the southern United States, and women 15 to 24 years of age (CDC, 2014b).

The number of antibiotic-resistant cases of gonorrhea in the United States has risen at an alarming rate. Penicillin-resistant gonorrhea was first identified in 1976 when 15 cases were reported (Phillips, 1976). By 1990, 64,972 resistant cases were reported (J. Blount, personal communication, January 18, 1991). Antibiotic-resistant *N. gonorrhoeae* has continued to develop exponentially, with gonorrhea becoming resistant to every antibiotic used for treatment, starting with penicillin and moving through sulfonamides, tetracycline, and fluoroquinolones, (CDC, 2013a). In 2012, the CDC revised its treatment guidelines and no longer recommended oral cephalosporins, specifically cefixime, as a first-line treatment for gonorrhea (CDC, 2012g), in an effort to preserve the last remaining treatment option (CDC, 2013a). At this time, combination therapy of ceftriaxone IM along with either oral doxycycline or azithromycin is the most reliably effective treatment for uncomplicated gonorrhea (CDC, 2012g). The injection route versus the previously recommended oral cefixime may make treatment more challenging due to patient fear of injection and health care facilities having to stock injectable medication (CDC, 2013a).

The increase in antibiotic-resistant infections is partially attributed to the indiscriminate or illicit use of antibiotics as a prophylactic measure by persons with multiple sexual partners. To ensure proper treatment and cure, those diagnosed with gonorrheal infection should return for health care if symptoms persist, have their partners of the previous 60 days evaluated for infection, and remain sexually abstinent until antibiotic therapy is completed (CDC, 2010b).

The development of PID is a risk for women who remain asymptomatic and do not seek treatment. PID is a serious infection involving the fallopian tubes (salpingitis) and is the most common complication of gonorrhea, but may also result from chlamydia infection. Its symptoms include fever, abnormal menses, and lower abdominal pain, but PID may not be recognized because the symptoms vary among women. PID can result in ectopic pregnancy and infertility related to fallopian tube scarring and occlusion. It may also cause stillbirths and premature labor (CDC, 2010b).

## Syphilis

Syphilis is caused by a member of the treponemal group of spirochetes called *Treponema pallidum*. It infects moist mucous or cutaneous membranes and is spread through direct contact, usually by sexual contact or from mother to fetus. Transmission via blood transfusion may occur if the donor is in the early stages of disease (Heymann, 2014).

Syphilis rates in the United States declined between 1990 and 2000, but then increased between 2001 and 2009. Rates increased again in 2012 (CDC, 2014d). The highest rates are among men having sex with men, but in recent years the number of infected women has increased.

The clinical signs of syphilis are divided into primary, secondary, and tertiary infections. Latency, a period when an individual is free of symptoms but has serologic evidence, may occur early or late in the infection. Latency that occurs during the first year of infection is called early latency. Late latency may occur after this first year. During latency, the possibility of relapse remains (CDC, 2010b).

### Primary Syphilis

When syphilis is acquired sexually, the bacteria produce infection in the form of a chancre at the site of entry. The lesion begins as a macula, progresses to a papule, and later ulcerates. If left untreated, this chancre persists for 3 to 6 weeks and then in most cases disappears (Heymann, 2014).

### Secondary Syphilis

Secondary syphilis occurs when the organism enters the lymph system and spreads throughout the body. Signs include rash, lymphadenopathy, and mucosal ulceration. Symptoms of secondary syphilis may include skin rash, lymphadenopathy, and lesions of the mucous membranes (CDC, 2010b).

## Tertiary Syphilis

Tertiary syphilis can lead to blindness, congenital damage, cardiovascular damage, or syphilitic psychoses. A further complication can be the development of lesions of the bones, skin, and mucous membranes, known as gummatous lesions. Tertiary syphilis usually occurs several years after initial infection and is rare in the United States because the disease is usually cured in its early stages with antibiotics. Tertiary syphilis is a major problem in developing countries.

## Congenital Syphilis

When primary and secondary syphilis rates increase, so do the rates of congenital syphilis (CS), which increased 23% in 2008 (CDC, 2010a). Syphilis is transmitted transplacentally and, if untreated, can cause premature stillbirth, blindness, deafness, facial abnormalities, crippling, or death. Signs include jaundice, skin rash, hepatosplenomegaly, or pseudoparalysis of an extremity. Treatment consists of penicillin given intravenously or intramuscularly (CDC, 2010a).

## Chlamydia

Chlamydia infection results from the bacterium *Chlamydia trachomatis*. It infects the genitourinary tract and rectum of adults and causes conjunctivitis and pneumonia in neonates. Transmission occurs when mucopurulent discharge from infected sites, such as the cervix or urethra, comes into contact with the mucous membranes of a noninfected person. Like gonorrhea, the infection is often asymptomatic in women, where up to 70% may experience no symptoms (Heymann, 2014). If left untreated, chlamydia can result in PID. When symptoms of chlamydial infection are present in women, they include dysuria, urinary frequency, and purulent vaginal discharge. In men, the urethra is the most common site of infection, resulting in non-gonococcal urethritis (NGU). The symptoms of NGU are dysuria and urethral discharge. Epididymitis is a possible complication (CDC, 2013p). The CDC recommends annual chlamydial screening of all sexually active women younger than 26 (CDC, 2014a). Older women with new or more than one sex partner and all pregnant women should also be tested (CDC, 2014g).

Chlamydia is the most common reportable infectious disease in the United States, and in 2012 a total of 1,422,976 cases of genital chlamydial infection were reported. Between 1992 and 2012, the rate of reported chlamydia infection increased from 182.3 to 456.7 cases per 100,000 population, reflecting increased screening rates, an emphasis on case reporting, and more sensitive testing (CDC, 2014a). Prevention is important because chlamydia can cause PID, ectopic pregnancy, infertility, and neonatal complications. Women under 25 years of age are the most commonly infected with chlamydial infection because of inconsistent use of barrier contraceptives, multiple sexual partners, and a history of infection with other STDs (CDC, 2014g). The high frequency of chlamydial infections in individuals infected with gonorrhea requires that effective treatment for both organisms be given when a gonorrheal infection is identified (CDC, 2010b).

## Herpes Simplex Virus (Genital Herpes)

Herpes simplex viruses (HSV-1 and HSV-2) cause genital herpes, and an increasing number of genital herpes infections are caused by HSV-1 (CDC, 2013c). The majority of genital herpes infections are caused by HSV-2, and these herpes infections are more likely to be recurrent (Buttaro, 2013).

As is true for other viral STDs, there is no cure for herpes infection, and it is considered a chronic disease. The virus is transmitted through direct exposure and infects the genitalia and surrounding skin. After the initial infection, the virus remains latent in the sacral nerve of the central nervous system and may reactivate periodically with or without visible vesicles.

Signs and symptoms of HSV infection include the presence of painful lesions that begin as vesicles and ulcerate and crust within 1 to 4 days. The first episode is typically longer and is usually characterized by more lesions than seen in subsequent infections. Lesions may occur on the vulva, vagina, upper thighs, buttocks, and penis and have an average duration of 11 days (Figure 14-3). The vesicles can cause itching and pain and may be accompanied by dysuria or rectal pain. Although the ability to pass the infection to others is higher with active lesions, some individuals can spread the virus even when they are asymptomatic. There can be a prodromal phase before lesions develop that includes tingling and paresthesia at the site (Heymann, 2014).

HSV-2 occurs in 16.2% of American adolescents and adults (CDC, 2013c). This prevalence is likely underrated because HSV-1 infections are rising, and a large number of people have no symptoms, thus HSV is difficult to identify. The consequences of genital herpes are of particular concern for women and their children. HSV-2 infection is linked with the development of cervical cancer. There is also an increased risk of fatal newborn infection during vaginal delivery with active lesions (Heymann, 2014). A pregnant woman who has active lesions at the time of giving birth should have a cesarean delivery before the rupture of amniotic membranes to avoid fetal contact with the herpetic lesions, whereas those who have no clinical evidence of herpes lesions should be delivered vaginally. A small number of infants are infected in utero. The clinical infection

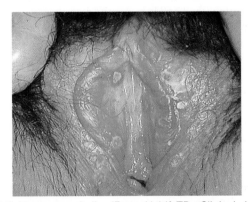

**FIG 14-3** Herpes genitalis. (From Habif TP: *Clinical dermatology: a color guide to diagnosis and therapy*, ed 5. St Louis, 2010, Mosby.)

in infants may present as liver disease, encephalitis, or infection limited to the skin, eyes, or mouth (Heymann, 2014).

## Human Papillomavirus Infection

Human papillomavirus (HPV) results in genital warts. Specific types of HPV cause cervical cancer, which is the second most common cancer worldwide (Heymann, 2014). HPV is the most common STD in the United States (CDC, 2014f). Transmission of HPV occurs through direct contact with warts that result from HPV and can infect the mouth, genitals, and anus. Genital warts are most commonly found on the penis and scrotum in men, and on the vulva, labia, vagina, and cervix in women. They appear as textured surface lesions, with what is sometimes described as a cauliflower appearance. The warts are usually multiple and vary between 1 mm to 1 cm in diameter. They may be difficult to visualize, so careful examination is required (Buttaro et al, 2013).

Since 2006, two FDA-licensed vaccines have been developed, bivalent and quadrivalent, both of which stimulate the immune system to block cancer-causing HPV infection before it occurs. The quadrivalent vaccine has the added benefit of preventing anogenital warts (CDC, 2014f). The recommended age for vaccination in both girls and boys is 11 to 12 years old, but it can be given in those aged 9 to 26 years old (CDC, 2014c). Complete vaccination coverage is an issue, however. In 2012, first dose vaccination rates for adolescent girls was low at 53.8%, and this dropped to 33.4% for all three doses. Experts recommend several strategies to increase vaccination rates in adolescent girls and boys, such as a reminder/recall system to increase vaccination rates and consideration of use of schools as a vaccination site. In some areas, requiring HPV vaccination for school entry has been successful, but this practice is not widely utilized to date (CDC, 2014f).

Once HPV infection occurs, the goal of therapy is to eliminate the warts. Genital warts spontaneously disappear over time, as do skin warts. However, because the condition is worrisome for the client and HPV may lead to the development of cervical neoplasia, treatment of the warts through surgical removal, laser therapy, or cytotoxic agents is often done (Buttaro, 2013).

Complications of HPV infection may be especially serious for women. The link between HPV infection and cervical cancer has been established and is associated with specific types of the virus. Other cancers attributed to HPV include vaginal, anal, and oropharyngeal (CDC, 2014f). Pap smears are vitally important because they allow for microscopic examination of cells to detect HPV, which can be surgically removed if detected early (Heymann, 2014). HPV infection is exacerbated in both pregnancy and immune-related disorders, which are believed to result from a decrease in cell-mediated immune functioning. HPV may infect the fetus during pregnancy and can result in a laryngeal papilloma that can obstruct the infant's airway. Genital warts may enlarge and become friable during pregnancy, and therefore surgical removal may be recommended. One challenge of HPV prevention is that condoms do not necessarily prevent infection. Warts may grow where barriers, such as condoms, do not cover and skin-to-skin contact may occur.

## HEPATITIS

Viral hepatitis refers to a group of infections that primarily affect the liver. These infections have similar clinical presentations but different causes and characteristics. Brief profiles of the types of hepatitis are presented in Table 14-4.

### Hepatitis A Virus

Hepatitis A virus (HAV) is most commonly transmitted through the fecal–oral route. Sources may be water, food, feces, or sexual contact. The virus level in the feces appears to peak 1 to 2 weeks before symptoms appear, making individuals highly contagious before they realize they are ill (Heymann, 2014).

The vaccine for hepatitis A infection has been available since 1995, and since that time the incidence has steadily declined (CDC, 2011). The vaccine makes HAV a completely preventable disease. Persons most at risk for HAV infection are travelers to countries with high rates of the disease, children living in areas with high rates of HAV infection, injection drug users, MSM, and persons with clotting disorders or chronic liver disease. Since routine childhood vaccination was recommended in 1996, the overall hepatitis A rate has declined 53%, from 2,979 cases reported in 2007 to 1,398 in 2011 (CDC, 2011).

Hepatitis A is found worldwide. In developing countries where sanitation is inadequate, epidemics are not common because most adults are immune from childhood infection. In countries with improved sanitation, outbreaks are common in daycare centers whose staff must change diapers, among household and sexual contacts of infected individuals, and among travelers to countries where hepatitis A is endemic. In many outbreaks, one individual is the source of an infection that may spread in the community. In other cases, hepatitis A is spread through food contaminated by an infected food-handler, contaminated produce, or contaminated water. The source of infection may never be identified in many outbreaks (Heymann, 2014).

The clinical course of hepatitis A ranges from mild to severe and often requires prolonged convalescence. Onset is usually acute, with fever, nausea, lack of appetite, malaise, and abdominal discomfort followed by jaundice after several days.

Vaccination and appropriate sanitation and personal hygiene remain the best means of preventing infection. The HAV vaccine is recommended for those who travel frequently or who spend long periods in countries where the disease is endemic. In cases of exposure through close contact with an infected individual or contaminated food or water, an injection of prophylactic immunoglobulin (IG) is indicated. IG should be given as soon as possible, but can be given within 2 weeks of exposure. Candidates for hepatitis A vaccine are listed in Box 14-2 (CDC, 2013d).

### Hepatitis B Virus

The number of new cases of hepatitis B virus (HBV) has steadily declined since HBV vaccination became available. In 2011 a total of 2,890 acute hepatitis B cases were reported, down 36% overall since 2007 (CDC, 2011). The groups with the highest prevalence are users of injection drugs, persons with

## TABLE 14-4  Viral Hepatitis Profiles

|  | Hepatitis A | Hepatitis B | Hepatitis C |
|---|---|---|---|
| Incubation period | Average, 28 days; range, 15-50 days | Average, 90 days; range, 60-150 days | Average, 45 days; range, 14-180 days |
| Mode of transmission | Fecal–oral, contaminated food/water, sexual | Bloodborne, sexual, perinatal | Primarily bloodborne; also sexual and perinatal |
| Incidence | Estimated number of new infections: 17,000 in 2010 in the United States. Reported in the U.S. in 2011: 1,398 | Estimated 38,000 cases/yr in United States in 2010. Reported in the U.S. in 2011: 2,890 | Estimated 16,500 cases/yr in United States in 2011. Reported in the U.S. in 2011: 1,229 |
| Chronic carrier state? | No | Yes, 5% of adult cases; 90% of infants; 25-50% of children aged 1-5 years | Yes, 75-85% or more of cases |
| Diagnosis | Serologic test (anti-HAV), viral isolation | Serologic tests (e.g. HBsAg), viral isolation | Serologic tests (anti-HCV) |
| Sequelae | No chronic infection | Chronic liver disease; liver cancer | Chronic liver disease; liver cancer |
| Vaccine availability | Yes, vaccination of all children at one year, children in areas of high disease rates recommended; travelers to endemic regions; men who have sex with men; injection and noninjection drug users. | Yes, vaccination of infants recommended; All children who have not been already immunized; individuals with exposure risks; men who have sex with men; people with end stage renal disease, people with HIV infection | No |
| Control and prevention | Good hygiene (e.g., handwashing); proper sanitation | Pre-exposure vaccination; reduce exposure risk behaviors | Screening of blood/organ donors; reduce exposure risk behaviors |

FROM: Centers for Disease Control and Prevention: *Viral hepatitis surveillance, United States*, 2011. Available at http://www.cdc.gov/hepatitis/Statistics/2011Surveillance/PDFs/2011HepSurveillanceRpt.pdf. Accessed February 13. 2014.
Centers for Disease Control and Prevention: *Hepatitis B FAQs for health professionals*, 2012a. Available at http://www.cdc.gov/hepatitis/HBV/HBVfaq.htm#overview. Accessed February 14. 2014.
Centers for Disease Control and Prevention: *Hepatitis A for health professionals: hepatitis A vaccination*, 2013d. Last updated. Available at http://www.cdc.gov/hepatitis/HAV/HAVfaq.htm#vaccine. Accessed February 14, 2014.
Centers for Disease Control and Prevention: *Hepatitis C information for health professionals: testing recommendations for chronic hepatitis C infection*, 2013e. Available at http://www.cdc.gov/hepatitis/hcv/guidelinesc.htm. Accessed February 17, 2014.

## BOX 14-2  Recommendations for Administration of Hepatitis A Vaccine or Ig After Exposure

- All household or sexual contacts of persons with HAV
- Persons who have shared illicit drugs with someone with HAV
- All staff and attendees of daycare centers if a case of HAV occurs among children or staff
- Household members whose children attend a daycare center where two or more families are infected
- Food-handlers who have a coworker infected with HAV; patrons in unhygienic situations or involvement where food is not heated

STDs or multiple sex partners, immigrants and refugees and their descendants who came from areas where there is a high endemic rate of HBV, health care workers, clients on hemodialysis, and inmates of long-term correctional institutions (Buttaro, 2013).

The HBV is spread through blood and body fluids and, like HIV, is a bloodborne pathogen. It has the same transmission properties as HIV, and thus individuals should take the same precautions to prevent spread of both HIV and HBV. A major difference is that HBV remains alive outside the body for a longer time than does HIV and thus has greater infectivity. The virus can survive for at least 1 week dried at room temperature on environmental surfaces, and thus infection control measures are paramount in preventing transmission from client to client (Heymann, 2014).

Infection with HBV results in either acute or chronic HBV infection. The acute infection is self-limited, and individuals develop an antibody to the virus and successfully eliminate the virus from the body. They subsequently have lifelong immunity against the virus. Symptoms range from mild, flu-like symptoms to a more severe response that includes jaundice, extreme lethargy, nausea, fever, and joint pain. Any of these more severe symptoms may result in hospitalization. A second possible outcome from infection is chronic HBV infection, which more likely occurs in persons with immunodeficiency (Heymann, 2014). Chronically infected individuals are unable to rid their bodies of the virus and remain lifelong carriers of the hepatitis B surface antigen (HBsAg). As carriers, they are able to transmit the HBV to others. They may develop hepatic carcinoma or chronic active hepatitis. The signs and symptoms of chronic hepatitis B include anorexia, fatigue, abdominal discomfort, hepatomegaly, and jaundice (Heymann, 2014).

Strategies for preventing HBV infection include immunization, prevention of nosocomial occupational exposure, and prevention of sexual and injection drug–use exposure. Vaccination is recommended for persons with occupational risk, such as health care workers, and for infants. The series of vaccines required for protection from HBV consists of three intramuscular injections, with the second and third doses administered 1 and 6 months after the first (CDC, 2014e). Pregnant women should be tested for HBsAg; if the mother is positive, newborns require hepatitis B immune globulin in addition to the hepatitis B vaccine within 12 hours of birth, and then at 1 and 6 months thereafter (CDC, 2014e). In instances in which the individual is not protected by vaccination and exposure to HBV occurs, hepatitis B immune globulin is given as soon as possible (within 24 hours is optimal) and the hepatitis B vaccine given (CDC, 2012a).

## OSHA Regulations

The Occupational Safety and Health Administration (OSHA) mandates specific activities to protect workers from HBV and other bloodborne pathogens. Potential exposures for health care workers are needlestick injuries and mucous membrane splashes. The OSHA standard requires employers to identify the risk of blood exposure to various employees. If employees perform work that involves a potential exposure to others' body fluids, employers are mandated to offer the HBV vaccine to the employee at the employer's expense, and to offer annual educational programs on preventing HBV and HIV exposure in the workplace. Employees have the right to refuse the vaccine. Employees may decline the vaccine for a variety of reasons including thinking they are not at risk since they are married or in a monogamous relationship, that the vaccine is too new to have adequate information about it, or that there may be side effects to the vaccine (CDC, 2013b).

## Hepatitis C Virus

Hepatitis C virus (HCV) infection is the most common chronic bloodborne infection in the United States (USPSTF, 2014). The HCV is transmitted when blood or body fluids of an infected person enter an uninfected person. Those groups at highest risk include health care workers and emergency personnel who are accidentally exposed, infants who are born to infected mothers, those born between 1945 and 1965 (CDC, 2012d), and 1-time or chronic injection drug users, particularly those who share needles or other drug-use equipment (Hande, 2014). Others at risk include hemodialysis patients (from dialysis equipment shared with infected persons) and recipients of donor organs and blood products before 1992 (USPSTF, 2014). The greatest risk factor is past or current injection drug use, with a hepatitis C prevalence rate of 50% (USPSTF, 2014).

During the 1980s, HCV spread rapidly. It is estimated that 2.7 to 3.9 million people are infected in the United States, and they are often unaware that they have hepatitis C. Although those born between 1945 and 1965 represent only 27% of the population, they account for a disproportionate 75% of all hepatitis C cases in the United States (CDC, 2012d). Chronic liver disease from hepatitis C is the most common indication for liver transplants, representing 30% of all transplants (USPSTF, 2014).

The clinical signs of hepatitis C may be so mild that an infected individual does not seek medical attention. The incubation period ranges from 2 weeks to 6 months. Clients may experience fatigue and other nonspecific symptoms. Although some have spontaneous resolution of the infection, 50% to 80% develop chronic liver disease. HCV infection may lead to cirrhosis or hepatocellular carcinoma (Heymann, 2014). Hepatitis C infection is related to about half of hepatocellular carcinoma cases, which have increased threefold (USPFTF, 2014).

Primary prevention of HCV infection includes screening of blood products and donor organs and tissue; risk reduction counseling and services, including obtaining injection drug use (IDU) history; and infection control practices. Secondary prevention strategies include testing of high-risk individuals, including those who seek HIV testing, and appropriate medical follow-up of infected clients. HCV testing should be offered to persons who received blood or an organ transplant before 1992; persons who have been on dialysis for many years; persons with signs and symptoms of liver disease; persons born between 1945 and 1965; and persons who received clotting factor before 1987. Routine testing for HCV is not recommended for health care workers, pregnant women, household contacts of HCV-positive persons, or the general population (CDC, 2013e).

## Non-ABC Hepatitis

Hepatitis viruses exist that are structurally unrelated to hepatitis A, B, or C. All are very uncommon in the United States, representing less than 5% of total cases (CDC, 2009b). Hepatitis D (HDV), called Delta hepatitis, can be acute or chronic and can only exist in people who are already infected with hepatitis B, either as a co-infection or as a superinfection. In the United States, between 1.5% and 7.2% of HBV cases had serologic evidence of HDV co-infection (CDC, 2009b). It is possible to become a chronic carrier in 70% to 80% of cases. Although there is no vaccination for HDV, infection can be prevented by being vaccinated for HBV (CDC, 2013f).

Hepatitis E virus (HEV) is an acute hepatitis infection that is transmitted through the fecal–oral route. Because it is not a chronic infection, one cannot become a chronic carrier for HEV. Although there is no hepatitis E vaccination, HEV can be prevented by protecting water systems from fecal contamination (CDC, 2012b).

Another type of hepatitis virus is hepatitis G (GB virus C). This type of virus has been isolated from patients with post-transfusion hepatitis, but has not been found to be the cause of either acute or chronic hepatitis (CDC, 2009b).

## TUBERCULOSIS

Tuberculosis is a mycobacterial disease caused by *Mycobacterium tuberculosis*. Transmission usually occurs through exposure to the tubercle bacilli in airborne droplets from persons with pulmonary tuberculosis who talk, cough, or sneeze. Common symptoms are cough, fever, hemoptysis, chest pains, fatigue, and weight loss. The incubation period is 4 to 12 weeks. The most critical period for development of clinical disease is the first 6 to 12 months after infection. About 5% of those initially infected may develop pulmonary tuberculosis or extrapulmonary involvement. The infection in about 95% of those initially infected becomes latent, but in about 10% of otherwise healthy individuals, it may be reactivated later in life. The chance of reactivation of latent infections increases in immunocompromised persons, substance abusers, underweight and undernourished persons, and persons with diabetes, silicosis, or gastrectomies (Heymann, 2014).

## Epidemiology

The WHO (2013) reported 8.6 million new cases of TB worldwide in 2012, and 1.3 million deaths due to TB. Prevalence is more difficult to determine, but WHO has reported 12 million prevalent cases in 2012, a number that has fallen dramatically since 1990. Worldwide, the Southeast Asia and Western Pacific Region accounts for 58% of the cases, and Africa accounts for 25% in 2012. India and China are the countries with the highest number of cases in the world (WHO, 2013). TB infection prevalence in Africa reflects the infection with HIV, where 37% of TB cases are co-infected with HIV (WHO, 2013). In the United States, the incidence of TB increased between 1985 and 1992, but since then has shown a steady rate of decline (CDC, 2013n). Of the new cases, 59% are foreign-born persons living in the United States, with Asians and Hispanics being the most common ethnic groups, representing 30% and 28% of national TB cases. Half of all new cases are concentrated in four states: New York, Florida, Texas, and California (CDC, 2013n). Table 14-5 shows TB case rates in the United States by race/ethnicity.

Worldwide, TB drug resistance is a significant issue. This can be caused by people not completing the full course of treatment, provider prescription error, poor quality drugs, or lack of TB drug availability. Types of drug-resistant TB include multidrug resistant TB (MDRTB), defined by resistance to rifampin and isoniazid, and extremely drug-resistant TB (XDRTB), which is MDRTB plus added resistance to fluoroquinolones and at least three injectable second-line drugs (e.g., amikacin, kanamycin, and capreomycin) (WHO, 2013). Drug-resistant TB is a significant concern to people with weak immune systems, such as HIV-infected individuals.

To prevent TB, the CDC works with public health agencies in other countries to improve screening and reporting of cases and to improve treatment strategies. This includes coordination of treatment for infected individuals who migrate to the United States. This coordination is particularly significant between Mexico and the United States (WHO, 2013).

### TABLE 14-5 U.S. Tuberculosis (TB) Case Rates by Ethnicity and Sex, 2012

| Ethnicity/Sex | Number of Cases | TB Case Rate Per 100,000 |
|---|---|---|
| Asian | 2,957 | 18.9 |
| Native Hawaiian/other Pacific Islander | 64 | 12.3 |
| Black/African American | 2,234 | 5.8 |
| Hispanic/Latino | 2,790 | 5.3 |
| American Indian/Alaska Native | 146 | 6.3 |
| White | 1,572 | 0.8 |
| Multiple Race | 148 | 2.5 |
| Female | 3,914 | 2.5 |
| Male | 6,028 | 3.9 |
| Total population | 9,945 | 3.2 |

Fr: Centers for Disease Control and Prevention: *Reported tuberculosis in the United States, 2012.* Atlanta: U.S. Department of Health and Human Services, CDC, October, 2013. Available at http://www.cdc.gov/tb/statistics/reports/2012/pdf/report2012.pdf.

## Diagnosis and Treatment

The standard and preferred TB screening test is the Mantoux tuberculin skin test (TST) (CDC, 2012f). The TST, previously referred to as the purified protein derivative (PPD) test, is used for initial screening. It can be followed by chest radiography for persons with a positive skin reaction and pulmonary symptoms. Persons who are immunosuppressed by drugs or who have diseases such as advanced tuberculosis, measles, or chicken pox may not have the ability to mount an immune response to the TST, so the result may be a false-negative skin test reaction resulting from cutaneous anergy (nonreaction due to weakened immune system). A second issue with the TST is that a positive result may come from an earlier TST or BCG vaccination boosting one's ability to respond to the infection, and not reflecting a recent infection. Therefore, it is difficult to determine if the infection is old or recent. A blood test (in vitro gamma release interferon assays or IVGRA) is available and is increasingly used for providing clinical care in lieu of the TST (CDC, 2012e; Buttaro, 2013). One example is the QuantiFeron-TB blood test to detect *M. tuberculosis* infection. Diagnosis can also be made through stained sputum smears and other body fluids to determine the presence of acid-fast bacilli (for presumptive diagnosis), and culture of the tubercle bacilli for definitive diagnosis. The following How To box describes how to read a TST.

---

**HOW TO How to Perform a Tuberculin Skin Test (TST)**

**Apply and Read the TST**
- *For the Mantoux test, inject 0.1 mL containing 5 tuberculin units of purified protein derivative PPD tuberculin.*
- *Read the reaction 48 to 72 hours after injection.*
- *Measure only induration, not redness.*
- *Record results in millimeters.*

**Interpret the TST (Buttaro, 2013)**

*Test is positive if the induration is greater than or equal to 5 mm in the following:*
- *Immunosuppressed clients*
- *Persons known to have HIV infection*
- *Persons whose chest radiograph is suggestive of previous TB that was untreated*
- *Close contacts of a person with infectious TB*
- *Organ transplant recipients*
  *Test is positive if the induration is greater than or equal to 10 mm in the following:*
- *Persons with certain medical conditions, such as diabetes, alcoholism, or drug abuse*
- *Persons who inject drugs (if HIV negative)*
- *Foreign-born persons from areas where TB is common*
- *Children under 4 years old*
- *Residents and staff of long-term care facilities, jails, and prisons*
  *Test is positive if the induration is greater than or equal to 15 mm in the following:*
- *All persons more than 4 years of age with no risk factors for TB*

---

(CDC, 2003; CDC, 2012e; Buttaro, 2013)
Fr: Heymann D: Control of Communicable Diseases Manual, Washington, DC, 2008, American Public Health Association.

Clients with TB should be treated promptly with the appropriate combination of multiple antimicrobial drugs. Effective drug regimens used in the United States include isoniazid, and in some instances, rifampin. Treatment regimens for persons with active symptomatic infection may be different from the regimens used for persons with latent TB infection or with HIV (Buttaro, 2013). Treatment failure may be due to clients' poor adherence in taking the medication, which can result in drug resistance. Nurses usually administer TSTs and provide education on the importance of compliance to long-term therapy. They may also be involved in directly observed therapy (DOT) and contact investigations of cases in the community.

## NURSE'S ROLE IN PROVIDING PREVENTIVE CARE FOR COMMUNICABLE DISEASES

From prevention to treatment, the nurse functions as a counselor, educator, advocate, case manager, and primary care provider. Appropriate interventions for primary, secondary, and tertiary prevention are reviewed in the following sections (see Levels of Prevention box). In the following discussion of primary prevention, the nursing process is applied to the care of clients with communicable diseases. Nurses are in an ideal position to affect the outcomes of communicable diseases, and their influence begins with primary prevention.

### LEVELS OF PREVENTION

**Primary Prevention**
- Provide community education about prevention of communicable diseases to well populations.
- Vaccinate for hepatitis A virus (HAV) or hepatitis B virus (HBV).
- Provide community outreach for education and needle exchange.

**Secondary Prevention**
- Administer tuberculin skin test (TST).
- Test and counsel for human immunodeficiency virus (HIV).
- Notify partners and trace contacts.

**Tertiary Prevention**
- Educate caregivers of persons with HIV about standard precautions.
- Maintain long-term directly observed therapy (DOT) for tuberculosis treatment.
- Identify community resources for providing supportive care (e.g., funds for purchasing medications).
- Set up support groups for persons with genital herpes.

### Primary Prevention

Primary prevention consists mainly of activities to keep people healthy before the onset of disease. This begins with assessing for risk behavior and providing relevant intervention through education on how to avoid infection, mostly through healthy behaviors.

### Assessment

To assess the risk of acquiring an infection, the nurse takes a history that focuses on risk behaviors and potential exposure, which varies with the specific organism by its mode of transmission. The specific questions that must be asked can be

especially challenging when STDs are the object of the study. In these situations, the nurse should obtain a sexual and IDU history for clients and their partners. The sexual history provides information that leads to the need for specific diagnostic tests, treatment modalities, and partner notification. It also facilitates evaluation of risk factors and is necessary for the nurse to be able to provide relevant education for the client's lifestyle.

Assessing a client's risk of acquiring an STD should be done with all sexually active individuals. Such risk assessments should be included as baseline assessment data for those attending all clinics and those who receive school health, occupational health, public health, and home nursing services.

A thorough sexual history requires obtaining personal and sensitive information. It includes information about the types of relationships, the number of sexual partners and encounters, and the types of sexual behaviors practiced. The confidential nature of the information and how it will be used should be shared with the client to establish open communication and goal-directed interaction. Most clients feel uneasy disclosing such personal information. The nurse can ease this discomfort by remaining supportive and open during the interview to facilitate honesty about intimate activities. The nurse serves as a model for discussing sensitive information in a candid manner. When discussing precautions, direct and simple language should be used to describe specific behaviors. This encourages the client to openly discuss sexuality during this interaction and with future partners.

Nurses who are uncomfortable discussing topics such as sexual behavior or sexual orientation are likely to avoid assessing risk behaviors with the client. They will, consequently, be ineffective in identifying risks and helping clients modify risky behaviors. Nurses need to be adept at helping clients prevent and control STDs. Nurses can gain confidence in conducting sexual risk assessments by understanding their own values and feelings about sexuality and realizing that the purpose of the interaction is to improve the client's health. The nurse's comfort in discussing sexual behavior can be improved by using role playing to practice assessments of sexual and IDU behavior, and by contracting with clients to make behavior changes.

Identifying the number of sexual and injection drug–using partners and the number of contacts with these partners provides information about the client's risk. The chance of exposure decreases as the number of partners decreases, so people in mutually monogamous relationships are at low risk for acquiring STDs. You can gather this information by asking, "How many sex (or drug) partners have you had over the past 6 months?" Try to avoid basing assumptions about the sexual partner or partners on the client's sex, age, ethnicity, or any other factor. Stereotypes and assumptions about who people are and what they do are common problems that keep interviewers from asking the questions that lead to obtaining useful information. For example, it should not be taken for granted that a homosexual man always has more than one partner. Be aware also that the long incubation of HIV and the subclinical phase of many STDs lead some monogamous individuals to assume erroneously that they are not at risk.

## EVIDENCE-BASED PRACTICE

Vaccination to prevent transmission of HPV has been recommended for several years for young men as well as women, with primary vaccination recommended for boys at 11-12 years and secondary vaccination to catch those never vaccinated through age 26. There is an emphasis on vaccination because half of new HPV infections occur in young people between the ages of 15 and 24.

In this study, nurse researchers surveyed 735 male college students (ages 18-25) who were sexually active (previously or currently) with men, women, or both, and examined their vaccination rates, personal perceptions of risk for sexually transmitted infections, and barriers to vaccination. Researchers collected both quantitative and qualitative data from the student participants, consisting of demographic data, vaccination rates, data about sexual practices, and qualitative data about perspectives on the HPV vaccination, such as why they had not received it, or why they may not have completed the three-dose vaccination.

The researchers found that, although the student participants engaged in risky sexual practices such as high number of lifetime sexual partners (mean 6.3) and over half either never using condoms (10%) or sometimes using condoms (41%), 93% of participants did not view themselves as being at risk for sexually transmitted infections. Multivariate analysis revealed that participants who always wore condoms were more likely to have received the vaccine, and the older the participant was, the less likely he was to have received the vaccine.

Quantitative data about the HPV vaccination focused on barriers to obtaining the vaccine, such as cost and inconvenience. Many participants had not heard of either HPV itself or the vaccine, or did not know that men could get the vaccine. The male participants also did not know about the link between oropharyngeal cancer and HPV for men, and only some participants knew about the link between cervical cancer and HPV for women.

### Nurse Use

This study highlights the importance of education and awareness about HPV and the HPV vaccination for both men and women. Nurses can play a large role in information dissemination and vaccination promotion effort.

Fontenot HB, Fantasia HC, Charyk A, et al: Human papillomavirus (HPV) risk factors, vaccination patterns, and vaccine perceptions among a sample of male college students. *Journal of American College Health* 62(3):186–192, 2014. DOI: 10.1080/07448481.2013.872649.

It is important to identify whether the person has sexual contact with men, women, or both. This information can be obtained by simply asking, "Do you have sex with men, women, or both?" This lets the client know that the nurse is open to hearing about these behaviors, and thus the nurse is more likely to obtain information that is relevant to sexual practices and risk. Women who are exclusively lesbian are at low risk for acquiring STDs, but bisexual women may transmit STDs between male and female partners. In addition, it is possible for men to have sexual contact with other men and not label themselves as homosexual. Therefore, education to reduce risk that is aimed at homosexual men will not be heeded by men who do not see themselves as homosexual. In such situations the nurse can ask, "When was the last time you had sex with another man?"

Certain sexual practices are more likely to result in exposure to and transmission of STDs. Dangerous sexual activities include all unprotected intercourse (anal, oral, or vaginal), oral–anal contact, and insertion of finger or fist into the rectum.

These practices introduce a high risk of transmission of enteric organisms or result in physical trauma during sexual encounters. The nurse can obtain information about sexual encounters by asking, "Can you tell me the kinds of sexual practices in which you engage? This will help determine what risks you may have and the type of tests we should do." Clients who engage in genital–anal, oral–anal, or oral–genital contact will need throat and rectal cultures for some STDs as well as cervical and urethral cultures.

### HOW TO  How to Effectively Obtain a Client's Sexual History

*To be most effective, the nurse obtaining a client's sexual history should do the following:*
- *Remain supportive and open to facilitate honesty.*
- *Use terms the client will understand (be prepared to suggest multiple terms).*
- *Speak candidly so the client will feel comfortable talking.*
- *Ask open-ended questions in a nonthreatening and nonjudgmental manner.*
- *Acknowledge that many people are uneasy disclosing personal information.*
- *Use the Five P's Approach (CDC, 2010b). Sample questions in each category are:*
  - *Partners: "In the past 2 months, how many partners have you had sex with?"*
  - *Prevention of pregnancy: "What are you doing to prevent pregnancy?"*
  - *Protection from STDs: "What do you do to protect yourself from STDs and HIV?"*
  - *Practices: "To understand your risk for STDs, I need to understand the kind of sex you've had recently."*
  - *Past history of STDs: "Have you ever had an STD?"*

Drug use is linked to STD transmission in several ways. Drugs such as alcohol put people at risk because they can lower inhibitions and impair judgment about engaging in risky behaviors. Addictions to drugs may cause individuals to acquire the drug or money to purchase the drug through sexual favors. This increases both the frequency of sexual contacts and the chances of contracting STDs. Thus, the nurse should obtain information on the type and frequency of drug use and the presence of risk behaviors.

The administration of immunizations is another example of primary prevention, because they prevent infection. Of the diseases presented here, vaccines are available for human papillomavirus and hepatitis A and B.

### Interventions

Interventions to prevent infection are aimed at preventing specific infections. These interventions can take several forms and include things such as education on how to prevent infection or the availability of vaccines. For example, on the basis of the information obtained in the sexual history and risk assessment just described, the nurse can identify specific education and counseling needs of the client. The nursing interventions focus on contracting with clients to change behavior and reduce their risk in regard to sexual practice.

## Sexual Behavior

Sexual abstinence is the best way to prevent STDs. However, for many people, sexual abstinence is not realistic and providing instruction about how to make sexual behavior safer is critical. Safer sexual behavior includes masturbation, dry kissing, touching, fantasy, and vaginal and oral sex with a condom.

If used correctly and consistently, properly fitted condoms can prevent both pregnancy and most STDs because they prevent the exchange of body fluids during sexual activity. Condom failure may occur from incorrect use rather than condom failure. Thus, information about proper use and how to communicate about them with a partner is also necessary. The nurse has many opportunities to convey this information during counseling. Most agency protocols recommend the use of latex condoms. Some may be lubricated with nonoxynol-9, a spermicide. If used frequently, nonoxynol-9 may result in genital lesions, which may provide openings for viruses to enter the body.

Condom use may be viewed as inconvenient, messy, or decreasing sensation. Moreover, alcohol consumption may accompany sexual activity, which may also decrease condom use. The nurse can help clients become more skilled in discussing safer sex through role modeling and practicing communication skills through role play. Role-playing scenarios with partners who are reluctant to use condoms can help individuals prepare for situations before they occur.

Female condoms are a barrier to body fluid contact and therefore protect against pregnancy and STDs. The main advantage of the female condom is that its use is controlled by the woman. The FC2 Female Condom is the only female condom that is FDA approved for use in the United States. Since it is made of nitrile it is also useful if a latex sensitivity develops to male condoms. Symptoms of latex allergy include penile, vaginal, or rectal itching or swelling after use of a male condom or diaphragm. The female condom consists of a sheath over two rings, with one closed end that fits over the cervix. The condoms are often free at public health clinics, or can be purchased in boxes of multiple condoms, making the overall cost per condom less than $1.50 each. Figure 14-4 provides instructions on its insertion.

Clients should understand the importance of knowing the risk behavior of their sexual partners, including a history of IDU and STDs, sexual preference, and any current symptoms. Each sexual partner is potentially exposed to all the STDs of all the persons with whom the other partner has been sexually active.

## Drug Use

IDU is risky because the potential for injecting bloodborne pathogens, such as HIV, HBV, and HCV exists when needles and syringes are shared. During IDU, small quantities of drugs are repeatedly injected. Blood is withdrawn into the syringe and is then injected back into the user's vein. Individuals should be advised against using injectable drugs and sharing needles, syringes, or other drug paraphernalia (a.k.a. works) (CDC, 2014i). If equipment is shared, it should be in contact with full-strength bleach for 30 seconds, and then rinsed with water

**1** Use your thumb and middle finger, and squeeze the ring toward the bottom so that it becomes thin and narrow. If you squeeze the inner ring near the top, when you insert it, your hand will be in the way.

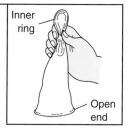

**2** Push the inner ring into your vaginal canal, behind your pubic bone. You will feel the female condom slide into place. IF you can feel the inner ring, or IF it causes any pain or discomfort, the ring is not up high enough near the cervix. Don't worry, you can't push it too far inside.

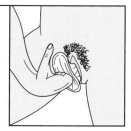

**3** Next, take your index finger, put it inside the condom, and push the condom up higher into the vagina. This way, the outer ring will be closer to the outside of your vagina. YES, it has to be on the outside of you, because HE has to go inside the condom.

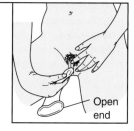

**4** The condom is in place.
Be sure that:
• Your partner puts his penis inside of the female condom
• Enough lubricant so the penis slips easily inside and out
• A new female condom for each sex act

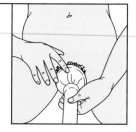

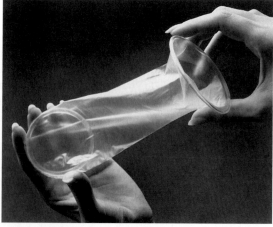

FIG 14-4 Insertion and positioning of the female condom. (Reproduced from The Female Health Company, Chicago, IL.)

several times to prevent injecting bleach (CDC, 2004). This is a last-resort option.

People who inject drugs are difficult to reach for health care services. Effective outreach programs include using community peers, increasing accessibility of drug treatment programs combined with HIV testing and counseling, and encouraging long-term repeat contacts after completion of the program.

## Community Outreach

Because of the illegal nature of injectable drugs and the poverty associated with HIV, many people at risk have neither the inclination nor the resources to seek health care. Nurses may work to establish programs within communities because the opportunities for counseling on the prevention of HIV and other STDs are increased by bringing services into the neighborhoods of those at risk. Workers go into communities to disseminate information on safer sex, drug treatment programs, and discontinuation of drug use or safer drug use practices (e.g., using new needles and syringes with each injection). Some programs provide sterile needles and syringes, condoms, and literature about testing services.

## Community Education

Education of well populations about prevention of communicable diseases by a nurse educator is an example of primary prevention. Relevant information about the modes of transmission, testing, availability of vaccines, and early symptoms can be provided to groups in the community. Providing accurate health information to large numbers of people is vital for preventing the spread of STDs. Nurses can provide educational sessions to community groups about HIV and other STDs. Such educational sessions are most effective in settings where groups normally meet and may include schools, businesses, and churches.

When addressing groups about HIV infection, it is important to discuss the number of people infected with HIV, the number of people living with AIDS, modes of transmission of the virus, how to prevent infection, testing services, common symptoms of illness, the need for a compassionate response to those afflicted, and available community resources. Teaching about other STDs can be incorporated into these presentations because the mode of transmission (sexual contact) is the same. Other information on these diseases can include the distribution and incidence in society, and the consequences of the infection for individuals and families.

## Evaluation

Evaluation is based on the extent of vaccination within a population, whether risky behavior has changed to safe behavior, and, ultimately, whether illness is prevented. Condom use can be evaluated for consistency of use if the client is sexually active. Other behaviors, such as abstinence or monogamy, can be evaluated for their implementation. At the community level, behavioral surveys can be done to measure reported condom use and condom sales, and measures of disease incidence and prevalence can be calculated to evaluate the effectiveness of intervention.

## Secondary Prevention

Secondary prevention includes screening for diseases to ensure their early identification, treatment, and follow-up with contacts to prevent further spread. In general, client teaching and counseling should include education about avoiding self-reinfection, managing symptoms, and preventing the infection of others.

## Testing and Counseling for HIV

Universal testing for HIV infection should be routine for all clients aged 15 to 65 years (USPSTF, 2013). Younger adolescents and older adults who are at increased risk should be screened as well (CDC, 2013q; USPSTF, 2013). Therefore, routine HIV testing should be a part of all annual physicals, labs for every pregnancy, and all hospital visits, without securing special permission. Clients can decline or "opt out" of HIV testing, but the benefits of testing are considerable. For persons who have engaged in high-risk behavior, the nurse should recommend annual HIV testing (Box 14-3). Individuals with the following characteristics are considered at risk and should be offered HIV testing: those with a history of STDs (which are transmitted through the same behavior and may decrease immune functioning), multiple sex partners, or IDU; those who have unprotected intercourse (i.e., without using a condom or pre-exposure prophalyaxis [PrEP]) (CDC, 2013m); those who have intercourse with someone who has another partner and those who have had sex with a prostitute; men with a history of homosexual or bisexual activity; and those who have been a sexual partner to anyone in one of these groups.

Testing enables clients to benefit from early detection and treatment, as well as risk reduction education. If HIV infection is discovered before the onset of symptoms, early monitoring of the disease process and CD4 lymphocyte counts or viral loads is indicated. In addition, prophylactic therapy with antiretroviral therapy and/or antibiotics may begin in order to delay the onset of symptomatic illness.

### BOX 14-3 Who Should Be Advised to Receive HIV Testing and Counseling?

For clients in all health care settings:
- HIV screening is recommended for clients in all health care settings after the client is notified that testing will be performed unless the patient declines (opt-out screening).
- Persons at high risk for HIV infection should be screened for HIV at least annually.
- Separate written consent for HIV testing should not be required; general consent for medical care should be considered sufficient to encompass consent for HIV testing.
- Prevention counseling should not be required with HIV diagnostic testing or as part of HIV screening programs in health care settings.

For pregnant women:
- HIV screening should be included in the routine panel of prenatal screening tests for all pregnant women.
- HIV screening is recommended after the client is notified that testing will be performed unless the client declines (opt-out screening).
- Separate written consent for HIV testing should not be required; general consent for medical care should be considered sufficient to encompass consent for HIV testing.
- Repeat screening in the third trimester is recommended in certain jurisdictions with elevated rates of HIV infection among pregnant women.

From Centers for Disease Control and Prevention: Revised recommendations for HIV testing of adults, adolescents, and pregnant women in health-care settings, *MMWR Morbid Mortal Wkly Rep* 55(RR-14), 2006.

---

**BOX 14-4    Responsibilities of Persons Who Are HIV Infected**

- Have regular medical evaluations and follow-ups.
- Do not donate blood, plasma, body organs, other tissues, or sperm.
- Take precautions against exchanging body fluids during sexual activity.
- Inform sexual or injection drug–using partners of the potential exposure to HIV, or arrange for notification through the health department.
- Inform health care providers of the HIV infection.
- Consider the risk of perinatal transmission and follow up with contraceptive use.

---

*Post-test Counseling.* Persons who have a negative test should be counseled about risk reduction activities to prevent any future transmission. Clients should understand that the test may not be truly negative because it does not reveal infections that may have been acquired within the several weeks before the test. Evidence of HIV antibody takes from 6 to 12 weeks to develop. Newer immunoassay tests can produce results in as little as three weeks (CDC, 2013q)

Clients must be aware of the ways viral transmission occurs, and how to avoid infection. All clients who are antibody positive should be counseled about the need to reduce their risks and notify partners. If the client is unwilling or hesitant to notify past partners, the nurse will do partner notification (or contact tracing), as described later in this chapter. Clients should seek treatment from their primary health care provider so physical evaluation can be performed and, if indicated, antiviral or other therapies begun. Box 14-4 describes the responsibilities of individuals who are HIV positive.

Psychosocial counseling is indicated when positive HIV test results precipitate acute anxiety, depression, or suicidal ideation. The client should be informed about available counseling services. The person should be cautioned to consider carefully who should be informed of the test results. Many individuals have told others about their HIV-positive test, only to experience isolation and discrimination. Plans for the future should be explored, and clients should be advised to avoid stress, drugs, and infections in order to maintain optimal health.

### Partner Notification and Contact Tracing

Partner notification, also known as contact tracing or disclosure, is an example of a population-level intervention aimed at controlling communicable diseases. Partner notification programs usually occur in conjunction with reportable disease requirements and are carried out by most health departments. It involves confidentially identifying and notifying exposed individuals of clients who are found to have reportable diseases, especially sexually transmitted diseases.

Individuals diagnosed with a reportable STD are asked to provide the names and locations of all partners so that these individuals can be informed of their exposure, receive counseling, and obtain the necessary referral and/or treatment. The originally diagnosed (index case) clients may be encouraged to notify their partners (can be sexual and/or injection drug partners) and to encourage them to seek treatment. If the client agrees to do so, suggestions on how to inform their partners

---

**▶▶ LINKING CONTENT TO PRACTICE**

This chapter emphasizes the epidemiology and prevention of selected communicable diseases, as well as the public health nursing services provided to clients. The Council on Linkages Between Academia and Public Health Practice (2010) Domains and Core Competencies are addressed through activities in caring for clients with communicable diseases. Examples of how these eight domains are used in providing nursing care to clients with communicable disease are as follows:

*Domain #1, Analytic/Assessment Skills,* is achieved through the review of the incidence and prevalence rates of communicable diseases to determine population health status.

*Domain #3, Communication Skills,* is applied when PHNs teach how to prevent and treat infections.

*Domain #4, Cultural Competency Skills,* is met through understanding the various social and behavioral factors that make health care acceptable to diverse populations (groups of people who are diverse in terms of culture, socioeconomic status, education level, race, gender, age, ethnicity, sexual orientation, profession, religious affiliation, and mental/physical capability).

From Public Health Foundation, Council on Linkages: *Core Competencies for Public Health Professionals,* 2008. Available at http://www.phf.org/link/corecompetencies.htm. Accessed March 2010.

---

and how to deal with possible reactions may be explored. In some instances, clients may feel more comfortable if the nurse notifies those who are exposed. If clients contact their partners about possible infection, the nurse contacts health care providers or clinics to verify positive test results or microscopic findings and treatment of the index case.

If the originally diagnosed client prefers not to participate in notifying partners, the public health nurse contacts the partners by phone, certified delivery letter, or home visit, depending on the nature of the individual circumstances, and counsels them to seek evaluation and treatment. Many times the client is treated for the sexually transmitted infection at the health department. At this appointment, the client is offered literature regarding the STD for which they need treatment, receives risk-reduction counseling, and is offered testing for the other STDs. The identity of the infected client who names sexual and injection drug–using partners cannot be revealed. Maintaining confidentiality is critical with all STDs.

### Tertiary Prevention

Tertiary prevention can apply to many of the chronic viral STDs and TB. For viral STDs, much of this effort focuses on managing symptoms and maintaining psychosocial support. Many clients report feeling contaminated and thus feel lower self-worth. Support groups may be available to help clients cope with chronic STDs, such as genital herpes or genital warts.

### Directly Observed Therapy

In **directly observed therapy** (DOT) programs for TB medication nurses observe and document individual clients taking their TB drugs. When clients prematurely stop taking TB medications, there is a risk of the TB becoming resistant to the medications. This can affect an entire community of people who are susceptible to this airborne disease. Health professionals share in the responsibility of adhering to treatment, and

DOT ensures that TB-infected clients have adequate medication. Thus, DOT programs are aimed at the population level to prevent antibiotic resistance in the community and to ensure effective treatment at the individual level. Many health departments have DOT home health programs to ensure adequate treatment (CDC, 2012c). Directly observed treatment, short course (DOTS) is a variation applied worldwide to combat multidrug-resistant TB (WHO, 2010a).

The management of AIDS in the home may include monitoring physical status and referring the family to additional care services for maintaining the client in the home. Case management is important in all phases of HIV infection. It is especially important to ensure that clients have adequate services to meet their needs. This may include ensuring that medication can be obtained through identifying funding resources, maintaining infection control standards, reducing risk behaviors, identifying sources of respite care for caretakers, or referring clients for home or hospice care. Nursing interventions include teaching families about managing symptomatic illness by preventing deteriorating conditions such as diarrhea, skin breakdown, and inadequate nutrition.

### Standard Precautions

It is important to teach caregivers about infection control in the home. Clients, families, friends, and others may express concerns about the transmission of HIV. Whereas fear may be expressed by some, others who are caring for loved ones with HIV may not take adequate precautions, such as glove wearing, because of concern about appearing as though they do not want to touch a loved one. Others may believe myths that suggest they cannot be infected by someone they love.

Standard precautions must be taught to caregivers in the home setting. All blood and articles soiled with body fluids must be handled as if they were infectious or contaminated by bloodborne pathogens. Gloves should be worn whenever hands might touch nonintact skin, mucous membranes, blood, or other fluids. A mask, goggles, and gown should also be worn if there is potential for splashing or spraying of infectious material during any care. All protective equipment should be worn only once and then disposed of. If the skin or mucous membranes of the caregiver come in contact with body fluids, the skin should be washed with soap and water, and the mucous membranes should be flushed with water as soon as possible after the exposure. Thorough handwashing with soap and water—a major infection control measure—should be conducted whenever hands become contaminated and whenever gloves or other protective equipment (e.g., mask, gown) is removed. Soiled clothing or linen should be washed in a washing machine filled with hot water using bleach as an additive and dried on a hot-air cycle of a dryer.

## PRACTICE APPLICATION

Yvonne Jackson is a 20-year-old woman who visits the Hopetown City Health Department's maternity clinic. Examination reveals she is at 14-weeks' gestation. She is single but has been in a steady relationship for the past 6 months with Ramón. She states that she has no other children. A routine test taken during the initial prenatal visit is an HIV test; the results are positive.

Ms. Jackson is shocked and emotionally distraught about the positive test results. Understanding that the client will not be able to concentrate on all of the questions and information that need to be covered, the nurse prioritizes essential information to obtain and provide during this visit.

A. List the relevant factors to consider on the basis of this information.
B. What questions do you need to ask with regard to controlling the spread of HIV to others?
C. What information is most important to give to Ms. Jackson at this time?
D. What follow-up does the nurse need to arrange for this client?
**Answers can be found on the Evolve site.**

## KEY POINTS

- Nearly all communicable diseases discussed in this chapter are preventable because they are transmitted through specific, known behaviors.
- STDs are among the most serious public health problems in the United States. Not only is there an increased incidence of drug-resistant gonococcal infection, but other STDs, such as HPV (genital warts), HIV, and HSV (genital herpes), are associated with cancer.
- STDs affect certain groups in greater numbers. Factors associated with risk include being less than 25 years of age, being a member of a minority group, living in an urban setting, being poor, and using crack cocaine.
- The increasing incidence, morbidity, and mortality of specific communicable diseases highlight the need for nurses to educate clients about ways to prevent communicable diseases.
- Many STDs do not produce symptoms in clients.
- Aside from death, the most serious complications caused by STDs are pelvic inflammatory disease, infertility, ectopic pregnancy, neonatal morbidity and mortality, and neoplasia.
- Hepatitis A is often silent in children, and children are a significant source of infection to others; thus, the use of the vaccination in children has caused a reduction in the number of cases.

## KEY POINTS—cont'd

- Hepatitis C is the most common bloodborne pathogen in the United States.
- The emergence of multidrug-resistant TB has prompted the use of directly observed therapy (DOT) to ensure adherence with drug treatment regimens.
- Early detection of communicable diseases is important because it results in early treatment and prevention of additional transmission to others. Treatment includes effective medications, stress reduction, and proper nutrition.
- Partner notification, or contact tracing, is done by identifying, contacting, and ensuring evaluation and treatment of

persons exposed to sexual and injectable drug–using partners. Contact tracing is also conducted with TB and HAV.

- HIV infection has created an entirely new group of people needing health care. This rapidly growing population is straining a health care system that is already unable to meet the needs of many.
- Most of the care (both home and outpatient) that is provided for HIV is done within the community setting, which reduces direct health care costs but increases the need for financial support of home and community health services.

## CLINICAL DECISION-MAKING ACTIVITIES

1. Identify sources of TB treatment in your community. Is there a DOT program available through the health department or home health agency? What factors make TB infection a difficult problem?
2. To whom does one report communicable diseases, such as HAV, in your community? How is this information given?
3. Identify the number of reported cases of AIDS and the number of reported cases of HIV infection within your state

and locale (if reportable in your state). How are the cases distributed by age, sex, geographic location, and ethnicity?
4. Identify the location(s) of HIV testing services in your community. Are the test results anonymous or confidential? Describe how and to whom the results are reported.
5. Form small groups and role play a nurse–client interaction involving risk assessment and counseling regarding safer sex and injection drug–using practices.

## REFERENCES

Buttaro T, Trybulski J, Polgar Bailey P, et al: *Primary Care: A Collaborative Practice*, ed 4. St Louis, 2013, Mosby.

Centers for Disease Control and Prevention (CDC): *Mantoux Tuberculin Skin Test: Facilitator Guide*, 2003. Available at: http://www.cdc.gov/tb/education/mantoux/images/mantoux.pdf.

Centers for Disease Control and Prevention: *IDU/HIV Prevention: Syringe Disinfection for Injection Drug Users*, 2004. Available at: http://www.cdc.gov/idu/facts/disinfection.pdf. Accessed February 24, 2014.

Centers for Disease Control and Prevention: Revised surveillance case definitions for HIV infection among adults, adolescents, and children aged <18 months and for HIV infection and AIDS among children aged 18 months to <13 years—United States, 2008. *MMWR Morb Mortal Wkly Rep* 57(RR–10):2008.

Centers for Disease Control and Prevention: Guidelines for the prevention and treatment of opportunistic infections among HIV-exposed and HIV-infected children. *MMWR Morb Mortal Wkly Rep* 58(RR–11):2009a.

Centers for Disease Control and Prevention: *Guidelines for Viral Hepatitis Surveillance and Case Management*, 2009b. Available at: http://www.cdc.gov/hepatitis/

statistics/surveillanceguidelines.htm#nonabc. Accessed March 14, 1014.

Centers for Disease Control and Prevention: Congenital syphilis—United States. *MMWR Morb Mortal Wkly Rep* 59(14):2010a. Available at: http://www.cdc.gov/mmwr/preview/mmwrhtml/mm5914a1.html.

Centers for Disease Control and Prevention: Sexually transmitted diseases treatment guidelines, 2010. *MMWR Morb Mortal Wkly Rep* 59(RR–12):2010b.

Centers for Disease Control and Prevention: *Viral Hepatitis Surveillance*. United States, 2011. Available at: http://www.cdc.gov/hepatitis/Statistics/2011Surveillance/PDFs/2011HepSurveillanceRpt.pdf. Accessed February 13. 2014.

Centers for Disease Control and Prevention: *Hepatitis B FAQs for Health Professionals*, 2012a. Available at: http://www.cdc.gov/hepatitis/HBV/HBVfaq.htm#overview. Accessed February 14, 2014.

Centers for Disease Control and Prevention: *Hepatitis E Information for Health Professionals*, 2012b. Available at: http://www.cdc.gov/hepatitis/HEV/index.htm. Accessed March 12, 2014.

Centers for Disease Control and Prevention: *Menu of Suggested Provisions for State Tuberculosis*

*Prevention and Control Laws*, 2012c. Available at: http://www.cdc.gov/tb/programs/Laws/menu/treatment.htm#2. Accessed March 1, 2014.

Centers for Disease Control and Prevention: Recommendations for the identification of chronic hepatitis C virus infection among persons born 1945-1965. *MMWR Morb Mortal Wkly Rep* 61(RR04):1–18, 2012d. Available at: http://www.cdc.gov/mmwr/preview/mmwrhtml/rr6104a1.htm. Accessed February 14, 2014.

Centers for Disease Control and Prevention: *Testing for Tuberculosis*, 2012e. Available at: http://www.cdc.gov/tb/publications/factsheets/testing/TB_testing.htm. Accessed February 21, 2014.

Centers for Disease Control and Prevention: *Tuberculin Skin Testing*, 2012f. Available at: http://www.cdc.gov/tb/publications/factsheets/testing/skintesting.htm. Accessed February 21, 2014.

Centers for Disease Control and Prevention: Update to CDC's Sexually Transmitted Diseases Treatment Guidelines 2010: oral cephalosporins no longer a recommended treatment for Gonococcal infections. *MMWR Morb Mortal Wkly Rep* 61(31):2012g.

Centers for Disease Control and Prevention: *CDC Fact Sheet: Gonorrhea Treatment Guidelines*,

2013a. Available at: http://www.cdc.gov/nchhstp/newsroom/docs/Gonorrhea-Treatment-Guidelines-FactSheet.pdf. Accessed March 12, 2014.

Centers for Disease Control and Prevention: CDC guidance for evaluating health-care personnel for hepatitis B virus protection and for administering post-exposure management. *MMWR* 62(10):2013b.

Centers for Disease Control and Prevention: *Genital Herpes: CDC Fact Sheet*, 2013c. Available at: http://www.cdc.gov/std/Herpes/STDFact-herpes-detailed.htm. Accessed February 12, 2014.

Centers for Disease Control and Prevention: *Hepatitis A for Health Professionals: Hepatitis A Vaccination*, 2013d. Available at: http://www.cdc.gov/hepatitis/HAV/HAVfaq.htm#vaccine. Accessed February 14, 2014. Last updated.

Centers for Disease Control and Prevention: *Hepatitis C Information for Health Professionals: Testing Recommendations for Chronic Hepatitis C Infection*, 2013e. Available at: http://www.cdc.gov/hepatitis/hcv/guidelinesc.htm. Accessed February 17, 2014.

Centers for Disease Control and Prevention: *Hepatitis D Information for Health Professionals*, 2013f. Available at: http://www.cdc.gov/hepatitis/HDV/index.htm. Accessed March 12, 2014.

Centers for Disease Control and Prevention: *HIV/AIDS: How Can I Tell if I'm Infected with HIV? What are the Symptoms?* Atlanta, 2013g, USDHHS, CDC. Available at: http://www.cdc.gov/hiv/basics/whatishiv.html. Accessed January 31, 2014.

Centers for Disease Control and Prevention: *HIV Among Transgender People*, 2013h. Available at: http://www.cdc.gov/hiv/risk/transgender/. Accessed February 24, 2014.

Centers for Disease Control and Prevention: *HIV Among Youth*, 2013i. Available at: http://www.cdc.gov/hiv/risk/age/youth/. Accessed January 24, 2014.

Centers for Disease Control and Prevention: *HIV Cost-Effectiveness*, 2013j. Available at: http://www.cdc.gov/hiv/prevention/ongoing/costeffectiveness/#BasicModel. Accessed January 24, 2014.

Centers for Disease Control and Prevention: *HIV in the United States: at a Glance*, 2013k. Available at: http://www.cdc.gov/hiv/statistics/basics/ataglance.html. Accessed February 1, 2014.

Centers for Disease Control and Prevention: *HIV Surveillance Report: Diagnoses of HIV Infection and AIDS in the United States and Dependent Areas 2011*, vol 23, 2013l. Accessed at: http://www.cdc.gov/hiv/topics/surveillance/resources/reports/. Published, February 2013. Accessed February 22. 2014.

Centers for Disease Control and Prevention: *Pre-exposure Prophylaxis*, 2013m. Available at: http://www.cdc.gov/hiv/prevention/research/prep/. Accessed March 12, 2014.

Centers for Disease Control and Prevention: *Reported Tuberculosis in the United States, 2012*. Atlanta, 2013n, U.S. Department of Health and Human Services, CDC. Available at: http://www.cdc.gov/tb/statistics/reports/2012/pdf/report2012.pdf. Accessed February 18, 2014.

Centers for Disease Control and Prevention: *State Laboratory Reporting Laws: Viral Load and CD4 Requirements*, 2013o. Available at: http://www.cdc.gov/hiv/policies/law/states/reporting.html. Accessed January 31, 2014.

Centers for Disease Control and Prevention: *STD Surveillance Case Definitions*, 2013p. Available at: www.cdc.gov-std-stats-CaseDefinitions-2014.pdf. Accessed February 14, 2014.

Centers for Disease Control and Prevention: *Testing: HIV Basics/HIV/AIDS*, 2013q. Available at: http://www.cdc.gov/hiv/basics/testing.html. Accessed January 31. 2014.

Centers for Disease Control and Prevention: *2012 Sexually Transmitted Diseases Surveillance: Chlamydia*, 2014a. Available at: http://www.cdc.gov/std/stats12/chlamydia.htm. Accessed February 22, 2014.

Centers for Disease Control and Prevention: *2012 Sexually Transmitted Diseases Surveillance, Gonorrhea*, 2014b. Available at: http://www.cdc.gov/std/stats12/gonorrhea.htm. Accessed February 8, 2014.

Centers for Disease Control and Prevention: *2012 Sexually Transmitted Diseases Surveillance: Other Sexually Transmitted Diseases*, 2014c. Available at: http://www.cdc.gov/std/stats12/other.htm. Accessed February 12, 2014.

Centers for Disease Control and Prevention: *2012 Sexually Transmitted Diseases Surveillance, Syphilis*, 2014d. Available at: http://www.cdc.gov/std/stats12/syphilis.htm. Published January, 2014. Accessed February 8, 2014.

Centers for Disease Control and Prevention: *2014 Recommended Combined Immunization Schedule Aged 0 Through 18 Years*. United States, 2014e. Available at: http://www.cdc.gov/vaccines/schedules/downloads/child/0-18yrs-combined-schedule-bw.pdf. Accessed February 14, 2014.

Centers for Disease Control and Prevention: CDC grand rounds: reducing the burden of HPV-associated cancer and disease. *MMWR* 63(4):2014f.

Centers for Disease Control and Prevention: *Chlamydia Fact Sheet*, 2014g. Available at: http://www.cdc.gov/std/chlamydia/STDFact-chlamydia-detailed.htm. Accessed February 11, 2014.

Centers for Disease Control and Prevention: *HIV Among African Americans*, 2014h. Available at: http://www.cdc.gov/hiv/risk/racialethnic/aa/facts/index.html. Accessed February 22, 2014.

Centers for Disease Control and Prevention: *HIV Prevention*, 2014i. Available at: http://www.cdc.gov/hiv/basics/prevention.html. Accessed February 24, 2014.

Centers for Disease Control and Prevention, Health Resources and Services Administration, National Institutes of Health, American Academy of HIV Medicine, Association of Nurses in AIDS Care, International Association of Providers of AIDS Care, National Minority AIDS Council, Urban Coalition for HIV/AIDS Prevention Services: *Recommendations for HIG Prevention with Adults and Adolescents with HIV in the United States*, 2014, Summary for Clinical Providers. Available at: http://stacks.cdc.gov/view/cdc/26063.

The Council on Linkages Between Academia and Public Health Practice: *Core Competencies for Public Health Professionals*, 2010. Available at: http://www.phf.org/programs/corecompetencies.

Fair C, Ginsburg B: HIV-related stigma, discrimination, and knowledge of legal rights among infected adults. *J HIV/AIDS Social Serv* 9(1):77–79, 2010. Available at: http://dx.doi.org/10.1080/15381500903583470. Accessed January 25, 2014.

Fontenot HB, Fantasia HC, Charyk A, et al: Human papillomavirus (HPV) risk factors, vaccination patterns, and vaccine perceptions among a sample of male college students. *J Am College Health* 62(3):186–192, 2014. doi:10.1080/07448481.2013.872649.

Hande K: Hepatitis C screening and guideline update. *J Nurse Practitioners* 10(1):64–66, 2014.

Heymann D: *Control of Communicable Diseases Manual*, ed 20. Washington, DC, 2014, American Public Health Association.

Panel on Opportunistic Infections in HIV-Exposed and HIV–Infected Children: *Guidelines for the Prevention and Treatment of Opportunistic Infections in HIV-Exposed and HIV–Infected Children*, 2013. Available at: aidsinfo.nih.gov/contentfiles/lvguidelines/oi_guidelines_pediatrics.pdf. Accessed March 16, 2014.

Panel on Antiretroviral Therapy and Medical Management of HIV-Infected Children: *Guidelines for the Use of Antiretroviral Agents in Pediatric HIV Infection*, 2014. Available at: http://aidsinfo.nih.gov/contentfiles/lvguidelines/pediatricguidelines.pdf. Accessed March 12, 2014.

Phillips I: Beta-lactamase producing penicillin-resistant gonococcus. *Lancet* 2:656, 1976.

UNAIDS: *AIDS Epidemic Update 2013, UNAIDS Fact Sheet*, 2013, UNAIDS publication. Available at: http://www.unaids.org/en/media/unaids/contentassets/documents/epidemiology/2013/gr2013/20130923_FactSheet_Global_en.pdf. Accessed January 31, 2014.

UNAIDS: *UNAIDS World AIDS Day Report*, 2012. Available at: http://www.unaids.org/en/media/unaids/contentassets/documents/epidemiology/2012/gr2012/jc2434_worldaidsday_results_en.pdf. Accessed January 31, 2014.

United States Department of Health and Human Services (USDHHS) Health Resources and Services Administration: *HIV/AIDS Programs: Legislation*. Washington, D.C., 2014a. Available at: http://hab.hrsa.gov/abouthab/legislation.html. Accessed January 25, 2014.

United States Department of Health and Human Services (USDHHS), Health Resources and Services Administration: *The HIV/AIDS Program: Part B-AIDS Drug Assistance Program*. Washington, DC, 2014b. Available at: http://hab.hrsa.gov/abouthab/partbdrug.html. Accessed January 25, 2014.

United States Department of Justice (USDJ): *Questions and Answers: The Americans with Disabilities Act and Persons with HIV/AIDS*. Washington, DC, 2012, USDJ. Available at: http://www.ada.gov/aids/ada_q&a_aids.pdf. Accessed February 4, 2014.Draft pg. 16.

United States Preventive Services Task Force (USPSTF): *Screening for HIV: U.S. Preventive Services Task Force Recommendation Statement*, 2013. Available at: http://www.uspreventiveservicestaskforce.org/uspstf13/hiv/hivfinalrs.pdf. Accessed March 12, 2014.

United States Preventive Services Task Force (USPSTF): *Final Recommendation Statement: Hepatitis C: Screening*. U.S. Preventive Services Task Force. 2014. Available at: http://www.uspreventiveservicestaskforce.org/Page/Document/RecommendationStatementFinal/hepatitis-c-screening. Accessed December 2014.

World Health Organization (WHO): *The Stop TB Strategy*. Geneva, 2010a, WHO Press. Available at: http://www.who.int/tb/publications/2010/strategy_en.pdf?ua=1. Accessed March 1, 2014.

World Health Organization (WHO): *WHO Recommendations on the Diagnosis of HIV Infection in Infants and Children*. Geneva, 2010b, WHO Press. Available at: http://whqlibdoc.who.int/publications/2010/9789241599085_eng.pdf?ua=1. Accessed February 4, 2014.

World Health Organization (WHO): *Global Tuberculosis Report 2013*. Geneva, 2013, WHO Press. Available at: http://apps.who.int/iris/bitstream/10665/91355/1/9789241564656_eng.pdf?ua=1. Accessed February 19, 2014.

# 15

# Evidence-Based Practice

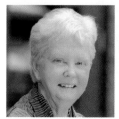

## Marcia Stanhope, PhD, RN, FAAN

Dr. Marcia Stanhope is currently an Associate of the Tufts and Associates Search Firm, Chicago, Ill. She is also a consultant for the nursing program at Berea College, Kentucky. She has practiced community and home health nursing, has served as an administrator and consultant in home health, and has been involved in the development of two nurse-managed centers. At one time in her career, she held a public policy fellowship and worked in the office of a U.S. Senator. She has taught community health, public health, epidemiology, policy, primary care nursing, and administration courses. Dr. Stanhope formerly directed the Division of Community Health Nursing and Administration and served as Associate Dean of the College of Nursing at the University of Kentucky. She has been responsible for both undergraduate and graduate courses in population-centered nursing. She has also taught at the University of Virginia and the University of Alabama, Birmingham. During her career at the University of Kentucky she appointed to the Good Samaritan Foundation Chair and Professorship in Community Health Nursing, and was honored with the University Provost's Public Scholar award. Her presentations and publications have been in the areas of home health, community health and community-focused nursing practice, as well as primary care nursing.

## ADDITIONAL RESOURCES

Ⓔ **Evolve Website http://evolve.elsevier.com/Stanhope**
- Healthy People 2020
- WebLinks—Of special note see the links for these sites:
  - Guidelines for Clinical Preventive Services
  - National Guideline Clearinghouse
  - Partners in Informational Access for the Public Health Workforce
  - National Center for Health Statistics

- Quiz
- Case Studies
- Glossary
- Answers to Practice Application
- Appendix
  - Focus on Quality and Safety Education for Nurses

## OBJECTIVES

*After reading this chapter, the student should be able to do the following:*

1. Define *evidence-based practice*.
2. Understand the history of evidence-based practice in health care.
3. Analyze the relationship between evidence-based practice and the practice of nursing in the community.
4. Provide examples of evidence-based practice in the community.
5. Identify barriers to evidence-based practice.
6. Apply evidence-based resources in practice.

## KEY TERMS

evidence-based medicine, p. 343
evidence-based nursing, p. 343
evidence-based practice, p. 343
evidence-based public health, p. 343
grading the strength of evidence, p. 348
integrative review, p. 347

meta-analysis, p. 347
narrative review, p. 347
randomized controlled trial (RCT), p. 345
research utilization, p. 343
systematic review, p. 347
*— See Glossary for definitions*

## CHAPTER OUTLINE

**Definition of Evidence-Based Practice**
**History of Evidence-Based Practice**
**Paradigm Shift in Use of Evidence-Based Practice**
**Types of Evidence**
**Factors Leading to Change**

**Barriers to Evidence-Based Practice**
**Steps in the Evidence-Based Practice Process**
    Approaches to Finding Evidence
    Approaches to Evaluating Evidence
**Approaches to Implementing Evidence-Based Practice**

Emphasis on evidence-based practice (EBP) is a standard to be met in health care delivery in the United States. It is a relevant approach to providing the highest quality of health care in all settings, which will result in improved health outcomes. EBP is important for all professionals who work in social and health care environments, regardless of the client or the setting with which professionals are dealing, including public health nurses who work with populations. Emphasis on EBP has resulted from increased expectations of consumers, changes in health care economics, increased expectations of accountability, advancements in technology, the knowledge explosion fueled by the Internet, and the growing number of lawsuits occurring when there is injury or harm as a result of practice decisions that are not based on the best available evidence (Makic et al, 2014). Nurses at all levels have an opportunity to improve the practice of nursing and client outcomes.

The Institute of Medicine has set a goal that by 2020, the best available evidence will be used to make 90% of all health care decisions, yet most nurses continue to be inconsistent in implementing EBP. An even greater concern in public health is that the field is lagging behind in developing evidence-based guidelines for the community setting. It is important to recognize that regardless of the level of education, undergraduate or graduate, nurses can be involved in the development, implementation, and evaluation of the effects of EBP (Florin et al, 2012; Gerrish and Cooke, 2013; Mattila et al, 2013; Merrill et al, 2013; Sprayberry, 2014).

Comprehensive databases are available through various Internet sites to assist nurses in applying the most recent best evidence to their clinical practice, like the Cochrane Library Database, the Centers for Disease Control and Prevention: Guide to Community Preventive Services, and others. (See the WebLinks for this chapter on the book's Evolve website.)

## DEFINITION OF EVIDENCE-BASED PRACTICE

The term *evidence-based* was first attributed to Gordon Gyatt, a Canadian physician at McMaster University in 1992 (Evidence Based Medicine Working Group, 1992). The term was first applied in medicine to begin the development of new ways of guiding professional decision making by using the best available evidence. Because the concept was developed in medicine, some of the first definitions focused on evidence-based medicine.

The definition of evidence-based medicine by Sackett and associates (Sackett et al, 1996) became the industry standard. Sackett et al (1996) defined evidence-based medicine as "the conscientious, explicit, and judicious use of current best

evidence in making decisions about the care of individual clients" (p. 71). Without current best external evidence, they said, "practice risks become rapidly out of date, to the detriment of clients" (Sackett et al, 1996, p. 72). A more succinct definition was proposed as the conscientious use of the current best evidence in making decisions about patient care (Sackett et al, 2000).

Adapting the definition by Sackett et al (1996), Rychetnik et al (2003) defined evidence-based public health as "a public health endeavor in which there is an informed, explicit, and judicious use of evidence that has been derived from any of a variety of science and social science research and evaluation methods" (p. 538). Brownson et al (2009) expanded the definition of evidence-based public health to include "making decisions on the basis of the best available evidence, using data and information systems, applying program planning frameworks, engaging the community in decision making, conducting evaluations, and disseminating what has been learned" (p. 175).

In a position statement on EBP, the Honor Society of Nursing, Sigma Theta Tau International, defined evidence-based nursing as "an integration of the best evidence available, nursing expertise, and the values and preferences of the individuals, families, and communities who are served" (Honor Society of Nursing, Sigma Theta Tau International, 2005). The definition of EBP continues to be broadened in scope and now includes a life-long problem-solving approach to clinical practice, integrating both external and internal evidence to answer clinical questions and to achieve desired client outcomes (Melnyk and Fineout-Overholt, 2011). *External evidence* includes research and other evidence such as reports and professional guidelines for example, whereas *internal evidence* includes the nurse's clinical experiences and the client's preferences.

Applied to nursing, evidence-based practice includes the best available evidence from a variety of sources including research studies, nursing experience and expertise, and community leaders. Culturally and financially appropriate interventions need to be identified when working with communities. The use of evidence to determine the appropriate use of interventions that are culturally sensitive and cost-effective is essential.

## HISTORY OF EVIDENCE-BASED PRACTICE

During the mid to late 1970s, there was growing consensus among nursing leaders that scientific knowledge should be used as a basis for nursing practice. During that time, the Division of Nursing in the U.S. Public Health Service began funding research utilization projects. Research utilization has been defined as

## EVIDENCE-BASED PRACTICE

Chronic diseases are considered a major disease burden in the United States, accounting for 75% of all medical care costs, and 7 of 10 deaths per year. Diabetes is one of the chronic diseases considered to have a major public health impact. To meet the *Healthy People 2010* goal of eliminating racial and ethnic disparities, the CDC created a demonstration project called REACH. Community projects were funded to develop, implement, and evaluate community action plans to improve health care and outcomes for racial and ethnic groups. One funded project was the Charleston and Georgetown, South Carolina Diabetes Coalition. The coalition is described as a community campus partnership with the Medical College of South Carolina and community agencies, organizations, and neighborhoods. The project serves about 12,000 African Americans with diabetes.

To implement the project, the coalition looked at the Chronic Care Model and after a systematic review of the literature, decided to expand the model and developed the Community Chronic Care Model. The goals of the project were to use community-based participatory actions to decrease disparities, improve health systems using the continuous quality improvement process, educate and empower communities, and build and sustain interpersonal and interorganizational links among communities and health professionals to improve diabetes outcomes and eliminate disparities. Local coalitions were developed, funds were provided to sustain diabetes activities, two new health facilities were opened in areas of need, and free medications were offered as samples.

One of the specific health outcomes was to reduce amputations among African American males. The University's college of nursing participated by developing and marketing a self-paced foot care educational program to train professionals in foot care. Lay educators were trained and health professionals provided patient care to the uninsured. A center for community health partnerships was established in the college of nursing and is a part of the ongoing plans for the college.

### Nurse Use

Nurses can be active in establishing small groups of partners in the community to develop a plan to meet a health care need, or participate in larger coalitions like this one. The focus on developing projects to meet needs and improve health care outcomes must be based on the evidence that shows these partnerships are needed to solve the health care need and improve health care outcomes (Jenkins et al, 2010).

Jenkins C, Pope C, Magwood G: Expanding the chronic care framework to improve diabetes management: The REACH Case Study. *Prog Community Health Partnersh* 4(1):65–79, Spring 2010.

"the process of transforming research knowledge into practice" (Stetler, 2001, p. 272) and "the use of research to guide clinical practice" (Estabrooks, Winther, and Derksen, 2004, p. 293).

Three projects funded by the Division of Nursing received the most attention and were the most influential in shaping nursing's view of using research to guide practice: the Nursing Child Assessment Satellite Training Project (NCAST) (Barnard and Hoehn, 1978; King, Barnard, and Hoehn, 1981), the Western Interstate Commission for Higher Education (WICHE) Regional Program for Nursing Research Development (WICHEN) (Krueger, 1977; Krueger, Nelson, and Wolanin, 1978; Lindeman and Krueger, 1977), and the Conduct and Utilization of Research in Nursing Project (CURN) (Horsley, Crane, and Bingle, 1978; Horsley et al, 1983). Using very different approaches and methods, each project tested interventions to facilitate research use in practice.

Although nursing continued to focus on research utilization projects, medicine also began to call for physicians to increase their use of scientific evidence to make clinical decisions. In the late 1970s, David Sackett, a medical doctor and clinical epidemiologist at McMaster University, published a series of articles in the *Canadian Medical Association Journal* describing how to read research articles in clinical journals. The term *critical appraisal* was used to describe the process of evaluating the validity and applicability of research studies (Guyatt and Rennie, 2002). Later, Sackett proposed the phrase "bringing critical appraisal to the bedside" to describe the application of evidence from medical literature to client care. This concept was used to train resident physicians at McMaster University and evolved into a "philosophy of medical practice based on knowledge and understanding of the medical literature supporting each clinical decision" (Guyatt and Rennie, 2002, p. xiv).

With Gordon Guyatt as Residency Director of Internal Medicine at McMaster, the decision was made to change the program to focus on "this new brand of medicine" that Guyatt eventually called *evidence-based medicine* (Guyatt and Rennie, 2002, p. xiv). Guyatt and Rennie described the goal of evidence-based medicine as being "aware of the evidence on which one's practice is based, the soundness of the evidence, and the strength of inference the evidence permits" (2002, p. xiv).

## PARADIGM SHIFT IN USE OF EVIDENCE-BASED PRACTICE

In 1992 the Evidence-Based Medicine Working Group published an article in the *Journal of the American Medical Association* expanding the concept of evidence-based medicine and calling it a *paradigm shift*. A paradigm shift simply means a change from old ways of knowing to new ways of knowing and practicing. Ways of knowing in nursing have included the empirical knowledge, or the science of nursing; the aesthetic knowledge, or the art of nursing; personal knowledge, or interpersonal relationships and caring; and ethical knowledge, or moral and ethical codes of conduct usually established by professional organizations (Bradshaw, 2010; Sandström et al, 2011). Nursing practice in the past often focused less on science and more on the other four ways of knowing described here.

According to the Working Group (Evidence-Based Medicine Working Group, 1992), the old paradigm viewed unsystematic clinical observations as a valid way for "building and maintaining" knowledge for clinical decision making (p. 2421). In addition, principles of pathophysiology were seen as a "sufficient guide for clinical practice" (p. 2421). Training, common sense, and clinical experience were considered sufficient for evaluating clinical data and developing guidelines for clinical practice. The Working Group cited developments in research over the past 30 years as providing the foundation for the paradigm shift and a "new philosophy of medical practice" (p. 2421).

The new paradigm, evidence-based medicine, acknowledged clinical experience as a crucial, but insufficient, part of clinical decision making. Systematic and unbiased recording of clinical observations in the form of research will increase confidence in the knowledge gained from clinical experience. Principles of pathophysiology were seen as necessary but not sufficient knowledge for making clinical decisions. The Working Group emphasized that physicians needed to be able to critically appraise the research literature in order to appropriately apply research findings in practice. Knowledge gained from authoritative figures was also deemphasized in the new paradigm (Working Group, 1992).

In the years since the Working Group began, the term *evidence-based practice* has been proposed as a term to integrate all health professions. The underlying principle was that high-quality care is based on evidence rather than on tradition or intuition (Beyers, 1999).

Nurses have always used various resources for problem solving. Intuition, trial and error, tradition, authority, institutional standards, prior knowledge, and clinical experience have often been used as the basis for decision making in clinical settings. However, not all of these resources are reliable and all have not consistently produced desired outcomes (Bradshaw, 2010; Sandström et al, 2011). A procedure performed based on intuition or trial and error might be performed successfully sometimes and not at other times. For example, tradition and authority, which comes from texts and policy and procedure manuals, can lead to faulty clinical decision making.

Institutional standards are developed by accrediting agencies (e.g., The Joint Commission), by licensing agencies, and by professional organizations. These standards have been developed in the past primarily by expert opinion and past experiences. The standards may not reflect the best practices in the current environment or from the literature.

Although prior knowledge gained in educational programs, through continuing education, or through experience can be a good teacher, it can also contain bias and quickly become outdated unless a nurse participates in constantly refreshing knowledge. For example, just because a nurse has experience in successfully performing an intervention a certain way today does not mean it is the best way or that it will be successful every time and in the future unless practices are changed based on the most current data.

When EBP was first emphasized in medicine, the focus was on the answer to clinical questions concerning an individual client problem in order to provide the best diagnosis to implement the best treatment. When nursing became involved in EBP, the focus seemed to shift to answering a clinical question about a health problem experienced by a group of clients (Levin et al, 2010).

The current nursing literature on EBP is primarily associated with applications in the acute and primary care settings and little is reported about its use in community settings. However, the basic principles of EBP can be applied at the individual level or at the community level. Although definitions of EBP vary widely in the literature, the common thread across disciplines is the application of the best available evidence to improve practice (Makic et al, 2014).

EBP has been described as both a process and a product (Bradshaw, 2010; Sandström et al, 2011; Scott and McSherry, 2009). The product is the use of evidence to make practice changes, whereas the process is a systematic approach to locating, critiquing, synthesizing, translating, and evaluating evidence upon which to base practice changes. Systematic reviews of research evidence can potentially assist nurses in putting evidence into practice. Systematic reviews, also known as evidence summaries, provide reliable evidence-based summaries of past research, making it easier for health care professionals to stay current on best practices without having to read a lot of research papers (Holly, Salmond, and Saimbert, 2011).

Scott and McSherry (2009) engaged in a process using an extensive literature review to arrive at a definition of evidence-based nursing and to differentiate the definition from evidence-based practice. Based on their review they arrived at the following definition: evidence-based nursing is a process whereby evidence, nursing theory, and the nurse's clinical expertise are evaluated and used, in conjunction with the client's involvement, to make critical decisions about the best care for the client. Continuous evaluation of the implementation of care is essential to make clinical decisions about client care for the best possible outcomes. In Chapter 9 there is extensive discussion of an example of how public health nurses have developed and used evidence on which to base population-centered nursing.

## TYPES OF EVIDENCE

No matter which definition of EBP is supported, what counts as evidence has been the issue most hotly debated. A hierarchy of evidence, ranked in order of decreasing importance and use, has been accepted by many health professionals. The double-blind **randomized controlled trial (RCT)** generally ranks as the highest level of evidence followed by other RCTs, nonrandomized clinical trials, quasi-experimental studies, case-controlled reports, qualitative studies, and expert opinion (Russell-Babin, 2009). Some nurses would argue that this hierarchy ignores evidence gained from clinical experience. However, the definition of evidence-based nursing presented previously indicates that clinical expertise as evidence, when used with other types of evidence, is used to make clinical decisions. Also in the hierarchy of evidence, expert opinion can be gained from nonresearch–based published articles, professional guidelines, national guidelines, organizational opinions, and panels of experts, as well as the nurse's clinical expertise.

Because it is difficult to find or perform RCTs in the community, other types of evidence have been highlighted as the best evidence in public health literature on which to base evidence-based public health practice: scientific literature found in systematic reviews, scientific literature used or quoted in one or more journal articles, public health surveillance data, program evaluations, qualitative data obtained from community members and other stakeholders, media/marketing data such as the results of a media campaign to reduce smoking, word of mouth, and personal/professional experience (Brownson et al, 2009; Jacobs et al, 2012).

Within public health practice, guidelines for finding and using evidence include the following:
- Engaging the community in assessment and decision making;
- Using data and information systems systematically;

- Making decisions on the basis of the best available peer-reviewed evidence (both quantitative and qualitative);
- Applying program planning frameworks (often based in health behavior theory);
- Conducting sound evaluation; and
- Disseminating what is learned (Jacobs et al, 2012).

## FACTORS LEADING TO CHANGE

EBP represents a cultural change in practice. It provides an environment to improve both nursing practice and client outcomes. Nursing is known for providing care based on environmental and client assessments; critical observations; development of questions or hypotheses to be explored; collecting data from the environment through community or organizational assessments, or from the client through history, physical assessment, and review of past heath records; analyzing the data to develop plans of care, whether for the individual client, family, group or community; and drawing conclusions upon which to base care for the purpose of improving client outcomes (Gerrish and Cooke, 2013). However, several factors have been identified in the literature that support implementation of EBP or that will need to be overcome for nursing and other disciplines to successfully implement EBP. These factors include the following:

- Knowledge of research and current evidence
- Ability to interpret the meaning of the evidence
- Individual professional's characteristics, such as a willingness to change, or personal viewpoints about the quality and credibility of evidence
- Commitment of the time needed to implement EBP and to engage in education and directed practice
- The hierarchy of the practice environment and the level of support of managers and the ability to engage in autonomous practice,
- The philosophy of the practice environment and the willingness to embrace EBP
- The resources available to engage in EBP, such as amount of work, proper equipment, computer-based EBP programs, and information systems
- The practice characteristics, such as leadership and colleague attitudes
- Links to outside supports such as teaching facilities like a teaching health department or a university
- Political constraints and the lack of relevant and timely public health practice research (Asadoorian Hearson, Satyanarayana, and Ursel, 2010; Brownson et al, 2009; Gerrish and Cooke, 2013)

## BARRIERS TO EVIDENCE-BASED PRACTICE

Although a community agency may subscribe in theory to the use of EBP, actual implementation may be affected by the realities of the practice setting. Community-focused nursing agencies may lack the resources needed for its implementation in the clinical setting, such as time, funding, computer resources, and knowledge. Nurses may be reluctant to accept findings and feel threatened when long-established practices are questioned. Cost can also be a barrier if the clinical decision or change will require more funds than the agency has available. Compliance can be a barrier if the client will not follow the recommended intervention. Public health departments are moving toward EBP and are seeking accreditation through the national public health accreditation board. The accreditation process began in 2011. As of March 2014, 31 public health departments had achieved national accreditation (Public Health Accreditation Board, 2014).

## STEPS IN THE EVIDENCE-BASED PRACTICE PROCESS

EBP is a philosophy of practice that respects client values. Melnyk and associates (2010) have described a seven-step EBP process:

0. Cultivating a spirit of inquiry
1. Asking clinical questions
2. Searching for the best evidence
3. Critically appraising the evidence
4. Integrating the evidence with clinical expertise and client preferences and values
5. Evaluating the outcomes of the practice decisions or changes based on evidence
6. Disseminating EBP results

Yes, their first step is step zero. This process was initially described as a five-step process by others (Dawes et al, 2004; Dicenso et al, 2005; Craig and Smyth, 2007). The unique features of the Melnyk et al (2010) model are the emphasis on the spirit of inquiry and the sharing of the results of the process.

Step zero involves a curiosity about the interventions that are being applied. Do they work, or is there a better approach? In public health nursing, for example, are there better parenting outcomes if the parents attend classes at the health department? Or are home visits to new mothers and babies more effective for achieving a healthy baby? Step one requires asking questions in a "PICOT" format.

Although Melnyk et al have developed a specific process for the PICOT, the process was first described by Sackett (1996), who discussed the need to define the (P)opulation of interest, the (I)ntervention or practice strategy in question, the population or intervention to be used for (C)omparision, the (O)utcome desired, and the (T)ime frame. Step two involves searching for the best evidence to answer the question. This step involves searching the literature. In the case of the previous example, a literature search would focus on a search of key terms like *public health nursing, parenting of new babies, parenting classes,* and *home visits.* Step three requires a critical appraisal of the evidence found in step two.

To appraise the literature found, Melnyk suggests asking three questions about each of the articles found in the literature search: (1) the validity, (2) the importance, and (3) whether or not the results of the article will help you as a nurse provide quality care for your clients. Step four is the step in which the evidence found is integrated with clinical expertise and client values. Institutional standards and practice guidelines, as well as cost of care and support of the health care environment to implement the findings, are all factors considered in this step.

Step five requires an evaluation of the outcomes of practice decisions and changes that were based on the answers to the first four steps. The goal in evaluation is a positive change in quality of care and health care outcomes. In the example of group parenting classes versus home visits to new mothers and babies, current literature suggests improved quality and health care outcomes with home visits (The Pew Center, 2010).

Step six is disseminating outcomes of the results to others, to colleagues, to the employing agency's administration, to faculty and other students, and through a poster or podium presentation of student nurse organizations or professional organizations. Professional organizations often sponsor student presentations for undergraduates as well as graduate students. Sharing of information is most important because it prevents each individual nurse from trying to find the best answer to the same question answered by someone else, and it gives us the basis for asking new questions. Sharing makes practice more efficient and improves quality and health care outcomes.

In a busy community practice setting, it is often difficult for nurses to access evidence-based resources. Using evidence-based clinical practice guidelines is one way for nurses to provide evidence-based nursing care in an efficient manner. Clinical practice guidelines are usually developed by a group of experts in the field who have reviewed the evidence and made recommendations based on the best available evidence. The recommendations are usually graded according to the quality and quantity of the evidence. The Public Health Practice Reference is an example of practice guidelines developed for population-centered nurses' use (AHRQ, 2014).

## Approaches to Finding Evidence

Returning to the previous example, the clinical question has been stated and the population has been defined as new mothers and babies. Two interventions will be compared. The outcome is stated as healthy babies and the time frame may be 6 months or 1 year, or another time at which the outcomes of the interventions will be evaluated.

Four approaches are described that allow the nurse to read research/nonresearch evidence in a condensed format. The first, a systematic review, is "a method of identifying, appraising, and synthesizing research evidence. The aim is to evaluate and interpret all available research that is relevant to a particular research question" (Cochrane Library, 2014). A systematic review is usually done by more than one person and describes the methods used to search for and evaluate the evidence. Systematic reviews can be accessed from most databases, such as Medline and CINAHL.

The Cochrane Library is an electronic database that contains regularly updated evidence-based health care databases maintained by the Cochrane Collaboration, a not-for-profit organization (http://www.cochrane.org). The Cochrane Library is composed of three main branches: systematic reviews, trials register, and methodology database. The Cochrane Library publishes systematic reviews on a wide variety of topics. Systematic reviews differ from traditional literature review publications in that systematic reviews require more rigor and contain less opinion of the author. Systematic reviews for public

health can be found in the Guide to Community Preventive Services, the Cochrane Public Health Group, the Center for Reviews and Dissemination, and the Campbell Collaboration (Box 15-1).

---

**HOW TO** Develop an Evidence-Based Practice Guide to a Community Preventive Service

- *Form a development team, preferably an interprofessional team, to choose a topic based on a community issue that needs to be addressed.*
- *Develop a structured approach to organize, group, select, and evaluate the interventions from the literature that work to address the issue.*
- *Select the interventions the group wishes to evaluate for use.*
- *Assess the quality of the evidence found in the literature.*
- *Summarize the findings.*
- *Make recommendations.*
- *Write a protocol or step-by-step guide to resolving the community issue.*

*From Task Force on Community Preventive Services:* Guide to community preventive services. *2007. Available at http://www.thecommunityguide.org/diabetes/default.htm. Accessed September 26, 2010.*

---

The second approach, meta-analysis, is a specific method of statistical synthesis used in some systematic reviews, where the results from several studies are quantitatively combined and summarized (GWU, 2014). A well-designed systematic review or meta-analysis can provide stronger evidence than a single randomized controlled trial.

The integrative review is a form of a systematic review that does not have the summary statistics found in the meta-analysis because of the limitations of the studies that are reviewed (e.g., small sample size of the population). Narrative review is a review done on published papers that support the reviewer's particular point of view or opinion and is used to provide a general discussion of the topic reviewed. This review does not often include an explicit or systematic review process.

Undergraduate students often perform narrative reviews. However, it is important to learn the process for systematic reviews, especially the use of the results of systematic reviews. Reading systematic reviews that have been completed is helpful in answering the question related to the EBP process.

What counts as evidence has also been argued in the public health literature (Earle-Foley, 2011). RCTs, which are the highest level of evidence used to make clinical decisions, are appropriate for evaluating many interventions in medicine, but are often inappropriate for evaluating public health interventions. For example, an RCT can be designed ethically to test a new medication for diabetes, but not for a smoking cessation intervention. In a smoking cessation intervention, subjects could not be assigned randomly to smoking or nonsmoking groups because a smoking cessation intervention is not appropriate for someone who does not smoke. In this situation, a case-control study would be most appropriate (see Chapter 12). Today there are many community-based clinical trials assisting in finding answers to the questions of which population-level intervention has the best outcomes. (Visit the CDC website to review these trials.)

---

**BOX 15-1  Resources for Implementing Evidence-Based Practice**

The following resources can assist nurses in developing evidence-based nursing practice:

1. The *Evidence-Based Practice for Public Health Project* at the University of Massachusetts Medical School Library has developed a website for evidence-based practice in public health (http://library.umassmed.edu/ebpph/). Many bibliographic databases, such as Medline, do not list all the journals of interest to public health workers. The project provides access to numerous databases of interest concerning public health. From the project's website, nurses can access free public health online journals and databases.

2. The *Agency for Healthcare Quality and Research (AHRQ)* developed clinical guidelines based on the best available evidence for several clinical topics, such as pain management. The guidelines are accessible via the agency's website (http://www.ahrq.gov) and serve as a resource to nurses involved in individual client care.

3. The *National Guideline Clearinghouse* (http://www.guideline.gov/), an initiative of the AHRQ, is an online resource for evidence-based clinical practice guidelines. AHRQ also supports Evidence-Based Practice Centers, which write evidence reports on various topics.

4. *PubMed* (http://www.pubmed.gov/) is a bibliographic database developed and maintained by the National Library of Medicine. Bibliographic information from Medline is covered in PubMed and includes references for nursing, medicine, dentistry, the health care system, and preclinical sciences. Full texts of referenced articles are often included. Searches can be limited to type of evidence (e.g., diagnosis, therapy) and systematic reviews.

5. The *Cochrane Database of Systematic Reviews* is a collection of more than 1000 systematic reviews of effects in health care internationally. These reviews are accessible at a cost via the website (http://www.cochrane.org). Nurses may also have free access from a medical library.

6. The *Evidence-Based Nursing Journal* (http://ebn.bmjjournals.com/) is published quarterly. The purpose of the journal is to select articles reporting studies and reviews from health-related literature that warrant immediate attention by nurses attempting to keep pace with advances in their profession. Using predefined criteria, the best quantitative and qualitative original articles are abstracted in a structured format, commented on by clinical experts, and shared in a timely fashion. The research questions, methods, results, and evidence-based conclusions are reported. The website for the journal is http://www.evidencebasednursing.com.

7. The Honor Society of Nursing, Sigma Theta Tau International, sponsors the online peer-reviewed journal *Worldviews on Evidence-Based Nursing* that publishes systematic reviews and research articles on best evidence that supports nursing practice globally. The journal is available by subscription (http://www.nursingsociety.org/).

8. The *Task Force on Community Preventive Services* is an independent, nonfederal task force appointed by the director of the Centers for Disease Control and Prevention. Information about the Task Force may be found at the website http://www.thecommunityguide.org. The Task Force is charged with determining the topics to be addressed by the CDC's Community Guide and the most appropriate means to assess evidence regarding population-based interventions. The Task Force reviews and assesses the quality of available evidence on the effects of essential community preventive services. The multidisciplinary Task Force determines the scope of the Community Guide that will be used by health departments and agencies to determine best practices for preventive health in populations.

9. The *U.S. Preventive Services Task Force (USPSTF)* is an independent panel of private-sector experts in prevention and primary care. The USPSTF conducts rigorous, impartial assessments of the scientific evidence for the effectiveness of a broad range of clinical preventive services, including screening, counseling, and preventive medications. Its recommendations are considered the "gold standard" for clinical preventive services. The mission of the USPSTF is to evaluate the benefits of individual services based on age, gender, and risk factors for disease; make recommendations about which preventive services should be incorporated routinely into primary medical care and for which populations; and identify a research agenda for clinical preventive care. Recommendations of the USPSTF are published as the *Guide to Clinical Preventive Services*. The guide is available online at http://www.ahrq.gov/clinic/uspstfix.htm.

10. The *Centers for Disease Control and Prevention* (www.cdc.gov) publishes guidelines on immunizations and sexually transmitted diseases. Guidelines are developed by experts in the field appointed by the U.S. Department of Health and Human Services and the CDC.

11. *Cochrane Public Health Group (PHRG),* formerly the health promotion and public health field, aims to work with contributors to produce and publish Cochrane reviews of the effects of population-level public health interventions. The PHRG undertakes systematic reviews of the effects of public health interventions to improve health and other outcomes at the population level, not those targeted at individuals. Thus, it covers interventions seeking to address macroenvironmental and distal social environmental factors that influence health. In line with the underlying principles of public health, these reviews seek to have a significant focus on equity and aim to build the evidence to address the social determinants of health. (Visit http://www.ph.cochrane.org/.)

12. *Center for Reviews and Dissemination (CRD)* is part of the National Institute for Health Research and is a department of the University of York. CRD, which was established in 1994, is one of the largest groups in the world engaged exclusively in evidence synthesis in the health field. CRD undertakes systematic reviews evaluating the research evidence on health and public health questions of national and international importance. (Visit http://www.york.ac.uk/inst/crd/index.htm.)

13. *Campbell Collaboration,* named after Donald Campbell, was founded on the principle that systematic reviews on the effects of interventions will inform and help improve policy and services. The collaboration strives to make the best social science research available and accessible. Campbell reviews provide high-quality evidence of what works to meet the needs of service providers, policy makers, educators and their students, professional researchers, and the general public. Areas of interest include crime, justice, education, and social welfare. (Visit http://www.campbellcollaboration.org/.)

---

## Approaches to Evaluating Evidence

One approach used in evaluating evidence is **grading the strength of evidence**. When evidence is graded, the evidence is assigned a "grade" based on the number and type of well-designed studies, and the presence of similar findings in all of the studies. Grading evidence has been debated so strongly that in 2002 the Agency for Healthcare Research and Quality (AHRQ) commissioned a study to describe existing systems used to evaluate the usefulness of studies and strength of evidence. The report reviewed 40 systems and identified three domains for evaluating systems for the grading of evidence: quality, quantity, and consistency. The *quality* of a study refers to the extent to which bias is minimized. *Quantity* refers to the number of studies, the magnitude of the effect, and the sample size. *Consistency* refers to studies that have similar findings, using similar and different study designs (Haine-Schlagel et al, 2014). An example of how the U.S. Preventive Services Task

## HOW TO Develop an Evidence-Based Protocol

*Evidence-based protocols are a recognized approach to providing quality client care. Such protocols enhance the abilities of providers and can reduce health care errors. The following are steps to developing a protocol:*

- *Identify the problem.*
- *Identify stakeholders.*
- *Form a team of others to help develop the protocol.*
- *Develop an action plan with project goals and a timeline.*
- *Review the available evidence.*
- *Examine current practice and identify gaps as well as best practices.*
- *Develop the protocol focusing on gaps.*
- *Initiate the approval process with the setting.*
- *Evaluate current practices and modify as needed.*
- *Educate others who will use the protocol.*
- *Implement the protocol.*
- *Evaluate protocol for safety, effectiveness, and adherence (McEuen and Gardner, 2010).*

*From McEuen JA, Gardner KP, Barnachea DF, et al: An evidence-based protocol for managing hypoglycemia. AJN 110(7): 40–45, 2010.*

Force 2003 graded the strength of evidence for the *Guidelines for Clinical Preventive Services* can be found at the website at the end of this chapter.

As indicated, many frameworks exist for evaluating the strength and the usefulness of the evidence found in the literature and other sources, such as professional standards. A popular framework was developed by the Agency for Healthcare Quality. Fineout-Overholt et al (2010) have also developed an approach for evaluating evidence. Although these approaches vary in the factors they evaluate, the best approach to choose is one that not only evaluates the strength, but also the usefulness of the evidence. Table 15-1 provides an example of an approach for evaluating evidence.

The strength of the literature is measured by the type of evidence it represents. For example, the RCT is the evidence that has the greatest strength upon which to make a clinical decision. In contrast, opinion articles, descriptive studies, and professional reports of expert committees have less strength. The usefulness of the evidence is measured by whether the evidence is valid, whether it is important, and whether it can be used to assist in making practice decisions or changes in the community environment and with the population of interest to improve outcomes (Scott and McSherry, 2009).

The best RCT conducted in a hospital setting on using an intervention to prevent falls may not be applicable at all in a community setting. Therefore, although it may be a strong study with outcomes that improve health, it may not have the usefulness for applicability in the community because of the setting in which it was conducted.

Shaughnessy, Slawson, and Bennett (1994) proposed criteria for evaluating the usefulness of evidence, calling the process *patient oriented evidence that matters* (POEM). In general, the reader should ask the following questions: "What are the results? (Are they important?) Are the results valid? How can the results be applied to client care?" (p. 489). Application of POEM (2014) can be found at www.essentialevidenceplus.com. Brownson et al (2009) proposed that the following questions be asked for EBP (plus suggested application examples):

- What is the size of the public health problem? What is the need for improved health outcomes for new mothers and babies in our community?
- Can interventions be found in the literature to address the problem (e.g., home visits or parenting classes)?

## TABLE 15-1 Typology for Classifying Interventions by Level of Scientific Evidence

| Type/ Category | Strength/How Established | Considerations for the Level of Scientific Evidence—Quality | Quantity/Consistency Data Source Examples |
|---|---|---|---|
| Evidence-based I | Peer review via systematic or narrative review | Based on study design and execution<br>External validity<br>Potential side benefits or harms<br>Costs and cost-effectiveness | *Community Guide*<br>Cochrane reviews<br>Narrative reviews based on published literature |
| Effective II | Peer review | Based on study design and execution<br>External validity<br>Potential side benefits or harms<br>Costs and cost-effectiveness | Articles in the scientific literature<br>Research-tested intervention programs (123)<br>Technical reports with peer review |
| Promising III | Written program evaluation without formal peer review | Summative evidence of effectiveness<br>Formative evaluation data<br>Theory-consistent, plausible, potentially high-reach, low-cost, replicable | State or federal government reports (without peer review)<br>Conference presentations |
| Emerging IV | Ongoing work, practice-based summaries, or evaluation works in progress | Formative evaluation data<br>Theory-consistent, plausible, potentially high-reaching, low-cost, replicable<br>Face validity | Evaluability assessments<br>Pilot studies<br>NIH CRISP database<br>Projects funded by health foundations |

From Brownson RC, Fielding JE, Maylahn CM: Evidence-based public health: a fundamental concept for public health practice. *Annu Rev Public Health* 30:175–201, 2009.

- Is the intervention useful in this community, with this population, or with populations at risk (e.g., the low income or uninsured)?
- Is the intervention the best one or are there other ways to address the problem considering cost and potential health outcomes for the population? (Assess cost and health outcomes of both of the interventions before choosing, including the nurses available to make home visits or who have the skills to teach the parenting class.)

Several variables are considered important in determining the quality of evidence used to make clinical decisions (Polit and Beck, 2011):

- *Sample selection:* Sample selection should be as unbiased as possible. For example, a sample is randomly selected when each subject has an equal chance of being selected from the population of interest. Random selection offers the least bias of any type of sample selection. Other types of sample selection such as convenience sampling contain researcher or evaluator bias.
- *Randomization:* When testing an intervention, randomly assign participants to either the intervention or control group. This type of assignment is less biased than if participants are allowed to choose the group they want to join.
- *Blinding:* The researcher or evaluator should not know which participants are in the experimental (treatment) group or which are in the control group. The researcher or evaluator is "blinded" as to who is receiving the treatment and who is not receiving the treatment.
- *Sample size:* The sample size should be large enough to show an effect of the intervention. In general, the larger the sample size, the better.
- *Description of intervention:* The intervention should be described in detail and explicitly enough that another person could duplicate the study if desired.
- *Outcomes:* The outcomes should be measured accurately.
- *Length of follow-up:* Depending on the intervention, the participants should be followed for a long enough period of time to determine if the intervention continued to work or if the results just happened by chance.
- *Attrition:* Few subjects should have dropped out of the study.
- *Confounding variables:* Variables that could affect the outcome should be accounted for either by statistical methods or by study measurements.
- *Statistical analysis:* Statistical analysis should be appropriate to determine the desired outcome.

## APPROACHES TO IMPLEMENTING EVIDENCE-BASED PRACTICE

The first step toward implementing EBP in nursing is recognizing the current status of one's own practice and believing that care based on the best evidence will lead to improved client outcomes (Melnyk et al, 2010). Since EBP is a relatively new concept, many practicing nurses are not familiar with the application of EBP and may lack computer and Internet skills necessary to implement EBP. Also, implementation will be successful only when nurses practice in an environment that supports evidence-based care. Public health nurses consider EBP a process to improve practice and outcomes and use the evidence to influence policies that will improve the health of communities.

---

**QSEN FOCUS ON QUALITY AND SAFETY EDUCATION FOR NURSES**

**Targeted Competency: Evidence-Based Practice**
Integrate best current evidence with clinical expertise and client and family preferences and values for delivery of optimal interventions.
Important aspects of EBP include:
- **Knowledge:** Describe EBP to include the components of research evidence, clinical expertise and client and family values
- **Skills:** Locate evidence reports related to clinical practice topics and guidelines
- **Attitudes:** Value the need for continuous improvement in clinical practice based on new knowledge

*Evidence-Based Practice Question*
As a nurse in the community you are working within a Native American community that has a high prevalence of diabetes. As you visit with clients in their homes, you notice that many have a standardized "Diabetes Care" handout they received from the same primary care clinic. Your clients comment that the nutritional recommendations are unrealistic in the context of their regular diet. You decide to initiate a focus group with clients who attend the diabetes clinic at the health department to customize nutritional diabetic guidelines for this community.
1. Go to The National Guideline Clearinghouse website at http://www.guideline.gov. This website is an initiative of the Agency for Healthcare Research and Quality and is a reservoir for evidence-based clinical guidelines.
2. On the home page, type "diabetes" in the search box.
3. The second result is: Guideline Synthesis: Nutritional Management of Diabetes Mellitus.
4. Review the various areas of the guidelines: Medical Nutritional Therapy, Carbohydrates, Protein, Fiber, Sucralose, Alcohol Consumption, Dietary Fat and Cholesterol, Micronutrients, Nutritional Interventions for Preventing and Managing Complications, and Physical Activity and Weight Management.
5. What baseline data might you gather from your focus group participants to be best informed in how to tailor the evidence-based recommendation for this community?
6. What might be effective strategies in writing up the community-specific guidelines and distributing them that might enhance their adoption?

*Answer*
- Understanding the common elements of this community's diet is a good place to start. What are common carbohydrates, proteins, sources of sugar, dietary fat, and cholesterol that are commonly consumed?
- How does the common diet compare to the National Clearinghouse Guidelines? Are there healthy sources of carbohydrates, healthy fats that are part of the diet that can be emphasized?
- What are common patterns in the community around alcohol consumption? Would educational efforts around the deleterious effects of alcohol on diabetes be helpful?
- Writing up community-based guidelines with assistance from leaders in the community would be a helpful strategy. You could include healthy recipes from community leaders in your guidelines.
  Your community-based guidelines might be distributed at a community celebration or gathering by members of the community who helped develop them.

Prepared by Gail Armstrong, PhD(c), DNP, ACNS-BC, CNE, Associate Professor, University of Colorado Denver College of Nursing.

# CURRENT PERSPECTIVES

## Cost Versus Quality

Much of the pressure to use EBP comes from third-party payers and is a response to the need to contain costs and reduce legal liability. Nurses must question whether the current agenda to contain health care costs creates pressure to focus on those research results that favor cost saving at the expense of quality outcomes for clients. Outcomes include client and community satisfaction and the safety of care. Costs can be weighed against outcomes when EBP is used to show the best practices available to reduce possible harm to clients (Makic et al, 2014; Asadoorian et al, 2010).

 **LEVELS OF PREVENTION**

### *Using Evidence-Based Practice*

According to evidence collected by the Task Force on Community Preventive Services, the following are interventions supported by the literature at each level of prevention:

**Primary Prevention**
Extended and extensive mass media campaigns reduce youth initiation of tobacco use.

**Secondary Prevention**
Client reminders and recalls via mail, telephone, e-mail, or a combination of these strategies are effective in increasing compliance with screening activities such as those for colorectal and breast cancer.

**Tertiary Prevention**
Diabetes self-management education in community gathering places improves glycemic control.

From Task Force on Community Preventive Services: *National Center for Chronic Disease Prevention and Health Promotion.* Available at http://www.cdc.gov. Accessed December 26, 2010.

## Individual Differences

EBP cannot be applied as a universal remedy without attention to client differences. When EBP is applied at the community level, best evidence may point to a solution that is not sensitive to cultural issues and distinctions and thus may not be acceptable to the community. Ethical practice in communities requires attention to community differences.

## Appropriate Evidence-Based Practice Methods for Population-Centered Nursing Practice

Gaining a number of perspectives in a situated community is important for nurses using EBP. Nursing has a legitimate role to play in interprofessional community-focused practice and can contribute to its evidence base. Nurses are obliged to ensure that the evidence applied to practice is acceptable to the community. Establishing an EBP culture depends on the use of both qualitative and quantitative research approaches, or the best evidence available at the time. For example, a quantitative research study of a community health center could provide information about patterns of client use, the cost of various services, and the use of different health care providers. However,

when quantitative research is combined with qualitative research, the nurse can gain an understanding of *why* clients use or do not use the services and help the health center be both clinically effective and cost-effective. Evidence from multiple research methods has the potential to enrich the application of evidence and improve nursing practice (Blakely et al, 2013).

The rising cost of health care will demand a more critical look at the benefits and costs of EBP. Finding resources to implement EBP will continue to be a challenge requiring creative strategies. An emphasis on quality care, equal distribution of health care resources, and cost control will continue. Implementing EBP can assist nurses in addressing these issues in the clinical setting. However, EBP can save money by providing the best care possible.

As nurses implement EBP in an environment focused on cost savings, the potential for governments, managed care organizations, or other health care agencies to endorse reimbursement of health care options solely on the basis of cost, without allowing for individual variation or considering environmental issues, will continue to be a concern. Nurses must use caution in adopting EBP in a prescriptive manner in different community environments. One aspect of the new health care reform act (PL 111-148) addresses the development of task forces on preventive services and community preventive services to develop, update, and disseminate EBP recommendations of the use of community preventive services. In addition, grant programs to support EBP delivery in the community are addressed in the Affordable Care Act of 2010.

Although the Internet is one source of evidence data (see Box 15-1), there may be a lack of quality indicators to evaluate the myriad websites claiming to contain evidence-based information. It is essential to evaluate the quantity of the information on the website, whether it comes from a reputable agency or scholar, and whether the source of the website has a financial interest in the acceptance of the evidence presented. (Refer to Chapter 16 on health education, which discusses the Internet as a source of data and how to evaluate its usefulness and reliability.)

## *HEALTHY PEOPLE 2020* OBJECTIVES

*Healthy People 2020* objectives offer a systematic approach to health improvement. See the Healthy People 2020 box for the most recent objectives to improve clients' understanding of EBP and how they can contribute to health care decisions.

## EXAMPLE OF APPLICATION OF EVIDENCE-BASED PRACTICE TO PUBLIC HEALTH NURSING

Chapter 9 describes the Intervention Wheel, a population-based practice model for public health nursing. The model consists of three levels of practice at the community, systems, and individual/family levels. It also consists of 17 public health interventions for improving population health. The model was originally developed using a qualitative grounded theory process but did

## LINKING CONTENT TO PRACTICE

It is important for nurses to acknowledge and understand EBP. They can participate by applying EBP or they can add to the research base for public health through active programs of research, participating in systematic reviews, or reviewing the best evidence available to them by reading published systematic reviews. Nurses can demonstrate leadership in supporting EBP by becoming change agents, fostering a cultural change in the practice environment, and assisting nurses who do not know how to use EBP to make a difference in practice.

For example, nurses who have recently graduated are knowledgeable about the use of evidence in practice. The new nurses can assist nurses who have been out of school for a while to find sources of evidence upon which to base their practice, such as referring them to the *Guide to Community Preventive Services*. Using evidence in practice will demonstrate its value, but implementation can be difficult because of the sheer volume of evidence and increasing

population needs. Sharing knowledge and engaging in teamwork can help to overcome these barriers.

Nurses have an important role to play in developing and using clinical guidelines for community practices. Use of a community development model and engaging in community partnerships will ensure that the community's perspective is included (see Chapter 18).

Nurses active in EBP can devote attention to understanding how best to incorporate the guidelines into practice demonstrating practice excellence. EBP offers the opportunity for shared decision making because it can help nurses focus their thinking, observe process outcomes, and thus improve care for clients by communicating with leaders and other nurses what they have observed. Participation in EBP offers continuing professional growth and a feeling of value, recognition for contributions, and respect from peers and administrators (Bradshaw, 2010; Sandström et al, 2011).

From Bradshaw WG: Importance of nursing leadership in advancing evidence-based nursing practice. *Neonatal Netw* 29(2):117–122, 2010; Sandström B, Borglin G, Nilsson R, et al: Promoting the implementation of evidence-based practice—a literature review focusing on the role of nursing leadership. *Worldviews Evid Based Nurs* Fourth quarter:212–223, 2011.

## ♥ HEALTHY PEOPLE 2020

Information access is important to assure clients and communities have the correct information to make EBP health care decisions. The *Healthy People 2020* objectives related to providing resources are as follows:
- HC/HIT-6.3: Increase the proportion of persons who use electronic personal health management tools.
- HC/HIT-4: Increase the proportion of patients whose doctor recommends personalized health information resources to help them manage their health.

- HC/HIT-12: Increase the proportion of crisis and emergency risk messages, intended to protect the public's health, that demonstrate the use of best practices.
- HC/HIT-11: Increase the proportion of meaningful users of health information technology.
- HC/HIT-13: Increase the social marketing in health promotion and disease prevention U.S. Department of Health and Human Services, 2010.

From U.S. Department of Health and Human Services: *Healthy People 2020: Roadmap to Improving All Americans' Health.* Washington, DC, 2010, U.S. Government Printing Office.

not include a systematic review of evidence to support the interventions or their application to practice. Initially, the model was developed from an extensive analysis of the actual work of 200 practicing public health nurses working in a variety of settings. The 17 interventions grew out of this analysis, as did the three levels of practice. The authors indicated that the original intent was to provide a description of the scope and breadth of public health nursing practice.

Because of the positive response to the Intervention Wheel, the decision was made to complete a systematic review of the evidence supporting the use of the Intervention Wheel. The goal was to examine the evidence underlying the interventions and the levels of practice. The systematic review involved answering six questions, a comprehensive search of literature, a survey of 51 BSN programs in five states, and a critique (by five graduate

students) of the 665 pieces of evidence found in the literature review for rigor (strength and usefulness). After limiting the final review to 221 sources of evidence, each source was independently rated by at least two members of a 42-member panel of practicing public health nurses and educators. The 42-member panel met to reach consensus on the outcomes of the reviews. The outcomes were field-tested with 150 practicing nurses, and then critiqued by a national panel of 20 experts.

The Intervention Wheel presented in Chapter 9 is the result of this systematic review and critique (Keller et al, 2004). Although this critique may appear overwhelming, the undergraduate or graduate student may be involved in such a systematic critique as one of many participants contributing to the outcome of such a review. Table 15-2 applies some of the interventions to the core functions of public health.

## PRACTICE APPLICATION

A nurse who is the director of a public health clinic is in the process of analyzing how best to expand services to operate as a full-time clinic in the most cost-effective and clinically effective manner. The director gathers evidence from the literature on public health clinics in rural settings to evaluate cost and clinical effectiveness of various models. The nurse also considers evidence from the following sources in the decision-making

process: client satisfaction research data, knowledge of clinic staff, expert opinion of community advisory board members, evidence from community partners, and data on service needs in the state. Having examined the evidence, the nurse decides that incremental (step-by-step) growth toward full-time status is warranted. Evidence of needs in the community and analysis of statistical data indicate that the addition of wellness services

## TABLE 15-2 Core Public Health Functions and Related Evidence-Based Nursing Interventions

| Core Functions | Related Nursing Interventions |
|---|---|
| Assessment | Diagnose and investigate health problems and hazards in the community.<br>Mobilize community partnerships to identify and solve health problems.<br>Link people to needed health services.<br>Use evidence-based practice for new insights and innovative solutions to health problems. |
| Policy development | Inform, educate, and empower communities about health issues.<br>Develop policies and plans using evidence-based practice that supports individual and community health efforts. |
| Assurance | Monitor health status to identify community health problems.<br>Enforce laws and regulations that protect health and ensure safety.<br>Ensure the provision of health care that is otherwise unavailable.<br>Ensure a competent public health and personal health care workforce.<br>Use evidence-based practice to evaluate effectiveness, accessibility, and quality of personal and population-based services. |

## ▌ PRACTICE APPLICATION—cont'd

for children is a priority and a pediatric nurse practitioner is hired as a first step to assist the public health nurses while planning for full-time status continues.

A. Evaluation of the evidence gathered demonstrates which of the following?
1. Effectiveness of the intervention in communities
2. Application of the data to populations and communities
3. Existence of positive or negative health outcomes
4. Economic consequences of the intervention
5. Barriers to implementation of the interventions in communities

B. Explain how this example applies principles of EBP.
**Answers can be found on the Evolve site.**

## ▌ KEY POINTS

- Evidence-based practice was developed in other countries before its use in the United States.
- The Institute of Medicine has indicated that by 2020, 90% of all health care should be evidence based.
- EBP is a paradigm shift in health care and nursing.
- EBP is both a process and a product.
- Application of EBP in relation to clinical decision making in population-centered nursing concentrates on interventions and strategies geared to communities and populations rather than to individuals.
- Nurses at all levels have an opportunity to improve the practice of nursing and client outcomes.
- The EBP process has seven steps.
- Approaches to EBP include systematic review, meta-analysis, integrative review, and narrative review.
- Evaluating the strength and usefulness of evidence is essential to finding the best evidence on which to make practice decisions.
- Cost and quality of care are issues in EBP.
- EBP includes interventions based on theory, expert opinions, provider knowledge, and research.
- Use of a community development model and community partnership model involves community leaders in making decisions about best practices in their community.
- The Intervention Wheel is an example of a result of EBP.
- Health care reform supports EBP.

## ▌ CLINICAL DECISION-MAKING ACTIVITIES

1. Give an example of how undergraduates can be involved in EBP.
2. Explain how the nurse's knowledge of the community relates to EBP. Give examples.
3. What are the barriers to implementing EBP? How can these barriers be resolved?
4. Is the cost or quality of care more important in EBP? Debate this issue with classmates.
5. When working with a community to improve its health, is it more important to consider the perspectives of the community or those of the provider when defining health problems? Elaborate.
6. Invite the director of nursing from the local health department to speak to your class. Ask if evidence is used to develop nursing policies and practice guidelines. If not, why not?
7. Explain how you can apply evidence to your practice.

# REFERENCES

AHRQ: *National Guideline Clearinghouse.* Wash, DC, 2014, USDHHS. Available at: www.AHRQ.gov. Accessed on 9/19, 2014.

Application of POEM. 2014. Available at www.essentialevidenceplus .com. Accessed 9/19/2014.

Asadoorian J, Hearson B, Satyanarayana S, et al: Evidence-based practice in healthcare: an exploratory cross-discipline comparison of enhancers and barriers. *J Healthcare Qual* 32(3):15–22, 2010.

Barnard K, Hoehn R: *Nursing Child Assessment Satellite Training: Final Report.* Hyattsville, MD, 1978, DHEW, Division of Nursing.

Beyers M: About evidence-based nursing practice. *Nurs Manag* 30:56, 1999.

Blakely T, Bruggink S, Dziadosz G, et al: Combining evidence-based practices for improved behavioral outcomes—a demonstration project. *Community Ment Health J* 49(4):396–400, 2013.

Bradshaw WG: Importance of nursing leadership in advancing evidence-based nursing practice. *Neonatal Netw* 29(2):117–122, 2010.

Brownson RC, Fielding JE, Maylahn CM: Evidence-based public health: a fundamental concept for public health practice. *Annu Rev Public Health* 30:175–202, 2009.

Cochrane Library: *Cochrane handbook for systematic reviews of interventions.* At: www.cochrane .org/resources/handbook/index.htm. Accessed 9/19/2014.

Craig JV, Smyth RL: *The Evidence-Based Practice Manual for Nurses*, ed 2. Edinburgh, 2007, Churchill Livingstone Elsevier.

Dawes M, Davies P, Gray A, et al: *Evidence-Based Practice: a Primer for Health Care Professionals*, ed 2. London, 2004, Churchill Livingstone Elsevier.

Dicenso A, Guyatt G, Ciliska D, editors: *Evidence-Based Nursing: a Guide to Clinical Practice.* St Louis, 2005, Elsevier Mosby.

Earle-Foley V: Evidence-based practice: issues, paradigms, and future pathways. *Nurs Forum* 46(1):38–44, 2011.

Estabrooks CA, Winther C, Derksen L: Mapping the field: a biliometric analysis of the research utilization literature in nursing. *Nurs Res* 53:293–303, 2004.

Evidence-Based Medicine Working Group: Evidence-based medicine: a new approach to teaching the practice of medicine. *JAMA* 268:2420–2425, 1992.

Fineout-Overholt E, Malnyk B, Stillwell SB, et al: Critical appraisal of the evidence: part 1: an introduction to gathering, evaluating, and recording the evidence. *AJN* 110(7):47–52, 2010.

Florin J, Ehrenberg A, Wallin L, et al: Educational support for research utilization and capability beliefs regarding evidence-based practice skills—a national survey of senior nursing students. *J Adv Nurs* 68(4):888–897, 2012.

Gerrish K, Cooke J: Factors influencing evidence-based practice among community nurses. *JCN* 27(4):98–101, 2013.

Guyatt G, Rennie D, editors: *Users' guides to the medical literature: a manual for evidence-based clinical practice.* Chicago, 2002, AMA.

GWU: *Himmelfarb Library.* Wash DC, 2014, George Washington University. Accessed at: http://himmelfarb.gwu.edu/tutorials/studydesign101/metaanalyses.html. on 9/19/2014.

Haine-Schlagel R, Fettes D, Garcia A, et al: Consistency with evidence-based treatments and perceived effectiveness of children's community-based care. *Community Ment Health J* 50(2):158–163, 2014.

Holly C, Salmond SW, Saimbert MK: *Comprehensive Systematic Review for Advanced Nursing Practice.* New York, 2011, Springer Publishing Company.

Honor Society of Nursing, Sigma Theta Tau International: *Position statement on evidence-based nursing,* Indianapolis, IN. 2005. Available at: http://www.nursing society.org. Accessed December 26, 2010.

Horsley JA, Crane J, Bingle JD: Research utilization as an organizational process. *J Nurs Admin* 8:4–6, 1978.

Horsley JA, Crane J, Crabtree MK, et al: *Using Research to Improve Nursing Practice: A Guide.* San Francisco, 1983, Grune & Stratton.

Jacobs JA, Jones E, Gabella BA, et al: Tools for implementing an evidence-based approach in public health practice. *Prev Chronic Dis* 9:110324, 2012. DOI: http://dx.doi.org/10.5888/pcd9.110324. Accessed 9/19/2014.

Jenkins C, Pope C, Magwood G: Expanding the chronic care framework to improve diabetes management: The REACH Case Study. *Prog Community Health Partnersh* 4(1):65–79, 2010.

Keller L, Strohschein S, Lia-Hoagbert B, et al: Population-based public health interventions: practice-based and evidence-supported. Part I.

*Public Health Nurs* 21(5):453–468, 2004.

King D, Barnard KE, Hoehn R: Disseminating the results of nursing research. *Nurs Outlook* 29:164–169, 1981.

Krueger JC: Utilizing clinical nursing research findings in practice: a structured approach. *Commun Nurs Res* 9:381–394, 1977.

Krueger JC, Nelson AH, Wolanin MO: *Nursing Research: Development, Collaboration and Utilization.* Germantown, MD, 1978, Aspen.

Levin RF, Keefer JM, Marren J, et al: Evidence-based practice improvement: merging 2 paradigms. *J Nurs Care Qual* 25(2):117–126, 2010.

Lindeman CA, Krueger JC: Increasing the quality, quantity, and use of nursing research. *Nurs Outlook* 25:450–454, 1977.

Makic MBF, Rauen C, Watson R, et al: Examining the evidence to guide practice—challenging practice habits. *Crit Care Nurse* 34(2):28–30, 32–46, 2014.

Mattila L, Rekola L, Koponen L, et al: Journal club intervention in promoting evidence-based nursing—perceptions of nursing students. *Nurse Educ Pract* 13(5):423–428, 2013.

Melnyk B, Fineout-Overholt E, Stillwell SB, et al: The seven steps of evidence-based practice. *AJN* 110(1):51–53, 2010.

Melnyk BM, Fineout-Overholt E: *Evidence-Based Practice in Nursing and Healthcare: A Guide to Best Practice,* ed 2. Philadelphia, 2011, Lippincott. Williams & Wilkins.

Merrill KC, Macintosh J, Mandleco B, et al: Overview—innovative methods to create a spirit of inquiry in undergraduate nursing students. *Commun Nurs Res* 46:184, 2013.

Pew Center on the States: *The case for home visiting,* May 2010. Available at: www.pewcenter onthestates.org. Accessed September 17, 2010.

Polit DF, Beck CT: *Nursing Research: Generngating and Assessing Evidence for Nursing Practice,* ed 9. New York, 2011, Lippincott, Williams & Wilkins.

Public Health Accreditation Board: *Accredited health departments,* PHAB press release. 2014. Available at: http://www.phaboard.org/news-room/accredited-health-departments/. Accessed May 21, 2014.

Russell-Babin K: Seeing through the clouds in evidence-based practice. *Nurs Manag* 40(11):26–32, 2009.

Rychetrik L, Hawe P, Waters E, et al: A glossary for evidence based public health. *J Epidemiol*

*Community Health* 58:538–545, 2003.

Sackett DL, Rosenberg WMC, Gray J, et al: Evidence-based medicine: what it is and what it isn't. *Br Med J* 312:71–72, 1996.

Sackett DL, Straus SE, Richardson WS, et al: *Evidence-Based Medicine: How to Practice and Teach EBM.* London, 2000, Churchill Livingstone.

Sandström B, Borglin G, Nilsson R, et al: Promoting the implementation of evidence-based practice—a literature review focusing on the role of nursing leadership. *Worldviews Evid Based Nurs* Fourth quarter:212–223, 2011.

Scott K, McSherry R: Evidence-based nursing: clarifying the concepts for nurses in practice. *J Clin Nurs* 18:1085–1095, 2009.

Shaughnessy AF, Slawson DC, Bennett JA: Becoming an information master: a guidebook to the medical information jungles. *J Fam Pract* 39:489–499, 1994.

Sprayberry LD: Transformation of America's healthcare system—implications for professional direct-care nurses. *Medsurg Nurs* 23(1):61–66, 2014.

Stetler CB: Updating the Stetler model of research utilization to facilitate evidence-based practice. *Nurs Outlook* 49:272–279, 2001.

Task Force on Community Preventive Services: *Guide to community preventive services.* 2007. Available at: http://www.thecommunityguide .org/diabetes/default.htm. Accessed September 26, 2010.

Task Force on Community Preventive Services: *National Center for Chronic Disease Prevention and Health Promotion.* 2010. Available at: www.cdc.gov. Accessed August 6, 2010.

Titler MG, Steelman VJ, Budreau G, et al: The Iowa model of evidence-based practice to promote quality care. *Crit Care Nurs Clin North Am* 13:497–509, 2001.

U.S. Department of Health and Human Services: *Healthy People 2020: Roadmap to Improving All Americans' Health.* Washington, DC, 2010, U.S. Government Printing Office.

U.S. Preventive Services Task Force: *Task force ratings: strength of recommendations and quality of evidence, 2000-2003.* Available at: http://www.ahrq.gov/clinic/prevenix. htm.

# 16

# Changing Health Behavior Using Health Education with Individuals, Families, and Groups

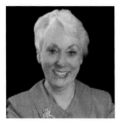

*Jeanette Lancaster, PhD, RN, FAAN*
Dr. Lancaster is Professor and Dean Emerita of Nursing at the University of Virginia. She has edited this book with Dr. Marcia Stanhope through its previous eight editions.

## ADDITIONAL RESOURCES

(e) **Evolve Website http://evolve.elsevier.com/Stanhope**
- *Healthy People 2020*
- WebLinks
- Quiz

- Case Studies
- Glossary
- Answers to Practice Application

## OBJECTIVES

*After reading this chapter, the student should be able to do the following:*
1. Describe the ways in which people learn.
2. Identify the steps and principles that guide community health education.
3. Discuss the importance of understanding the needs of learners including their cultural background, educational and health literacy level, and their motivation to learn and change behavior.

4. Describe how nurses can work with groups to promote the health of individuals and communities.
5. Examine types of health education including written, spoken, and the growing area of social media.
6. Explore ethical issues that arise in the practice of health education.

## KEY TERMS

affective domain, p. 358
andragogy, p. 363
change, p. 357
cognitive domain, p. 358
cohesion, p. 369
democratic leadership, p. 372
education, p. 357
established groups, p. 372
ethics, p. 356
evaluation, p. 367
formal groups, p. 368
goals, p. 359
group, p. 369
health belief model, p. 366

health education, p. 357
health literacy, p. 365
informal groups, p. 368
learning, p. 357
long-term evaluation, p. 368
maintenance functions, p. 369
maintenance norms, p. 370
motivational interviewing, p. 361
norms, p. 370
objectives, p. 359
patriarchal leadership, p. 371
pedagogy, p. 363
precaution adoption process model, p. 367
process evaluation, p. 367

One of the best ways to manage health care costs is for people to stay healthy. Nurses are in an ideal role to help individuals, families, and groups learn about health education and health promotion in order to change their behavior. Nurses can help clients by (1) educating across all three levels of prevention: primary, secondary, and tertiary; and (2) working with individuals, families, groups, and communities. The goal is to assist clients to attain optimal health, prevent health problems, identify and treat health problems early, and minimize disability. Education allows individuals to make knowledgeable health-related decisions, assume personal responsibility for their health, change behavior if needed, and cope effectively with alterations in their health and lifestyles. The Levels of Prevention box provides an example of how to use these three prevention levels in health education.

## LEVELS OF PREVENTION

### Related to Community Health Education

**Primary Prevention**
Provide education at health fairs about diet, exercise, or environmental hazards.

**Secondary Prevention**
Provide both education and health screenings at health fairs for such health issues as early diagnosis and treatment of diabetes and hypercholesterolemia in order to shorten the duration and severity of the disease.

**Tertiary Prevention**
Provide education in rehabilitation centers to teach ways to increase function to individuals who have been in an accident that left them with either an amputation or some paralysis.

This chapter discusses ways to develop individual, group, and community health promotion programs. Specific content in the chapter includes information about how people learn; the sequence of actions that a nurse follows when developing an educational program; the process of making change; literacy, especially health literacy; and the ethics related to health education. The role of groups in health promotion is also presented. Many of the objectives of *Healthy People 2020* address the importance of health promotion, and selected objectives are cited in this chapter.

## *HEALTHY PEOPLE 2020* OBJECTIVES FOR HEALTH EDUCATION

As mentioned in other chapters, *Healthy People 2020* lists national health needs and outlines goals and objectives designed to improve health. The *Healthy People 2020* educational objectives emphasize the importance of educating various populations (based on age and ethnicity) about health promotion activities in the priority areas of unintentional injury; violence; suicide; tobacco use and addiction; alcohol or other drug use; unintended pregnancy, human immunodeficiency virus/acquired immunodeficiency syndrome (HIV/AIDS), and sexually transmitted disease (STD); unhealthy dietary patterns; and inadequate physical activity (U.S. Department of Health and Human Services [USDHHS], 2010).

In designing, implementing, and evaluating health education activities, it is useful to understand the primary health problems in the community as well as education principles related to both learning and teaching. Also, effective educational programs are built on the premise that the best approach is to teach what people think they want to learn and in ways that facilitate their learning. For this reason, a core public health principle relates to asking the learners to participate in identifying their learning needs. Then health education programs are designed to meet the health need or problem in that population. In general, these programs involve educating individual members of the population about health promotion, illness prevention, and treatment. For example, in a community where childhood and adolescent asthma is a problem, a community-based asthma education and training program can be developed. If childhood obesity is a major health concern, a program to educate children in their schools and parents and other caregivers in an after-school program about healthy eating, cooking, and exercise may be useful.

To develop a community-based education program, nurses need to follow a set of steps. Typical steps that are discussed in detail throughout the chapter include the following: (1) *identify* a population-specific learning need for the community health client; (2) *select* one or more learning theories to use in the education program; (3) *consider* which educational principles are most likely to increase learning and choose those that are most appropriate and feasible; (4) *examine* educational issues, such as population-specific or cultural concerns, identify barriers to learning, such as limited literacy or limited or lack of health literacy, and choose the most appropriate teaching and learning strategies based on the age, gender, education, and learning needs of the learners; (5) *design and implement* the educational program, using carefully chosen strategies; and (6) *evaluate* the effects of the educational program. The steps used in designing educational programs parallel those of the nursing process.

## EDUCATION, LEARNING, AND CHANGE

When helping people change their behavior, remember that people can most easily change knowledge. The next step is to help people change their attitudes, and the most difficult area to change is behavior. For this reason, nurses provide people with health information so they can improve their decision-making abilities and thereby decide if they will change their behavior. There is a difference between education and learning and between knowing and doing. **Education** is an activity "undertaken or initiated by one or more agents that is designed to effect changes in the knowledge, skill, and attitudes of individuals, groups, or communities" (Knowles et al, 2005, p. 10). Education emphasizes the provider of knowledge and skills. In contrast, **learning** emphasizes the recipient of knowledge and skills and the person(s) in whom a change is expected to occur. Remember that learning involves change.

Change is not easy for most people. To **change** means to move away from one way of thinking, believing, and acting and move toward a new way. Thompson (2010) describes understanding and managing organizational change. Although much of the change regarding health education is directed toward clients, not organizations, the steps he uses also apply to health education. They are as follows: (1) identify the need for change—and this means that the client or clients being served need to believe that they need to make a change; (2) plan how to implement the change—and this step includes explaining the basis for the change, the benefits of the change, and seeking ideas from those being served about the best way to make an identified change; (3) implement the change; and (4) evaluate whether the change made a difference in health. Fielding (2013) offers a similar approach toward health education, consisting of the following five steps: (1) understanding the problem, (2) understanding what works, (3) agreeing on the approach or action, (4) implementing the plan, and (5) evaluating the effect. As nurses work with clients to make health changes, it is important to watch for resistance or reverting back to past behaviors.

## HOW PEOPLE LEARN

People learn in a variety of ways. Some people learn better by hearing a message; others learn by observing and/or participating in what is being taught. Learners accept information on the basis of many factors including what they already know, what they believe, and the culture in which they have been raised; as well as how well they can understand and relate to the information that they receive. What a person hears is filtered through his past experiences, the social groups to which he belongs, assumptions, values, level of attention and knowledge, and the respect he has for the person communicating the information. In some cultures, elders are considered to be valued sources of information. In other cultures, people value individuals with more education than they have. Also, because social groups play a critical role in the development of understanding or learning, concepts related to groups are discussed later in this chapter. Effective **health education** is a competency that is included in many documents that describe the role of public health professionals, including nurses. The Linking Content to Practice box illustrates the relationship between health education and selected standards, expectations, and competencies in public health.

A variety of educational principles can be used to guide the selection of health information for individuals, families, communities, and populations. Three of the most useful categories of educational principles include those associated with the nature of learning, the educational process, and the skills of effective educators.

## The Nature of Learning

One way to think about the nature of learning is to examine the cognitive (thinking), affective (feeling), and psychomotor (acting) domains of learning. Each domain has specific behavioral components that form a hierarchy of steps, or levels. Each level builds on the previous one. Understanding these three learning domains is crucial in providing effective health education (Bloom et al, 1956). First, consider assumptions about how adults learn. Specifically, adults are motivated to learn when (1) they think they need to know something, (2) the new information is compatible with their prior life experiences, (3) they value the person(s) providing the information, and (4) they believe they can make any necessary changes that are implied by the new information (Knowles et al, 2005).

### Cognitive Domain

The cognitive domain includes memory, recognition, understanding, reasoning, application, and problem solving and is divided into a hierarchical classification of behaviors. Learners master each level of cognition in order of difficulty (Bloom et al, 1956). Start by assessing the cognitive abilities of the learners. This is especially important when learners have a limited level of literacy either of the language used in the instruction or of the content that is presented. A later section discusses both literacy in general and health literacy in particular. Teaching above or below a person's level of understanding can lead to frustration and discouragement. It is therefore important to be sensitive to the value of the cognitive domain in learning. The

cognitive domain consists of the following components (Bloom et al, 1956):

1. *Knowledge:* Requires recall of information
2. *Comprehension:* Combines recall with understanding
3. *Application:* In which new information is taken in and used in a different way
4. *Analysis:* Breaks communication down into parts in order to understand both the parts and their relationships to one another
5. *Synthesis:* Builds on the first four levels by assembling them into a new whole
6. *Evaluation:* In which learners judge the value of what has been learned

### Affective Domain

The affective domain includes changes in attitudes and the development of values. For affective learning to take place, nurses consider and attempt to influence what learners feel, think, and value. Because the attitudes and values of nurses may differ from those of their clients, it is important to listen carefully to detect clues to feelings or misperceptions that learners have that may influence learning. It is difficult to change deeply rooted attitudes, beliefs, interests, and values. To make such changes, people need support and encouragement from those around them. Affective learning, like cognitive learning, consists of a series of steps that the learner takes:

1. *Knowledge:* Receives the information
2. *Comprehension:* Responds to the information received
3. *Application:* Values the information
4. *Analysis:* Makes sense of the information
5. *Synthesis:* Organizes the information
6. *Evaluation:* Adopts behaviors consistent with new values

### Psychomotor Domain

The psychomotor domain includes the performance of skills that require some degree of neuromuscular coordination and emphasizes motor skills (Bloom et al, 1956). Clients are taught a variety of psychomotor skills including bathing infants, changing dressings, giving injections, measuring blood glucose levels, taking blood pressures, walking with crutches, as well as many skills related to health promotion exercises.

In teaching a skill, first show clients how to do a task requiring the skill being taught. You can use pictures, a model, or a device, or via a live demonstration, video, CD, or the Internet. Next, have clients practice through a repeat demonstration to validate that what is being taught was actually learned. Also, if the teaching is being done in a class, participants may learn by observing one another master a task. Psychomotor learning is dependent on learners meeting three conditions (Bloom et al, 1956; Dembo, 1994). The learner must have the following:

- The *necessary ability:* This will include both cognitive and psychomotor ability. For example, you may find that a person with Alzheimer's disease can follow only one-step instructions. Thus, you need to tailor your education plan to that person.
- A *sensory image* of how to carry out the skill: For example, when teaching a group of women how to cook heart-healthy foods, ask the women to describe their kitchen and how they would actually go about the cooking process.

- *Opportunities to practice* the new skills: Provide practice sessions during the program to help the client adapt the skill to the home or work environment where the skill will be performed.
- *The following Quality and Safety Education for Nurses box describes the importance of clear and appropriate communication.*

## (QSEN) FOCUS ON QUALITY AND SAFETY EDUCATION FOR NURSES

### *Targeted Competency: Client-Centered Care*

Important aspects of client-centered care include the following:

**Knowledge:** Integrate understanding of multiple dimensions of client-centered care: information, communication, and education

**Skills:** Communicate client values, preferences, and expressed needs to other members of the health care team

**Attitudes:** Respect and encourage individual expression of client values, preferences, and expressed needs

#### Client-Centered Care Question

Providing health information in a way that is not understandable or useful to the recipient is a poor form of client-centered communication. If you were teaching a group of four women about wound care after surgery, what steps would you take to assure that the message the women received was the message that you intended to send?

*Answer:* In general, you would begin by providing the needed information by describing each step; you might include an easy-to-understand handout in the language that the four women understand, or you might give them a CD to take home with them that has the information on it. Next you would demonstrate how to clean the wound. Then you would ask each woman to repeat the cleaning process that you just demonstrated. Finally, you would ask each woman if she had the facilities and supplies to clean the wound at home; and then you would ask if they each had any questions or concerns that you might answer. What else would you do?

Source: Cronenwett L, Sherwood G, Barnsteiner J, et al: Quality and safety education for nurses. *Nurs Outlook* 55:122–131, 2007.

In assessing a client's ability to learn a skill, be sure to evaluate intellectual, emotional, and physical ability, and then teach at the level of the learner's ability. Some clients do not have the intellectual ability to learn the steps that make up a complex procedure. Others may have cultural beliefs that conflict with healthy behaviors. Another client may be tremulous or have poor eyesight, making him incapable of learning insulin self-injection.

## THE EDUCATIONAL PROCESS

The educational process builds on an understanding of education, learning, and how people learn. The five steps of the educational process (identify educational needs, establish educational goals and objectives, select appropriate educational methods, implement the educational plan, and evaluate the educational process) are discussed next.

### Identify Educational Needs and Develop Goals and Objectives

Begin with a needs assessment to learn about health education needs. The steps of such an assessment are listed in Box 16-1.

### BOX 16-1  Steps of a Needs Assessment

1. Identify what the client wants to know. (Consider *Healthy People 2020* educational objectives.)
2. Collect data systematically about learning needs, readiness to learn, and barriers to learning.
3. Analyze assessment data that have been collected and identify cognitive, affective, and psychomotor learning needs.
4. Think about what will increase the client's ability and motivation to learn.
5. Assist the client to prioritize learning needs.

Once you identify the needs, prioritize them to meet the most important needs first. Consider the many factors that influence a person's learning needs and the ability to learn including demographic, physical, geographic, economic, psychological, social, and spiritual factors. Consider also the learner's knowledge, skills, and his or her motivation to learn, as well as what resources are available to support or prevent learning. Resources include printed, audio or visual materials, equipment, agencies, and other individuals. Barriers for the presenter include lack of time, skill and/or confidence, money, space, energy, and organizational support.

When you have identified the learning needs, develop the goals and objectives for the educational program. **Goals** are broad, long-term expected outcomes such as, "Each child in the third-grade class will participate in 30 minutes of daily physical exercise, 4 days per week for 2 months." Program goals should deal directly with the clients' overall learning needs. Regarding the third graders, their learning need is to know how important exercise is to their health and level of fitness.

**Objectives** are specific, short-term criteria that need to be met as steps toward achieving the long-term goal such as, "Within 2 weeks, each of the children will be able to demonstrate at least two exercises that they have learned." Objectives are written statements of an intended outcome or expected change in behavior and should define the minimal degree of knowledge or ability needed by a client. Objectives must be stated clearly and defined in measurable terms, and they typically imply an action (Knowles et al, 2005).

### Select Appropriate Educational Methods

Educational methods should be chosen to facilitate the efficient and successful accomplishment of program goals and objectives. The methods should also be appropriately matched to the client's strengths and needs as well as those of the presenter. Choose the simplest, clearest, and most succinct manner of presentation and avoid complex program designs. Try to vary the methods in order to hold the attention of the learners and to meet the needs of different learners. Educators also need to be able to deliver presentations, lead group discussions, organize role plays, provide feedback to learners, share case studies, use media and materials, and, where indicated, administer examinations. You will want to think about what content to include, how to organize and sequence the information, what your rate of delivery will be, whether or not you need to include repetition, how much practice time should be included, how you will evaluate the effectiveness of the teaching, and ways that you can provide reinforcement and rewards. The Internet and use of social media have created an entirely new way of providing health information. Sites such as Facebook, YouTube, and Twitter have large numbers of users (Bernhardt et al, 2013). Data from the Pew Internet & American Life Project (Pew Charitable Trusts, 2013) show that laptop computers are used more often than desktop computers and that the use of music players, video game equipment, electronic book readers, and tablet computers has grown rapidly. The most explosive growth has been in the use of mobile phones. These new forms of access to information affect the way in which health education is developed and delivered.

It is important to consider the ethical issues involved in using various forms of teaching tools, especially when using social media. According to the Pew Internet & American Life Project (Pew Charitable Trusts, 2013), 60% of patients seek both support and information online. Of 3,014 survey respondents, 77% said that they used Google, Bing, or Yahoo to find health information. Remember, not all websites are developed by health care professionals, nor have they all been peer reviewed. Also, when nurses use patient cases or data to illustrate a health education point, it is important to clearly understand the guidelines of the Health Insurance Portability and Accountability Act (HIPAA) and avoid privacy ethical violations of the ethics code. When nurses use social media to provide health education, they should consult the *ANA's Principles for Social Networking and the Nurse* (American Nurses Association, 2011) and the National Council of State Boards of Nursing's *White Paper: A Nurse's Guide to the Use of Social Media* (National Council of State Boards of Nursing, 2011). It is essential to protect the privacy of patients and their health data when making presentations in person or via social media or any other medium (Lachman, 2013).

When choosing educational methods, consider age, gender, culture, hearing, sight or developmental disabilities or special learning needs, educational level, knowledge of the subject, and size of the group. For example, clients with a visual impairment need more verbal description than those with no impairment in sight. Persons who have hearing impairments or language deficits need more visual material and speakers or translators who can use sign language or speak their native language. Also, when the learners have limitations in attention and concentration, the educator will need to use creative methods and tools to keep them focused. For example, you might include frequent breaks; simple surroundings with few or no distractions; use of small group interactions to keep learners involved and interested; and the use of hands-on equipment such as mannequins, models, interactive games, and other materials and devices that the learner can physically manipulate. Try to involve the learner appropriately, actively, and creatively in learning. Interactive educational programs may be more effective than noninteractive ones. Interactive strategies include discussion, small group work, games, and role-playing, whereas noninteractive strategies include lectures, videos, or demonstrations. The mnemonic TEACH is a useful way to teach clients. The steps are as follows:

*Tune in:* Listen before you start teaching. The client's needs should direct the content.

*Edit information:* Teach necessary information first. Be specific.

*Act on each teaching moment:* Teach whenever possible. Develop a good relationship.

*Clarify often:* Make sure your assumptions are correct. Seek feedback.

*Honor the client:* Respect the client as a partner, share responsibility, and build on the client's experience.

The goal of nurses who use *Healthy People 2020* as a guide in educating clients is to foster healthy communities mainly through primary and secondary prevention. Health fairs are a popular way to provide primary and secondary health education. The objectives of holding health fairs are to increase awareness by providing health screenings, activities, information and educational materials, and demonstrations. A health fair can target a specific population or focus on a specific health issue, as well as target a range of groups and cover a variety of health education and health promotion topics. The fair can be held in many locations and can be either inside or outside. The How To box lists guidelines to assist nurses who chair, co-chair, or serve on a planning committee for a health fair.

---

**HOW TO** Plan, Implement, and Evaluate a Health Fair
- *Form a planning committee (2-12 people who represent the groups that will be part of the health fair). Possibilities include health professionals, representatives from health agencies, schools, churches, employers, the media, and the target audience.*
- *Identify the target group; develop a theme.*
- *Establish goals, expected outcomes, and screening activities consistent with the needs and wishes of the target group. Your primary goal might be to improve the health of a specific population such as workers at one plant or children in one school. You might have secondary goals such as reduced health care costs for the workers and reduced absenteeism for the children.*
- *Develop a timeline and schedule.*
- *Choose a site and consider the site logistics: Do this about 1 year ahead. Think about the size of the site you will need and the traffic flow from one booth or demonstration to another, whether parking is available and free or low cost, and whether there are toilets and places to get food and drinks. If the site is inside, consider adequate exits; the possible risks to children, the elderly, or handicapped people; and other safety and security issues. You may need to create maps: one for how to get to the fair and another one to help attendees get from one table, exhibit, or screening station to another. Be sure to include on the map the location of amenities such as toilets and food vendors.*
- *Plan for supplies that you will need: Tables, chairs, electronic equipment, and accessories such as extension cords, office supplies, sign-in sheets (and what information should be included), release forms for screenings, name tags, bags for attendees to gather the educational information, and evaluation forms. Set your budget. Obtain these supplies in advance.*
- *Recruit and manage exhibitors: Do this about 4 months ahead. Develop a list of possible exhibitors and sponsors, and contact them via letter, fax, e-mail, telephone, or in person. Follow-up with a confirmation letter (or fax) that outlines the details of the health fair.*
- *Publicize the health fair: The planning committee will have many good ideas about how to publicize in the specific community.*

*Examples might include fliers/posters, memos, brochures, e-mail blasts, local print, or radio/television.*

- *On the day of the fair: Greet health care professionals, agency representatives, sponsors, and members of the population being served.*
- *Evaluate the health fair: By exhibitors, participants and volunteers. You will need a specific form for each of these groups.*
- *Between 1 week and 1 month after the fair: Send thank-you letters to health care professionals, sponsors, and agencies, and pay bills associated with the fair.*

From Rice CA, Pollard JM: Health fair planning guide, Agri LIFE EXTENSION Texas A&M System, September 16, 2009. Available at http://fcs.

## Skills of the Effective Educator

The educator needs to understand the basic sequence of instruction. The following steps are useful in planning an educational program. Begin by (1) gaining the attention of the learners and helping them understand that the information being presented is important and helpful to them; (2) tell the learners the objectives of the instruction; (3) ask the learners to recall previous knowledge related to this topic of interest so that they link new knowledge with previous knowledge; (4) present the essential material in a clear, organized, and simple manner and in a way consistent with the learners' strengths, needs, and limitations; (5) help learners apply the information to their lives and situations; (6) encourage learners to demonstrate what they have learned, which will help you correct any errors and improve skills; and (7) provide feedback to help learners improve their knowledge and skills. When you use each of these steps you can help clients increase their learning experiences.

## Motivational Interviewing

Sometimes clients do not provide all of the information needed to help promote their health. It is important before developing an implementation plan to carefully assess the need. The goal in health education is to engage the clients in wanting to learn ways in which they can change their behavior. Pay attention to the words you use and avoid medical jargon. Instead, use conversational language. One tool to use in health education is "motivational interviewing" (MI), which is a tool designed to help clients state their motivations to change (Miller and Rose, 2009). It is a collaborative partnership between the teacher and the learner designed to help people make their own choices. It seeks to help clients resolve their ambivalence about change and uses the techniques of elaboration, affirmation, reflection, and summary to engage people in talking about change. MI often is used in conjunction with other communication techniques. MI has four essential steps: engaging, which includes person-centered, empathic listening; guiding, which includes a particular identified target for change; evoking of the client's own motivations for change; and planning (Motivational Interviewing Network of Trainers, 2013).

MI was initially designed to treat problem drinkers and is used often with individuals rather than groups. However, the principles can be applied to health education. For example, if a public health nurse determines that she has four women in a community group she leads who are overweight, eat high-calorie foods, and indicate they exercise little if any on a regular basis, how could the nurse use MI? First, the nurse needs to form a partnership with each of the women, in which she and the clients can communicate easily and in which each woman trusts the nurse. The nurse draws each woman out and learns what, if anything, each wishes to change. The nurse also learns about each one's motivation to change and ability to do so. Consider the client, Anna, and examine her motivation to change her eating and activity patterns. Anna says that her family will eat only fried foods, so to get her husband and children to eat a meal she fries their meats and vegetables. The family does eat fresh fruit and drink milk. Anna says that she gets exercise by walking to the bus stop en route to work and cleaning her home. She has not considered other forms of regular exercise. If you want to use MI with Anna and incorporate these principles in designing your nursing plan you could begin as follows:

1. Expressing empathy by trying to see the world through Anna's eyes
2. Building on Anna's strengths and helping her believe that she has the ability to make a change (self-efficacy)
3. Rolling with resistance when Anna is ambivalent about her ability to change
4. Developing discrepancy by helping Anna recognize that her current actions conflict with her expressed goals of eating healthy foods and exercising regularly

You could incorporate into your strategy the counseling skills that are part of MI: open-ended questions, affirmations, reflections, and summaries (OARS). These communication skills are useful in any nurse-client interaction. Open-ended questions refer to those that are not easily answered with yes or no or a short answer. These questions invite elaboration and more thinking about what is being asked. In helping Anna prepare healthier meals, ask her to describe the dinner she cooked the previous night. Affirmations are designed to recognize client strengths; they must be genuine and correct. Once Anna begins to explore the idea of preparing more nutritious food, you would affirm her progress and encourage her to continue working toward that goal. Reflections or reflective listening is possibly the most critical skill in that it conveys empathy because you are listening carefully. You can then guide Anna toward dealing with her ambivalence about change by examining the positive and negative aspects of the present situation. Using reflective listening, if Anna expresses concern or difficulty in her goal of preparing different meals, you can focus on her concern and possible ambivalence about sticking to the plan for change.

MI uses the term *change talk* to refer to statements by clients that they are motivated and willing to make change. An easy-to-use mnemonic is "DARN-CAT," which refers to the following:

| Preparatory Change Talk | Implementing Change Talk |
|---|---|
| **D**esire (I want to change) | **C**ommitment (I will make changes) |
| **A**bility (I can change) | |
| **R**eason (It's important to change) | **A**ctivation (I am ready, prepared, willing to change) |
| **N**eed (I should change) | **T**aking steps (I am taking actions to change) |

Apply the DARN-CAT mnemonic to the goal you and Anna have for her to learn ways to prepare more nutritious meals. Although MI is a set of skills that requires training to use completely, nurses can incorporate some of the MI techniques into their communication with clients. See the website www.motivationalinterviewing.org for more information on motivational interviewing.

## Develop Effective Health Education Programs

All programs, including sessions using MI skills, should include a clear message conveyed in a format appropriate to the learners and in an environment that is free from distractions and consistent with the message. Emotions such as anxiety, stress, anger, or fear can interfere with the listener actually hearing the message being sent. Also, provide information that is understandable to the listener. Use plain language and avoid jargon, multisyllable words, slang, and complex medical terms. Use words that the listener will know and recognize. For example, some people are more familiar with terms like *high blood pressure* and *high blood sugar levels* rather than *hypertension* and *increased glucose levels*. On the other hand, be careful not to oversimplify your terms if your audience is knowledgeable about health care. You want to avoid "talking down" or "over the head" of your listeners.

The type of learning format that you select will depend on the learners. If they are young, you will want an interactive format and many of your options will include the use of technology. You could use a game such as developing a bingo game with food groups to teach about healthy eating. The old adage "A picture is worth a 1000 words" still holds true. People tend to remember what they see or hear; a lively format rather than a passive one encourages learning. Most people have a short attention span, so you need to make your point quickly and directly. It may help to provide take-home written materials or a CD for further reminders and follow-up of what is taught. Because people often learn better when they are actively engaged in the learning, small group discussion, role-playing, and question-and-answer sessions may reinforce learning. See Box 16-2 for examples of types of learning formats.

Pontius (2013) offers many useful suggestions for developing both verbal and written messages. Her audience is composed of school nurses; however, her messages fit many areas of health education. For written material, first limit the content and make it relevant; use an active voice and conversational tone so that you engage the learner in the process; make the material easy to read and write the way you talk. You do not want to use a thesaurus to find terms to use, so say what you mean in understandable words. As has been mentioned, make the content relevant to the age, gender, and culture of the learner. For online and social media messages, send out one message at a time. Use 12-point print size for most people and 14 point for older people. Use bullets or numbers to easily catch the attention of the reader, and put your most important points early in the list. Leave some white space on the page and choose ink that contrasts clearly with the background of the paper. Use examples to show the desired behavior. Figure 16-1 shows a community

### BOX 16-2   Examples of Learning Formats

**Presentation:** This method can be used when the group is large and you want to be consistent in the message that is delivered to all participants. Remember, people tend to have a short attention span, so what can you do to keep them engaged? You might ask them to spend some time talking with one another in small groups and then have the group respond to questions, or ask attendees to write answers to questions and invite several to share their answers. The presentation can also be a webinar or similar electronic tool, including Skype.

**Demonstration:** Use the demonstration technique to show attendees how to perform a task. You could demonstrate insulin injection, heart-healthy food preparation, and exercise.

**Small Informal Group:** Because learners often learn as much from one another as from the instructor, small groups can be valuable. For example, in working with women in a shelter for abused women, participants may share actions they took to remove themselves safely from the violent environment. They might also be able to jointly plan how each might move to the stage of independent living outside the shelter.

**Health Fair:** See the How To box on ways to plan, implement, and evaluate a health fair. For example, you might offer a health fair in a senior center and have displays such as posters; videos; live demonstrations; handouts on such topics as reducing fat in selected recipes (including samples) and age-appropriate exercises for flexibility; as well as screenings for elevated blood pressure, glucose, or cholesterol or for osteoporosis and vision.

**Non-native Language Sessions:** You could adapt the health fair approach for a Hispanic group by holding the session in Spanish and providing all of the materials in Spanish. Then ask Spanish-speaking nurses to staff each of the stations for health learning.

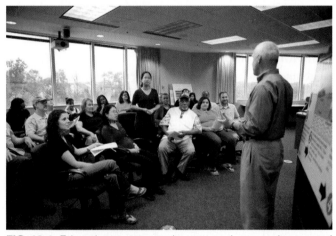

FIG 16-1 Educating a community group about environmental health issues and gathering their concerns. (From Centers for Disease Control and Prevention [2009]; courtesy Dawn Arlotta.)

group being educated, and Box 16-3 lists ways to design clear educational programs.

## EDUCATIONAL ISSUES

There are three important educational issues to consider when you are planning educational programs. First, different populations of learners require different teaching strategies. Second, be prepared to overcome barriers to learning. And

## BOX 16-3  Ways to Design Clear Educational Programs

1. Develop the content for your message.
2. Identify the most appropriate format and location for the program, taking into account your budget, location, and other available resources and constraints. See Box 16-2 for examples of formats.
3. Organize the learning experience to fit the audience; consider how to engage the learners in the process.
4. Plan how you will deliver the material, using the following points:
   - Limit the number of points that you wish to cover to the most important ones.
   - Begin with a strong opening and close with a strong ending; people remember most what is said first and last.
   - Fit your use of language to the learners; use an active voice and emphasize the positive. For example, "Many people are able to lose weight by reducing their intake by 500 calories a day and exercising 45 minutes at least four times a week."
   - Use examples, stories, and other vivid messages. Limit statistics and complex terminology.
   - Refer to trustworthy sources. In general, government, educational, or professional association sources are peer reviewed by professionals and dependable. The Centers for Disease Control and Prevention, National Cancer Institute, American Public Health Association, and the American Academy of Pediatrics are four examples of sites that offer useful information.
   - Use aids to highlight your message. For example, you might have posters, handouts, or CDs to give to attendees. You might also incorporate a clip from a website such as www.YouTube.com to emphasize your point. Be sure to verify that the content on the site is accurate; not all information is provided by professionals.
5. Don't forget to plan the evaluation when you are initially planning the program.

third, consider the appropriateness of using technology in the programs.

## Population Considerations Based on Age and on Cultural and Ethnic Backgrounds

Nurses are an important source of health education in the community. The increase in populations of varying cultural and ethnic backgrounds and the aging of baby boomers require that community health education cross age and cultural boundaries. In terms of age, children, adults, and older adults have different learning needs and respond to different educational strategies. In each age group, learners vary also in their cognitive ability, personality, and prior knowledge. Some people learn better with more direct instruction, supervision, and encouragement than do other people.

Learning strategies for children and individuals with little knowledge about a health-related topic are characterized as pedagogy. In the pedagogical model of learning, the teacher assumes full responsibility for making decisions about what will be learned, and how and when it will be learned. This form of learning is teacher directed. Learning strategies for adults, older adults, and individuals with some health-related knowledge about a topic are called andragogy. In andragogy, learners play an important role in deciding what they need and want to learn.

Andragogy is a more transactional way of learning than is the pedagogical model. Each model has useful elements (Knowles et al, 2005). For example, when learners are dependent and entering a totally new content area, they may require more pedagogical experiences. In addition to considering the age of the population to be educated, think about the learning needs of the population and use the pedagogical and andragogical principles that will best meet these needs. In educational programs for children, provide information that matches the developmental abilities of the group. The following age-specific strategies may help the nurse tailor educational programs for children.

- *With younger children use more concrete examples and word choices.* You might tell a group of 3-year-old children that it is good to brush their teeth two times a day. With 10-year-olds, you can explain to them the benefits of brushing their teeth and the risks of not brushing and talk about issues such as the care of their teeth with braces.
- *Use objects or devices, rather than just discuss ideas, to increase attention.* When teaching a group of children with asthma how to use inhalers, it is better to hand out inhalers to each participant and have them practice proper technique with the inhalers rather than just giving them a handout with instructions or demonstrating how to use an inhaler while they watch you.
- *Incorporate repetitive health behaviors into games to help children retain knowledge and acquire skills.* Singing songs while acting out healthy activities such as washing hands before eating helps children get in the habit of washing their hands and makes this health promotion behavior fun. For example, the time a child should wash his or her hands is about the same amount of time it takes to sing "Twinkle, Twinkle Little Star."

In thinking about culture, it is important to know that by 2050 approximately 50% of the U.S. population will consist of ethnic minorities such as Asians, African Americans, Hispanic Americans, Native Americans, and Pacific Islanders. Culture influences family structure and interactions as well as views about health and illness. These demographic changes present new challenges to nurse educators. Nurses need to understand the health belief systems of the ethnic populations being served and be familiar with populations who are prone to develop certain health problems. When presenting seminars or providing written, audio, or visual information, provide information in a culturally competent manner.

For example, in a rural farming area, there might be a large population of Mexican migrant crop workers. Knowing that this Spanish-speaking group is more likely to have tuberculosis than other segments of the community, nurses may visit the migrant worker camp to present information on tuberculosis such as prevention, symptom identification, early diagnosis, and treatment. An interpreter may accompany the nurses and provide oral content in Spanish. Written handouts can be in Spanish and designed to be read and understood on a second- or third-grade reading level.

Think also about the generation of the learner. The generation born between 1980 and the present time have always had digital media and access to the Internet and are called the *net generation* (Billings and Kowalski, 2004). They are connected and use mobile devices for many purposes including learning. They typically prefer to work in groups or teams, are active learners who seek innovation, want an immediate response to their questions, and are able to multitask. They like simulations and virtual reality forms of learning. *Generation X* members were born between 1960 and 1980, and they tend to be self-directed, like to work in teams, and may need to develop skills because they may not be as tech savvy as the net generation. Members of this group can tolerate delayed gratification; they want clear information with practical value; and they can engage in games and activities when appropriate. The *boomers*, born between 1940 and 1960, are accustomed to being dependent on the teacher, want to be in charge of their own learning, respond positively to feedback, and want to do a good job. They like to be connected to other people.

## Use of Technology in Learning

Many kinds of technologies such as computer games and programs, videos, CDs, and Internet resources can increase learning. These technologies may enable the learner to control the pace of instruction, offer flexibility in the time and location of learning, present an appealing form of education, and provide immediate feedback. You may want to use a variety of technological applications in your teaching. It is also important to be aware that people increasingly are using the Internet as a source of health information. Why do people use the Internet? A major benefit is its convenience: It is available 24 hours a day, 7 days a week, and there is no need to drive there, take public transportation, or find a parking place.

Educating people through the Internet has been shown to be more effective in fostering treatment adherence than in-person counseling, telephone counseling, or self-directed learning (Dauz et al, 2004). Clients may ask nurses to provide them with information about ways to evaluate the quality and reliability of this information. The following list provides some criteria for assessing the quality of Internet health information (Agency for Healthcare Research and Quality, 1999; VanBiervliet and Edwards-Schafer, 2004):

- *Authorship:* Are the authors and contributors listed with their credentials and affiliations?
- *Caveats:* Does the site clarify whether its function is to provide information or to market products?
- *Content:* Is the information accurate and complete, and is an appropriate disclaimer provided?
- *Credibility:* Does the site include the source, currency, relevance, and editorial review process for the information?
- *Currency:* Are dates listed for when the content was posted and updated?
- *Design:* Is the site accessible, capable of internal searches, easy to navigate, and logically organized?
- *Disclosure:* Is the user informed about the purpose of the site and about any profiling or collection of information associated with using the site?
- *Interactivity:* Does the site include feedback mechanisms and opportunities for users to exchange information?

- *Links:* Have the links been evaluated according to back-linkages, content, and selection? The Evidence-Based Practice box below describes the effective use of a smartphone app for health promotion.

### EVIDENCE-BASED PRACTICE

The authors describe the development and formative evaluation of a smartphone app that deals with physical activity promotion. They say that physical inactivity is the fourth leading risk factor for global mortality and that self-monitoring of physical activities levels can support a healthier life. Because the Internet is easily accessed by many people, the authors used "10,000 Steps," which is an online physical activity health program to encourage the use of step-counting pedometers to track daily exercise. Their goal was to evaluate the design and usability of this smartphone app. They used both qualitative (video-taping and having participants "think aloud") and quantitative (a four-item usability questionnaire that used a 5-point Likert-type scale followed by a semistructured interview) measures. During the project they made modifications to the app. The results showed that the design changes significantly reduced the time it took for participants to complete their tasks. The study demonstrates the relevance of testing the design and then modifying a smartphone app designed for health promotion.

#### Nurse Use

Smartphones and their apps are an innovative medium for the delivery of health messages and health care interventions. It is a good idea to test the app before launching it to work out any areas that could be improved in terms of ease of use.

Kirwan M, Duncan MJ, et al: Design, development, and formative evaluation of a smartphone application for recording and monitoring physical activity levels: the 10,000 Steps "iStepLog." *Health Educ Behav* 40:140–151, 2013.

## Barriers to Learning

Barriers to learning fall into two broad categories: one concerning the educator and the other concerning the learner.

### Educator-Related Barriers

Some common educator-related barriers to learning, together with strategies to minimize them, follow (Knowles et al, 2005):

- *Fear of public speaking:* Be well prepared, use icebreakers, recognize and acknowledge the fear, and practice in front of a mirror or video camera or with a friend.
- *Lack of credibility with respect to a certain topic:* Increase your confidence by carefully preparing for the talk so that you have included useful information and you understand the information; avoid apologizing for lack of expertise, and instead convey the attitude of an expert by briefly sharing your personal and professional background.
- *Limited professional experiences related to a health topic:* You may want to describe personal experiences (brief ones), share experiences of others, or use analogies, illustrations, or examples from movies, current news, or famous people.
- *Inability to deal with difficult people who need to learn health-related information:* One strategy that may help with handling difficult learners is to confront the problem learner directly. Other strategies include using humor, using small groups to foster participation of timid people, asking

disruptive people to give others a chance to speak, or, if this does not work, asking them to leave.

- *Lack of knowledge about how to gain participation:* You can foster participation by asking open-ended questions, inviting participation, and planning small group activities whereby a person responds based on the group rather than presenting his own information.

- *Lack of experience in timing a presentation so that it is neither too long nor too short:* Plan ahead and practice the presentation by speaking during the practice at the same pace that you will speak to the group.

- *Uncertainty about how to adjust instruction:* You can more easily adjust instruction when you know the participants' needs, request feedback, and redesign the presentation during breaks, based on what you have learned about the participants.

- *A sense of discomfort when learners ask questions:* Try to anticipate questions, concisely paraphrasing questions to be sure that you correctly understood the question, and recognizing that it is appropriate to admit that you do not know the answer to a question.

- *Lack of feedback from learners:* Solicit informal feedback during the program and at the end with program evaluation.

- *Concern about whether media, materials, and facilities will function properly:* Test the equipment before the program to make sure it runs and also that you know how to use it. Also, have back-up plans for how to get help if you have a problem.

- *Difficulty with openings and closings:* Strategies to foster successful openings and closings include developing several examples of openings and closings, memorizing the opening and closing, concisely summarizing information, and thanking participants for attending.

- *Overdependence on notes:* You may wish to use note cards or visual aids as prompts; also, practicing in advance is a proven way to increase skill at presenting.

## Learner-Related Barriers

Two of the most important learner-related barriers are low literacy and lack of motivation to learn information and make needed behavioral changes.

*Low Literacy Levels.* Nurses often deal with individuals and populations who are illiterate or who have low literacy levels. These individuals may be embarrassed to admit this deficit to health care providers and educators and may try to appear to understand when they really do not. Specifically, they may not ask questions to clarify information even when they do not understand it. As society becomes more multicultural, the problem of low literacy can increase due to limited use of the primary language as well as limited education. One of the Core Competencies for Public Health Professionals listed in the 2009 revisions by the Council on Linkages between Academia and Public Health Practice is to "assess the health literacy of populations served" (Council on Linkages, 2010). The next paragraphs describe the significance of this problem and the need for nurses to address health literacy.

The National Assessment of Adult Literacy (NAAL) is the largest literacy assessment study done in the United States. This assessment was first conducted in 1992. At that time, out of five levels in the assessment, 50% of American adults were in the top two levels and 50% were in the bottom three levels of literacy. The minimal standard needed to function in the workplace is that of level 3 proficiency. In 2003, the tool measured literacy in four levels: *Below Basic, Basic, Intermediate,* and *Proficient.* The literacy scales used in 2003 were as follows: prose literacy, document literacy, and quantitative literacy. Prose examples include searching, comprehending, and using information from editorials, news stories, brochures, and instructional materials. Document literacy refers to searching, comprehending, and using information from documents such as job applications, payroll forms, transportation schedules, maps, tables, and drug and food labels. Quantitative literacy is the ability to identify and perform computations such as balancing a checkbook, completing an order form, or determining the interest on a loan from an advertisement. The 2003 test is more than just a survey and actually asks the test takers to perform tasks to demonstrate their literacy (Kutner et al, 2006). The 2003 NAAL included information about health literacy, which is an important topic for nurses.

Health literacy is gaining considerable attention for many reasons including the costs of health illiteracy when people are unable to follow directions about health care. *Healthy People 2020* defines health literacy as "[t]he degree to which individuals have the capacity to obtain, process, and understand basic information and services needed to make appropriate health decisions" (USDHHS, 2010). Health literacy includes a range of abilities including being able to "read, comprehend, and analyze information; decode instructions, symbols, charts and diagrams; weigh risks and benefits; and, ultimately, make decisions and take action" (National Institutes of Health [NIH], 2014). "Literacy skills are a stronger predictor of an individual's health status than age, income, employment status, education level, or racial/ethnic group" (Weiss, 2007, p. 13). A person with limited literacy may be unable to understand instructions on prescription bottles, interpret health appointment cards, fill out health insurance forms, and read and understand self-care or hospital discharge instructions. What happens when someone has health illiteracy? A person with limited literacy may:

- Have a limited vocabulary and general knowledge and does not ask for clarification
- Focus on details and deal in literal or concrete concepts versus abstract concepts
- Select responses on a survey or questionnaire without necessarily understanding them
- Be unable to understand math (which is important in calculating medications)

In the past few years a great deal of federal and local attention has been paid to health literacy. Box 16-4 summarizes a sample of websites available to guide people in learning more about how to provide information in a way that learners who have varying levels of literacy can understand. The *Plain Writing Act of 2010* requires the federal government to write all new publications, forms, and publicly distributed documents in a "clear, concise, well-organized" manner and according to plain writing guides (see Public Law 111-274 at http://www.gpo.gov/

---

**BOX 16-4** Examples of Useful Websites for Health Education

- Centers for Disease Control and Prevention: Plan and Act: What Is the National Action Plan to Improve Health Literacy? (http://www.cdc.gov/healthliteracy/planact/index.html)
- Centers for Disease Control and Prevention: *Simply Put: A Guide for Creating Easy-to-Understand Materials* (http://www.cdc.gov/healthliteracy/pdf/Simply_Put.pdf)
- National Institutes of Health: *Health Literacy* (http://www.cdc.gov/healthliteracy/planact/index.html)
- www.motivational interviewing network of trainers (MINT): *Motivational Interviewing at http://www.motivationalinterviewing.org/*

---

**BOX 16-5** Excerpts from *Simply Put*

***A Guide for Creating Easy-to-Understand Materials***

**Make Your Message Clear**
1. Give the most important information first and limit the number of messages.
2. Tell audiences what they need to do and what they will gain from understanding and using material.
3. Choose your words carefully.

**Text Appearance Matters**
1. Use font sizes between 12 and 14 points; for headings use a font size at least 2 points larger than that in the main text.
2. Font style: Do not use all caps; limit use of light text on a dark background.

**Visuals Help Tell Your Story**
1. Choose the best type of visual for your material.
2. Use visuals to help communicate your messages in a culturally relevant and sensitive manner.
3. Make visuals easy for your audience to follow and understand and of high quality.
4. Sometimes drawings can help your audience understand.
5. Use realistic images to illustrate internal body parts or small objects.

**Layout and Design**
1. Design an effective cover.
2. Organize your messages so they are easy to act on and recall.
3. Organize ideas in the order that your audience will use them.
4. Make the text easy for the eye to follow and invite the audience into the text.

**Consider Culture**
1. Use terms that your audience uses and/or is comfortable with.
2. Target messages to each cultural or ethnic group or subgroup.

**Translations Take Your Message Further**
1. Messages that work well with an English-speaking audience may not work for audiences who speak another language.
2. Design material for minority populations based on subgroups and geographic locations.
3. Get advice from community organizations in the areas you wish to reach.
4. Carefully select your translator and avoid literal translations.
5. Use the back-translation method and field-test your materials with members of the intended audience.

**Test for Readability**
1. Reduce reading level before using formulas; test a document's readability level (CDC, 2010, pp. 5-27).

Source: Centers for Disease Control and Prevention (CD): *Simply Put: A Guide for Creating Easy-to-Understand Materials*, ed 3, Atlanta GA, 2010, CDC.

---

fdsys/pkg/PLAW-111publ274/pdf/PLAW-111publ274.pdf). Similarly, the National Institutes of Health has developed materials on health literacy and clear communication and calls attention to the enormous costs associated with health illiteracy and how clear, understandable communication is needed for health care professionals (NIH, 2014). An especially helpful document is *Simply Put: A Guide for Creating Easy-to-Understand Materials* developed by the Centers for Disease Control and Prevention (2009). This 43-page guide is filled with information on how to create materials that will increase knowledge or change beliefs, attitudes, and behaviors by sending messages that are clear, relevant, and appropriate for the intended audience. Box 16-5 summarizes key sections in the guide.

Nurses may use pictures including comic books, slides and videos including YouTube presentations, and models in educating clients with low literacy. Some people learn better in a series of educational sessions. For example, at the first session, identify learning capacity and provide a small amount of foundational information. During subsequent sessions, new information that builds on existing knowledge and skills is provided and evaluated. Give additional information when you believe that the information has been understood and can be incorporated into learners' lives. To evaluate whether a person has limited health literacy, listen for the following clues: "I forgot my reading glasses," "I can read this when I get home," or "I will talk about this with my family—may I take the instructions home?" These comments may be quite straightforward or be a clue that the person actually cannot read the material.

Some people do not engage in learning because they have low levels of motivation to do so. Although adults respond to some external motivators, the most powerful motivators are internal. People are motivated to learn if they value the information and feel that they will benefit from the outcome, if they think they can follow through on what is being taught, and if it will improve their situation in life or increase their self-esteem (Ota et al, 2006).

As discussed in Chapter 17, models can be used to structure health education and health promotion plans. One model, the health belief model (HBM), is an individual-level model. This model can be useful in planning programs in which the motivation of learners might be a concern. Specifically, the HBM was one of the first theories of health behavior. As is discussed in Chapter 17, it began in an interesting way when people failed to use free chest x-rays in the 1950s. A group of social psychologists were asked to try to explain the failure to use this screening. Specifically, what would motivate people to seek health care?

As discussed in Chapter 17, the HBM includes six components that attempt to answer the question of what motivates an individual to do something. These components are as follows: (1) perceived susceptibility ("Will something happen to me?"),

Health first.

(2) perceived severity ("If something does happen to me, will it be a big problem?"), (3) perceived benefits ("If I do what is suggested, will it really help me?"), (4) perceived barriers ("Assuming I do what is suggested, will there be barriers that will be unpleasant, costly, and so forth?"), (5) cues to action ("What might motivate me to actually do something?"), and (6) self-efficacy ("Can I really do this?"). This model has been applauded and criticized. It does offer guidance in planning health education programs in that it reminds nurses to think carefully about what motivates people to change. To understand motivation, it is important to learn (1) how the people involved feel about the health problem, (2) whether they think it is serious, (3) whether they believe that action on their part will make a difference, and (4) whether they think that they can both manage the barriers and actually perform the action.

Consider the following example of how the HBM might be applied to a person in the community who has recently been diagnosed with diabetes. The person, June, is 25 years old and was diagnosed 2 months ago with diabetes mellitus. She has found it difficult to follow the recommendations of the public health nurse who has seen her in the community clinic. When the nurse asked June what seemed to be getting in the way of her complying, June said that she had asked herself these questions:

1. If I do not follow the nurse's advice about diet, exercise, and taking my insulin, will something really happen to me?
2. If I do not follow the advice and something does happen, will it really be a problem?
3. On the other hand, if I take my medicine, eat a diet that will keep my diabetes under control, exercise as recommended by the nurse, and take my insulin according to the nurse's directions, will I really reduce the seriousness of my disease?
4. How much will it cost me to purchase the foods in order to follow the diet? How much time will it take each week to exercise as recommended? Will it hurt me to give myself insulin injections?
5. I did see that my friend, Sue, who was diagnosed about 2 years ago with diabetes was careful about what she ate at the party, and she did talk about her exercise program where she walks 50 minutes 5 days a week. Sue did look better than she did when I saw her last year.
6. Is it possible for me to take care of myself like Sue does?

Two additional models that are especially useful in health promotion are discussed in Chapter 17. They are the transtheoretical model (TTM) and the precaution adoption process model (PAPM). Both models deal with change that occurs in stages and over time.

Further details about health promotion models can be found in Chapter 17.

## Evaluation of the Educational Process

Evaluation is as important in the educational process as it is in the nursing process. Evaluation provides a systematic and logical method for making decisions to improve the educational program. You will need to evaluate the educator, the process, and the product.

Feedback to the *educator* provides the person an opportunity to modify the teaching process and enables the educator to better meet the learner's needs. The learner's evaluation of the educator occurs continuously throughout the educational program. The educator may receive written or verbal feedback from learners. Educators can get feedback by using return demonstrations to see what learners have mastered (Palazzo, 2001).

The educator should assume that inadequate learner responses reflect an inadequate program, not an inadequate learner. If the evaluation reveals that the learning objectives are not being met, the nurse must determine why the instruction is not effective. At this point, the educator will want to present the material creatively and meaningfully in new ways that will increase learner retention and the learner's ability to apply the new knowledge. Ultimately, the educator must assume responsibility for the success or failure of the educational process and the development of learner knowledge, skills, and abilities.

### Process Evaluation

Process evaluation examines the dynamic, ongoing components of the educational program. It follows and assesses the movements and management of information transfer and attempts to make sure that the objectives are being met. Use process evaluation throughout the educational program to determine whether goals and objectives are being met and the time required for their accomplishment. Ongoing evaluation also allows the teacher to correct misinformation, misinterpretation, or confusion (Palazzo, 2001).

Periodically review program goals and objectives, and ask whether the desired health behavior change is really necessary. Such a question inevitably leads back to the original learning objectives and enables the nurse to rethink the practicality and merit of each of the objectives. If teaching seems not to be working, re-examine the factors that influence learner readiness and motivation. Process evaluation uses information gathered from the educator as well as from learner evaluations and assesses the dynamics of their interactions (Knowles, 1990).

## THE EDUCATIONAL PRODUCT

The educational product is the outcome of the educational process, and the product can be measured both qualitatively and quantitatively. For example, a qualitative assessment should answer the question, "How well does the learner appear to understand the content?" A quantitative assessment should answer the question, "How much of the content does the learner retain?" Thus, the quality of the product is measured by improvement and increase, or the lack thereof, in the learner's knowledge, skills, and abilities related to the content of the educational program. Selected outcomes for the population of interest need to be identified when the educational program is conceived. Measurement of changes in these outcomes determines the effectiveness of the program. In nursing, the educational product is assessed as a measurable change in the health or behavior of the client.

## Evaluation of Health and Behavioral Changes

Many approaches, methods, and tools are used to evaluate health and behavioral changes. Examples include questionnaires, rating scales, surveys, checklists, skills demonstrations, testing, subjective client feedback, and client repeat demonstration. Whether you use qualitative or quantitative strategies depends on the expected educational outcome. Evaluation of outcomes measured includes changes in knowledge, skills, abilities, attitudes, behavior, health status, and quality of life. Approaches to evaluating health education effects will vary, depending on the situation. For example, when considering a client's ability to perform a psychomotor skill such as changing a dressing, observing the client doing the skill is the most appropriate means of evaluation.

If evaluation of the educational product shows positive changes in health status and health-related behaviors, the educator can expect good results in similar health educational programs. If evaluation shows no changes or negative changes in health status and health-related behaviors, then re-examine and modify the program to attain better results in the future.

It is important to evaluate short-term health and behavioral effects of health education programs and to determine whether they are really caused by the educational program. Short-term objectives are often easy to evaluate (Babcock and Miller, 1994). For example, a short-term evaluation of whether a client can perform a return demonstration of a process being taught requires minimal energy, expense, or time; skill mastery can be determined within a matter of minutes. If the short-term objective is not met, the nurse determines why and identifies possible solutions so that successful learning can occur. If the short-term objective is met, the nurse can then focus on long-term evaluation designed to assess the lasting effects of the education program.

The goal of health education is to help clients make lasting behavioral changes that will improve their overall health status. Long-term follow-up with clients is a challenging task. Long-term evaluation is geared toward following and assessing the status of an individual, family, community, or population over time. The tools of evaluation are designed to assess whether specific goals and objectives were met. Also, monitor the extent and direction of client changes in health status and health behaviors (Kleinpell and Mick, 2001).

Often, for nurse educators, the goal of long-term evaluation is an analysis of the effectiveness of the education program for the entire community, not the health status of a specific client. Nurses track the achievement of community objectives over time, but not that of the individual community members. Thus, in a changing population, long-term evaluation of the results of an education program is still possible. The percentage of objectives and goals met by sampling the target population gives valid statistics for program assessment, even though the population of individuals may have experienced a complete turnover (Kleinpell and Mick, 2001).

For example, a nurse notes that according to annual health department data, 60% of all pregnant women in the nurse's catchment area received some prenatal care. Wanting to increase this percentage to 100%, the nurse tries an educational intervention in which radio and television stations make public service announcements (PSAs) about the importance and availability of prenatal services.

After 1 year, the nurse discovers that 80% of all pregnant women now receive prenatal care. The nurse continues to use PSAs the next year because good results are evident. However, the long-term goal of the education program to influence the behavior of 100% of the pregnant women in the community has not yet been met. The nurse enlists volunteers to put informational posters in shopping malls, grocery stores, public transportation stops, laundries, and public transportation vehicles. In the second year after implementing the revised educational program, again using the statistics from the health department, the nurse finds that 95% of all pregnant women in the target area now receive prenatal care. The nurse can now evaluate and modify a community educational program over time to increase the rate, range, and consistency of progress made toward meeting the long-term goals of the project. It will be important and often difficult to keep track of clients; e-mail, telephone calls, and text messages may be useful.

Because health education is often conducted in the community in groups rather than provided to one person at a time, the use of groups in health education is discussed.

## GROUPS AS A TOOL FOR HEALTH EDUCATION

People are part of a variety of groups, and each can influence health behavior and support useful or poor health practices. Groups are an effective and powerful medium by which to initiate and implement changes for individuals, families, organizations, and the community. People naturally form groups in the home, and groups in the community dramatically influence the community's health. They may form for a clearly stated purpose or goal, or they may form naturally as shared values, interests, activities, or personal characteristics attract individuals to each other.

Community groups represent the collective interests, needs, and values of individuals; they provide a link between the individual and the larger social system. Throughout life, group membership influences thoughts, choices, behaviors, and values as people socialize and interact. Through groups, people may express personal views and relate them to the views of others. Groups serve as communication networks and can help organize various aspects of communities.

Community groups may be informal or formal. Formal groups have a defined membership and a specific purpose. They may or may not have an official place in the community's organization. In informal groups, the ties between members are multiple, and the purposes are unwritten yet understood by members. These groups often form spontaneously when participants have a common interest or need. You can find out about what formal and informal groups exist in a community by reading the local newspaper, listening to public service information on the radio or television, reading items on the Internet, and asking residents about the groups to which they belong. Nurses often serve as a catalyst for forming new groups or by creating linkages among groups that currently exist.

Group support often helps people make needed health changes. Skillful use of group methods can help a person analyze the problem, sustain motivation for change, experience support during vulnerable periods, and receive quick interpersonal feedback. The discomfort associated with change can be reduced through the relationships with others in beneficial groups. Many of the *Healthy People 2020* priorities can be addressed in health promotion and disease prevention groups, where individuals learn healthier behaviors and gain support from others in changing from risky to healthy lifestyle choices. For example, groups may support physical activity and fitness, sound nutrition, and safe sexual practices. Through group support, individuals may conquer smoking, drug abuse, or abusive relationships. They may identify and reduce exposure to environmental hazards and promote safer physical settings for all. Also, one of the core competencies for public health professionals is to "use group processes to advance community involvement" (Council on Linkages, 2010, p. 10).

## Group: Definitions and Concepts

An understanding of several group concepts facilitates group work in the community. Some of the core concepts answer the following questions: (1) What is a group? (2) What is the purpose of the group? (3) How do groups develop and function? (4) What are their stages? and (5) What roles do members typically play in the group?

### Definitions

A **group** is a collection of interacting individuals who have common purposes and are influenced by one another. Groups form for a variety of reasons. Families are an example of a community group. Families share kinship bonds, living space, and economic resources. They have many purposes such as teaching their members as well as providing psychological support and socialization. Groups also form in response to community needs, problems, or opportunities. For example, community residents may form a neighborhood association to protect their health and welfare. Community groups occur spontaneously because of mutual attraction between individuals and obvious and keenly felt personal needs such as those for socialization and recreation. Health-promoting groups may form when people meet to work together to support one another in achieving health goals such as weight loss, exercise, dealing with loss, and giving up smoking, gambling, or drinking.

### Concepts

Groups need to identify a clear purpose. Having a clear purpose helps in establishing criteria for member selection and determining the action plan. For example, a clear statement of purpose proved valuable in forming a new group in one city's housing development. The local department of social services had received numerous reports of child abuse and neglect. Routine home visits for well-child care documented high stress between parents and their offspring, and some parents requested teaching and guidance from the nurse in child discipline. The

nurse proposed that a parent group address this community need, and she chose this purpose for the group: dealing with kids for child and parent satisfaction. The purpose indicated both the process (to help parents deal with children) and the desired outcome (satisfaction for parents and children). As potential members were approached, this statement of group purpose helped them decide if they wanted to join.

**Cohesion** is the attraction between individual members and between each member and the group. Individuals in a highly cohesive group identify themselves as a unit, work toward common goals, endure frustration for the sake of the group, and defend the group against outside criticism. Attraction increases when members feel accepted and liked by others, see similar qualities in one another, and share similar attitudes and values. Group effectiveness also improves as members work together toward group goals while still satisfying the needs of individual members.

Members' traits that increase group cohesion and productivity include the following: (1) compatible personal and group goals, (2) attraction to group goals, (3) attraction to some members of the group, (4) a mix of leading and following skills, and (5) good problem-solving skills.

Groups have both task and maintenance functions. A **task function** is anything a member does that deliberately contributes to the group's purpose. Members with task-directed abilities become more attractive to the group. These traits include strong problem-solving skills, access to material resources, and skills in directing. Of equal importance are abilities to affirm and support individuals in the group. These functions are called **maintenance functions** because they help other members stay with the group and feel accepted. Other maintenance functions are the ability to help people resolve conflicts and create social and environmental comfort. Both task and maintenance functions are necessary for group progress. Naturally, those members who provide these functions are attractive, and an abundance of such traits within the membership tends to increase group cohesion.

The following group members' traits may decrease cohesion and productivity: (1) a sense of conflict between personal and group goals, (2) lack of interest in group goals and activities, (3) poor problem-solving and communication abilities, (4) lack of both leadership and supporter skills, (5) disagreement about types of leadership, (6) aversion to other members, and (7) behaviors and attributes that others do not understand.

Usually, the more alike group members are, the stronger a group's attraction, whereas differences tend to decrease attractiveness. Members' perceptions of differences can create marked competition and jealousy. At the same time, personal differences can increase group cohesion if they support complementary functioning or provide contrasting viewpoints necessary for decision making. Cohesive factors are complex and many factors influence member attraction to each other and to the group's goal. High group cohesion positively affects productivity and member satisfaction. The following example illustrates factors that influence group cohesion. A nurse initiated a group for clients who had been treated for burns. Ten residents, all from one town, had been discharged after a month in the local burn unit. The stated purpose for the group was to teach coping skills to assist members in the difficult transition from hospital to home. Each person had been treated for extensive burns in an intensive care treatment center; each had relied heavily on health care workers for physical, social, and emotional rehabilitation; and each had faced the challenge of resuming work and family roles. Individuals shared some similar experiences and hopes for the future but varied in the amount of trauma and stress experienced. They also differed widely in psychological readiness for return to ordinary daily routines. One woman in the group was able to return quickly to her job as a cashier in a large supermarket. The strength of her determination to overcome public reaction to her scars, coupled with an ability to "use the right words" and an empathy for others, distinguished her from others in the group. These differences proved attractive to other members, inspiring them to work toward a return to their own roles in life. These members saw her differences as attainable.

This group's cohesion was provided by the members' attraction to the common purpose of returning to successful life patterns and managing relationships with others. Members also believed that interaction with others with similar burn experiences could help them reach that goal. This example shows that certain member experiences such as crises or traumas may help individuals identify with each other and may increase member attraction.

Being different from the general population and similar to the other group members can be positive for some members and negative for others. Some members may not want to be identified by an aversive characteristic such as disfigurement. Empathy for another's pain, learned only through mutual experience, may provide a person with a required perspective for problem solving or affirming another's view. This group was effective, and the nurse helped members use common experiences and learn from their differences.

Members' attraction to the group is influenced by factors such as the group programs, size, type of organization, and position in the community. Attraction to the group is increased when members view goals clearly and see group activities as effective.

The concept of cohesion helps to explain group productivity. Some cohesion is necessary for people to remain with a group and accomplish the set goals. Attractiveness positively influences members' motivation and commitment to work on the group task. Group cohesion may be increased as members better understand the experiences of others and identify common ideas and reactions to various issues. Nurses facilitate this process by pointing out similarities, contrasting supportive differences, or helping members redefine differences in ways that make those dissimilarities compatible.

Norms are standards that guide, control, and regulate individuals and communities. Group norms set the standards for group members' behaviors, attitudes, and perceptions. Norms suggest what a group believes is important, what it finds acceptable or objectionable, or what it perceives as of no consequence. This commonly held view of what ought to be motivates members to use the group for their mutual benefit (Northen and Kurland, 2001). All groups have norms and mechanisms to accomplish conformity. Group norms serve three functions: (1) to ensure movement toward the group's purpose or tasks; (2) to maintain the group through various supports to members; and (3) to influence members' perceptions and interpretations of reality.

Although certain norms keep the group focused on its task, some diversion can be present if members respect goals and feel committed to return to them. The task norm is the commitment to return to the central goals of the group, and its strength determines the group's ability to adhere to its work.

Maintenance norms create group pressures to affirm members and maintain their comfort. Individuals in groups seem most productive and at ease when their psychological and social well-being is nurtured. Maintenance behaviors include identifying the social and psychological tensions of members and taking steps to support those members at high-stress times. For example, maintenance norms often refer to things such as scheduling meetings at convenient times and in an accessible and comfortable space with parking as well as seating, refreshments, and toilets.

Groups also have reality norms, where members reinforce or challenge and correct their ideas of what is real. Groups can examine the life situations confronting individuals and help to make sense of them. As individuals gather information, attempt to understand that information, make decisions, and consider the facts and their implications, they can take responsible action, not only in relation to themselves and their group, but also for the community. Group (task, maintenance, and reality) norms combine to form a group culture. Although working with a group does not mean dictating its norms, the nurse can support helpful rules, attitudes, and behaviors. Norms form when these rules, attitudes, and behaviors become part of the life of the group, independent of the nurse. Reality norms influence each member to see relevant situations in the same way the other members see them. For example, suppose a group of individuals with diabetes defines an uncontrolled diet as harmful; members may try to influence one another to maintain diet control. The nurse's role in this group is to provide accurate information about diet and the disease process while continually displaying a belief that health through diet control is attainable and desirable.

Group members with similar backgrounds may have a limited scope of knowledge. For example, women in a spouse abuse group may believe that men are exploitive and harmful on the basis of common childhood and marriage experiences. Such a stereotypical view of men could be reinforced by similar perceptions in other members; this might lead to continuing anger or fear of interactions with men, and a hostile or helpless approach to family affairs. Nurses or group members who have known men in loving, helpful, and collaborative ways can describe their different and positive perceptions of men, thereby adding information and challenging beliefs. The health and condition of members improve as their perceptions of reality are based on a more complete range of data. Nurses bring an important perspective to groups in which similar backgrounds limit the understanding and interpretation of personal concerns.

---

**BOX 16-6  Examples of Group Role Behavior**

(There are many examples; this is a representative list of the types of roles members assume.)
- **Follower:** Seeks and accepts the authority or direction of others
- **Gatekeeper:** Controls outsiders' access to the group
- **Leader:** Guides and directs group activity
- **Maintenance specialist:** Provides physical and psychological support for group members, thereby holding the group together
- **Peacemaker:** Attempts to reconcile conflict between members or takes action in response to influences that disrupt the group process and threaten its existence
- **Task specialist:** Focuses or directs movement toward the main work of the group

---

**BOX 16-7  Examples of Leadership Behaviors**

- **Advising:** Introducing direction on the basis of knowledgeable opinion
- **Analyzing:** Reviewing what has occurred as encouragement to examine behavior and its meaning
- **Clarifying:** Verifying the meanings of interaction and communication through questions and restatement
- **Confronting:** Presenting behavior and its effects to the individual and group to challenge existing perceptions
- **Evaluating:** Analyzing the effect or outcome of action or the worth of an idea according to some standard
- **Initiating:** Introducing topics, beginning work, or changing the focus of a group
- **Questioning:** Generating analysis of a view or views by questions that support examination
- **Reflecting behavior:** Providing feedback on how behavior appears to others
- **Reflecting feelings:** Naming the feelings that may be behind what is said or done
- **Suggesting:** Proposing or presenting an idea to a group
- **Summarizing:** Restating discussion or group action in brief form, highlighting important points
- **Supporting:** Giving the kind of emotionally comforting feedback that helps a person or group continue ongoing actions

---

The role structure of a group refers to the expected ways in which members behave toward one another. The role that each person assumes serves a purpose in the group. Examples of roles are leader, follower, task specialist, maintenance specialist, evaluator, peacemaker, and gatekeeper. Box 16-6 includes descriptions of each of these group roles.

## Stages of Group Development

Tuckman (1965) developed a model of the stages of group development that has remained useful over time. He contended that any group, regardless of its type or setting, went through four stages: forming, storming, norming, and performing. In 1977 Tuckman and Jensen determined that there was actually a fifth stage: adjourning. This model can be used for health-related groups to identify in what stage the group is and what may be the next stage. Specifically, in the "forming" stage, members become acquainted with one another and the leader, become oriented to the group, and try to determine what their behaviors should be in relation to one another and to the goal of the group. In the "storming" stage, members begin to express their own individuality, which may run counter to that of others, and they may express hostility to one another and polarize because of interpersonal issues. In the third, or "norming," stage, members start to accept one another; develop some cohesion, norms, and roles; and become comfortable in expressing their opinions and offering ideas. Members begin to trust one another and their interaction takes on more depth. In the fourth stage, "performing," the group uses its interpersonal structure to accomplish its goals, and group energy is directed toward the tasks. In the fifth stage, "adjourning," the group engages in separating from one another.

Leadership is a complex concept. It consists of behaviors that guide or direct members and determine and influence group action. Positive leadership defines or negotiates the group's purpose, selects and helps implement tasks that accomplish the purpose, maintains an environment that affirms and supports members, and balances efforts between task and maintenance. An effective leader pays attention to communications and interactions among the members. Attention is paid to both spoken words and body language, and this information provides continuous feedback about the members and the group process. By paying close attention to communications and interactions, members detect changing group needs, and they can take responsibility and pride in their own involvement. One or more members may lead the group or many may share leadership. Shared leadership may increase productivity, cohesion, and satisfying interactions among members.

After initiating or establishing a group, nurses may facilitate leadership within and among members, frequently relinquishing central control and encouraging members to determine the ultimate leadership pattern for their group. In some settings and circumstances, a single authority seems necessary (e.g., when members have limited skills or limited time, or when groups claim discomfort with shared responsibility for leading). A leadership style that shares leading functions with other group members is effective when there are many alternatives and when issues of values and ethics are involved in the group's action. Examples of leadership behaviors are shown in Box 16-7. Leadership can be described as patriarchal (paternal), or democratic. Each of these styles has a particular effect on members' interaction, satisfaction, and productivity. Groups may reflect one or a combination of styles.

A patriarchal or paternal style is seen when one person has the final authority for group direction and movement. A person using **patriarchal leadership** may control members through rewards and threats, often keeping them in the dark about the goals and rationale behind prescribed actions. Paternal leaders win the respect and dependence of their followers by parent-like devotion to members' needs. The leader controls group movement and progress through interpersonal power. Patriarchal and paternal styles of leadership are authoritarian. These styles are effective for groups such as a disaster team in which immediate task accomplishment or high productivity is the goal. Group morale and cohesiveness are typically low under sustained authoritarian styles of leadership, and members may not learn how to function independently. Also, issues of authority and control may disrupt productivity if the group members challenge the power of the leader.

Democratic leadership is cooperative in nature and promotes and supports members' involvement in all aspects of decision making and planning. Members influence each other as they explore goals, plan steps toward the goals, implement those steps, and evaluate progress.

## Choosing Groups for Health Change

Nurses choose the type of group that will be used after studying the overall needs of the community and its people. Such a study is based on client contacts, expressed concerns from various community spokespersons, health statistics for the area, available health resources, and the community's general well-being. These data point to the community's strengths and critical needs.

The nurse can identify goals for the community and for various groups through media reports, from community informants, and from colleagues. Goals may include visions for change as perceived by the people living and working in the local community. Data may be organized according to the opinions and behaviors of the identified groups. Such information about community groups and assessment data are used with community representatives to plan desired interventions. Alliances or coalitions unite diverse interest groups who share a common interest in perceived threats to community health, and nurses may work with groups both for community analysis and vehicles for change.

Deciding whether to work in established groups or to begin new ones is based on the clients' needs, the purpose of existing groups, and the membership ties in existing groups. There are advantages to using established groups for individual health change. Membership ties already exist, and the existing structure can be used. It is not necessary to find new members because compatible individuals already form a working group. Established groups usually have operating methods that have proved successful; an approach for a new goal is built on this history. Members are aware of each other's strengths, limitations, and preferred styles of interaction and may be comfortable working with and may be able to influence one another. If you choose to work with an established group, be sure to determine whether the new focus is compatible with the existing group purposes. Figure 16-2 shows a breakout session during a community forum.

Groups can be used during a community assessment for information. Groups such as health-planning groups, better business clubs, women's action groups, school boards, and neighborhood councils are excellent information resources because part of their purpose is to determine and respond to community needs. In addition, they are already established as part of the community structure. When a group representing one community sector is selected for community health intervention, the total community structure is studied. Groups reflect existing community values, strengths, and norms.

How might nurses help established groups to work toward community goals? The same interventions recommended for

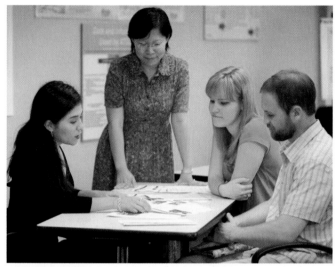

FIG 16-2 Breakout session in a community forum on environmental health concerns. (From Centers for Disease Control and Prevention [2009]; courtesy Dawn Arlotta.)

groups formed for individual health change can be used for groups focused on community health. Such interventions include the following:
- Building cohesion through clarifying goals and individual attraction to groups
- Building member commitment and participation
- Keeping the group focused on the goal
- Maintaining members through recognition and encouragement
- Maintaining member self-esteem during conflict and confrontation
- Analyzing forces affecting movement toward the goal
- Evaluating progress

When nurses enter established groups, they need to assess the leadership, communications, and normative structures. This facilitates group planning, problem solving, intervention, and evaluation. The following example illustrates working with a community group. A nurse was asked to meet with a neighborhood council to help them study and "do something about" the number of homeless living on the streets. Residents knew this nurse from a local clinic and from his consulting work at a shelter for the homeless in an adjacent community. In their invitation to the nurse, council members said "our intent is to be part of the solution rather than part of the problem." The nurse accepted the invitation to visit. He learned that this council had addressed neighborhood concerns for 20 years—protecting zoning guidelines, setting up a recreational program for teens, organizing an after-school program for latchkey children, and generally representing the homeowners of the area. The neighborhood was made up of low-income families who took great pride in their homes. After meeting with the council and listening to their description of the situation, the nurse agreed to help and joined the council.

As the first step in addressing the problem, the council conducted a comprehensive problem analysis on the homeless situation. All known causes and outcomes of homeless persons on the street were identified, and the relationships between each factor and the problem were documented from literature and from the local history. The nurse brought expertise in health planning and knowledge of the homeless and their health risks. He suggested negotiation between the council and the local coalition for the homeless, recognizing that planning would be most relevant if homeless individuals participated. The council was cohesive and committed to the purpose, had developed working operations, and did not need help with group process. They made adjustments in their usual group operation to use the knowledge and health-planning skills of the nurse. Interventions for the homeless included establishing temporary shelters at homes on a rotating basis, providing daily meals through the city council or churches, and joining the area coalition for the homeless.

This example shows how an established, competent group addressed a new goal successfully by building on existing strengths in partnership with the nurse. Community groups, because of their interactive roles, are logical and natural ways for people who work together for community health change. As the decision-making and problem-solving capabilities of community groups are strengthened, the groups become more able representatives for the whole community. Nurses improve the community's health by working with groups toward that goal.

How can the nurse enter existing groups and direct their attention to individual health needs? One nurse employed by an industrial firm noted the harmful effect of managerial stress on several individuals. They had elevated blood pressure, stomach pain, and emotional tension. The nurse learned that the employees with stress were all members of a jogging team that met weekly for conversation in addition to regular workouts. High-level health had been a value shared by all team members, but although jogging was seen as an enjoyable and health-promoting activity, they had never talked about a shared purpose for improved health. The nurse saw a need for stress reduction, thought that the individuals at risk could achieve stress reduction if supported through a group process from valued friends, and proposed that a new purpose be added to the jogging team's activities. All in the group readily accepted and began to focus more on their stress levels as they jogged.

When it is neither desirable nor possible to use existing groups, the nurse can initiate a selected membership group. Choose members who have common health needs or concerns. For instance, individuals with diabetes can meet to discuss diet management and physical care and to share problem-solving remedies; community residents can meet for social support and rehabilitation after treatment for mental illness; or isolated older adults can meet to socialize, eat nutritious meals, and exercise.

Consider members' attributes when composing a new group. Members are attracted to others from similar backgrounds, with similar experiences, and with common interests and abilities. Members' behavior is influenced by the membership, purpose, attraction, norms, leadership, and group structure, and by memories of prior groups. Select members so that common ties or interests balance out dissimilar traits. Try to have members with expressive and problem-solving skills and

others who serve in supportive roles; try to have a mix of people with both task and maintenance functions, and others who can develop these skills.

The size of the group influences effectiveness; generally, 8 to 12 is a good number for group work focused on individual health changes. Groups of up to 25 members may be effective when their focus is on community needs. Large groups often divide and assign tasks to subgroups, with the original large groups meeting less frequently for reporting and evaluation. Setting member criteria can facilitate recruitment and selection of the most appropriate members for any group. The criteria usually suggest a mixture of member traits, allowing for balance for the processes of decision making and growth.

## Managing the Community Group

As soon as the group forms, begin to work on the stated purpose. Help members interact by paying attention to maintenance tasks of attending, eliciting information, clarifying, and recognizing contributions of members. Begin by talking about what brought each person to the group. Encourage each one to participate; recognize and support them as they take on leadership functions. The new group begins to take shape in the early sessions as members try out familiar roles and test their individual abilities. The core competency skills for communication recommended by the Public Health Foundation (Council on Linkages, 2010) are useful to nurses working with community groups. Box 16-8 lists these competencies. Subsequent steps are then planned not only according to the nurse's skill and preference, but also according to the group composition and the skills brought by members.

Conflict is normal in human relations. People may see conflict as the opposite of harmony and try to guard against it. This is an unfortunate view because the tensions of difference and potential conflict actually help groups work toward their purposes. Conflict occurs when members feel obstructed or irritated by one or more other group members (Northen and Kurland, 2001). Conflict signals that antagonistic points of view must be considered and that one must reexamine beliefs and assumptions underlying relationships. Some people are

---

**BOX 16-8  Core Competencies for Communication Skills of Educators**

**Communication Skills**
- Communicates effectively both in writing and orally, including via e-mail
- Solicits input from individuals and organizations
- Advocates for public health programs and resources
- Leads and participates in groups to address specific issues
- Uses the media, varied technologies, and community networks to convey information
- Effectively presents accurate demographic, statistical, programmatic, and scientific information for professional and lay audiences

**Attitudes**
- Listens to others in an unbiased manner
- Respects points of view of others
- Promotes the expression of diverse opinions and perspectives

concerned about security, control of self and others, respect between parties, and access to limited resources. In groups, members may express frustrations about trust, closeness and separation, and dependence and independence. These themes of interpersonal conflict operate to some extent in all interactions and are not unique to groups.

People tend to repeat the same patterns of behavior in conflicts. Sometimes the pattern works; other times it does not. The best approach is to match the response style to the situation (Sportsman and Hamilton, 2007), which requires personal awareness and awareness of others. Specifically, when you respond with avoidance, forcing with power, capitulation, and exclusion of a member, the behaviors fail to satisfy the concerns of participants. Assertiveness (attempting to satisfy one's own concerns) and cooperativeness (attempting to satisfy the concerns of others) can be positive responses to conflict. Behaviors that reflect either assertiveness or cooperativeness and that may satisfy the frustrated parties include confrontation, competition, compromise, reconciliation, and collaboration. Resolving conflict within groups depends on open communication among all parties, diffusion of negative feelings and perceptions, concentration on the issues, and use of fair procedures and a structured approach to the process.

Conflict can be overwhelming, especially when members view the expression of controversy as unacceptable or unremitting. Conflict suppressed over time tends to build up and finally explode out of proportion to the current frustration. A group that repeatedly avoids expressing conflict becomes fragile, is unable to adapt and helpless to face challenges. Conflict may be destructive if contentious parties fail to respect the rights and beliefs of others.

Approaches for acknowledging conflict and solving problems that respect others and represent self-concerns are first learned in families and other small groups. These lessons teach people to embrace conflict as a natural occurrence that supports growth and change. Other people learn to avoid conflict or to disregard others in the promotion of self. Teams that try to be harmonious and avoid conflict may hinder collaboration and personal growth (Gerow, 2001).

It is important to evaluate individual and group progress toward health goals. Early in the planning, specify the action steps that should be taken to meet the goals. These small steps may be responses to learning objectives (listed as action steps designed to support facilitative forces and deal with resistive forces), or they may reflect the group's problem-solving plan. The action steps and the indicators of achievement are discussed and written in a group record. Recognition of accomplishments in the group and of the group is built into the group's evaluation system. Recognition may include concrete rewards such as special foods and drinks, or it may be the personal expression of joy and member-to-member approval. Celebration for group accomplishments marks progress, rewards members, and motivates each person to continue.

## Implementing the Educational Plan

Once educational methods have been selected, they should be implemented through management of the educational process. Implementation entails the following: (1) control over starting, sustaining, and stopping each method and strategy in the most effective and appropriate time and manner; (2) coordination and control of environmental factors, the flow of the presentation, and other contributory parts of the program; and (3) keeping the materials logically related to the core theme and overall program goals (Knowles, 1990). Administrative and political support is essential to successful program implementation.

Educators must be flexible and modify educational methods and strategies to meet unexpected challenges that confront both the educator and the learner. External influences (such as time limitations, expense, and administrative and political factors) and learner needs require an ongoing evaluation of their impact on the educational program. Implementation is a dynamic element in the educational process.

## PRACTICE APPLICATION

During Kristi's BSN student public health practicum at a local health department, the health department got many calls from people wanting information about H1N1 virus. For Kristi's community health intervention project, she decided to do an educational piece on this topic. What is her best course of action?

A. Develop a poster presentation to have on display at the health department.

B. Make an educative pamphlet to mail to anyone calling with questions.

C. Work with the health department staff to develop a community forum presentation and information brochures on H1N1.

D. Develop an in-service program for health department staff on potential spread of the virus and ways to prevent its spread.

**Answers can be found on the Evolve site.**

## KEY POINTS

- Health education is a vital part of nursing because the promotion, maintenance, and restoration of health rely on clients' understanding of health care topics.
- Nurse educators identify learning needs, consider how people learn, examine educational issues, design and implement educational programs, and evaluate the effects of the educational program on learning and behavior.

- Nurses often use the *Healthy People 2020* educational objectives as a guide to identifying community-based learning needs.
- Education and learning are different. Education is the establishment and arrangement of events to facilitate learning. Learning is the process of gaining knowledge and expertise and results in behavioral changes.

## KEY POINTS—cont'd

- Three domains of learning are cognitive, affective, and psychomotor. Depending on the needs of the learner, one or more of these domains may be important for the nurse educator to consider as learning programs are developed.
- Nine principles associated with community health education are gaining attention, informing the learner of the objectives of instruction, stimulating recall of prior learning, presenting the stimulus, providing learning guidance, eliciting performance, providing feedback, assessing performance, and enhancing retention and transfer of knowledge.
- Often theory can guide the development of health education programs. Two useful ones are the health belief model (HBM) and the transtheoretical model (TTM), the latter discussed in connection with the precaution adoption process model (PAPM).
- Principles that guide the effective educator include message, format, environment, experience, participation, and evaluation.
- Educational issues include population considerations, barriers to learning, and technological issues.
- Two important learner-related barriers are low literacy, especially health literacy, and lack of motivation to learn information and make the needed changes.
- The five phases of the educational process are identifying educational needs, establishing educational goals and objectives, selecting appropriate educational methods, implementing the educational plan, and evaluating the educational process and product.
- Evaluation of the product includes the measurement of short- and long-term goals and objectives related to improving health and promoting behavioral changes.
- Working with groups is an important skill for nurses. Groups are an effective and powerful vehicle for initiating and implementing healthful changes.

- A group is a collection of interacting individuals with a common purpose. Each member influences and is influenced by other group members to varying degrees.
- Group cohesion is enhanced by commonly shared characteristics among members and diminished by differences among members.
- Cohesion is the measure of attraction between members and the group. Cohesion or the lack of it affects the group's function.
- Norms are standards that guide and regulate individuals and communities. These norms are unwritten and often unspoken and serve to ensure group movement to a goal, to maintain the group, and to influence group members' perceptions and interpretations of reality.
- Some diversity of member backgrounds is usually a positive influence on a group.
- Groups also go through a set of stages in order to form, operate, and adjourn.
- Leadership is an important and complex group concept. Leadership is described as patriarchal (or paternal), or democratic.
- Group structure emerges from various member influences, including members' understanding and support of the group purpose.
- Conflicts in groups may develop from competition for roles or member disagreement about the roles ascribed to them.
- Health behavior is greatly influenced by the groups to which people belong and for which they value membership.
- An understanding of group concepts provides a basis for identifying community groups and their goals, characteristics, and norms. Nurses use their understanding of group principles to work with community groups toward needed health changes.

## CLINICAL DECISION-MAKING ACTIVITIES

1. Think about an educational interaction that you had with each type of client (individual, family, community, and population) that did not seem to go well. For each type of client and on the basis of how people learn, identify what might have been the problem. Develop a plan for ways in which the interaction could have been improved, based on how people learn.
2. Recall a learning experience in which the message, format, environment, experience, participation, or evaluation was unsatisfactory. Then develop a plan for how the problem could have been overcome and turned from a negative or neutral learning situation into a positive one.
3. Review the phases of the educational process. Apply this process to a population of individuals with hypertension, a community in which tuberculosis is on the rise, and families with a child who has attention deficit disorder.
4. Select one of the *Healthy People 2020* educational objectives and design a population-specific education program to meet that objective. Consider how people learn, educational issues,

educational process including teaching strategies, and evaluation procedures that you would use.

5. Consider three groups of which you are a member. What is the stated purpose of each group? Are you aware of unstated but clearly understood purposes? What is the nature of member interaction in each group? How do purpose and interaction differ in the three groups?
6. Observe two working groups in session, from the community, a health care agency, or a school. Notice the attractiveness of each group through the eyes of its members.
7. List actions that nurses may take to assist groups in various aspects of their work, such as member selection, purpose clarification, arrangements for comfort in participation, and group problem solving.
8. Observe a nurse working with a health promotion group. Does the nurse function in the way you anticipated? What nursing behavior facilitates the group process? List the areas of skill and knowledge that groups consisting of community residents would most likely expect of the nurse.

# REFERENCES

Agency for Healthcare Research and Quality: *Assessing the Quality of Internet Health Information*. 1999. from: http://www.ahrq.gov/research/data/infoqual.html. Retrieved January 2015.

American Nurses Association (ANA): *Scope & Standards of Practice: Public Health Nursing*. Silver Spring, MD, 2007, ANA.

American Nurses Association (ANA): *ANA's Principles for Social Networking and the Nurse*. Silver Spring, MD, 2011, ANA.

Babcock DE, Miller MA: *Client Education: Theory and Practice*. St. Louis, MO, 1994, Mosby.

Bernhardt JM, Chaney JD, Chaney BH, et al: New media for health education: a revolution in progress. *Health Educ Behav* 40:129–132, 2013.

Billings D, Kowalski K: Teaching learners from varied generations. *J Contin Ed Nurs* 35:104–105, 2004.

Bloom BS, Englehart MO, Furst EJ, et al: *Taxonomy of Educational Objectives: The Classification of Educational Goals—Handbook 1: Cognitive Domain*. White Plains, NY, 1956, Longman.

Centers for Disease Control and Prevention: *Simply Put: A Guide for Creating Easy-to-Understand Materials*, ed 3. Atlanta, GA, 2010, Centers for Disease Control and Prevention.

Council on Linkages between Academia and Public Health Practice: *Core Competencies for Public Health Professionals*. Washington, DC, 2010, Public Health Foundation. from: www.phf.org. Retrieved January 2015.

Dauz E, Moore J, Smith CE, et al: Installing computers in older adults' home and teaching them to access a patient education web site: a systematic approach. *Comput Inform Nurs* 22:266–272, 2004.

Dembo MH: *Applying Educational Psychology*, ed 5. White Plains, NY, 1994, Longman.

Fielding JE: Health education 2.0: the next generation of health education practice. *Health Educ Behav* 40:513–519, 2013.

Gerow SJ: Teachers in school-based teams: contesting isolation in schools. In Sockett HT, DeMulder EK, DePage PC, et al, editors: *Transforming Teacher Education: Lessons in Professional Development*. Westport, CT, 2001, Bergin & Garvey.

Kirwan M, Duncan MJ, Vandelanotte C, et al: Design, development and formative evaluation of a smartphone application for recording and monitoring physical activity levels: the 10,000 steps "iStepLog." *Health Educ Behav* 40:140–151, 2013.

Kleinpell RM, Mick DJ: Evaluating outcomes. In Fulter TT, Foreman MD, Walker M, editors: *Critical Care Nursing of the Elderly*, ed 2. New York, 2001, Springer, pp 179–196.

Knowles M: *The Adult Learner: A Neglected Species*, ed 4. Houston, 1990, Gulf.

Knowles MS, Holton EF III, Swanson RA: *The Adult Learner: The Definitive Classic in Adult Education and Human Resource Development*, ed 6. London, 2005, Elsevier/Butterworth Heinemann.

Kutner M, Greenberg E, Jin Y, et al: *The Health Literacy of America's Adults: Results from the 2003 National Assessment of Adult Literacy (NCES 2006-483)*. Washington, DC, 2006, U.S. Department of Education, National Center for Education Statistics. from: http://nces.ed.gov/pubs2006/2006483.pdf. Retrieved December 2014.

Lachman CD: Social media: managing the ethical issues. *Med Surg Nurs* 22:326–329, 2013.

Miller WR, Rose GS: Toward a theory of motivational interviewing. *Am Psychol* 64:527–537, 2009.

Motivational Interviewing Network of Trainers (MINT): *Motivational Interviewing*. Fairfax, VA, 2013, MINT. from: http://www.motivationalinterviewing.org/YES. Retrieved January 2015.

National Council of State Boards of Nursing (NCSBN): *White Paper: A Nurse's Guide to the Use of Social Media*. Chicago, 2011, NCSBN. from: https://www.ncsbn.org/Social_Media.pdf. Retrieved January 2015.

National Institutes of Health (NIH): *Health Literacy*. 2014. from: http://www.nih.gov/clearcommunication/healthliteracy.htm. Retrieved January 2015.

Northen H, Kirland R: *Social Work with Groups*, ed 3. New York, 2001, Columbia University Press.

Ota C, DiCarlo C, Burts D, et al: Training and the needs of adult learners. *J Extension* 44(6):2006. from: http://www.joe.org/joe/2006december/tt5.php. Retrieved January 2015.

Palazzo M: Teaching in crisis: patient and family education in critical care. *Crit Care Nurs Clin North Am* 13:83–92, 2001.

Pew Charitable Trusts: *Pew Internet & American Life Project*. Washington, DC, 2013, Pew Charitable Trusts. from: www.pewinternet.org. Retrieved January 2015.

Pontius BJ: Health literacy: Part 2. *NASN School Nurse* 28:246–252, 2013.

Rice CS, Pollard JM: *Health Fair Planning Guide*. College Station, TX, 2011, Texas A&M AgriLife Extension Service, Family Development and Resource Management. from: http://fcs.tamu.edu/health/hfpg/Health-Fair-Planning-Guide-with-Appendix.pdf. Retrieved January 2015.

Sportsman S, Hamilton P: Conflict management styles in the health professions. *J Prof Nurs* 23:157–166, 2007.

Thompson JM: Understanding and managing organizational change: implications for public health management. *J Public Health Manage Pract* 16:167–173, 2010.

Tuckman BW: Developmental sequence in small groups. *Psychol Bull* 63:384–399, 1965.

Tuckman BW, Jensen MAC: Stages of small-group development revisited. *Group Organ Manag* 2:419–427, 1977.

UnitedHealthcare: *Health Fair Planning Guide: Wellness Toolkit*. 2010. from: https://uhctools.com/assets/Health%20Fair%20Planning%20Guide.pdf. Retrieved January 2015.

U.S. Department of Health and Human Services (USDHHS): *Healthy People 2020*. 2010. from: http://www.healthypeople.gov. Retrieved January 2015.

VanBiervliet A, Edwards-Schafer P: Consumer health information on the web: trends, issues, and strategies. *Dermatol Nurs* 16:519–523, 2004.

Weiss BD: *Removing Barriers to Better, Safer Care: Health Literacy and Patient Safety: Help Patients Understand. Manual for Clinicians*, ed 2. Chicago, 2007, American Medical Foundation, p 13.

# Building a Culture of Health through Community Health Promotion

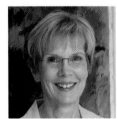

## *Pamela A. Kulbok, DNSc, RN, PHCNS-BC, FAAN*

Pamela A. Kulbok earned her BS and MS from Boston College and her doctorate at Boston University and did postdoctoral work in psychiatric epidemiology at Washington University in St. Louis. She was a U.S. Navy nurse; has worked in a visiting nurse service; and has directed a hospital-based home health agency. She is the Theresa A. Thomas Professor of Primary Care Nursing, Professor of Public Health Sciences, and Chair of the Department of Family, Community, and Mental Health Systems at the University of Virginia, School of Nursing. Dr. Kulbok is a Robert Wood Johnson Foundation, Executive Nurse Fellow (2102-2015). She was the Principal Investigator of an interprofessional, cross-institution, community-based participatory research project to design a youth substance use prevention program and of a series of studies of youth nonsmoking behavior. She has taught undergraduate and graduate courses in public health nursing, health promotion research, and nursing knowledge development. She was Co-Chair of the American Nurses Association (ANA) workgroup that revised the *Public Health Nursing: Scope and Standards of Practice* (2013), a member of the American Public Health Association (APHA) PHN Section, Definition Task Force that updated the *Definition of Public Health Nursing* (2013), President of the Association of Community Health Nursing Educators, and Chair of the Quad Council of Public Health Nursing Organizations. She was a member of the ANA—Congress on Nursing Practice and Economics. She is Fellow in the Center for Health Policy at the University of Virginia.

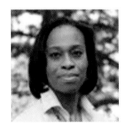

## *Nisha Botchwey, PhD, MCRP, MPH*

Nisha Botchwey earned her doctorate degree at the University of Pennsylvania and completed her Masters of Public Health at the University of Virginia. She taught Urban and Environmental Planning and Public Health at the University of Virginia. She is an Associate Professor of City and Regional Planning in the College of Architecture at the Georgia Institute of Technology. Dr. Botchwey specializes in public health and the built environment and community engagement. She teaches Public Health and the Built Environment, Community Engagement and the Citizen Participation and Health Impact Assessment, courses subscribed by community design and public health students from Emory and Georgia State University. Dr. Botchwey is author of *Health Impact Assessment in the United States* (Springer, 2014). She is also Director of the *Built Environment and Public Health Clearinghouse* (www.bephc.gatech.edu), an online resource supported by the Centers for Disease Control and Prevention and the National Prevention Strategy, offering training resources and multisector community building for public health, planning, architecture, transportation engineering, and health impact assessment. Dr. Botchwey is co-lead of the *Atlanta Dashboard*, an interactive tool that collects, analyzes, and displays quality of life and health data at the sub-county level to aid in evidence-based decision making. Dr. Botchwey is Co-Director of the National Academy of Environmental Design's Research Committee, a member of the Centers for Disease Control and Prevention's Advisory Committee to the Director, and an NSF ADVANCE Woman of Excellence Faculty award recipient.

## ADDITIONAL RESOURCES

ⓔ **Evolve Website http://evolve.elsevier.com/Stanhope**
- Healthy People 2020
- WebLinks—Of special note see the links for these sites:
  - National Prevention Strategy
  - MAP-IT: A Guide To Using Healthy People 2020 in Your Community

- Quiz
- Case Studies
- Glossary
- Answers to Practice Application

## OBJECTIVES

*After reading this chapter, the student should be able to do the following:*

1. Describe a culture of health and community health promotion in the context of the ecologic model and social determinants of health (SDOH).
2. Analyze participatory approaches and the interrelationships among communities, populations, and interprofessional health care providers in the application of community health promotion strategies.
3. Describe evidence-based practice using the integrative model of community health promotion at multiple levels of the client system: individual, family, aggregate, and community.
4. Analyze nursing and interprofessional roles that are essential to build a culture of health through community health promotion.

## INTRODUCTION

The Robert Wood Johnson Foundation (RWJF) (2013) recently introduced the idea of a culture of health. Recognizing that health and health care are in the forefront of national debate and dialogue about health reform, nurses and other providers are questioning the foundation of our health care system. There is a significant shift away from acceptance of the status quo, and toward building a culture of health. Such a shift puts emphasis on the pursuit of long, healthy lives for all Americans and is consistent with the national health vision and goals proposed in *Healthy People 2020* (U.S. Department of Health and Human Services [USDHHS], 2014a) and the National Prevention Strategy (National Prevention Council [NPC], 2011). The RWJF foresees "… a vibrant American culture of health: where good health flourishes across geographic, demographic, and social sectors; where being healthy and staying healthy is an esteemed social value; and everyone has access to affordable, quality health care" (2013). While most people recognize the need to exercise regularly, maintain their weight at recommended levels, and manage stress in their lives, modifiable health behaviors remain the major contributors to deaths in the United States (U.S.) (National Center for Health Statistics [NCHS], 2012). For example, tobacco use remains the leading cause of premature deaths in the United States, with 480,000 deaths annually attributed to cigarette smoking (USDHHS, 2014b). Nurses,

other health professionals, and the public recognize that initiating and maintaining a healthy lifestyle is difficult and requires different approaches directed toward individuals, families, communities, populations, and the environments in which they live.

In this chapter, we describe the historical underpinnings of health and health promotion for communities and populations including the concepts of community and social determinants of health (SDOH). In addition, we describe community health promotion models and frameworks including those specific to public health nursing and health promotion models from the social sciences. These concepts and models and the ways they are related are critical to building a culture of health and determine the nature of nursing practice with communities and populations. We emphasize an ecologic approach to community health promotion and population health, which integrates multilevel interventions to promote the health of the public. The integrative model of community health promotion (Laffrey and Kulbok, 1999) can help nurses plan care for clients including communities and populations. The model synthesizes knowledge from public health, nursing, and the social sciences. The chapter describes studies that illustrate community-based participatory research (CBPR) and multilevel interventions. Applications of the integrative model of community health promotion show that the way nurses view these concepts is important in their approach to practice.

# HISTORICAL PERSPECTIVES, DEFINITIONS, AND METHODS

## Health and Health Promotion

Health is the key term in the process of building a culture of health through community health promotion. Beginning with Nightingale's efforts to discover and use the laws of nature to enhance humanity, nursing has taken an active role in promoting the health of communities and populations. The way one defines health shapes the process of nursing and health care, including making decisions about what to assess, with what level of client, and how to evaluate the outcomes of care. For example, health from a medical perspective as alleviating an individual's illness symptoms, involves assessment of the duration, intensity, and frequency of specific symptoms. Intervention focuses on symptom relief and treatment of the cause of symptoms. Evaluation consists of determining the extent of symptom alleviation. On the other hand, health defined from an ecologic or environmental perspective as maximizing a community's physical recreation opportunities, may involve assessment of existing recreation facilities, accessibility to the population, and beliefs and knowledge related to recreation and land use in the community as resources for healthy living.

The holistic or ecologic view of health is not new. The ancient Greeks viewed health as the influence of environmental forces on human well-being and healing from illness. Scientific medicine emerged slowly and in the twentieth century, professional care took precedence over self-care. During the last five decades, the concept of self-care as derived from a positive idea of health has reemerged to compete with professional care. Some proponents of self-care emphasize lay diagnosis and self-treatment, whereas others focus on teaching people how to work with their health care providers. As a result, health care system changes include the renegotiation of roles and emphasize collaboration between consumers and providers, as well as recognition of the health impact of the conditions in which people live.

Many health professionals believe that individuals are in a position to produce health. This idea is not new. In 1974, Fuchs suggested that the "greatest potential for improving health lies in what we do and don't do for and to ourselves" (p. 55). In the political arena, LaLonde introduced a similar idea in *A New Perspective on the Health of Canadians* (1974). LaLonde identified four major determinants of health: human biology, environment, lifestyle, and health care. In 1976, policy makers in the United States reinforced these determinants of health and supported efforts to improve health habits and the environment as the best hope of achieving any significant extension of life expectancy (U.S. Department of Health, Education and Welfare [USDHEW], 1976, p. 69). The fundamental ideas of these landmark documents about the determinants of health emerged during the era of social ecology (Bronfenbrenner, 1977 and 1979). Box 17-1 lists some landmark initiatives in health promotion and disease prevention.

The ecosocial or social-ecological perspective, initially presented by Bronfenbrenner in 1977, described human-environment interaction and health outcomes over a life span.

---

### BOX 17-1    Landmark Health Promotion/Disease Prevention Initiatives

1974—LaLonde's *A New Perspective on the Health of Canadians*
1976—Forward Plan for Health, FY 1978-1982
1979—*Healthy People: The Surgeon General's Report on Health Promotion and Disease Prevention*
1989—Guide to Clinical Preventive Services (USPSTF, 1989)
1990—*Healthy People 2000*
1994—Put Prevention into Practice (PPIP)
2000—*Healthy People 2010: Understanding and Improving Health and Objectives for Improving Health,* ed 2 (supersedes Jan 2000 conference edition)
2002—Progress reviews of *Healthy People 2010* initiated
2005—Guide to Community Preventive Services: What Works to Promote Health? (TFCPS, 2005)
2009—*Healthy People 2020* Framework
2010—*Healthy People 2020* Objectives
2012—Guide to Clinical Preventive Services (USPSTF, 2011)

Sources: Task Force on Community Preventive Services: *The Guide to Community Preventive Services-What Works to Promote Health,* New York, 2005, Oxford University Press. U.S. Preventive Services Task Force: *Guide to Clinical Preventive Services: Report of the U.S. Preventive Services Task Force,* Baltimore, 1989, Lippincott, Williams & Wilkins. U.S. Preventive Services Task Force: *Guide to Clinical Preventive Services, 2012: Recommendations of the U.S. Preventive Services Task Force.* October 2011. Agency for Healthcare Research and Quality, Rockville, MD. Available at http://www.ahrq.gov/professionals/clinicians-providers/guidelines-recommendations/guide/index.html. Accessed April 26, 2014.

---

The environments are described as the micro-, meso-, and macro-system levels. McLeroy et al (1988) translated these levels of the ecologic model to actionable layers of influence that include intrapersonal (characteristics of the individual), interpersonal (formal and informal social networks and social support systems), institutional (social institutions), community (mediating institutions, relationships and power), and public policy (multilevel laws and policies).

The U.S. Public Health Service established the first national objectives involving disease prevention, health protection, and health promotion strategies in the surgeon general's *Healthy People* report. Disease prevention strategies focus on services such as family planning and immunizations delivered in clinical settings. Health protection strategies include environmental measures to improve health and quality of life. Health promotion strategies focus on achieving well-being through community and individual lifestyle change measures (USDHEW, 1979).

As described in Chapter 2, the health objectives for the nation outlined in *Healthy People 2020* build on initiatives that have been pursued since 1980. Designed for use by individuals, communities, states, and professional organizations, these health objectives provided a guide for community and population programs to improve health. The release of *Healthy People 2020* in 2010 included a national vision, mission, and overarching goals. The four goals emphasized prevention, health equity, environments conducive to health for all, and healthy development across the life span. Information on *Healthy People 2020* objectives and action plans (USDHHS, 2014c) is available at http://www.healthypeople.gov/2020/default.aspx.

## DETERMINANTS OF POPULATION HEALTH

**FIG 17-1** Determinants of Population Health (From Centers for Disease Control and Prevention: *Social determinants of health.* Available at http://www.cdc.gov/socialdeterminants/faq.html#b. Accessed April 26, 2014.)

The **National Prevention Strategy** (NPS) published through the U.S. Surgeon General's Office by the National Prevention Council (NPC, 2011) seeks to "improve the health and quality of life for individuals, families, and communities by moving the nation from a focus on sickness and disease to one based on prevention and wellness" (NPC, 2011, p. 7). To realize this vision for children, youth, adults and the elderly, the NPS targets interventions in multiple settings. These include healthy and safe community environments, clinical and community preventive services, empowered people, and elimination of health disparities. A focus on safe and healthy communities recognizes the power of the social, economic and environmental factors that have a stronger influence on health and well-being than does the health care setting (see Figure 17-2 for National Prevention Strategy).

This idea that the health of communities and populations is shaped by multiple determinants has been reinforced in the national (Institute of Medicine [IOM], 2003) and international (World Health Organization [WHO], 2014a) health policy literature. The current focus is on determinants of population health (Figure 17-1), which include genes and biology, health behaviors, medical care, total ecology, and social/societal characteristics (Centers for Disease Control and Prevention [CDC], 2014a; IOM, 2006). In Figure 17-1, genes, biology, and health behavioral choices account for 25% of population health; and social determinants of health including medical care, the physical and social environment account for the remaining 75%. Although recent trends reveal improvement in determinants of population health such as healthier living conditions and a decrease in smoking, these positive trends are associated with persistent socioeconomic disparities worldwide (WHO, 2014a) (see Healthy People 2020 box).

### Definitions of Health

The WHO (1948) reflected a holistic perspective in its classic definition of health as a state of complete physical, mental, and social well-being, and not merely the absence of disease and infirmity. Terris expanded the WHO definition: "Health is a state of physical, mental and social well-being and the ability to function and not merely the absence of illness and infirmity" (Terris, 1975, p. 1038). By deleting "complete" and adding "ability to func-

## ♥ HEALTHY PEOPLE 2020

### *Tobacco Use*

Selected objectives from *Healthy People 2020* that pertain to tobacco use:
- TU-1: Reduce tobacco use by adults.
- TU-2: Reduce tobacco use by adolescents.
- TU-3: Reduce the initiation of tobacco use among children, adolescents, and young adults.
- TU-6: Increase smoking cessation during pregnancies.
- TU-7: Increase smoking cessation by adolescent smokers.
- TU-11: Reduce the proportion of nonsmokers exposed to secondhand smoke.

From U.S. Department of Health and Human Services: *Healthy People 2020.* Available at http://www.healthypeople.gov/2020/default.aspx. Accessed January 15, 2011.

function," Terris placed the WHO definition in a realistic context, providing a useful framework for health promotion.

Smith (1981), a nursing scholar, suggested that the "idea of health" directs nursing practice, education, and research. She defined health along a continuum, allowing for "more" or "less" health. Smith proposed four models of health, ordered from narrow and concrete to broad and abstract: clinical health, or absence of disease; role performance health, or ability to perform one's social roles satisfactorily; adaptive health, or flexible adaptation to the environment; and eudaemonistic health, or self-actualization and attainment of one's human potential.

**Population health** is a term widely used in several IOM reports and in contemporary health care policy. Recently, the IOM Roundtable on Population Health Improvement defined population health as "the health outcomes of a group of individuals, including the distribution of such outcomes within the group" (Kindig and Stoddart, 2003, p. 381). Though not a part of the definition itself, population health outcomes are the product of multiple determinants of health, including genetics, behaviors, public health, medical care, and environmental and social factors (Adler et al, 2013; IOM, 2014).

It is important for nurses and health care providers to reflect on their own definition of health and recognize how their definition influences the care they provide. Likewise, it is equally important for nurses to assess clients' personal health definitions. Only through knowledge of their own health definition, together with assessment of clients' health definitions, can nurses create interventions tailored to achieve the clients' health goals. Nurses and health care providers who emphasize health promotion and population health that is congruent with the beliefs, health definitions, and goals of the population also acknowledge the importance of illness prevention. Nurses must strive to understand health policies and the consequences of these policies on vulnerable populations whose living conditions may include few determinants of good health.

### Definitions of Health Promotion

**Health promotion** is an aim of nursing and health care, although explicit definition of health promotion and differentiation from disease prevention or health maintenance is rare. **Leavell and Clark (1965)** strongly influenced the evolution of health promotion and disease prevention strategies through their classic definitions of primary, secondary, and tertiary levels of prevention that were rooted in the biomedical model of health and epidemiology. The application of preventive measures, according to Leavell and Clark, corresponds to the natural history or stages of disease (see Chapter 12). Primary preventive measures apply to "well" individuals in the prepathogenesis period to promote their health and to provide specific protection from disease. Secondary preventive measures apply to diagnosis or to treatment of individuals in the period of disease pathogenesis. Tertiary prevention addresses rehabilitation and the return of people with chronic illness to a maximal ability to function (see Levels of Prevention box).

## LEVELS OF PREVENTION

### Diabetes

**Primary Prevention**
For a person with identified risk factors for diabetes, the goal is to maintain a normal weight, to exercise regularly, and to reduce the intake of carbohydrates.

**Secondary Prevention**
Have regular blood glucose level testing done and be alert for any symptoms of the onset of diabetes. If the blood glucose level indicates that the client has diabetes, begin treatment.

**Tertiary Prevention**
For a person diagnosed with diabetes, monitor blood glucose levels and maintenance of a diabetic diet, regular exercise, and medication.

Even though primary, secondary, and tertiary levels of prevention had their origins in the medical model, Leavell and Clark (1965) moved beyond the medical model. They conceptualized primary prevention as two distinct components: health promotion and specific protection. Health promotion focuses on positive measures such as education for healthy living and promotion of favorable environmental conditions as well as periodic examinations including, for example, well-child developmental assessment and health education. Specific protection includes measures to reduce the threat of specific diseases or injury, such as hygiene, immunizations, use of seat belts, and the elimination of workplace hazards.

Health promotion and specific protection, when used as subconcepts of primary prevention, stem from a definition of health as the absence of disease. However, health promotion and specific protection strategies are not the same. Some terms used to describe health promotion are linked to a positive view of health (e.g., *health habits or health practices*), whereas other terms are linked to the negative view of the absence of disease (e.g., *disease or illness prevention*). Using the terms *health promotion, health protection,* and *disease prevention* interchangeably, as indicators of preventive behavior, leads to confusion (Kulbok et al, 1997). Interestingly, similar confusion exists today in the field of health education regarding definition of the terms *health behavior, health education,* and *health promotion* (Simons-Morton, 2013). As interprofessional practice opportunities increase, public health nurses need to have clear definitions in mind when they use terms associated with community health promotion.

The WHO described health promotion as a process that enables individuals to increase control over and improve their health (WHO, 2014b). According to the 1986 Ottawa Charter, health promotion combines both individual- and community-level strategies to build healthful public policy, create supportive environments, strengthen community action, develop personal skills, and reorient health services. Health is a resource for daily living. For individuals or communities to realize physical, mental, and social well-being, they must become aware of and learn to use the social and personal resources available within their environment.

There is considerable evidence supporting a positive view of health underlying health promotion activities directed toward individuals, communities, and populations. The WHO's definition of health promotion as a process and the current focus on an ecologic approach to determinants of population health are grounded in the perspective of positive health. These approaches view health promotion in the context of a holistic healthy lifestyle, as well as involving simultaneous interaction with the social and physical environments. Clearly, health promotion and population health are consistent with the goals of public health nursing.

*Disease Oriented versus Process and Environmentally Oriented Health and Health Promotion.* Nurses have long recognized the importance of an emphasis on wellness and health promotion in health care. In public health nursing (PHN) practice, it is clear that many factors, beyond illness, affect the health of individuals, communities, and populations. The biomedical model, in which health is defined as absence of disease, does not explain why some populations exposed to illness-producing stressors remain healthy, whereas others, who appear to be in health-enhancing situations, become ill. Viewing clients from the perspective of the biomedical model alone makes it difficult to identify health potential beyond the absence of disease in the individual. For example, most at-risk populations such as the frail elderly have at least one diagnosed chronic disease. Limiting the definition of health potential to the absence of disease, nurses would never perceive this population as healthy. Defining health as the absence of disease is a pessimistic and individual-level definition; nursing actions can help older and chronically ill persons become healthier if a broader definition of health is used.

Laffrey, Loveland-Cherry, and Winkler (1986) describe two perspectives from which the key concepts of nursing science (e.g., person, health, environment) and nursing can be viewed. The first is the disease-oriented perspective that views health objectively, and defines it as the absence of disease as discussed previously. This perspective assumes that humans are composed of organ systems and cells; in this instance, health care focuses on identifying what is not working properly with a given system and repairing it. In this context, health behavior begins with patient compliance with health professionals' recommendations. The second perspective defines health subjectively as a process, not as a presence or absence. In this health-oriented perspective, humans are complex and ever-changing systems, and are interconnected with others and the environment. Health behavior within this latter health-oriented perspective involves a holistic view of lifestyle and interaction with the environment and not simply compliance with a prescribed regimen.

*Lifestyle Changes*

Both perspectives support the aims and processes of population-focused nursing. The disease-oriented approach directs nursing toward illness prevention, risk appraisal, risk reduction, prompt treatment, and disease management of individuals. However, the health-oriented approach directs nursing practice toward promotion of positive health for a larger segment of the population. Defining health broadly as the life process, taking into account the mutual and simultaneous interaction of humans and their environment, views illness as a potential manifestation of that interaction. Because positive health does not exclude any part of the life process (it includes illness prevention and illness care), it goes beyond the disease perspective to include positive and holistic health (Laffrey and Kulbok, 1999).

## Community

Another concept essential to building a culture of health through community health promotion is community. The emphasis on community as the target of practice gained increased attention since the mid-1970s when the U.S. and Canadian governments and health researchers attributed declining mortality and morbidity rates to better standards of living, such as sanitation, clean air and water, and wider availability of healthy foods. Again, these approaches were consistent with emerging ideas about social ecology during the same period. The IOM's seminal report on the future of public health highlighted the importance of community in its statement that the "mission of public health is to assure conditions in which people can be healthy by generating organized community effort to prevent disease and promote health" (National Research Council [NRC], 1988, p. 7). (See Chapter 18 for more on the concept of community.)

As discussed previously, national health goals emphasize that environment and community are central to achieving health. *Healthy People in Healthy Communities: A Community Planning Guide Based on Healthy People 2010* (USDHHS, 2001) (Box 17-2), outlines practical recommendations for coalition building, creating a vision, and measuring outcomes to improve the health of communities. Communities can tailor these recommendations to their own local needs, and health professionals in public and private organizations can work together with community members to develop programs that fit the needs and resources of their own communities. The National Prevention Strategy also offers recommendations on what can be done to improve population health in specified contexts and across goal areas (NPC, 2011). Nurses participate in this collaborative and interprofessional process through community assessments, community development activities, and identification of key persons in the community with whom to build partnerships for health programs. Nurses working with nonprofit hospitals can also directly engage in improving health of communities through completion of a Community Health Needs Assessment (CHNA) as required under the Affordable Care Act (Rosenbaum, 2013).

One of the four overarching goals of the *Healthy People 2020 Framework* is to create social and physical environments that promote good health for all (USDHHS, 2014d). Community-wide program planning provides a strategy to achieve this goal. *Healthy People 2020* highlighted a community framework called

---

### BOX 17-2   *Healthy People 2010:* A Strategy for Creating a Healthy Community

To achieve the goal of improving health, a community must develop a strategy supported by many individuals who are working together. The MAP-IT technique helps you to map out the path toward the change you want to see in your community. This guide recommends that you MAP-IT—that is, **m**obilize, **a**ssess, **p**lan, **i**mplement, and **t**rack.

Mobilize individuals and organizations that care about the health of your community into a coalition.

Assess the areas of greatest need in your community, as well as the resources and other strengths that you can tap into to address those areas.

Plan your approach: start with a vision of where you want to be as a community; then add strategies and action steps to help you achieve that vision.

Implement your plan using concrete action steps that can be monitored and will make a difference.

Track your progress over time.

From U.S. Department of Health and Human Services: A strategy for creating a healthy community: MAP-IT. In Healthy people in healthy communities: A community planning guide using Healthy People 2010, Washington, DC, 2001, U.S. Government Printing Office.

---

### BOX 17-3   Milio's Propositions for Improving Health Behavior

- Health status of populations is a function of the lack or excess of health-sustaining resources.
- Behavior patterns of populations are related to habits of choice from actual or perceived limited resources and related attitudes.
- Organizational decisions determine the range of personal resources available.
- Individual health-related decisions are influenced by efforts to maximize valued resources in both the personal and societal domains.
- Social change is reflective of a change in population behavior patterns.
- Health education will impact behavior patterns minimally without new health-promoting options for investing personal resources.

Modified from Milio N: A framework for prevention: changing health damaging to health-generating life patterns, *Am J Public Health* 66:435, 1976.

---

MAP-IT (USDHHS, 2014e) as a guide to using *Healthy People 2020* in your community (see http://healthypeople.gov/2020/implement/mapit.aspx). MAP-IT stands for Mobilize, Assess, Plan, Implement, and Track; and communities can use the guide to evaluate public health interventions designed to implement the goals of *Healthy People 2020*.

Nurses and interprofessional health care providers have many opportunities to participate in community-wide health care. To address community problems, these professionals need to integrate concepts of health and illness, individual and population, public health and health care, health promotion and disease prevention, and ecology and environmental health. This integration means that nurses must consider the complex relationship between personal and environmental forces that affect health. Over 35 years ago, Milio (1976) offered a set of propositions for improving health behavior by considering personal choices in the context of available societal resources. These propositions (Box 17-3) remain relevant today. They constitute a fitting model for health promotion that addresses both personal and societal resources for this and future decades.

## COMMUNITY HEALTH PROMOTION MODELS AND FRAMEWORKS

Numerous models and frameworks have community health promotion as the goal. The following sections provide brief descriptions of models specific to community and/or health promotion that are useful to public health nurses practicing at a basic or advanced level.

### Public Health Nursing Community Models and Frameworks

Although theoretical frameworks developed within nursing and other health disciplines are traditionally oriented toward individuals, there is increasing recognition of the importance of community and person–environment interactions that go beyond social cognitive theory and other interpersonal frameworks (USDHHS, 2005) in promoting health. PHN defined community as "… persons in interaction, being and experiencing together, who may or may not share a sense of common purpose" (ANA, 2013, p. 65). Nurses realize that the community is more than the sum of the individuals, families, aggregates, and organizations within it and that interaction is essential for any real change to occur. The following are examples of public health nursing models focused on interventions with communities or populations.

Chopoorian (1986) was among the first to acknowledge that nurses could strengthen their position with communities by focusing on the social, economic, and political structures that make up the community, as well as the social relations and patterns of everyday life in the community. Within this perspective, interventions targeted to public health policy can have far-reaching health benefits. Shuster and Goeppinger (2012) asserted that definitions of *community* vary widely and that nurses working with communities learn quickly that there are many different types. Shuster and Goeppinger highlighted the importance of person, place, and function, as well as interaction among systems within a community. Nurses must examine the complexity and dynamic nature inherent in the process of community building, rather than viewing the community as a geographic, racial, or cultural group that is static.

Despite the ideal, it is not easy to integrate the concept of the community as client into practice. Consequently, the provision of care to individuals *in the community* may still overshadow nursing practice and health promotion directed *to the community*. Bekemeier and Jones (2010), in a study of local public health agency (LPHA) functions, leadership, and staffing, reported that the proportion of nursing staff in an LPHA related strongly to provision of services involving individual-level care. They found that the staff nurses were most likely to perform individual-family interventions, and that both the staff nurses and the managers rated individual-family interventions as more important than community- or system-level interventions. These findings suggest that there is an ongoing need to expand "… education and outreach to nurses regarding their roles and responsibilities to assure environmental health protection, community assessment, and health improvement planning" (Bekemeier and Jones, 2010, p. E16).

Anderson and McFarlane (2000, 2010) and Salmon (1993, 2009) developed system models based on the assumption that assessing the various components of the system (i.e., individual, family, community, and society) facilitates a healthy community. Anderson and McFarlane's community-as-partner model includes eight major community subsystems. The basic core of the community, according to these authors, is its people, described by their demographic characteristics and their values, beliefs, culture, religion, laws, and more. Within the community system, the people interact with the other subsystems. A community health assessment must include information about the subsystems and the pattern of interactions among the subsystems and of the total community with the systems external to it.

Salmon's model (1993, 2009) focused on the public health mission of organized efforts to protect, promote, and restore health. It embraces multiple determinants of health and is consistent with the IOM's perspective on population health (IOM, 2014). According to Salmon's model, nursing includes health promotion, illness prevention, and health protection strategies. Systems models provide important guidance for assessing communities and populations and indicate that system-level interventions require participation with relevant subsystems. However, systems models may not provide the guidance needed for intervention development.

Keller et al (1998, 2004) proposed a population-based intervention model based on the scope of PHN practice that crosses multiple levels of care; this model defines the population-focused underpinning of PHN practice and provides guidance for PHN interventions at the individual, community, and system levels. The model was later termed the "Intervention Wheel" (Keller et al, 2004, p. 453). The Intervention Wheel includes community, systems, and individual/family levels of practice. (See Chapter 9 for more information on the Intervention Wheel.) It is population based and identifies 17 public health interventions. The models proposed by Anderson and McFarlane (2000, 2010), Salmon (1993, 2009), and Keller et al (1998, 2004) focus on stability and equilibrium. They emphasize protecting the community from specific disease risks; less attention is directed toward factors that promote an optimally healthy community. A few of the classic community-wide epidemiologic studies focused on multilevel interventions or community health promotion are described next.

### Influential Multilevel Community Studies

Two significant community studies of health risks, morbidity, and mortality are the Framingham Heart Study, initiated in 1949, and the Human Population Laboratory's longitudinal survey in Alameda County, California, initiated in the early 1970s. The Framingham Heart Study followed 5209 adults over their life span to identify factors contributing to coronary heart disease (CHD). Collecting periodic health assessments and morbidity and mortality data, major risk factors associated with CHD mortality were identified (e.g., elevated systolic blood pressure, elevated serum cholesterol level, and cigarette smoking). The investigators used health risk appraisals to relate the risk factors in well individuals to the probability of future cardiovascular disease (Lieb et al, 2009). The Framingham study continues today (see http://www.framinghamheartstudy .org/).

The Alameda County study measured the relationships of health and social behaviors to mortality in a community sample of 6928 individuals over 4 years. The behaviors included eating three meals daily, eating breakfast, sleeping 7 to 8 hours a night, using alcohol moderately, exercising regularly, not smoking, maintaining a desirable weight-to-height ratio, and maintaining social networks. There was a positive relationship between smoking and excessive alcohol use and mortality. There was an inverse relationship between physical exercise, 7 to 8 hours of sleep, optimal weight in relation to height, and social networks and mortality (Berkman and Breslow, 1983). These findings led to the emphasis on social and environmental variables, in addition to personal behaviors, in strategies for community health promotion.

Findings from these early large-scale surveys prompted a number of public health multilevel intervention programs. Examples include the Stanford Five-City Heart Disease Prevention program (Farquhar et al, 1990), the North Karelia study (Puska et al, 1983), the Pawtucket Heart Health program (Lasater et al, 1984), the Minnesota Heart Health program (Luepker et al, 1994), and the Dutch Heart Health Community Intervention (Ronda et al, 2005). These programs provided beginning scientific evidence for the implementation of community-level risk reduction programs, although the results were modest and often not statistically significant. However, these studies made major contributions to theory and practice in building community partnerships, establishing social marketing, developing behavior change strategies, and evaluating health programs. Results of these studies make it clear that multiple levels of intervention are necessary to reach the community in a meaningful way. Nurses have close relationships with individuals, families, high-risk groups, organizations such as schools, congregations and workplaces, and other health care professionals. They can contribute to health promotion by participating in community projects such as the ones described here. It is important that nurses develop health programs and document improved outcomes for high-risk groups with whom they interact.

## Health Promotion Models and Frameworks

There are a variety of theoretical approaches that can be used to help public health nurses design and implement health promotion programs for individuals and communities. The National Cancer Institute's seminal document, *Theory at a Glance* (USDHHS, 2005), organized these health promotion models and frameworks into three levels, which are consistent with the ecologic perspective used in this chapter. The first level is intrapersonal or individual, including models focused on knowledge, attitudes, personal beliefs and values. The second level is interpersonal, including models that emphasize processes and groups such as family, friends, and peers who may

provide support. The third level is community, which includes institutional structures and policies that may enhance or inhibit health behavior. Brief descriptions of selected models and frameworks are provided in the following sections.

### Individual Health Promotion Models

There are several intrapersonal or individual level models including the health belief model, the theory of reasoned action and the theory of planned behavior, the stages of change or transtheoretical model, and the precaution adoption process model (Edberg, 2013). The **health belief model (HBM)** can be used to plan programs to increase an individual's motivation to take a positive health action. Specifically, the HBM was one of the first theories of health behavior. It began in the 1950s, when the U.S. Public Health Service sent mobile units to communities to provide chest x-rays as a way to screen for tuberculosis (Rosenstock, 1974). The chest X-rays were free, convenient, and painless, yet people did not take advantage of the service. A group of social psychologists tried to explain the failure to use this screening, or more specifically, to determine what would motivate people to seek health care.

The HBM includes six components that attempt to determine what motivates an individual to adopt a health behavior. These components are (1) perceived susceptibility ("Will something happen to me?"); (2) perceived severity ("If something does happen to me, will it be a big problem?"); (3) perceived benefits ("If I do what is suggested, will it really help me?"); (4) perceived barriers ("If I do what is suggested, will there be barriers that will be unpleasant or costly?"); (5) cues to action ("What might motivate me to take the recommended action?"); and (6) self-efficacy ("Can I really do this?"). This model has been praised and criticized. It provides guidance in planning health promotion programs because it reminds nurses to think carefully about what motivates people to change. To understand motivation, it is important to learn (1) how people involved feel about the health problem, (2) whether they think the problem is serious, (3) whether they think that action on their part will make a difference, and (4) whether they think they can both manage the barriers and actually perform the action (Edberg, 2013; USDHHS, 2005).

The **transtheoretical model (TTM) or stages of change (SOC)**, and the precaution adoption process model (PAPM) are discussed together because they both deal with the process of change that occurs in stages and over time. The TTM or SOC has six stages:

1. **Precontemplation**, in which the person does not plan to change; this may be because the person does not know there is a problem or does not want to do anything about it. For example, a person may not know that potential exposure to radon, a cancer-causing radioactive gas that he cannot see, smell or taste in his home, is a health risk.

2. **Contemplation**, in which the person begins thinking about making a change in the future and examines the pros and cons of doing so. The person may have heard about home radon exposure on the local news and is considering whether his home may have unsafe levels of radon and whether he should test for radon.

3. **Preparation**, in which the person intends to do something. In the example about radon exposure, the person might contact the environmental office of the local health department for advice about radon testing.

4. **Action** occurs when the person actually buys a radon-testing kit and uses it in his home.

5. **Maintenance** is when the person decides to test for radon and to take measures to reduce radon to acceptable levels.

6. **Termination** is when the person has adopted and sustained the behavior change process. For most behaviors, this stage is rarely accomplished and individuals stay in the maintenance stage (Edberg, 2013; USDHHS, 2005).

Although the terms used are slightly different, the intent of the PAPM is much like that of the TTM or SOC. The stages are (1) unaware of the issue, (2) unengaged by the issue, (3) deciding about acting, (4) deciding not to act, (5) deciding to act, (6) acting, and (7) maintenance. You can apply the cooking example later in this chapter to these stages, as well (Edberg, 2013).

### Interpersonal Health Promotion Models

Interpersonal-level models generally involve interaction between individuals and the social environment. These models focus on the reciprocal or mutual nature of interaction; that is, the person's thoughts, feelings or actions are influenced by and also exert influence on his or her immediate environment. The social environment typically involves family, friends, peers, co-workers, health providers and others (USDHHS, 2005). Social learning theory, social cognitive theory, social network theory, and social support (Edberg, 2013) are examples of interpersonal-level frameworks that are useful for health promotion. Social cognitive theory (SCT) is one of the commonly used interpersonal theories. It evolved from Bandura's social learning theory (SLT), which proposed that individuals learned from their own behaviors and from observations of the behaviors of others and the benefits of those behaviors. Bandura expanded SLT by adding the construct of self-efficacy, which addresses the degree of confidence individuals have in their ability to perform a behavior (Edberg, 2013; USDHHS, 2005).

Continuing with the example of radon exposure, an individual would need to believe that he was capable of obtaining a radon test kit, understanding the directions for radon testing, and using it properly to test radon levels in his home. Note that there are incremental, small steps involved in a behavior seemingly as simple as using a radon testing kit. Bandura stressed the importance of understanding the target behavior in order to plan potential strategies to assist an individual in the process of behavior change. In addition to understanding the target behavior, change strategies based on SCT include (1) verbal persuasion, (2) role modeling, (3) positive affective response, and (4) positive reinforcement of the behavior. Strategies that public health nurses can use to change behavior include (1) communication skills to persuade a person to test his home for radon, (2) modeling the radon testing behavior, (3) emphasizing the positive emotional response associated with reducing the health risk for his family, and (4) providing positive encouragement and affirmation when the person has completed the radon testing in his home.

### Community Health Promotion Models

The social ecological model is another model used to guide public health nursing interventions for community health promotion (USDHHS, 2005; Edberg, 2013). The social ecological model (SEM) guides health promotion as well as illness prevention interventions. According to this model, health care and health-related behavior are a function of individual, interpersonal, organizational, community, and population factors. Thus, interventions are specific to each of these levels. In one of the first comprehensive studies using the SEM to assess factors related to the uptake of influenza vaccine, researchers examined vaccine uptake during the 2009 H1N1 pandemic. Of the 2079 adults surveyed, only 18.4% reported that they received the 2009 H1N1 vaccine. The results indicated that variables at all SEM levels influenced acquiring the vaccination: intrapersonal level explained 53%; interpersonal explained 47%; institutional level explained 34%; and, the policy and community levels each explained 8% of the variance related to influenza vaccine uptake. Together the SEM levels explained 65% of the variance in vaccine uptake. This data indicated that interventions aimed at multiple levels might be more effective than those targeting a single level (Kumar et al, 2013) (see Evidence-Based Practice box).

### EVIDENCE-BASED PRACTICE

A study of leisure time physical activity (LTPA) in black adults, which used the social ecological model, helped to clarify relationships between LTPA and social-ecological factors such as self-efficacy, self-regulation, social support, outcome expectations, and policy beliefs (Li et al, 2012). The results suggested that self-regulation and intention to organize personal time for routine PA may yield successful results and that a PA intervention may succeed if participants in the intervention include people in their close network who support each other. In addition, the results suggested that planning policies to enhance the built environment and satisfy the community have the potential for wide-reaching effect on PA levels of African Americans. Several other major community-wide studies have drawn on concepts such as those presented in these models.

Li K, Seo DC, Torabi MR, et al: Social-ecological factors of leisure-time physical activity in black adults. *Am J Health Behav* 36:797–810, 2012.

## THE ECOLOGIC APPROACH TO COMMUNITY HEALTH PROMOTION

### Ecologic Perspectives on Population Health

Because individuals ultimately make decisions to engage in healthy or risky behaviors, lifestyle improvement efforts have focused typically on the individual as the target of care. Following the health belief model (Rosenstock, 1974), individuals generally concentrate on immediate personal rewards or threats when deciding whether to engage in specific behaviors; in this context, they may convince themselves that their immediate personal risks from certain behaviors such as smoking are low, or that the immediate rewards outweigh the risks. However, from a public health perspective, smoking in the United States has resulted in more than 480,000 deaths annually in the United

Institute of Hlth = Local?

States, approximately 20% of all deaths (USDHHS, 2014b). Though still alarming, the percent of American adults who smoke today is 18%, down from 43% in 1964. However, we continue to increase spending on smoking-related medical care for adults, $132 billion in 2014, and lose more money in worker productivity costs, $157 billion, a 50% increase from just six years ago (CDC, 2008; USDHHS 2014b). Therefore, it is clear that health behaviors extend beyond the individual or the intrapersonal and the interpersonal levels, having multiple determinants both internal and external to individuals and communities, as well as determinants within the society.

For example, adolescents' decisions not to smoke are associated with their individual attributes (e.g., positive self-image), family characteristics (e.g., parent–child connectedness), aggregate characteristics (e.g., peer influence), and community factors (e.g., living in a tobacco-growing region) (Kulbok et al, 2008a). As a result, interventions to initiate or maintain healthy behaviors have greater potential for success when directed systematically toward the multiple targets of the individual, family, group, community, and society—that is, when they use an ecologic approach to community health promotion.

## The Social Determinants of Health

Current trends in public health and health promotion emphasize the ecologic perspective on interaction between individuals and the environment. The ecologic approach also addresses the SDOH (McQueen, 2009) through social networks, organizations, neighborhoods, and communities (Navarro et al, 2007). According to the World Health Organization (WHO), SDOH "are the conditions in which people are born, grow up, live, work and age, including their health. These circumstances are in turn shaped by a wider set of forces: economics, social policies, and politics" (2010, p. 1). The WHO is an important contributor to defining and developing strategies to address the SDOH, and has outlined ten components of SDOH. (Box 17-4 lists the 10 components.)

There is increasing awareness that to achieve lasting gains in population health, assessments and interventions must be directed to multiple levels of the client system like those outlined in the SDOH. For example, a multilevel analysis of depressive symptoms in a national sample of 18,473 adolescents in the United States (Wight et al, 2005) showed that individual, family, aggregate, and community characteristics accounted for significant differences in adolescent depression. The American Academy of Pediatrics (2005) issued a statement urging pediatricians to increase their partnerships with communities in developing programs to improve child health. Examples of pediatrician–community partnerships (Sanders et al, 2005) include establishing a child health consultant program, working with a community to repair and fund sites to facilitate safe physical activity for children, developing dance programs for overweight and obese adolescent girls, and arranging a program for community leaders to learn about the Medicaid enrollment process. Traditional interventions that target only an individual's risk or illness are not as effective as interventions and programs developed using an ecologic approach that can affect all levels of the client system that contribute to good or ill health

**BOX 17-4   The Social Determinants of Health**

1. *The Social Gradient:* Life expectancy is shorter and most diseases are more common further down the social ladder in each society.
2. *Stress:* Stressful circumstances—making people feel worried, anxious, and unable to cope—are damaging to health and may lead to premature death.
3. *Early Life:* The health impact of early development and education lasts a lifetime.
4. *Social Exclusion:* Hardship and resentment, poverty, social exclusion, and discrimination cost lives.
5. *Work:* Stress in the workplace increases the risk of disease. People who have more control over their work have better health.
6. *Unemployment:* Job security increases health, well-being, and job satisfaction. Higher rates of unemployment cause more illness and premature death.
7. *Social support:* Friendship, good social relations, and strong supportive networks improve health at home, at work, and in the community.
8. *Addiction:* Individuals turn to alcohol, drugs, and tobacco and suffer from their use, but use is influenced by the wider social setting.
9. *Food:* Because global market forces control the food supply, healthy food is a political issue.
10. *Transport:* Healthy transport means less driving and more walking and cycling, backed up by better public transport.

From World Health Organization: *Social Determinants of Health*, Geneva, 2010. Available at http://www.who.int/socialdeterminants/thecommission/finalreport/keyconcepts/en/index.html. Accessed January 2, 2010.

(Navarro et al, 2007). More studies are needed to design and test these ecologic, multilevel community health interventions.

Farley and Cohen (2005) introduced the curve-shifting principle. This principle complements the ecologic model and calls for targeting health interventions at the population level. They built on representations of the relationship between individual and group behavior (Rose, 1992), with individual behavior being the foundation of the total population distribution. The median of this normal distribution represents prevailing social norms that govern health behavior. Traditional approaches to health behavior interventions for public health problems like obesity focus on the intrapersonal and interpersonal levels for high-risk populations—people at the extremes of the population curve. Although treating high-risk populations may be effective for selected individuals and may move them closer to the center or the prevailing social norm, this approach does little to prevent others from becoming the extremes of the distribution. Therefore, a focus on the total population, not just the high-risk group, with efforts to change the social norm so that everyone is consuming less sugar or participating in more hours of moderate to vigorous physical activity, exemplifies the curve-shifting principle.

Consider another example of the curve-shifting principle that involves the built environment. The built environment includes the physical parts of the environment where we live and work (e.g., homes, buildings, streets, open spaces, and infrastructure) (CDC, 2013). Prentice and Jebb (1995) were among the first to report the association between obesity and the built environment by measuring inactivity, car ownership, and television viewing.

Instead of simply teaching children the importance of walking and biking to school, the Safe Routes to Schools initiative improved the environment and the walkability of areas near schools, which correlates with increased local resident walking (Owen et al, 2004). Increased walking among local adult residents is evidence that "… increasing neighborhood walkability may affect people in the larger community, not just schoolchildren" (Watson et al, 2008, p. 5). As a result, the population living nearest to walkable areas will walk more, thereby shifting the population social norms about walking and biking, including to school. People's behavior will change based on targeted interventions to the environment in which they live, a concept advanced by B.F. Skinner (1978), a behavioral psychologist in the 1950s. In following this curve-shifting principle in health promotion and illness prevention, the ecologic model works at the population level to shift social norms governing health behavior and ultimately health outcomes.

## AN INTEGRATIVE MODEL FOR COMMUNITY HEALTH PROMOTION

Laffrey and Kulbok (1999) developed an integrative model for community health promotion to guide nursing and health care. The intent of the model was threefold. First, the model assists nurses to see the continuity of care at multiple levels. Second, it helps nurses describe their own areas of expertise within the complex health care system. Third, the model provides a basis for collaboration and partnership among nurses, other health care providers, and the population. Each of these collaborators brings expertise to the client system. Important assumptions underlying the model include the need for integration of care in the complex health care system; the inseparable nature of individuals, families, aggregates, and community systems; and the maximization of health potential through health promotion interventions. In addition, the model builds upon complementary health and disease perspectives described previously (Figure 17-2). The health perspective focuses on promoting health as a dynamic and positive quality of life and includes the promotion of physical, mental, emotional, functional, spiritual, and social well-being considered in the context of ecologic and environmental factors. The disease perspective includes both the care and prevention of illness (disease and disability) and focuses on reducing risks and threats to health. Although some clinical strategies may be similar in the two perspectives, their ultimate goals differ fundamentally. The difference in these two perspectives is seen in the specific purpose of nursing and health care, as it is applied to health promotion, illness prevention, or illness care.

The integrative model (Laffrey and Kulbok, 1999) includes two dimensions: client system and focus of care. The client system is multidimensional with nursing and health care targeting the multiple levels of clients. The simplest level of the client system is its most delimited target, the individual. When the individual is the client, the environment includes the family, the broader aggregate, and the community of which the individual is a part. The nurse and health care provider are concerned with how these environments affect the individual's health.

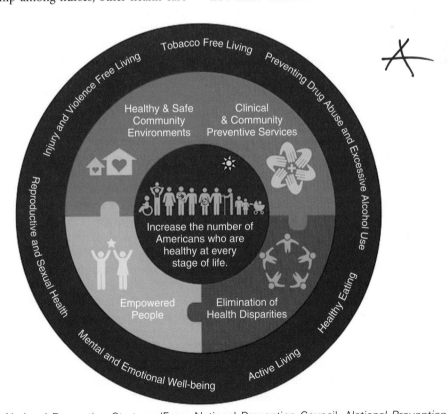

**FIG 17-2** National Prevention Strategy (From National Prevention Council, *National Prevention Strategy*, Washington, DC, 2011, U.S. Department of Health and Human Services, Office of the Surgeon General. Available at http://www.surgeongeneral.gov/initiatives/prevention/strategy/. Accessed on May 16, 2014.)

Each succeeding level of the client system is more complex, since the client can also be the family, an aggregate, or the community. The aggregate and community make up the environment for the family, and the community is the environment for the aggregate. Examples of different types of assessments and interventions appropriate at each level of client within the system are discussed later in this chapter. It is important to remember that community-oriented care is holistic in nature and is population focused in that it addresses multiple levels of clients and multiple levels of care within the total system. The integrative model of community health promotion is consistent with the ecologic approach described earlier, which addresses SDOH through social networks, organizations, neighborhoods, and communities (Navarro et al, 2007).

Focus of care in the integrative model includes health promotion, illness (disease or disability) prevention, and illness care. Each focus is appropriate for some aspects of nursing and health care. It is even more important to remember that the goal of health care is a healthier community, achieved through health promotion interventions. No matter where care begins, it ultimately leads to health promotion of the community. It underscores the need for nurses and health care providers to have a good understanding of care requirements at all client levels. The individual, family, aggregate, and community each have characteristics, strengths, and health needs that are unique and that differ from those at the other levels.

## INTERPROFESSIONAL APPLICATION TO NURSING AND PUBLIC HEALTH

The integrative community health promotion model reflects the basic beliefs and values of holistic nursing and health care practice and is consistent with the current emphasis on building a culture of health (RWJF, 2013) and the ecologic perspective on multiple determinants of health (IOM, 2014; WHO, 2014a). The model depicts continuity and expansiveness of the client systems and foci of care. Health promotion is the central axis, or core, of the model. At its narrowest focus, individuals receive illness care. According to the model, at the broadest level of care, nurses work with community leaders, other community residents, and health professionals to plan programs to promote optimal health for the community and its people. The goals of nursing and health care actions in the integrative model, at any client level from the individual to the community, are to identify health potential and achieve maximal health. To achieve these goals it is essential to have an active partnership between the nurse, health care providers, and the client system. By facilitating an active partnership with the client system, whether the focus of care is health promotion, illness prevention, or illness care, nurses involve clients in each step of the process of managing care from the assessment of their health needs and resources to implementation and evaluation of outcomes. In the following sections, strategies such as community-based participatory research and Photovoice that are useful in interprofessional community health promotion interventions are discussed.

## Community-Based Participatory Research (CBPR)

The aim of PHN is to create partnerships with individuals, families, groups, and communities to promote their health. Community-based participatory research, grounded in epistemology and critical social theories (Minkler and Wallerstein, 2008), provides the philosophical and theoretical basis for forming partnerships and for collaboration with the community. Researchers have used CBPR to conduct ecologic, community, and environmental assessments. This approach to community assessment allows understanding of sociocultural contexts, systems, and meaning through a collaborative research process. In CBPR, partnerships are active and community members are involved in assessing, planning, implementing, and evaluating change. Both professionals and community residents determine health needs and plan interventions. As residents increase their awareness, they are better able to determine what they want for themselves, their families, and their community and they are more likely to take leadership roles in program development, using health professionals as consultants.

Just as early PHN roles extended beyond disease prevention and illness care to encompass advocacy, community organizing, health education, political and social reform (Kulbok and Glick, 2014), contemporary PHN roles emphasize collaboration with community organizations and community members. Recently, Kulbok, Thatcher, Parks, and Meszaros (2012) examined emerging PHN roles that address complex, multicausal, community problems. They utilized a community participatory and ethnographic community assessment model and provided a PHN exemplar from their CBPR project, Youth Substance Use Prevention in a Rural County. The project involved an interprofessional team (i.e., the community participatory research team [CPRT]), including an advanced practice public health nurse, a human development specialist, a psychologist, an architecture and urban planning specialist, a nurse anthropologist, graduate students, and youths, parents, and leaders from the rural community. The CPRT used community participatory strategies, Geographic Information Systems (GIS) mapping, and Photovoice to design a substance use prevention program in a rural tobacco-growing county in the South. The CPRT completed a comprehensive community and environmental assessment of the county, its rural ecology, context, and culture, and reviewed evidence-based prevention programs as the foundation for designing and implementing a youth substance use prevention program that was acceptable, effective, relevant, and sustainable by the rural county.

In another example of a CBPR project, the community residents of the East Side Village Health Worker Partnership (ESVHWP) on Detroit's East Side developed a community-based program titled Healthy Eating and Exercising to Reduce Diabetes (HEED) (Schulz et al, 2005). The purpose was to increase community awareness about diabetes and prevention. Community groups and individuals with expertise in diabetes served as the project steering committee. They developed training protocols and recruited and trained community advocates. After training completion, the HEED advocates developed activities to promote healthy diets and physical activity. The advocates and other community residents identified important barriers to healthy dietary choices, such as lack of access to grocery stores and fresh produce. Members of the HEED project established a monthly mini-market at a community site with a few retail outlets carrying high-quality produce. The project was successful in fostering a strong interest among participants in healthy cooking demonstrations and cooking techniques. Subsequently, the HEED project joined forces with another community initiative to obtain funding to expand the mini-markets and food demonstrations.

The Physical Activity and Neighborhood Resources in High School Girls study (Pate et al, 2008) followed an ecologic model based on the social cognitive theory for adolescent females in urban, suburban, and rural communities. Researchers hypothesized that physical activity is influenced by a comprehensive set of personal, social, and physical environmental factors. Using GIS mapping, mixed regression models on BMI, and environmental variables, as well as 3-day physical activity recall, they found that the physical environment explained less than 5% of the variance in physical activity among adolescent girls. However, after adjusting for race, BMI, socioeconomic status (SES), and household income, there was an association between churches and vigorous physical activity. An additional study by Botchwey (2007) showed that up to 80% of congregations and faith-based organizations offer health services to their community, with a greater variety of services than secular non-profit organizations. Therefore, as nurses work with communities, it is important to consider the social and physical components of the environment, especially those actively engaged in health promotion.

## Photovoice Method and Projects

Photovoice is a novel method used in CBPR projects that integrates the strengths of social support and engagement, building local capacity to identify and address community concerns. Wang and Burris (1997) developed this methodology in 1997 by expanding the use of "photo novella" (Wang and Burris, 1994) as a means to empower communities while gathering qualitative data. It is a grassroots community method of gathering information by using photography. By using Photovoice participants photograph, contemplate, and then verbalize stories or simple descriptions about their photo(s) taken in response to a particular prompt, thereby allowing their voices to be heard. This process prevents written text from hindering communication and is effective in a society that uses oral tradition to preserve its culture (Riley et al, 2004). Health care researchers have used Photovoice as an assessment tool (Lacson, 2007; Strecher, 2004; Thompson et al, 2008).

This study by Kulbok et al (2008b) addressed gaps in the youth tobacco prevention literature. The purpose was to identify attitudes, beliefs, values, strategies, and shared meanings associated with tobacco-free behaviors of rural-dwelling male adolescents and their parents. The study examined differences in the meaning attached to nonsmoking and nonuse of smokeless tobacco among groups of African American and white male adolescents and their parents from two tobacco-growing counties in Virginia. In addition, the study assessed whether a modified Photovoice method would enhance the contribution of male adolescent participants and parents in individual and group interviews. Photovoice is a qualitative approach that uses images to promote effective ways of sharing beliefs about a specific topic. Researchers have used Photovoice to facilitate group conversations and to encourage participants to share their thoughts among themselves. In this study, Photovoice was a concrete way for youth and parents to express their perceptions about being tobacco-free, amplified through photographs that respond to questions about this topic. This approach was particularly effective with the male adolescents, who were hesitant to share their thoughts and feelings, and had a hard time articulating their thoughts.

The Ngudo Nga Zwinepe (NNZ) Learning through Photos projects use Photovoice to understand water perceptions and innovations as well as health in the Limpopo Province of rural South Africa where water resources are scarce and frequently contaminated (Cunningham et al, 2009). In one Photovoice project, community members took pictures documenting their perception of water and their water system. In contrast to the researchers' expectations, there was little mention of the deleterious health effects of contaminated water. Instead, the participants listed infrastructure/storage, community, money, and food as their top priorities; health/hygiene ranked fifth overall. Photovoice provided data to characterize the water priorities of this community and to implement an intervention that meets the community's primary concerns in the shorter term while developing educational strategies regarding the health risks of contaminated water.

The projects described in the previous paragraphs show the importance of multiple approaches to reaching the population. In multilevel intervention approach to community-oriented programs, it is important to pay attention to all client levels (i.e., individual, family, aggregate, and community). For example, in nutritional programs, it is important to address the individual, the household, grocery store accessibility and environment, the community, and the food environment. No one individual can address all of these levels, but there is increasing emphasis on working in teams and in developing partnerships consisting of residents, health providers, and other professionals outside the health field as specified through the National Prevention Strategy. In addition, it is important to frame and initiate interventions based on participants' priorities, not the priorities of experts. This approach promotes increased buy-in to projects and the necessary compliance by community participants to adhere to healthy behaviors. Nurses have many opportunities to work with and to lead these multidisciplinary teams to conduct assessments, develop strategies with the community and its populations, and facilitate the empowerment of community residents and recommended change. It is increasingly important that nurses integrate these intervention strategies with the epidemiologic evidence base for practice.

## APPLICATION OF THE INTEGRATIVE MODEL FOR COMMUNITY HEALTH PROMOTION

In the previous sections we described the importance of multiple levels of nursing and health care aimed at health promotion and illness prevention of individuals, families, aggregates, and the total community. In the remainder of this chapter, we present an example using the integrative model to apply these concepts.

## Obesity and the Built Environment

### Illness Care

In this case example (Table 17-1), a young woman recently diagnosed with obesity is referred for care. The nurse's immediate goal is to provide care that will help this client resolve her illness. Obesity rates have doubled over the last 20 years, with 16.9% of children ages 2 to 19 years and 34.9% of U.S. adults considered obese (Ogden et al, 2014). These rates are the result of a built environment that promotes increased unhealthy food consumption and decreased physical activity. Our built environment includes all of the places we live, work, learn, worship, and play and that are created or modified by people. According to the CDC, in order for people to make healthy choices to combat obesity, both policy and environmental changes are needed to assure affordable healthy food and safe places for activities (CDC, 2014b). Therefore, teaching the client about the effects and side effects of her medications, and how to monitor her weight, nutrition, and physical activity at home, are important interventions. Since predisposing genetic, lifestyle, and environmental factors related to obesity exist, it is important to give family members information about this illness, including early recognition of signs and symptoms for themselves. Other important aspects of illness care include assessing the prevalence of obesity among high-risk aggregates in the community and teaching obesity prevention and treatment classes in community-wide settings that high-risk groups frequent. An example is providing cooking classes in churches to at-risk women in the community. At the community level, it is important to assess whether there are adequate and available providers and resources for healthy food and safe physical activity in the community.

### Illness/Disease Prevention

Prevention care is also addressed at the individual level by teaching measures such as healthy nutrition, progressive

exercise, and lifestyle techniques to prevent additional weight gain. Healthy nutrition and regular moderate to vigorous exercise are important preventive measures for all family members. Aggregate-level preventive interventions include providing showers at workplaces to encourage exercise before or during the workday. Community intervention examples include year-long multimedia campaigns to provide intensive education to the community about prevention of obesity.

### Health Promotion

Health promotion can motivate a person to adopt a less sedentary and more active lifestyle. Health promotion includes encouraging individuals to adopt a health-promoting lifestyle and helping them to become aware of their own power and self-efficacy to do so. Nurses can encourage families to make health-promoting activities a part of their daily lives. This might include taking walks, swimming together, or joining an

## TABLE 17-1 Community Health Levels of Care: Obesity and the Built Environment

| | CLIENT SYSTEM | | | |
|---|---|---|---|---|
| **Focus of Care** | **Individual** | **Family** | **Aggregate** | **Community** |
| Illness care | Administer medications Monitor weight as well as adherence to nutrition and physical activity recommendations of individual client in the home setting | Teach family members about nutrition and physical activity practices to lose weight and prevent the onset of obesity-related diseases | Assess prevalence of obesity in the community Teach obesity classes community-wide in settings that high-risk groups frequent | Assess community for accessibility and adequacy of healthy food and safe physical activity venues in the local environment |
| Illness/disease prevention | Teach nutrition, progressive exercise, and lifestyle techniques to prevent additional weight gain | Teach nutrition and importance of regular exercise to all family members to prevent additional cases of obesity | Develop classes about obesity risk reduction for targeted high-risk groups and their community | Participate in community-wide multimedia education for obesity risk reduction |
| Health promotion | Empower individual to adopt a less sedentary and more active health promotion lifestyle | Plan with family to incorporate health promotion activities into lifestyle | Provide group education (classes) regarding benefits of regular exercise and healthy eating | Work with community leaders and citizens to establish safe physical activity space and healthy food options |

intergenerational baseball or bowling team in which families compete with other families. Aggregates can also benefit from heart-healthy classes or activities that are culturally specific to particular subgroups, such as older Hispanic women or African American teenage girls. These activities can include stress management, well-balanced nutrition, exercise, dance classes, sports, or any other topic that can promote heart health. When looking at the total community, an example of a health promotion intervention is participating in a coalition to plan for supermarkets and community gardens, as well as parks or recreation areas within the community that are safe and accessible to the population.

In summary, the concepts of health, health promotion, and community are inextricably linked; it is difficult to discuss one without including the others. It is also important that nurses examine their definitions and beliefs about each concept as the basis for their practice. The essence of public health is the ability to see the totality of community while addressing its component parts and, at the same time, to see the total needs for health promotion, health protection, illness and disease prevention, and illness care and management. The integrative relationship among these components distinguishes public health nursing from nursing in more circumscribed settings, such as hospitals and clinics.

## ►► LINKING CONTENT TO PRACTICE

In this chapter, we describe the origins of the integrative model of community health promotion (Laffrey and Kulbok, 1999) and its application in public health nursing practice. The integrative model addresses the multiple determinants of population health and is consistent with the ecologic framework (IOM, 2014) and social determinants of health (SDOH) (Commission on Social Determinants of Health [CSDH], 2008; WHO, 2014a). The ecologic approach provides a basis for understanding population health and the challenges of building a culture of health (RWJF, 2013). It emphasizes that multiple social determinants of health influence the conditions that promote health on multiple levels (i.e., individual, family, aggregate, community, and society). The central focus of public health nursing practice is health promotion. Health promotion is also central and dominant in the integrative model of community health promotion. Public health nurses strive to improve the health status of communities and populations. Whether the client system is the family or a vulnerable population, and the focus of care is illness prevention or illness care, health promotion remains the central goal. No matter where public health nursing care begins, it ultimately leads to health promotion of the community and population health.

## ■ PRACTICE APPLICATION

A rural health outreach program serves migrant workers, their families, and other vulnerable populations in the local community. The program's goals include increased knowledge about risk factors, services, and self-care; improved community health; increased access and affordability of individual- and community-level health promotion services; and reduced barriers to health services. The program offers health promotion and disease prevention educational materials and classes in English and Spanish throughout the region in churches, schools, community centers, fire departments, and migrant camps. In addition, clinics in eight local sites across the county provide services. Clinic services include health risk assessments, disease screening, immunizations, health education, counseling, and referral. The program staff trained community health workers (CHWs) from the migrant community to deliver basic health education and resource information. Funding from a variety of public and private sources supports the program. It is essential that the program show effective outcomes if it is to sustain funding.

Mary Ann Jones, a nurse with a bachelor of science in nursing degree, works for the outreach program. She is a member of a group asked to evaluate whether the outreach program (including the eight clinics) is effective in meeting the stated objectives.

A. Using the integrative model for community health promotion as a guide, how might you organize a comprehensive approach to assessment and data collection?
B. What are sources of data you might use for assessing individual, aggregate, and community health indicators?
C. What is the value of interviewing rural residents, migrant workers, and clinic participants about their perceptions of health and the value of health services?
D. Who else can you interview to elicit important information about the usefulness of the outreach program?
E. How can you best use CHWs to increase participation and partnership among concerned health professionals, community residents, and migrant families and to sustain the program?

Be creative and comprehensive in your approach, and consider how you might build a culture of health using the ecologic perspective, the social determinants of health, and cultural factors associated with rural and migrant populations in the United States. Current spending limits on federal and state programs for health promotion and disease prevention require that nurses deal effectively with issues of outreach, sustainability, and success of community health programs.

**Answers can be found on the Evolve site.**

## ■ KEY POINTS

- The goals of a culture of health for America are for good health across geographic, demographic, and social sectors; for being healthy and staying healthy as a social value; and for everyone to have access to affordable, quality health care.

- The idea of health shapes the process of population-focused nursing practice, from assessment of health-related needs of individuals, families, aggregates, and communities to evaluation of health outcomes.

## KEY POINTS—cont'd

- The National Prevention Strategy foresees a prevention-oriented society where public and private sectors value health for individuals, families, and society and work together to achieve better health for Americans.
- The greatest benefits in public health are likely to come from efforts to improve individual and family lifestyles through community and population interventions that address the social determinants of health including social conditions and the built environment.
- Public health nurses have a history of commitment to primary health care and to enhancing levels of wellness in communities and populations.
- When nurses examine their own definition of health, they recognize how this health definition directs the nursing care they provide.
- When nurses examine the client's definition of health, they are more likely to tailor care to the client's culture, needs, lifestyle, and social and physical environment.

- The Framingham Heart Study has provided more than 50 years of research about risk factors and lifestyle habits; Framingham researchers are currently studying how genes contribute to common disorders such as obesity, hypertension, and diabetes.
- The Stanford Heart Disease Prevention program, the North Karelia Project, the Pawtucket Heart Health program, and the Minnesota Heart Health program contributed to the scientific knowledge base for the design, implementation, and evaluation of community- and population-level risk-appraisal and risk-reduction programs.
- Public health nurses function beyond resolving a specific illness to preventing the illness and promoting optimal health for the individual, the family, the aggregate, and the total community. All of these levels are important to promote the health of the community and populations.

## CLINICAL DECISION-MAKING ACTIVITIES

1. Write your own definition of health, and interview a nurse, client, and physician about their definitions of health. How are these definitions similar or different? How do they "fit" with your understanding of what nurses and health care providers need to do to build a culture of health?
2. What are some challenges encountered when you consider different definitions of health and health promotion from a disease oriented versus an environmental or social-ecologically oriented perspective? Illustrate these challenges and opportunities with examples of strategies that are health promoting and will contribute to building a culture of health.
3. Discuss the importance of the built environment in community health promotion, and provide examples of environmental health promotion indicators for a specified community.

4. Develop a nursing care plan for addressing childhood obesity using the propositions of Milio (1976) as a frame of reference.
5. Use the integrative model for community health promotion and social determinants of health to identify the most important strategies in a community-wide plan for childhood obesity.
6. Illustrate community health levels of care including the client system and the focus of care:
   A. For teenage pregnancy: begin with community-level health promotion
   B. For childhood obesity: start with community-level illness prevention

## REFERENCES

Adler N, Bachrach C, Daley D, et al: Building the Science for a Population Health Movement. Discussion Paper. Washington, DC, 2013, Institute of Medicine. Available at: http://www.iom.edu/Global/Perspectives/2013/BuildingTheScience. Accessed on May 14, 2014.

American Academy of Pediatrics: Committee on Community Health Services: The pediatrician's role in community pediatrics. Pediatrics 115:1092–1094, 2005.

American Nurses Association: Public Health Nursing: Scope and Standards of Practice. Washington, DC, 2013, ANA.

Anderson ET, McFarlane J: Community-As-Partner: Theory and Practice in Nursing, ed 4.

Philadelphia, 2000, Lippincott Williams & Wilkins.

Anderson ET, McFarlane J: Community-As-Partner: Theory and Practice in Nursing, ed 6. Philadelphia, 2010, Lippincott Williams & Wilkins.

Bekemeier B, Jones M: Relationships between local public health agency functions and agency leadership and staffing: a look at nurses. J Public Health Manag Pract 16:E8–E16, 2010.

Berkman LF, Breslow L: Health and Ways of Living, the Alameda County Study. New York, 1983, Oxford University Press.

Botchwey N: The religious sector's presence in local community development. J Plan Educ Res 27(1):36–48, 2007.

Bronfenbrenner U: Toward an experimental ecology of human development. Am Psychologist 32:513–531, 1977.

Bronfenbrenner U: The Ecology of Human Development. Cambridge, MA, 1979, Harvard University Press.

Centers for Disease Control and Prevention: CDC's Built Environment and Health Initiative, 2013. Available at: http://www.cdc.gov/nceh/information/built_environment.htm. Accessed May 14, 2014.

Centers for Disease Control and Prevention: Overweight and obesity, 2014b. Available at: http://www.cdc.gov/obesity. Accessed May 14, 2014.

Centers for Disease Control and Prevention: Smoking-attributable

mortality, years of potential life lost, and productivity losses—United States, 2000-2004. MMWR Morb Mortal Wkly Rep 57(45):1226–1228, 2008.

Centers for Disease Control and Prevention: Social determinants of health, 2014a. Available at: http://www.cdc.gov/socialdeterminants/faq.html#b. Accessed April 26, 2014.

Chopoorian TL: Reconceptualizing the environment. In Moccia P, editor: New Approaches to Theory Development, Pub. No. 15-1992. New York, 1986, National League for Nursing.

Commission on Social Determinants of Health: Closing the Gap in a Generation: Final Report. Geneva, 2008, World Health Organization.

Cunningham T, Botchwey N, Dillingham R, et al: Understanding water perceptions in Limpopo Province: a Photovoice community assessment. *Environ Poll Public Health IEEE*, 2009.

Edberg M: *Essentials of Health Behavior: Social and Behavioral Theory in Public Health*, ed 6. 2013, Jones & Bartlett.

Farley T, Cohen W: *Prescription for a Healthy Nation: A New Approach to Improving Our Lives by Fixing Our Everyday World*. Boston, 2005, Beacon Press, Chapter 4.

Farquhar JW, Maccoby N, Wood PD, et al: Effects of community-wide education on cardiovascular disease risk factors: the Stanford Five-city Project. *JAMA* 264:359, 1990.

Fuchs V: *Who Shall Live?* New York, 1974, Basic Books.

Institute of Medicine: *The Future of the Public's Health in the 21st Century*. Washington, DC, 2003, The National Academies Press. Available at: http://www.nap.edu/catalog/10548.html. Accessed May 14, 2014.

Institute of Medicine: *The Impact of Social and Cultural Environment on Health. Defining the Social and Cultural Environment. Genes, Behavior, and the Social Environment: Moving Beyond the Nature/Nurture Debate*. Washington, DC, 2006, The National Academies Press.

Institute of Medicine: *Working definition of population health*. Roundtable on population health, 2014. Available at: http://www.iom.edu/Activities/PublicHealth/PopulationHealthImprovementRT.aspx. Accessed on March 9, 2014.

Keller LO, Strohschein S, Lia-Hoagberg G, et al: Population-based public health nursing interventions: a model for practice. *Public Health Nurs* 15:207, 1998.

Keller LO, Strohschein S, Lia-Hoagberg B, et al: Population-based public health nursing interventions: practice-based and evidence-supported. Part 1. *Public Health Nurs* 21:453–468, 2004.

Kindig D, Stoddart G: What is population health? *Am J Pub Health* 93(3):380–383, 2003.

Kulbok PA, Baldwin JH, Cox CL, et al: Advancing discourse on health promotion: beyond mainstream thinking. *Adv Nurs Sci* 20:12, 1997.

Kulbok PA, Glick DF: "Something must be done!": The history of public health nursing education 1900-1950. *Fam &Comm Health* 37(3):170–178, 2014.

Kulbok P, Meszaros P, Hinton I, et al: *Tobacco-Free Boys and Parents Use Photovoice to Tell Their Stories: Issues and Solutions [Abstract]*. San Diego, CA, October 25–29, 2008b, Proceedings of the 136th American Public Health Association, Annual Meeting.

Kulbok P, Rhee H, Hinton I, et al: Factors influencing adolescents' decisions not to smoke. *Public Health Nurs* 25:505–515, 2008a.

Kulbok PA, Thatcher E, Park E, et al: Evolving public health nursing roles: focus on community participatory health promotion and prevention. *OJIN: The Online Journal of Issues in Nursing* 17(2):1, 2012.

Kumar S, Quinn SC, Kim KH, et al: The social ecological model as a framework for determinants of 2009 H1N1 influenza vaccine uptake in the United States. *Health Educ Behav* 39:229–243, 2013.

Lacson RS: *tb. Tuberculosis. pv. Photovoice*, 2007. Available at: http://tbphotovoice.org/tbpv2/. Accessed June 30, 2008.

Laffrey SC, Kulbok PA: The integrative model for community health nursing: a conceptual guide to education, practice, and research. *J Holist Nurs* 17:88–103, 1999.

Laffrey SC, Loveland-Cherry CJ, Winkler SJ: Health behavior: evolution of two paradigms. *Public Health Nurs* 3:92–97, 1986.

LaLonde M: *A New Perspective on the Health of Canadians*. Ottawa, 1974, Government of Canada.

Lasater T, Abrams T, Artz L, et al: Lay volunteer delivery of a community-based cardiovascular risk factor change program: the Pawtucket experiment. In Matarazzo JD, et al, editors: *Behavioral Health: A Handbook of Health Enhancement and Disease Prevention*. Silver Spring, MD, 1984, Wiley.

Leavell HR, Clark EG: *Preventive Medicine for the Doctor in His Community: An Epidemiological Approach*, ed 3. New York, 1965, McGraw-Hill.

Li K, Seo DC, Torabi MR, et al: Social-ecological factors of leisure-time physical activity in black adults. *Am J Health Behav* 36:797–810, 2012.

Lieb W, Pencina ML, Lanier KJ, et al: Association of parental obesity with concentrations of select systemic biomarkers in nonobese offspring: The Framingham Heart Study. *Diabetes* 58(1):134–137, 2009.

Luepker RV, Murray DM, Jacobs JN, et al: Community education for cardiovascular disease prevention: risk factor changes in the Minnesota Heart Health Program. *Am J Public Health* 84:1383, 1994.

McLeroy KR, Bibeau D, Steckler A, et al: An ecological perspective on health promotion programs. *Health Educ Behav* 15(4):351–377, 1988.

McQueen DV: Three challenges for the social determinants of health pursuit. *Int J Public Health* 54:1–2, 2009.

Milio N: A framework for prevention: changing health-damaging to health-generating life patterns. *Am J Public Health* 66:435, 1976.

Minkler M, Wallerstein N, editors: *Community-Based Participatory Research for Health*, ed 2. San Francisco, 2008, John Wiley & Sons.

National Center for Health Statistics: *Health, United States, 2011: With Special Feature on Socioeconomic Status and Health*. Hyattsville, MD, 2012.

National Prevention Council: *National Prevention Strategy*. Washington, DC, 2011, U.S. Department of Health and Human Services, Office of the Surgeon General.

National Research Council: *The Future of Public Health*. Washington, DC, 1988, The National Academies Press.

Navarro AM, Voetsch KP, Liburd LC, et al: Charting the future of community health promotion: recommendations from the National Expert Panel on Community Health Promotion. *Prev Chronic Dis* July 2007: [serial online]. Available at: http://www.cdc.gov/pcd/issues/2007/jul/07_0013.htm. Accessed January 3, 2011.

Ogden CL, Carroll MD, Kit BA, et al: Prevalence of childhood and adult obesity in the United States, 2011-2012. *JAMA* 311:806–814, 2014.

Owen N, Humpel N, Leslie E, et al: Understanding environmental influences on walking: review and research agenda. *Am J Prev Med* 27:67–76, 2004.

Pate RR, Colabianchi N, Porter D, et al: Physical activity and neighborhood resources in high school girls. *Am J Prev Med* 34:413–419, 2008.

Prentice AM, Jebb SA: Obesity in Britain; gluttony or sloth? *Br Med J* 311:437–439, 1995.

Puska P, Salonen JL, Nissinen JT, et al: Change in risk factors for coronary heart disease during 10 years of a community intervention programme (North Karelia Project). *Br Med J* 287:1840, 1983.

Riley RG, Manias E: The uses of photography in clinical nursing practice and research: a literature review. *J Adv Nurs* 48:397–405, 2004.

Robert Wood Johnson Foundation: *About the Culture of Health Blog*, 2013. Available at:: http://www.rwjf.org/en/blogs/culture-of-health/2013/05/about_culture_ofhea.html. Accessed March 8, 2014.

Ronda G, Van Assema E, Ruland E, et al: The Dutch heart health community intervention 'Hartslag Limburg': results of an effect study at organizational level. *Pub Health* 119:353–360, 2005.

Rose G: *The Strategy of Preventive Medicine*. New York, 1992, Oxford University Press.

Rosenbaum S: *Principles to Consider for the Implementation of a Community Health Needs Assessment Process*. 2013, The George Washington University School of Public Health and Health Services, Department of Health Policy. Available at: http://nnphi.org/CMSuploads/PrinciplesToConsiderForTheImplementationOfACHNAProcess_GWU_20130604.pdf. Accessed May 26, 2014.

Rosenstock I: Historical origins of the health belief model. *Health Educ Monog* 2(4):1974.

Salmon M: Editorial: Public health nursing: the opportunity of a century. *Am J Public Health* 83:1674–1675, 1993.

Salmon M: An open letter to public health nursing. *Public Health Nurs* 26:483–485, 2009.

Sanders LM, Robinson TN, Forster LQ, et al: Evidence-based community pediatrics: building a bridge from bedside to neighborhood. *Pediatrics* 115:1142–1147, 2005.

Schulz BJ, Zenk S, Odoms-Young A, et al: Healthy eating and exercising to reduce diabetes: exploring the potential of social determinants of health frameworks within the context of community-based participatory diabetes prevention. *Am J Public Health* 95:645–651, 2005.

Shuster G, Goeppinger J: Community as client: assessment and analysis. In Stanhope M, Lancaster J, editors: *Public Health Nursing: Population-Centered Health Care in the Community*, ed 8. St Louis, 2012, Mosby.

Simons-Morton B: Health behavior in ecological context. *Health Educ Behav* 40:6, 2013.

Skinner BF: *Why I am Not a Cognitive Psychologist in Reflections on Behaviorism and Society*. Englewood Cliffs, NJ, 1978, Prentice-Hall.

Smith JA: The idea of health: a philosophical inquiry. *Adv Nurs Sci* 3:43, 1981.

Strecher VJ: *Photovoice for tobacco, drug, and alcohol prevention among adolescents in South Africa [Abstract]*, 2004. Available at: http://apha.confex.com/apha/132am/techprogram/paper_84002.htm. Accessed January 3, 2011.

Task Force on Community Preventive Services: *The Guide to Community Preventive Services-What Works to Promote Health*. New York, 2005, Oxford University Press.

Terris M: Approaches to an epidemiology of health. *Am J Public Health* 65:1037–1038, 1975.

Thompson NC, Hunter EE, Murray L, et al: Experience of living with chronic mental illness: a Photovoice study [Abstract]. *Perspec Psych Care* 2008. Available at: http://findarticles.com/p/articles/

# Community As Client: Assessment and Analysis

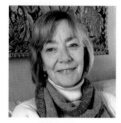

### Mary E. Gibson, PhD, RN

Dr. Mary E. Gibson was a public health nurse in Albemarle County, Virginia, early in her career. Since that time she has practiced in a variety of Maternal Child Health settings. Mary was involved in the Virginia Department of Health's early initiative to regionalize high risk pregnancies and has worked as an outpatient nurse, childbirth educator, Perinatal Outreach nurse including systems work with regional hospitals and nurses, and outreach education; and as a labor and delivery and perinatal nurse. Her master's degree concentration was community health. Her doctoral work at University of Pennsylvania focused on nursing history, and this continues to be her research focus. At the University of Virginia, Mary's teaching experience includes graduate level Community Assessment, undergraduate Obstetric and Neonatal Nursing and clinical undergraduate Community Health Nursing. She currently leads a local nonprofit's board that serves at-risk, underserved children and families.

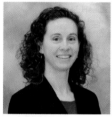

### Esther J. Thatcher, PhD, RN, APHN-BC*

As a BSN nursing student, Esther volunteered in El Salvador several times with a group called Nursing Students Without Borders. After graduating, she continued to work with Latinos as a migrant farmworker outreach nurse in rural Virginia. She then worked in adult Internal Medicine settings, where she became interested in preventing chronic diseases in underserved populations. Later, as a public health nurse, Esther reignited her interest in how community environments affect health outcomes. Her PhD research at the University of Virginia was to describe community influences on healthy food access in rural Appalachia. She is currently a postdoctoral fellow at University of North Carolina—Chapel Hill.

## ADDITIONAL RESOURCES

(e) **Evolve Website http://evolve.elsevier.com/Stanhope**
- Healthy People 2020
  - Centers for Disease Control and Prevention (provides numerous .pdf files for download)
  - Behavior Risk Factor Surveillance System (BRFSS) data
  - American Public Health Association: *The Guide to Implementing Model Standards*
  - The Community Guide

- Quiz
- Case Studies
- Glossary
- Answers to Practice Application

## OBJECTIVES

*After reading this chapter, the student should be able to do the following:*

1. Analyze the importance of community assessment in nursing practice.
2. Select and utilize a method and model for assessment of a community.
3. Appraise various online data sources for reliability and accuracy of information.
4. Utilize the nursing process to create a community assessment for a selected community.
5. Interpret concepts basic to community nursing practice: community, community client, community health and partnership for health.
6. Develop a prioritized community problem list and nursing diagnosis, and a care plan for a community.

## KEY TERMS

active participation, p. 400
aggregate, p. 398
coalitions, p. 399
community, p. 398

community as client, p. 398
community as partner, p. 407
community health, p. 399
community health workers, p. 401

---

*With gracious thanks to Elayne Kornblatt Phillips, MPH, PhD, RN, FAAN for careful reading and critique.
A special thanks to George Shuster for his contributions to this chapter through many editions of this text.

*"I believe that the community—in the fullest sense: a place and all its creatures—is the smallest unit of health and that to speak of the health of an isolated individual is a contradiction in terms."*

**Wendell Berry**

## INTRODUCTION

Communities are the environments where we live and work. Naturally, the community's ability to serve the needs of its members defines key aspects in the health of the community. The public health nurse (PHN) is in an ideal position to view the "community as client," and to begin to identify and work with the strengths present in the community and to help harness these strengths to meet the challenges faced by the community. Health is a broadly defined and interdependent concept. As defined by the World Health Organization, "Health is a state of complete physical, mental and social well-being and not merely the absence of disease or infirmity" (WHO, 1948). Therefore, the health of the community involves many aspects besides the absence of disease. The influence of environment, public

services and policies along with economics play a large role in the health of the community.

We use the nursing process from assessment through evaluation to promote a community's health. This process begins with community assessment (sometimes called community needs assessment)—one of the core functions of public health nursing—which involves getting to know the community inside and out. It is a logical, systematic approach to identifying community needs, clarifying problems, and identifying community strengths and resources. In this chapter we will clarify specific community concepts including community as client, provide a snapshot of the nurse's role in communities, and outline the process for undertaking a comprehensive community assessment using a hybrid of the nursing process.

## COMMUNITY DEFINED

"Boston Strong" was a phrase that spread quickly after the 2013 Boston Marathon bombing. Like many communities in the immediate aftermath of a major disaster, residents of Boston and beyond rallied together in a declaration of solidarity and shared community identity. The community spirit and hope implied in "Boston Strong" is an example of the comfort and reassurance that a strong community identity can provide to individuals (Lin, 2014). But what do we mean by *community*, and how might being part of a community influence a person's health?

There are many definitions of community. At its simplest, a community is a group of people that share something in common, such as geographic location, interests, or values (Obst & White, 2005, p. 127). The World Health Organization defines community as "a group of people, often living in a defined geographical area, who may share a common culture, values and norms, and are arranged in a social structure according to relationships which the community has developed over a period of time" (World Health Organization, 2004, p. 16). One study that aimed to define community among a diverse U.S. population reached the consensus definition of "a group of people with diverse characteristics who are linked by social ties, share common perspectives, and engage in joint action in geographical locations or settings" (MacQueen et al, 2001).

A community is a system, not just the sum of the characteristics of its inhabitants. In most definitions, the community includes three factors: people, place, and function. *People* are the community members or residents. An aggregate is a population or group of individuals who share common personal or environmental characteristics. *Place* can be a geographic location or other shared spaces such as the Internet. *Function* refers to the aims and activities of the community.

Community is a concept rather than simply a specific place, and individuals living in the same place may describe their community differently. When an organization asks a nurse to perform a community assessment, community usually refers to a specific population, an aggregate with specific characteristics that lives within the area that an organization serves, such as a school district, or a geographic area such as a county. However, it is important to remember that individuals within this defined area could view the community through a different lens. Understanding the many identities of community is part of the community assessment and is best done through talking with residents and stakeholders.

## COMMUNITY AS CLIENT

### Nursing Care of the Community As Client

Population-focused health care is highly relevant in our current health care environment, and the community as client is important to nursing practice for several reasons. The community is the client when the nursing focus is on the collective or common good of the population, instead of on individual health. When focusing on the community as client, direct clinical care can be a part of population-focused community health practice (Radzyminski, 2007). For example, sometimes direct nursing care is provided to individuals and family members because their health needs are common community-related problems. Changes in individual health will ultimately affect the health of the community (O'Donnell et al, 2009).

Improved health of the community remains the overall goal of nursing intervention. This is often accomplished through individual treatment; for example, addressing intimate partner violence, child or elder abuse is intended primarily to impact the effects of abuse on society and ultimately on the population as a whole. Similarly, treating a client for tuberculosis reduces the risk to other community members, thereby reducing the risk of an epidemic in the community. Since 1965, large-scale campaigns to encourage smoking reduction or cessation among groups and individuals, and laws that prohibit smoking in specific public spaces have resulted in significantly lower smoking rates in the adult population (42% in 1965 compared to 19% in 2011) (CDC, *Trends in Current Cigarette Smoking Among High School Students and Adults, United States*, 1965-2011).

Focusing on the community client highlights the complexity of the change process. Change for the benefit of the community client must often occur at several levels, ranging from the individual to society as a whole. For example, health problems caused by lifestyle, such as lack of exercise, overeating, and speeding, cannot be solved simply by asking individuals to choose health-promoting habits. Society must also provide healthy choices. Most individuals find changing their habits independently extremely difficult; indeed, sometimes impossible. The support of family members, friends, community health care systems and relevant social policies are necessary for success. Individuals who have lifestyle health problems are often blamed for their illness because of their choices (e.g., to smoke), often referred to as "blaming the victim." In his classic work, Ryan (1976) points out that the "victim" cannot always be blamed and expected to correct the problem without changes also being made in the helping professions and public policy. Figure 18-1 illustrates the continuum of care from the individual to global health.

Commitment to the health of the community client requires a process of change at each appropriate level on the continuum. One nursing role emphasizes individual and direct personal care skills, another nursing role focuses on the family as the unit of service, and a third centers on the community. The most successful change processes often arise from collaborative practice models that involve the community and nurses in joint decision making. (Bencivenga et al, 2008). Nurses must remember that collaboration means shared roles and a cooperative effort in which participants want to work together (Ndirangu et al, 2008). Participants must see themselves as part of a group effort and share in the process, beginning with planning and including decision making. This means sharing not only the power but also the responsibility for the outcomes of the intervention. Viewing the community as client and thus as the target of service means a commitment to two key concepts: (1) community health and (2) partnership. These two concepts form not only the *goal* (community health), but also the *means* of population-centered practice (partnership).

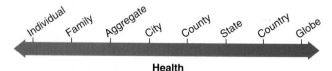

**FIG 18-1** Health on a population continuum.

## Community As Client

Population-centered practice seeks healthful change for the whole community's benefit (Radzyminski, 2007). Although the nurse may work with individuals, families or other groups, aggregates, or institutions, the resulting changes are intended to affect the whole community. For example, an occupational health nurse's target typically includes preventing illness and injury and maintaining or promoting the health of an entire company workforce. Because of this focus, the nurse might help an individual disabled worker become independent in activities of daily living. The nurse could also take action to make the whole community better able to support persons with disabilities. These actions might include promoting vocational rehabilitation services in the community and advocating for local policies that improve equal opportunities for disabled workers.

Community health nurses join professionals from many other fields in fulfilling the core public health functions: assessment, assurance, and policy development (National Research Council, 1988). The community assessment process described in this chapter is a key role of PHNs. The findings of the assessment process guide actions of *assurance*, or ensuring that all community members have access to high-quality health services. *Policy development* includes informing and mobilizing community members to advocate for business and government policies that improve health.

The community as client perspective guides decisions about allocation of resources and services to create the greatest benefit for the community. Sometimes this means spreading the benefit to as many people as possible in the community. For example, clean air and water are resources needed by everyone in a community. At other times, the community will experience the greatest benefit if resources are prioritized for groups within the community who are in high-risk categories. For example, supplies of vaccine for the 2009 H1N1 influenza pandemic were limited at first. Population groups at highest risk for complications from the disease were vaccinated before making the vaccine available to the general population (Shim, Meyers, & Galvani, 2011).

Two main ethical concepts that guide the community as client perspective are utilitarianism and justice. Utilitarianism means doing the greatest good for the greatest number of people. Distributive justice means treating people fairly, and distributing resources and burdens equitably among the members of a society. Social justice means ensuring that vulnerable groups are included in equitable distribution of resources. The outcome of social justice should be a reduction in health disparities between privileged and marginalized social groups. Nurses can use these concepts to carefully consider how to best allocate scarce resources, such as health services and funding, in ways that benefit the whole community. More information on ethics in community practice is found in other chapters of this book.

## Community Health

Community health is reflected in the health behaviors and subsequent outcomes of its residents and also by the ability of the community as a system to support healthy individuals. The socio-ecological model views individuals as having dynamic interactions with social and environmental features of communities, for example social networks, organizations such as schools and businesses, media, government policies, and natural and built environments (Richard, Gauvin, & Raine, 2011). Nurses caring for the community as the client identify effects that these complex community parts have on individuals' health; they work with all parts of a community to achieve the goal of a healthy community. Betty Neuman's Health Care Systems Model illustrates this system well (Neuman, 1980).

Neuman's model views systems as greater than the sum of their parts; the strength of each part of a community and the synergy between these parts contribute to the ability of its residents to be healthy. Community systems provide stability and protection from chronic or sudden stressors such as homelessness, health declines, disease outbreaks, or disasters. Another community model, Community-As-Partner, identifies major community systems as physical environment, health and social services, economy, transportation and safety, politics and government, communication, education, and recreation (Anderson & McFarlane, 2011).

The World Health Organization's (WHO) Healthy Cities program is an international leader in promoting health through community systems. It defines a healthy community as "one that is continually creating and improving those physical and social environments and expanding those community resources which enable people to mutually support each other in performing all the functions of life and developing to their maximum potential" (World Health Organization, 2014). The WHO describes four aims of healthy communities as (1) supporting individual health, (2) promoting quality of life, (3) distributing the resources needed for basic sanitation and hygiene, and (4) creating accessible health care services.

## Community Partnerships for Assessment

Partnering with community members is a key element of a successful community health program or intervention. Involving community members not only in the data collection process, but in all phases of the assessment, ensures that the data collected are more accurate and more relevant to the concerns of the community. Partnerships also promote community members' investment in the success of the assessment and in the resulting projects to improve community health. Therefore, successful strategies for improving community health must include community partnerships as the basic means or key for improvement. Some community assessment models feature community partnerships as a central activity, such as Mobilizing for Action through Planning and Partnerships (MAPP) (NACCHO, 2014).

Nurse-community partnerships can take many forms. A successful democratic partnership requires hard work from all parties and is usually achieved only through a long-term commitment to the process, wherein diverse community members and health care professionals share all resources and work equitably (D'Alonzo, 2010). Coalitions are formal partnerships in which individuals and organizations serve in defined capacities such as steering committees, advisory committees, and work groups. Coalitions are *active partnerships*, in which all participants share leadership and decision making to some degree. Unfortunately, some community health efforts view community residents only as sources of information and receivers of interventions; this limits residents to *passive participation.* Passive participation is the antithesis of the partnership approach most valued in nurse-community partnerships, in which all partners are actively involved in and share power in assessing, planning, and implementing needed community changes (Ndirangu et al, 2008; Timmerman, 2007).

Community members who are recognized as community leaders (whether professionals, pastors, government officials or interested citizens) possess credibility and skills that health professionals often lack. The community member–professional partnership approach specifically emphasizes active participation. O'Donnell (2009) wrote that partnership means the active participation and involvement of the community or its representatives in healthy change. For example, a partnership between Native American community members and academic researchers ensured the development of an effective ongoing program to address breast cancer disparities in this community (Christopher et al, 2008) (Box 18-1).

Partnership, as defined here, is an essential concept for nurses to know and use, as are the concepts of community, community as client, and community health. Experienced nurses know that partnership is important because health is not a static reality but is continuously generated through new and increasingly effective means of community member–professional collaboration. Other active professional service providers such as school teachers, public safety officers, and agricultural extension agents play a large part in the overall health of the community. Partnership in identifying strengths and problems and in setting goals is especially important because it brings commitment from all persons involved, an essential component of successful change (Biel et al, 2009).

Partnerships involving nurses working with community organizations offer one of the most effective means for interventions because they actively involve the community and build on existing community strengths. Nurses working with community groups and organizations can fulfill many different roles including media advocacy, political action, community-based health communication, social marketing, and outreach facilitation. Regardless of what roles nurses fulfill as their contribution to the partnership, they must remember to "start where the people are" (Severance & Zinnah, 2009).

Shoultz et al (2006) looked at the challenges and possible solutions in developing partnerships with communities. Community partnerships involve both influence and power. Nurses must focus on where and how health professionals and the community can work together, respecting voices of all community members. This approach requires nurses to do *with* rather than *to* the partner, while the partner's role throughout the process is active and empowered, not passive. Mutually determined goals and plans of action, and the assignment of roles and responsibilities, are negotiated. Through this model, community partners become more effective at working independently to solve their own problems and make their own decisions.

Prioritizing the problems through the lens of the participants may not match the identified priorities defined by other sources of data. In the language of community empowerment advocates, community participants must have an active role in the change process. The PHNs must work hard to include members of a setting, neighborhood, or organization while developing trust and providing the community with a central role throughout the process (Christopher et al, 2008; Hanks, 2006).

One historical example of a nurse-community partnership remains an inspiring story of this important work. Nancy Milio was a young, white PHN when she began working with an inner-city African American community in Detroit during the 1960s. Together, she and community members identified needs and designed a program to meet them. Milio's painstaking process of working *with* the community to create a Mom's and Tot's Center where mothers and children could access primary health care and child care is a sentinel example of community partnership. The true value of this partnership was demonstrated when the Detroit riots occurred in 1967, and the storefront where the clinic was located remained intact while surrounding structures burned; the local rioters had spared the clinic because it "belonged to the people" (Milio, 2000; DeGuzman & Keeling, 2012). Thus, working within the community to develop priorities and to create programs promotes longstanding ownership and at the same time assures the probability for sustainability.

## The Nurse's Role in the Community

The nurse's ability to establish credibility and trust in the community is important in doing a thorough community assessment. The nurse may be considered to be an *insider* if he or she grew up in the community, has personal ties to the people there or comes from a similar cultural or ethnic background. This insider status may increase community members' willingness to speak openly and partner with the nurse. However, sometimes this insider status can be a disadvantage if it compromises the nurse's impartiality or objectivity (Ochieng, 2010). Nurses who are new to the community or have few insider connections can increase their familiarity with the community and its residents through taking part in informal community activities, such as shopping, attending church, or participating in organizations. They can also partner with trusted insiders in the community, such as *gatekeepers* and *community health workers.*

**Gatekeepers** refer to formal or informal community leaders who create opportunities for nurses to meet diverse members of the community (Sixsmith, Boneham, & Goldring, 2003). Gatekeepers can confer credibility to the nurse. For example, a church pastor may act as a gatekeeper by introducing a nurse to the congregation, thus increasing the likelihood that the church members will trust the nurse enough to provide information or to serve as partners in the assessment and throughout any program planning, intervention, and evaluation.

**Community health workers** (CHW) are not professional or licensed health care providers but are community members from diverse backgrounds who receive training to do health outreach work. CHWs can assist nurses in doing community health assessments in several ways. They extend the reach of the nurse by being able to do many activities that are part of the community assessment process. They can also serve as gatekeepers, using their own insider status to engage community members in the assessment process.

## COMMUNITY ASSESSMENT

Community assessment put quite simply is taking detailed stock of a community both from the outside in and from the inside out for the purpose of identifying and analyzing conditions therein. Community assessment, sometimes called community needs assessment, is one of three core functions of public health. This process requires clinical judgment and critical appraisal of multiple types of data from a variety of sources, and it requires a clear knowledge and understanding of the community as client. People, place, and function are the foundational dimensions of a community and need to be defined as part of the assessment process. These dimensions guide the gathering of data. Data can be primary or secondary. **Primary data** are collected directly through interaction with community members, which may include community leaders or interested stakeholders. **Secondary data** are obtained through existing reports on the community including census, vital statistics, and numerical reports (e.g., morbidity and mortality information) or information from reference books.

There might be many reasons for conducting a community assessment but for public health nursing the purpose is usually to identify community health needs and to develop strategies to address them. The purpose of this section is to provide a clear method for completing a comprehensive community assessment, using the tools of the nursing process adapted to communities. CDC (2013) offers a clear set of common elements that constitute a community assessment (see Box 18-2). An example of Santa Cruz's very comprehensive and ongoing community assessment (2009) can be accessed at http://www.appliedsurveyresearch .org/projects_database/quality-of-life/santa-cruz-county -community-assessment-project-cap.html.

---

**BOX 18-2  Common Elements of Assessment and Planning Frameworks**

1. Organize and plan
2. Engage the community
3. Develop a goal or vision
4. Conduct community health assessment(s)
5. Prioritize health issues
6. Develop community health improvement plan [in this case Nursing Diagnosis]
7. Implement and monitor community health improvement plan
8. Evaluate process and outcomes

Source: CDC *Assessment and Planning Models, Frameworks and Tools* 2014A, www.cdc.gov/stltpublichealth/ch/assessment.html.

### Why Community Assessment?

Community assessments may be done for various reasons. For example, a PHN in a community may want to conduct an assessment to learn more about community needs or strengths, or may want to locate confirmation data to address a recognized community problem. Recently a new directive resulting from the Affordable Care Act requires charitable hospitals to perform a community needs assessment of their catchment area every three years and plan an implementation strategy to address any identified needs (Barnett, 2012).

In some cases administrators will perform these assessments, but PHNs are ideal choices to lead the community in this required activity. Public health personnel are the recognized experts in this arena. The recent formation of the Public Health Department Accreditation Board placed responsibility to implement standards for uniform performance with health departments in the United States. These standards include enhanced surveillance of community health services through regularly conducted community assessments (Riley, Bender, & Lownik, 2012).

Assessment is one of the three core functions of public health (CDC *Core Functions*, 2011). Public health nursing places assessment at the forefront of PHN competencies. The Quad Council of Public Health Nursing Organizations is a coalition that includes the Association of Community Health Nursing Educators (ACHNE), the Association of Public Health Nurses (APHN), the American Public Health Association—Public Health Nursing Section (APHA), and the American Nurses Association's Congress on Nursing Practice and Economics (ANA). In 2011, the Quad Council revised the core competencies for public health nursing and adopted a three-tiered structure describing the skills expected of nurses as the generalist, specialist, and executive levels of public health nursing practice (Swider et al, 2013). The **Public Health Nursing Competencies** include eight major domains: analytic and assessment skills, policy development/program planning skills, communication skills, cultural competency skills, community dimensions of practice skills, public health sciences skills, financial management and planning skills, and leadership and systems thinking skills. The domain of analytic and assessment skills (Table 18-1), details the competencies specific to community assessment across all tiers of public health nursing practice.

## TABLE 18-1   Public Health Nursing Competencies, Domain 1: Analytic and Assessment Skills

| Tier 1: Generalist | Tier 2: Specialist/Mid-Level | Tier 3: Executive/Senior-Level |
|---|---|---|
| 1. Identifies the determinants of health and illness of individuals and families, using multiple sources of data. | 1. Assesses the health status of populations and their related determinants of health and illness. Partners with populations, health professionals, and other stakeholders to attach meaning to collected data. | 1. Conducts comprehensive, in-depth system/organizational assessment as it relates to population health. |
| 2. Uses epidemiologic data and the ecological perspective to identify the health risks for a population. Identifies individual and family assets and needs, values and beliefs, resources, and relevant environmental factors. | 2. Develops public health nursing diagnoses for individuals, families, communities, and populations. Uses a synthesis of nursing, public health, and system science/theory when characterizing population-level health risks. Assures that assessments identify population assets and needs, values and beliefs, resources, and relevant environmental factors. Derives population diagnoses and priorities based on assessment data, including input from populations. | 2. Uses organizational and other theories to guide development of system-wide approaches to reduce population-level health risks. Designs systems that identify population assets and needs, values and beliefs, resources, and relevant environmental factors. |
| 3. Identifies variables that measure health and public health conditions. | 3. Utilizes a wide variety of relevant variables to measure health conditions for a community or population. | 3. Utilizes a comprehensive set of relevant variables within and across systems to measure health conditions. |
| 4. Uses valid and reliable methods and instruments for collecting qualitative and quantitative data from multiple sources. Develops a data collection plan using appropriate technology to collect data to inform the care of individuals, families, and groups. | 4. Develops a data collection plan using models and principles of epidemiology, demography, and biostatistics, as well as social, behavioral, and natural sciences to collect quantitative and qualitative data on a community or population. Uses methods and instruments for collecting valid and reliable quantitative and qualitative data. | 4. Develops systems that support the collection of valid and reliable quantitative and qualitative data on individuals, families, and populations. |
| 5. Identifies sources of public health data and information. Collects, interprets, and documents data in terms that are understandable to all who were involved in the process, including communities. | 5. Uses multiple methods and sources when collecting and analyzing data for a comprehensive community/population assessment. Assures that assessments are documented and interpreted in terms that are understandable to all who were involved in the process, including communities. | 5. Designs systems that assure that assessments are documented and interpreted in terms that are understandable to all who are involved in the process, including individuals, communities, and populations. Designs data collection system that uses multiple methods and sources when collecting and analyzing data to ensure a comprehensive assessment process. |
| 6. Uses valid and reliable data sources to make comparisons for assessment. | 6. Critiques the validity, reliability, and comparability of data collected for communities/populations. | 6. Designs systems to assure the validity, reliability, and comparability of data. Revises systems to assure optimal validity, reliability, and comparability of data. |
| 7. Identifies gaps and redundancies in data sources in a community assessment through work with individuals, families, and communities. | 7. Identifies gaps and redundancies in data sources used in a comprehensive community/population assessment. Examines the effect of gaps in data on PH practice/program planning. | 7. Identifies gaps and redundancies in sources of data used in a comprehensive organizational assessment. Strategizes with relevant others to address data gaps. |
| 8. Applies ethical, legal, and policy guidelines and principles in the collection, maintenance, use, and dissemination of data and information. | 8. Assures the application of ethical, legal, and policy principles in the collection, maintenance, use, and dissemination of data and information. | 8. Ensures information disseminated is understandable to the community and stakeholders. Establishes systems that incorporate ethical, legal, and policy principles into the collection, maintenance, use, and dissemination of data and information. |
| 9. Describes the public health nursing applications of quantitative and qualitative data. | 9. Synthesizes qualitative and quantitative data during data analysis for a comprehensive community/population assessment. Uses various data collection methods and qualitative and quantitative data sources to conduct a comprehensive, community/population assessment. | 9. Synthesizes qualitative and quantitative data during data analysis for a comprehensive organizational assessment. Uses multiple methods and qualitative and quantitative data sources for a comprehensive system/organizational assessment. |

**TABLE 18-1    Public Health Nursing Competencies, Domain 1: Analytic and Assessment Skills—cont'd**

| Tier 1: Generalist | Tier 2: Specialist/Mid-Level | Tier 3: Executive/Senior-Level |
|---|---|---|
| 10. Collects quantitative and qualitative data that can be used in the community health assessment process. Assesses data collected as part of the community assessment process to make inferences about individuals, families, and groups. | 10. Incorporates an ecological perspective when analyzing data from a comprehensive community/population assessment. Partners with groups, communities, populations, health professionals, and stakeholders to review and evaluate data collected. | 10. Incorporates ecological perspective when analyzing data from a comprehensive, system/organizational assessment as it relates to population health. |
| 11. Utilizes information technology to collect, analyze, store, and retrieve data related to public health nursing care of individuals, families, and groups. | 11. Utilizes information technology effectively to collect, analyze, store, and retrieve data related to care of communities and populations. | 11. Collaborates with others in the design of data collection processes and applications that facilitate the collection, use, storage, and retrieval of data. |
| 12. Practices evidence-based public health nursing to promote the health of individuals, families, and groups. | 12. Practices evidence-based public health nursing to promote the health of communities and populations. | 12. Practices evidence-based public health nursing to create and/or modify systems of care. Utilizes data to address scientific, political, ethical, and social public health issues. |
| 13. Uses available data and resources related to the social determinants of health when planning care for individuals, families, and groups. | 13. Collects data related to social determinants of health and community resources to plan for community-oriented and population-level programs. Analyzes those data. Incorporates the results of those analyses into program planning. | 13. Evaluates organization/system capacity to analyze the health status of the community/population effectively. Allocates organization/system resources to support the effective analysis of the health status of the community/population. |

From Swider SM, Krothe J, Ryes D, and Cravetz M (working group for the QUAD Council): The QUAD Council practice competencies for public health nursing, *Public Health* Nursing 30(6):519-526, 2013.

Assessing the health of the community requires a broad definition of health, including consideration of the economic, social, physical, and mental health of the population. Access to resources that provide for these broad needs and services will be part of the assessment process.

The PHN should place the assessment of community strengths as high on the list as recognized problems in the development of an assessment plan. It is important to value both in the assessment, planning, implementation, and evaluation process.

*…Healthy Communities initiatives are better served by assets-oriented methods than by standard "problem-focused" or "needs-based" approaches. An assets orientation allows community members to identify, support and mobilize existing community resources to create a shared vision of change, and encourages greater creativity when community members do address problems and obstacles (Sharpe et al, 2000).*

Communities have both resources and needs. We recommend a balanced approach to the assessment, highlighting community assets as well as problems to identify the community vehicles already present for positive change. Community strengths can later be called upon in the planning and intervention phases of the process to address the challenges the community faces. This strength-based approach may be better received by communities and funders, and promotes the inclusion of key informants and interested stakeholders; it can make strategic planning a part of the process.

## Data Sources
### Health Status Indicators

Measures of health status take more than one form. Numerical data put out by a recognized agency (such as the U.S. Census Bureau or Centers for Disease Control and Prevention, or Robert Woods Johnson Foundation) are referred to as *secondary* data (collected by someone else). Information that is gleaned from telephone surveys, personal interviews, or focus groups conducted by those who are assessing the community—any data derived from personal connections or key informants—are considered *primary* data (collected by the assessor[s]). Both types of data are required for the community assessment and both types of data will be included when analyzing the assessment data.

### Secondary Sources of Data

Even before setting foot in the community it is possible to learn a great deal about its residents' health status. Health indicators are numerical measures of health outcomes, such as morbidity and mortality, as well as determinants of health and population characteristics. Generally, these data are from *secondary* sources such as websites or printed materials. Table 18-2 lists several of these sources.

Creation of a set of health indicator data during a community health assessment serves several purposes. First, it creates a "snapshot" of health conditions that can guide the assessment team during the analysis and problem prioritization phases. Second, it is an important and easily comprehensible means of communicating the results of the assessment to the larger

| TABLE 18-2 | Frequently Used Secondary Sources for Health Indicator Data | |
|---|---|---|
| Behavioral Risk Factors Surveillance Survey (BRFSS) | http://www.cdc.gov/brfss/ | Wide variety of data on individuals' health status, health behaviors, and preventive health services |
| CDC Wonder | http://wonder.cdc.gov/ | Public health data on births, mortality, infectious diseases, cancer, and environment |
| County Health Rankings | http://www.countyhealthrankings.org/ | Collates county-level data on a wide range of health outcomes and health determinants |
| Dartmouth Atlas of Health Care | http://www.dartmouthatlas.org/data/region/ | Distribution and outcomes of health care services, in chart and map formats |
| Health Indicators Warehouse | http://www.healthindicators.gov/ | U.S. government website that gathers data from multiple sources and provides a search engine by topic, geography, and program |
| Local advocacy organizations | | Organizations that specialize in social issues such as homelessness, child abuse, or domestic violence |
| Robert Woods Johnson Foundation (RWJF) Data Hub | www.rwjf.org/en/research-publications/research-features/rwjf-datahub.html# | Provides access to data about health statistics by demographic breakdown. Statistics can be compared state to state. |
| State Cancer Profile | http://statecancerprofiles.cancer.gov/incidencerates/index.php | Incidence of cancer types by race/ethnicity, sex, and geography |
| U.S. Census | http://www.census.gov | Demographic and economic data |

community. Third, it is an effective way to compare the current health status in the community with the same community at different time points, with other communities, or with larger populations such as state or national data. Table 18-3 lists health indicators that are frequently included in community health assessments.

There are two important considerations for selecting which indicators to include in an assessment: the priorities of the community, and comparability to other data. Ideally, diverse community stakeholders should participate in identifying health indicators that address their interests or concerns. Stakeholders include anyone with a personal or occupational interest or concern in a community's life. If the health indicators will be compared with other assessments, then use similar measures when possible. For example, the total number of deaths in a community is different from the annual rate of deaths per 100,000 population. The box below gives additional tips on obtaining high-quality data.

### SECONDARY SOURCE DATA

*Questions to ask about data from secondary sources:*
1. *How current is the reported information?*
2. *When was the site last updated?*
3. *How credible is the data source?*
4. *Is an author identified?*
5. *Are demographic data reported about the people?*
6. *Are data reported about different community systems?*
7. *Is there any obvious bias in the reporting of data?*
8. *Are community voices represented?*

Shuster, G: Community as client" assessment and analysis. In Stanhope and Lancaster (editors), Public Health Nursing, Population-centered health care in the community, *ed 8, 2012* Elsevier, St. Louis, Mo.

*Healthy People 2020* and County Health Rankings are useful resources for health indicators. *Healthy People 2020* identifies national health priorities, providing baseline data as well as

health indicator goals. For example, the baseline rate of injury-related mortality was 59.7 deaths per 100,000 population and the *Healthy People 2014* goal rate is 53.7 deaths per 100,000 population (www.healthypeople.gov). The County Health Rankings report is updated annually, and provides county-level data for a wide variety of health indicators and also compares county rankings within and across states (www.countyhealthrankings.org).

### Primary Sources of Data

Primary data involve the researcher or community members at the community level. Various methods can be used to collect the data, such as participant observation, key informant interviews, surveys, town hall meetings, focus groups, Photovoice, spatial data, or windshield surveys. The researcher or the community members experience the events or interact directly with the community as a group, with individuals, or by observation.

Participant observation refers to the deliberate sharing in the life of a community, for example, participating in a local fair or festival or attending a political or social event. Just as you would assess a hospital patient's room upon entering and note details about the environment (family members, emotional tone, patient's level of consciousness, IV access or vital signs, cleanliness, organization), visiting or attending an event can be a window through which to view the community. In addition, participant observation can be a fun way to experience community events.

Key informants can be identified through formal or informal channels in the community. They might be leaders in a sector of the community such as a church congregation, civic club, governmental body or neighborhood. They need not hold any formal title, but are generally viewed as community leaders by other community members and often have a long history in the community. Meeting with key informants and identifying local issues, strengths, and concerns from their viewpoint constitutes an important component of the overall assessment. See How To box for more information.

## TABLE 18-3   Health Status Indicators: Frequently Recommended Health Metrics

| HEALTH OUTCOME METRICS | | HEALTH DETERMINANT AND CORRELATE METRICS | | | |
| --- | --- | --- | --- | --- | --- |
| Mortality | Morbidity | Health Care (Access & Quality) | Health Behaviors | Demographics & Social Environment | Physical Environment |
| **SUGGESTED DATA SOURCES** | | | | | |
| • CDC Wonder<br>• Health Indicators Warehouse | • BRFSS<br>• County Health Rankings<br>• State Cancer Profiles<br>• BRFSS<br>• CDC Wonder | • County Health Rankings<br>• Health Indicators Warehouse<br>• U.S. Census<br>• Dartmouth Atlas<br>• RWJF DataHub | • BRFSS<br>• County Health Rankings<br>• Health Indicators Warehouse<br>• RWJF DataHub | • U.S. Census<br>• County Health Rankings<br>• Local advocacy organization<br>• Health Indicators Warehouse<br>• RWJF DataHub | • County Health Rankings<br>• U.S. Census<br>• CDC Wonder |
| Mortality: Leading Causes of Death | Obesity | Health Insurance Coverage | Tobacco Use/ Smoking | Age | Air Quality |
| Infant Mortality | Low Birth Weight | Provider Rates (PCPs, Dentists) | Physical Activity | Sex | Water Quality |
| Injury-related Mortality | Hospital Utilization | Asthma-Related Hospitalization | Nutrition | Race/Ethnicity | Housing |
| Motor Vehicle Mortality | Cancer Rates | | Unsafe Sex | Income | |
| Suicide | Motor Vehicle Injury | | Alcohol Use | Poverty Level | |
| Homicide | Overall Health Status | | Seatbelt Use | Educational Attainment | |
| | STDs (chlamydia, gonorrhea, syphilis) | | Immunizations and Screenings | Employment Status | |
| | AIDS | | | Foreign-Born | |
| | Tuberculosis | | | Homelessness | |
| | | | | Language Spoken at Home | |
| | | | | Marital Status | |
| | | | | Domestic Violence and Child Abuse | |
| | | | | Violence and Crime | |
| | | | | Social Capital/Social Support | |

Adapted from CDC. (2013). Community health assessment for population health improvement: resource of most frequently recommended health outcomes and determinants. Retrieved May 3, 2014 from http://c.ymcdn.com/sites/www.cste.org/resource/resmgr/CrossCuttingI/FinalCHAforPHI508.pdf

**HOW TO  Identify a Key Informant**
- *Talking to key informants is a critical part of the community assessment.*
- *Key informants are not always people who have a formal title or position.*
- *Key informants often have an informal role within the community.*
- *County health department nurses and church leaders are often key informants. They also know many community members and can identify other key informants.*

*Shuster, G: Community as client" assessment and analysis. In Stanhope and Lancaster (editors),* Public Health Nursing, Population-centered health care in the community, *ed 8, 2012 Elsevier, St. Louis, Mo.*

Town hall meetings are opportunities for local constituents to come together, usually to discuss a particular issue or proposal that influences all members of the community. Many town hall meetings have been held recently, for example, to address the issue of health care reform. The following photo represents one town hall meeting held for that purpose in Hartford, Connecticut, in 2009. Political rallies and delegate forums are often held in this format.

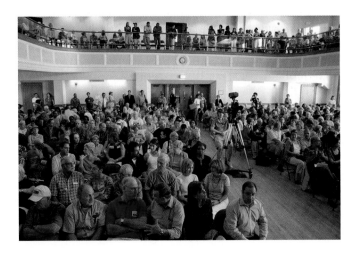

A **focus group** is similar to an interview, in that it collects data mainly through asking open-ended questions to participants but to a small group rather than an individual. Focus groups are useful for situations where the interaction between participants is likely to prompt discussions or generate ideas that individual interviews might not. Focus groups work well when the topic is not a sensitive one and participants feel comfortable speaking out about the issue with the group. For example, an assessment of the role of a parks and recreation department used focus groups to prompt discussions about individual experiences as well as perceptions about the larger community (Henderson et al, 2001).

Focus groups should be structured to balance a diversity of perspectives with opportunities for in-depth understanding of the chosen topics. The design of the question guide should address the goals for the data: for example, do you want to generate a free-flowing discussion of ideas or obtain specific information from each participant? Participants should be recruited through community channels such as churches, associations, and other places where people gather. An ideal number of participants is between six and eight, though smaller or larger groups can work in different circumstances (Rabiee, 2004).

Each focus group should be organized so that its participants are fairly homogenous in key characteristics. For example, in an assessment to compare different neighborhoods, each focus group might contain residents from one neighborhood. In an assessment of community barriers and resources for physical activity, focus groups might be divided among participants who identify themselves as exercisers, and non-exercisers (Lees et al, 2005). A typical format for a focus group is that one moderator leads the discussion, while an assistant takes written notes, and the session is often audio recorded. The recording is then transcribed and included in the analysis.

## Photovoice

**Photovoice**, also called photo elicitation, is a community assessment technique in which community members take photos to represent a topic or theme about community health. For example, a study on childhood obesity asked rural youth to take photos on the theme of assets and barriers to healthy diets and physical activity (Findholt, Michael, & Davis, 2010). Photovoice has been used with many types of community participants, but can be especially useful in working with groups that may be marginalized or have little power such as youths, the elderly, individuals living in poverty, or those involved in substance abuse. Photovoice is a way for participants to communicate powerful messages about their experiences, without the need for words.

Photography is a relatively easy group activity because devices to take photos are relatively common and inexpensive. Disposable cameras and the participants' cell phones are examples of devices with minimal added cost. Video, sound recording, and other forms of media can also be used in ways similar to Photovoice. For example, a group of New Orleans residents used Videovoice to create their own documentary to advocate for housing, education, and economic development after Hurricane Katrina (Catalani et al, 2013).

The basic process to incorporate Photovoice into a community assessment is as follows:

1. **Train participants:** Participants receive training in Photovoice methods, including the topic of interest, basic photography techniques, and ethical and safety issues. Participants may need to learn how to obtain written consent before photographing people, businesses, or other identifiable subjects. Training is especially important when the topic of interest is sensitive or illegal, such as substance abuse.
2. **Take photos:** Participants take the cameras into their communities and take photographs that reflect the topic. Equipment should be modified to fit the participants. For example, adolescents may be very comfortable with a variety of mobile devices, whereas older adults may prefer simpler cameras with modifications for low vision or manual dexterity (Novek et al, 2012).
3. **Display photos:** The photos are collected from the participants, and then printed or digitally projected for group participants, and sometimes members of the public, to view them.
4. **Discuss photos:** Viewing the photos is meant to spark discussions that provide additional information about the topic of interest. These discussions may take place as focus groups with the Photovoice participants. If the photos are displayed in public, the aim may be to raise awareness and to start conversations among diverse stakeholders.
5. **Analyze and report results:** The information gathered through these discussions, as well as the photos themselves, can be included in the data analysis phase. The photos can also be part of the report to the community about the findings of the community assessment (Catalani & Minkler, 2010).

Photovoice can be useful at different stages of a community assessment, but may be especially useful in the early stages of data collection. The "insider" knowledge gained through this type of activity can guide subsequent community assessment activities. For example, if the Photovoice topic is "barriers to healthy lifestyles" and the majority of photos focus on places that make pedestrian or bike travel difficult, then the later stages of the assessment should give additional attention to walkability and transportation.

## Spatial Data

*Everything is related to everything else, but near things are more related than distant things.*

### *Tobler's First Law of Geography (Sui, 2004)*

Most of the information gathered in a community assessment has a spatial component: it is located somewhere in the community. The location of places like health care services, food stores, schools, bus routes, factories, highways, bodies of water, and parks can affect residents' access to health benefits or exposure to health threats. Demographic data can also be spatial. We can look at a neighborhood or other area and learn about its residents, such as age, racial or ethnic background, health characteristics, income, home value, and crime rates. Having this information can be very helpful for assessing health resources

Access to health care is a national priority, especially in regions with an insufficient number of health care providers. Recruiting and retaining qualified health professionals can be a challenge in underserved communities, particularly inner cities and rural areas of the United States. Until recently, however, only limited research has been undertaken on the special challenges, problems, and opportunities of nursing practice—especially public health nursing in rural settings. This chapter presents major issues surrounding health care delivery in rural environments, which sometimes differs from that in urban or more populated settings. Common definitions for the term *rural* are discussed, as are its associated lifestyle, the health status of rural populations, barriers to obtaining a continuum of health care services, and public health nursing practice issues. Strategies are discussed to help nurses deliver more effective population-focused nursing services to clients who live in more isolated environments with sparser resources. This chapter describes rural public health nursing practice and can be used by students, nurses who practice in rural public health departments, and those who work in agencies located in urban areas that offer outreach services to rural populations in their catchment area.

## HISTORIC OVERVIEW

Formal rural nursing originated with the Red Cross Rural Nursing Service, which was organized in November 1912. The Committee on Rural Nursing was directed by Mabel Boardman (Chair), Jane Delano (Vice-Chair), and Annie Goodrich along with other Red Cross leaders and philanthropists (Bigbee and Crowder, 1985). Before the formation of the Red Cross Rural Nursing Service, care of the sick in a small community was provided by informal social support systems. When self-care and family care were not effective in bringing about healing, this task was assigned to healers, who often were women who lived in the local community. Historically, the health needs of rural Americans have been numerous, and although not necessarily unique, they are different from those of urban populations. Consistent problems of maldistribution of health professionals, poverty, limited access to services, ignorance, and social isolation have plagued many rural communities for generations.

The history of the Red Cross Rural Nursing Service shows a consistent movement away from its initial rural focus, as demonstrated by its frequent name changes. Unfortunately, concern for rural health is similarly often temporary and replaced by other areas of greater need. It can be hoped that health care

reform initiatives will ensure equitable access to care for rural and urban residents alike (NACRHHS, 2012).

## DEFINITION OF TERMS

### Rurality: A Subjective Concept

Everyone has an idea as to what constitutes rural as opposed to urban residence. However, the two cannot be viewed as opposing entities. With the increased degree of urban influence on rural communities, the differences may not be as distinct as they may have been even a decade ago (Bureau of the Census, 2011, 2012, 2013; Meckler & Chinni, 2014). In general, **rural** is defined in terms of the geographic location and population density, or it may be described in terms of the distance from (e.g., 20 miles) or the time (e.g., 30 minutes) needed to commute to an urban center. See Box 19-1 for selected terms and definitions.

Both urban and rural communities are highly diverse and vary in their demographic, environmental, economic, and social characteristics. In turn, these characteristics influence the magnitude and types of health problems that communities face. Urban counties, however, tend to have more health care providers in relation to population, and residents of more rural counties often live farther from health care resources (Bushy, 2013).

---

**BOX 19-1  Terms and Definitions**

**Farm residency:** Residency outside area zoned as "city limits"; usually infers involvement in agriculture

**Frontier:** Regions having fewer than six persons per square mile

**Large central:** Counties in large (1 million or more population) metro areas that contain all or part of the largest central city

**Large fringe:** Remaining counties in large (1 million or more population) metro areas

**Metropolitan county:** Regions with a central city of at least 50,000 residents

**Non-farm residency:** Residence within area zoned as "city limits"

**Micropolitan county:** Counties that do not meet SMSA (see below) criteria

**Rural:** Communities having fewer than 20,000 residents or fewer than 99 persons per square mile

**Small:** Counties in metro areas with fewer than 1 million people

**Standard metropolitan statistical area (SMSA):** Regions with a central city of at least 50,000 residents

**Suburban:** Area adjacent to a highly populated city

**Urban:** Geographic areas described as non-rural and having a higher population density; more than 99 persons per square mile; cities with a population of at least 20,000 but less than 50,000

Some equate the idea of rural with farm residency and urban with non-farm residency, whereas others consider *rural* to be a "state of mind." For the more affluent, rural may bring to mind a recreational, retirement, or resort community located in the mountains or in lake country where one can relax and participate in outdoor activities, such as skiing, fishing, hiking, or hunting. For the less affluent, the term can impose grim scenes. For example, some people may think of an impoverished Indian reservation as comparable to an underdeveloped country, and other people may think about a migrant labor camp with several families living in a one-room shanty with no access to safe drinking water or adequate sanitation.

Just as each city has its own unique features, also it is difficult to describe a "typical rural town" because of the wide population and geographic diversity. For example, rural towns in Florida, Oregon, Alaska, Hawaii, and Idaho are different from one another, and quite different from those in Vermont, Texas, Alabama, or California. Also, there can be vast differences between rural areas within one state. Still, descriptions and definitions for *rural* tend to be more subjective and relative in nature than those for *urban*.

For example, "small" communities with populations of more than 20,000 have some features that one may expect to find in a city. Then again, residents who live in a community with a population of less than 2000 may consider a community with a population of 5000 or 10,000 to be a city. Although some communities may seem geographically remote on a map, the residents who live there may not feel isolated. Those residents believe they are within easy reach of services through telecommunication and dependable transportation, although extensive shopping facilities may be 50 to 100 miles from the family home, obstetric care may be 150 miles away, or nursing services in the district health department in an adjacent county may be 75 or more miles away (Bolin & Bellamy, 2014; Gamm et al, 2003).

## RURAL-URBAN CONTINUUM

Frequently used definitions to describe rural and urban and to differentiate between them are provided by several federal agencies (Bureau of the Census, 2011; USDA, 2013a; 2013b) (see Box 19-1). These definitions, which in many cases are dichotomous in nature, fail to take into account the relative nature of ruralness. Rural and urban residencies are not opposing lifestyles. Rather, they must be seen as a rural-urban continuum ranging from living on a remote farm, to a village or small town, to a larger town or city, to a large metropolitan area with a *core inner city*. See Figure 19-1, which describes the continuum of rural-urban residency.

Several federal agencies classify U.S. counties and county equivalents (N = 3007) according to population density, specifically, metropolitan counties (84% of the total population) and non-metropolitan counties (16% of the total population) (USDA, 2013b). The terms metropolitan area and micropolitan area (metro and micro areas) refer to geographic entities primarily used for collecting, tabulating, and publishing federal statistics. Core-based statistical area (CBSA) is a collective term for both metro and micro areas. A metro area contains a core urban area of 50,000 or more population. A micro area contains an urban core of at least 10,000 (but less than 50,000) population. Each metro or micro area consists of one or more counties containing the core urban area. Likewise, adjacent counties have a high degree of social and economic integration (as measured by commuting to work) with their urban core (USDA, 2013b).

Demographically, micro areas contain about 60% of the total non-metro population, with an average of 43,000 people per county. In contrast, non-core areas, with no urban cluster of 10,000 or more residents, have on average about 14,000 residents. In general, lack of an urban core and low overall population density may place these counties at a disadvantage in efforts to expand and diversify their economic base. The designation

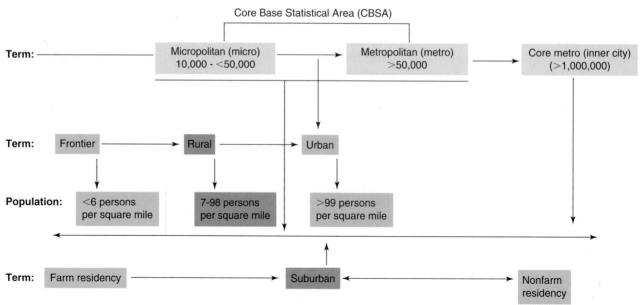

**FIG 19-1** The continuum of rural-urban residency.

of micro areas is an important step in recognizing non-metro diversity. The term also provides a framework to understand population growth and economic restructuring in small towns and cities that have received less attention than metro areas. Nationally and regionally, many measures of health, health care use, and health care resources among rural populations vary by the level of urban influence in a particular region.

Micro areas embody a widely shared residential preference for a small-town lifestyle—an ideal compromise between large highly populated urban cities and sparsely populated rural settings. As information about these places makes its way into government data and publications alongside metro areas in the coming years, hopefully the notion of "micropolitan" will draw increased attention from policy makers and the business community.

In the past two decades there has been a steady population shift from urban to less-populated regions of the United States. Demographers metaphorically refer to this demographic phenomenon as the "doughnut effect." That is to say, people are moving away from highly populated areas to outlying suburbs of urban centers. Most of the population growth has been in rural counties with a booming economy coupled with the geographic area to expand, such as in many western and southern states (USDA, 2013a, 2013b).

Clearly, a notable population shift will also affect the health status and lifestyle preferences of communities in which the shift occurs. As beliefs and values change over time, urban-rural differences narrow in some aspects and others became more pronounced. Depending on the definition that is used, the actual rural population might vary slightly. According to Bureau of the Census estimates (2011, 2012, 2013), almost 20% of all U.S. residents live in rural settings. In this chapter, rural refers to areas having fewer than 99 persons per square mile and communities having 20,000 or fewer inhabitants.

## CURRENT PERSPECTIVES

### Population Characteristics

Adding to the confusion about what constitutes rural versus urban residency are the special needs of the numerous underrepresented groups (minorities, subgroups) who reside in the United States. In general, there are a higher proportion of whites in rural areas than in urban areas. There are, however, regional variations, and some rural counties have a significant number of minorities. Little is documented on the needs and health status of special rural populations (AHCPR, 2013a, 2013b; Bolin & Bellamy, 2014; USDHHS, 2013). Anthropologists are quick to report that, within a group, there often exists a wide range of lifestyles. Consequently, even in the smallest or most remote town or village, a subgroup may behave differently and have different values about health, illness, and patterns of accessing health care. Also, a group's lifestyle may be associated with health problems that are different from those of the predominant cultural group in a given community. Background information on selected populations can be found in Chapters 7 and 32.

Demographically, rural communities include a higher proportion of younger and older residents. Nurses can expect to encounter more residents under the age of 18 and over 65 years of age in rural areas compared with an urban setting. Rural residents 18 years of age and older are more likely to be, or to have been, married than are their urban counterparts. As a group, rural adults are more likely to be widowed and have fewer years of formal education than urban adults (Meckler & Chinni, 2014; USDA, 2013a).

Although there are regional variations, rural families in general tend to be poorer than their urban counterparts. Comparing annual incomes with the standardized index established, more than one fourth of rural Americans live in or near poverty, and nearly 40% of all rural children are impoverished. Compared with those in metropolitan settings, a substantially smaller proportion of rural families are at the high end of the income scale. Accompanying the recent population shifts from urban to formerly rural areas, one can speculate that average income level might also change; however, no data are available at this time to substantiate this estimate. Regardless, level of income is a critical factor in whether a family has health insurance or qualifies for public insurance. Consequently rural families are less likely to have private insurance and more likely to receive public assistance or to be uninsured.

The working poor in rural areas are particularly at risk for being underinsured or uninsured. In working poor families, one or more of the adults are employed but still cannot afford private health insurance. Furthermore, their annual income is such that it disqualifies the family from obtaining public insurance. Several factors help explain why this phenomenon occurs more often in rural settings (Bushy, 2013). For example, a high proportion of rural residents are self-employed in a family business, such as ranching or farming, or they work in small enterprises, such as a service station, restaurant, or grocery store. Also, an individual may be employed in part-time or in seasonal occupations, such as farm laborer and construction, in which health insurance often is not an employee benefit. In other situations, a family member may have a preexisting health condition that makes the cost of insurance prohibitive, if it is even available to them. At present it remains to be seen if this situation will change with the recent health care reform. A few rural families fall through the cracks and are unable to access any type of public assistance because of other deterrents, such as language barriers, compromised physical status, the geographic location of an agency, lack of transportation, or undocumented worker status. Insurance, or the lack of it, has serious implications for the overall health status of rural residents and the nurses who provide services to them (AHCPR, 2013a, 2013b; NCHS, 2014).

### Health Status of Rural Residents

Even though rural communities constitute about one fourth of the total population, the health problems and the health behaviors of the residents in them are not fully understood. This section summarizes what is known about the overall health status of rural adults and children. The health status measures that are addressed are perceived health status, diagnosed chronic conditions, physical limitations, frequency of seeking medical treatment, usual source of care, maternal–infant health, children's health, mental health, minorities' health, and environmental and occupational health risks (Bolin & Bellamy, 2014; OSHA, 2013). Residents of rural areas suffer some of the same health problems as migrant farmworkers, as described in Chapter 34, including exposure to environmental factors and accidents.

## Perceived Health Status

In general, people in rural areas have a poorer perception of their overall health and functional status than their urban counterparts. Rural residents over 18 years of age assess their health status less favorably than do urban residents. Studies show that rural adults are less likely to engage in preventive behavior, which ultimately increases exposure to risk. Specifically, they are more likely to use tobacco products and self-report higher rates of alcohol consumption and obesity; furthermore, they are less likely to engage in routine physical activity during leisure time, wear seat belts, have regular blood pressure checks, have Pap smears, complete breast self-examinations, and have colorectal screenings. Ultimately, failure to participate in health-promoting lifestyle behaviors impacts the overall health status of rural residents, their level of function, physical limitations, degree of mobility, and level of self-care activities (American Legacy Foundation, 2013; Crosby et al, 2012; NCHS, 2014).

## Chronic Illness

Rural adults are more likely than urban adults to have one or more of the following chronic conditions: heart disease, chronic obstructive pulmonary disease, hypertension, arthritis and rheumatism, diabetes, cardiovascular disease, and cancer. Nearly half of all rural adults have been diagnosed with at least one of these chronic conditions, compared with about one fourth of non-rural adults. Also, the prevalence of diagnosed diabetes in rural adults is about 7 out of 100 as opposed to 5 out of 100 in non-rural environments. Rural adults are more likely to have cancer (almost 7%) compared with urban adults (about 5%). Although most cases of acquired immunodeficiency syndrome (AIDS) are still found in urban areas, the rate is increasing in some rural populations (Smalley, Warren, Rainer, 2012; South Carolina Research Center, 2013).

Rural-urban health disparities have been documented in health status (Box 19-2) and for health behaviors (Box 19-3). For example, there are disparities in the proportion of rural adults who receive medical treatment for both life-threatening illness and degenerative or chronic conditions compared with urban adults. The proportion of rural residents who receive these treatments is high in rural versus urban areas. Life-threatening conditions include malignant neoplasms, heart disease, cardiovascular problems, and liver disorders. Degenerative or chronic diseases include diabetes, kidney disease, arthritis, and chronic diseases of the circulatory, nervous, respiratory, and digestive systems. In essence, chronic health conditions, coupled with their poor health status, limit the physical activities of a larger proportion of rural residents than of their urban counterparts (Bolin & Bellamy, 2014; NCHS, 2014).

## Physical Limitations

Limitations in mobility and self-care are strong indicators of an individual's overall health status. Specific assessed measures on

---

**BOX 19-2  Disparities Among U.S. Urban (Metropolitan) and Rural (Micropolitan) Residents' Health Status**

Residents of fringe counties near large metro areas have the following:
- Lowest levels of premature mortality, partly reflecting lower death rates for unintentional injuries, homicide, and suicide
- Lowest levels of smoking, alcohol consumption, and childbearing among adolescents
- Lowest prevalence of physical inactivity during leisure time among women
- Lowest levels of obesity among adults
- Greatest number of physician specialists and dentists per capita
- Lowest percentage of the population without health insurance
- Lowest percentage of the population who had no dental visits

Residents in the most rural counties have the following:
- Highest death rates for children and young adults
- Highest death rates for unintentional and motor vehicle traffic–related injuries
- Highest death rates among adults for ischemic heart disease and suicide
- Highest levels of smoking among adolescents
- Highest levels of physical activity during leisure time among men
- Highest levels of obesity among adults
- Highest percentage of adults with activity limitations caused by chronic health conditions
- Fewest physician specialists and dentists per capita
- Least likely to have seen a dentist
- Highest percentage of the population without health insurance

From Centers for Disease Control and Prevention: *United States, 2001—Urban and Rural Chartbook*, Washington, DC. Available at http://www.cdc.gov/nchs/data/hus/hus01.pdf. Accessed December 22, 2010; Gamm L, Hutchison L, Dabney B, Dorsey A: *Rural Healthy People 2010: A Companion Document to Healthy People 2010* (Vol. I, II, III), 2003. Available at http://www.srph.tamhsc.edu/centers/rhp2010/publications.htm. Accessed June 28, 2005.

---

a national health survey included walking one block, walking uphill or climbing stairs, bending, lifting, stooping, feeding, dressing, bathing, and toileting. In fact, almost 10% of rural adults report at least three or more of these physical limitations, compared with about 6% of metropolitan adults. The increased prevalence of poor health status and impaired function is not necessarily attributable to the increased number of older adults found in rural areas. Similar patterns are evident in adults 18 to 64 years of age. Rural adults under 65 years of age are more likely than urban adults to assess their health status as fair to poor, and a greater percentage have been diagnosed with a chronic health condition (NCHS, 2014; USDHHS, 2013).

Based on data from national health surveys, the overall health status of rural adults leaves much to be desired. This is attributed to a number of factors, including impaired access to health care providers and services, coupled with other rural factors. Thus nurses who practice in rural areas are essential in providing a continuum of care to to their clients. Specifically, nurses can help clients have healthier lives by teaching them how to prevent accidents, engage in more healthful lifestyle behaviors, and reduce the risk of chronic health problems. Once clients in rural environments have been diagnosed with a long-term problem, nurses can help them manage chronic conditions to achieve better health outcomes and functioning (Gamm et al, 2003; Bolin & Bellamy, 2014).

## BOX 19-3 Rural-Urban Disparities: Lifestyle and Health Behaviors

- Residents in any rural areas are more likely to report fair to poor health status (19.5%) than were residents of urban counties (15.6%).
- Rural residents are more likely to report having diabetes (9.6%) versus urban adults (8.4%).
- Rates of diabetes are markedly higher among rural American Indians (15.2%) and African American adults (15.1%).
- Rural residents are more likely to be obese (27.4%) versus urban residents (23.9%).
- Rural black adults are particularly at risk for obesity; ranging from 38.9% in rural micropolitan counties to 40.7% in remote rural counties.
- Rural residents are less likely to meet CDC recommendations for moderate or vigorous physical activity (44%) versus urban residents (45.4%).
- Rural African American adults are less likely to meet recommendations for physical activity than other rural residents; this difference persists across all levels of rurality.

**Access to Health Care Services**
- Rural residents are more likely to be uninsured (17.8%) versus urban residents (15.3%).
- Hispanic adults are more likely to lack insurance, with uninsured rates ranging from 40.8% in rural micropolitan counties to 56.1% in small remote counties.
- Most rural residents (81%) and urban residents (79.4%) report having a personal health care provider. However, residents in remote rural counties were least likely to have a personal physician (78.7%).
- Rural white adults are more likely to have a personal health care provider than were other adults. Among Hispanic adults, the proportion with a

personal provider ranged from 60.4% in rural micropolitan counties to 47.7% in remote rural counties.
- Rural adults are more likely than urban adults to defer seeking health care because of cost (15.1% vs 13.1%)
- Rural adult African Americans, Hispanics, and American Indians are more likely to report having deferred care due to cost compared with white rural residents.

**Receipt of Preventive Services**
- Rural women are less likely (70.7%) than urban women (77.9%) to be in compliance with mammogram screening guidelines.
- Rural women are less likely (86%) than urban women (91.4%) to have had a Pap smear within the past 3 years.
- Rural residents over age 50 years are less likely (57.7%) to have had a colorectal screening versus urban counterparts (61.4%).

**Quality of Diabetes Care**
- The proportion of adults with diabetes who reported receiving at least two hemoglobin A1c tests within the past year was low among both rural (33.1%) and urban residents (35%).
- White rural residents with diabetes were more likely than African American or Hispanic residents to receive at least two hemoglobin A1c tests in the past year.
- Only 64.2% of rural and 69.1% or urban residents with diabetes reported receiving an annual dilated eye examination.

From Bennett K, Olatosi B, Probst J: Health disparities: a rural-urban chartbook, 2008. Available at http://rhr.sph.sc.edu/report/(73)%20Health%20Disparities%20A%20Rural%20Urban%20Chartbook%20-%20Distribution%20Copy.pdf. Accessed December 8, 2011.

## Patterns of Health Service Use

When the use of health care services is measured, it is found that more than three fourths of adults in rural areas received medical care on at least one occasion during a year. Despite their overall poorer health status and higher incidence of chronic health conditions, rural adults seek medical care less often than urban adults. In part, this discrepancy can be attributed to scarce resources and lack of providers in rural areas. Other reasons for this phenomenon are discussed later under Rural Health Care Delivery Issues and Barriers to Care (AHCPR, 2013a, 2013b; NACRHHS, 2012). Nurses must be especially thorough in their health assessment of rural clients who may not receive regular care for chronic health conditions.

## Availability and Access of Health Care

The ability of a person to identify a usual source of care is considered a favorable indicator of access to health care and a person's overall health status. Essentially, a person who has a usual source of care is more likely to seek care when ill and adhere to prescribed regimens. Having the same provider of care can enhance continuity of care, as well as a client's perception of the quality of that care. Rural adults are more likely than urban adults to identify a particular medical provider as their usual source of care. Rural adults are more likely to receive care from general practitioners and advanced practice registered nurses (APRNs) compared to urban adults who are more likely to seek care from a medical specialist. However, this trend may

be changing with health care reform, which emphasizes the importance of primary care (BHPR, 2013a, 2013b; Bushy, 2012; IOM, 2010; Krey, 2014).

Another measure of access to care is traveling time and/or distance to ambulatory care services. Rural persons who seek ambulatory care are more likely to travel more than 30 minutes to reach their usual source of care. Extended commuting time may also be a factor for residents in highly populated urban areas and those who must rely on public transportation. Once the person arrives at the clinic or physician's office, no differences between rural and urban residents are found in the waiting time to see the provider.

In general there is a maldistribution of health professionals among rural and urban counties. For instance, 1 out of 17 rural counties is reported to have no physician. Among rural respondents on national surveys, the ability to identify a usual site of care or a particular provider often stems from a community or county having only one, perhaps two, health care providers. The limited number of health care facilities is reinforced by the finding that nearly all rural residents who seek health care use ambulatory services that are provided in a physician's office as opposed to a clinic, community health center, hospital outpatient department, or emergency department (NACRHHS, 2012). One can speculate about the indicator of *usual place and usual provider*; that is to say, it suggests that rural residents are at least as well off as urban residents in regard to access to care. However, this finding may be related to the fact that rural physicians tend to live and practice in a particular community for decades, thus providing care to multigenerational families who seek care from this particular provider.

Moreover, in a **health professional shortage area (HPSA)**, a physician or a nurse practitioner may provide services to residents who live in surrounding counties. One or two nurses in a public health department usually offer a full range of services for all residents in a rural catchment area, which may span more than 100 miles from one end to the other end of a county or health district. Consequently, rural physicians and nurses frequently report, "I provide care to individuals and families with all kinds of conditions, in all stages of life, and across several generations." It should not come as a surprise that rural respondents who participate in national surveys are able to identify a usual source and a usual provider of health care (Woolston, 2010).

## Maternal–Infant Health

Reports in the literature conflict regarding pregnancy outcomes in rural areas. Overall, rural populations have higher infant and maternal morbidity rates, especially counties designated as HPSAs, which often have a high proportion of racial minorities. Here one also finds fewer specialists, such as pediatricians, obstetricians, and gynecologists, to provide care to at-risk populations. There are extreme variations in pregnancy outcomes from one part of the country to another, and even within states. For example, in several counties located in the north-central and intermountain states, the pregnancy outcome is among the finest in the United States. However, in several other counties within those same states, the pregnancy outcome is among the worst. Particularly at risk are women who live on or near Indian reservations, are migrant workers, and are of African American descent residing in rural areas in southeastern states (Bolin & Bellamy, 2014; Leipert, Leach & Thurston, 2012; USDHHS, 2013).

Public health nurses appreciate the interactive effects of socioeconomic factors, such as income level (poverty), education level, age, employment-unemployment patterns, and use of prenatal services, on pregnancy outcomes. There are other, less well-known health determinants, such as environmental hazards, occupational risks, and the cultural meaning placed on child-bearing and child-rearing practices by a community. The interaction effects of these multifaceted factors vary and often are difficult to measure (Nelson, 2009; Warren & Smalley, 2014).

## Health of Children

Reports on the health status of rural children show regional variations and conflicting data. Comparing rural children with urban children under 6 years of age on the measures of access to providers and use of services reveals the following (AHCPR 2013a, 2013b; Bolin & Bellamy, 2014; USDHHS, 2013):

- Urban children are less likely to have a usual provider but are more likely to see a pediatrician when they are ill.
- Like rural adults, rural children are more likely to be cared for by a general practitioner who is identified as their usual caregiver.

School nurses play an important role in the overall health status of children in the United States. The availability of school nurses in rural communities also varies from region to region. More specifically, in **frontier** and rural areas of the United States, school nurses usually are scarce. In part, this deficit can be attributed to limited resources associated with very low local tax revenues and shortages of health personnel in those counties. In other words, there are fewer taxpayers living in those large geographic areas. Some frontier areas have fewer than four persons per square mile and a few areas have fewer than two persons per square mile. Consequently, rural county commissioners, like their urban counterparts, are forced to prioritize the allocation of scarce resources, in particular for essential public services such as maintaining the infrastructures of utilities, roads, bridges, and education; supporting a financially suffering county hospital; hiring a county health nurse; and offering school health services. In rural communities there are fewer resources overall, yet certain public services must be provided to local residents—albeit in many situations with aging and outdated infrastructures.

Clearly, creativity is required by both community residents and local public health care providers to resolve health care and school nursing needs. Partnership arrangements, for example, have been negotiated by two or more counties that agree to share the cost of a "district" public health nurse. Other county commissioners have forged partnerships with an agency in an urban setting and contracted for specific health care services. In both of these situations, it is not unusual for the nurse to provide services to *all* children attending *all* schools in the health district's participating counties. In some frontier states, schools may be situated more than 100 miles apart and as many miles or more from the district health office. Because of the number of schools and distances between them, the county nurse may be able to visit each school only once or twice in a school term. Usually the nurse's visit is to update immunizations and perhaps teach maturation classes to students in the upper grades.

The health status of rural women, infants, and children is less than optimal. In part this can be attributed to inadequate preventive, primary, and emergency services to meet their particular health care needs. On one hand, scarce resources can pose a challenge to a nurse who provides care to rural residents, especially those in underserved areas. On the other hand, resource deficits encourage creativity and innovation; both of these behaviors are characteristic of nursing in general and of rural nurses in particular.

## Mental Health

Like many other measures of health, the facts about the mental health status of rural people are also ambiguous and conflicting (AHCPR, 2013a, 2013b; Crosby et al, 2012; NCHS, 2014). Stress, stress-related conditions, and mental illness are prevalent among populations who are economically deprived. Increasing federal regulations imposed on agriculture, timber, and marine- and mining-related industries in the past two decades led to many job losses in rural communities. The term *farm stress* is associated with the economic downturn in the agriculture industry as it affects an individual, family, and the community. This same term or diagnosis could be applied to other communities experiencing economic recessions in their predominate enterprises, such as marine-, automobile-, and timber-related industries. Economic factors also contribute to a family's being underinsured or uninsured. Interestingly, even if mental health services are available and accessible, rural residents delay seeking care when they have an emotional problem until there is an emergency or a crisis. This behavior is reflected in the lower number of annual visits for mental health services and chronic health conditions by rural residents.

Mental health professionals who serve rural populations report a persistent, endemic level of depression among residents in economically stressed rural areas. They speculate this condition is exacerbated by high levels of poverty, geographic isolation, and an insufficient number of mental health services. Depression may also contribute to the escalating incidence of accidents and suicides, especially among rural male adolescents and young men. These incidents have increased dramatically over the last decade and continue to rise within this group, to the point of being epidemic in some small communities. Likewise, the stigma associated with mental illness remains, especially in communities having fewer health care providers to educate the public about mental and behavioral health conditions (Smalley et al, 2012).

There are conflicting reports on the prevalence of interpersonal violence and alcohol and substance use among rural populations. These behaviors are less likely to be reported in areas where residents are related or personally acquainted. Over time, destructive coping behaviors in small, tight-knit communities may be accepted by local residents as "business as usual" for a particular family. Family problems may also be ignored if formal social services and public health services are sparse or nonexistent, or if residents do not trust the professionals who provide services at a local agency. In underserved rural areas, there are gaps in the continuum of mental health services, which, ideally, should include preventive education, anticipatory guidance, screenings, early intervention programs, crisis and acute care services, and follow-up care. As with other aspects of health care, nurses in rural areas play an important role in community education, case finding, advocacy, and case management of client systems experiencing acute and chronic emotional and behavioral health problems (Bushy, 2012, 2014; Smalley et al, 2012).

## Health of Minorities

As mentioned previously, a significant number of at-risk minority groups in rural America have some rather distinctive concerns (particularly children, older adults, Native Americans, Native Alaskans, Native Hawaiians, migrant workers, African Americans, and the homeless) (CDC, 2013b; NCFH, 2014; USDHHS, 2013). The rural homeless, for example, may be migrant farmworkers or local families whose homes were foreclosed. Sometimes the family may be allowed by law to continue living in the house that once was theirs. The family no longer has a means of livelihood and often remains hidden in the community with insufficient income to purchase food or other necessary services. The particular health problems of these at-risk groups are discussed in Chapters 7 and 27 through 38. Nurses

should be aware, however, that at-risk and underrepresented groups may experience some unique challenges associated with rural social structures, lifestyle, and sparse resources.

### Environmental and Occupational Health Risks

A community's primary industry or industries are a determinant in the local lifestyle, the health status of its residents, and the number and types of health care services it may need. For example, four high-risk industries identified by the Occupational Safety and Health Administration (OSHA) and found in predominantly rural environments are forestry, mining, marine-related fields, and agriculture. See Table 19-1 for a description of rural groups, their typical health care needs, and their health risks or conditions. Associated health risks of these industries are machinery and vehicular accidents, trauma, selected types of cancer related to environmental factors, and allergies and respiratory conditions associated with repeated exposure to toxins, pesticides, and herbicides (NCFH, 2014; NCHS, 2014; OSHA, 2013; USDA, 2013b).

For example, agriculture production industries such as farming and ranching are often owned and operated by a family. Small enterprises with a low number of employees do not fall under OSHA guidelines. For that reason safety standards are not enforceable on most farms and ranches, since these often are family enterprises. Moreover, small businesses, such as farms, are not covered under workers' compensation insurance. Additional concerns arise because family members participate in the farm or ranch work. This means that some adults and children may work with animals and operate dangerous machinery with minimal operating instructions on the hazards and on safety precautions. Also, many agriculture workers do not speak or read English. Consequently, agriculture-related accidents result in a significant number of deaths and long-term injuries, particularly among children and women. The morbidity and mortality rates associated with agriculture vary from state to state. The rising incidence of these injuries and deaths, however, has become a national concern. Nurses in rural settings can help address this problem by including farm safety content in school and community education programs (NCFH, 2014; OSHA, 2013).

In summary, it is risky to generalize about the health status of rural Americans because of their diversity coupled with conflicting definitions of what differentiates rural from urban residences. Many vulnerable individuals and families live in rural communities across the United States, but little is known about most of them. This information deficit therefore is a potential area of research for nurses who practice in rural environments.

## RURAL HEALTH CARE DELIVERY ISSUES AND BARRIERS TO CARE

Although each rural community is unique, the experience of living in a rural area has several common characteristics (Bushy & Winters, 2013; Hurme, 2009; Molinari & Bushy, 2012). Barriers to health care may be associated with these characteristics (e.g., whether services and professionals are available,

## TABLE 19-1    Select Health Care Needs, Risks/Conditions of Select Rural Aggregates

| Rural Aggregates | Health Care Needs | Health Risks/Conditions |
|---|---|---|
| Farmers/ranchers | Advanced life support/emergency services<br>Oral/dental care<br>Obstetric/perinatal/pediatric services<br>Mental/behavioral health services<br>Agricultural health nurses<br>Geriatric specialists | Agricultural chemicals and environmental hazards<br>Dermatitis<br>Stress/depression/anxiety disorders<br>Respiratory conditions (i.e., farmer's lung)<br>Accidents (vehicular/machinery)<br>Trauma-related chronic conditions<br>Dental caries/loss<br>Interpersonal/domestic violence |
| Native Americans | Advanced life support/emergency services<br>Oral/dental care<br>Obstetric/perinatal/pediatric services<br>Mental/behavioral health services<br>Culturally appropriate substance abuse treatment programs<br>Epidemiologists<br>Diabetes screening and educators<br>Community health workers/education | Infectious diseases (e.g., hepatitis, TB)<br>Sudden infant death syndrome (SIDS)<br>Interpersonal/domestic violence<br>Diabetes<br>Alcohol/substance abuse<br>Cirrhosis of the liver<br>Vehicular accidents<br>Hypothermic/environmental injuries<br>Trauma-related injuries/chronic conditions<br>Dental caries/loss |
| African Americans | Community nursing health promotion and screening services<br>Diabetes screening and educators<br>Hypertension screening/education<br>Prenatal and perinatal health care services<br>Oncology services (education/screening/follow-up interventions)<br>HIV/AIDS prevention education/screening/follow-up care<br>Mental/behavioral health services | Diabetes<br>Hypertension<br>Sickle cell anemia<br>Infectious diseases (e.g., hepatitis, HIV/AIDS)<br>Cancer (e.g., prostate, breast)<br>Dental caries/loss<br>Depression<br>Interpersonal/domestic violence |
| Migrant farmworkers | Environmental protection policies (safe drinking water/sanitation)<br>Community nursing/migrant health services (primary, secondary, tertiary prevention)<br>Diabetes screening and educators<br>Hypertension screening/education<br>Maternal/child services<br>Oncology services (education/screening/follow-up interventions)<br>Mental/behavioral health services | Infectious diseases (e.g., hepatitis, typhoid, TB, HIV/AIDS, STDs)<br>Exposure effects of pesticides/herbicides<br>Otitis media (children)<br>Substance abuse (alcohol, recreational drugs, imported medicinal/herbs)<br>Dental caries/loss<br>Interpersonal/domestic violence |
| Native Alaskans | Advanced life support/emergency care services<br>Medical transport services<br>Oral/dental care<br>Obstetric/perinatal/pediatric services<br>Mental/behavioral health services<br>Culturally appropriate substance abuse treatment programs<br>Epidemiologists<br>Diabetes screening and educators | Infectious diseases (e.g., hepatitis, TB)<br>Dental caries/loss<br>Depression<br>Interpersonal/domestic violence<br>Environmental health risks (e.g., exposure to toxic substances/contaminants, hypothermia)<br>Diabetes<br>Alcohol/substance abuse<br>Cirrhosis of the liver<br>Vehicular accidents/trauma/long-term chronic residual effects |
| Coal miners | Occupational Safety and Health Administration policy/standards<br>Mental/behavioral health services<br>Emergency/advanced life support services<br>Occupational health nurses<br>Grief counselors | Depression/substance abuse<br>Occupational-related accidents/trauma<br>Respiratory conditions (e.g., black lung, chronic obstructive pulmonary disease)<br>Interpersonal/domestic violence |

Adapted from: CDC (2013b). *Health disparities and inequalities report: United States 2013.* Available at http://www.cdc.gov/mmwr/pdf/other/su6203.pdf. Accessed March 28, 2014; Bolin & Bellamy, 2014; *Rural Healthy People 2020: a companion document to Healthy People 2020,* Vol I, II, III, College Station, TX, 2003, The Texas A&M University System Health Science Center, School of Rural Health, Southwest Rural Health Research Center. Available at http://www.srph.tamhsc.edu/centers/srhrc/rural-healthy-people-2020.html. Accessed March 28, 2014.

affordable, accessible, or acceptable to rural consumers). Box 19-4 lists common barriers to health care in rural areas.

Availability implies the existence of health services as well as the necessary personnel to provide essential services. Sparseness of population limits the number and array of health care

services in a given geographic region. Lacking a critical mass, the cost of providing special services to a few people often is prohibitive, particularly in frontier states where there are an insufficient number of physicians, nurses, and other types of health care providers. Consequently, where services and

## BOX 19-4   Characteristics of Rural Life

- More space; greater distances between residents and services
- Cyclical/seasonal work and leisure activities
- Informal social and professional interactions
- Access to extended kinship systems
- Residents who are related or acquainted
- Lack of anonymity
- Challenges in maintaining confidentiality stemming from familiarity among residents
- Small (often family) enterprises; fewer large industries
- Economic orientation to land and nature with industries that are extractive in nature (e.g., agriculture, mining, lumbering, marine-related; outdoor recreational activities)
- More high-risk occupations
- Town as center of trade
- Churches and schools as socialization centers
- Preference for interacting with locals (insiders)
- Mistrust of newcomers to the community (outsiders)

## BOX 19-5   Barriers to Health Care in Rural Areas

- Lack of health care providers and services
- Great distances to obtain services
- Lack of personal transportation
- Unavailable public transportation
- Lack of telephone services
- Unavailable outreach services
- Inequitable reimbursement policies for providers
- Unpredictable weather and/or travel conditions
- Inability to pay for care/lack of health insurance
- Lack of "know how" to procure publicly funded entitlements and services
- Inadequate provider attitudes and understanding about rural populations
- Language barriers (caregivers not linguistically competent)
- Care and services not culturally and linguistically appropriate

personnel are scarce, these must be allocated wisely. Accessibility implies that a person has logistical access to, as well as the ability to purchase, needed services. Affordability is associated with both availability and accessibility of care. It infers that services are of reasonable cost and that a family has sufficient resources to purchase these when needed. Acceptability of care means that a particular service is appropriate and offered in a manner that is congruent with the values of a target population. This can be hampered by a client's cultural preference and the urban orientation of health professionals (Bushy, 2013; NACRHHS, 2012). Box 19-5 lists barriers to health care in rural areas.

Providers' attitudes, insights, and knowledge about rural populations are also important. A patronizing or demeaning attitude, lack of accurate knowledge about rural populations, or insensitivity about the rural lifestyle on the part of a nurse can perpetuate difficulties in relating to those clients. Moreover, insensitivity fosters mistrust, resulting in rural clients' perceiving professionals as outsiders to the community. Some nurses in rural public health practice settings express feelings of professional isolation and community nonacceptance. To address disparate views, nursing faculty members should expose students to the rural environment and the people who live there. Clinical experiences must include opportunities to provide care to clients in their natural (e.g., rural) setting to gain accurate insight about a particular community.

To design population-focused programs that are available, accessible, affordable, and appropriate, nurses must implement interventions that mesh with clients' beliefs. This implies that a family and a community are actively involved in planning and delivering care for those who receive it. Nurses must have an accurate perspective on rural clients. Although the importance of forming partnerships and ensuring mutual exchange seems obvious, to date, most research about rural communities has been for policy or reimbursement purposes. Empirical data about rural family systems are sparse in terms of their health beliefs, values, perceptions of illness, and health care–seeking behaviors as well as what is deemed to be appropriate nursing care. Therefore, nurse scholars must assume a more active role in implementing research on the needs of rural populations for nursing services to expand the profession's theoretical base and subsequently implement community-oriented, empirically based clinical interventions (deValpine, 2014; Williams, 2012; Williams et al, 2012).

## NURSING CARE IN RURAL ENVIRONMENTS

### Theory, Research, and Practice

Information on nursing practice in small towns and rural environments is growing, and several themes have emerged as shown in Box 19-6. A nurse who practices in this setting can view each of these dimensions either as an opportunity or as a challenge.

Researchers from the University of Montana contend that existing theories do not fully explain rural nursing practice (Long & Weinert, 1989; Winters, 2013; Winters & Lee, 2009). Their focus has been on the key concepts pertinent to nursing theory (health, person, environment, and nursing/caring) and proposed relational statements that are relevant to clients and nurses in rural environments (see the Evidence-Based Practice box). Because the focus of their research was primarily with non-Hispanic whites living in the Rocky Mountain area, care must be taken about generalizing those findings to other geographic regions and minorities. These researchers propose that rural residents often judge their health by their ability to work. They consider themselves healthy, even though they may suffer from several chronic illnesses, as long as they are able to continue working. For the rural person, being healthy is the ability to be productive. Chronically ill people emphasize emotional and spiritual well-being rather than physical wellness.

Distance, isolation, and sparse resources characterize rural life and are seen in residents' independent and innovative coping strategies. Self-reliance and independence are demonstrated through their self-care practices and preference for family and community support. Community networks provide support but still allow for each person's and family's

## BOX 19-6    Characteristics of Nursing Practice in Rural Environments

- Variety/diversity in clinical experiences
- Broader/expanding scope of practice
- Generalist skills
- Flexibility/creativity in delivering care
- Sparse resources (e.g., materials, professionals, equipment, fiscal)
- Professional/personal isolation
- Greater independence/autonomy
- Role overlap with other disciplines
- Slower pace
- Lack of anonymity
- Increased opportunity for informal interactions with clients/coworkers
- Opportunity for client follow-up upon discharge in informal community settings
- Discharge planning allowing for integration of formal and informal resources
- Care for clients across the life span
- Exposure to clients with a full range of conditions/diagnoses
- Status in the community (viewed as prestigious)
- Viewed as a professional role model
- Opportunity for community involvement and informal health education

From Bushy A: Conducting culturally competent rural nursing research. In Merwin B, editor: *Annual Review of Nursing Research: Focus on Rural Health*, 26:221–236, 2008; Hurme E: Competencies for nursing practice in a rural critical access hospital, *Online J Rural Nurs Health Care* 9(2):67–81, 2009. Available at http://www.rno.org/journal/index.php/online-journal/article/viewFile/198/256. Accessed January 8, 2011; Nelson W, editor: *Handbook for Rural Health Care Ethics*, Lebanon, NH, 2009, Dartmouth. Available at http://dms.dartmouth.edu/cfm/resources/ethics/. Accessed January 8, 2011; Winters C, Lee H: *Rural Nursing: Concepts, Theory and Practice*, ed 3, New York, 2009, Springer Publishing.

## EVIDENCE-BASED PRACTICE

Nurse researchers at Montana State University proposed the following theoretical concepts and dimensions of rural nursing practice: (Long & Weinert, 1989; Winters, 2013; Winters & Lee, 2009).

- **Health:** Defined by rural residents as the ability to work. Work and health beliefs are closely related for rural Montana sample.
- **Environment:** Distance and isolation are particularly important for rural dwellers. Those who live long distances neither perceive themselves as isolated nor perceive health care services as inaccessible.
- **Nursing:** Lack of anonymity, outsider versus insider, old-timer versus newcomer. Lack of anonymity is a common theme among rural nurses who report knowing most people for whom they care, not only in the nurse–client relationship, but also in a variety of social roles, such as family member, friend, or neighbor. Acceptance as a health care provider in the community is closely linked to the outsider/insider and newcomer/old-timer phenomena. Gaining trust and acceptance of local people is identified as a unique challenge that must be successfully negotiated by nurses before they can begin to function as effective health care providers.
- **Person:** Self-reliance and independence in relationship to health care are strong characteristics of rural individuals. They prefer to have people they know care for them (informal services) as opposed to an outsider in a formal agency.

### Nurse Use

In working with rural residents, it is important to know how they define their health and their environment, because their definitions may differ from yours. Understand that you may not find acceptance and trust immediately; rural residents often trust informal caregivers more than those in a formal organization.

Long K, Weinert C: Rural nursing: developing a theory base, *Sch Inq Nurs Pract* 13(3):275–279, 1999; Winters C, Lee H: *Rural Nursing: Concepts, Theory and Practice*, ed 3. New York, 2009, Springer Publishing.

---

independence. Ruralites prefer and usually seek help through their informal networks, such as neighbors, extended family, church, and civic clubs, rather than seeking a professional's care in the formal system of health care, including services such as those provided by a mental health clinic, social service agency, or health department.

Although nursing is generally similar across settings and populations, there are some unique features associated with practice in a geographically remote area or in small towns where most people know one another. The following paragraphs highlight a few of the variations that nurses in rural practice report (Roberge, 2009; Winters, 2013; Woolston, 2010).

A nurse's professional and personal boundaries often overlap and are diffuse. It is not unusual for a nurse to have more than one work-related role in the community. For example, a nurse may work at the local hospital or in a physician's office and may also be actively involved in managing the family farm, a local grocery store, or pharmacy. For nurses, this means that many, if not all, clients they encounter are known also as neighbors, as friends of an immediate family member, or as part of one's extended family. Associated with social informality is a corresponding lack of anonymity in a small town. Some rural nurses say, "I never really feel like I am off duty because everybody in the county knows me through my work." In part, this can be attributed to nurses being highly respected and viewed by local

people as experts on health and illness. Often rural residents informally ask a nurse's advice before seeing a physician for a health problem. Rural residents may ask health-related questions when they see a local nurse (who may be a neighbor, friend, or relative) in a grocery store, at a service station, during a basketball game, or at church functions (Bushy, 2012).

Nurses in rural public health practice must make decisions about the care of individuals of all ages with a variety of health conditions. They assume many roles because of the range of services they provide in a rural health care facility and because of the scarcity of nurses and other health professionals. Nurses who work in rural areas need to have skills that include technical and clinical competency, adaptability, flexibility, strong assessment skills, organizational abilities, independence, interest in continuing education, sound decision-making skills, leadership ability, self-confidence, and skills in handling emergencies, teaching, and public relations. The nurse administrator is also expected to be a jack-of-all-trades (i.e., a generalist) and to demonstrate competence in several clinical specialties in addition to managing and organizing staff within the facility for which he or she is responsible (Hurme, 2009; Roberge, 2009; Woolston, 2010).

Rural nursing practice provides challenges, opportunities, and rewards. The way in which each factor is perceived depends on individual preferences and the situation in a given community. Challenges of rural practice sometimes include professional isolation, limited opportunities for continuing education, lack of other kinds of health personnel or professionals with whom one can interact, heavy workloads, an ability to function well in several clinical areas, lack of anonymity, and, for some, a restricted social life (Molinari & Bushy, 2012; Smalley et al, 2012; Warren & Smalley, 2014).

The most often cited opportunities and rewards in rural nursing practice are close relationships with clients and coworkers, diverse clinical experiences that evolve from caring for clients of all ages who have a variety of health problems, caring for clients for long periods of time (in some cases, across several generations), opportunities for professional development, and greater autonomy. Many nurses value the solitude and quality of life found in a rural community personally and for their own family. Others thrive on the outdoor recreational activities. Still others thoroughly enjoy the informal, face-to-face interactions coupled with the public recognition and status associated with living and working as a nurse in a small community. Disease prevention is also an important consideration in rural communities. The Levels of Prevention box shows the levels of prevention that nurse in a rural locale might use.

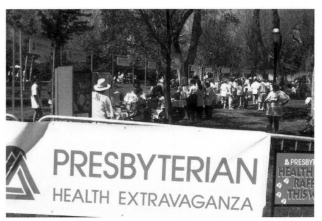

**FIG 19-2** A hospital-sponsored health fair is one example of a community event to provide health services to individuals in a rural area.

##  LEVELS OF PREVENTION

### *Rural Health*

**Primary Prevention**
- The public health nurse partners with a women's organization in a faith community located in a small Midwestern town to instruct members on meal planning as a strategy to offset the tendency to develop diabetes in family members.
- The public health nurse advocates for policy changes regarding sexual education content (to include information on contraception that goes beyond abstinence) in the schools with the district commissioners of education.

**Secondary Prevention**
- The public health nurse screens congregation members of the faith community in the Midwestern town for the presence of diabetes.
- The public health nurse partners with the local critical access hospital to offer free cholesterol, blood pressure, and blood sugar screening as well as the influenza vaccine to adults attending the annual county health fair.

**Tertiary Prevention**
- The public health nurse collaborates with the senior center in the small community town, which provides meals on a routine basis to the elderly, to reach individuals with a diagnosis of diabetes.
- The public health nurse provides consultation on diabetic nutrition, exercise habits, foot care, and, if needed, assists clients in obtaining medications through a mail-order pharmaceutical vendor.

Although most of the publications about rural health care and nursing focus on hospital practice, much of that information is applicable to both community agencies and community-focused nursing (Davis and Droes, 1993; Molinari and Bushy, 2012). There are some work-related stressors of nursing in rural communities. Case (1991) in the 1990s identified stressful experiences of nurses working in rural Oklahoma public health

departments as including: political/bureaucratic problems and intraprofessional and interpersonal conflicts associated with inadequate communication; unsatisfactory work environment and understaffing; difficult or unpleasant nurse–client encounters, such as with relatives who refuse to deliver needed care to clients, and with clients who are hostile, apathetic, dependent, or of low intelligence; fear for personal safety; difficulty locating clients, and clients falling through the cracks of the health care system. These same stressors continue to be cited by nurses who work in rural as well as urban public health agencies. Anecdotal reports describe specific stressors associated with geographic distance, isolation, sparse resources, and other environmental factors that characterize rurality.

Nursing in rural areas is characterized by physical isolation that may lend itself to any one of the following: professional isolation; scarce financial, human, and health care resources; and a broad scope of practice. Associated with personal familiarity with local residents, nurses often possess in-depth knowledge about clients and their families. Along with the acknowledged benefits, informal (face-to-face) interactions can significantly reduce a nurse's anonymity in the community and at times be a barrier to completing an objective assessment on a client. Like urban practice, rural community nursing as shown in Figure 19-2 takes place in a variety of locations, including homes, clinics, schools, occupational settings, and correctional facilities, and at community events such as county fairs, rodeos, civic and church-sponsored functions, and school athletic events.

### Research Needs

Recent empirical studies on rural nursing practice reinforce anecdotal reports by nurses (Bushy & Winters, 2013; Graves, 2009; Hurme, 2009; Merwin, 2006). Specific research topics of importance to nursing practice in rural environments include the following:

1. Most nurses indicate that they enjoy practicing in rural areas and are proud of what they do. They believe that their work deserves more recognition by professional nursing organizations. Also, the retention rate of nurses in some practice

settings is poor. The perspective of nurses who are dissatisfied with rural nursing provides a more complete picture of the rural experience. This information can be useful to a variety of people: other nurses who are considering rural practice, nurse managers in need of better screening tools to assess the fit between the nurse and the environment when interviewing applicants, planners of continuing nursing education programs, and faculty members who teach public health to undergraduate and graduate students.

2. More information is needed about the stressors and rewards of rural practice, in particular public health nursing. These data could lead to the development of stress management techniques to be used by nurses and their supervisors to retain nurses and to improve the quality of their workplace environment.

3. With the increasing number of rural residents in all regions of the United States, empirical data are needed on the particular nursing needs of rural client systems, especially under-represented groups, minorities, and other at-risk populations that vary by region and state.

4. A need also exists for the international perspective on the health of rural populations, and on nursing practice within the rural community. Australian, New Zealand, and Canadian nurse scholars have provided some insights into rural practice in these nations. Information is needed from less-industrialized nations as well as from those that are highly industrialized.

5. Technology increasingly is used in health care and seems to hold great potential in improving access to health care in rural and underserved areas. However, research is needed to determine the most efficient and effective way to meet the needs and preferences of rural clients, and to ensure quality.

6. Communication technology increasingly is used by institutions of higher learning to deliver educational programs to nurses who live and work some distance from campus. Empirical studies are needed to measure the most effective modalities to achieve desired learning outcomes and the impact on recruitment and retention of nurses in rural settings.

7. Rural–urban disparities in health status and health behaviors need closer examination from the nursing perspective. Evidence-based practice nursing guidelines are needed that take into consideration the rural context and preferences of residents who obtain health care in these settings.

## Preparing Nurses for Rural Practice Settings

Nurses in rural practice need broad knowledge about nursing including health promotion, primary prevention, rehabilitation, obstetrics, medical-surgical specialties, pediatrics, planning and implementing community assessments, and understanding the public health risks and needs for emergency preparedness in a particular state. A community's demographic profile and its principal industry(ies) can provide a snapshot of local social determinants that can affect health. Using demographic information, a nurse can anticipate the particular nursing skills that will be needed to care for clients in a catchment area (U.S.A. Center for Rural Health Preparedness, n.d.). In rural areas

nurses use their knowledge of resources and their ability to coordinate formal and informal services to coordinate a continuum of services for clients even when resources are sparse and fragmentation exists in the health care delivery system.

Technology has great potential for connecting rural public health providers and consumers with resources outside of their community. The concept of *telehealth* is an expansion of the term *telemedicine*. Essentially, telemedicine more narrowly focuses on the curative aspect of health care, whereas telehealth encompasses preventive, promotive, and curative aspects of health care and can include delivery of education/information to a more distant site. Telehealth uses a variety of technology solutions such as a health care provider communicating by e-mail with clients, ordering medications from a pharmacy, consulting with other health care providers, or accessing advanced or continuing education offered by a university located some distance from the receiving site. More specifically, telecommunication technology could be as simple as nurses in two or more different public health settings consulting over the telephone or via computer video conferencing coordinating local health fairs, or as complex as nurse scholars collaborating with international peers on a community health–focused research project or a medical specialist located at a health science center using complex robotic surgical technology on a client who is located in another country. Regardless of the practice setting, the nurse must be computer literate and be proficient in using the communication technology that is available in that community. Increasingly, the Internet is linking nurses in rural public health practice with nursing colleagues, educators, and researchers in urban-based academic settings, thereby addressing often-cited concerns associated with professional isolation (ANCC, 2013; Molinari & Bushy, 2012; Bushy & Winters, 2013).

## FUTURE PERSPECTIVES

It is important for all people involved in providing health care in rural areas to understand the possible problems they might encounter when trying to provide the continuum of needed services in an area with a disproportionally high number of underserved persons. Those who should be involved include residents, their elected representatives, the administrators of public and private health care agencies, and members of the media. The media need to focus on public health as well as hospital care and the lack of primary care providers in rural areas (deValpine, 2014). As discussed later, both case management and community-oriented primary health care (COPHC) are effective models for dealing with some of the care deficits and resolving rural health disparities.

## Scarce Resources and a Comprehensive Health Care Continuum

The current fragmented health care system makes it difficult to provide a comprehensive continuum of care to populations living in areas having scarce resources, such as money, personnel, equipment, and ancillary services. In rural communities, the most critically needed services are usually preventive services, such as health screening clinics, nutrition counseling, and

**BOX 19-7 Health-Related Priorities for Many Rural Communities**

- Access to care
- Cancer (screening, early intervention, oncology services)
- Diabetes (prevention, screening, tertiary care)
- Maternal–infant and children services
- Mental illness and behavioral health services
- Nutrition/obesity
- Drugs, alcohol, and substance abuse
- Use of tobacco products
- Education and an array of community-based programs
- Public health infrastructures
- Immunizations and infectious diseases
- Injury and violence prevention
- Family planning
- Environmental and occupational health
- Emergency medical services infrastructures
- Long-term care/assistive living facilities

From Bennett K, Olatosi B, Probst J: *Health Disparities: A Rural- Urban Chartbook*, 2008. Available at http://rhr.sph.sc.edu/report/(7-3)%20Health%20Disparities%20A%20Rural%20Urban%20Chartbook%20-%20Distribution%20Copy.pdf. Accessed January 8, 2011; Gamm L, Hutchison L, Dabney B, et al: *Rural Healthy People 2010: A Companion Document to Healthy People 2010*, Vol I, II, III, College Station, TX, 2003, The Texas A&M University System Health Science Center, School of Rural Health, Southwest Rural Health Research Center. Available at http://www.srph.tamhsc.edu/centers/rhp2010/publications.htm. Accessed January 8, 2011.

wellness education (Bolin and Bellamy, 2014; Gamm et al, 2003). Box 19-7 lists several health related priorities for rural communities.

Although the nursing needs vary by community, there is generally a need in most rural areas for the following:

- School and parish nurses
- Family planning services
- Prenatal and postpartum services
- Resources for individuals diagnosed with HIV/AIDS and their families
- Emergency medical services
- Resources for families of children with special needs, including those who are physically and mentally challenged
- Mental health services
- Resources for older adults (especially the frail elderly and those with declining mental capacity) to include a continuum of residential and respite services, including adult day care, hospice, homemaker assistance, and provision of nutritional meals along with public transportation for those who remain at home

Providing a continuum of care has been further hindered by the closure of many small hospitals in the past two decades. Of those that remain, many report financial problems that could lead to closure (NACRHHS, 2012). A shortage or the absence of even one provider, most often a physician or nurse, could mean that a small hospital must close its doors. Closure of the hospital has a ripple effect on the health of local residents, other health care services, recruitment and retention of health

professionals, as well as on economic development efforts in a small community (USDA, 2013a, 2013b; USDHHS, 2013).

The short supply and increasing demand for primary care providers in general, and nurses in particular, will continue for some time. To help solve this problem, elected officials and policy developers need nurses, especially those in advanced practice roles, to provide vital services in underserved areas. In an effort to effectively respond to this opportunity, nurses must be creative to ensure delivery of appropriate and acceptable services to at-risk and vulnerable populations who live in rural and underserved regions. Nurses must be sensitive to the health beliefs of clients, and then plan and provide nursing interventions that mesh with the community's cultural values and preferences.

### *Healthy People 2020* National Health Objectives Related to Rural Health

Because the demographic profile varies from community to community, each state has variations in the health status of its population. *Healthy People 2020* has important implications for nurses in that a significant number of at-risk populations cited in that policy-guiding document live in rural areas across the United States (Bolin and Bellamy, 2014; AHCPR, 2013a, 2013b). Consequently, priority objectives vary, depending on population mix, health risks, and health status of residents in the state.

**♥ HEALTHY PEOPLE 2020**

These selected objectives pertain to residents of both rural and urban areas:
- AHS-3: Increase the proportion of persons with a usual primary care provider.
- IVP-13: Reduce motor vehicle crash–related deaths.
- MHMD-9: Increase the proportion of adults with mental disorders who receive treatment.
- HDS-2: Reduce coronary heart disease deaths.
- IVP-1: Reduce fatal and nonfatal injuries.

From U.S. Department of Health and Human Services: *Healthy People 2020*, 2010. Available at http://www.healthypeople.gov/2020/default.aspx. Accessed January 9, 2011.

At the local level, communities have been using *Healthy People* as a guide for action and to identify objectives and establish meaningful goals. The three-volume *Rural Healthy People 2010: A Companion Document to Healthy People 2010* focused on the particular concerns relative to vulnerable populations in rural environments (Gamm et al, 2003). A parallel rural compendium is being developed for *Healthy People 2020* (Bolin and Bellamy, 2014).

The Center for Disease Control's (CDC, 2013a) *Healthy Communities Initiative* mobilized rural as well as urban communities to focus on chronic disease prevention. Individuals and groups at the local level collaborated with state health departments, the CDC, and other organizations to implement programs that promote and support good health in their community. This CDC initiative is a useful tool for state and local officials and health care planners to use to tailor *Healthy People* objectives to fit a community's specific needs, both rural and urban. Translating national objectives highlighted in *Healthy People 2020* (USDHHS, 2013) into achievable community health goals requires integration of the following components to ensure that services will be acceptable and appropriate for rural clients:

- Health statistics must be meaningful and understandable, and they must include appropriate process and outcome objectives that can be readily measured.
- Strategies must be designed that involve the public, private, and voluntary sectors of the community to achieve agreed-on local objectives.
- Coordinated efforts are needed to ensure that the community works together to achieve the goals.

Consider, for example, general objectives in developing a health plan for a rural county having a large population of young people. *Healthy People 2020* objectives for the county should target women of child-bearing age, children, and adolescents. Priority objectives should include offering accessible prenatal care programs, improving immunization levels, providing preventive dental care instructions, implementing vehicular accident prevention and firearm safety programs, and educating teachers and health professionals for early identification of cases of interpersonal violence. On the other hand, consider a rural county that has a higher number of residents over the age of 65 years, compared with the national average. Priority objectives in the health plan should target health risks and problems of older adults in that community. Specific objectives might include developing health-promoting programs to prevent chronic health problems, or establishing community programs to meet the needs of those having chronic illness, specifically cardiovascular disease, diabetes, hypertension, and accident-related disabilities; or, organizing a partnership to build progressive/assistive care residential facilities in the community. In general, the objectives in *Healthy People 2020* are pertinent to people living in all areas and not unique to rural residents. The *Healthy People 2020* box illustrates selected objectives that fit people in rural as well as more urban areas.

When implementing community-focused health plans that emerge from *Healthy People 2020*, consideration must always be given to the rural context, such as sparse population, geographic remoteness, scarce resources, personnel shortages, and physical, emotional, and social isolation. In addition to being actively involved in empowering the community and planning and delivering care, nurses play an important role in representing their community's perspective to local, state, regional, and national health planners and to their elected officials.

## BUILDING PROFESSIONAL-COMMUNITY-CLIENT PARTNERSHIPS IN RURAL SETTINGS

Health care reform initiatives are focusing on cutting costs while improving access to care with equitable quality for all citizens, especially vulnerable and underserved populations. State and local grassroots organizations must be actively involved for health care reform to succeed in rural areas. Specifically, professional-client-community partnerships are essential to accomplish reform at the local level. As seen in the Linking

Content to Practice box, nursing practice in rural areas is comprehensive and incorporates skills from nursing and public health. Two models have been found to be particularly useful for nurses in rural environments: case management and Community-Oriented Primary Health Care (COPHC).

### ⟫ LINKING CONTENT TO PRACTICE

As discussed, practice in rural areas relies on excellent nursing and public health skills in assessment, communication, cultural competency, problem solving, coalition building, coordination, and policy development, among others. Documents that guide the practice include the American Nurses Association Standards of Nursing Practice, the core competencies as identified by the Council on Linkages, and the Quad Council Public Health Nursing Competencies. As one example of the congruence, consider assessment. The Council on Linkages' Core Competency of "Assess the health status of populations and their related determinants of health and illness" under their analytic assessment skills is then elaborated on by the Quad Council as a public health nursing skill of "Conducts thorough health assessments of individuals, families, communities and populations" and the public health nursing practice standard under assessment of "the public health nurse collects comprehensive data pertinent to the health status of populations" (p. 15). The relationship among these three sets of standards continues through all phases of the public health care provision process.

From American Nurses Association: *Public Health Nursing: Scope and Standards of Practice*, Silver Spring, MD, 2007, Available at http://www.nursebooks.org; Public Health Foundation: *Council on Linkages: Core Competencies for Public Health Professionals*, 2008, Washington, DC, Author. Available at http://www.phf.org/link/index.htm. Accessed June 24, 2010; Quad Council: *Public Health Nursing Competencies*, 2009. Available at http://www.astdn.org/publication squadcouncilphncompetencies.htm. Accessed January 17, 2011.

### Case Management

Case management is a client-professional partnership that can be used to arrange a continuum of care for rural clients, with the case manager tailoring and blending formal and informal resources. Collaborative efforts between a client and the case manager allow clients to participate in their plan of care in an acceptable and appropriate way, especially when local resources are few and far between. The Practice Application at the end of this chapter demonstrates how nursing case management can allow an older adult resident to stay at home in a rural environment if adequate supports can be provided. Outcomes are often remarkably different when case management is used. Additional information on case management is found in Chapter 22.

### Community-Oriented Primary Health Care

COPHC is an effective model for delivering available, accessible, and acceptable services to vulnerable populations living in medically underserved areas. This model emphasizes flexibility, grassroots involvement, and professional-community partnerships. It blends primary care, public health, and prevention services, which are offered in a familiar and accessible setting. As shown in Box 19-8 the COPHC model is interprofessional, uses a problem-oriented approach, and mandates community involvement in all phases of the process (Graves, 2009; Molinari & Bushy, 2012).

---

### BOX 19-8   Community-Oriented Primary Health Care (COPHC): A Partnership Process

The steps in the COPHC process include the following:
- Define and characterize the community.
- Identify the community's health problems.
- Develop or modify health care services in response to the community's identified needs.
- Monitor and evaluate program process and client outcomes.

---

8. Identify potential funding sources needed to implement the program.
9. Establish the community's health care priority list, and involve many community members in considering and selecting their health care options.
10. Incorporate business principles in marketing the program.
11. Measure the health system's local economic impact.
12. Educate residents about the important role the local health care system plays in the economic infrastructure of the community and the consequences of a system failure.
13. Develop local leadership and support for the community's health system through training and providing experience in decision making.

*From McGinnis P: Rural Policy Development: A Community Leadership Development Approach, Kansas City, MO, 2003, National Rural Health Association.*

Building professional-community partnerships is an ongoing process. At various times, nurses, other health professionals, and community leaders must assume the role of advocate, change agent, educator, expert, or group facilitator to gain both active and passive support from the community. Partnerships involve give-and-take negotiations by all participants to reach consensus. Essentially, the process begins with professionals gaining entrance into a community, establishing rapport and trust with local people, and then working together to empower the community to resolve mutually defined problems and goals. As mentioned previously and discussed also in Chapter 20, the *Healthy Communities Initiative* is an excellent resource for developing, defining, and responding to the stated goals. Because of the importance of churches and schools in a rural community, leaders from those institutions often are key players in building provider-community partnerships. The organizational phase is a priority because it forms the foundation for all other activities related to planning, implementing, and evaluating community initiatives.

As was described for case management, professional-community partnerships allow more effective identification of existing informal support systems that are accepted by rural residents. The goal is to integrate community preferences with new or existing formal services. Public input should be encouraged early in the planning process and must continue throughout the process to allow the community to feel that it has ownership in the project. This strategy can go a long way to address local residents viewing the process as outsiders bringing another bureaucratic program into town. Strategies that nurses can use to enhance the building of partnerships in rural environments are listed in the How To Build Professional-Community-Client Partnerships box.

### HOW TO   Build Professional-Community-Client Partnerships
1. Gain the local perspective.
2. Assess the degree of public awareness and support for the cause.
3. Identify special interest groups.
4. List existing services to avoid duplication of programs.
5. Note real and potential barriers to existing resources and services.
6. Generate a list of potential community volunteers and professionals who are willing to assist with the project.
7. Create awareness among target groups of a particular program (e.g., individuals, families, seniors, church and recreation groups, health care professionals, law enforcement personnel, and members of other religious, service, and civic clubs).

Partnership models, such as case management and COPHC, have proven to be highly effective in areas with scarce resources and an insufficient number of health care providers. Individuals and communities who are informed, active participants in planning are more likely to develop consensus about the most appropriate solution for local problems. Subsequently, involved participants are more likely to use and support that system after it is implemented. Partnership models enhance the ability of rural communities to do what they historically have done well (i.e., assume responsibility for the services and institutions that serve their residents). Knowledge about partnership models and the skills to effectively implement them are useful for nurses who coordinate services that are accessible, available, and acceptable for rural populations in their catchment area.

---

### (QSEN) FOCUS ON QUALITY AND SAFETY EDUCATION FOR NURSES

**Targeted Competency: Quality Improvement**
Use data to monitor the outcomes of care processes and use improvement methods to design and test changes to continuously improve the quality and safety of health care systems.
Important aspects of quality improvement include:
- **Knowledge:** Explain the importance of variation and measurement in assessing quality of care.
- **Skills:** Use quality measures to understand performance.
- **Attitudes:** Value measurement and its role in good client care.

**Quality Improvement Question:**
Examine health statistics and demographic data in your geographic area to determine which vulnerable groups are predominant. Look on the web for examples of agencies you think provide services to these vulnerable groups. If the agency has a web page, read about the target population they serve, the types of services they provide, and how they are reimbursed for services. Learn about different agencies and share results during class. Based on your findings, identify gaps or overlaps in services provided to vulnerable groups in your community. Which data do these agencies collect to demonstrate the efficacy of their services? How could you deal with these gaps and overlaps to help clients receive needed services?

Prepared by Gail Armstrong, DNP, ACNS-BC, CNE, Associate Professor, University of Colorado Denver College of Nursing.

## PRACTICE APPLICATION

Mrs. Jones, an 89-year-old widow, was diagnosed over 10 years ago with progressive congestive heart failure. She continues to live in her beloved home of 60+ years in spite of being on continuous oxygen the last 3 years. She also has "bad knees" and gets around her house and yard with the use of a walker. Her husband of more than 60 years suddenly died 4 years ago of a heart attack while working on their farm. Their two married daughters live in California and Arkansas. The Midwestern town where she lives has about 1000 residents. The nearest hospital is more than 60 miles away from this town. Mrs. Jones's 82-year-old widowed sister, Lydia Thomas, lives a few blocks from her. Their 76-year-old brother recently entered the county nursing home located in a town 20 miles away.

Even with her dyspnea and physical limitations, Mrs. Jones is able to live alone with her dog and cat, and insists that she will not relinquish her independent lifestyle as has her brother. Yet, in the past year she has been hospitalized three times: for a bad chest cold, for a kidney infection, and after a neighbor found her lying unconscious by the picnic table in her yard. Her doctor says this episode was related to a "heart problem."

Upon being discharged from the hospital, Crystal Moore, the local home health nurse, was assigned to visit Mrs. Jones. Ms. Moore's office is based in the County Senior Center near the nursing home where the brother is a resident. He is also a client of Ms. Moore and she visits him every Wednesday. The nurse provides outreach services to all the residents in the county referred to her by a large homehealth agency located in the city 70 miles away. As a case manager, she works closely with the hospital's discharge planners to arrange a continuum of care for clients in the county. Nursing-related activities include coordinating formal and informal services for clients, including biomedical supplies, oxygenation, nutrition, hydration, pharmacological care, arranging for personal care, homemaker assistance, writing checks, home maintenance, emergency respite services, and home delivery of meals.

A. Describe the nursing roles that Ms. Moore uses in coordinating a continuum of care for Mrs. Jones in terms of nutrition, oxygenation, pharmaceutical and biomedical equipment, transportation, and homemaker assistance.

B. Identify formal health care and support resources that can be accessed for Mrs. Jones.

C. Identify informal support resources that might be available in the small community that could help to ensure that Mrs. Jones is safe.

D. Identify three outcomes for Mrs. Jones that can be achieved by using nursing care (case) management.

E. Select a rural community in your geographic area. Create hypothetical situations, or select real clients with real health problems (e.g., an older adult with Alzheimer's disease, a middle-aged person with cancer requiring end-of-life care, a child who is dependent on technology as a result of a farm accident). Prepare a list of services and referral agencies in that community that could be used to develop a continuum of care for each of these cases. How are these the same as, or different from, the case described in this chapter?

F. How could a public or home health nurse who is new to the community learn about formal and informal resources that could be accessed to develop a continuum of care for a rural resident for whom she cares?

**Answers can be found on the Evolve site.**

## KEY POINTS

1. There is wide diversity in the demography, economy, and geography of rural communities.
2. Not all rural communities are based on an agricultural economy; most are not!
3. Although many are struggling, not all rural communities are suffering economically. Some rural communities only need more extensive economic development for sustainability.
4. Some rural towns are located in urban counties.
5. There are wide variations in the health status of rural populations, depending on genetic, social, environmental, economic, and political factors.
6. There is a higher prevalence of working poor in rural America than in more populated areas.
7. There are rural-urban health disparities. Rural adults 18 years and older overall are in poorer health than their urban counterparts; nearly 50% have been diagnosed with at least one major chronic condition. However, they average one less physician visit each year than healthier urban counterparts.

8. More than 26% of rural families are below the poverty level; more than 40% of all rural children younger than 18 years of age live in poverty.
9. General practitioners and nurse practitioners are usual providers of care for rural adults and children.
10. Rural residents must often travel more than 30 minutes to access a health care provider.
11. Nurses must take into consideration the belief systems and lifestyles of a rural population when planning, implementing, and evaluating community services.
12. Barriers to rural health care include the lack of availability, affordability, accessibility, and acceptability of services.
13. Partnership models, particularly case management and community-oriented primary health care (COPHC), are effective models to provide a comprehensive continuum of care in environments with scarce resources.

## CLINICAL DECISION-MAKING ACTIVITIES

- Compare and contrast the terms *urban, suburban, rural, frontier, farm, non-farm residency,* and *metropolitan* and *micropolitan areas.*
- Describe residency as a continuum, ranging from farm residency to core metropolitan residency.
- Discuss economic, social, and cultural factors that affect rural lifestyle and the health care–seeking behaviors of residents who live there.
- Identify factors that affect the accessibility, affordability, availability, and acceptability of services in the health care delivery system.
- Compare and contrast the health status and lifestyle behaviors of rural and urban residents.
- Summarize key nursing concepts in terms of practice in the rural context.

- Examine the characteristics of rural community nursing practice and describe how these might differ from those of practice in more populated settings.
- Compare and contrast challenges, opportunities, and benefits of living and practicing as a nurse in the rural environment.
- Evaluate case management and community-oriented primary care as partnership models that can help nurses enhance the continuum of care for clients living in an environment with sparse resources.
- Propose potential areas for rural nursing research activities. Specify research questions that focus on the professional and clinical concerns of public health nurses who practice in the rural context.

## REFERENCES

Agency for Health Care Policy and Research (AHCPR): *National healthcare disparities report*, 2013a. Available at: http://nhqrnet.ahrq.gov/inhqrdr/reports/nhdr. Accessed March 28, 2014.

Agency for Health Care Policy and Research (AHCPR): Chapter 10, Priority Populations. In *National healthcare disparities report*, 2013b. Available at: http://www.ahrq.gov/research/findings/nhqrdr/nhdr12/chap10a.html#chap10ref30. Accessed March 28, 2014.

American Legacy Foundation: *Tobacco Facts Sheet: Youth and Tobacco*. Washington, DC, 2013, Author. Available at: http://www.legacyforhealth.org/content/download/568/6824/file/LEG-FactSheet-Youth_and_Tobacco-AUGUST2013.pdf. Accessed March 28, 2014.

American Nurses Association Credentialing Center (ANCC): *Pathway to excellence program*, 2013. Available at: http://www.nursecredentialing.org/Pathway/AboutPathway. Accessed on March 28, 2014.

Bigbee J, Crowder E: The Red Cross Rural Nursing Service: an innovation of public health nursing delivery. *Publ Health Nurs* 2(2):109, 1985.

Bolin J, Bellamy G: *Rural Healthy People: 2020*. 2014, Southwest Rural Health Research Center, Texas A & M Health Science Center, School of Rural Public Health. Available at: http://www.srph.tamhsc.edu/centers/srhrc/images/rhp2020#rhp2020. Accessed March 28, 2014.

Bureau of the Census: *Population distribution and change 2000-2010*, 2011. Available at: http://www.census.gov/prod/cen2010/briefs/c2010br-01.pdf. Accessed March 28, 2014.

Bureau of the Census: *Annual estimates of the resident population for incorporated places, April 1, 2-10 to July 1, 2012*, 2012. Available at: http://www.census.gov/popest/data/cities/totals/2012/SUB-EST2012-3.html. Accessed March 28, 2014.

Bureau of the Census: *2010 Census interactive website*, 2013. Available at: http://www.census.gov/2010census/. Accessed March 28, 2014.

Bureau of Health Professions (BHPR): *Shortage Designation: HPSAs, MUAs, MUPs*. Washington, DC, 2013a. Available at: http://www.hrsa.gov/shortage/. Accessed March 18, 2014.

Bureau of Health Professions (BHPR): *The U.S. nursing workforce: trends in supply and education*, 2013b. Available at: http://bhpr.hrsa.gov/healthworkforce/supplydemand/nursing/nursingworkforce/nursingworkforcefullreport.pdf. Accessed March 28, 2014.

Bushy A: The rural context and nursing practice. In Molinari D, Bushy A, editors: *The Rural Nurse: Transition to Practice*. New York, 2012, Springer.

Bushy A: Health disparities in rural populations across the lifespan. In Winters C, editor: *Rural Nursing: Concepts, Theory and Practice*, 4 ed. New York, 2013, Springer Publishing.

Bushy A, Winters C: Nursing workforce development, clinical practice, research and nursing theory: Connecting the dots. In Winters C, editor: *Rural Nursing: Concepts, Theory and Practice*, ed 4. New York, NY, 2013, Springer Publishing.

Bushy A: Rural health care ethics. In Warren J, Smalley K, editors: *Rural Health: Best Practices and Preventive Modes*. New York, NY, 2014, Springer.

Case T: Work stresses of community health nurses in Oklahoma. In Bushy A, editor: *Rural Nursing*, vol 2. Newbury Park, CA, 1991, Sage.

Centers for Disease Control and Prevention (CDC): *Healthy communities program: an overview*, 2013a. Available at: http://www.cdc.gov/nccdphp/dch/programs/healthycommunities program/overview. Accessed March 28, 2014.

Centers for Disease Control (CDC): *Health disparities and inequalities report: United States 2013*, 2013b. Available at: http://www.cdc.gov/mmwr/pdf/other/su6203.pdf. Accessed March 28, 2014.

Crosby R, Wendell M, Vanderpool R, et al: *Rural Populations and Health: Determinants, Disparities and Solutions*. Hoboken, NJ, 2012, Wiley.

Davis D, Droes N: Community health nursing in rural and frontier counties. *Nursing Clin N Am* 28:159, 1993.

deValpine M: Extreme nursing: A qualitative assessment of nurse retention in a remote setting. *Int Electronic J Rural Remote Health* *Res, Educ, Pract Policy*, 2014. Available at: http://www.rrh.org.au/articles/showabstractearlynthamer.asp?ArticleID=2859. Accessed March 28, 2014.

Gamm L, Hutchison L, Dabney B, et al: *Rural Healthy People 2010: A Companion Document to Healthy People 2010*, vol I, II, III. College Station, TX, 2003, The Texas A&M University System Health Science Center, School of Rural Health, Southwest Rural Health Research Center. Available at: http://www.srph.tamhsc.edu/centers/rhp2010/publications.htm. Accessed March 28, 2014.

Graves B: Community-based participatory research: toward eliminating rural health disparities. *Online J Rural Nurs Health Care* 9(1):12–14, 2009. Available at: http://rnojournal.binghamton.edu/index.php/RNO/article/viewFile/98/80. Accessed March 28, 2014.

Hurme E: Competencies for nursing practice in a rural critical access hospital. *Online J Rural Nurs Health Care* 9(2):67–81, 2009. Available at: http://rnojournal.binghamton.edu/index.php/RNO/article/viewFile/88/72. Accessed March 28, 2014.

Institute of Medicine (IOM): *The future of nursing: leading change: advancing health*, 2010. Available at: http://www.nap.edu/catalog.php?record_id=12956. Accessed March 28, 2014.

Krey A: ACA and migrants: challenges and opportunities. *Migrant Clinician Network (MCN) Streamline* 20(1):5–6, 2014. Available at: http://www.migrantclinician.org/services/publications/

streamline.html. Accessed March 28, 2014.

Leipert B, Leach B, Thurston W, editors: *Rural Women's Health*. Toronto, 2012, University of Toronto Press.

Long K, Weinert C: Rural nursing: developing a theory base. *Scholarly Inquiry Nurs Pract* 3:99–113, 1989.

Meckler L, Chinni D: City vs. country: how where we live deepens the nation's political divide. Differences between rural and urban America. *Wall St J* 2014. Available at: http://online.wsj.com/news/articles/SB10001424052702303636404579395532755485004?mg=reno64-wsj&url=http%3A%2F%2Fonline.wsj.com%2Farticle%2FSB10001424052702303636404579395532755485004.html. Accessed March 28, 2014.

Merwin B, editor: *Annual Review of Nursing Research: Focus on Rural Health*, vol 26. New York, 2006, Springer.

Mississippi State University-Extension Service: *A Community Report of Oktibbeha County: Smart Aging—Healthy Future*. Mississippi State, MS, 2012. Available at: http://msucares.com/health/smart_aging/community_reports.html. Accessed March 28, 2014.

Molinari D, Bushy A, editors: *The Rural Nurse: Transition to Practice*. New York, 2012, Springer.

National Advisory Committee on Rural Health and Human Services (NACRHHS): *The 2011 report to the secretary: rural health and human services issues*, 2012. Available at: http://www.hrsa.gov/advisorycommittees/rural/2011secreport.pdf. Accessed March 28, 2014.

National Center for Farmworkers' Health (NCFH): *Farmworkers' health*, 2014. Available at: http://www.ncfh.org/. Accessed March 28, 2014.

National Center for Health Statistics (NCHS): *Summary health statistics for U.S. adults, National Health Interview Survey 2012*, 2014. Available at: http://www.cdc.gov/nchs/data/series/sr_10/sr10_260.pdf. Accessed March 28, 2014.

Nelson W, editor: *Handbook for Rural Health Care Ethics*. Lebanon, NH, 2009, Dartmouth. Available at: http://dms.dartmouth.edu/cfm/resources/ethics/. Accessed March 28, 2014.

Occupational Safety and Health Administration (OSHA): *Safety and Health Topics: Agricultural Operations*. Washington, DC, 2013, OSHA. Available at: https://www.osha.gov/dsg/topics/agriculturaloperations/index.html. Accessed March 28, 2014.

Roberge C: Who stays in rural nursing practice? An international review of the literature on factors influencing rural nurse retention. *Online J Rural Nurs Health Care* 9(1):82–93, 2009. Available at: http://

www.thefreelibrary.com/Who+stays+in+rural+nursing+practice%3f+An+international+review+of+the...-a0201712846. Accessed March 28, 2014.

Smalley K, Warren J, Rainer J, editors: *Rural Mental Health: Issues, Policies, and Best Practices*. New York, 2012, Springer Publishing Company.

South Carolina Rural Research Center: *Key facts. HIV in rural America*, 2013. Available at: http://rhr.sph.sc.edu/report/(11-1)Fact%20Sheet%20HIV%20AIDS%20in%20Rural%20America.pdf. Accessed March 28, 2014.

U.S.A. Center for Rural Public Health Preparedness, n.d. Available at http://usacenter.org/training.html. Accessed March 28, 2014.

U.S. Department of Agriculture (USDA): *Rural America at a glance: 2013 edition*, 2013a. Available at: http://www.ers.usda.gov/publications/eb-economic-brief/eb24.aspx#.UyHkNvldWMJ. Accessed March 28, 2014.

U.S. Department of Agriculture (USDA): *Rural classifications 2013*, 2013b. Available at: http://ers.usda.gov/topics/rural-economy-population/rural-classifications.aspx#.Uwt0qeNdXTo. Accessed March 28, 2014.

U.S. Department of Health and Human Services (USDHHS): *Healthy People 2020*, 2013. Available at: http://www

.healthypeople.gov/2020/default.aspx. Accessed March 12, 2014.

Warren J, Smalley K, editors: *Rural Health: Best Practices and Preventive Modes*. New York, NY, 2014, Springer.

Williams M: Rural professional isolation: An integrative review. *Online J Rural Nurs Health Care* 12(2):2012. Available at: http://rnojournal.binghamton.edu/index.php/RNO/article/view/51. Accessed March 28, 2014.

Williams M, Andrews J, Zanni K, et al: Rural nursing: searching for the state of the science. *Online J Rural Nurs Health Care* 12(2):102–117, 2012. Available at: http://rnojournal.binghamton.edu/index.php/RNO/article/view/117. Accessed March 28, 2014.

Winters C, Lee H: *Rural Nursing: Concepts, Theory and Practice*, ed 3. New York, 2009, Springer Publishing.

Winters C, editor: *Rural Nursing: Concepts, Theory and Practice*, ed 4. New York, 2013, Springer Publishing.

Woolston C: Lonesome doc: medicine in a small town. *AARP Bulletin*, June 10, 2010. Available at: http://www.aarp.org/health/doctors-hospitals/info-06-2010/medicine_in_a_small_town.html. Accessed March 28, 2014.

# Promoting Health Through Healthy Communities and Cities

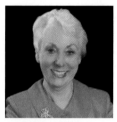

### Jeanette Lancaster, PhD, RN, FAAN

Dr. Lancaster is Professor and Dean Emerita of Nursing at the University of Virginia. She has edited this book with Dr. Marcia Stanhope through its previous eight editions.

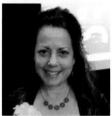

### Loren Kelly, RN, MSN

Ms. Loren Kelly is a Clinician Educator at the University of New Mexico College of Nursing. She is also the Interprofessional Education Coordinator for the College at the University of New Mexico Health Sciences Center. She earned her BA in Political Science from the State University of New York at Potsdam; the Associate degree in Nursing at Castleton State College in Castleton, CT, her MSN in Community Health Nursing from the University of New Mexico, College of Nursing.

## ADDITIONAL RESOURCES

ⓔ **Evolve website http://evolve.elsevier.com/Stanhope**
- *Healthy People 2020*
- WebLinks
- Quiz
- Case Studies
- Glossary
- Answers to Practice Application

## OBJECTIVES

*After reading this chapter, the student should be able to do the following:*

1. Discuss the history of the Healthy Communities and Cities movement.
2. Discuss the Centers for Disease Control and Prevention Healthy Communities Program.
3. Describe the core concepts and principles that guide the development of a healthy community program.
4. Describe the steps used when working with communities in the Healthy Communities and Cities process.
5. Apply the steps in working with Healthy Communities and Cities to the concepts of health promotion.
6. Explain the role nurses can assume in working with Healthy Communities and Cities.

## KEY TERMS

appropriate technology, p. 444
Community Health Promotion Model, p. 450
community participation, p. 444
equity, p. 444
health promotion, p. 444
Healthy Communities and Cities (HCC), p. 442

healthy public policy, p. 445
international cooperation, p. 444
multisectoral cooperation, p. 444
primary health care, p. 444
—*See Glossary for definitions*

The Healthy Communities and Cities (HCC) initiative, or movement, began with the World Health Organization (WHO) in 1986 with the signing of the Ottawa Charter for Health Promotion. The initiative has grown and changed since 1986. This initiative, originally called *Healthy Cities,* has assumed a healthy communities focus in recent years. Some locales use the term *healthy communities and cities,* whereas other locales talk about *healthy municipalities and cities,* and still others use the term *healthy communities.* The Centers for Disease Control and Prevention (CDC) in the United States initiated work in this area in 2003, and called their program the *steps program.* The CDC program is now called *Healthy Communities.* The term *healthy communities* is used in this chapter; however, reference is made to other terms in order to describe the history of the movement and to refer to specific programs that use a term other than *healthy communities and cities.* The goal of this movement is to promote health through community engagement and collaboration to activate and diffuse local changes that support good health. The premise is that community members must be involved in identifying the need for health programs and in developing programs to meet those needs. Building healthy communities relies on broad-based participation to make systems change in communities that can improve the health of the residents. The overall goals are to build community capacity, prevent chronic diseases, reduce health risk factors and attain health equity.

This chapter provides an introduction to the history of the HCC movement and to the basic terminology related to the movement. It describes various models in which communities have structured their programs both in the United States and selected other countries. Key facilitators and barriers to the Healthy Communities process are discussed, as is the role for nurses in supporting the development and sustainment of healthy communities.

## HISTORY OF THE HEALTHY COMMUNITIES AND CITIES MOVEMENT

HCC is found in many regions of the world. The movement began in 1986 when the WHO's Ottawa Charter became the first worldwide action plan for health promotion. At that time, the delegates to the conference declared that the following broad categories were prerequisites to health: peace, shelter, education, food, income, a stable ecosystem, sustainable resources, social justice, and equity. This is a much different approach to viewing health than the individualistic approach that holds that each person is responsible for his or her own health. Although 1986 seems to be in the distant past, the

areas for action that were determined by the *Ottawa Charter for Health Promotion* are highly relevant today (WHO, 1986). They are as follows:

- *Building healthy public policy:* Many countries around the world have begun to recognize the need to integrate health considerations into policy making and programming across sectors to achieve better health and health equity. One example of this is the Health in All Policies (HiAP) approach to improve population health. What this means is that health and equity must be embedded into governmental decision making at local, state, and national levels for collaboration across all of the sectors that influence health. Intersectoral collaboration includes policies in the areas of education, housing, transportation, land use, and neighborhood safety to promote health equity.
- *Creating supportive environments:* For example, when communities are being revitalized or developed, places should be designated as "green areas," and made accessible to the public with parks, walking or bike paths, and fitness facilities. Both work and leisure should be a source of health for people. See Chapter 17, Integrating Multilevel Approaches to Promote Community Health for a discussion of how the environment, especially the built environment affects health.
- *Strengthening community action:* The Ottawa Charter states (and this continues to hold true) that health promotion is most effective in communities when residents are fully engaged in the development and implementation of programs. This requires a "tried and true" public health approach in which nurses listen to and respond to the needs of the community. Community members need to be involved in setting priorities, making decisions, planning strategies, and implementing them in order to attain better health.
- *Developing personal skills:* This includes providing information and teaching people the skills that they need in order to be healthy, such as regular and competent hand washing, choosing the right foods, engaging in regular age-appropriate exercise, and learning to avoid risk factors and increase their protective factors. This step increases the options available to people so they can have more control over their own health and their environments.
- *Reorienting health services:* This involves health care systems emphasizing health promotion and prevention, beyond providing clinical and curative services. Individuals, community groups, health practitioners, health care institutions, and the government share responsibility for health promotion (WHO, 2010). The following Quality and Safety Education for Nurses box describes the importance of safety in community care.

## QSEN FOCUS ON QUALITY AND SAFETY EDUCATION FOR NURSES

As described in earlier chapters of the text, including Chapter 2: History of Public Health and Public Health Nursing, there are six Quality and Safety in Nursing competencies. All of the competencies could easily apply to Healthy Communities and Cities. However, safety is especially important for a healthy community program. Safety is an important competency for public health nurses who work in rural, suburban, and urban areas and for nurses who care for clients and communities in developed and less-developed countries. Aspects of community safety include but are not limited to the following:

1. **Knowledge:** Learn about the potential threats to safety including from the physical and social environments including those at home, school, and at worksites.
2. **Skills:** If a safety threat is identified, such as toxic materials from a factory being channeled into a water source, organize appropriate community leaders, workers, and volunteers to work toward reducing the pollution.
3. **Attitudes:** Be aware of the various conflicting points of view and goals in a situation in which industrial pollution affects the health of the community.

### Safety Question

If you think that a particular industry is emitting noxious chemicals into the air or water of the community, how do you get specific information to inform your actions?

**Answer:** Start by going to the Environmental Protection Agency (EPA) website (http://www.epa.gov) and search for pollutants by categories including ZIP code, address, or facility name. See Envirofacts Multisystem Search User Guide at http://www.epa.gov/enviro/facts/multisystem_user_guide.html.

As discussed in Chapter 17, health promotion is a process designed to help people increase control over, and improve, their health. Health promotion is not just the responsibility of the health sector but rather includes individuals, families, groups, and communities. Strategies and programs should be customized to meet local needs and take into account different cultural needs, economies, customs, resources, and priorities. The original goals of the Ottawa Conference continue to be areas of concern, and work must continue to achieve the goals. Chapter 4 also addresses, from a global health perspective, the need for a healthy community approach in selected countries around the world.

HCC began in the United States in 1988, with Healthy Cities Indiana and the California Healthy Cities project. Healthy Cities Indiana adapted the European experiences to the American context. The concept of Healthy Communities was used to include localities that were not cities but rather smaller communities such as towns or counties. In recent years, many U.S. communities have initiated the HCC process with the result that thousands of communities have taken local action to promote health. Several of these communities are featured in the chapter as examples of what a focus on health promotion at the community level would look like.

In other parts of the world, HCC has different names, including Healthy Islands, Healthy Villages, and, in Latin America, Healthy Municipalities and Communities. In addition, national networks have developed in Australia, Canada, Costa Rica, Iran,

and Egypt. Other regional networks have been developed in Francophone Africa, Latin America, Southeast Asia, and the western Pacific. Particular attention is given later in the chapter to Healthy Municipalities and Communities in the Pan American Health Organization (PAHO) region, since PAHO's work is long-standing and well developed and has demonstrated effective results.

Some claim that the concept of a healthy community or city is not new (Hancock, 1993). It is based on the belief that the health of the community is largely influenced by the environment in which people live and that health problems have multiple causes: social, economic, political, environmental, and behavioral. The HCC process has been applied to rural and metropolitan areas. The HCC process engages local residents in action and is based on the premise that when people have the opportunity to work out their own locally defined health problems they will find sustainable solutions to those problems. This concept is integral to good public health practice, which is to engage those for whom programs are being developed in the identification of need for, planning, implementing, and evaluating the programs. The *Healthy People 2020* process is consistent with the way healthy communities and cities have developed their priorities and plans. One of the four goals of *Healthy People 2020* is to create physical and social environments that promote good health for all. This goal relies on an ecologic perspective that says that health and health behaviors are determined by many influences including personal, organizational, environmental, and policy factors. Many of the goals of *Healthy People 2020* will be challenging to meet in light of the poor economic conditions in the United States and many other countries. For example, it is difficult to increase the income of low-income persons in an era in which people continue to lose their jobs and where unemployment, especially unemployment of youth, is high. See the Healthy People 2020 box for objectives that relate to healthy communities and cities.

### ♥ HEALTHY PEOPLE 2020

#### *Selected Goals That Pertain to Healthy Communities*

- ECBP-8: Increase the proportion of worksites that offer a comprehensive employee health promotion program to their employees.
- ECBP-9: Increase the proportion of employees who participate in employer-sponsored health promotion activities.
- ECBP-11: Increase the proportion of local health departments that have established culturally appropriate and linguistically competent community health promotion and disease prevention programs.
- PA-13: Increase the proportion of trips made by walking.
- PA-1: Reduce the proportion of adults who engage in no leisure-time physical activity.
- PA-4: Increase the proportion of the nation's public and private schools that require daily physical education for all students.
- OSH-9: Increase the proportion of employees who have access to workplace programs

From U.S. Department of Health and Human Services, Healthy People 2020, Washington, DC, 2010, U.S. Government Printing Office.

## DEFINITION OF TERMS

There are many definitions of a healthy community. The *Healthy People 2010* document described a healthy community as one that included those elements that enable people to maintain a high quality of life and productivity (USDHHS, 2000). To expand on this definition, consider what was stated in the document *Healthy People in Healthy Communities: A Community Planning Guide Using Healthy People 2010*: that a healthy community would include access to health care services that include both treatment and prevention for all community members; the community would be safe; and there would be adequate roads, schools, playgrounds, and other services to meet the needs of the people in the community; and that the environment would be healthy and safe (USDHHS, 2001).

The CDC defines a healthy place as one that is "designed and built to improve the quality of life for all people who live, work, worship, learn, and play within their borders—where every person is free to make choices amid a variety of healthy, available, accessible, and affordable options" (CDC, 2014, p. 201). The CDC also points out that a healthy community is one that continuously creates and improves both the physical and social environments and expands community resources to enable people to mutually support each other in carrying out essential life functions as well as in developing to their maximum potential. A healthy community seeks to improve the quality of life of its people and does this through collaboration, partnerships, diverse and extensive citizen ownership, and partnership in the process.

The principles of primary health care (WHO and UNICEF, 1978) and the Ottawa Charter for Health Promotion (WHO, 1986) were instrumental in the development of the Healthy Cities movement. Primary health care refers to meeting the basic health needs of a community by providing readily accessible health services. Because health problems transcend international borders, international cooperation is important to ensure health. The principles of primary health care include equity, health promotion, community participation, multisectoral cooperation, appropriate technology, and international cooperation.

Equity implies providing accessible services to promote the health of populations most at risk for health problems (e.g., the poor, the young, older adults, minorities, the homeless, and immigrants and refugees). As discussed in Chapter 17, health promotion and disease prevention focus on providing community members with a positive sense of health that strengthens their physical, mental, and emotional capacities. Individuals within communities become involved in health promotion through community participation, whereby well-informed and motivated community members participate in planning, implementing, and evaluating health programs. Multisectoral cooperation is the coordinated action by all parts of a community, from local government officials to grassroots community members. Appropriate technology refers to affordable social, biomedical, and health services that are relevant and acceptable to individuals' health, needs, and concerns.

## ASSUMPTIONS ABOUT COMMUNITY PRACTICE

There are different models of community practice, and the assumptions that professionals have about communities shape the implementation of the HCC process. The classic work of Rothman and Tropman (1987) describing these different models and some of the key assumptions continue to be relevant today, as shown in the examples used in this chapter. The key models for community practice include the following:

1. Locality development is a process-oriented model that emphasizes consensus, cooperation, and building group identity and a sense of community.
2. Social planning stresses rational-empirical problem solving, usually by outside professional experts. Social planning does not focus on building community capacity or fostering fundamental social change.
3. Social action, on the other hand, aims to increase the problem-solving ability of the community with concrete actions that attempt to correct the imbalance of power and privilege of an oppressed or disadvantaged group in the community.

Effective models of community practice use a partnership between citizens and professionals in which there is delegated power and citizen control (Rothman and Tropman, 1987). A partnership approach, considered a bottom-up approach, incorporates the concepts of a multisectoral approach as well as community participation. A partnership approach contrasts with the top-down approaches in which professionals and experts tell the citizens what to do rather than involve and ask them.

## HEALTHY COMMUNITIES AND CITIES IN THE UNITED STATES

In the following paragraphs, HCC initiatives in various regions of the United States are discussed. These examples show the different models of community practice that are being implemented. Specifically, the CDC's Healthy Communities Program emphasizes policy, systems, and environmental changes that focus on chronic diseases and that encourage people to be more physically active, eat a healthy diet, and not use tobacco. The rationale is based on the fact that about 50% of Americans are affected by chronic disease, and these diseases account for 7 of the 10 leading causes of death in the country. Also, there are many direct and indirect costs associated with being obese and overweight. Many chronic diseases are preventable. By preventing a chronic disease from occurring, people can enjoy a higher quality of life, communities have a decreased burden of illness, and both the state and federal governments are able to reduce the amount they spend on health care (CDC, 2011). Some examples of chronic diseases cited by the CDC include the fact that heart disease and stroke account for 30% of all deaths in the United States; that nearly 26 million Americans have diabetes; and one of every 3 adults and 1 of 5 children aged 6-19 in the United States are obese (CDC, 2011, p. 2). The CDC said also that more than half of all adults fail to meet recommendations for aerobic physical activity based on the *2008 Physical Activity Guidelines for Americans*; that tobacco is the single most preventable cause of disease, disability, and death; and that excessive alcohol use is the third leading cause of death related to lifestyle (CDC, 2011, p. 2).

These chronic disease facts support the priority that the CDC has placed on funding projects that will interrupt chronic diseases in communities around the country. Since 2003, the CDC's Healthy Communities Program has funded more than 330 rural, urban, and tribal communities to support their goals. Specifically, their programs include Strategic Alliances for Health Communities, ACHIEVE (Action Communities for Health, Innovation, and EnVironmental ChangE), REACH U.S., Pioneering Healthy Communities (in collaboration with the YMCA of the USA), and Steps Communities (CDC, 2014). Also, Communities Putting Prevention to Work (CPPW) is a locally driven program that supports 50 communities as they tackle obesity and tobacco use. The CDC (2014) says that over 50 million people, or one in six Americans, live in a city, town, county or tribal community that benefits from these programs.

The CDC has also developed a set of "tools for community action" that can be used in developing healthy communities. Some of these tools are as follows:

1. Community Health Online Resource Center: formerly the Community Health Resources Database: see http://cdc.gov/ DCH_CHORC/ to find assistance in planning, implementing, and evaluating community health interventions and programs that address their focus on chronic disease.
2. The Community Guide: see http://www.thecommunity guide.org/index.html to find evidence-based public health and community health interventions.
3. Community Health Assessment and Group Evaluation (CHANGE) Tool: Community leaders can use this tool to see what local policy, systems, and environmental strategies are currently in place in their communities and identify areas where health strategies are needed. CHANGE assists communities to define and prioritize areas for their own improvement. See http://www.cdc.gov/nccdphp/dch/ programs/healthycommunitiesprogram/tools/change/pdf/ changeactionguide.htm. Accessed August 15, 2014.
4. Action Guides: *The Community Health Promotion Handbook: Action Guides to Improve Community Health* (Partnership for Prevention, 2008). In collaboration with the Partnership for Prevention program, the CDC has developed a set of "how-to" guides for five community-level health promotion strategies related to its chronic disease prevention target areas of diabetes self-management, physical activity, and tobacco-use cessation. See http://www.prevent.org/ Initiatives/Action-Guides.aspx for a listing of specific guides. Also, see the CDC website for the other five guides to help communities develop health programs.

Given the usefulness of the CDC *Community Health Promotion Handbook*, further discussion is warranted here. The recommendations for the five guides that the CDC chose came from the Task Force on Community Preventive Services (TFCPS, 2005). The handbooks primarily target public health

professionals but also can be used by community leaders. The Task Force on Community Preventive Services continually updates its recommendations. See www.uspreventiveservicetask force.org. The current task force is called the U.S. Preventive Services Task Force (USDHHS, 2014). This guide provides health professionals with an authoritative source for making decisions about preventive services. The guides build on a socio-ecological model that recognizes that social and physical environments affect health and health behavior. This model divides the environment into five areas that affect health behavior: individual, interpersonal, organizational, community, and policy. Using the *Handbook* relies on the same process used in the assessment of a community. In other words, before deciding which of the five areas to target in your work, follow these steps:

1. Conduct a needs assessment and set health priorities.
2. Find out what social and environmental factors may affect each health priority as well as what options are available for dealing with the chosen health priorities.
3. Think about the acceptability (to the community) and the feasibility (are resources available, etc.) to implement the project(s).

As you work with the action guides, remember to take small steps and do first things first; involve the appropriate people and do not be reluctant to make changes as you go based on what you learn and the outcomes you have (Partnership for Prevention, 2008).

## HEALTHY COMMUNITIES AND CITIES AROUND THE WORLD: SELECTED EXAMPLES

As mentioned earlier, PAHO in collaboration with the WHO has a long-standing involvement in developing healthy communities that they call the Healthy Municipalities and Communities Movement. The mission of this movement is to "strengthen the implementation of health promotion activities at the local level, making health promotion a high priority of the political agenda; fostering the involvement of government authorities and the active participation of the community, supporting dialogue, sharing knowledge and experiences and stimulating collaboration among municipalities and countries" (PAHO, 2012). Other key concepts in their approach include multisectoral partnerships to improve social and health conditions and advocacy for developing healthy public policy, maintaining healthy environments, and promoting healthy lifestyles. PAHO believes that creating a healthy municipality involves a process that relies on strong political commitment and support that is aligned with equally strong communities who are determined to achieve their goals and who participate actively in the process of goal achievement (PAHO, 2012).

PAHO recommends a participatory development framework to gain commitment from the mayor, local government (all sectors), and representatives of community groups and organizations. PAHO has found this process to be the most effective in the Americas. The phases are as follows:

1. Aspects in the initial phase of the process
   - Meet with local government authorities and community leaders to gain their perspectives about such things as

healthy spaces and health promotion and to request that they make a public statement as well as a joint declaration of their commitment.
- Create an intersectoral, community planning committee.
- Conduct a needs assessment including analysis of problems and needs.
- Build consensus and decide on priorities for action.
2. Steps in the planning process
   - Train the committee and task forces to ensure that they understand the concept of healthy community, the settings approach to health promotion, and participatory methods including needs assessment, planning, evaluation, and health education.
   - Develop an action plan.
   - Mobilize resources needed to implement the plan and develop a detailed work plan.
3. Moments in the consolidation phase of the process
   - Implement activities that are included in the plan. Examples might be establishing health-promoting schools, workplaces, markets, hospitals, and other healthy environments.
   - Evaluate the results as well as the quality of participation.
   - Share knowledge and experiences with others.

PAHO notes that the steps that work in its region may be somewhat different from those that have been successful in Canada, the United States, and Europe. Later in this chapter, the 20 steps that PAHO says have been used by these other countries are cited as a way for nurses and other public health workers to develop a healthy community strategy. Interestingly, PAHO has found that it must start its process by gaining support from the mayor of the community and from other community leaders. These individuals must understand the concept of health promotion and the healthy municipalities process before they will offer their support. PAHO has also found that it must have a strong and knowledgeable support group who can envision a healthy municipality and convey that vision to opinion leaders (PAHO, 2012).

There are many excellent examples of Healthy Communities and Cities around the world. PAHO says that in some countries in their region, such as Mexico, Costa Rica, Chile, and Cuba, national networks have been established and been producing good results for many years (PAHO, n.d.). A few examples are highlighted here with information on how to locate their websites and learn more about the work being done around the world.
- *Ontario (Canada) Healthy Communities Coalition:* They focus on "What makes a healthy community." Their website, www.ohcc-ccso.ca, is filled with useful resources.
- *Horsens, Denmark:* One of their key foci is on "safe community Horsens." Their website, www.horsenssundby.dk, is in Danish, but the button to choose English is clearly marked and they provide an overview of the work they are doing.
- *Community Builders of New South Wales, Australia:* They have an interactive electronic clearinghouse for persons involved in community level, social, economic, and environmental renewal, including community leaders, community and government workers, volunteers, program managers,

academics, policy makers, youth, and seniors. They include rural and regional communities (www.communitybuilders .nsw.gov.au).
- *Association for Community Health Improvements:* This organization's website includes many healthy community tools and organizations in the United States and internationally. Similarly, www.healthycommunities.org hosts a website with valuable information about healthy communities and extensive links to other sites.

Selected examples of healthy communities in the United States are discussed later in this chapter. Also see Chapter 4 for examples of Healthy Cities Toronto, Canada, and Chengdu, China.

## DEVELOPING A HEALTHY COMMUNITY

What do people want from a healthy community? We know that each community is different and its challenges, goals, resources, competencies, problem-solving skills, and practices are different. As discussed throughout the chapter, many organizations in the United States and other countries have worked to help communities become healthier (Figure 20-1). One of these organizations in the United States is the National Civic League (2007). (See www.communitycommons.org/tag/nation-civic-league). In 2014, the National Civic League partnered with Community Commons to celebrate 25 years of Healthy Communities and to spread the ideas and insights in published and new online media. They emphasize the complexity of developing healthy communities and have identified five principles that they think should be applied in community work if the goal is to find solutions using a broad-based inclusive process. These principles are as follows:
1. A broad definition of health that goes beyond the absence of disease to address the root problems in communities and

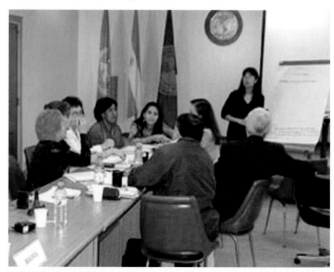

**FIGURE 20-1** Community participation for developing a healthy community involves a representative community planning committee. (From CDC, Pulsenet News, 2004. Available at: http://www.cdc.gov/pulsenet/newsletter/Spring_2004.htm. Accessed January 10, 2011.)

includes economy, education, parks and recreation, arts, mental health, and community spirit and unity.

2. A collaborative, consensus-based approach to problem solving that involves a diverse group of citizens from the community.

3. An assets-based approach to problem solving that defines people and relationships by their skills and abilities rather than their needs and deficits.

4. Addressing challenges at a systems level in the community rather than implementing another short-term, low-impact project.

5. Creating a shared vision for the future that captures the hopes and dreams of the community and that guides collaborative work.

Other principles will guide the development and implementation of a healthy community. Examples of useful principles include the following:

- The whole is greater than the sum of the parts; in other words, most communities have limited resources, and no one agency can do all that is needed. However, if agencies work together, the outcome of the whole can be much bigger than the outcome of the aid provided by one agency.

- A change in one part of the system affects the others. For example, if the public transportation workers in a large city go on strike and there is no public transportation for many days, many areas of the community will be affected.

- Collaboration is central to the development of a healthy community.

- All systems have feedback loops whereby information from one area is fed back to the whole and provides an opportunity for change or "course correction." For example, you might establish a helping program for dependent older adults where daycare is provided at low cost. This would enable the family members with whom the elder lives to provide safe care while they worked. However, if the family has no transportation of their own and the facility is not accessible by public transportation, the program would not be as helpful as hoped.

The National Civic League also asked hundreds of communities across the country "What would your community look like if it were a really healthy place to live?" The replies shown in Box 20-1 come as no surprise. You might ask yourself that

BOX 20-1 **What Is a Healthy Community?**

- A clean and safe environment
- A diverse and vibrant economy
- Good housing for all
- Good roads and good public transportation
- Parks, playgrounds, and recreational facilities
- People who respect and support each other
- A place that promotes and celebrates its cultural and historical heritage
- A place where citizens and government share power and where citizens feel a sense of belonging
- A place that has affordable health care for all
- A place that has good schools
- A place that has and supports strong families

same question before looking at Box 20-1 and see how close your replies are to those of the respondents.

This chapter indicates that a healthy community has involvement, inclusiveness, cooperation, and collaboration, among other qualities. Collaboration can help make the best use of resources, reduce duplication and competition, increase effectiveness, and develop more sustainable resources. It is like a recipe in that each agency in the collaboration brings one or more ingredients to the product. Putting all the ingredients together leads to a better product. Collaboration involves doing things differently than in the past and developing different kinds of partnerships and relationships. Organizations that work together effectively have generally achieved three things:

1. High levels of trust
2. Serious time commitment from the partners
3. A diminished need to protect their own turf (Torres & Margolin, 2003)

Collaboration requires the same mix of behaviors and goals as those associated with the development of a healthy community—that is, a group of participants including those who are paid and volunteers who bring different skills and talents to the process and who work together to do the following:

1. Address a specific problem or opportunity
2. Work on a broad agenda of mutually beneficial goals
3. Provide a forum to discuss and respond to community concerns, interests, and resources
4. Recognize that there are roles in a partnership and they will be different from the role the person had in the parent organization.

As mentioned earlier, Indiana and California have the longest history of Healthy Communities and Cities in the United States. Healthy Cities Indiana began as a pilot program in 1988 with a grant from the W.K. Kellogg Foundation as a collaborative effort among Indiana University School of Nursing, Indiana Public Health Association, and six Indiana cities. On the basis of this project's success, the W.K. Kellogg Foundation funded the dissemination phase, called CITYNET-Healthy Cities, in cooperation with the National League of Cities through their network of 19,000 local officials (Flynn, Rider, & Ray, 1991). This was an extensive project that initially involved six cities (Gary, Fort Wayne, New Castle, Indianapolis, Seymour, and Jeffersonville). Activities in these cities focused on problems of diverse populations. For example, actions were consistent with local priorities that included problems of children, teen parents, the homeless, access to health care, crime and violence, and older adults. Action was also taken on the broader environmental policy issues, including management of solid waste and promotion of air quality. For each of these projects, the Community Health Promotion process was followed, thereby providing a broad base of community participation at all stages of community planning. This was a process developed at Indiana University School of Nursing, and it was consistent with many of the other U.S. and international processes for implementing healthy community initiatives.

An early example of the use of the Community Health Promotion process was the New Castle Healthy City community

# REFERENCES

American Nurses Association: *Scope & Standards of Practice*, ed 2. Silver Springs, MD, 2013, Public Health Nursing, ANA.

Ashton J: *Creating Healthy Cities*, paper presented at Healthy Cities Indiana Network Session. Seymour, IN, May 1989.

California Endowment: *Overview Strategic Vision 2010-2020: Building Healthy Communities*. 2010, author. Available at: www.csun.edu/alliance/Wellness-Coreteam/Documents/CA%20Endowment%20Building%20Healthy%20Communities.pdf. Accessed August 15, 2014.

Center for Civic Partnerships: *CA Healthy Cities and Communities Program*. 2014. Available at: http://www.civicpartnerships.org/#!ca-healthy-cities-and-communities-progra/cjhg. Accessed August 16, 2014.

Centers for Disease Control and Prevention: *Principles of Community Engagement (Electronic Version)*. Atlanta, 1997 and ed 2, 2011. Available at: http://www.cdc.gov. Accessed August 16, 2014.

Centers for Disease Control and Prevention: *Healthy communities: Preventing chronic disease by activating grassroots change: at a glance*. 2011. Available at: www.cdc.gov/chronicdisease/resources/publications/AAGHealthy_communities.htm. Accessed February 2, 2015.

Centers for Disease Control and Prevention: *About healthy places*. 2014. Available at: www.cdc.gov/healthyplaces. Accessed August 16, 2014.

Columbus Regional Hospital: *Healthy communities initiative*. 2014. Available at: www.crh.org/community-involvement/

healthy-communities.aspx. Accessed August 15, 2014.

Flynn BC: Partnership in Healthy Cities and Communities: a social commitment for advanced practice nurses. *Adv Pract Nurs Q* 2:1, 1997.

Flynn BC, Rider MS, Ray DW: Healthy Cities: the Indiana model of community development in public health. *Health Educ Q* 18:331, 1991.

Hancock T: The evolution, impact, and significance of the Healthy Cities/Healthy Communities movement. *J Public Health Policy* 14:5, 1993.

National Civic League: *Healthy Communities Initiatives*. Denver CO, 2007, author.

Pan American Health Organization: *Healthy Municipalities & Communities: Mayors' Guide for Promoting Quality of Life*. Washington, DC, n.d., PAHO. Available at: http://www.paho.org/english/ad/sde/hs/mayors-guide.htm. Accessed August 16, 2014.

Pan American Health Organization: *Healthy Municipalities and Communities*. Washington, DC, 2012, PAHO. Available at: http://www.paho.org/hq/index.php?option=com_content&view=category&layout=blog&id=4535&Itemid=39554. Accessed August 15, 2014.

Partnership for Prevention: *The Community Health Promotion Handbook: Action Guides to Improve Community Health*. Washington, DC, 2008, Partnership for Prevention.

Quad Council of Public Health Nursing Organizations: *Public Health Nursing Competencies*. Wheat Ridge, CO, 2011, Quad Council.

Rothman J, Tropman JE: Models of community organization

and macro practice: their mixing and phasing. In Cox FM, Tropman ME, Rothman J, et al, editors: *Strategies of Community Organization*, ed 4. Itasca, IL, 1987, Peacock.

Roussos ST, Fawcett SB: A review of collaborative partnerships as a strategy for improving community health. *Annu Rev Public Health* 21:369–402, 2000.

Sanneh EJ, Hu AH, Njai M, et al: Making basic health care accessible to rural communities: A case study of Kiang West District in rural Gambia. *Public Health Nursin* 31(2):126–133, 2013.

Task Force on Community Preventive Services: *The guide to community preventive services: Social environment and health*. 2005. Available at: http://www.thecommunityguide.org/library/book/Front-Matter.pdf. Accessed August 16, 2014.

Torres GW, Margolin FS: *Collaboration Primer: Proven Strategies, Consideration, and Tools to Get You Started*. Chicago, 2003, Health Research & Educational Trust. Available at: www.hret.org.

U.S. Department of Health and Human Services: *Healthy People 2000: National Health Promotion and Disease Prevention Objectives*. Washington, DC, 1991, USDHHS.

U.S. Department of Health and Human Services: *Healthy People in Healthy Communities 2010*. Atlanta, 2000, USDHHS, Centers for Disease Control and Prevention, National Center for Chronic Disease Prevention and Health Promotion (electronic version). Available at: http://www.healthypeople.gov/2010/publications/healthycommunities2001/

default.htm?visit=1. Accessed August 16, 2014.

U.S. Department of Health and Human Services: *Healthy People in Healthy Communities: A Community Planning Guide Using Healthy People 2010*. Washington, DC, February 2001, U.S. Government Printing Office.

U.S. Department of Health and Human Services. Agency for Healthcare Research and Quality. AHRQ. The Guide to Clinical Preventive Services, 2014. Recommendations of the U.S. Preventive Services Task Force. AHRQ Pub. No. 14-05158, May 2014.

U.S. Department of Health and Human Services: *Healthy People 2020*. Washington, DC, 2010, USDHHS.

U.S. Preventive Services Task Force: 2014. http://www.uspreventiveservicestaskforce.org. Accessed January 27, 2015.

Veazie MA, Teufel-Shone NI, Silverman GS, et al: Building community capacity in public health: the role of action-oriented partnerships. *J Public Health Manag Pract* 7:21–32, 2001.

World Health Organization: *United Nations Children's Fund: Primary Health Care*. Geneva, Switzerland, 1978, WHO, UNICEF.

World Health Organization: *Ottawa Charter for Health Promotion*. Copenhagen, Denmark, 1986, WHO Regional Office for Europe.

World Health Organization: *About WHO. Ottawa Charter for Health Promotion, 1986*. Copenhagen, Denmark, 2010, WHO Regional Office for Europe.

# The Nurse-led Health Center: A Model for Community Nursing Practice

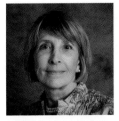

## Katherine K. Kinsey, PhD, RN, FAAN

Dr. Katherine K. Kinsey is the Nurse Administrator and Principal Investigator of the Philadelphia Nurse-Family Partnership (NFP), the Mabel Morris Family Home Visit Program, and other special projects including early childhood initiatives. Dr. Kinsey earned the BS from Millersville University in Pennsylvania and the BSN and MSN from the University of Pennsylvania School of Nursing. She earned the PhD from the Graduate School of Education with a speciality in Health Professions Education also from the University of Pennsylvania. Dr. Kinsey previously directed a nationally recognized academic-based nurse-managed health center. She is a past chairperson of the American Public Health Association, Public Health Nursing Section. Dr. Kinsey serves on several nonprofit boards and is the president of the Kingsley Family Foundation, which is dedicated to improving the well-being of vulnerable, underserved populations.

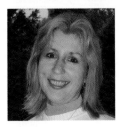

## Mary Ellen T. Miller, PhD, RN

Dr. Mary Ellen T. Miller is an Associate Professor at De Sales University School of Nursing in Center Valley, PA, and teaches in the undergraduate, graduate, and doctoral nursing programs. She earned the BSN and MSN from LaSalle University and the PhD from Temple University. Both universities are in Philadalphia, Pennsylvania. Dr. Miller serves as Chair of the Wellness Center Committee of the National Nursing Center Consortium. Previously, she served as the Associate Director of Public Health Programs for an academic nursing center. Dr. Miller has published works about nurse-managed centers and presents regionally and nationally on topics related to her work, as well as about student involvement with community service and learning, and about nurse-managed wellness centers.

## ADDITIONAL RESOURCES

## OBJECTIVES

*After reading this chapter, the student should be able to do the following:*

1. Describe key characteristics of nurse-led center models.
2. Explain community collaboration.
3. Identify interventions that address *Healthy People 2020* goals.
4. Determine the feasibility of establishing and sustaining a nurse-led center.
5. Describe the roles and responsibilities of the advanced practice nurse in a nurse-led center.
6. Discuss the future of population-centered nursing practice, education, and research.

## KEY TERMS

Considerable data document that nurse-led health centers (NLHC) improve health outcomes. The nurse-led health center (NLHC) model increases access to care; provides a more comprehensive approach to health and illness; decreases racial, ethnic, and geographic disparities in health status; and can potentially reduce the overall costs of health care. NLHCs, as safety net providers, reach out to and engage underserved, vulnerable populations in public health and primary health care initiatives. This chapter describes NLHCs and their origins, evolution, and future directions. Emphasis is placed on the *Healthy People 2020* framework, community collaboration, and multilevel interventions to improve access and reduce health disparities. This chapter describes nursing roles and responsibilities in delivering client-centered, community-based services, managing center operations, and expanding initiatives for practice, research, and education in public health and primary care settings. Economic, social, political, national health care reform, and global factors influencing NLHC operations and population-centered nursing practice are discussed.

## WHAT ARE NURSE-LED HEALTH CENTERS?

### Overview and Definition

The terms *nurse-led health center, nursing center, nurse-managed health center,* and *nurse-managed health clinic* are interchangeable in this chapter and are used to describe this model of health care. The citations in this ninth edition of *Public Health Nursing: Population-Centered Health Care in the*

*Community* include historical references noted in earlier editions and current references regarding the evolution of NLHCs. The references frame the decades-long NLHC movement. However, the ways in which we gain knowledge is changing. The introduction of new Internet-based technology and communication venues regarding public health programs and NLHCs will grow exponentially (Khan et al, 2010). Access to NLHCs initiatives, public health practice examples, and career opportunities are now featured on social media websites, wikis, and blog communities. These venues, and others still in the research and development phases, will add rich content as NLHCs continue to transition into mainstream health care provider status.

In the past, the most frequently cited and referenced definition of nurse-led health centers was the one developed by the American Nurses Association (ANA) Nursing Centers Task Force in the mid-1980s and shown in Box 21-1. However, the Nurse-Managed Health Clinic Investment Act of 2009 (Senate Bill 1104/House of Representatives Bill 2754) of the 111th Congress provides a more current and functional definition of nurse-managed health clinics with an amendment to Title III of the Public Health Service Act (42 U.S.C. 241 et sez.) as seen in Box 21-2.

NLHC provide unique opportunities to improve the health status of individuals, families, and communities through direct access to nurses and nursing models of care (Lancaster, 1999). All NLHCs possess characteristics that reflect the values, beliefs, and scientific knowledge and skills inherent in nursing models of care. Furthermore, each is guided, managed, and primarily staffed by nurses, thus ensuring that decision making and ultimate accountability for this model of care rest with professional nurses (Kinsey and Gerrity, 2005).

The NLHC is supported by the ANA seminal position paper titled *Health Promotion and Disease Prevention* (ANA, 1995). The paper recognizes health promotion strategies as pivotal points of any health care system designed to control costs and reduce human suffering. It acknowledges nursing's scope of practice and underscores its efforts to focus on disease prevention interventions (ANA, 1995).

Nurse-led center models combine human caring, scientific knowledge about health and illness, and understanding of family and community characteristics, interests, assets, needs, and goals for health promotion, disease prevention, and disease management. NLHC models de-emphasize illness-oriented and institutional care that has dominated health care since World War II and subscribe to a holistic perspective on improving personal, community, and societal well-being.

## Nurse-led Models of Care

NLHCs are strategically positioned to improve the health and well-being of vulnerable populations (Kinsey, 1999) and reduce

health disparities by providing access to comprehensive primary health care and health promotion and disease prevention services (Hansen-Turton, Miller, & Greiner, 2009). Interdisciplinary staff achieves success through shared vision, positive attitudes, and respect for team members (Phillips, 2009). Social determinants of health (Wilensky & Satcher, 2009) as well as the integration of time, tact, talent, trust, caring, personal respect, equity, and social justice perspectives serve as the foundation from which health is viewed as essential for everyday life (Plowfield, Wheeler, & Raymond, 2005). Efforts of the center focus on enhancing people's capacity to meet their personal, family, and community responsibilities and interests and typically include the following:

- *Community-based culturally competent care* that is accessible, acceptable, and responsive to the populations being served
- A *holistic approach* to care based on complex and interrelated bio-psychosocial factors
- *Interorganizational and interdisciplinary collaboration* that crosses health and human service systems and increases opportunities for comprehensive and seamless services among care providers, agencies, and payers
- *Multilevel interventions* that acknowledge organizational, environmental, health, economic, and social policy contributions to health, health problems, and issues of access to care
- *Community partnerships* in establishing and supporting the center's health efforts
- *Relationship-based practice* with individuals, families, organizations, and communities that fosters understanding of context, interests, and needs for health care

Nurse-led center models combine people, place, approach, and strategy in everyday life to develop appropriate health interventions. Advanced practice nurses (APNs) work in close partnership with the communities they serve to provide public health programs, community-wide health education, and primary health care services. They establish relationships with families, community representatives, policy makers, and others in designing, implementing, and evaluating appropriate health intervention strategies, services, and programs (Zimmerman, Mieczkowski, & Wilson, 2002; Hansen-Turton, Miller, & Greiner, 2009).

A nurse-led center's *health* and *community* orientation builds strong connections to the population served. These strong relationships with community leaders, residents, and clients foster a deep awareness of local factors that influence daily life (Lundeen, 1999). This orientation builds on Lillian Wald's community work more than a century ago. Wald's work to establish The Henry Street Visiting Nurse Service and a cadre of public health nurses who treated social and economic problems—not just infections, diseases, and providing care to the chronically ill—is part of the nursing center legacy (Fee & Bu, 2010). Figure 21-1 depicts the opening of a nurse-led center.

## TYPES OF NURSE-LED HEALTH CENTERS

There are many types of nurse-led centers. Each has a "personality" of its own (Gerrity and Kinsey, 1999). A center should be

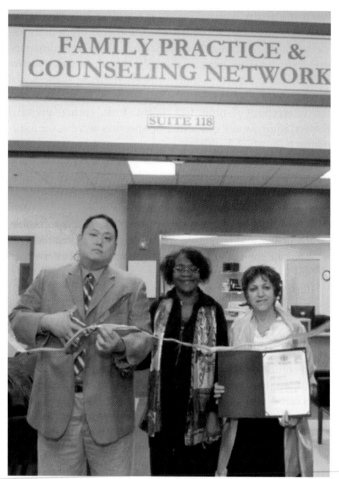

**FIG 21-1** Donna Torrisi, MSN, Nurse-Managed Health Center Director with community leaders at the 2008 Grand Opening of the Family Practice and Counseling Health Annex, Philadelphia, PA. (From Family Practice and Counseling Network Clients, Philadelphia, PA.)

---

| BOX 21-3 Nurse-led Center Typologies |
| --- |

**Service Model**
- *Wellness centers:* Provide health promotion and disease prevention programs
- *Comprehensive primary care centers:* Provide health-oriented primary care and public health programs
- *Special care centers:* Provide programs targeting specific health conditions (such as diabetes) or population groups (such as the frail elderly)

**Organizational Structure**
- *Academic nurse-led center:* Housed within a school of nursing
- *Free-standing center:* Independent center with its own governing board
- *Subsidiary:* Part of larger health care systems, home-health agencies, community centers, senior centers, schools, and others
- *Affiliated center:* Legal partnership association with health, human services, or other organization

**Internal Revenue Service Designation**
- *501(c)3:* Non-profit business
- *Proprietary:* Incorporated as a for-profit business

**Reimbursement Mechanism**
- *Fee-for-service:* Payment at time of service; may include sliding-fee scale
- *HMO provider:* Payment at contracted rates by health maintenance organization
- *Federally Qualified Health Center (FQHC):* Federal designation that allows cost-based reimbursement per encounter
- *Third-party reimbursement:* Client billing to public program or commercial/private insurance
- *Contributions:* Individual donations, philanthropic gifts, fund-raising activities to support a program

---

based on community assets and perceived needs with a clearly stated mission and vision as well as its commitment to community well-being, contributing to its profile (Hansen Turton, Miller, & Greiner, 2009). Organizational structure (academic, non-academic), federal tax status (profit or nonprofit), and reimbursement systems (fee for service, sliding scale fee rates, or no charge) also define centers. Other types will evolve as a result of national health care legislation. The legislative initiatives include maximizing federally qualified health center services; increasing access to primary health care for people of all ages; introducing new public health, preventive health, and home visiting programs; and implementing and using electronic medical records. To date, most nurse-led centers fit into the types described in Box 21-3.

## Wellness Centers

Wellness centers focus on health promotion, disease prevention, and management programs. APNs and others provide outreach and public awareness services, health education, immunizations, family assessment and screening services, home visiting, and social support (Hansen-Turton, Miller, & Greiner, 2009). Public health education and support programs may include smoking cessation (Lakon, Hipp, & Timberlake, 2010) and management of chronic conditions such as diabetes, asthma, and hypertension. Many centers also provide dental, behavioral health, environmental health risk reduction, and parenting education (Hansen-Turton, Bailey, Torres, & Ritter, 2010). "Enabling" services help people access language translation, registration for entitlement programs, transportation vouchers, and specialty services. *Healthy People 2020* goals and objectives provide direction to services planned, implemented, and evaluated through the wellness center model.

These centers complement existing primary care services. The staff maintains strong relationships with local health care providers in community health centers, clinics, private practices, long-term care facilities, and other organizations. In general, financial support for center programs comes from public health department and other service contracts, foundation grants, fee for services, voluntary contributions, and shared resources from affiliated organizations (Hansen-Turton, Miller, & Greiner, 2009). In addition, these centers often serve as venues for community service learning activities for graduate and undergraduate students from multiple disciplines. Nursing centers extend learning beyond the classroom and into the community, providing a legitimate experience whereby students apply theoretical content to a community setting (Miller & Guigliano, 2006).

## Special Care Centers

Some nurse-led centers focus on a particular demographic group or on those with special health care needs. Special care centers provide services and specialized health knowledge and skills to a particular group, and they are an adjunct to comprehensive primary health care models. Examples of special care centers are those that focus on the needs of people with diabetes or HIV/AIDS, adolescent mothers, the frail elderly, and support services for people with mental disorders (Alakeson, Frank, & Katz, 2010). Other centers are the hub for public health nursing practice in home and community settings. These include Nurse-Family Partnership models across the nation as well as other early childhood home visiting models including Parents As Teachers and Early Head Start.

## Comprehensive Primary Health Care Centers

In many communities, nurse-led centers offer comprehensive primary health care. In addition to the health and wellness programs described previously, these centers also serve as the primary care (medical) home for families in the communities where they are located. In the centers, nurse practitioners, other advanced practice nurses, and allied health professionals provide both physical and behavioral health care services. These centers address the needs of individuals and families across the life span, ensuring access to specialized health care as indicated. Public health nurses and community workers provide outreach, social support, and an array of public health programs. Public health programs include health education, screening, immunizations, lead poisoning prevention, home visitation such as in the Nurse-Family Partnership, environmental health initiatives, and other preventive community-based health services (Figure 21-2).

Comprehensive primary health care centers face the challenge of establishing systems for documenting clinical care and utilization patterns. These systems include demographic profiles, accounting support, billing mechanisms, reimbursement

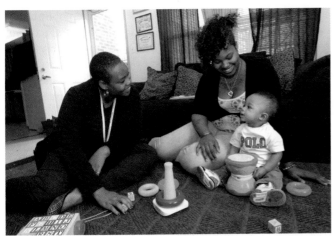

FIG 21-2 Investing in the future: public health nurses and programs like Nurse-Family Partnership, Early Head Start, Parents As Teachers, and others improve family health and mother-child (or maternal–child) well-being. (Used with permission of Philadelphia Inquirer Copyright © 2010. All rights reserved.)

protocols, quality improvement strategies, and client satisfaction measures (Sherman, 2005). Nursing centers must meet standards established by government, insurers, health maintenance organizations, and other payers.

Increasingly, the Bureau of Primary Health Care (BPHC) of the U.S. Department of Health and Human Services (USDHHS) designates nurse-led primary health centers as federally qualified health centers (FQHCs). Their purposes are to (1) provide population-based comprehensive care in medically underserved areas and (2) maintain the appropriate mission, organizational, and governance structure according to the FQHC designation. These designations include community health center, public housing center, homeless center, or school-based center.

The FQHC designation is important from a number of perspectives. Most importantly, it supports a primary care center's efforts to serve low-income and uninsured populations and remain fiscally solvent. FQHCs receive federal grant funds from the Health Resources and Services Administration (HRSA) to support operational expenses. They also receive cost-based payment for services provided to Medicare and Medicaid patients, Federal Tort Claim coverage, and 340b drug pricing, and they have the option to participate in the National Health Services Corps.

Many nurse-led centers need to overcome internal and external organizational hurdles to initiate the FQHC application process and receive funding approval (Torrisi & Hansen-Turton, 2005). The National Nursing Centers Consortium (NNCC), with offices in Pennsylvania, Washington, DC, and California, provides regional training for the FQHC application processes. The recent passage of the Nurse-Managed Health Clinic Investment program by the 111th Congress holds great potential for additional NLHC-affiliated academic institutions to be eligible for FQHC status.

Many NLHCs are in nonprofit academic settings. They are housed within or closely affiliated with schools of nursing. These NLHCs actively integrate service, education, and research in their model. They build on public health and primary care nurse practitioner educational programs, draw on the knowledge and skills of faculty, and provide rich learning experiences for nursing students at all levels. Furthermore, they use the knowledge, skills, and resources of other schools of health professions, business, communications, and law to expand the center's service capacity (Shiber & D'Lugoff, 2002). Academic nursing centers have documented benefits to communities served, specifically regarding the strengths of nurse practitioners and the centers' ability to provide outreach to the community (Pohl et al, 2007).

One example of an academic nurse-led center is the Lewis and Clark Community College Nurse-Managed Health Center located in Godfrey, Illinois. The college also has a mobile health unit. This NLHC was the first to open to the public on a U.S. community college campus. The center provides nonemergency, low-cost primary care services and partners with the Southern Illinois Healthcare Foundation for referrals and specialty care. Nursing students have clinical rotations through the NLHC and its mobile unit. Students and faculty are involved in client education and illness prevention services. This model introduces students to the expanding roles and responsibilities of APNs in community settings and career options (Weller, 2010).

Other centers may be affiliated with freestanding organizations, subsidiaries of health care or other human services organizations, or sponsored by an affiliate of such entities. Each of these organizational arrangements requires carefully established legal agreements. To conduct business, these organizations must become incorporated; apply to the Internal Revenue Service (IRS) for a tax status designation; and receive a Statement of Tax Status Determination. Organizations are generally categorized as a nonprofit (501(c)3) entity or some form of proprietary (for-profit) organization. The majority of nursing centers are with nonprofit organizations; others fit within a proprietary business model, and others operate as subsidiaries of established organizations. In all cases, staff must be familiar with the particular laws and regulations associated with the IRS tax status under which they operate.

Another way to describe nurse-led centers involves the health care system's financial reimbursement methods that support services and programs. These include fee-for-service, designated HMO provider, Medicaid provider, Medicare provider, and FQHC status. Each designation requires a center to possess certain characteristics, meet a set of standards, and possess identification numbers that allow them to participate in billing and reimbursement systems.

Regardless of the type of center, a wide array of social determinants, personal, social, educational, economic, and environmental concerns, indicate the need for and expansion of nursing centers. Increasing population density and diversity, challenging community conditions, and long-standing and emerging health problems indicate the role such models of care can play (Kinsey, 2002). The 2010 national health reform law, the **Patient Protection and Affordable Care Act**, holds the potential for NLHCs to work with like entities to help improve the nation's health. This law and the 2013-2014 "roll-out" focuses on reforming the health care system, increasing disease prevention initiatives and access to services, and containing or reducing health care expenditures (Thorpe & Ogden, 2010). The national commitment to build integrated delivery systems offers nurse-led centers and academic health systems new opportunities to demonstrate effectiveness, efficiency, and cost savings (Dentzer, 2010).

With the anticipation of NLHCs expansion grants, it is essential to work with like-minded individuals and groups to share knowledge, resources, and lessons learned. Several organizations dedicated to the promotion and sustainability of NLHCs are in place to support its members through these expansion phases. The NNCC is one nationally recognized organization dedicated to this work. As of 2014, NNCC represents more than 250 members and is the largest national repository of member nurse-led health centers. Its members represent organizations, programs within parent organizations, freestanding entities, and individuals invested in the nurse-managed center model. (A current membership list is available at http://www.nncc.us). Members have the benefits of NNCC monthly newsletters, grant updates, current legislative and advocacy work, and its Annual National Conference. NNCC reaches out to nonprofit organizations and individuals interested in establishing or expanding a nurse-led (clinic) model.

The Consortium often links members with potential members to share expertise and consult on program design and implementation. See the Linking Content to Practice box.

> ## ▶▶ LINKING CONTENT TO PRACTICE
>
> This chapter discusses the ways in which nurses provide primary care and public health services within the context of a nurse-led center. The skills of assessment, planning, implementation, evaluation, and policy development are integral to this role. In order to effectively practice in a nurse-led center, nurses use the standards of nursing practice from many specialty areas as well as the core competencies for both public health nursing and public health. Specifically, the nurse working in this setting would incorporate the following core competencies from the Quad Council of Nursing (QCN) *Public Health Nursing* (2011) and the American Association of Colleges of Nursing (AACN), supplement to the 2010 *Essentials of Baccalaureate Nursing Education for Professional Nursing Practice* titled *Recommended Baccalaureate Competencies and Curricular Guidelines for Public Health Nursing* (2013). The QCN competencies are built on those of the Council on Linkages (PHF, 2014) and their core competencies for public health professionals. For example, Domain #1 in both documents describes analytic assessment skills and Competency #1 is "conducts thorough health assessments of individuals, families, communities and populations." There are 10 additional skills that nurses would use from this domain in nursing centers. As has been discussed throughout this chapter, nurses working in nursing centers use the policy process in providing care. Domain #2 is that of policy development/program planning skills and each of the 11 competencies/skills are used in a nursing center. The AACN supplemental competencies are based on the nine essentials from the original AACN recommendations and focus on primary and secondary prevention strategies in population health, including interprofessional collaboration.

From Public Health Foundation, Council on Linkages: *Core competencies for public health professionals, Washington DC*, 2009, PHF; Quad Council: *Domains of practice*, 2009. Available at http:www.sphtc.org/phncompetenciesfinalcomb.pdf. Accessed July 29, 2010.

## THE FOUNDATIONS OF NURSE-LED CENTER DEVELOPMENT

The foundations for integrating primary care and public health services through the NLHC model include the perspective of the World Health Organization (WHO) and the *Healthy People 2020* systematic approach to improving individual and community health. The WHO's definition of health and its framework to address global health supports an NLHC's integration of primary care and public health services in community settings (WHO, 1978).

The *Healthy People* initiative has framed the nation's health promotion and disease prevention agenda since 1980. Its framework, vision, mission, goals, and objectives are developed to achieve better health for all by 2020. *Healthy People* represents a collaborative federal, public, and stakeholder process and accounts for global and national environmental, social, demographic changes, and trends such as the increasing older populations. *Healthy People* accommodates the escalating technological influences on personal and population health status, and incorporates anticipated changes in the U.S. sickness-oriented health system. Chapter 2 describes the history of *Healthy People*, and chapters throughout the text apply the objectives of *Healthy People 2020* to their content. The concept of *Healthy People 2020* builds on shared responsibility to improve the nation's health. Communities, individuals, and systems have the potential for change, yet no one person or organization can do this alone. Powerful, productive partnerships among diverse people and groups and long-term commitments to community collaboration are needed to achieve *Healthy People 2020* goals. NLHCs can help to achieve the goals and objectives of *Healthy People 2020* and would emphasize those goals and objectives that fit the target populations' needs. For example, an NLHC associated with an elementary school where more than 40% of the students are obese would select *Healthy People 2020* objectives relative to childhood nutrition, physical activity, and exercise. The NLHC would also implement communication strategies that address the need to reduce childhood obesity in school-age children.

## Community Collaboration

Nurse-led centers and APNs are well positioned to guide and facilitate community collaboration and engagement (Keefe, Leuner, & Laken, 2000; Bechtel & Ness, 2010; Thompson & Feeney, 2004). Productive collaboration requires staff expertise and commitment from many to change communication patterns, professional agendas, and speak in a common voice to generate positive community transformation (Cross & Prusak, 2002). The community transformations occur through policy, legislative, and funding changes that improve the health status of many and help design the patient-centered medical homes that include NLHCs (Landon et al, 2010).

Individuals, families, groups, organizations, policy makers, and staff are involved in the process. Referred to as stakeholders, each entity brings a unique perspective. Their particular knowledge and skills enhance the community's efforts to address critical needs, solve problems, and recognize unique strengths and resources. Stakeholders facilitate or undermine strategic efforts to improve health. It is impossible to fully know and address issues and concerns in a community without having all perspectives heard and every stakeholder respectful of different opinions and experiences (Bechtel & Ness, 2010). The following Healthy People 2020 box lists a sample of goals that affect nurse-led centers.

> **♥ HEALTHY PEOPLE 2020**
>
> The following objectives are examples that pertain to the work of nurses in nurse-led centers:
> - ECBP-3.3: Advocating for personal, family, and community health (skills).
> - HC/HIT-2: Increase the proportion of persons who report that their health care providers have satisfactory communication skills.
> - AHS-7: Increase the proportion of persons who receive appropriate evidence-based clinical preventive services.
> - MICH-10: Increase the proportion of pregnant women who receive early and adequate prenatal care.
> - MICH-21: Increase the proportion of infants who are breastfed.
>
> From U.S. Department of Health and Human Services: *Healthy People 2020: understanding and improving health*, Washington, DC, 2010, U.S. Government Printing Office

Collaboration takes time, effort, and resources. It requires nurturing and support to make it work. Relationships among

people and organizations serve as the foundation for the collaborative process and for community change. Relationships begin with introductions and open discussion to listen to and learn from one another. From this, relationships grow toward a collective willingness to work together toward a common purpose, sharing *risks, responsibilities, resources,* and *rewards* along the way. The seminal definition of collaboration developed by Mattessich and Monsey (1992) describes the work involved; they view collaboration as a relationship entered into by two or more groups to achieve common goals that are well defined and beneficial to all. There must be a respectful commitment to these goals with mutual accountability and authority that allows for shared responsibilities, resources, and successes. See Resource Tool 21.A: Factors Influencing the Success of Collaboration.

Nurse-led center staff needs to have skills in networking, coordination, and cooperation in order to collaborate (Hansen-Turton, Miller, & Greiner, 2009). A number of basic agreements and interview strategies help set the stage for a long-term process of discussion, decision making, and action (Rollnick, Miller, & Butler, 2008). Once established, they are reviewed and rigorously adhered to throughout the life of the collaboration. These agreements are as follows:

- Regular meetings where diverse perspectives are heard and respected
- A mutually agreed on decision making process
- Consistent and accurate communications so all participants have the necessary information to make decisions
- Agreement by all participants to support collaborative decisions once they are made—within the groups or organizations they represent and publicly in the community

Mattessich and Monsey (1992) have identified six critical elements that contribute to the success of a collaborative endeavor: the environment, membership characteristics, process and structure of the group, communication patterns, purpose of the collaboration, and resources within and outside the group.

Perhaps the most important feature in community collaboration is the capacity of those involved to enhance the capacity of *another* person, group, or organization to achieve the common purpose. For instance, rather than the nurse-led center serving as the lead organization, different participating organizations will serve from time to time in the leadership role, or hold greater responsibility, or perhaps receive additional funds to achieve the common purpose to which they all have subscribed. This cooperation allows participants to achieve a mutual benefit (Goffee & Jones, 2001).

Each nurse-led center develops its philosophy, goals, and activities through a process of community collaboration, community assessment, and strategic planning. Strategic planning recognizes multiple levels of intervention required for bringing about and sustaining change. Often, community collaboration and assessment are concurrent activities.

## Community Assessment

Nurse-managed centers must conduct periodic community assessments. This chapter reemphasizes the importance of data and analysis of community needs and assets in determining the

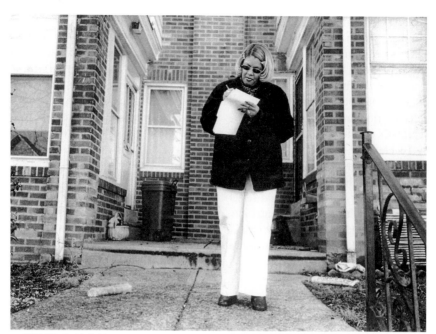

**FIG 21-3** Neighborhood walks provide insight into the community's health.

type of nursing center to establish or expand. Through the assessment process, nurses learn both the community's formal and informal infrastructure and the communication networks through which everyday life takes place (Baker, White, & Lichtveld, 2001). Neighborhood walks, bus rides, car trips, and discussions with elected officials, administrators of health care systems, public health department staff, and community members provide insight into the community's health and the many other influencing factors. Figure 21-3 depicts a nurse doing a neighborhood walk. Also, historical, ethnographic multimedia news features add context to the community assessment (Anderson, 1999).

Assessment activities identify community assets and health problems. For example, there may be a rich network of block captains who serve as leaders and communication liaisons with the community. There may be a local community college that can provide space and support for meetings. If high rates of childhood asthma are discovered, there may be human service organizations that can help in disease prevention and management efforts (Kawachi & Berkman, 2003).

As nurses conduct individual interviews and focus groups, develop surveys, review health care data, and examine social determinants of health (social, educational, employment, economic, housing, and others), they gather detailed information about the overall well-being of the community. These sources of information build an understanding of the community and its traditions, strengths, interests, concerns, problems, needs, and preferences. The assessment process includes sharing current health data, historical trends, and future projections with the community. Center staff can discuss the findings, share perspectives and ideas, and encourage involvement in the collaborative process. From this, the nursing center's overall direction, services, and programs emerge (Anderko, 2000).

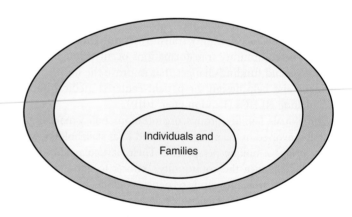

Sociopolitical systems
**FIG 21-4** Multilevel intervention model.

## Multilevel Interventions

As the community and the center work together for comprehensive community health, a multilevel approach is needed. Some behavioral decisions or changes occur at the individual and family level. However, for comprehensive community health improvement, strategies are needed at organizational, community, and sociopolitical levels. Nursing center staff may focus their efforts on system issues, community capacity, and family and individual health care access concurrently. Alternatively, the staff may concentrate programmatic efforts solely at the individual or family level and later address system and community issues. There is no one approach. Figure 21-4 presents the "big picture" perspective that the majority of center interventions take place in community rather than institutional settings. In the twenty-first century, innovative and disruptive preventive health models are challenging the status quo of institutionally driven primary care practices (Lawrence, 2010).

APNs involved in public health and nurse-managed center services are strategically positioned to communicate, adapt, and influence change to improve and support individual, population, and community health outcomes (Vermeulen, Puranam, & Gulati, 2010). The multilevel intervention approach helps people enter the health care system earlier, with greater ease and confidence, and continue in care long enough to realize positive outcomes (Berkman & Lochner, 2002). This approach also recognizes that one size (static, rote services) does not meet all the needs and interests of the target population.

Nurses keep in mind the prevention levels that improve the health of the public. *Primary, secondary,* and *tertiary prevention* are not terms the general population understands. In fact, the idea of prevention at different levels requires thoughtful investigation and analysis. One of multiple national resources regarding prevention levels and agendas is Partnership for Prevention (www.prevent.org). The Levels of Prevention box is one example that a NMHC might use.

---

### 📄 LEVELS OF PREVENTION

#### *Nursing Center Application*

**Primary Prevention**
Assess home for lead dust; educate family on lead poisoning prevention strategies.

**Secondary Prevention**
Conduct blood lead level screenings on a regular basis for children younger than age 6.

**Tertiary Prevention**
Treat child who has an elevated blood lead level with appropriate therapies and eliminate environmental lead toxicity exposures.

---

The foundations of nursing center development are rooted in public health nursing history and the evolution of the nursing profession (Fee & Bu, 2010). Other chapters in this text provide historical details and factors that have influenced nursing education, practice, service, and research throughout the twentieth century.

Most nursing center models as currently known emerged from academic nursing programs in the 1970s through 2000s. At that time, opportunities did not exist within the traditional health care system for faculty or their nurse practitioner students to apply their knowledge and skills in a nursing framework of care. Bold ideas in the schools of nursing at the University of Wisconsin-Milwaukee, Arizona State University, Columbia University, and others established practice settings that simultaneously provided health care to the community and learning experiences for students. Many of the academic centers focused on the underserved populations in nearby communities. Over time, centers have achieved national recognition as essential safety net providers to vulnerable populations (Sherman, 2005).

The success of these early efforts supported the establishment of other academic nursing centers across the nation. Interest in this model of practice grew rapidly among community service organizations, schools, churches, public housing facilities, and others (Bellack & O'Neil, 2000). Although there continues to be no historical or current databank regarding the absolute number of nursing centers that have been developed, NNCC surveys document that models have been developed in every state, and in urban, suburban, and rural communities. Some nurse-managed centers have curtailed services or closed because of factors such as funding challenges, changes in institutional commitment, scarcity of qualified advanced practice nurses, and population losses resulting from natural catastrophes (Pohl et al, 2010).

Resource Tool 21.B highlights the evolution of nursing centers over the past century, and lists educational, political, legislative, and funding factors that have influenced the development and sustainability of nursing centers. This evolutionary trend will be altered with the implementation of the Patient Protection and Affordability Care Act and committed funding to NLHCs.

## THE TEAM OF A NURSE-LED CENTER

Nurses, including APNs, other health and allied health professionals, support staff, and the community at large, comprise the nurse-led center team. The center type and its services determine staff patterns and roles, responsibilities, and reporting lines. Every center must have an organizational chart that clearly shows staffing positions and reporting responsibilities. The organizational framework must be dynamic in nature and adaptive to new community-focused initiatives.

A fundamental premise to any NLHC is that the community in which the model is placed has the most power and influence on model development and team composition. The demand for services will be community driven. A rural NLHC model may have different staff needs than one situated in a distressed urban area (Jacobson, 2002).

A center's success also relates to how well the team works together to ensure the delivery of high-quality health care to target populations (Heifetz & Linsky, 2002). Positive collegial and professional relationships set the tone for the work. Critical center clinical and management positions are briefly highlighted in the following section. Resource Tool 21.C presents actual or potential nurse-led center positions and extensive descriptions of staff and adjunct roles.

### Director: Nurse Executive

The director or nurse executive is an APN who is committed to the NLHC model. The roles and responsibilities of the nurse executive are dynamic and diverse. The director has a current knowledge of the target community, the ability and willingness to work with many community organizations and groups, and a background in organizational planning, administration, and fiscal management. The nurse executive is responsible for oversight of contracts and grants, annual reports, and development of the advisory board or board of directors. Other responsibilities include hiring and retention of highly qualified staff.

Directors are visionary leaders and planners. They constantly use data, collaborative feedback, existing resources, and partnerships to modify and adjust the overall direction of the nursing center (Salmon, 2007; Torrisi & Hansen-Turton, 2005). As NLHCs have evolved and third-party reimbursement opportunities for nurse practitioner services increase, APN practitioners have assumed leadership positions in center practices. Likewise, advanced practice public health nurses have led the NLHC movement and employed nurse practitioners as advanced practice providers. For the most part, public health nurse directors have implemented a holistic service model. This model incorporates public health service and community-based programs that complement the primary care services.

There are NLHCs that started with public health programs and then established primary health care services. These public health programs include maternal–child home visitation funded by Title V federal funds, Nurse-Family Partnership (NFP), and Environmental Protection Agency (EPA) grants focusing on lead poisoning prevention, asthma triggers prevention, and many others. Other centers started with primary health care services at one location and later on incorporated client-centered public health services.

## Advanced Practice Nurses

Advanced practice nurses (APNs) have additional education and training beyond their basic nursing program and are certified or licensed in a specialty area such as women's health nurse practitioner. They provide an expanded level of health services to individuals and families. These nurses are responsible for the oversight of clinical staff as well as program services and outcome measures.

Nurses with advanced preparation in community or public health nursing are essential to the advancement of NLHCs and integrated health services (Dentzer, 2010). These nurses use nursing and public health principles to promote and sustain the health of populations in neighborhood and community settings. Their work is diverse. Nurses are responsible for assessing populations' needs and interests in health care, developing grant proposals to expand services, and managing contracts for preventive and early intervention programs in community settings. Nurses implement group health education classes and screenings, and provide individual case management in community and home settings. Health advocacy is an essential component of their work (ANA, 2007).

In comprehensive primary care centers, nurse practitioners provide on-site services. As APNs, nurse practitioners can be generalists (i.e., family nurse practitioners who provide services to people of all ages) or specialists. The specialist nurse practitioner has skills with particular age groups (e.g., pediatric, adolescent, or geriatric) or skills developed to meet the interests and needs of particular population groups such as women's health; menopausal health; and wound, ostomy, and continence management (Horrocks, Anderson, & Salisbury, 2002).

Naylor and Kurtzman's article in *Health Affairs* (2010) discusses nursing workforce issues, and the need to support the work of APRNs in primary care settings. In 2008, APRNs represented about 8% of the 3.1 million licensed registered nurses in the United States (ANA, 2011). The majority of APNs

practice in primary care and public health settings. These settings include FQHCs, local and state health departments, NLHCs, and convenient care clinics (retail clinics).

National health reform legislation supports increasing the advanced practice workforce in primary care patient–centered medical homes. As discussed in Chapter 5, on March 23, 2010, the Patient Protection and Affordable Care Act was signed into law. The act makes a significant investment of $50 million to expand nurse-managed health centers to serve vulnerable, at-risk populations. In addition, it also supports faculty scholarship programs to expand nursing school enrollment and student loan repayment programs.

## Other Staff

Community health workers are essential staff in many NLHCs. Typically, they are neighborhood residents who have completed high school or 2-year associate degree programs and who want to work with others in their community. The workers are trained in community outreach, family case management, or on-site services (Rosenthal et al, 2010).

The operations of any center require support staff. Staff members include a business or operations manager and data operations personnel. A parent organization may dedicate a portion of staff lines, including human resources and public relations, to assist the director and senior staff. The operations manager handles contracts and grant budgets, advertising for staff, personnel hires, and billing. Personnel management, staffing patterns, and site management including data collection are also responsibilities of an operations manager.

Data operations personnel are essential. Client-based and population-based outcomes are necessary for program evaluation, proposal development, and funding purposes. Rapid changes in technology related to billing and reporting requirements, and federal regulations regarding protection of information about an individual's health care status, require data operations personnel on site or as consultants. In today's litigious society, the operation of any NLHC involves ensuring privacy of client records and securing access to computerized data.

At present and into the future, information systems (IS) and technology support (TS) personnel must be in place to meet the escalating expectation to institute and effectively use a computerized client-centered database. Computerized systems require upgrades and maintenance. Also, as hardware and software programs become obsolete and new programs are introduced, staff will need training and support to adapt to new data systems.

Staff may also be needed for public relations and multimedia campaigns to gain support as the center expands. Other multidisciplinary providers are engaged in nursing center work and share responsibility in outreach and educational campaigns. Provider representation is diverse. Staff includes physician collaborators, family therapists, mental health counselors, students, faculty, administrators, and clinical social workers. Other professionals include dentists, podiatrists, lactation specialists, and clinicians with interests in holistic health (Lutz, Herrick, & Lehman, 2001).

## Educators, Researchers, Students, and Other Members

The education and research roles held by faculty, staff, and consultants are essential if the NLHC model is to advance in today's health care system (AACN, 2002). The opportunity for faculty involvement through clinical training of students as well as community-focused research programs is evident and promising for community collaboration and well-being (Greiner & Knebel, 2003).

NLHC programs are client and student oriented. Nursing students can learn about the intersection of health care economics, service, education, and research (Thies & Ayers, 2004). Students also have opportunities to promote social justice while engaging in community service learning activities with underserved, vulnerable populations (Hansen-Turton, Miller, & Greiner, 2009; Thompson & Feeney, 2004). If the center is part of a school of nursing, faculty roles include clinical oversight of graduate and undergraduate students assigned to the center or involved in related community projects, such as adult influenza inoculation campaigns.

Other members include community advocates, board of directors/advisory board members, and organizational partners. Community advocates are frequently known as key stakeholders. Community voices are often the most influential and listened to by elected officials and their staff.

Every NLHC should have a board of directors or advisory board. The organizational structure of a center as part of a larger institution or a freestanding entity dictates the type of board members that govern or advise staff on the direction of the center. A board of directors has oversight responsibilities, including fiscal management, for the NLHC model. An advisory board guides the work of an NLHC but holds no fiduciary or voting responsibilities. The board should represent diverse professions and occupations and be knowledgeable about the target community and its residents.

In addition, organizational partners are valued members. Centers that develop and maintain organizational relationships will benefit through service agreements and contracts with one or more of the partners.

## THE BUSINESS SIDE OF NURSE-LED CENTERS: ESSENTIAL ELEMENTS

Nurses who work in nursing centers are committed to working with diverse people in noninstitutional settings. The nurses use community characteristics, population profiles, health indexes, epidemiologic findings, and positive working relationships with professionals and the public at large to develop the model (Hansen-Turton, Miller, & Greiner, 2009). The model requires careful planning and structure to be a successful education, service, and business enterprise. During the planning and implementation phases, interrelated elements must be considered. Resource Tool 21.D outlines essential elements in nursing center development. These elements serve as an annual checklist to measure growth of a nursing center and guide sound decisions regarding sustainability and future planning.

## Start-up and Sustainability

In planning and establishing a nursing center (Schultz, Krieger, & Galea, 2002), nurses and others need to seek expert advice and support. This includes having financial advisors. It is important to remember that this work is a business enterprise in which the art and science of nursing is practiced. Final decisions about establishing a nursing center are made after exploration of the following essential areas:

1. Organizational goals, commitments, and resources
2. Community interests, assets, and needs
3. Feasibility study, internal and external to the parent organization
4. Strategic plan
5. Business plan
6. Information management plan and resources
7. Existing social policy and health care financing
8. Legal and regulatory considerations
9. Mission, vision, and commitment of the lead organization

The initial work of assessing the interests, resources, and capacity of an organization to undertake the nursing center model is interrelated yet separate. For example, conduct a feasibility study before developing a business plan and incorporate elements of the feasibility study into the business plan. A strategic plan builds on feasibility data as well as economic principles and practices. Planners must also consider workforce needs, personnel management, public information and outreach campaigns, community capacity, and the health care environment relative to funding streams. In 2015 and beyond, any feasibility study must analyze the national health care reform legislation dollars committed, and funded programs. As a cautionary note, dollars committed do not guarantee funding at that level. Regardless of the federal funding level, there will be widespread competition for program support.

### Feasibility Study

A feasibility study identifies the strengths, limitations, and capacity of an organization and the community to support the establishment and continuation of a nursing center. It requires interviews with key individuals, surveys and data collection, focus groups, and community forums. It is necessary to consider epidemiologic, environmental, and other community assessments as well as data from public health agencies. Local agencies and tertiary care institutions can provide data about health needs and gaps in care for targeted groups. The study must consider legal and regulatory policies. States vary in their regulations for APNs, particularly nurse practitioners. The planners must investigate required professional credentialing, site accreditation, state Medicaid waivers, physician collaborative agreements, and any local or state requirements (Naylor & Kurtzman, 2010). The overall processes of community collaborations, assessment, and feasibility studies support the development of business plans, strategic plans, and timelines.

A sound business plan considers all aspects of establishing a nursing center and describes the development and direction of the nursing center and how goals will be met (see the How To Develop a Business Plan box). A business plan is built on the known or more predictable sources of funding at the time the plan is developed. In today's uncertain economic health care environment, it may be necessary to modify the business plan at a moment's notice (Torrisi & Hansen-Turton, 2005). Legislative changes and reimbursement regulations can significantly alter the business plan. In addition, no grant allocation should ever be included in the business plan until the grant is awarded.

---

**HOW TO** Develop a Business Plan

1. Cover page includes date, name, address, and phone number(s) of the person(s) responsible for the nursing center and any consultants to the business plan.
2. Executive summary. This is a one- or two-page overview of the center and the plan.
3. Table of contents.
4. Description of the business plan that details what the center is and what services it will provide.
5. Survey of the industry. This summarizes the past, present, and future of the local and regional health care market.
6. Market research and analysis. This description outlines existing competition and the potential market share and identifies target groups.
7. Marketing plan. This details how the center will reach its targeted clients.
8. Organizational chart with a description of the management team.
9. List of supporting professional staff (e.g., accountants).
10. Operations plan. This describes how and where services will be provided.
11. Research and development. This projects program improvement and opportunities for new initiatives.
12. Overall schedule. The timeline establishes the start date and development phase of the nursing center.
13. Critical risks and problems. This examines the internal and external threats to the center and how these will be addressed.
14. Financial plan. The fiscal projections for the first 3 to 5 years are presented. A budget, cash flow forecast, and break-even point are included.
15. Proposed funding. Specific sources are listed that can provide funding.
16. Legal structure of the center. This describes the status of the center, such as free-standing, a corporation, or part of a larger organization.
17. Appendixes and supporting documents

---

The strategic plan complements the business plan. A strategic plan looks into the future and guides the work of the nursing center in that direction. Strategic plans have a regular timeline and may change as indicated by local, national, and global events. Strategic planning meetings are periodically scheduled to review and refine the plan. The plan includes goals, objectives, and target timelines for implementation and evaluation of projected and ongoing services. The strategic plan should answer these questions: (1) What resources will the center need after start-up? (2) What economic and legislative factors may influence center productivity and sustainability? (3) What will be the center's core functions in 5, 7, and 9 years? (4) How can the staff move the center in the appropriate direction? (5) How will staff process and handle change?

Feasibility studies, business plans, and strategic plans lay the foundation for strong nursing centers. These components are crucial to the day-to-day functioning of a newly opened nursing center and reflect the abilities of the management team to build community coalitions and collaboratives. In addition, the management team must be knowledgeable about federal regulations, acts, and funding changes, especially Medicaid and Medicare reimbursement, and grant opportunities. One resource tool that should be on site for reference is the NNCC Guide: *Nurse-Managed Wellness Centers: Developing and Maintaining Your Center, a National Nursing Center Consortium Guide and Toolkit* (Hansen-Turton et al, 2009).

Once the community assessment, feasibility study, business plans, and organizational networking are completed, it is important for key people to ask the following questions:

- Why would the organization want to do this?
- What will be the immediate and long-term outcomes for the organization and the community at large?
- Can the investment (that is, staff, money, time, and space) be made?
- Does the community truly want and need a nursing center model?

The organization cannot drive the desire for the nursing center. The center must be person- and community-centric, not provider-centric. If the establishment of a nursing center is solely done from the organization's vantage point, the possibility of long-term sustainability may be jeopardized. The final question is the most critical one: Does the community truly want and need a nursing center model? No assessment, study, or plan can ignore this question. If the answer is not clear, more time must be invested to find out if there is a match in need, interest, and a center's potential capacity. For example, if the community is focused on helping young women move from public assistance into jobs and the immediate need is daycare, a nursing center that offers linkages with daycare providers and on-site physical examinations and childhood immunizations will be an essential community resource. However, if the nursing center offers only senior citizen services, the immediate and expressed community need was ignored.

The establishment of a nursing center is warranted if the model reflects the needs, interests, and strengths of the target population and is economically feasible. There should be long-term commitments by all involved in the planning process, including any parent organization. The parent organization's mission, vision, and commitment influence the viability of the nursing center model. Planners must determine the support of the parent organization before investing the time, effort, and collaborative work necessary to develop the model. If there is uncertainty at the administrative level, it is foolhardy to move forward until there is strong and documented commitment from the organization that matches the community commitment.

It is challenging for those involved in the planning process to forecast programs, determine service patterns, integrate outcome measures, and project costs. The planning process over time can be difficult. Planners may not devote sufficient time to the matter of nursing center revenue sources (Torrisi & Hansen-Turton, 2005). If money matters are not thoroughly considered, any nursing center's future will be compromised and may not withstand the stresses of changing funding streams, political decisions, and policy changes (Kinsey & Gerrity, 2005).

The business plan provides information that forecasts the minimum funding necessary to begin a nursing center and project income 1, 3, and 5 years from inception. A break-even analysis is essential. A business plan must be periodically modified when legislation regarding Medicaid and Medicare reimbursement rates occurs. In addition, a business plan must accommodate a state's reimbursement parameters for APNs.

Potential income sources include fee-for-service, commercial reimbursement, and self-pay. Fee-for-service may be the most viable of economic strategies. Commercial reimbursement includes private health care insurers with established fee schedules. Clients without a source of health insurance are characterized as self-pay. Costs and charges for services must be established. Nursing centers located in medically underserved areas or working with medically underserved populations (migrants) have sliding-fee schedules based on published federal poverty guidelines. Managed care contracts with particular insurance companies, particularly Medicaid contractors, are other sources of income; however, the monthly Medicaid reimbursements do not cover the cost of providing health care to the most vulnerable and underserved in society (Torrisi & Hansen-Turton, 2005). Cost-effectiveness and quality care are key concerns as providers deal with the instability of reimbursement rates and the variable number of underinsured people seeking a medical home.

Financial support for nursing centers may also come from foundations, charitable contributions, private giving, and fund-raising. Fund-raising can take the form of direct mailings, pledges, and events that raise money. Grants are a source of initial and ongoing funding. The funding organization generally releases guidelines of what the organization will fund. The guidelines are frequently released as a request for proposals (RFP). A proposal developed in response to the RFP specifies how the nursing center would meet the goals of the granting organization in the given timeline. The description of services and client outcomes must be presented in relation to the RFP guidelines.

Nursing centers have agreements and contracts in place for specific services. Agreements and contracts may have different language as well as reporting and fiscal management requirements; however, the basic premise is similar. The nursing center enters into a written agreement to provide services to a select population group or develop a program that targets a specific area. For example, a center may have an agreement with the American Cancer Society to develop a cancer education program for minority seniors in a low-income senior housing complex. The agreement is for a defined time period, has target goals and objectives, and outlines staff assignments and expectations, but there is no budget related to the program. A contract is a legal document that lists the purchase of services, reporting requirements, invoicing, and expected client outcomes. An example would be a city health department that issues a contract to a nursing center to immunize 100 adults against influenza for a specified sum per vaccine. Each nursing center may have one or many contracts and agreements; however, a nursing center should enter into each arrangement with clear understanding of the business side of the model. Any contract or agreement should be fiscally sound and not deplete center resources.

## EVIDENCE-BASED PRACTICE

Evidence-based practice represents the clinical application of particular nursing (health care) interventions and documented client and population outcome data over time (Deaton, 2002). Trends in health care services, client responses, and changes in community characteristics must be documented and summarized periodically (Oros et al, 2001). Assessments of sources of ill health, including noncommunicable conditions, and community influences on economic, environmental, behavioral, and physical health are conducted periodically and reported (Lancaster, 2005). Outcome measurements include client use of on-site services, childhood and adult immunizations patterns, pregnancy outcomes, emergency department and hospital use, and other health indexes including client satisfaction and quality-of-life measures.

The cost of collecting and documenting outcome measures must be included in the NLHC budget (Tudor, 2005; Bates & Bitton, 2010). Measurement instruments require technological support and staff expertise and ongoing monitoring and analyses (Garrett & Yasnoff, 2002; Browne et al, 2010). The Patient Protection and Affordable Care Act includes the prevention and wellness national strategy to fund and support evidence-based and community-based services. This act should provide support to NLHCs with defined outcome measures and electronic medical records (EMRs) in place (Forrest & Whelan, 2000).

Defined outcome measures (evidence) will enable NLHC staff to determine program effectiveness and cost savings associated with clinical outcomes (Resick et al, 2011). The challenge is how to define the criteria, develop measurements and collection methods, compare the evidence with broader community findings, interpret the data to funders, and disseminate findings to the wider health care community. Nursing center staff can use a variety of forums to share findings including professional conferences and publications, popular press, multimedia venues, and testimonies at public hearings (Callahan & Jennings, 2002).

### Evidence-based Practice Model

In the twenty-first century health care market, research focusing on evidence-based practices demonstrating meaningful client and family outcomes will drive grant calls and investment decisions by public and private entities. An outstanding example relevant to advanced practice nurses and nurse-led models of care was published online July 7, 2014 in the *Journal of the American Medical Association (JAMA) Pediatrics*. Dr. David Olds et al reported on the *Effect of Home Visiting by Nurses on Maternal and Child Mortality*. He and colleagues found that the

Nurse-Family Partnership reduces preventable death among both low-income mothers and their first-born children living in urban, disadvantaged neighborhoods. Primarily African American low-income mothers and children residing in Memphis, Tennessee, were engaged in a randomized, clinical trial of this early intervention program for more than two decades (1990-2011). In earlier studies, mothers participating in the NFP program, when compared with those in the control group, were found to have received better prenatal care; reduced short-interval second pregnancies; decreased use of public assistance programs; and had less substance abuse. Their nurse-visited children, compared to children not receiving nurse home visits, were less likely to be hospitalized with injuries through age two years; more likely to be school ready; and less likely to reveal depression, anxiety, and substance abuse at age 12. This study reports on the findings that mothers in the control groups who did not receive nurse home visits were nearly three times more likely to die than mothers receiving nurse home visits. The relative reduction in maternal mortality was even greater for deaths related to external causes including drug overdose, suicide, and homicide. Children in the control group not receiving nurse home visits had a mortality rate of 1.6% for preventable causes such as sudden infant death syndrome, unintentional injuries, and homicide. There were zero preventable deaths among nurse-visited children.

For more than 37 years, Dr. Olds and colleagues continued to study the long-lasting maternal and early childhood outcomes of those involved in Nurse-Family Partnership. NFP is the most rigorously studied maternal and early childhood health program of its kind. The data demonstrate that NFP public health nurse home visitors, in partnership with their enrolled mothers, contribute to multigenerational health and family stabilization. These outcomes also have measurable economic and societal benefits that reduce long-term social service expenditures. The Nurse-Family Partnership National Service Office (www.nursefamilypartnership.org) helps communities and nurse-led models of practice implement and sustain this evidence-based public health program. The Philadelphia Nurse-Family Partnership is highlighted later in this chapter.

## Health Insurance Portability and Accountability Act (HIPAA)

Staff committed to evidence-based practice, outcome measures, EMRs, data collection, and analyses must be knowledgeable about the Health Insurance Portability and Accountability Act (HIPAA). HIPAA, which is Public Law 104-191 passed by the 104th Congress to protect the privacy of individually identified health data referred to as protected health information (PHI). The regulations took into consideration the shift to paperless, electronic medical records. Electronic records increase the potential for individuals to access, use, and disclose sensitive personal health data. The act enables consumers to have more control over their health information, establishes boundaries about the use and release of health records, sets safeguards about provider protection of private health information and penalizes violations of same, and enables consumers to obtain and/or make informed decisions about how their health

information is used and disclosed. According to current regulations, all staff must monitor and keep secure client records, have mechanisms to transfer client information securely and appropriately, and strictly adhere to client confidentiality (Thorpe & Ogden, 2010).

Nurses in NLHCs are required to comply with HIPAA regulations, as well as be responsive to and report public health threats such as tuberculosis, disease outbreaks related to food contaminations, and influenza. Reference resources for staff include the HIPAA website of the Office for Civil Rights (http://www.hhs.gov/ocr/hipaa/) (USDHHS, 2010b) and the CDC website on Privacy Rule guidelines (http://www.cdc.gov/privacy rule) (CDC, 2010b). Other chapters further detail public health responsiveness and HIPAA documentation challenges.

## Outcomes and Quality Indicators

Quality health indicators and related performance measures are priorities in any type of nursing center (Stryer, Clancy, & Simpson, 2002). These data are presented to the nursing center's board, funders, and the community at large and document the center's contributions to the health and welfare of the community. Outcome measures and quality indicators can be preset, or staff may determine that there are outcome measures that were not predetermined, but at time of review have meaningful results. For example, the nurse practitioners may have set up a callback system that improves timely use of primary care services. This can now be documented through client satisfaction, adherence to advised health practices, and changes in health behaviors. Such outcomes can be considered quality indicators that emerged from the day-to-day practices.

Center staff must carefully consider and determine what outcome measures and quality indicators have meaning for the community and the health care system. Despite a staff tendency to want to measure everything, begin with particular indicators and measures and incrementally add as information is indicated. Excessive measures consume staff time and resources and valid measurements may not emerge.

The Quality Care Task Force of the NNCC has developed *Guidelines for Quality Management for Nursing Centers with Standards for Community Nursing Centers*. This publication is a vital tool for staff and can be accessed at www.nncc.us. The standards assist nursing centers to assess growth and development and areas that need improvement. The standards also include quality indicators, population groups, performance targets, and measures. The indicators are grouped into the areas of prevention, utilization, client satisfaction, functional status, symptom severity, and others.

Utilization of the standards and select indicators and associated processes enable a nursing center to document evidence-based practice. References used to develop the standards include the National Committee for Quality Assurance (NCQA) (Gingerich, 2000). An example of evidence-based practice follows; also refer to Table 21-1.

The Philadelphia Nurse-Family Partnership (NFP) serves first-time low-income parents and their children through an intensive public health nurse home visit model. This replication model is based on the most rigorously tested program of its kind

## TABLE 21-1   Examples of Quality Health Indicators for Nursing Centers

| Indicator | Population | Performance Targets | Measure |
|---|---|---|---|
| **Prevention**<br>Annual influenza vaccine | High-risk groups: Age 65 or those with heart or lung disease and other chronic conditions | *Healthy People 2020* = 90% age 65+<br>*Healthy People 2020* = 60% high-risk ages 18-64 years | Client self-report and/or clinical records/audit |
| **Utilization**<br>Mammogram within past 2 years | HEDIS: Women age 52-69 years<br>*Healthy People 2020:* Women 40 years and older | HEDIS 2001 = 81%<br>*Healthy People 2020* = 70% | Client self-report and/or clinical records/audit |
| **Client Satisfaction**<br>Client satisfaction, annual | 100 consecutive clients per quarter | Performance targets to be determined by individual nursing center and/or health care plan | Surveys |
| **Functional Status**<br>Quality-of-life indicator | Adults age 18 years and older | Determined by individual nursing center and related to baseline indicators and improvement goals | Screen using Short Form 12 or 36 |

(www.nursefamilypartnership.org). Philadelphia's NFP was established July 1, 2001. It is the largest countywide site in the Commonwealth of Pennsylvania and was formed to reduce child abuse and neglect in high-risk Philadelphia neighborhoods. Eligible low-income women are enrolled during pregnancy. Each woman receives intensive home visit services until the child reaches age 2 (program graduation). The Philadelphia NFP adheres to the national NFP model of nurse home visitation. NFP goals are to improve pregnancy outcomes, improve children's health and development, and improve families' economic self-sufficiency over time. NFP is based on the primary prevention and early intervention model developed by Dr. David Olds and colleagues (Eckenrode et al, 2010). Advanced practice public health nurses receive extensive education in NFP protocols, maternal-infant-toddler assessment measures, and motivational interviewing strategies. As of 2014, NFP nationally serves over 29,000 women in 43 states, the US Virgin Islands and six tribal communities.

On July 21, 2010, Health and Human Services Secretary Kathleen Sebelius announced the Affordable Care Act Initial Funding for Maternal, Infant, and Early Childhood Home Visiting (MIECHV) State Grants to fund evidence-based home visiting programs that improve the well-being of families with young children. In 2012, Philadelphia NFP and its complementary Mabel Morris Family Home Visit Program received a MIECHV federal expansion grant award and increased enrollment from 400 pregnant adolescent and adult women in any given year to 650. Data released in July 2014 summarize participant demographics and health and employment outcomes from 2001 to 2014 ($N = 4012$). Upon enrollment, the median age of clients was 18 years (range, 10 to 45 years). The median education was eleventh grade. Ninety-three percent of the population was unwed with 72% unemployed and from 2010 to present a decline in median annual incomes to $7,500. Ninety-two percent of the population was of African American or Hispanic heritage. Cumulative data document the following outcomes: there was a 19% reduction in smoking during pregnancy, a statistically significant (63%) reduction in marijuana use, and a statistically significant (62%) reduction in domestic violence during pregnancy. Seventy-five percent of mothers initiated breastfeeding with 13.5% breastfeeding at 12 months of infancy. Upon graduation when children turn 2 years, 93% of the toddlers were fully immunized. Of the mothers who entered the program without high school or GED diplomas, 60% were still in school and 40% completed education, with 17% pursuing higher education. Philadelphia NFP mothers during the first year postpartum entered the workforce earlier than national counterparts and remained employed. The Mabel Morris Family Home Visit program complements the NFP model as it uses the Parents As Teachers curriculum and enrolls pregnant and parenting families and follows the youngest child until age 5. This program enables graduating NFP families to continue with home visit services if needed. Nurse home visitors also staff this program and are involved in extensive Parents As Teachers training. This model focuses on positive parenting education emphasizing parents as the child's first teacher and school readiness at age five for each child.

The Philadelphia NFP reflects NFP National Service Office findings across the nation. It is a cost-effective nurse home visit program proven to be of great benefit for low-income, first-time at-risk mothers and their first-borns (NFP, 2014). Dr. Ted Miller of the Pacific Institute for Research and Evaluation prepared a report analyzing to date NFPs costs, outcomes and return from investment. NFP programs in Pennsylvania have an average cost per family of $8,327 and Miller's model predicts that by a child's 18th birthday the benefits to society of NFP are estimated to be $59,972, which represents a $7.20 return on investment for every dollar invested in Nurse-Family Partnership (Maternal and child health program, 2014).

The momentum to support evidence-based home visitation programs will continue beyond this decade. Forty-nine states, the District of Columbia, and five territories were awarded funds to create and support successful home visiting programs, such as Nurse-Family Partnerships and Parents As Teachers Home Visit models (USDHHS, 2010a).

This is an opportune time for APNs interested in public health and prevention initiatives to explore employment options in NLHCs that host nurse-family partnerships and other maternal-child-family health services. Throughout the nation, there is great momentum in the health and economic sectors to create social impact bonds that would sustain early childhood initiatives demonstrating measurable, long-term personal and family outcomes. The cost savings to society are measurable and investors want to make wise investment decisions that have "payouts." Nurses committed to prevention work in community settings are on the cusp of new careers in early childhood programs.

## Quality Improvement

The evidence-based practice application exemplifies what nurses can do to measure outcomes, strive to improve those outcomes given particular standards, and make meaningful contributions to the public's health. Accurate data collection, measurement methods, summary statistics, and preparation of evidence-based practice reports are fundamental standards in any NLHC.

As the nursing center model continues to grow throughout the nation, the potential to collectively summarize data and outcomes will further strengthen this movement. Through collaboration and the pooling of data, this model will continue to move into the mainstream health care system (Christensen,

Bohmer, & Kenagy, 2000; Naylor & Kurtzman, 2010). However, the staff must be as committed to data as to the provision of quality services. Data will enable the staff to clearly understand what goals are in place, and if areas are to be improved, they can develop action plans to improve services and client outcomes (Campbell, 2000). The concurrent emphasis on service and data can stress staff and the capacity of any nursing center to effectively and efficiently manage services and technology (Bates & Bitton, 2010). The Quality and Safety in Nursing Education box describes how to use data to improve care.

## Technology and Information Systems

Currently, technology and information systems are essential for data collection and analyses. Available technologies need to be used to collect, collate, and analyze data and to support the provision of quality health care services (Shortliffe, 2005; DesRoches, Campbell, & Vogeli, 2010). Technology and information systems will continue to change and adapt to accommodate existing health care legislation, HIPAA, *Healthy People 2020*, public health mandates, and unfolding global and national events. Continual reinforcement about the confidentiality of client records is critical (Callahan & Jennings, 2002). Transfer of information must be carefully monitored, and the use of computers and the entering and retrieval of data by staff will be delineated by role and responsibility and passwords. One resource tool that should be on site for reference is the National

---

**QSEN  FOCUS ON QUALITY AND SAFETY EDUCATION FOR NURSES**

### *Quality and Safety Focus*

**Targeted Competency: Quality Improvement**
Use data to monitor the outcomes of care processes and use improvement methods to design and test changes to continuously improve the quality and safety of health care systems.

Important aspects of quality improvement include:
- **Knowledge:** Recognize that nursing and other health professions students are parts of systems of care and care processes that affect outcomes for patients and families
- **Skills:** Seek information about outcomes of care for populations served in care setting
- **Attitudes:** Value own and others' contributions to outcomes of care in local care settings

**Quality Improvement Question**
Nursing centers are established to address a specific health need in a community. You are a public health nurse who has been invited to help develop a new nursing center whose primary aim is to provide primary care to a newly insured group prevalent in your community: previously uninsured young adults. This population is newly insured because of the Affordable Care Act of 2010. As you begin to research this population, you come to appreciate the importance of this target population. In your research you discover that an important aspect of the success of the Affordable Care Act is the inclusion of young adults (age 19 to 29). According to 2013 statistics collected by The Commonwealth Fund, this population has historically been uninsured at higher rates than any other age group, not because of a lack of desire for health coverage

but because they have lacked access to affordable health coverage—only 64 percent of young adults had health insurance coverage in 2010. Additionally, 41 percent of all young adults and 60 percent of uninsured young adults said they did not receive needed health care because of the cost of care. Half of uninsured young adults also reported medical debt or problems paying medical bills, while 29 percent of insured young adults reported these problems due to the lack of sufficient health care coverage (Collins, Robertson, Garber & Doty, 2013).

The new Nursing Center is funded by a local large university (whose many graduates stay in the community), the local, large regional university hospital, and a large regional charity organization. Consider the following questions in the development of this important community-based resource:
- Knowing that quality improvement is data driven work, what data will you need to track to demonstrate an improvement in providing primary care to your target population?
- How will you gather data about current barriers to access to care for your target population?
- How might you involve your financial stakeholder partners in ensuring that your nursing center is providing more accessible care to your target population?
- Since ongoing monitoring of relevant data is vital to assessing whether a nursing center is meeting its stated goal for its target population, how will you educate the staff of the nursing center about the importance of these data? Develop bullet points for ongoing education/motivation of the nursing center staff.

Collins SR, Robertson R, Garber T, Doty MM: *Insuring the future: current trends in health coverage and the effects of implementing the Affordable Care* Act, New York, 2013, The Commonwealth Fund.
Prepared by Gail Armstrong, PhD(c), DNP, ACNS-BC, CNE, Associate Professor, University of Colorado Denver College of Nursing.

Nursing Center Consortium Guide: *Community and Nurse-Managed Health Centers: Getting Them Started and Keeping Them Going* (Torrisi & Hansen-Turton, 2005).

## EDUCATION AND RESEARCH

Nursing centers provide many education and research opportunities. Clinical assignments through the nursing center model enable students at all levels to work with skilled clinicians, develop positive community collaboratives, and build their skills to become professionals. These students often develop an interest in working with underserved populations in medically underserved areas of the nation. Students are assets to the nursing center model. Faculty brings skills that enable nursing center staff to develop and implement programs that integrate faculty-student contributions and enable the programs to engage more of the target population.

It is necessary to carefully coordinate, supervise, and evaluate student education in nursing centers. A faculty liaison enables students to have a resource within the educational system as well as a link with the center. Student schedules must also be coordinated with nursing center timelines. A year-round nursing center that provides 24-hour coverage of services must accommodate academic schedules and students moving in and out of clinical assignments. Nursing center staff and faculty must work to maintain ongoing communication with clients and community agencies about student rotations, program assignments, and student projects. Students should be encouraged to share their work with the community because learning is a mutual exchange of goods and services. In addition, in any nursing center model nothing is done in isolation (Shiber & D'Lugoff, 2002).

Research in nursing centers provides the opportunity to gain answers to questions and to share the findings with colleagues and the public (Sherman, 2005). It is important to answer questions about individual and population health status, client outcomes over time, roles and capacities to address health promotion with the existing health system, and the value and affordability of care (Gladwell, 2005). Centers offer many opportunities for educational research.

Each center needs a research or program evaluation agenda. Resource Tool 21.E displays the WHO's priorities for a common nursing research agenda. The research focus includes identification and clarification of client needs, particularly those not engaged in an existing health system; description of nursing interventions and linkages with consumer needs and resources; demonstration of effective interventions that produce appropriate outcomes; and cost analysis and documented cost-effectiveness of services (Hirschfeld, 1998).

Over the past three decades, nursing center research has principally focused on the development and characteristics of nursing centers (Sherman, 2005). Descriptive data have been collected about clients, types of services, the financial supports, and community relationships. However, more than descriptive clinical studies are needed. Research efforts are underway to capture and name the unique features of nursing models of care and link them with health outcomes. For example, the significance of

psychosocial interventions inherent in nursing practice is being examined, such as listening to, supporting, and interpreting information for clients. Client satisfaction studies document the perceived value by those who use nursing centers. Factors associated with access to services are being examined. These include availability, timeliness, acceptability, and affordability of services. Environmental conditions, such as housing, transportation, criminal activities, and welfare-to-work transitions that influence health care access and use patterns are being examined. Resource Tool 21.F presents a template for research in NLHCs.

### Program Evaluation

Program evaluation is an essential organizational practice in NLHCs, and research questions emerge from program evaluation. The evaluation process is a systematic approach to improve and account for public health and primary care actions. Evaluation is thoroughly integrated in routine program operations. The process drives community-focused strategies, allows for program improvements, and identifies the need for additional services.

Program evaluation separates what is working from what is not and enables clinicians, faculty, and students to ask difficult questions and handle pressing challenges (Schultz, Krieger, & Galea, 2002). Resources are available to nursing center staff to enhance their understanding and application of program evaluation in their particular setting. Resources include courses offered through the Centers for Disease Control and Prevention (CDC) Public Health Training Network, The Community Toolbox (http://www.cdc.gov/eval/framework.index.htm), and other resources updated by the CDC Evaluation Working Group (2010a). These resources enable nursing center staff to implement the six essential program evaluation steps in the context of their model and in their particular community. The essential steps are outlined in Box 21-4.

## POSITIONING NURSE-LED HEALTH CENTERS AND ADVANCED PRACTICE NURSES FOR THE FUTURE

The future for nurse-led health centers is promising. The advent of the Affordable Care Act and consumer demand is changing the traditional Western model of health care. NLHCs continue to be strategically positioned to meet these changing demands and needs. Consumers are seeking alternative sources of care such as acupuncture, meditation, and mindfulness training. They are also presenting with health stressors related to the

> **BOX 21-4 Essential Program Evaluation Steps**
> - Engaging stakeholders
> - Describing the program
> - Focusing the evaluation design
> - Gathering credible evidence
> - Justifying conclusions
> - Ensuring use and sharing lessons learned

# 22

# Case Management

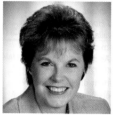

## Ann H. Cary, PhD, MPH, RN, FNAP

Dr. Ann H. Cary began practicing public health nursing as a home-health nurse in New Orleans, Louisiana, where she executed case management functions daily. She has served on national workgroups to establish the standards of practice for public health nurses and case managers and created certification examinations for case managers; authored numerous articles on case management issues, taught baccalaureate and graduate-level courses in case management, and directed graduate programs in case management and continuity of care. She is the Dean of the School of Nursing and Health Studies at the University of Missouri, Kansas City, MO. In Kansas City, she also serves on a variety of non-profit and interprofessional foundation and community boards whose missions are to increase access, coordinated care, and quality delivery for clients; and, to prepare health care leaders of the future to assure population health.

## ADDITIONAL RESOURCES

Ⓔ **Evolve Website http://evolve.elsevier.com/Stanhope**
- *Healthy People 2020*
- WebLinks
- Quiz
- Case Studies
- Glossary
- Answers to Practice Application

## OBJECTIVES

*After reading this chapter, the student should be able to do the following:*

1. Define *continuity of care, care management, case management, care coordination, transitional care, integrated care, social determinants of health,* and *advocacy.*
2. Describe the scope of practice, roles, and functions of a case manager.
3. Compare and contrast the nursing process with processes of case management and advocacy.
4. Identify methods to manage conflict, as well as the process of achieving collaboration.
5. Define and explain the legal and ethical issues confronting case managers.

## KEY TERMS

accountable care organizations, p. 477
advocacy, p. 489
affirming, p. 491
allocation, p. 493
amplifying, p. 490
assertiveness, p. 494
autonomy, p. 497
beneficence, p. 497
brainstorming, p. 492
care coordination, p. 481
care management, p. 478
care maps, p. 485
case management plans, p. 485
case manager, p. 485
clarifying, p. 491
collaboration, p. 494
cooperation, p. 494
coordinate, p. 481

critical pathways, p. 478
dashboard indicators, p. 477
demand management, p. 479
disease management, p. 478
distributive outcomes, p. 493
fidelity, p. 497
information exchange process, p. 490
informing, p. 490
integrative outcomes, p. 493
justice, p. 497
life care planning, p. 486
Medical/Health Home or Patient/Client-Centered Medical Home model, p. 481
negotiating, p. 493
nonmaleficence, p. 497
patient engagement, p. 483
population management, p. 477
problem-purpose-expansion method, p. 492

## CHAPTER OUTLINE

**Definitions**
**Concepts of Case Management**
  Case Management and the Nursing Process
  Characteristics and Roles
  Knowledge and Skill Requisites
  Tools of Case Managers
**Evidence-Based Examples of Case Management**
  Historical Evidence
  Contemporary Evidence

**Essential Skills for Case Managers**
  Advocacy
  Conflict Management
  Collaboration
**Issues in Case Management**
  Legal Issues
  Ethical Issues

Since the Patient Protection and Affordable Care Act (ACA) was initiated in 2010, the health care industry continues to re-evaluate systems that attempt to integrate financing, management, quality, and service delivery models. Challenges abound for clients and providers as they attempt to coordinate care, transition clients among providers and systems, access and share information and documentation about clients and communities, and navigate the complexity of integrated care to optimize quality and access while managing costs. The new models of health care financing provide incentives to value care outcomes over the volume of care provided. Delivery of care is now organized through a network of providers, such as negotiated contracts with hospitals and other levels of care, physicians, nurse practitioners, pharmacies, ancillary health services, and outpatient centers.

Managing the health of populations served by the integrated systems is essential (Newman et al, 2014). These include **accountable care organizations** (ACOs). Nurse case managers and nurse care managers will play a pivotal role in innovative systems of delivery (Institute of Medicine [IOM], 2011). **Population management** includes wellness and health promotion, illness prevention, acute and subacute care, chronic disease, rehabilitation, end-of-life care, care coordination, and community engagement. Case managers are at the core of population health strategies to improve the community outcomes (Noonan, 2014). Population health management can maintain and improve the physical and psychosocial status of clients through cost-effective and customized solutions, such as coordinating and transitioning of care to reduce gaps and costs; supporting evidence-based practices; selecting quality care that is culturally competent; and providing disease management and self-management educational programming (Case Management Society of America [CMSA], 2009; Noonan, 2014). Examples include planning and health delivery strategies for adolescents in a school system or the chronic disease management of elderly in a rural community (Huber, 2010; McKesson Corporation, 2014).

Like the earlier concept described by the American Hospital Association (AHA, 2003-2004), the ACA endorses the use of integrated systems to realize the following important consequences on the focus of care:

- Emphasis is on population health management across the continuum, rather than on episodes of illness for an individual.
- Management has shifted from inpatient care as the point of management to primary care providers as points of entry.
- Care management services and programs provide access and accountability for the continuum of health.
- Successful outcomes are measured by systems performance and pay for performance for providers to meet the needs of populations.

The contemporary focus of integrated health systems defines the nature of the client as a population in addition to that as an individual. In these systems, population management involves the following activities:

- Assessing the needs of the client population through health histories (and, in the future, genograms), claims, use-of-service patterns, and risk factors; and communicating through interoperable information systems to ascertain patterns, trends, and responses to health programming in a population
- Creating benefits and network designs to address these needs
- Selecting dashboard indicators to measure performance
- Prioritizing actions to produce a desired outcome with available resources
- Selecting evidence-based programs related to wellness, prevention, health promotion, and demand management; patient/client engagement; and educating the population about them
- Instituting evidence-based care management processes that assure transitional and coordinated care across the health continuum for a population aggregate
- Deploying case managers within a variety of delivery and insurance systems to clients and providers
- Evaluating provider patterns of performance and client dashboard indicators for impact

Establishing a relationship between financing, managing, delivering, and coordinating services is critical to reach the goal of population management—that is, achieving health outcomes at the population level. The *Healthy People 2020* goals are to attain both quality of life and increase years of healthy life, achieve health equity and eliminate health disparities, and create social and physical environments as a social mandate for health care. In the second decade of the twenty-first century, case management will be an essential intervention to positively influence the leading health indicators, chronic disease outcomes, and focus areas of *Healthy People 2020* (USDHHS 2010).

Establishing evidence-based strategies for all functions is critical to the success of case management for individuals and populations. Using the current best evidence blended with clinical expertise is a critical skill of the case manager (American Nurses Association [ANA], 2013; Lamb, 2013; CMSA, 2010). In their practice, nurse case managers have the following core values: increasing the span of healthy life, reducing disparities in health among Americans, and promoting access to care and to preventive services. Many of the interventions nurses use with clients and health care systems will further the *Healthy People 2020* objectives. These include case management interventions to minimize fragmented care and promote quality transitions of care; incorporate standardized practice tools and adherence guidelines; improve safety of care; and use interprofessional teams to deliver services.

In the Intervention Wheel model for public health nursing practice, the nursing actions of case management, collaboration, and advocacy comprise 3 of 17 evidence-based interventions for individuals, families, and populations served by public health nurses (Keller et al, 2004; and see Chapter 9). These three concepts and practice arenas for public health nurses are more fully described in this chapter. Case management incorporates many of the *Quad Council Competencies for Public Health Nursing* (Quad Council, 2011) because it involves individual and family care as well as community resources, population health, interprofessional teams, and policy implementation.

> **♥ HEALTHY PEOPLE 2020**
>
> Case management strategies offer opportunities for nurses to help meet the following *Healthy People 2020* objectives for target populations:
>
> **Access to Care**
> - **AHS-2:** Increase the proportion of insured persons with coverage for clinical preventive services
> - **AHS-3:** Increase the proportion of persons with a usual primary care provider
> - **AHS-6:** Reduce the proportion of individuals who experience difficulties or delays in obtaining necessary medical care, dental care, or prescription medications
> - **ECBP-14 and -14.1:** Increase the inclusion of clinical prevention and population content in undergraduate nursing, including counseling training for health promotion and disease prevention
> - **SA-9:** Increase the portion of persons who are referred for follow-up for substance abuse problems
>
> *AHS,* Access to health services; *ECBP,* educational and community-based programs; *SA,* substance abuse.
> From USDHHSS: Healthy People 2020: A roadmap for health, Washington, DC, 2010, U.S. Government Printing Office.

## DEFINITIONS

Care management is a health care delivery process that helps achieve better health outcomes by anticipating and linking populations with the services they need more quickly (CMSA, 2010). It is an enduring process in which a population manager establishes systems and processes to monitor the health status, resources, and outcomes for a targeted aggregate of the population. The population manager is the tactical architect for a population's health in the delivery system. According to a report by McKesson Corporation (2014), nurse care managers are predicted to hold the primary responsibility for the care management process in health systems. Building blocks that are used by the manager include risk analysis; data mapping; predictive modeling; dashboard indicators; monitoring for health processes, indicators, and unexpected illnesses; epidemiologic investigation of unexpected illnesses; development of multidisciplinary action plans and programs for the population; and identifying case management triggers or events (e.g., when dramatic results are obtained by prevention or early intervention) that indicate the need for early referrals of high-risk clients (ANA, 2013; Stricker, 2014).

Care management strategies were initially developed by health maintenance organizations (HMOs) in the late 1970s to manage the care of different populations. The purpose was to promote quality and ensure appropriate use and costs of services. Typically these involved clients with reduced self-care capacity and whose diseases and treatments were intense (Michaels and Cohen, 2005). Care management strategies include utilization management, critical pathways, case management, disease management, and demand management.

Utilization management attempts to promote optimal use of services to redirect care and monitor the appropriate use of provider care/treatment services for both acute and community/ambulatory services. Providers are offered multiple options for care with different economic implications. Through the use of utilization management, clients who have repetitive readmissions (i.e., they fail to respond to care) are often referred to care management programs.

Critical pathways and maps, which were initiated in the early 2000s, are tools that specify activities providers may use in a timely sequence to achieve desired outcomes for care. The outcomes are measurable, and the pathway tools strive to reduce variation in client care. Today, agencies are more likely to call these clinical paths, evidence-based practice protocols, clinical decision supports or guidelines, or case management plans of care.

Care management services are used for clients with specific diagnoses who may have high-use patterns, noncompliance issues, cost caps (e.g., no more than $10,000 to $20,000 can be spent on their case), or threshold expenses.

Disease management constitutes systematic activities to coordinate health care interventions and communications for populations with disease conditions in which client self-care efforts are significant (CMSA, 2010). For example, diabetes, asthma, and depression are typically targeted by providers and insurers. These programs have evolved largely as initiatives in managed care organizations (Huber, 2010) and will be a focus of accountable care organizations (ACOs). Demand management seeks to control use by providing clients with correct information and education strategies to make healthy choices, to use healthy and health-seeking behaviors to improve their health status, and to make fewer demands on the health care system (Tufts Managed Care Institute, 2011).

In contrast to care management—which was developed as a population approach to manage care after the aegis of individual case management—case management comprises the activities implemented with individual clients/families in the system. In the latest Standards of Practice for Case Management, case management is defined as "a collaborative process of assessment, planning, facilitation, care coordination, evaluation, and advocacy for options and services to facilitate an individual's and family's comprehensive health needs through communication and available resources to promote quality cost-effective outcomes. Related activities…include care coordination; complex condition management; population health management through wellness, disease and chronic care management; and promoting transitions of care services" (CMSA, 2010, p. 224).

The case manager builds on the basic functions of the traditional nurse's role and adapts new competencies for managing transitions among health care facilities, such as wellness and prevention, and interprofessional teams. The complexity of care and the publishing of the ICD-10s bring more in-depth documentation requirements to the scope of the case manager's activities but the essence remains: accountability, collaboration, advocacy, care coordination, and professionalism (Owen, 2014).

Case management is provided by the disciplines of nursing, social work, and rehabilitation counseling, to name a few. Research by Park and colleagues (2009) found that common knowledge exists for case management providers from the disciplines of nursing, social work, and rehabilitation counseling: case recording and documentation, conflict resolution strategies, negotiation, ethics, relevant legislation, interpersonal communication, and roles and functions required in various settings. Figure 22-1 illustrates the unified knowledge domains for professionals in case management and emphasizes the fluidity of common knowledge used by case managers regardless of discipline.

Treiger (2013) indicates that the challenges of academic preparation for future case managers will be to prepare them in interprofessional case management programs rather than through the lens of a particular clinical practice. In addition, case managers in case management programs are expanding their clinical expertise to embrace the process of disease management, a successful strategy for population outcomes. Specialty case management in advanced nursing practice is a critical

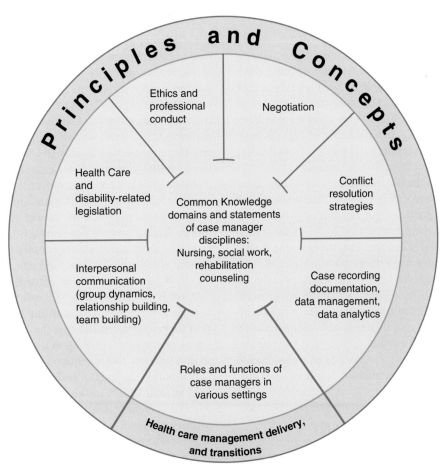

FIG 22-1 Evidence-based knowledge of case managers from disciplines of nursing, social work, and rehabilitation counseling. (Courtesy of Ann H. Cary.)

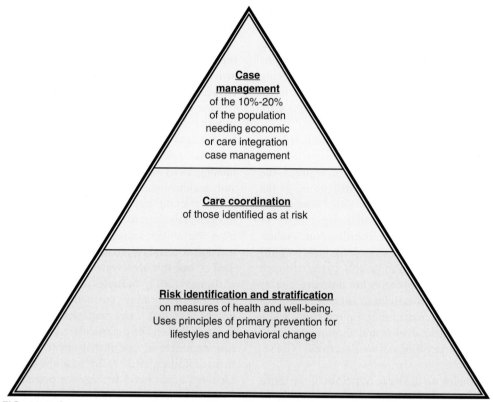

FIG 22-2 Case management model. (From Coggeshall Press: *Case Management Model.* Coralville, IA, 2008, Coggeshall Press; as cited in Huber, 2010.)

role in this field (Treiger, 2013). In implementing case management, advance practice nurses work with clients or community aggregates as well as systems managing disease and outcomes, whereas nurses with bachelor's degrees more often focus on care at the individual level. Treiger (2013) also observes that there are many individuals working under the title of case manager who fail to perform the full scope of roles and functions, leading to the question of title protection for case managers.

This chapter describes the nature and process of case management for individual and family clients. Case management has a rich tradition in public health nursing as practiced by Lillian Wald and now is frequently found in hospitals, transitional and long-term care, home and hospice care, and health insurance companies. Case management is at the top of the care management pyramid, reserved for a subset of the population. In Figure 22-2, Coggeshall Press (2008) illustrates a case management model pyramid that recognizes the tenets of risk stratification and case finding, coordination, and ultimately case management of a smaller proportion of clients in the population. This model recognizes the interchange of public health and populations at risk for service intensity resulting from economic or care integration needs.

## CONCEPTS OF CASE MANAGEMENT

Reviewing multiple or historical definitions of case management helps to demonstrate the complex process and the concept of case management over time. Weil and Karls, in 1985, described

case management as a "set of logical steps and process of interacting within a service network which ensures that a client receives needed services in a supportive, effective, efficient and cost-effective manner" (p. 4). Case management was defined by the American Hospital Association (1986) as the process of planning, organizing, coordinating, and monitoring services and resources needed by clients, while supporting the effective use of health and social services. Secord (1987) defined case management as a systematic process of assessing, planning, and coordinating the service, referrals, and monitoring that meets the multiple needs of clients. Bower (1992) described the continuity, quality, and cost containment aspects of case management as a health care delivery process, the goals of which are to provide quality health care, decrease fragmentation, enhance the client's quality of life, and contain costs.

A focus on collaboration is important in the National Case Management Task Force definition. The definition emphasizes a collaborative process between the case manager, the client, and representatives of other agencies and provider groups. The process includes assessments, plans, implementation, coordination, monitoring, and the evaluation of options and services to meet an individual's health needs. Effective communication is essential to identify available resources to promote quality, cost-effective outcomes (CMSA, 2010; Mullahy, 2010; Stricker, 2013).

As a competency, case management was defined in the public health nursing literature as the "ability to establish an appropriate plan of care based on assessing the client/family and coordinating the necessary resources and services for the client's benefit" (Muller and Flarery, 2003, p. 230). Case management has been a term prevalent in the social work literature as well as in public health nursing beginning in the mid-1900s. Knowledge and skills required to achieve this competency include the following:

- Knowledge of community resources and financing mechanisms
- Written and oral communication and technology-enhanced documentation
- Proficient negotiating and conflict-resolving practices
- Critical-thinking processes to identify and prioritize problems from the provider and client viewpoints
- Application of evidence-based practices and outcomes measures

Case management practice is complex as evidenced by the need to coordinate activities of multiple providers, payers, and settings throughout a client's continuum of care. Care coordination, one function of case management, is the deliberate organization of client care activities between two or more participants involved in a client's care to facilitate the appropriate delivery of health care services…and involves the marshaling of personnel and resources to carry out all required patient care activities… managed by the exchange of information among participants for different aspects of care (McDonald et al, 2010). For example, in a contemporary model of primary care practice, the Medical/Health Home or Patient/Client-Centered Medical Home model provides accessible, continuous, coordinated, comprehensive care and is managed centrally by a physician/nurse practitioner with the active involvement of nonphysician practice staff. Care provided must be assessed, planned, implemented, adjusted, and evaluated on the basis of goals designed by many disciplines as well as goals of the client, the family, significant others, and community organizations. Although likely employed and located in one setting, the nurse as case manager will be influencing the selection, monitoring, and evaluation of care provided in other settings by formal and informal care providers.

With the increased use of electronic care delivery through telehealth activities, case management activities are now handled via iTablets, phones, e-mail, and fax, and through video visits with the electronic monitoring of physiological status at a client's residence from a case manager who is located elsewhere. Case managers may also deliver care to a global network of clients located in different countries. A challenging problem is the fragmentation of services and miscommunication handoffs, which can result in overuse, underuse, gaps in care, and miscommunication. These can result in costly client outcomes and quality issues in hand-offs and transitions from provider to provider. Health information technology and electronic health records are benefiting collaborative care team communication, real-time data, and timely adjustments in care.

Case management, including the care coordination function, is part of a wider concept of transitions of care illuminated by the National Transitions of Care Coalition (NTOCC, 2011). Transitional care services bridge the gaps among diverse services, providers, and settings through the systematic application of evidence-based interventions that improve communication and transfer of information within and across services, enhancing

post–acute care follow-up, and decreasing gaps in care by the use of a single consistent provider (cited in ANA, 2013, p. 19). To advance knowledge on the outcomes of transitions of care, NTOCC has developed a number of tools and resources for case managers to assure effective communication between clients, caregivers, and providers, and published a compendium of transition models in practice that provides evidence of cost savings and lower 30-day hospital readmission rates and emergency room visits. The Transitional Care Bundle includes seven essential interventions: medication management, transition planning, client/family engagement and education, information transfer, follow-up care, provider engagement, and shared accountability across providers (Lattimer, 2013). Research indicates that the models employing the "Transitions" concept are currently ensuring higher quality and health care savings (http://www.ntocc.org/portals/0/Tangiblesavings.pdf).

Case management differs between urban and rural settings. In the rural setting, where the distance between populations is more expansive, there are fewer organized community-based systems and communication and distance are often a greater challenge. Furthermore, the economics, pace and style of life, values, and social organization all differ. In a study referenced in Stanton and Dunkin (2009), rural residents identified four barriers to access to care that confront case managers in rural areas: lack of proximity to providers, limited services, scarcity of providers, and reduced availability of emergency and acute care services. Transportation, both for nurses and for clients, and lack of health insurance and benefits were documented challenges to rural clients of case managers.

In a study of rural Veterans Affairs (VA) mental health patients who received case management services, Mohamed, with Neale and Rosenheck (2009) and Mohamed, with colleagues Rosenheck and Cuerdon (2010) found that intensive case management services were characterized as slightly less frequent, less intensive, and less recovery oriented than services delivered to the urban VA population. Travel distances and times were longer for rural case managers. Case management service intensity was related to premature termination of services for the veteran populations. Because case management is part of a transitional care model and coordination of care can reduce readmissions and promote safety, appropriate delivery of case management is essential to support The Joint Commission's National Safety Goals (2009) as well as the National Quality Strategy (AHRQ, 2013).

## Case Management and the Nursing Process

The nurse views the process of case management through the broader health status of the community. Clients and families receiving service represent the microcosm of health needs within the larger community. Through a nurse's case management activities, general community deficiencies in quality and quantity of health services are often discovered. For example, the management of a severely disabled child by a nurse case manager may uncover the absence of respite services or parenting support and education resources in a community. While managing the disability and injury claims within a corporation, the nurse may discover that alternative care referrals

| TABLE 22-1 | The Nursing Process and Case Management | |
|---|---|---|
| **Nursing Process** | **Case Management Process** | **Activities** |
| Assessment | • Case finding<br>• Identification of incentives for target population<br>• Screening, selection and intake<br>• Determination of eligibility<br>• Assessment of challenges, opportunities, and problems | • Develop networks with target population<br>• Disseminate written materials<br>• Seek referrals<br>• Apply screening tools according to program goals and objectives<br>• Use written and on-site screens<br>• Apply comprehensive assessment methods (physical, social, emotional, cognitive, economic, and self-care capacity)<br>• Obtain consent for services if appropriate |
| Diagnosis | • Identification of problem/opportunity and challenges | • Hold interprofessional, team, family, and client conferences<br>• Determine conclusion on basis of assessment<br>• Use interprofessional team |
| Planning for Outcomes | • Problem prioritizing<br>• Planning to address care needs<br>• Identification of resource match | • Validate and prioritize problems with all participants<br>• Select evidence-based interventions<br>• Develop goals, activities, time frames, and options<br>• Create case management plan<br>• Gain client's consent to implement<br>• Have client choose options |
| Implementation | • Advocating for client interests<br>• Frequent monitoring to assess alignment with goals and changing nature of client needs | • Contact providers<br>• Coordinate care activities<br>• Negotiate services and price<br>• Adjust as needed during implementation<br>• Document processes and monitor progress |
| Evaluation | • Measuring attainment of activities and goals of service delivery plan<br>• Continued monitoring and follow-up of client status during service<br>• Reassessment<br>• Bringing closure to care when client needs are achieved or change<br>• Appropriate discharge to ensure effective transitional care and termination of case management processes | • Ensure quality of transitional communication and coordination of service delivery<br>• Monitor for changes in client or service status<br>• Follow up as needed<br>• Examine outcomes against goals<br>• Examine needs against service<br>• Examine costs<br>• Examine satisfaction of client, providers, and case manager<br>• Examine best practices and outcomes for this client |

for home-health visits and physical therapy are generally underused by the acute care providers in the community. Through a nurse's case management of brain-injured young adults, the absence of community standards and legislative policy for helmet use by bicyclists and motorcyclists may be revealed, stimulating advocacy efforts for changing community policy. Case management activities with individual clients and families will reveal the broader picture of health services and health status of the community. *Community assessment, policy development,* and *assurance activities* that frame core functions of public health actions are often the logical next step for a nurse's practice. When observing lack of care or services at the individual and family intervention levels, the nurse can, through case management, intervene at the community level to make changes. Clearly, the core components of case management and the nursing process are complementary (Table 22-1).

Secord's classic illustration of case management (1987) remains an appropriate picture of the process that nurses use. The CMSA model (2010) is a contemporary illustration of the case manager's process in the continuum of care (Figure 22-3) and Table 22-1 also compares the case management process and nursing process.

## Characteristics and Roles

Case management can be labor intensive, time consuming, and costly. Because of the rapid growth in the nature of complexity in clients' problems managed by the case manager, the intensity and duration of activities required to support the case management function may soon exceed the demands of direct caregiving. Managers and clinicians in community health are exploring methods to make case management more efficient including the use of providers who can perform to the limit of their licenses, auxiliary case management providers/services, and evidence-based practices. These provider characteristics, which incorporate the four CMSA activities (previously noted in the Concepts of Case Management section), are used today (CMSA, 2010):

1. The technical/intellectual qualifications to understand and evaluate specific diagnoses, generally requiring clinical credentials (and experience), financial resources, health information technology knowledge and analyses, and risk arrangements
2. Capability in language and terminology (able to understand and then to explain to others in simple terms)
3. Assertiveness, diplomacy, and negotiation skills with people at all levels

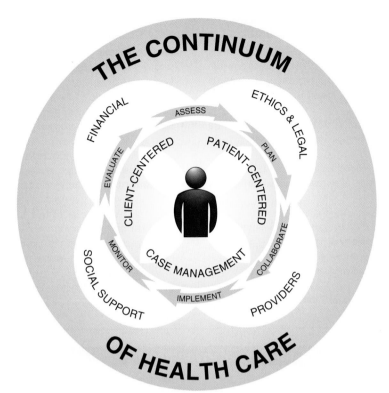

**FIG 22-3** The continuum of care case management model. (From Case Management Society of America [CMSA]: *Standards of Practice for Case Management.* Little Rock, AR, 2010, CMSA, p. 5.)

4. The ability to *assess* situations objectively and to *plan* appropriate case management services
5. Knowledge of available clinical evidence and resources as well as their strengths and weaknesses
6. The ability to act as *advocate* for the client and payer in models relying on third-party payment
7. The ability to act as a counselor or *facilitator* to clients to provide support, understanding, information, and intervention
8. Interprofessional team player

In 1998, Cary described the roles of case managers in the practice setting. These roles are clearly affirmed today by the CMSA (2010) (Box 22-1). The roles demanded of the nurse as case manager are greatly influenced by the forces that support or detract from the role. Figure 22-4 presents factors that demand the attention of both the nurse and the system during the case management process.

## Knowledge and Skill Requisites

Nurses, as in other disciplines, are not automatically experts in the role of case manager. First, they develop and refine the knowledge and skills that are essential to implementing the role successfully. Knowledge domains useful for nurses in systems desiring to implement quality case management roles are found in Box 22-2 (Cary, 1998; Stanton and Dunkin, 2009; Treiger, 2013).

When a nurse seeks a case manager position, some of the skills and knowledge will need to be acquired through academic and continuing education programs, literature reviews, onboarding, orientation, and mentoring experiences. Basic nursing education may need to be updated, and practical experiences in case management may be required. Treiger (2013) recommends that case managers pursue advanced education in case management. In fact, professional development activities for case managers in public health have been demonstrated to contribute to job satisfaction (Schutt et al, 2010). Finally, title protection for case managers is an issue under discussion in the literature in order to ensure credibility of services provided by professional, skilled case managers.

## Tools of Case Managers

The six "rights" of case management are right care, right time, right provider, right setting, right price/value, and right outcomes. How does the nurse judge the effectiveness of case management? Three tools are useful for case management practice: case management plans, disease management, and life care planning tools. An underlying principle for the use of each of these tools is the need to use robust evidence as the basis for the selection of activities; technology and health information systems and analytics are now the drivers of these tools.

Technology supports the delivery of processes used by the case manager. The technology sector is refining software in the areas of documentation, decision support, dashboard tools, predictive modeling, workflow automation, reporting capabilities, electronic health records, **patient engagement** strategies and social media, and remote monitoring (Carneal and Pock,

### BOX 22-1    Case Manager Roles

- **Broker:** Acts as an agent for provider services that are needed by clients to stay within coverage according to budget and cost limits of health care plan
- **Client advocate:** Acts as advocate, provides information, and supports benefit changes that assist member, family, primary care provider, and capitated systems
- **Consultant:** Works with providers, suppliers, the community, and other case managers to provide case management expertise in programmatic and individual applications
- **Coordinator:** Arranges, regulates, and coordinates needed health care services for clients at all necessary points of services. Effectively participates and leads interprofessional teams
- **Educator:** Educates client, family, and providers about case management process, delivery system, community health resources, and benefit coverage so that informed decisions can be made by all parties
- **Facilitator:** Supports all parties in work toward mutual goals
- **Liaison:** Provides a formal communication link among all parties concerning the plan of care management
- **Mentor:** Counsels and guides the development of the practice of new case managers

- **Monitor/reporter:** Provides information to parties on status of member and situations affecting client safety, care quality, and client outcome, and on factors that alter costs and liability
- **Negotiator:** Negotiates the plan of care, services, and payment arrangements with providers; uses effective collaboration and team strategies
- **Researcher:** Accesses and applies evidence-based practices for programmatic and individual interventions with clients and communities; participates in protection of clients in research studies; initiates/collaborates in research programs and studies; accesses real-time evidence for practice
- **Standardization monitor:** Formulates and monitors specific, time-sequenced critical path and care map plans (see page 485) as well as disease management protocols that guide the type and timing of care to comply with predicted treatment outcomes for the specific client and conditions; attempts to reduce variation in resource use; targets deviations from standards so adjustments can occur in a timely manner; uses dashboards and predictive modeling to anticipate outcomes
- **Systems allocator:** Distributes limited health care resources according to a plan or rationale

### BOX 22-2    Knowledge Domains for Case Management

- Standards of practice for case management
- Evidence-based practice guidelines for specific health and disease conditions and communities
- Knowledge of health care financial environment and the financial dimension of client populations managed by nurses
- Clinical knowledge, skill, and maturity to direct quality timing and sequencing of care activities
- Care resources for clients within institutions and communities: facilitating the development of new resources and systems to meet clients' needs
- Transition planning for ideal timing, sequencing, and levels of care
- Management skills: communication, delegation, persuasion, use of power, consultation, problem solving, conflict management, confrontation, negotiation, management of change, marketing, group development, accountability, authority, advocacy, ethical decision making, and profit management

- Teaching, counseling, and education skills
- Program evaluation and research
- Performance improvement techniques
- Peer and team consultation, collaboration, and evaluation
- Requirements of eligibility and benefit parameters by third-party payers
- Legal and ethical issues
- Information management systems: clinical and administrative
- Health care legislation/policy
- Technical information skills, interoperable information systems, dashboard monitoring, data management and analysis, predictive modeling software, facile use of EHRs
- Outcomes management and applied research

*EHRs,* Electronic health records.

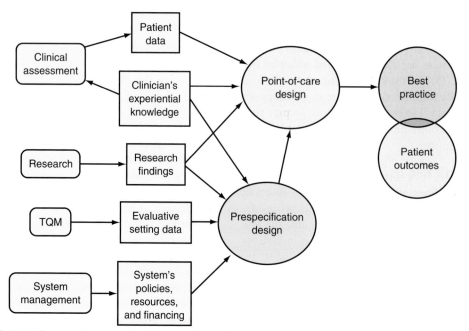

**FIG 22-4** Factors that require the attention of the nurse and client in the case management process. *TQM,* total quality management.

2014; Stricker, 2014; Treiger, 2013). For example, health information technology (HIT) allows the case manager to access real-time data to improve timeliness of decisions or program changes for any number of adjustments in care protocols to ensure optimal outcomes. Data analytic software and dashboards allow for rapid decisions for clinical, administrative, and financial outcomes. Dashboard functions typically include (1) manipulation of report data, (2) access to information, (3) observing individual/population trends, and (4) observing trends in large datasets (Stricker, 2014). These data-reporting tools can vary from off-the-shelf, to customized, to simple Excel spreadsheets—each with their own advantages and gaps.

Historically, case management plans have evolved through various titles and methods (e.g., critical paths, critical pathways, care maps, multidisciplinary action plans, nursing care plans). Regardless of the title given, standards of client care, standards of nursing practice, and clinical guidelines using evidence-based practices for case management serve as core foundations of case management plans. Likewise, in interprofessional action plans, core professional standards of each discipline guide the development of the standard process.

As early as 1985, the New England Medical Center (Boston, MA) instituted a system of critical path development to guide the case management process in the acute care setting. This method of designing structures and processes of care laid the groundwork for the critical paths, care maps, and clinical decision tools now used in the industry. A *critical path* was described as a case management tool composed of abbreviated versions of discipline-specific processes; it was used to achieve a measurable outcome for a specific client "case" (Zander et al, 1987). The critical path detailed the essential and sequential activities in care, so that the expected progress of the client was known at a point in time. Outcomes from critical paths included satisfaction, client competency, continuity of care, continuity of information, and costs and quality of care. However, one criticism was that critical paths may not be evidence based (Renholm et al, 2002).

At that time the prevailing method of establishing critical paths was by internal, "expert knowledge" from a specific institution, the result being that they could not be applied generally or tested under systematic, scientific methods. In the New England model, key incidents included consults, tests, activities, treatments, medication, diet, discharge planning, and teaching. The paths showed the differences between clients' progress. However, the paths were generally not revised unless a body of evidence was found to adjust the expected actions.

Care maps became the second generation of critical pathways of care. Rather than give definitions, as early as in 2001 Brown discussed the "various types of evidence that must be accessed, interpreted, and integrated into care design" (p. 3). Brown proposed the best practice health care map (BPHM) as a model for providing quality clinical care within an interprofessional practice. This model discussed all the components of knowledge development and care planning activities that must occur to have positive client outcomes. The author noted that care designed in advance takes the form of "clinical guidelines, care maps, decision algorithms, and clinical protocols for specified populations of clients" (Brown, 2001, p. 3). The "prespecification design" of the BPHM entailed these preplanning courses of care. Brown (2001) stressed the importance of incorporating research findings and clinical experience when developing prespecified plans. Furthermore, the author emphasized that at the point of care, these prespecified plans must be adapted to the individual client or population. The Brown BPHM was (1) client centered, (2) scientifically based, (3) population-outcomes based, (4) refined through quality assessment and compared with other maps, (5) individualized to each client, and (6) compatible with the larger system of health care in the United States.

Such activities today are more likely referred to as case management plans, care maps, and integrated clinical pathways and are the foundation for the methods to establish standardized, evidence-based case management plans. Clinical paths today are defined as structures of care based on interventions translated from evidence for use with clients; include detailed steps in a course of care; are based on pilot applications; and are modified (Kinsman et al, 2010). In the electronic health record (EHR) critical paths become the centerpiece of communication and interprofessional team processes for the case manager (Hyde and Murphy, 2012). Care guidance formats (critical paths, care maps) are integrated into the EHR to be used by the case manager to provide clinical decision support. They may appear as prompts, checklists, references, for example, that will auto-populate a documented service and remind providers as to the array of procedures to be implemented. Case managers need to ensure that any "guidance care plans" embrace the unique needs of the client and care in order to optimize outcomes of care for clients.

Adaptation of any standardized case management plan to each client's characteristics is a crucial skill for the process and outcome of care. These plans link multiple provider interventions to client responses and offer reasonable predictions to clients about health outcomes. Institutions report that sharing case management plans with clients empowers the clients to assume responsibility for monitoring and adhering to the plan of care. Self-responsibility by clients incorporates autonomy and self-determination as the core of case management. For the nurse employed as a case manager, ample opportunity exists to apply and revise critical path/map care guidance prototypes for a target population experiencing acute and chronic health problems.

Disease management is an organized program of coordinated health care interventions that use consensus-driven performance measures and scientifically based evaluations in clinical outcomes for populations with conditions in which client self-care efforts are critical (CMSA, 2010; URAC, 2014). This approach focuses on the natural progression of a disease in high-risk populations. Disease management programs may contain many of the following components (Disease Management Association of America [DMAA], 2008, 2010):

- Selection of high-risk patients, with a focus on a singular disease state (diabetes, asthma, congestive heart failure [CHF])
- Financial and risk-sharing arrangements between payers and providers

- Programs for monitoring the use of clinical paths and evidence-based guidelines to assess outcomes and costs
- Protocols for clinical, financial, and administrative processes
- Services to educate clients and promote self-management skills, including the use of motivational interviewing techniques.
- Enhanced quality through evidence-based decision support and other registry technologies
- Support for provider/client relationships and plans of care
- Evaluation of clinical, humanistic, and economic outcomes to address the goal of improving overall health

---

**HOW TO** Apply Telehealth Interventions for Clients

*To learn more about telehealth interventions for clients, case managers can do the following:*

- *Make it a point to learn how telehealth works in your community and in the industry.*
- *Examine the evidence base for telehealth as an option for the types of clients you are servicing when considering available resources.*
- *Seek continuing education to prepare you on the art and science of telehealth application and client receptivity. Read the literature on e-communication and monitoring impact effectiveness.*
- *Be aware of the strengths and weaknesses of this delivery and plan to adjust the delivery model to optimize effectiveness for your clients.*
- *Seek networking opportunities with professional organizations and other case managers about the uses of telehealth.*
- *Examine the clinical guidelines and practice algorithms for telehealth adoption, application, and use.*
- *Sharpen your personal interaction and program evaluation skills to better assist in decision making about the use of telehealth services.*

---

From *Hagan L, Morin D, Lepine R: Evaluation of telenursing outcomes: satisfaction, self-care practices, and cost savings.* Public Health Nurs *17:305–313, 2000.*

---

The philosophy of disease management can give clients the tools needed to better manage their lives (Newman et al, 2014; CMSA, 2010). Clients with chronic diseases may benefit from a disease management approach. The goals are to interrupt the continued development of a disease and prevent future disease and complications through secondary and tertiary prevention interventions. Promotion of wellness is necessary for success. For specific client populations that consume a disproportionate share of resources, disease management programs allocate the correct resources in an efficacious manner. Disease management programs may reduce emergency department visits, result in fewer inpatient days and rehospitalizations, greater client satisfaction, and reduced school absences (NTOCC, 2011; Sidorov, 2010). As the science of disease management evolves to predict direct relationships between outcomes and protocols of care, case managers will need to demonstrate cost-effective, optimal clinical care across the continuum—a goal of care management for populations. In fact, disease management is viewed as a top strategy by employers. The Joint Commission (TJC)

certifies and URAC accredits disease management organizations and programs on the basis of their respective standards (see websites www.jointcommission.org and www.urac.org). This may influence the choice of programs a case manager selects to use with clients.

Opponents of the use of disease management programs cite the study by McCall and Cromwell (2011), which described a comparison of eight commercial disease management programs used with Medicare populations and using a nurse call center approach. This comparative evaluation study revealed only modest improvement in quality of care measures with no significant reduction in utilization of acute care services or costs. Some of the possible explanations included that clients had complex comorbidities that required more than a singular disease approach; social determinants and environmental factors may not have been adequately addressed in the plans; and the inclusion of high-risk with low-risk patients could have diluted the significance of the results. Clearly, more research with innovative models that can capture the true nature and intensity of client needs in a disease management program will be necessary to inform the use or discontinuance of this approach in the future.

**Life care planning** is another tool used in case management. A life care plan assesses the current and future needs of a client for catastrophic or chronic disease over a life span. The life care plan is a customized, medically based document that provides an organized plan to estimate reasonable and necessary current and future medical and nonmedical needs of clients with associated costs and frequencies of goods and services. Typically these needs incorporate medical, financial (income), psychological, vocational, built environment, and social costs during the remaining life of the client (Sambucini, 2013). Life care plans are typically used for clients experiencing catastrophic illness or adverse events resulting from professional malpractice or accidents/injuries or those who have sustained an injury when younger and subsequently have changes in requirements as they age. For example, conditions may include spinal cord injury, traumatic brain injury, chronic pain, amputation, cerebral palsy, and burns. Life care plans are also used to set financial rewards, which can be used to secure resources for care in the future and create a lifetime care plan. A systematic process like the nursing process is used and interprofessional input is required.

The American Association of Nurse Life Care Planners (AANLCP) has published a *Code of Professional Ethics and Conduct for Nurse Life Care Planners with Interpretive Statements* (2012a) as well as the *Nurse Life Care Planners Standards of Practice with Interpretive Statements* (2012b). Nurse life care planners have access to academic course work, continuing education activities, and a published *A Core Curriculum for Nurse Life Care Planning* (Apuna-Grummer and Howland, 2013). There is also a certification examination for nurse life care planners that awards the designation of Certified Nurse Life Care Planner (CNLCP) as a specialty designation (www.cnlcp.org).

The first phase of the plan is crafted to include a thorough assessment of the client, financial/billing agreements, an information release signed by the client, and a targeted date for report completion. Development of the plan is the second phase. Plans are based on a number of factors: social and cultural situation, leisure activities, educational and employment status, medical history, physical and psychological abilities, current status, assistance required for completing activities of daily living, and regulatory requirements.

---

**| HOW TO Ensure High-Quality Care**

*The following actions can ensure high-quality care for clients and have implications for case managers in their practice:*

- *Provide access to easily understood information for each client based on his or her needs and health literacy level.*
- *Remember that the client is the source of control and that patient/family engagement is critical.*
- *Provide access to appropriate specialists with coordination and communication transparency.*
- *Ensure continuity of care for those with chronic and disabling conditions (transition care).*
- *Provide access to emergency services when and where needed.*
- *Disclose financial incentives that could influence medical decisions and outcomes.*
- *Prohibit "gag clauses" (which mean that providers cannot inform clients of all possible treatment options).*
- *Provide antidiscrimination protections.*
- *Provide internal and external appeal processes to solve grievances of clients.*
- *Make decisions on the basis of evidence.*

*McClinton DH: Protecting patients. Contin Care 17:6, 1998; Institute of Medicine (IOM): Crossing the Quality Chasm: A New Health System for the 21st Century. Washington, DC, 2001, National Academies Press.*

---

The following can ensure high-quality care for clients and have implications for case managers in their practice:

- Provide access to easily understood information for each client based on their needs and health literacy level
- The client is the source of control and patient/family engagement is critical.
- Provide access to appropriate specialists with coordination and communication transparency.
- Ensure continuity of care for those with chronic and disabling conditions (transition care).
- Provide access to emergency services when and where needed.
- Disclose financial incentives that could influence medical decisions and outcomes.
- Prohibit "gag clauses" (which mean that providers cannot inform clients of all possible treatment options).
- Provide antidiscrimination protections.
- Provide internal and external appeal processes to solve grievances of clients.
- Decision making is evidence based.
- The plan includes projected costs and resources needed for the frequency and duration of treatments, equipment, supplies, and future evaluations.
- The execution of a life care plan is typically managed by a case manager who will work with the life care planner, especially when re-evaluation of the plan is necessary (AANLCP, 2013).

All of these tools/programs, in coordination, constitute population health management strategies to educate clients and promote self-management, provide nurse coaching support, promote safe care transitions, improve care management and coordination, and enhance quality (DMAA, 2010).

## EVIDENCE-BASED EXAMPLES OF CASE MANAGEMENT

### Historical Evidence

Carondelet Health at St. Mary's Hospital in Tucson, Arizona, developed a community nursing network in which enrollees are distributed among a number of community health centers. Professional nurse case managers assisted older clients to attain healthier lifestyles and maintain themselves in the community. Nurses were successful in delivering economical services per month for Medicare enrollees. Through nurse case management services, this nursing HMO was reported to have reduced the number of inpatient days per 1000 enrollees by one third, at an average cost of $900 per day, for a savings of $300,000 for every 1000 enrollees (ANA, 1993; American Nurses Foundation [ANF], 1993). These strengths have been critical to allow the model to evolve to provide group and telephonic case management and automated standardized care instruments. Future endeavors will capitalize on the advances in information technology to capture clinical and cost data in a timely manner for decision support (Cohen and Cesta, 2005).

Community-based statewide programs in New Jersey used case management methods to promote early identification, selection, evaluation, diagnosis, and treatment of children who are potentially physically compromised. Local case management units provided coordinated and comprehensive care. Collaboration with existing local and regional agencies serving children supported this process. The nurse case manager (1) provided counseling and education to parents and children about identifying problems and increasing their knowledge, (2) developed individual plans incorporating multidisciplinary services (education, social issues, medical development, rehabilitation), (3) obtained appropriate community services, (4) acted as a family resource in crises and service concerns, (5) facilitated communication between child and family, and (6) monitored services for outcomes. Interprofessional teams include nurses and social workers (with master's degrees) for larger caseloads. A recommended caseload was 300 to 350 children per case manager (Bower, 1992).

A national study of 2437 people who tested positive for human immunodeficiency virus (HIV) and who had case managers demonstrated that, regardless of the model, these clients were more likely to use life-prolonging HIV medications and meet the needs for income, health insurance, home care, and supportive emotional counseling than those without case management. Having contact with a case manager was not significantly related to use of outpatient care, hospital admission, or emergency department visits. Case managers in this study included social workers, nurses, and acquired immunodeficiency syndrome (AIDS) service organization staff (Katz et al, 2001).

Liberty Mutual Insurance Company had used case management principles for more than 30 years in workers' compensation cases and expanded services for employees whose conditions were noted as chronic or catastrophic. Case managers coordinated all clients, providers, and services to reduce expenses caused by lack of coordination; failure to use beneficial alternatives; and duplication and fragmentation of services (Bower, 1992).

---

### ⟫ LINKING CONTENT TO PRACTICE

Important guidance in developing a community-based case management program can be found in the United States. Case management is a key component of federally financed and many state-financed health delivery options. The experiences of states over the past two decades provide testimony to the importance of case management for populations at risk. For older clients, state-derived case management provides objective advice and assistance with care needs. It also provides access to interprofessional providers and services. For payers (federal, state, clients), case management serves as a way to ensure that funds are allocated appropriately to those in greatest need. Case management serves a policy assurance and accountability function for communities. The PACE (Program of All-Inclusive Care for the Elderly) program addresses the needs of chronically ill seniors who wish to remain in their homes rather than be admitted to nursing homes and are enrolled in a managed care model of medical and support services, case management, medications, respite, hospital, and nursing home care when necessary. PACE prevents institutionalization in nursing homes, uses a strong social model of health care delivery, and case manages transitions of clients between delivery systems and providers. Studies (Wieland et al, 2013; Fretwell and Old, 2011) have demonstrated cost savings with PACE programs compared with nursing home costs. The PACE model has been permanently recognized as a provider type under both Medicare and Medicaid and has grown to 104 programs operating in 31 states (National PACE Association, 2014).

---

Within the states, the types of agencies designated to conduct case management are often district offices of state government, area agencies on aging, county social services departments, and private contractors. States maintain the oversight responsibilities for case management agencies to (1) ensure they are complying with program standards, contracts, reporting, and fiscal controls, (2) identify emerging problems and issues to be resolved by additional state policies, and (3) provide on-site technical assistance and consulting to improve performance. States' payment methods for case management include daily/monthly rates, hourly/quarterly rates, capped rates for services, and capped aggregate rates to cover both case management and provider costs (Health Resources and Services Administration [HRSA], 2004; U.S. Department of Health and Human Services [USDHHS], 2008).

The models of case management vary today as they did in the recent past. In 1999, Taylor described three models by their focus: client, system, and social service. *Client-focused models* are concerned with the relationship between case manager and client to support continuity of care and to access providers of care. *System-focused models*, in contrast, address the structure and processes of using the population-based tools of disease management and case management plans to offer care for client populations. The *social service models* provide services to clients

to assist them in living independently in the community and in maintaining their health by eliminating or reducing the need for hospital admissions or long-term care.

These models offer a solution to unnecessary health care expenses by reducing costs and accessing appropriate health care services. Imagine the impact on health status if these saved expenses were shifted to primary prevention and health promotion activities.

## Contemporary Evidence

Reducing the rate of readmission within 30 days of hospital discharge is a quality goal in health care. For psychiatric clients, the risk of rehospitalization is greatest and most costly during this time. Kolbasovsky (2009) replicated a model of intensive case management (ICM) in the United States that had been successful in Europe in reducing 30-day readmission rates (Burns et al, 2001, 2007) and found that ICM significantly reduced readmissions and the associated costs of 305 clients at a cost of $41.39 per member during the 30-day period. Had these persons been rehospitalized, the hospital psychiatric costs would have been $1528.14 per member. The nature of the case management activities included transitional and coordination of aftercare, monitoring of symptoms, medication and treatment adherence, education of client and families, motivational interviewing to detect barriers, linkages to community-based resources, treatment refill reminders, alcohol screening, and brief interventions.

In a randomized controlled trial of 450 clients post–cardiac bypass surgery, case management intervention by nurses using telephone-based collaborative care improved the mental and physical health of persons experiencing depression after cardiac bypass in an 8-month case management intervention. Case management activities included education about post–cardiac surgery depression, self-management skills, assessing and monitoring of treatment and medication adherence, interprofessional weekly case conferences, and routine communication with persons and primary care providers to ensure the provision of coordinated, consistent care. The case manager used ongoing telephone support, encouragement of client preferences, self-management workbooks, coaching, and electronic support for care guidelines and protocols. Outcomes included increased mental health scores, improved physical and functional status, and fewer readmissions among males with subsequent cost savings (AHRQ, 2010a).

Using a managed care model of enrollment, the Care One program at the University of New Mexico Health Sciences Center provides intensive case management and care coordination to medically complex, costly clients who lack health insurance. Among the top 1% of high-cost clients, all were offered enrollment in a case management service with an interprofessional team of providers who help persons in this population to navigate the system, access available financial assistance, and use appropriate community resources. Each person meets with the entire team to assess and prioritize needs, goals, and subsequent steps, and to schedule medical appointments. Activities also include securing financial resources; counseling and assistance to complete paperwork; scheduling appointments, reminders, and follow-ups; behavioral health counseling; medication management; and access to community resources to support health. Case management resulted in 80% fewer hospital admissions, a 60% decline in emergency room visits, and consistently high client satisfaction scores (AHRQ, 2010b).

## EVIDENCE-BASED PRACTICE

A successful pilot program led to the execution of a randomized controlled trial—After Discharge Care Management of Low Income Frail Elderly (AD-LIFE)—for community-based elderly. The care management model uses the integration of medical and social care to improve the outcomes of low-income and chronically and functionally impaired elderly after hospital discharge. AD-LIFE uses an interprofessional team, comprehensive geriatric assessment, and care management by a team nurse. Throughout the first year after hospital discharge, the nurse works with the area Agency on Aging social services program, performs a hospital and home assessment, uses a client goal-setting approach, creates a plan for development of self-care skills, and provides care planning for chronic illnesses and geriatric syndromes (e.g., incontinence, depression, nutrition, skin problems, and memory impairment). The interprofessional team can access specialists, and the primary care provider performs frequent evaluations and revises care plans as needed.

Ninety-two percent (92%) of the 118 clients had the need for at least one medical or social intervention. Half were taking 5 to 10 prescription drugs, 40% were living alone, 28% had congestive heart failure, 28% had diabetes, and many were unable to perform some ADLs or experienced geriatric syndrome. About 70% of clients said the care management program improved their health, allowed them to more easily access health care services, and provided them with a greater understanding of their disease(s). Hospital admissions decreased and the care cost savings were $1000 per client per month.

- As a nurse working in public health, aspects of this program could be built on to design an interprofessional program for community-based clients with Alzheimer's disease, people living with AIDS, chronically ill or disabled children, or clients with unstable psychiatric conditions.

### Nurse Use
Postdischarge care management that integrates medical, nursing, and socially and culturally proficient care can improve outcomes of the low-income elderly as well as other groups named above. It is important to identify the interprofessional team members who could be assembled to conduct the program with each client group, to identify measures of success for each of the programs, and to relate the case management process to *Healthy People 2020* objectives that could be addressed for each of these client groups.

From Wright K, Hazelett S, Jarjoura D, Allen K: The AD-LIFE trial. *Home Healthcare Nurse* 25(5):308–314, 2007.

The impact of using a nurse case manager (NCM) and community health worker (CHW) team on diabetic control, emergency room (ER) visits, and hospitalizations among urban African Americans with type 2 diabetes in a randomized controlled clinical trial comparing intensive case management with minimal case management revealed the positive effects of the intensity of case management services on outcomes. Intensive services included mailings and telephone calls about preventive screenings, culturally tailored care provided by the NCM and CHW team, and evidence-based clinical algorithms with feedback to the primary care providers. Those clients receiving intensive case management were 23% less likely to have ER visits, and this effect was strongest for clients who received the

most nurse and community health worker visits for their care (Gary et al, 2009). Culturally tailored interventions are essential to approaching health equity outcomes.

In a 2012 study with 83 clients in an urban setting, most of whom were uninsured, a community-based case management program with clients experiencing one or more chronic diseases yielded impressive results: acute outpatient encounters decreased by 62% and inpatient admissions by 53%. Primary care visits increased by 162% with an overall reduction in aggregate costs of 41%—from $16,208 preintervention to $9541 postintervention (Glendenning-Napoli et al, 2012).

## ESSENTIAL SKILLS FOR CASE MANAGERS

Three skills are essential to the role performance of the case manager: advocacy, conflict management, and collaboration.

### Advocacy
Case managers report that they are first and foremost client advocates (Barefield, 2003; Stanton and Dunkin, 2009; CMSA, 2010). The definition of nursing includes advocacy: "Nursing is the protection, promotion and optimization of health and abilities, prevention of illness and injury, alleviation of suffering through the diagnosis and treatment of human response, and advocacy in the care of individuals, families, communities and populations" (ANA, 2010, p. 6). For nurses, advocacy involves a number of activities, ranging from exploring self-awareness to lobbying for health policy. Advocacy is essential for practice with clients and their families, communities, organizations, and colleagues on an interprofessional team. The functions of advocacy require scientific knowledge, expert communication, facilitating skills, and problem-solving and affirming techniques.

As the *Guide to the Code of Ethics for Nurses* (ANA, 2008) states, "The nurse, in all professional relationships, practices with compassion and respect..." (p. 4). This means the nurse has the obligation to move beyond his or her own personal feelings of agreement or disagreement to respond compassionately. However, this goal is a contemporary one; the perspective regarding the advocacy function has shifted through history. The nurse advocate has been described in earlier writings as one who acted on behalf of or interceded for the client (Nelson, 1988). An example of the nurse interacting on behalf of the client is the nurse who calls for a well-child appointment for a mother visiting the family planning clinic when the mother is capable of making an appointment on her own.

The advocate role evolved to that of mediator and is described as a response to the complex configuration of social change, reimbursement, and providers in the health care system (Tahan, 2005). Mediating is an activity in which a third party attempts to provide assistance to those who may be experiencing a conflict in obtaining what they desire. The goal of the nurse advocate as mediator is to assist parties to understand each other on many levels so that agreement on an action is possible. In the example of a nurse as case manager for an HMO, mediating activities between an older adult client and the payer (the HMO) could accomplish the following results: the client may understand the options for community-based skilled nursing care, and the payer may understand the client's desires for a less restrictive environment for care, such as the home. The case manager as mediator does not decide the plan of action but facilitates the decision-making processes between the client and the payee so that the desired care can be reimbursed within the options available.

In contemporary practice, nurse advocates place the client's rights as the highest priority. The goal of promoter for the client's autonomy and self-determination may result in an optimal degree of independence in decision making. For example, when a group of young pregnant women is the collective "client" (the aggregate), the nurse advocate's role may be to inform the group of the benefits and consequences of breastfeeding their infants. However, if the new mothers decide on formula feeding, the nurse advocate should support the group and continue to provide parenting, infant, and well-child services. This example shows a different perspective of the nurse as advocate. It notes that the nurse's role as advocate may demand a variety of functions that are influenced by the client's physical, psychological, social, and environmental abilities. Advocacy can result in clients becoming their own "client expert" in problem solving, decision making, maximization of resources, partnership development with providers, and ultimately appropriate interventions (Burton et al, 2010).

The advocacy role aims to achieve client engagement—a process in which clients are invested in their health and care through programs that provide information and tools to empower them to take control and evaluate their care (ANA, 2013). The nurse adapts the advocacy function to the client's dynamic capabilities as the client moves from one health state to another. Even clients who desire access to more substantial health promotion activities can benefit from a partnership with the nurse advocate. Case managers are called to mediate between client needs and payer requirements/economic constraints without becoming a barrier to quality care. Examples of advocacy in such cases might include promoting a client's (as an aggregate) access to on-site physical fitness programs in the occupational setting, or supporting parents' and students' concerns about the high-fat content of vending machine food in the school system. With the cost of health care exceeding $2.7 trillion annually and consumers assuming a larger financial portion of the care they choose, the promoter role of advocacy for those clients capable of autonomy is expected to increase.

## Process of Advocacy

The goal of advocacy is to promote self-determination in a client. The client may be an individual, family, peer, group, or community. The classic process of advocacy has been historically defined by Kohnke (1982), Mallik and Rafferty (2000), and Smith (2004) to include informing, supporting, and affirming. All three activities are more complex than they may initially seem, and they require self-reflection by the nurse as well as skill development. It is often easier for the nurse to inform, support, and affirm another person's decision when it is consistent with the nurse's values. When clients make decisions within their value systems that are different from the nurse's values, the advocate may feel conflict about contributing to the process of

**LINKING CONTENT TO PRACTICE**
*Advocacy: Text Link to Public Health Nursing*

The clinical practice skill of advocacy as an inherent concept in the practice of case management. Of the 16 interventions by public health nurses described in the Wheel of Intervention model (see Chapter 9), both advocacy and case management are described in accordance with best practices and operational definitions of 2 of the 16 interventions. Advocacy can be applied at the community, systems, individual, or family level. In fact, when a public health nurse advocates for clients at any of these levels, the source of conflict and collaboration will likely come from competing values, that is, those of the client and any of these other levels of population values. For example:
- a client may want access to unlimited treatment, financial values may pose a source of conflict as the system attempts to justify the comparative effectiveness or costs.
- Family members may pose conflicting values for the nature of care they wish a family member to receive, even as the client refuses care.
- Communities can divert budget allotments to needs that are in competition for other population services such as community policing, health care access, and environmental services.

The nurse as advocate must listen carefully to his or her client in order to truly represent the interest of the client and encourage "win-win" processes and outcomes for the client. Advocacy occurs in all three of the core functions of public health: assessment, policy development, and assurance.

informing, supporting, and affirming those decisions. Promoting self-determination in others demands that the nurse have a philosophy of free choice once the information necessary for decision making has been discussed.

*Informing.* Knowledge is essential, but it is not enough to make decisions that affect outcomes. Interpreting knowledge is affected by the client's values and the meanings assigned to the knowledge. Interpreting facts is the result of both objective and subjective processing of information. Subjective processes greatly influence client decisions.

Informing clients about the nature of their choices, the content of those choices, and the consequences to the client is not a one-way activity. The information exchange process is composed of interactions that reflect three subprocesses: amplifying, clarifying, and verifying. Amplifying occurs between the nurse and the client to assess the needs and demands that will eventually frame the client's decision. Information is exchanged from both viewpoints. Although the exchange may be initiated at the objective, factual level, it is likely to proceed to incorporate the subjective perspectives of both parties.

The tone of the amplifying process can direct the remainder of the information exchange. It is important to relate with clients in a manner that reflects the advocate's endorsement of the client's self-determination. Setting aside the time necessary to listen to clients is critical. Clients will sense they are part of a mutual process if the nurse can engage them during the information exchange with a message that says, "I respect your needs and desires as I share my knowledge with you." Nonverbal behaviors, including using direct eye contact, sitting at the client's level, arriving and concluding at a prescribed time, and using verbal patterns that foster exchange (e.g., open-ended statements, questions, probes, reflections of feelings, paraphrasing), convey the nurse's desire to promote the client's ability to self-determine. Recent research indicates that clients' race and ethnicity may influence how providers and clients communicate with one another, thus contributing to disparities in health. Active communication among clients and providers has been linked to better treatment compliance and health outcomes (Schraeder and Shelton, 2011).

A client may not desire to exchange information because of lack of self-esteem, fear of the information, or inability to comprehend the content of the communication. In such a case, the focus is to understand the client's desire to be given no information and to express to the client the consequences of such inaction. The nurse may invite the client to ask for the information exchange at a later time, when the client is ready, and can periodically check with the client whether information exchange and amplifying are desired. In these cases, the nurse should document the implemented nursing actions to reflect the guidelines just discussed. This can reduce the basis for lawsuits and misunderstanding by other parties.

**Clarifying** is a process in which the nurse and client strive to understand meanings in a common way. Clarifying builds on the breadth and depth of the exchange developed during amplifying to determine whether the nurse and client understand each other. During this process, misunderstandings and confusions are examined. The goal of clarifying is to avoid confusion between the nurse and the client. To foster clarifying, nurses can use certain verbal prompts such as the following:

- "What do you understand about…?"
- "Please tell me more about how you…"
- "I don't think I am clear. Let me explain the situation in another way."
- "As an example,…"
- "What other information would be helpful so that we both understand?"

**Verifying** is the process used by the nurse advocate to establish accuracy and reality in the informing process. Low health literacy is a challenge for 90 million Americans who have difficulty understanding and acting on health information. Peterson and colleagues (2011) report that 40% of whites and 41% of those from Asia and the Pacific Islands living in the United States are proficient in reading English. In contrast, 13% of African American, 5% of Hispanic, and 18% of Native American U.S. students are proficient in reading English. Reading/literacy proficiency varies by ethnicity/race (Baer et al, 2009). In 2014, a *Public Broadcasting Newshour* publication cited the Department of Education as revealing that about 1 in 10 people in the United States has a proficient level of health literacy (Gorman, 2014).

If the nurse discovers that a client is misinformed, the nurse may return to the clarifying or amplifying stage and begin the process again. Verifying produces the chance for the advocate and client to examine "truth" from their points of view, which may include knowledge, intuition, previous experiences, and anticipated consequences.

Promoting a client's self-determination may take the advocate and client through the information exchange process several times, as new dimensions, or obstacles, to an issue develop. Information exchange is a critical process for advocacy and is applicable to all advocacy clients: individuals, families, groups, and communities (see the How To Box).

---

**| HOW TO   Provide for Information Exchange between Nurse and Client**

*1. Assess the client's present understanding of the situation. Have you considered your client's literacy level? Health literacy level? Cultural and ethnic values? Age and any disabilities that would interfere with learning?*

*2. Provide correct information.*

*3. Communicate on the client's literacy level, making the information as understandable as possible. Use interpreters and translators where needed.*

*4. Use a variety of media sources and teach-back methods to increase the client's comprehension.*

*5. Discuss other factors that affect the decision, such as financial, legal, and ethical issues.*

*6. Discuss the possible consequences of a decision.*

---

***Supporting.*** The second major process, **supporting**, involves upholding a client's right to make a choice and to act on it. People who are aware of clients' decisions fall into three general groups: supporters, dissenters, and obstructers. Supporters approve and support clients' actions. Dissenters do not approve and do not support clients. Obstructers cause difficulties when clients try to implement their decisions.

In 1998, Cary noted that the nurse advocate needs to implement several actions to fulfill the supporting role. Important interventions are assuring clients that they have the right and responsibility to make decisions, and reassuring them that they do not have to change their decisions because of others' objections.

***Affirming.*** The third process in the advocacy role is **affirming**. It is based on an advocate's belief that a client's decision is consistent with the client's values and goals. The advocate validates that the client's behavior is purposeful and consistent with the choice that was made. The advocate expresses a dedication to the client's mission, and a purposeful exchange of new information may occur so that the client's choice remains possible. Recognizing that a client's needs may fluctuate with changing resources, the affirming activity must encourage a process of re-evaluation and rededication to promote client self-determination.

The importance of affirming activities cannot be emphasized strongly enough. Many advocacy activities stop with assuring and reassuring, but affirming is often critical in promoting a client's self-determination. Table 22-2 compares the nursing process with the advocacy process.

The advocate's role in the decision-making process is *not* to tell the client that an option is correct or right. The advocate's role is to provide the opportunity for information exchange, and to arm clients with tools that can empower them in making the best decision from their point of view. Enabling clients to make an informed decision is a powerful tool for building self-confidence. It gives clients the responsibility for selecting the options and experiencing the success and consequences of their decisions. Clients are empowered in their decision making when they recognize that although some events are beyond

### TABLE 22-2   Comparison of Nursing Process and Advocacy Process

| Nursing Process | Advocacy Process |
| --- | --- |
| Assessment/ diagnosis | • Exchange information<br>• Gather data<br>• Illuminate values |
| Planning/outcome | • Generate alternatives and consequences<br>• Prioritize actions |
| Implementation | • Make decisions<br>• Support the client<br>• Assure<br>• Reassure |
| Evaluation | • Affirm<br>• Evaluate<br>• Reformulate |

their control, other events are predictable and can be affected by decisions they can make.

Nurses can promote client decision making by using the information exchange process, promoting the use of the nursing process, incorporating written techniques (e.g., contracts, lists), using reflecting and prioritizing techniques, and using role playing and sculpturing to "try on" and determine the "fit" of different options and consequences for the client. By engaging clients in the information-sharing process and assisting them to recognize the progression of activities they experience as they build their informed decision-making base, the nurse advocate is providing clients the opportunity to empower themselves with skills that can strengthen their autonomy and confidence in the future.

Advocacy is a complex process that maintains a delicate balance between doing for the client and promoting autonomy. The process is influenced by the client's physical, emotional, and social capabilities. The goal of advocacy is to promote the maximal degree of client self-determination, given the client's current and potential status; for most clients, this goal can be realized. When clients are comatose, unborn, or legally incompetent, nurse advocates have unique functions. The advocate's role is usually determined by the legal system; however, in some cases, nurses must decide what roles they will play. These are areas requiring intensive self-exploration, research, and collaboration with professionals, family members, and significant others. We are reminded that every encounter with a client is an opportunity to serve in the advocacy role (Mahlin, 2010).

### Skill Development

Skills needed by the nurse advocate are not unique to their profession. Nursing demands scientific, technical, relationship, and problem-solving knowledge and skills. Advocacy applies nursing skills of communication and competency to promote client self-determination.

Knowledge of nursing and other disciplines as well as of human behavior is essential for the advocacy role in establishing authority, promoting authenticity, and developing skills. The capacity to be assertive for personal rights and the rights of others is essential.

### Systematic Problem Solving

The nursing process—assessment, diagnosis, planning, implementing, and evaluating—is an example of a method of problem solving that can be used in the advocacy role. Advocates can be particularly helpful with clients in identifying values and generating alternatives.

*Illuminating Values.* People's values affect their behavior, feelings, and goals. In the process of amplifying, clarifying, and validating, the advocate understands a client's values. Through the process of self-revelation, an emerging value (such as environment, people, cost, or quality) may become more apparent to a client. This can have an effect in two ways. The client may be able to focus on actions on the basis of the value, or the value may confuse the decision process. The nurse can assist the client in prioritizing action and clarifying the value. Values can also change as new or relevant data are processed. The advocate's role is to assist clients in discovering their values. This process can be particularly demanding in the information exchange and affirming process.

*Generating Alternatives.* Clients and advocates may feel limited in their options if they generate solutions before completely analyzing the problems, needs, desires, and consequences. Several techniques can be used to generate alternatives, including brainstorming and a technique known as the problem-purpose-expansion method. In brainstorming, the nurse, client, professionals, or significant others generate as many alternatives as possible, without placing a value on them. Brainstorming creates a list that can then be examined for the critical elements the client seeks to preserve (e.g., environmental preferences, degree of control). The list can be analyzed according to the consequences and the effect of the alternatives on self and others.

The classic problem-purpose-expansion method, as described by Volkema (1983) and later expanded on by Heslin and Moldoveanu (2002) and Winston and Albright (2012), is a way to broaden limited thinking. It involves restating the problem and expanding the problem statement so that different solutions can be generated. If problem formulation yields to solution generation too early, important dimensions of the problem may go undetected and opportunities are missed. For example, if the problem statement is to convince the insurance company to approve a longer length of service, the nurse and client have narrowed their options. However, if the problem statement is to improve the client's convalescence and safety, several solutions and options are available, such as the following:

- Obtaining skilled nursing facility placement
- Obtaining home-health skilled services
- Arranging physician home visits
- Paying for custodial care
- Paying for private skilled care
- Obtaining informal caregiving

### Impact of Advocacy

Advocacy empowers clients to participate in problem-solving processes and decisions about health care. Clients try to understand changing opportunities in the health care system for access, use, and achieving continuity of care. Nurse advocates promote client self-determination and management of behavior as it relates to health and the adherence to therapeutic regimens. Clients are part of larger systems: the family, the work environment, and the community. Each system interacts with the client to shape the available options through resources, needs, and desires. Each system also exhibits both confirming and conflicting goals and processes that need to be understood for client self-determination to be successful. For example, the practice of advocacy among minority groups may involve the ability to focus attention on the magnitude of problems caused by diseases affecting minority clients. Whether the client is an individual, family, group, or community, the advocacy function can promote the interest of self-determination, which influences the progress of societies.

Advocacy is not without opposition. Clients and advocates may find barriers to services, vendors, providers, and resources. A community may experience a shortage in nursing home beds or providers, a childcare facility may experience staffing shortages, a family may not have the money to keep a child at home, and a client may find that the school system cannot fund a full-time nurse for its clinic. The reality of scarce resources creates a difficult barrier for advocates. However, events such as these often stimulate a community's self-determination and lead to innovative actions to correct gaps in service (see the Levels of Prevention box).

## LEVELS OF PREVENTION

### Case Management

| Levels of Prevention | Strategy |
|---|---|
| Primary | Use information exchange process to increase health literacy in order to use the health care system, adopt health promotion strategies that will maintain health, and engage in health education to create and maintain healthy lifestyles |
| Secondary | Use case finding and dashboard data to identify existing health problems in your caseload and the population served by your agency. Timely, holistic assessments and interventions can slow disease trajectories and promote healing and health |
| Tertiary | Monitor and adjust the use of prescription medications and adherence to treatment to reduce the risk of complications. Use models such as the CMSA Case Management Adherence Guidelines at http://www.csma.org to prevent subsequent consequences of issues in medication compliance as part of the treatment plan. Institutionalize this model in your agency |

### Allocation and Advocacy: Complements or Conundrum?

Whereas advocacy holds a traditional role in the nursing profession, allocation is a staple of market competition. Nurses perform allocation roles when they triage clients or perform the gatekeeping and rationing functions. Nurses often reflect that clinical judgments are influenced by their values and ethics as well as organizational demands (ANA, 2008). When working in organizations, nurses experience allocation demands at the

systems level through budgetary decisions and staffing assignments. At the clinical level, demands relate to implementing treatment protocols. When nurses act as client advocates by clarifying a client's desires or needs, they can conflict with systems procedures for allocation of limited resources within these systems. Case managers need to balance efficient use of resources.

Nurses who shoulder both advocacy and allocation responsibilities may benefit from a clear understanding of their personal and professional values. A systematic procedure for mediating conflict between the two competing responsibilities is also helpful (Cary, 1998; Fink-Samnick and Muller, 2010).

### Conflict Management

Case managers help clients manage conflicting needs and scarce resources. Techniques for managing conflict include a range of active communication skills. These skills are directed toward learning all parties' needs and desires, detecting their areas of agreement and disagreement, determining their abilities to collaborate, and assisting in discovering alternatives and activities for reaching a goal. Mutual benefit with limited loss is a goal of conflict management.

Conflict and its management vary in intensity and energy in a number of ways. The effort needed to manage a conflict depends on various factors: the existing evidence to support facts and the objective and subjective perceptions of the parties involved.

Negotiating is a strategic process used to move conflicting parties toward an outcome. The outcome can vary from one in which one party gains benefit at the other's expense (distributive outcomes) or in which mutual advantages override individual gains (integrative outcomes) (Thompson et al, 2010).

The process of negotiating can be characterized in three stages: prenegotiating (preparing and discussing), negotiating (discussing, proposing, bargaining), and aftermath (closing, renegotiating, willingness to negotiate again). Prenegotiating activities are designed to have parties agree to collaborate. Parties must see the possibility of agreeing and the costs of not agreeing (Lee and Lawrence, 2013). Preparations must be made as to time, place, and ground rules concerning participants, procedures, and confidentiality.

The negotiation stage consists of phases in which parties must develop trust, credibility, distance from the issue (to limit the feeling of "one best way"), and the ability to retain personal dignity. Bazarman (2005) and Lee and Lawrence (2013) agree that stages occur in negotiation:

*Phase 1:* Establishing the issues and agenda. This is accomplished by identifying, clarifying, presenting, and prioritizing the issues.

*Phase 2:* Advancing demands and uncovering interests. Negotiations center on presenting parties' interests and differentiating parties' demands and positions on the conflict.

*Phase 3:* Bargaining and discovering new options. Debates include gathering facts, based on reasoning, that will generate understanding and promote relearning. Bargaining reduces differences on issues by giving or removing rewards or desired objects. Creating new solutions or options through brainstorming, reflective thinking, and problem-purpose-expansion techniques is important in achieving options that provide mutual benefits.

*Phase 4:* Working out an agreement. This may involve settling on some but not all points. Parties can agree to re-examine the issues later, and steps for implementing and follow-up must be clarified.

The aftermath of negotiation is the period following an agreement in which parties are experiencing the consequences of their decisions and will discern the degree to which they are willing to work together in the future (Thompson et al, 2010). The reality of their decisions may lead to re-evaluating their values. In a conflict situation, parties engage in behaviors that reflect the dimensions of assertiveness and cooperation. **Assertiveness** is the ability to present one's own needs. **Cooperation** is the ability to understand and meet the needs of others. Each person uses a primary and secondary orientation to engage in conflict (Box 22-3).

Clearly, flexibility in conflict management behavior can facilitate an outcome that meets the client's goals. Helping parties navigate the process of attaining a goal requires effective personal relations, knowledge of the situation and alternatives, and a commitment to the process.

## Collaboration

In case management, the activities of many disciplines (social workers, nurses, physicians, insurers, physical therapists, etc.) are needed for success. Clients, the family, significant others, payers, and community organizations contribute to achieving the goal. **Collaboration** is achieved through a developmental process. Collaboration is a dynamic, highly interactive, and interdependent process in which people work together, sharing resources and even a vision for a goal (Morales Arroyo, 2003). Androwich and Cary (1989) found that collaboration occurs in a sequence and is reciprocal and can be characterized by seven stages and activities (Figure 22-5).

The goal of communication in the collaborative development process is to amplify, clarify, and verify all team members' points of view. Although communication is essential in collaboration, it is not sufficient to result in or maintain collaboration. Although the collaboration model recognizes the contributions of joint decision making, one member of the team should be accountable to the system and to the client. This team member should be responsible for monitoring the entire process (see the following QSEN box.

---

**QSEN FOCUS ON QUALITY AND SAFETY EDUCATION FOR NURSES**

**Targeted Competency: Teamwork and Collaboration**—Function effectively within nursing and interprofessional teams, fostering open communication, mutual respect, and shared decision making to achieve quality client interventions and outcomes.

Important aspects of teamwork and collaboration include:

**Knowledge:** Describe scopes of practice and roles of health care team members

**Skills:** Clarify roles and accountabilities under conditions of potential overlap in team member functioning

**Attitudes:** Value the perspectives and expertise of all health team members

**Teamwork and Collaboration Question**
Observe a typical workday of a nurse in community health or public health nurse, noting the types of activities that are done in coordination and case management and the amount of time spent in these areas. Interview several staff members to determine whether they perceive that the amount of their time spent in case management is changing. To what degree are the staff members involved in care management activities? Ask about colleagues with whom case managers collaborate. Besides primary care physicians, which health care team members are often involved in managing clients' care across time and across settings? What skills are needed by the case management nurse to best facilitate these interdisciplinary teams?

Prepared by Gail Armstrong, PhD(c), DNP, ACNS-BC, CNE, Associate Professor, University of Colorado Denver College of Nursing.

---

Case managers encounter conflict on a daily basis. Competing needs, resources, organizational demands, and professional role boundaries present opportunities and pitfalls for conflict management and collaboration (Box 22-4). Providers report that in the collaborative role of serving as advocates for clients, they encounter competing expectations by other providers in the system—even other case managers (Sands, 2013).

Teamwork and collaboration clearly demand knowledge and skills about clients, health status, resources, treatments, and community providers. The ability to assess clients' and families' complex needs involves knowledge of intrapersonal, interpersonal, medical, nursing, and social dimensions. Demonstrating team member and leadership skills in facilitating a goal-directed group process is essential. It is unlikely that any single professional possesses the expertise required in all dimensions. It is likely, however, that the synergy produced by all can result in successful outcomes.

## ISSUES IN CASE MANAGEMENT

### Legal Issues

Case managers today face pressure to control costs, to use evidence-based guidelines for practice, and to reduce risks for

---

**BOX 22-3 Categories of Behaviors Used in Conflict Management**

**Accommodating:** Individual neglects personal concerns to satisfy the concerns of another.

**Avoiding:** Individual pursues neither his or her concerns nor another's concerns.

**Collaborating:** Individual attempts to work with others toward solutions that satisfy the goals of both parties.

**Competing:** Individual pursues personal concerns at another's expense.

**Compromising:** Individual attempts to find a mutually acceptable solution that partially satisfies both parties.

Modified from Volkema RJ, Bergmann TJ: Conflict styles as indicators of behavioral patterns in interpersonal conflicts, J Social Psychol 135: 5-15, 2001; CPP: *History and Validity of the Thomas-Kilmann Conflict Mode Instrument (TKI).* Mountainview, CA, CPP, Inc. Available at http://www.cpp.com/products/tki/tkiinfo.aspx. Retrieved June 14, 2010.

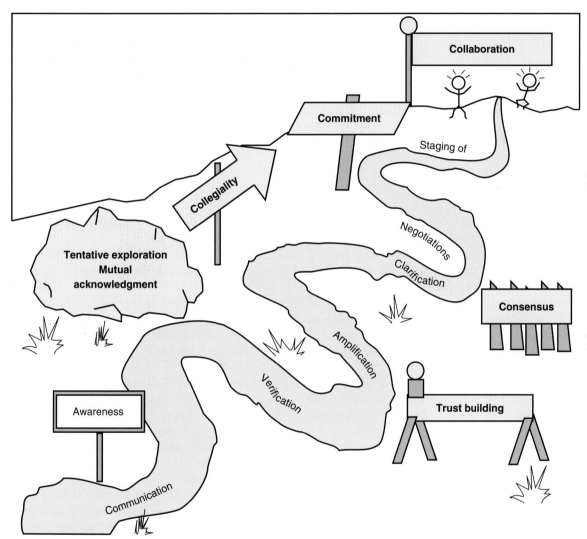

**FIG 22-5** Collaboration is a sequential yet reciprocal process. (From Androwich I, Cary AH: *A Collaboration Model: A Synthesis of Literature and a Research Survey.* Paper presented at the Association of Community Health Nurse Educators Spring Institute, Seattle, June 1989.)

---

**BOX 22-4  Stages of Collaboration**

1. Awareness
   - Make a conscious entry into a group process; focus on goals of convening together; generate a definition of collaborative process and what it means to team members.
2. Tentative exploration and mutual acknowledgment
   - Exploration: Disclose professional skills for the desired process; disclose areas where contributions cannot be made; disclose values reflecting priorities; identify roles and disclose personal values, including time, energy, interest, and resources.
   - Mutual acknowledgment: Clarify each member's potential contributions; verify the group's strengths and areas needing consultation; clarify members' work style, organizational supports, and barriers to collaborative efforts.
3. Trust building
   - Determine the degree to which reliance on others can be achieved; examine congruence between words and behaviors; set interdependent goals; develop tolerance for ambiguity.
4. Collegiality
   - Define the relationships of members with each other; define the responsibilities and tasks of each; define entrance and exit conditions.
5. Consensus
   - Determine the issues for which consensus is required; determine the processes used for clarifying and making decisions to reach consensus; determine the process for re-evaluating consensus outcomes.
6. Commitment
   - Realize the physical, emotional, and material actions directed toward the goal; clarify procedures for re-evaluating commitments in light of goal demands and group standards for deviance.
7. Collaboration
   - Initiate a process of joint decision making reflecting the synergy that results from combining knowledge and skills.

Modified from Cary A, Androwich I: A collaboration model: a synthesis of literature and a research survey, paper presented at the Association of Community Health Nurse Educators Spring Institute, Seattle, June 1989; Mueller WJ, Kell B: Coping with conflict, Englewood Cliffs, NJ, 1972, Prentice Hall.

---

legal liability. They are vulnerable to legal risks because of inadequate preparation, changing legislation and policy, health systems changes, the advent of new workers and the absence of title protection, insufficient support, and role expectations. Liability concerns of case managers exist when the following three conditions are met: (1) the provider had a duty to provide reasonable care, (2) a breach of contract occurred through an act or an omission to act, and (3) the act or omission caused injury or damage to the client. Case managers must strive to reduce risks, practice wisely within acceptable practice standards, and limit legal defense costs through professional insurance coverage. Areas of risk are adapted from Hendricks and Cesar (2003), Cunningham (2007), Llewellyn and Leonard (2009), and Sambucini (2013):

1. Liability for managing care
   a. Inappropriate design or implementation of the case management system
   b. Failure to obtain all pertinent records on which case management actions are based
   c. Failure to have cases evaluated by appropriately experienced and credentialed clinicians
   d. Failure to confer directly with the treating provider (physician or nurse practitioner) at the onset and throughout the client's care
   e. Substituting a case manager's clinical judgment for that of the medical provider
   f. Requiring the client or his or her provider to accept case management recommendation instead of any other treatment
   g. Harassment of clinicians, clients, and family in seeking information, and setting unreasonable deadlines for decisions or information
   h. Claiming orally or in writing that the case management treatment plan is better than the provider's plan
   i. Restricting access to otherwise necessary or appropriate care because of cost
   j. Referring clients to treatment furnished by providers related to the case management agency without proper disclosure
   k. Connecting case managers' compensation to reduced use and access of services
   l. Inappropriate delegation of care
   m. Inappropriate use of clinical practice guidelines
2. Negligent referrals
   a. Referral to a practitioner known to be incompetent
   b. Substituting inadequate treatment for an adequate but more costly option
   c. Curtailing treatment inappropriately when treatment was actually needed
   d. Referral to a facility or practitioner inappropriate for the client's needs
   e. Transfer to another facility that lacks care requirements
   f. Communication and transition handoff failures
3. Experimental treatment and technology
   a. Failure to apply the contractual definition of "experimental" treatment found in the client's insurance policy
   b. Failure to review sources of information referenced in the applicable insurance policy (e.g., Food and Drug Administration, or published medical literature)
   c. Failure to review the client's complete medical record
   d. Failure to make a timely determination of benefits in light of timeliness of treatment
   e. Failure to communicate coverage determined to be needed, to the insured client or participant
   f. Improper economic considerations determining the coverage
   g. Failure to understand and retrieve information from HIT sources.

4. Confidentiality/security
   a. Failure to deny access to sensitive information that is awarded special protection by federal or state law
   b. Failure to protect access to computerized medical records
   c. Failure to adhere to regulatory provisions (e.g., Health Insurance Portability and Accountability Act provisions [http://hipaa.cms.gov]; Americans with Disabilities Act)
5. Fraud and abuse
   a. Making false statements of claims or causing incorrect claims to be filed
   b. Falsifying the adherence to conditions of participation of Medicare and Medicaid
   c. Submitting claims for excessive, unnecessary, or poor-quality services
   d. Engaging in remuneration, bribes, kickbacks, or rebates in exchange for referral
   e. Upcoding intensity of care or intervention requirements

Legal citations relevant to case management and managed care include negligent referrals, provider liability, payer liability, breach of contract, denial of care, and bad faith. As in any scope of nursing practice and with the potential growth in tort reform, it behooves the nurse to seek preventive education on contemporary practice and legal trends to lower exposure to legal liability.

Sambucini (2013) notes that court cases and federal and state tort reforms influence the legal considerations of case managers generally. When courts find that cost considerations affect medical care decisions, all parties to the decision will be liable for resulting damages. Guidelines to reduce risk exposure include the following:

1. Clear documentation of the extent of client participation in decision making and reasons for decisions
2. Records demonstrating accurate and complete information on interactions and outcomes
3. Use of reasonable care in selecting referral sources, which may include verifying of licensure of providers
4. Written agreements when arrangements are made to modify benefits other than those in the contract
5. Good communication with clients
6. Informing clients of their rights of appeal
7. Applying the ethical guidelines of case management (Valiant and Jensen, 2012)

## Ethical Issues

Case managers as nursing professionals are guided in ethical practice by the *Code of Ethics for Nursing* (ANA, 2008; to be revised for publication in 2015) and *Code of Professional Conduct for Case Managers* (Commission for Case Management Certification [CCMC], 2005), by performance indicators for ethics in the *Standards of Practice for Case Management* (CMSA, 2010), and by the contract expressed in *Nursing's Social Policy Statement* (ANA, 2010).

By integrating these guidelines and philosophies, nursing practice is ideally suited to preserve the ethical principles of autonomy, beneficence, fidelity, justice, nonmaleficence, and veracity in case management processes. Numerous authors,

notably Hendricks and Cesar (2003), McCollom (2004), Llewellyn and Leonard (2009), Fink-Samnick and Muller (2010), and Apuna-Grummer and Howland (2013), describe how case managers may confront dilemmas in these areas:

- Case management may hamper a client's autonomy, or the individual's right to choose a provider, if a particular provider is not approved by the case management system. If a new provider must be found who can be approved for coverage, continuity of care may be disrupted.
- Beneficence, or doing good, can be impaired when excessive attention to containing costs supersedes the nurse's duty to improve health or relieve suffering.
- Fidelity is defined as faithfulness to the obligation of duty (www.merriam-webster.com/dictionary), in this case to the client by keeping promises and remaining loyal within the nurse-client relationship (www.merriam-webster.com/dictionary. Accessed July 7, 2014). Duty to clients to secure benefits on their behalf and to limit unnecessary expenditures can create dilemmas when the goals are not uniform.
- Justice as an ethical principle for case managers considers equal distribution of health care with reasonable quality. Tiers of quality and expertise among provider groups can be created when quality providers refuse to accept reimbursement allowances from the managed system, leaving less experienced or lower quality providers as the caregiver of choice for clients being managed.
- Nonmaleficence is defined as doing no harm. When case managers incorporate outcomes measures, evidence-based practice, and monitoring processes in their plans of care, this principle is addressed.
- Veracity, or truth telling, is absolutely necessary to the practice of advocacy and building a trusting relationship with clients. Clients particularly complain that in the changing health care system, payers do not seem to be able to provide comprehensive yet inexpensive options for care.

Three of the most common legal dilemmas have been historically classified as conflicts in advocacy, priorities, and duties (Hendricks and Cesar, 2003; Mahlin, 2010). For example, a case manager may advocate for many perspectives—clients, organizations, and society—that are not harmonious. When considering priorities in values, the case manager will ultimately be considering personal, professional, organizational, and client values. Selecting which values to honor can result in violating the values of the other, and asking the question "Whose best interests can be served?" may create a dilemma. Finally, conflicts in duties can result when placing the best interest of a client first adversely affects the other party.

Standards of practice and care, codes of ethics, licensure laws, credentialing through certification, and organizational policies and procedures (e.g., ethics committees, risk management units) offer the case manager information and support in managing ethical conflicts and dilemmas in the case management system. Maintaining familiarity with ethical issues published in the case management literature can offer specific assistance for practicing case managers (Tables 22-3 and 22-4).

## TABLE 22-3   Credentialing Resources for Case Managers (Individual Certification Options)

| Organization | Website | Credentials |
|---|---|---|
| American Nurses Credentialing Center | http://www.nursecredentialing.org | Nurses: RN-BC, for Registered Nurse-Board Certified for Case Management |
| Case Management Administrators | http://www.ptcny.com | CMA-C, for Case Management Administrator-Certified |
| Certification of Disability Management Specialists Commission | http://www.cdms.org | Interprofessionals: CDMS, for Certified Disability Management Specialist |
| Commission for Case Manager Certification | http://www.ccmcertification.org | Interprofessionals: CCM, for Certified Case Manager |
| Certification Board for Certified Nurse Life Care Planners | http://www.ptcny.com | CNLCP, for Certified Nurse Life Care Planner (specialty certification for nurses who are life care planners) |
| National Academy of Certified Care Managers | http://www.naccm.net | Interprofessionals: CLM, for Certified Long-term Care Manager |
| Rehabilitation Nursing Certification Board | http://www.rehabnurse.org/certification | CRRN, for Certified Rehabilitation Registered Nurse |

## TABLE 22-4   Websites for Case Management Resources

| Resource | Website | Details |
|---|---|---|
| URAC | www.urac.org | Accredits disease management, case management, and health plan programs and other services. Supports efforts for clinical benchmarking, quality of care, chronic care evidence-based models |
| America's Health Insurance Plans | http://www.ahip.org | Trade association representing health insurance industry |
| American Nurses Credentialing Center | http://www.nursecredentialing.org | Offers review course materials for nurse case managers |
| American Medical Association | http://www.ama-assn.org | Includes continuing medical education unit (CEU) programs |
| Case Management Society of America | http://www.cmsa.org | Specialty organization for case managers |
| Centers for Medicare and Medicaid Services | http://www.cms.gov | Oversees execution of rules and regulations for clients of state and federally funded services |
| Center Watch Clinical Trial Listing Service | http://www.centerwatch.com | Global source for clinical trials information |
| Centers for Disease Control and Prevention | http://www.cdc.gov | Provides education, training, and research for disease, emergency preparedness, environmental health, traveler health, workplace safety and health, population health, and healthy living |
| The Joint Commission (TJC) | http://www.jointcommission.org | Accredits health care–related delivery organizations and disease-specific care programs |
| Medscape | http://www.medscape.org | Features clinical updates and education for professionals |
| National PACE Association | http://www.npaonline.org | Provides information on models and locations of PACE services for the elderly |
| National Transitions of Care Coalition (NTOCC) | http://www.ntocc.org | Provides information on transitions of care models and outcomes |
| National Committee for Quality Assurance | http://www.ncqa.org | Publishes HEDIS performance indicators for provider systems and accredits managed care organizations. Provides certification of disease management, utilization management, and credentialing verification organizations. Also ACOs, case management and patient-centered medical homes (among other organizations) |
| National Library of Medicine | http://www.nlm.nih.gov | Global medical library |
| *NurseWeek* | http://www.nurse.com | Provides information links to other sites and nursing professional education course work |
| Oncology | http://www.oncolink.upenn.edu | Oncology links |
| *Online Journal of Issues in Nursing* | http://www.nursingworld.org | Publication on issues in nursing |
| Commission on Accreditation of Rehabilitation Facilities | http://www.carf.org | Accredits services globally that may be used by case management clients such as adult day care, assisted living, behavioral health, disability rehab, addiction and substance abuse rehabilitation, employment and community services, and medical rehabilitation |

*ACO,* Accountable care organization; *HEDIS,* Healthcare Effectiveness Data and Information Set.

## PRACTICE APPLICATION

During her regularly scheduled visit to a blood pressure clinic in a local apartment cluster, a Hispanic resident, Mrs. B., 45 years old, complained of feeling dizzy and forgetful. She could not remember which of her six medications she had taken during the last few days. Her blood pressure readings on reclining, sitting, and standing revealed gross elevation. The nurse and Mrs. B. discussed the danger of her present status and the need to seek medical attention. Mrs. B. called her physician from her apartment and agreed to be transported to the emergency department.

In the emergency department, Mrs. B. manifested the progressive signs and symptoms of a cerebrovascular accident (a CVA, or stroke). During hospitalization, she lost her capacity for expressive language and demonstrated hemiparesis and loss of bladder control. Her cognitive function became intermittently confused, and she was slow to recognize her physician and neighbors who came to visit. The utilization review/discharge planning nurse at the hospital contacted the case manager from the health department to screen and assess for the continuum of care needs as early as possible, because Mrs. B. lived alone and family members resided out of town.

It became apparent that family caregiving in the community could only be intermittent because family members lived too far away. Mrs. B. had residual functional and cognitive deficits that would demand longer-term care.

As the case manager contracted by the plan, place the following actions in the correct sequence to construct a case management plan:

**A.** Discuss with the family their schedule of availability to offer care in the client's home.

**B.** Discuss their cultural values in caring for family members.

**C.** Call the client and introduce yourself, as a prelude to working with her.

**D.** Obtain information on the scope of services covered by the benefit plan for your client.

**E.** Arrange a skilled nursing facility site visit for the client and family.

**Answers can be found on the Evolve site.**

## KEY POINTS

- An important role of the nurse is that of client advocate.
- The goal of advocacy is to promote the client's self-determination.
- When performing in the advocacy role, conflicts may emerge about the full disclosure of information, territoriality, accountability to multiple parties, legal challenges to clients' decisions, and competition for scarce resources.
- The functions of advocacy and allocation can pose dilemmas in practice.
- Amplification, clarification, and verification are three communication skills necessary in the advocacy process.
- Additional skills important to fulfilling the role of client advocate include the helping relationship, assertiveness, and problem solving.
- Problem solving is a systematic approach that includes understanding the values of each party and generating alternative solutions.
- Brainstorming and the problem-purpose-expansion method are two techniques to enhance the effectiveness of problem-solving skills.
- During conflict, negotiations can move conflicting parties toward an outcome.
- Prenegotiation, negotiation, and aftermath are three phases of managing a conflict.
- Each individual has a predominant orientation when engaging in conflict: competing, accommodating, avoiding, collaborating, or compromising.
- Collaboration may result by moving through seven stages: awareness, tentative exploration and mutual acknowledgment, trust building, collegiality, consensus, commitment, and collaboration.
- Care management is a strategic program to maintain the health of a population enrolled in a delivery system.

- Continuity of care is a goal of nursing practice. It requires making linkages with services and information systems to improve the client's health status.
- As the structure of the health care system moves toward delivering more services in the community, the achievement of continuity of care will present a greater challenge.
- Case management is typically an interprofessional process in which the client is the focus of the plan.
- Documentation and use of dashboards for case management activities and outcomes are essential to nursing practice.
- Case management is a systematic process of assessment, planning, service coordination, referral, monitoring, and evaluation that meets the multiple service needs of clients.
- A nurse's scope of practice includes advocacy, allocation, and case management functions.
- Nurses functioning as advocates and case managers need to be aware of the ethical and legal issues confronting these components of their practice.
- Standardization of care for predictable outcomes can be achieved through critical paths, disease management protocols, dashboards, clinical guidelines, interprofessional action plans, and a caring-based practice in which processes of diagnosis and treatment are applied to the human experiences of health and illness.
- Nurses are guided by a philosophy of caring and advocacy.
- Nurses have a high regard for client self-determination, independence, and informed choice in decision making.
- Recognizing that responses to illness and disability may limit independence and self-determination, nurses focus on the rights of individuals, families, and communities to define their own health and evidence-based guidelines for practice.
- Telehealth application provides expansive alternatives within resource delivery options but must be customized for clients.

## CLINICAL DECISION-MAKING ACTIVITIES

1. Observe a typical work day of a nurse working with a population, noting the types of activities that are done in coordination, transition care, case management, and documentation as well as the amount of time spent in these areas. Interview several staff members to determine whether they perceive that their time spent in case management is changing. To what degree are the staff members involved in care management activities? What are the top three legal and ethical issues they encounter in their practice? What do the nurses report as their greatest sources of satisfaction and dissatisfaction in their jobs?

2. Initiating, monitoring, and evaluating resources are essential components of nursing practice. Describe a client situation and the case management process that might occur in the following practices:
   A. A school nurse in an elementary school and one in a high school working with brain-injured students
   B. An occupational health nurse in a hospital and one in a manufacturing plant
   C. A nurse working in a well-child clinic
   D. A case manager employed by a managed care organization
   E. A care manager employed in a health benefits corporation

3. Explain how the case management processes affected client outcome in each of these situations.

4. The values and beliefs held by a nurse influence the nurse's ability to be an advocate for clients. Analyze your values and beliefs about rationing health care and describe how they may affect your ability to be a client advocate. How did you develop your values and beliefs?

5. Read one of the following and respond to the respective questions: Fink-Samnick E, Muller LS: Case management across the life continuum: ethical obligations versus best practice. *Prof Case Manag* 15:153-156, 2010. Discuss your reactions to the mini case studies and the statement, *Allocation always works within the mixed interests of the individual and other stakeholders.* What values do you hold and how do they frame your reactions?
   A. What are the mixed values of individuals?
   B. What are the mixed values of other stakeholders (providers, policy makers, insurers)?
   C. What are the mixed values of society in the United States? What are the mixed values of society in underdeveloped nations? How are the mixed values different or similar in these three situations (A-C)? How does your answer affect client outcomes?
   Or read: Sands JR: Where was care coordination? *CMSA Today* 8:14-17, 201.
   A. Name three problems the author described as her aunt transitioned between levels of care in the hospital.
   B. Name three problems the author experienced with the manner in which case management was delivered.
   C. What changes would you make as the manager of the case management office to the manner in which case management and coordination was delivered in the future? What criteria would you use to judge if the change was effective?
   D. Which of the categories of legal risks exist based on the story the authors tells?

## REFERENCES

Agency for Healthcare Research and Quality (AHRQ): *Nurse-Led, Telephone-Based Collaborative Care Improves Mental and Physical Health of Depressed Clients after Cardiac Bypass Surgery* [Health Care Innovations Exchange], 2010a. From: https://innovations.ahrq.gov/profiles/nurse-led-telephone-based-collaborative-care-improves-mental-and-physical-health-depressed. Retrieved January 2015.

Agency for Healthcare Research and Quality (AHRQ): *Intensive Case Management Reduces Inpatient Admissions and Emergency Department Visits among Costly, Medically Complex Clients without Insurance* [Health Care Innovations Exchange], 2010b. From: https://www.innovations.ahrq.gov. Retrieved January 2015.

Agency for Healthcare Research and Quality (AHRQ): *Annual progress report to Congress: National strategy for quality improvement in health care.* 2013, Available at: www.ahrq.gov/workingforquality/nqs/nqs2013annlrpt.htm.

American Association of Nurse Life Care Planners (AANLCP): *Code of Professional Ethics and Conduct for Nurse Life Care Planners with Interpretive Statements.* AANLCP membership guide. 2012a. From: www.AANLCP.org. Retrieved January 2015.

American Association of Nurse Life Care Planners (AANLCP): *Nurse Life Care Planners: Standards of Practice with Interpretive Statements.* AANLCP membership guide. 2012b. From: www.AANLCP.org. Retrieved January 2015.

American Association of Nurse Life Care Planners (AANLCP): *A core curriculum for nurse life care planners.* Bloomington Indiana, October 2013, Universe LLC.

American Hospital Association (AHA): *Glossary of Terms and Phrases for Health Care Coalitions.* Chicago, 1986, AHA Office of Health Coalitions and Private Sector Initiatives.

American Hospital Association (AHA): *Guide to the Health Care Field.* Chicago, 2003-2004, AHA.

American Nurses Association (ANA): *Managed Care: Cornerstone for Health Care Reform—A Fact Sheet.* Washington, DC, 1993, ANA.

American Nurses Association (ANA): *Guide to the Code of Ethics for Nurses.* Silver Spring, MD, 2008, Nursesbooks.org.

American Nurses Association (ANA): *Nursing's Social Policy Statement,* ed 3. Silver Spring, MD, 2010, Nursesbooks.org.

American Nurses Association (ANA): *Framework for Measuring Nurses' Contributions to Care Coordination.* Silver Spring, MD, 2013, ANA.

American Nurses Foundation (ANF): *America's Nurses: An Untapped Natural Resource.* Washington, DC, 1993, ANF.

Androwich I, Cary AH: *A Collaboration Model: A Synthesis of Literature and a Research Survey.* Paper presented at the Association of Community Health Nurse Educators Spring Institute. Seattle, June 1989.

Apuna-Grummer D, Howland WA, editors: *A Core Curriculum for Nurse Life Care Planning.* Bloomington, IN, 2013, iUniverse.

Baer J, Kutner M, Sabatini J: *Basic Reading Skills and the Literacy of America's Least Literate Adults: Results from the 2003 National Assessment of Adult Literacy (NAAL) Supplemental Studies* (NCES 2009-481). Washington, DC, 2009, National Center for Education Statistics, Institute of Education Sciences, U.S. Department of Education.

Barefield F: Working case managers' view of the profession. *Case Manager* 14:69–71, 2003.

Bazarman MH, editor: *Negotiating, Decision Making and Conflict Management.* Cheltenham, UK, 2005, Edward Elgar Publishing United.

Bower KA: *Case Management by Nurses.* Washington, DC, 1992, American Nurses Association.

Brown SJ: Managing the complexity of best practice health care. *J Nurs Care Qual* 15:1–8, 2001.

Burns T, Catty J, Dash M, et al: Use of intensive case management to reduce time in hospital in people with severe mental illness: systematic review and meta-regression. *BMJ* 335:336–342, 2007.

Burns T, Fioritti A, Holloway F, et al: Case management and assertive community treatment in Europe. *Psychiatr Serv* 52:631–636, 2001.

Burton J, Murphy E, Riley P: Primary immunodeficiency disease: a model for case management of chronic disease. *Prof Case Manag* 15:5–14, 2010.

Carneal G, Pock R: Six year of study reveals the impact of IT on the practice of case management. *CMSA Today* 2:16–17, 2014.

Cary AH: Advocacy or allocation. *Nurs Connect* 11:1–7, 1998.

Case Management Society of America (CMSA): *Case Management Model Act: Supporting Case Management Programs.* Little Rock, AR, 2009, CMSA. From: http://www.cmsa.org/portals/0/pdf/publicpolicy/cmsa_model_act.pdf. Retrieved January 2015.

Case Management Society of America (CMSA): *Standards of Practice for Case Management.* Little Rock, AR, 2010, CMSA. From: http://www.cmsa.org/portals/0/pdf/memberonly/StandardsOfPractice.pdf. Retrieved January 2015.

Coggeshall Press: *Case Management Model.* Coralville, IA, 2008, Coggeshall Press. as cited in Huber, 2010.

Cohen EL, Cesta TG: *Nursing Case Management,* ed 4. St. Louis, 2005, Elsevier.

Commission for Case Management Certification (CCMC): *Code of Professional Conduct for Case Managers.* St. Paul, MN, 2005, CCMC.

CPP: *History and Validity of the Thomas-Kilmann Conflict Mode Instrument (TKI).* Mountain View, CA, CPP, Inc. From: https://www.cpp.com/products/tki/tki_info.aspx. Retrieved January 2015.

Cunningham B: Powell SK, Tahan HA, editors: *CMSA Core Curriculum for Case Management.* Philadelphia, 2007, Lippincott, Williams & Wilkins.

Disease Management Association of America (DMAA): *The Care Continuum Alliance.* Washington, DC, 2008, DMAA.

Disease Management Association of America (DMAA): *Organization Calls for MLR to Recognize Population Health as Aspect of Clinical Care.* Washington, DC, 2010, DMAA. From: http://www.dmaa.org/news_releases/2010/pressrelease_043010.asp. Retrieved January 2015.

Fidelity [Def. 2]. (n.d.). *Merriam-Webster Online.* In Merriam-Webster. From: http://www.merriam-webster.com/dictionary/fidelity. Retrieved January 2015.

Fink-Samnick E, Muller LS: Case management across the life continuum: ethical obligations versus best practice. *Prof Case Manag* 15:153–156, 2010.

Fretwell MD, Old JS: The PACE program: home-based care for nursing home–eligible individuals. *N C Med J* 72:209–211, 2011.

Gary TL, Batts-Turner M, Yeh HC, et al: The effects of a nurse case manager and a community health worker on diabetic control, emergency department visits, and hospitalizations among urban African Americans with type 2 diabetes mellitus. *Arch Intern Med* 169:1788–1794, 2009.

Glendenning-Napoli A, Dowling B, Pulvino J, et al: Community-based case management for uninsured patients with chronic diseases: effects on acute care utilization and costs. *Prof Case Manag* 17:267–275, 2012.

Gorman A: *Many new patients overwhelmed by health care jargon. Kaiser Health News* 2014. From: http://www.pbs.org/newshour/rundown. Retrieved January 2015.

Hagan L, Morin D, Lepine R: Evaluation of telenursing outcomes: satisfaction, self-care practices, and cost savings. *Public Health Nurs* 17:305–313, 2000.

Health Resources and Services Administration (HRSA): *Health Systems and Financing Group: Medicaid Case Management Services by State, archived Webcast.* 2004. From: http://www.hrsa.gov/financeMC/webcast-Sept1-Case-Mgmt-by-State-040825.htm. Retrieved January 2015.

Hendricks AG, Cesar WJ: How prepared are you? Ethical and legal challenges facing case managers today. *Case Manager* 14:56–62, 2003.

Heslin PA, Moldoveanu M: What's the "real" problem here? A model of problem formulation. Presented at Managing the Complex IV: Conference on Complex Systems and the Management of Organizations, Fort Myers, FL, December 2002.

Huber DL: *Leadership and Nursing Care Management,* ed 4. St. Louis, 2010, Elsevier.

Hyde E, Murphy B: Computerized clinical pathways: piloting a strategy to enhance quality patient care. *Clin Nurse Spec* 26:277–282, 2012.

Institute of Medicine (IOM): *Crossing the Quality Chasm: A New Health System for the 21st Century.* Washington, DC, 2001, National Academies Press.

Institute of Medicine (IOM): *The Future of Nursing: Leading Change, Advancing Health.* Washington, DC, 2011, National Academies Press.

Katz MH, Cunningham WE, Fleishman JA, et al: The effects of case management on unmet needs and utilization of medical care and medications among HIV-infected persons. *Ann Intern Med* 135:557–565, 2001.

Keller LO, Strohschein S, Lia-Hoagberg B, et al: Population-based public health interventions: innovations in practice, teaching and management, Part II. *Public Health Nurs* 21:469–487, 2004.

Kinsman L, Rotter T, James E, et al: What is a clinical pathway? Development of a definition to inform the debate. *BMC Med* 8:31, 2010.

Kohnke MF: *Advocacy: Risk and Reality.* St. Louis, 1982, Mosby.

Kolbasovsky A: Reducing 30 day inpatient psychiatric recidivism and associated costs through intensive case management. *Prof Case Manag* 14:96–105, 2009.

Lamb G: *Care Coordination: The Game Changer.* Silver Spring, MD, 2013, Nursesbooks.org.

Lattimer C: Working to improve transitions of care. *CMSA Today* 5:12–14, 2013.

Lee R, Lawrence P: *Organizational Behavior: Politics at Work.* New York, NY, 2013, Routledge.

Llewellyn A, Leonard M: *Case Management Review and Resource Manual,* ed 3. Silver Spring, MD, 2009, Nursesbooks.org.

Mahlin M: Individual patient advocacy, collective responsibility and activism within professional nursing associates. *Nurs Ethics* 17:247–254, 2010.

Mallik M, Rafferty AM: Diffusion of the concept of advocacy. *J Adv Nurs* 32:399–404, 2000.

McCall N, Cromwell J: Results of the Medicare health support disease management pilot program. *NEJM* 365:1704–1712, 2011.

McClinton DH: Protecting patients. *Contin Care* 17:6, 1998.

McCollom P: Advocate versus abdicate. *Case Manager* 15:43–45, 2004.

McDonald KM, Sundaram V, Bravata DM, et al: Care coordination. In Shojania KG, McDonald KM, Wachter RM, et al, editors: *Closing the Quality Gap: A Critical Analysis of Quality Improvement Strategies.* 2007. Technical Review 9 (prepared by Stanford-UCSF Evidence-Based Practice Center under Contract No. 290-02-0017). From: http://www.ahqr.gov/research/findings/evidence-based-reports/caregap.pdf. Retrieved January 2015.

McDonald KM, Schultz E, Albin L, et al: *Care Coordination Atlas.* version 3 (prepared by Stanford University under contract to Battelle on Contract No. 290-04-0020). AHRQ Publication No. 11-0023-EF. Rockville, MD, 2010, Agency for Healthcare Research and Quality. From: http://www.ahrq.gov/professionals/systems/long-term-care/resources/coordination/atlas/care-coordination-measures-atlas.pdf. Retrieved January 2015.

McKesson Corporation: *How Care Management Evolves with Population Management—A White Paper.* 2014. From: http://www.healthleadersmedia.com/content/SPR-300965/How-Care-Management-Evolves-with-Population-Management.* Retrieved January 2015.

Michaels C, Cohen EL: Two strategies for managing care. In Cohen EL, Cesta TG, editors: *Nursing Case Management,* ed 4. St. Louis, 2005, Elsevier.

Mohamed S, Neale M, Rosenheck RA: VA intensive mental health case management in urban and rural areas: veteran characteristics and service delivery. *Psychiatr Serv* 60:914–921, 2009.

Mohamed S, Rosenheck R, Cuerdon T: Who terminates from ACT and why? Data from the National VA Mental Health Intensive Case Management Program. *Psychiatr Serv* 61:675–683, 2010.

Morales Arroyo MA: *The physiology of collaboration: an investigation of library-museum-university partnerships.* Dissertation. August 2003. From: http://digital.library.unt.edu/ark:/67531/metadc4303/?q=%22physiology%20of%20collaboration%22. Retrieved January 2015.

Mullahy C: *The Case Manager's Handbook,* ed 4. Sudbury, MA, 2010, Jones & Bartlett.

Muller LS, Flarery DL: Defining advanced practice nursing. *Lippincotts Case Manag* 8:230–231, 2003.

National PACE Association: *Who, What and Where is PACE?* 2014. From: http://www.npaonline.org/website/article.asp?id=12&title=Who,_What_and_Where_Is_PACE? Retrieved January 2015.

National Transitions of Care Coalition (NTOCC): *Improved Transitions of Patient Care Yield Tangible Savings.* 2011. From: http://www.ntocc.org/portals/0/Tangiblesavings.pdf. Retrieved January 2015.

Nelson ML: Advocacy in nursing. *Nurs Outlook* 36:136–141, 1988.

Newman MB, Kowlsen T, Beckworth V: An integrated approach: the impact of health care reform from a managed care perspective. *CMSA Today* 1:20–23, 2014.

Noonan P: The case manager's role in population health. *CMSA Today* 3:16–17, 2014.

Owen M: Going forward: what is case management? *Prof Case Manag* 19:143–144, 2014.

Park EJ, Huber DL, Tahan HA: The evidence base for case management practice. *West J Nurs Res* 31:693–714, 2009.

Peterson PE, Woessmann L, Hanushek EA, et al: *Globally Challenged: Are US Students Ready to Compete?* PEPG report #11-03. 2011. Harvard Kennedy School. From: http://www.hks.harvard.edu/pepg/PDF/Papers/PEPG11-03_GloballyChallenged.pdf. Retrieved January 2015.

Quad Council: *Quad Council Competencies for Public Health Nursing.* 2011. From: http://www.achne.org/files/Quad%20Council/QuadCouncilCompetenciesforPublicHealthNurses.pdf. Retrieved January 2015.

Renholm M, Leino-Kilpi H, Suominen T: Critical pathways: a systematic review. *J Nurs Adm* 32:196–202, 2002.

Sambucini A: History and evolution of the nurse life care planning specialty. In Apuna-Grummer D, Howland WA, editors: *A Core*

*Curriculum for Nurse Life Care Planners.* Bloomington, IN, 2013, iUniverse.

Sands JR: Where was care coordination? *CMSA Today* 8:14–17, 2013.

Schraeder C, Shelton PS: *Comprehensive Care Coordination for Chronically Ill Adults.* West Sussex, UK, 2011, John Wiley & Sons.

Schutt RK, Fawcett J, Gall GB, et al: Case manager satisfaction in public health. *Prof Case Manag* 15:124–134, 2010.

Secord LJ: *Private Case Management for Older Persons and Their Families.* Excelsior, MN, 1987, Interstudy.

Sidorov J: *TRICARE saves taxpayers millions on chronic illness disease management [Disease Management Care Blog].* 2010. From: http://diseasemanagementcareblog.blogspot.com/2010/06/tricare-saves-taxpayers-millions-on.html. Retrieved January 2015.

Smith AP: Patient advocacy: roles for nurses and leaders. *Nurs Econ* 22:88–90, 2004.

Stanton MP, Dunkin J: A review of case management functions related to transitions of care at a rural nurse managed clinic. *Prof Case Manag* 14:321–327, 2009.

Stricker P: Collaborative care teams and the benefits of communicating across disciplines. *CMSA Today* 4:20–23, 2013.

Stricker P: Data analytics: a critical tool. *CMSA Today* 4:20–23, 2014.

Tahan HA: Essentials of advocacy in case management. *Lippincotts Case Manag* 10:136–145, 2005.

Taylor P: Comprehensive nursing case management: an advanced practice model. *Nurs Case Manag* 4:2–10, 1999.

The Joint Commission (TJC): *2009 National Patient Safety Goals for Ambulatory Care.* Oakbrook Terrace, IL, 2009, TJC.

Thompson LL, Wang J, Gunia BC: Negotiation. *Annu Rev Psychol* 61:491–515, 2010.

Treiger TM: Case management today and its evolution into the future. *CSMA Today* 7:16–20, 2013.

Tufts Managed Care Institute: *Demand Management: Introduction and References.* 2011. From: http://jobfunctions.bnet.com/abstract.aspx?docid=102064. Retrieved January 2015.

URAC: *Disease Management.* At: https://www.urac.org/accreditation-and-measurement/accreditation-programs/all-programs/disease-management/. Retrieved January 2014.

U.S. Department of Health and Human Services (USDHHS): *Redefining Case Management.* Rockville, MD, 2008, USDHHS, HRSA, HIV/AIDS Bureau.

U.S. Department of Health and Human Services: *Healthy People 2020: A Roadmap for Health.*

Washington, DC, 2010, U.S. Government Printing Office.

Valiant C, Jensen S: Ethical and legal issues: ten guidelines the professional case manager cannot afford to ignore. *CCMC Issue Brief* 3(4):2012. From: http://ccmcertification.org/sites/default/files/downloads/2012/41%20-%20Ethics%20issue%20brief.pdf. Retrieved January 2015.

Volkema RJ: *Problem-Purpose-Expansion: A Technique for Reformulating Problems* [unpublished manuscript]. Madison, WI, 1983, University of Wisconsin.

Weil M, Karls JM: Historical origins and recent developments. In Weils M, et al, editors: *Case management in Human Service Practice.* San Francisco, 1985, Jossey-Bass.

Wieland D, Kinosian B, Stallard E, et al: Does Medicaid pay more to a program of all-inclusive care for the elderly (PACE) than for fee-for-service long term care? *J Gerontol A Biol Sci Med Sci* 68:47–55, 2013.

Winston W, Albright S: *Practical Management Science*, ed 4. Mason, OH, 2012, South-Western.

Wright K, Hazelett S, Jarjoura D, et al: The AD-LIFE trial. *Home Healthc Nurse* 25:308–314, 2007.

Zander K, Etheredge ML, Bower KA: *Nursing Case Management: Blueprints for Transformation.* Waban, MA, 1987, Winslow Printing Systems.

# Public Health Nursing Practice and the Disaster Management Cycle

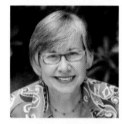

### Sharon A. R. Stanley, PhD, RN, FAAN

Dr. Sharon Stanley was Chief Nurse of the American Red Cross, 2009 – 2013. She has worked in public health for over 30 years and her leadership positions in disaster include National Director of Disaster Health and Mental Health, American Red Cross; Chief of Disaster Planning, Ohio Department of Health; and Director, Ohio Center for Public Health Preparedness, The Ohio State University. Colonel Stanley retired from the U.S. Army Reserve in 2007 with 34 years of service, 12 of them on active duty to include Desert Storm and Operation Iraqi Freedom. She is the recipient of numerous awards, including the Order of Medical Military Merit, the Surgeon General's "A" proficiency designator, the 2013 Florence Nightingale Medal of Honor, induction into the 2013 Ohio Veterans Hall of Fame, and the 2011 Association of State and Territorial Directors of Nursing (ASTDN) Recognition Award

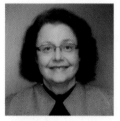

### Sharon L. Farra, PhD, RN

Dr. Sharon Farra has practiced nursing for over 30 years and is experienced in emergency and disaster preparedness, response, and recovery. She is an Assistant Professor at Wright State University, where she is leading evaluation efforts for a national disaster health certificate program. A Regional Nurse Leader with the American Red Cross, Dr. Farra serves on the Clinton County Red Cross Board and volunteers with the Medical Reserve Corps. As a nurse educator she has designed, developed, and launched disaster courses for health care providers, to include nurses and allied health professionals. Her research concentration is in disaster training, including innovative teaching methods integrating virtual reality simulation and interprofessional triage.

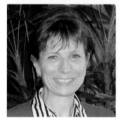

### Susan B. Hassmiller, PhD, RN, FAAN

Dr. Susan Hassmiller is the Senior Advisor for Nursing at the Robert Wood Johnson Foundation in Princeton, New Jersey, and Director of the Future of Nursing: Campaign for Action. The Foundation provides support to improve the health and health care for all Americans. Dr. Hassmiller has taught public health nursing at the university level and has dedicated her career to the care and prevention of disease in vulnerable populations. She is a former member of the National Board of Governors for the American Red Cross, having served as the Chair of Chapter and Disaster Services. She is Chair of the Central New Jersey Chapter of the American Red Cross. She is a 2002 recipient of both the national American Red Cross Ann Magnussen Award and the regional American Red Cross Clara Barton Award, both recognizing her outstanding leadership in the field of nursing and disaster services. She is the 2009 recipient of the Florence Nightingale Medal of Honor, the highest award in nursing presented by the International Committee of Red Cross in Geneva, Switzerland. She oversees the annual Susan Hassmiller American Red Cross Award, which provides recognition to a Red Cross chapter that has made outstanding contributions in providing disaster health services involving nurses as leaders.

## ADDITIONAL RESOURCES

Ⓔ **Evolve Website http://evolve.elsevier.com/Stanhope**
- *Healthy People 2020*
- Glossary
- Answers to Practice Application

## OBJECTIVES

*After reading this chapter, the student should be able to do the following:*

1. Discuss how disasters, both human-made and natural, affect people and their communities.
2. Differentiate disaster management cycle phases to include prevention (mitigation and protection), preparedness, response, and recovery.
3. Examine the nurse's role in the disaster management cycle.
4. Describe competencies for public health nursing practice in disasters.
5. Explain how the community works together to prevent, prepare for, respond to, and recover from disasters.
6. Identify organizations where nurses can volunteer to work in disasters.

The authors wish to acknowledge the manuscript review and consultation of a review committee, which included Linda MacIntyre, PhD, RN, Chief Nurse, American Red Cross; Barbara J. Polivka, PhD, RN, Shirley B. Powers Endowed Chair & Professor, School of Nursing, University of Louisville; and Janice Springer, DNP, RN, Public Health Nurse Consultant and Division Disaster Health Services Advisor, American Red Cross.

---

*"Wherever disaster calls there I shall go. I ask not for whom, but only where I am needed."*
**From Creed of the Red Cross Nurse, *by Lona L. Trott, RN, 1953***

Around the world, people are experiencing unprecedented disasters from natural causes, such as hurricanes and earthquakes to human-made disasters such as oil spills and terrorism.

Disasters, whether human-made or natural, are inevitable, but there are ways to help communities prepare for, respond to, and recover from disaster. This chapter describes the disaster management cycle phases of prevention, preparedness, response, and recovery as well as the public health nurse's role.

## DEFINING DISASTERS

A disaster is any natural or human-made incident that causes disruption, destruction, and/or devastation requiring external

assistance. Although natural incidents such as earthquakes or hurricanes trigger many disasters, predictable and preventable human-made factors can further affect the disaster. On March 11, 2011, northeastern Japan was rocked by a 9.0 magnitude earthquake that was quickly followed by a tsunami (see Figure 23-1). These dual natural disasters caused an estimated death toll of 20,000, but there was a third, human-made component to complete the incident triad: a nuclear reactor crisis. An independent parliamentary investigation later found the Fukushima nuclear disaster to be the result of a mix of several human-made factors (Inajima et al, 2012). Box 23-1 lists examples of natural and human-made disasters.

In the disaster response phase, the incident type and timing predict subsequent injuries and illnesses. If there is prior warning (e.g., in hurricanes or slow-rising floods), the impact brings fewer injuries and deaths. Disasters resulting with little or no advance notice such as earthquakes or bioterrorism could have more casualties because those affected have little time to make evacuation preparations or to obtain adequate

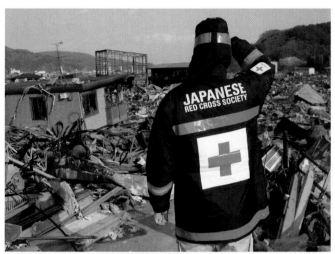

**FIG 23-1** A week after the earthquake struck and tsunami surged through northeast Japan, a Japanese Red Cross volunteer surveys the damage to Ōtsuchi in Iwate Prefecture. (Courtesy of the American Red Cross Disaster Online Newsroom, Washington, DC. From: http://newsroom.redcross.org. Retrieved January 2015.)

---

### BOX 23-1   Types of Disasters

| Natural | Human-Made |
|---|---|
| Hurricanes | Conventional warfare |
| Tornadoes | Unconventional warfare (e.g., |
| Hailstorms |    nuclear, chemical) |
| Cyclones | Transportation accidents |
| Blizzards | Structural collapse |
| Drought | Explosions/bombing |
| Floods | Fires |
| Mudslides | Hazardous materials incident |
| Avalanches | Pollution |
| Earthquakes | Civil unrest (e.g., riots) |
| Volcanic eruptions | Terrorism (chemical, biological, |
| Pandemics and epidemics |    radiological, nuclear, explosives) |
| Lightning-induced forest fires | Cyber attacks |
| Tsunamis | Airplane crash |
| Thunderstorms and lightning | Radiological incident |
| Extreme heat and cold | Nuclear power plant incident |
| | Critical infrastructure failure |
| | Water supply contamination |

From U.S. Department of Health and Human Services: *Healthy People 2020: A Roadmap to Improve all Americans Health.* Washington, DC, 2010, USDHHS.

---

treatment. Individuals can also be injured attempting to prepare for the disaster or while evacuating. Public health disasters can create needs across a widespread region. In a pandemic, pressing and competing health needs occur within a close time frame, producing a public health surge. In the disaster recovery phase, the immediate threat shifts to adjusting to a new normal in the affected community or region.

## DISASTER FACTS

Disasters can affect one family at a time, as in a house fire, or they can kill thousands and result in economic losses in the

millions, as with floods, earthquakes, tornadoes, hurricanes, tsunamis, and bioterrorism. The American Red Cross reports that it responds to a disaster in the United States every 8 minutes, resulting in response to more than 70,000 incidents each year (American Red Cross, 2014).

The number of reported natural and human-made disasters continues to rise worldwide, yet the number of lives lost has declined over the past couple of decades. The increase in the number of lives saved in a disaster may be explained by better forecasting and early warning systems (International Federation of Red Cross and Red Crescent Societies [IFRC], 2013).

Around the globe in 2012, the reported numbers of people (139 million) affected by disasters were the lowest of the decade after previous peaks in 2003, 2010, and 2011. Flooding, the largest number impacted in China, accounted for the majority of that influence, with droughts in Kenya, Sudan, and Ethiopia and elsewhere affecting 28 million people. Typhoon Bopha affected 6.3 million people in the Philippines and an earthquake in Guatemala affected 1.3 million people (IFRC, 2013).

In 2013 alone, there were more than 60 major disaster declarations in the United States with another 5 emergency declarations and more than 25 fire management assistance declarations (Federal Emergency Management Agency [FEMA], 2014a). An additional explanation on how a disaster declaration is made is presented later in this chapter, but the point is that disaster incidents are a regular occurrence. Hurricane names such as Katrina (2005) and Sandy (2012) and tornado pathways in Joplin, Missouri (2011) and Norman, Oklahoma (2013) are familiar to all. Yet, the latest report card for our nation's emergency care environment in disaster preparedness grades our overall system with a C− for 2014, dropping from a C+ in 2009 (American College of Emergency Physicians [ACEP], 2014). The report states that this is due, in large part, to state variation. For example, although the average number of health professionals registering in the volunteer system (the Emergency System for Advance Registration of Volunteer Health Professionals [ESAR-VHP]) is 279.6 nurses per 1 million people overall, that number is 0 per 1 million in Mississippi and 1069 per 1 million in the District of Columbia (ACEP, 2014).

Disaster disproportionably strikes at-risk individuals, whether their day-to-day risk is physical, emotional, or economic. Disasters in less developed communities can also destroy decades of progress in a matter of hours, in a manner that rarely happens in more developed countries. The poor, elderly, ethnic minorities, people with disabilities, and women and children in developing communities are excessively affected and least able to rebound (World Health Organization, 2011). Unfortunately, by 2050, the percentages of population areas more vulnerable to disasters will increase. Eighty percent of the world's population will live in developing countries, with 46% living in tornado and earthquake zones, near rivers, and on coastlines (United Nations Development Programme, 2012; Dilley et al, 2005).

The monetary cost of disaster recovery efforts also rose sharply. The cost in more developed countries is higher because of the extent of material possessions and complex infrastructures, including technology. In the United States, increases in

**TABLE 23-1   Total Amount of Disaster Estimated Damage by Continent, Level of Human Development,* and Year (2003-2012), in Millions of U.S. Dollars (2012 Prices)**

|  | 2003 | 2004 | 2005 | 2006 | 2007 | 2008 | 2009 | 2010 | 2011 | 2012 | Total |
|---|---|---|---|---|---|---|---|---|---|---|---|
| Africa | 6,908 | 2,041 | 40 | 261 | 726 | 977 | 185 | 62 | 1,038 | 929 | 13,167 |
| Americas | 26,653 | 80,081 | 202,343 | 8,128 | 17,520 | 68,679 | 15,873 | 81,821 | 69,222 | 103,582 | 673,902 |
| Asia | 29,558 | 80,603 | 32,496 | 26,776 | 38,268 | 126,230 | 18,926 | 40,149 | 280,093 | 28,004 | 701,102 |
| Europe | 22,917 | 2,216 | 18,481 | 2,767 | 24,403 | 4,971 | 12,954 | 18,949 | 2,998 | 24,201 | 134,856 |
| Oceania | 740 | 671 | 258 | 1,465 | 1,592 | 2,683 | 1,846 | 17,562 | 20,982 | 855 | 48,654 |
| *Very high human development* | *57,046* | *136,241* | *219,861* | *14,599* | *56,928* | *73,209* | *30,734* | *107,799* | *303,136* | *126,978* | *1,126,530* |
| *High human development* | *27,996* | *13,575* | *16,190* | *15,420* | *16,373* | *123,141* | *11,450* | *27,395* | *65,394* | *25,945* | *342,878* |
| *Medium human development* | *1,255* | *15,094* | *17,493* | *9,374* | *8,461* | *6,682* | *7,351* | *14,925* | *5,658* | *4,241* | *90,534* |
| *Low human development* | *479* | *704* | *73* | *4* | *747* | *509* | *249* | *8,423* | *145* | *406* | *11,739* |
| Total: | 86,776 | 165,613 | 253,617 | 39,396 | 82,509 | 203,540 | 49,784 | 158,542 | 374,333 | 157,570 | 1,571,681 |

From International Federation of Red Cross and Red Crescent Societies (IFRC): *World Disasters Report 2012: Focus on Technology and the Future of Humanitarian Action.* Geneva, Switzerland, 2013, IFRC, p. 233.
*Source:* EM-DAT, The International Disaster Data Base. Centre for Research on the Epidemiology of Diseases, CRED. At the University of Louvain, Belgium.
*See also UNDP. United Nations Development Programme. Human Development Reports. At www.hdr.undp.org for details and any later reports.
*Notes:* Some totals in Table 23-1 may not correspond, due to rounding.
Damage assessment is frequently unreliable. Even for existing data, methodologies are not standardized and the financial coverage can vary significantly. Depending on where the disaster occurred and who reported it, estimations may vary from zero to billions of U.S. dollars.
The total amount of damage reported in 2012 was the fifth lowest of the decade. In the Americas and in Europe, the amount of damages was the second highest of the decade and the fifth highest in Africa. In Asia and Oceania, however, the amount of reported damages was, respectively, the third and fourth lowest of the decade. The Americas accounted for almost 66% of damage and Europe for 15%, higher than their respective 43 and 9% average for the decade.
The contribution of very high human development countries to the total amount of damages climbed to 80%, an amount greater than their 72% average for the decade. Inversely, high human development countries accounted for only 16% of damage (decade average, 22%). The two costliest disasters in 2012 occurred in the United States. Hurricane Sandy cost U.S.$ 50 billion and a drought in the Southwest and Midwest regions cost U.S.$ 20 billion. Two earthquakes that hit Italy's Ferrara region cost more than U.S.$ 15 billion.

population and development in areas vulnerable to natural disasters, especially coastal areas, have led to sharply increased insurance payouts (see Table 23-1).

## NATIONAL DISASTER PLANNING AND RESPONSE: A HEALTH-FOCUSED OVERVIEW

There is a concerted national effort to provide guidance to state and local planning regions to assist with the coordinated and successful responses and recovery efforts in all-hazard disasters and catastrophes. Many documents have been written at the national level, some of which are reviewed in this chapter.

The reader may ask: "Isn't this all beyond what an individual nurse should have to know?"

As the single largest profession within the health care network, nurses must understand the national disaster management cycle. Without nursing integration at every phase, communities and clients lose a critical part of the prevention network, and the multidisciplinary response team loses a first-rate partner. Actually, it matters greatly how the nation dials 911, and it matters to individuals as well as communities,

regions, and the country as a whole. It also matters globally, beyond our own borders. Our national response is not just about the United States, but our international ability to assist other nations in their times of need.

The U.S. Department of Homeland Security (DHS) was created through the Homeland Security Act of 2002 (DHS, 2002), consolidating more than 20 separate agencies.

Presidential Policy Directive 8: National Preparedness (PPD-8) was signed and released by President Barack Obama on March 30, 2011. PPD-8 replaced Homeland Security Presidential Directive 8 from the Bush era, and guides how the nation, from the federal level to private citizens, can "prevent, protect against, mitigate the effects of, respond to, and recover from those threats that pose the greatest risk to the security of the Nation" (DHS, 2011). The National Preparedness Guidelines (NPG) (DHS, 2007a) and the National Response Plan (NRP), which provide a national doctrine for preparedness that includes the National Response Framework (NRF), was promulgated in January 2008. The second edition of the National Response Framework, updated in 2013, provides context for how the whole community works together and how response efforts relate to other parts of national preparedness (DHS, 2013). Each of the five frameworks covers one mission area: Prevention, Protection, Mitigation, Response, or Recovery. In that framework there are also 15 emergency support functions. **Emergency Support Function 8: Public Health and Medical** provides coordinated federal assistance to supplement state, local, and tribal resources in response to public health and medical care needs (FEMA, 2013a).

Homeland Security Presidential Directive 5 (HSPD-5) created the **National Incident Management System** (NIMS), a unified, all-discipline, and all-hazards approach to domestic incident management (Naval Postgraduate School [NPS], 2014; FEMA, 2013c). The NIMS was established to provide a common language and structure enabling all those involved in disaster response to communicate with each other more effectively and efficiently.

Two national preparedness documents specifically guide disaster health preparedness, response, and recovery: **Homeland Security Presidential Directive (HSPD) 21: Public Health and Medical Preparedness** and the **National Health Security Strategy** (NHSS). HSPD-21 established a national strategy that enables a level of public health and medical preparedness sufficient to address a range of possible disasters. It did so through four critical components of public health and medical preparedness: (1) biosurveillance, (2) countermeasure distribution, (3) mass casualty care, and (4) **community resilience** (NPS, 2014). The NHSS is updated every 4 years and focuses on the national goals for protecting people's health in the case of disaster in any setting. National health security is achieved when "the Nation and its people are prepared for, protected from, respond effectively to, and able to recover from incidents with potentially negative health consequences" (U.S. Department of Health and Human Services [USDHHS], 2013a, p. 2). The NHSS was directed by the 2006 Pandemic and All-Hazards Preparedness Act (PAHPA), an act to improve the nation's ability to detect, prepare for, and respond to a variety of public health emergencies. The PAHPA was re-enacted in 2013 and is now called the **Pandemic and All-Hazards Preparedness Reauthorization Act** (PAHPRA). The PAHPRA funds public health and hospital preparedness programs, medical countermeasures under the BioShield Project, and enhances the authority of the Food and Drug Administration (FDA) (USDHHS, March 2014).

In discussing community resiliency and impact of health care reform on public health preparedness, Vinter and colleagues (2010) state: "Comprehensive health reform presents a rare opportunity to further strengthen our nation. However, even with health reform, there are still major gaps in our public health preparedness. Addressing these underlying weaknesses in our health system will not be easy or cheap, but failure to address these concerns could prove extremely costly" (p. 340).

Our national system of homeland security includes public health preparedness and response as a core part of its national strategies. Some of the strategy documents introduced in this section are covered in greater detail throughout the chapter. Every aspect of disaster management involves the practice of public health nursing.

## *HEALTHY PEOPLE 2020* OBJECTIVES

Because disaster affects the health of people in many ways, disaster incidents have an effect on almost every *Healthy People 2020* objective. For example, although Access to Health Services and Public Health Infrastructure comprise two important *Healthy People 2020* topic areas with subsequent objectives, they become even more significant when individual and community needs escalate in disaster (USDHHS, 2010). Disasters also play a direct role in the objectives related to environmental health, food safety, immunization and infectious disease, and mental health and mental disorders. Public health professionals, such as those who work at the Centers for Disease Control and Prevention (CDC), study the effect that disasters have on population health and continuously develop new prevention strategies. Other organizations, such as the American Psychological Association and the American Red Cross, work with communities in the preparedness, response, and recovery phases of a disaster and to revise and align the *Healthy People 2020* objectives related to mental health.

---

 **HEALTHY PEOPLE 2020**

### *Objectives Related to Preparedness*

- **PREP-1:** Reduce the time necessary to issue official information to the public about a public health emergency.
- **PREP-2:** Reduce the time necessary to activate designated personnel in response to a public health emergency.
- **PREP-3:** Increase the proportion of Laboratory Response Network (LRN) laboratories that meet proficiency standards.
  - **PREP-3.1:** Increase the proportion of LRN biological laboratories that meet proficiency standards for Category A and B threat agents (http://www.bt.cdc.gov/agent/agentlist-category.asp).
  - **PREP-3.2:** Increase the proportion of LRN chemical laboratories that meet proficiency standards for chemical threat agents.
- **PREP-4:** Reduce the time for state public health agencies to establish after-action reports and improvement plans following responses to public health emergencies and exercises.

From U.S. Department of Health and Human Services (USDHHS): *Healthy People 2020*. Washington, DC, 2014 (updated 2015), USDHHS. Retrieved January 2015 from http://www.healthypeople .gov/2020/topicsobjectives2020/objectiveslist.aspx?topicId=34

---

## THE DISASTER MANAGEMENT CYCLE AND NURSING ROLE

Disaster management includes four stages: prevention (including mitigation and protection), preparedness, response, and recovery. Figure 23-2 shows the disaster emergency management cycle. Nurses have unique skills for all aspects of disaster including assessment, priority setting, collaboration, and addressing both preventive and acute care needs. In addition, public health nurses have a skill set that serves their community well in disaster, including health education and disease screening, mass clinic expertise, an ability to provide essential public health services, community resource referral and liaison work, population advocacy, **psychological first aid**, **public health**

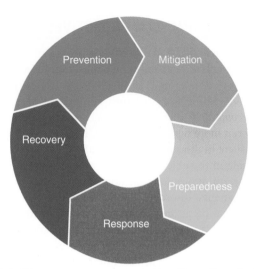

**FIG 23-2** Disaster management cycle. (From Ontario Agency for Health Protection and Promotion (Public Health Ontario). Public health emergency preparedness: an IMS-based workshop. Base scenario. Toronto, ON: Queen's Printer for Ontario; 2015 July. (p. 7))

**triage**, and **rapid needs assessment**. Nurses have served worldwide in disaster care for more than a century. They continue to provide a significant resource to both the employee and the volunteer disaster management workforce, and their numbers are unmatched by any other profession. In addition, nurses work closely with the **interprofessional** health team, community leaders, and organizations, engaging with and advocating for clients as needed across the disaster management cycle.

The World Association for Disaster and Emergency Medicine (WADEM) includes a nursing section. The Nursing Section of WADEM represents nurses from all countries to strengthen and improve the practice and knowledge of disaster nursing. The Nursing Section purposes are as follows (WADEM, 2013):

- Define nursing issues for public health care and disaster health care.
- Exchange scientific and professional information relevant to the practice of disaster nursing.
- Encourage collaborative efforts enhancing and expanding the field of nursing disaster research.
- Encourage collaboration with other nursing organizations.
- Inform and advise WADEM of matters related to disaster nursing.

The International Council of Nurses (ICN) also hosts a disaster-focused response network and published a framework of disaster nursing competencies in 2009 (ICN, 2013).

## Prevention (Mitigation and Protection)

All-hazards mitigation (prevention, protection) is an emergency management term for reducing risks to people and property from natural hazards before they occur. The ability to provide primary prevention through national missions of prevention, mitigation, or protection can include structural measures, such as protecting buildings and infrastructure from the forces of wind and water, and nonstructural measures, such as land development restrictions. These primary prevention

measures implemented at the local government level achieve effectiveness, in an all-hazards approach to threats. Of course, prevention also includes human-made hazards and the ability to deter potential terrorists, detect terrorists before they strike, and take decisive action to eliminate the threat (DHS, 2007b). Prevention activities for terrorism may include heightened inspections; improved surveillance and security operations; public health and agricultural surveillance; and testing, immunizations, isolation, or neutralizing **CBRNE threats (chemical, biological, radiological, nuclear, and explosive)**.

The nurse may be involved in many roles in the primary prevention of disaster. As community advocates, nurses promote environmental health by identifying environmental hazards and serving on the public health team for mitigation purposes. Public health nurses in particular are involved with organizing and participating in mass prophylaxis and vaccination campaigns to prevent, treat, or contain a disease. The nurse should be familiar with the region's local cache of pharmaceuticals and how the **Strategic National Stockpile** (SNS) (described later in this chapter) will be distributed. Once federal and local authorities agree that the SNS is needed, medicine delivery to any state in the United States occurs within 12 hours (CDC, 2012c). State and local emergency planners then ensure **points of dispensing** (POD), to provide prophylaxis to the entire population within 48 hours.

In terms of human-made disaster prevention, the nurse should be aware of high-risk targets and current vulnerabilities and what can be done to eliminate or mitigate the vulnerability. Targets may include military and civilian government facilities, health care facilities, international airports and other transportation systems, large cities, and high-profile landmarks. Terrorists might also target large public gatherings, water and food supplies, banking and finance, information technology, postal and shipping services, utilities, and corporate centers.

## Preparedness
### Role of the Public Health Nurse in Personal and Professional Preparedness

Public health nurses play a key role in community preparedness, but they must accomplish the critical elements of personal and professional preparedness first.

*Personal Preparedness.* Disasters by their nature require nurses to respond quickly. Public health nurses without plans in place to address their own needs, to include family and pets, will be unable to fully participate in their disaster obligations at work or in volunteer efforts (Figure 23-3). In addition, the nurse assisting in disaster relief efforts must be as healthy as possible, both physically and mentally. Disaster workers who do not practice self-health are of little service to their family, clients, and community (see the How To box entitled *Be Red Cross Ready*). Disaster kits should be made for the home, workplace, and car. There are emergency supplies specific to nursing that should be prepared and stored in a sturdy, easy-to-carry container (see the accompanying How To box). Important documents should always be in waterproof containers. Nurses should consider several contingencies for children and older adults with a plan to seek help from neighbors in the event of being

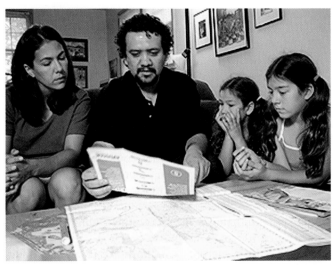

**FIG 23-3** Personal preparedness. Public health nurses need to develop their own disaster plan as a part of their community disaster activities. (Courtesy of the Wichita Falls Health District [Wichita Falls, TX]. From: http://tx-wichitafalls2.civicplus.com/index.aspx?NID=1301. Retrieved January 2015.)

called to a disaster. Many public shelters do not allow pets inside and other arrangements must be made. At present, local emergency management agencies include pet management in the local disaster plans and so should the pet owner (FEMA, 2014c).

One way a nurse can feel assured about family member protection is by working with them to develop the skills and knowledge necessary for coping in disaster. For example, long-term benefits occur by involving children and adolescents in activities such as writing preparedness plans, exercising the plan, preparing disaster kits, becoming familiar with their school emergency procedures and family reunification sites, and learning about the range of potential hazards in their vicinity to include evacuation routes. This strategy also offers children and adolescents an opportunity to express their feelings.

*Professional Preparedness.* Every state needs a qualified workforce of public health nurses for solutions for today's public health problems that include natural disasters and the threat of terrorism. Public health nurses, in turn, need "dedicated, resourceful, and visionary leaders" (ASTDN, 2008, p. 4). Chief public health nurse officers at the state level develop and maintain a strong public health nursing workforce and practice, especially when those nurses are scattered throughout state and local systems.

Disaster management in the community is about population health: The core public health functions of *assessment, policy development*, and *assurance* hold as true in disaster as in day-to-day operations. Operating in the chaos of disaster surge, however, demands a flexible and proficient practice base in each of public health's 3 core functions and 10 essential services (see http://www.cdc.gov/nphpsp/essentialservices.html).

Just as the mission of public health and its core functions and essential services do not change in disaster, neither does the practice of public health nursing. The public health nurse must be prepared to advocate for the community in terms of a

## HOW TO   Be Red Cross Ready

**1. Get a Kit**

*Consider the following when assembling or restocking your kit to ensure that you and your family are prepared for any disaster:*
- *Store at least 3 days of food, water, and supplies in your family's easy-to-carry preparedness kit. Keep extra supplies on hand at home in case you cannot leave the affected area.*
- *Keep your kit where it is easily accessible.*
- *Remember to check your kit every 6 months and replace expired or outdated items.*

**2. Make a Plan**

*When preparing for a disaster, always:*
- *Talk with your family.*
- *Plan.*
- *Learn how and when to turn off utilities and how to use life-saving tools such as fire extinguishers.*
- *Tell everyone where emergency information and supplies are stored. Provide copies of the family's preparedness plan to each member of the family. Always ensure that information is up to date and practice evacuations, following the routes outlined in your plan. Don't forget to identify alternative routes.*
- *Include pets in your evacuation plans.*

**3. Get Informed**

*There are three key parts to becoming informed:*
- *Get Info: Learn the ways you would get information during a disaster or an emergency.*
- *Know Your Region: Learn about the disasters that may occur in your area.*
- *Action Steps: Learn first aid from your local Red Cross chapter.*

**Emergency Supplies That Nurses Should Have Ready**
- *Identification badge and driver's license*
- *Proof of licensure and certification (e.g., RN, CPR/AED, First Aid)*
- *Pocket-size reference books (e.g., nursing protocols and intervention standards)*
- *Blood pressure cuff (adult and child) and stethoscope*
- *Gloves, mask, other personal protective equipment (PPE) for general care*
- *First aid kit with mouth-to-mouth cardiopulmonary resuscitation (CPR) barrier*
- *Radio with batteries and cell phone charger*
- *Cash, credit card*
- *Important papers and contact information in hard copy*
- *Sun protection*
- *Sturdy shoes with socks*
- *Medical identification of allergies, blood type*
- *Medications for self*
- *Weather-appropriate clothing to include rain gear*
- *Toiletries*
- *Watch, cell phone, PDA with pre-entered emergency numbers*
- *Flashlight, extra batteries*
- *Record-keeping materials, including pencil/pen*
- *Map of area*

*(Courtesy of the American Red Cross. Retrieved January 2015 from http://www.redcross.org/flash/brr/english-html/default.asp)*

focus on population-based practice. The number of public health nurses available to get the job done is small when compared with those with generic or other specialty nurse preparation. Also, disaster produces conditions that demand an aggregate-care approach, increasing the need for public health nursing involvement in community service during disaster and catastrophe.

The Public Health Nursing Intervention Wheel (Chapter 9) is a population-based practice model that encompasses 3 levels of practice (community, systems, and individual/family) and 16 public health interventions. Each intervention and practice level contributes to improving population health, providing a practice foundation. This Wheel holds true to public health nursing interventions whether the nurse is working in day-to-day or in disaster operations.

Interprofessional disaster care teams need nurses with disaster and emergency management training and experience. Although the majority of disaster work is not high tech, the knowledge one needs for CBRNE disasters must be developed to include access to a ready cache of information related to nursing care. The following sites provide useful information:

- CDC: *Emergency Preparedness and Response: A to Z Index* (http://www.bt.cdc.gov/agent)
- National Library of Medicine: *Disaster Information Management Research Center* (http://disaster.nlm.nih.gov/)
- Unbound Medicine: *Relief Central* (http://relief .unboundmedicine.com/relief/ub/)
- National Library of Medicine: *WISER—Wireless Information System for Emergency Responders* (http://wiser.nlm.nih.gov/) (see Box 23-2 for further information)

Depending on the job and possible volunteer assignments, it is expected that nurses know how to use **personal protective equipment** (PPE), operate specialized equipment needed to perform specific activities, and safely perform duties in disaster environments.

Professional preparedness also requires that nurses become aware of and understand emergency and disaster plans at their workplace and in their community. Nurses should review the disaster history of the community, understanding how past disasters have affected the community's health care delivery system. It is important for nurses to understand and gain the competencies needed to respond in times of disasters *before* disaster strikes.

Box 23-3 displays core disaster competencies for those working in public health. Disaster competencies for public health nursing practice have been proposed in a set of 25 competencies categorized into preparedness, response, and recovery (Polivka et al, 2008). The preparedness competencies focus on personal preparedness and on comprehending disaster preparedness terms, concepts, and roles. The competencies also define the role of the public health nurse in a surge event. Response phase competencies include the ability to provide a rapid needs assessment, outbreak investigation and surveillance, public health triage, risk communication, and technical skills such as mass dispensing. Recovery competencies include after-action participation, disaster plan modifications, and

---

### BOX 23-2   Nurses and Technology

#### *Hazardous Material Information Delivered via Wireless*

WISER (Wireless Information System for Emergency Responders) is a system designed to assist emergency responders in hazardous material incidents. Developed by the National Library of Medicine, WISER provides a wide range of information on hazardous substances, including substance identification support, physical characteristics, human health information, and containment and suppression guidance. By inputting a substance's physical properties and entering an individual's symptoms, WISER can help narrow the range of substances that may be involved. It provides detailed information about hazardous substances, health effects, treatment, personal protective equipment, toxicity, the emergency resources available, and the surrounding environmental conditions. In January 2014, WebWISER version 4.5 was released. This new release integrates Chemical Hazards Emergency Medical Management (CHEMM) content and updates the Emergency Response Guidebook (ERG) content to 2012. It also now includes hospital provider and preparedness profiles. WISER is available as a standalone application on Microsoft Windows PCs, Apple's iOS devices (iPhone, iPad, and iPod touch), Google Android devices, BlackBerry devices (Internet connectivity required), Windows Mobile devices, and Palm OS PDAs.

From National Library of Medicine: *About WISER.* Bethesda, MD, 2014, National Library of Medicine. From: http://wiser.nlm.nih.gov/about.html. Retrieved January 2015.

---

### BOX 23-3   Core Competencies for Disaster Medicine and Public Health

**1.0:** Demonstrate personal and family preparedness for disasters and public health emergencies.

**2.0:** Demonstrate knowledge of one's expected role(s) in organizational and community response plans activated during a disaster or public health emergency.

**3.0:** Demonstrate situational awareness of actual/potential health hazards before, during, and after a disaster or public health emergency.

**4.0:** Communicate effectively with others in a disaster or public health emergency.

**5.0:** Demonstrate knowledge of personal safety measures that can be implemented in a disaster or public health emergency.

**6.0:** Demonstrate knowledge of surge capacity assets, consistent with one's role in organizational, agency, and/or community response plans.

**7.0:** Demonstrate knowledge of principles and practices for the clinical management of all ages and populations affected by disasters and public health emergencies, in accordance with professional scope of practice.

**8.0:** Demonstrate knowledge of public health principles and practices for the management of all ages and populations affected by disasters and public health emergencies.

**9.0:** Demonstrate knowledge of ethical principles to protect the health and safety of all ages, populations, and communities affected by a disaster or public health emergency.

**10.0:** Demonstrate knowledge of legal principles to protect the health and safety of all ages, populations, and communities affected by a disaster or public health emergency.

**11.0:** Demonstrate knowledge of short- and long-term considerations for recovery of all ages, populations, and communities affected by a disaster or public health emergency.

From National Center for Disaster Medicine and Public Health (NCDMPH): *Resources for Core Competencies in Disaster Health.* Bethesda, MD, 2014, NCDMPH. From: http://ncdmph.usuhs.edu/KnowledgeLearning/2013-CompetenciesResources.htm. Retrieved January 2015.

---

**BOX 23-4** **Websites Providing Education and Training Opportunities**

**Public Health Workforce Development Centers**
- Centers for Disease Control and Prevention: http://www.bt.cdc.gov/training/
- Heartland Centers for Public Health and Community Capacity Development: http://www.heartlandcenters.slu.edu/
- National Public Health Training Centers Network, HRSA: http://bhpr.hrsa.gov/grants/publichealth/trainingcenters/index.html
- Northwest Center for Public Health Practice: http://www.nwcphp.org/training

**Government and Other Nurse-Specific Courses**
- American Red Cross Disaster Health and Sheltering Course for Nursing Students: http://www.drc-group.com/library/exercise/osc/OSC-DHS-FactSheet.pdf
- Emergency Management Institute: http://training.fema.gov/
- Federal Emergency Management Agency (FEMA) Training: http://www.fema.gov/prepared/train.shtm
- National Nurse Emergency Preparedness Initiative: http://www.nnepi.org/

**Public Health Organizations**
- American Public Health Association (APHA): http://www.apha.org
- Association of Public Health Nurses (APHN): http://www.phnurse.org/
- Association of Schools of Public Health (ASPH): http://www.asph.org
- National Association of County and City Health Offices (NACCHO): http://www.naccho.org
- Public Health Foundation (PHF): http://www.phf.org

**BOX 23-5** **Volunteer Opportunities in Disaster Work**

- American Red Cross (ARC): http://www.redcross.org
- Buddhist Compassion Relief (Tzu Chi): http://www.tzuchi.org/
- Certified Emergency Response Team (CERT): https://www.citizencorps.gov/cert/
- Citizen Corps: http://www.citizencorps.gov/
- Disaster Medical Assistance Team (DMAT): http://www.phe.gov/Preparedness/responders/ndms/teams/Pages/dmat.aspx
- Medical Reserve Corps (MRC): http://www.medicalreservecorps.gov/HomePage
- National Voluntary Organizations Active in Disaster (NVOAD): http://www.nvoad.org
- One Nurse at a Time: http://onenurseatatime.org/volunteer/
- The Salvation Army: http://www.salvationarmyusa.org/usn/www_usn_2.nsf

**BOX 23-6** **Trust for America's Health (TFAH): Bioterrorism and Public Health Preparedness**

Health emergencies pose some of the greatest threats to our nation, because they can be difficult to prepare for, detect, and contain. Important progress has been made to improve emergency preparedness since September 11, 2001. However, while there has been significant progress toward improving public health preparedness over the past 10 years, particularly in core capabilities, there continue to be persistent gaps in the country's ability to respond to health emergencies, ranging from bioterrorist threats to serious disease outbreaks to extreme weather events.

In the 10th annual *Ready or Not? Protecting the Public from Diseases, Disasters, and Bioterrorism* report, 35 states and Washington, DC, scored a 6 or lower on 10 key indicators of public health preparedness.

Along with its annual report on public health preparedness, TFAH also offers a series of recommendations to further strengthen America's emergency preparedness.

*What do you think about the recommendations through a public health nursing lens?*

From Trust for America's Health: *TFAH Initiatives—Bioterrorism and Public Health Preparedness.* 2012. From: http://healthyamericans.org/report/101/. Retrieved January 2015.

---

coordinating efforts to address the psychosocial and public health impact. See Box 23-4 for education and training opportunities.

Nurses who seek increased participation or who seek a better understanding of disaster management can become involved in any number of community organizations. The **National Disaster Medical System** (NDMS) provides nurses the opportunity to work on specialized teams such as the **Disaster Medical Assistance Team** (DMAT). The **Medical Reserve Corps** (MRC) and the **Community Emergency Response Team** (CERT) provide opportunities for nurses to support emergency preparedness and response in their local jurisdictions. The American Red Cross offers training in disaster health services and disaster mental health for both local response and national deployment opportunities. In the Red Cross, nurses and nursing students can join a local disaster action team (DAT); act as a liaison with local hospitals; plan health services support for shelter sites; participate on an interprofessional team for optimal service delivery; address the logistics of health and medical supplies; and teach disaster nursing in the community. A list of opportunities is shown in Box 23-5.

The importance of being adequately trained and properly associated with an official response organization to serve in a disaster cannot be overstated. In a disaster, many untrained and ill-equipped individuals rush in to help. Spontaneous volunteer overload, leading to role conflict, anger, frustration, and helplessness, adds to the burden in an already tense situation. The World Trade Center attacks of September 11, 2001, brought many qualified but unassociated responders to the site. "Many well-intentioned local physicians in shirt sleeves and light footwear proceeded to the area and attempted to find victims, risking further injuries to themselves and getting in the way of structured rescue protocols. ... [They were] prohibited from participating in rescue operations within any area designated as a disaster by the Fire Department of New York" (Crippen, 2002). After the bombing of the Alfred P. Murrah building in Oklahoma City in 1995, a nurse who rushed into the building to rescue people became the only fatality who was not killed or injured in the initial blast and collapse (Oklahoma City National Memorial & Museum, 2010). See Box 23-6 for more on the importance of national preparedness.

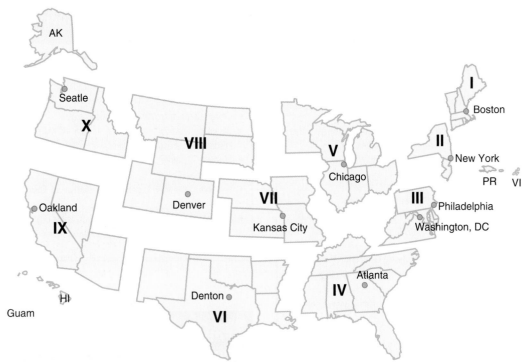

FIG 23-4 The 10 FEMA regions. (Courtesy of the Federal Emergency Management Agency [FEMA]: *Regional Operations.* Washington, DC, 2014, FEMA. From: http://www.fema.gov/regional-operations. Retrieved January 2015.)

## Community Preparedness

Presidential Policy Directive (PPD)-8 emphasizes that true preparedness is a *whole* community event. PPD-8 urges the strengthening of our nation's security and resilience through an integrated set of guidance, programs, and processes to implement the national preparedness goal, described earlier in this chapter (DHS, 2011).

This planning and implementation require a coordinated response that involves many stakeholders, including first and foremost the general public. Community preparedness also involves all levels of government, public health agencies, hospitals, first responders, emergency management, health care providers within the community, schools and universities, the private sector, and business and nongovernmental organizations (NGOs) such as the Red Cross. Mutual aid agreements and prior planning help to bridge perceived and actual barriers; establish relationships before the incident at the local, regional, state, and national levels; and ensure seamless service. Sometimes barriers involve regulatory authority and jurisdictional boundaries; sometimes the barriers involve organizational control versus the common good.

Emergency management is responsible for developing and coordinating emergency response plans within their defined area, whether local, state, federal, or tribal. The Federal Emergency Management Agency (FEMA) coordinates comprehensive, all-hazard planning at the national level, assuring a menu of exercises and plan templates to address plausible incidents in any given community. Emergency management personnel at the state and local levels work closely with their communities

and response partners, providing opportunities to train, exercise, evaluate, and update disaster plans. Stronger predisaster partnerships, which include all stakeholders, produce a more coordinated response. Figure 23-4 shows FEMA regions across the nation.

Disaster planning involves simplicity and realism with back-up contingencies because (1) the disaster will never be an "exact fit" for the plan, and (2) all plans must be implementation ready, no matter who is present to start them (DHS, 2007a). The following Quality and Safety Education for Nurses box describes safety guidelines for the nurse's family.

Finally, the community must have an adequate warning system and an evacuation plan that includes measures to remove those individuals who hesitate to leave areas of danger. Some people refuse to leave their homes over fear that their possessions will be lost, destroyed, or looted. They also do not want to leave pets behind. Also, some people mistakenly believe that experience with a particular type of disaster is enough preparation for the next one. This faulty belief was demonstrated in New York City during Hurricane Sandy in October 2012, fueled by a false sense of security after Hurricane Irene in August 2011. Sandy killed at least 125 people, including 60 in New York—48 of them in New York City (Huffington Post, 2012). The nurse's visibility in the community can help develop the trust and credibility needed to help in contingency planning for evacuation. In December 2014 nurses were rated the highest on honesty and ethics in a ranking of professions. Their ranking of 80% was compared to medical doctors at 65% and clergy at 4 percent (www.gallup.com/poll/1654/Honesty-Ethics-Professions.aspx).

## (QSEN) FOCUS ON QUALITY AND SAFETY EDUCATION FOR NURSES

**Targeted Competency: Safety:**
Minimize risk of harm to clients and providers through both system effectiveness and individual performance. Selected knowledge, skills, and attitudes are cited below in order to develop a disaster safety plan:

**Knowledge**
Examine human factors and other basic safety design principles as well as commonly used unsafe practices (such as workarounds and dangerous abbreviations). Specific steps might be:
1. Learn how you can get information during the disaster or emergency.
   a. Determine what types of disasters are most likely to happen.
   b. Learn about warning signals in your community.
   c. Ask about postdisaster pet care (shelters usually will not accept pets).
   d. Review the disaster plans at your workplace, school, and other places where your family spends time.
   e. Determine how to help older adult or disabled family members or neighbors.
   f. WHAT should you do?

**Skills**
Demonstrate effective use of strategies to reduce risk of harm to self or others.
1. Create a disaster plan:
   a. Talk with your family and create two places to meet, including outside your home and outside your neighborhood. Give each member of the family a copy of the plan.
   b. Discuss the types of disasters that are most likely to happen, and review what to do in each case and make a plan.
   c. Choose an out-of-state friend to be your family contact; this person will verify the location of each family member. After a disaster, it may be easier to call long distance than to make local calls.
   d. Review evacuation plans, including care of pets. Have alternative routes for evacuation.
2. Complete this checklist:
   a. Post emergency phone numbers next to telephones.
   b. Teach everyone how and when to call 911.

c. Determine when and how to turn off water, gas, and electricity at the main switches.
   d. Check adequacy of insurance coverage for yourself and your home.
   e. Locate and review the use of fire extinguishers.
   f. Install and maintain smoke detectors.
   g. Conduct a home hazard hunt and fix potential hazards.
   h. Stock emergency supplies and assemble a disaster supplies kit.
   i. Acquire first aid and cardiopulmonary resuscitation (CPR) certification.
   j. Locate all escape routes from your home. Find two ways out of each room.
   k. Find safe spots in your home for each type of disaster.
3. Practice and maintain your plan:
   a. Review the plan every 6 months.
   b. Conduct fire and emergency evacuation drills.
   c. Replace stored water every 3 months and stored food every 6 months.
   d. Test and recharge fire extinguishers according to manufacturer's instructions.
   e. Test your smoke detectors monthly and change the batteries at least once a year.
   f. WHAT more should you do?

**Attitudes**
Appreciate the cognitive and physical limits of human performance.
1. Monitor your personal reactions to the disaster and seek assistance if the stress of the losses and the potential work to re-establish a new normal seem overwhelming. Monitor also the reactions of your colleagues and the clients you serve and provide or refer to others anyone who needs stress management intervention.

**Safety Question**
To prepare more effectively for the event of a future disaster, list the steps that you would take to ensure the safety of your family, including any pets you may have.

---

Nurses should be involved in identifying and educating communities about what effect the disaster might have on them, including helping at-risk populations to address preparedness planning. In addition to identifying high-risk individuals in neighborhoods, locations of congregate concern include schools, college campuses, residential centers, prisons, hospitals, and high-rise buildings. During Hurricane Sandy even the health care facilities did not have consistency in evacuation decisions and risk assessment (Powell et al, 2012). Nurses can greatly assist in community preparedness given their knowledge of the community's diversity such as non–English-speaking groups, the immunocompromised, children, older adults with functional and access needs, and the physically and mentally challenged.

### The National Health Security Strategy and Community Resilience

The NHSS, mentioned earlier in this chapter, as part of the nation's national planning has been instrumental in bringing the concept of community resilience into all preparedness operations. The NHSS is designed to achieve two goals: (1) build community resilience and (2) strengthen and sustain health and emergency response systems (U.S. Department of Health and Human Services (USDHHS), 2013a). Some maintain, though, that the concept of community resilience is not fully defined at our national level and accountability measures to examine resilience pre- and postdisaster are lacking (Uscher-Pines et al, 2013). Community resilience is a policy issue in all levels of planning (federal, state, and local) because limited resources postdisaster demand whole community resilience in order to move back into normalcy. Healthier communities, by default, will have better bounce-back ability.

Community resilience is defined as the sustained ability of a community to withstand and recover from adversity (Chandra et al, 2011). Healthy individuals, families, and communities with access to health care and protective, preventive knowledge that can be used to launch timely action become some of our nation's strongest assets in disaster incidents. A recent Rand publication dedicated to advancing operational implementation of community resilience developed a list of resilience indicators after carefully researching the existing literature and national disaster policy documents and conducting focus groups with communities recently affected by disasters (Chandra et al, 2011):

- Engagement at the community level, including a sense of cohesiveness and neighborhood involvement or integration
- Partnership among organizations, including integrated pre-event planning, exercises, and agreements
- Sustained local leadership supported by partnership with state and federal government
- Effective and culturally relevant education about risks
- Optimal community health and access to quality health services
- Integration of preparedness and wellness
- Rapid restoration of services and social networks
- Individual-level preparedness and self-sufficiency
- Targeted strategies that empower and engage vulnerable populations
- Financial resiliency of families and businesses, and efficient leveraging of resources for recovery

## Disaster and Mass Casualty Exercises

Although practice will not ensure a perfect response to disaster, disaster and mass casualty drills and exercises are extremely valuable components of preparedness. After the exercise, the lessons learned through after-action reports are used to update disaster plans and subsequent operations. Exercise categories include discussion-based simulations or "tabletops" and operations-based events such as drills, functional, and full-scale exercises (FEMA, 2013b). The latter operation types involve escalating scope and scale testing of the disaster preparedness and response network, using a specific plan. In addition, implementation of virtual reality (VR)-based training for disaster preparedness and response, conducted either independently or combined with other training formats, is growing within the exercise community. For example, a virtual reality preparedness research project led through the University of Minnesota Preparedness Emergency Response Research Center focuses on an immersive simulation workshop that is designed especially for health science students in public health, medicine, nursing, pharmacy, veterinary medicine, and dentistry at the university. The researchers propose that engaging interprofessional health students in realistic simulated disaster response scenarios will improve system performance and quality disaster response through the acquisition of knowledge and team-based skills (University of Minnesota School of Public Health, 2014).

National Level Exercise 2009 (NLE09) was the first major exercise conducted by the U.S. government that focused exclusively on terrorism prevention and protection, as opposed to incident response and recovery. NLE09 was designated a Tier I National Level Exercise. These exercises started out as the Top Officials exercise series [TOPOFF]) but now incorporate the whole community, with an understanding that the practice must reach all levels of the public, private, and government sectors to be effective.

The National Exercise Program (NEP) serves to test and validate core capabilities. Participation in exercises, simulations or other activities, including real world incidents, helps organizations validate their capabilities and identify shortfalls, pulling in their partners and stakeholders including citizen participation (FEMA, 2014b). An annual Capstone Exercise, formerly titled the National Level Exercise (NLE), is conducted every 2 years as the final component of each NEP progressive exercise cycle. The Capstone Exercise for 2014 examined the nation's collective ability to coordinate and conduct risk assessments and implement National Frameworks and associated plans to deliver core capabilities (FEMA, 2014b).

Most exercises conducted in hospitals, communities, colleges, counties, or regions are much smaller in scope and scale than the Capstone Exercises. The Homeland Security Exercise and Evaluation Program (HSEEP) was developed to help states and local jurisdictions improve overall preparedness with all natural and human-made disasters. It provides a standardized methodology and terminology for exercise design, development, conduct, evaluation, and improvement planning and assists communities to create exercises that will make a positive difference before a real incident (FEMA, 2013b). HSEEP is the national standard for all exercise development and implementation.

Whether conducted as drills, tabletops, functional, or full-scale scenarios, and whether the scope is local or national in nature, nurses and other health care providers must be included as a part of the exercise's planning, response, and after-action activities. Nurses, as client and community advocates, are essential players in the exercise and preparedness arena.

---

**❚ HOW TO    Conduct a Disaster Exercise**

**Formidable Footprint: A National Community/Neighborhood Exercise Series**

*A team of national, regional, state, and local agencies and organizations has undertaken an effort to develop, conduct, and evaluate a recurring series of disaster exercises entitled "Formidable Footprint."*

*This series of exercises serves as an opportunity for community and faith-based organizations along with governmental agencies to assess their capability to prepare for, respond to, and recover from a variety of natural disasters that affect communities and neighborhoods across the United States. There is no charge to participate in one or several of the neighborhood exercises, provided by the Disaster Resistant Communities (DRC) Group.*

*In addition, DRC provides the Disaster Health and Sheltering Course through nursing faculty and to their nursing students through the American Red Cross National Student Nurse Program.*

Wherever and whenever you get to practice nursing in disaster response and recovery, you become a better-prepared health team member.

---

*From Disaster Resistant Communities Group:* Formidable Footprint—A National Community/Neighborhood Exercise Series, *2014. Retrieved January 2015 from http://www.drc-group.com/project/footprint.html.*

## Response

The first level of disaster response occurs at the local level with the mobilization of a team of responders such as the fire department, law enforcement, public health, and emergency services. If the disaster exceeds local resources, the county or city emergency management agency (EMA) will coordinate activities through an Emergency Operations Center (EOC). The EOC provides central functions at a strategic level to oversee the emergency situation. In general, local responders within a county sign a regional or statewide mutual aid agreement to allow the sharing of needed personnel, equipment, services, and supplies.

The initial scope of disaster assessment is usually measured in dollars, health risk, injury, and/or lives lost. The more destruction and lives at risk, the greater the degree of attention and resources provided at the local, regional, and state levels. When state resources and capabilities are overwhelmed, governors may, through provisions provided in the Robert T. Stafford Disaster Relief and Emergency Assistance Act (FEMA, 2013e), request federal assistance under a presidential disaster or emergency declaration. If the event is considered an incident of national significance (a potential or high-impact disaster), appropriate response personnel and resources are provided.

In a mass casualty incident, the goal is to maximize the number of lives saved and to do the greatest good for the greatest number of individuals. These circumstances could lead to changes in the usual standards of health and medical care in the affected locality or region. Rather than doing everything possible to save every life, crisis standards of care enable the health care operations necessary to allocate scarce resources in a different manner to save as many lives as possible (Institute of Medicine [IOM], 2012). Crisis standards need to be explored and discussed with all community stakeholders in the preparedness phase. Community engagement is key to this process.

### National Response Framework

As previously discussed, the NRF was written to provide an approach to domestic incidents in a unified, well-coordinated manner, enabling all responding entities the ability to work together more effectively and efficiently. The online component of the NRF Resource Center (http://www.fema.gov/national-response-framework) contains supplemental materials including annexes, partner guides, and other supporting documents and learning resources. The framework involves the entire community and is scalable, flexible, and adaptable to the given situation. It is a living document that is revised every 18 months in response to evolving conditions, and real-world applications (DHS, 2013).

The NRF includes the 15 emergency support functions (ESFs) (FEMA, 2014d):

**ESF #1:** Transportation
**ESF #2:** Communications
**ESF #3:** Public Works and Engineering
**ESF #4:** Firefighting
**ESF #5:** Information and Planning
**ESF #6:** Mass Care, Emergency Assistance, Temporary Housing and Human Services
**ESF #7:** Logistics
**ESF #8:** Public Health and Medical Services
**ESF #9:** Search and Rescue
**ESF #10:** Oil and Hazardous Materials
**ESF #11:** Agriculture and Natural Resources
**ESF #12:** Energy
**ESF #13:** Public Safety and Security
**ESF #14:** Long-Term Community Recovery
**ESF #15:** External Affairs/Standard Operating Procedures.

Each ESF includes a coordinator function, and the primary and support agencies that work together to coordinate and deliver federal capabilities. Specifically, the ESFs provide the structure for coordinating federal interagency support to align with state, regional, and local capabilities. The NRFs also include support annexes, incident specific annexes, and partner guides.

ESF-8, Public Health and Medical Services, provides guidance for medical and mental health personnel, medical equipment and supplies, assessment of the status of the public health infrastructure, and monitoring for potential disease outbreaks (FEMA, 2013a). The ESF-8 primary coordinating agency is the U.S. Department of Health and Human Services; supporting agencies include the DHS, the American Red Cross, the Department of Defense, and the Department of Veterans Affairs. The National Disaster Medical System (NDMS) is part of ESF-8.

### National Incident Management System

The National Incident Management System (NIMS) is the national platform for disaster response and it includes universal protocols and language. The NIMS identifies concepts and principles that answer how to manage emergencies from preparedness to recovery regardless of their cause, size, location, or complexity. "NIMS provides a consistent, nationwide approach and vocabulary for multiple agencies or jurisdictions to work together to build, sustain and deliver the core capabilities needed to achieve a secure and resilient nation" (FEMA, 2013c, p. 1).

No matter what type of nursing practice or which agency a nurse chooses, they will come into direct contact with NIMS, which includes the Incident Command System (ICS). Figure 23-5 displays basic ICS operations. The NIMS includes varying levels of education and training, with many organizations requiring a base level of familiarization to comply with federal funding requirements.

A well-developed training program promotes nationwide NIMS implementation, producing an adequate number of trained and qualified emergency management/response personnel. The Emergency Management Institute (EMI) is the premier emergency management training institution, training more than 2 million students annually. The mission of EMI is to "directly supports the implementation of the National Incident Management System (NIMS), the National Response Framework (NRF), the National Disaster Recovery Framework (NDRF), and the National Preparedness Goal (NPG) by conveying necessary knowledge and skills to improve the nation's capa-

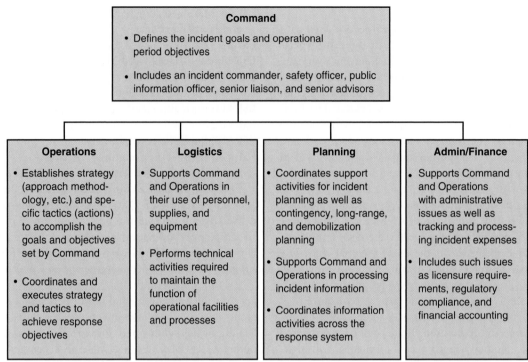

**FIG 23-5** Incident Command System (ICS). (Courtesy of U.S. Department of Health and Human Services, Washington, DC. From: http://www.phe.gov/Preparedness/planning/mscc/handbook/chapter1/Pages/emergencymanagement.aspx. Retrieved January 2015.)

bility" (FEMA, 2012, paragraph 1). EMI is located at the National Emergency Training Center in Emmitsburg, Maryland, and offers a broad range of both onsite and online courses related to all phases of the disaster cycle. Some of the NIMS-related training offered includes the following online courses (FEMA, 2013c):

- IS-100.HCb: Introduction to the Incident Command System for Healthcare/Hospitals
- IS-200.HCa: Applying ICS to Healthcare Organizations
- IS-700.a: National Incident Management System (NIMS), An Introduction
- IS-701.a: NIMS Multiagency Coordination System
- IS-800.b: National Response Framework, An Introduction

### Response to Biological Incidents

Biological agents pose a high risk to public health because only small amounts of the agents are needed to affect thousands of people and some of the agents are easy to conceal, transport, and disseminate. The CDC is an excellent source of biological agent information, including the latest agent fact sheets for health (CDC, 2014a). Important information provided includes the methods of transmission and communicability period. Through the Pandemic and All-Hazards Preparedness Reauthorization Act (PAHPRA), several biodefense programs exist to help public health professionals mount a proactive response to these events (USDHHS, 2013b):

- *BioWatch* is an early warning system for biothreats that uses an environmental sensor system to test the air for biological agents in several major metropolitan areas.

- *BioSense* is a data-sharing program to facilitate surveillance of unusual patterns or clusters of diseases in the United States. It shares data with local and state health departments and is a part of the BioWatch system.
- *Project BioShield* is a program to develop and produce new drugs and vaccines as countermeasures against potential bioweapons and deadly pathogens.
- *Cities Readiness Initiative* is a program to aid cities in increasing their capacity to deliver medicines and medical supplies during a large-scale public health emergency such as a bioterrorism attack or a nuclear accident.
- *Strategic National Stockpile (SNS)* is a CDC-managed program with the capacity to provide large quantities of medicine and medical supplies to protect the public in a public health emergency to include bioterrorism. The SNS is deployed through a combination of a state-level request and the public health system.

Some of the most important lessons from live biological incidents and exercises involve communication. In an effort to keep the public health community informed, the CDC developed the Public Health Information Network (PHIN). The PHIN provides for the electronic exchange of information among governmental agencies. It focuses on six components that help ensure information access and sharing: early event detection, outbreak management, connecting laboratory systems, countermeasure and response administration, partner communications and alerting, and cross-functional components, and is critical to information exchange (CDC, 2014b).

## How Disasters Affect Communities

One Health recognizes that the health of humans is connected to the health of animals and the environment, and the One Health concept integration in disaster preparedness and response requires interprofessional efforts at global, national, and local levels (CDC, 2013). The spread of infectious diseases and the relationships among humans, animals, and the environment are at the core of One Health. For example, animals serve as early warning signs of potential human illness; an example is that birds often die of West Nile virus before humans get sick with West Nile virus fever.

The first goal of any disaster response is to re-establish sanitary barriers as quickly as possible (Veenema, 2012). Water, food, waste removal, vector control, shelter, and safety are basic needs. Difficult weather conditions such as extreme heat or cold can hamper efforts, especially if electricity is affected. Continuous monitoring of the environment proactively addresses potential hazards. Disease prevention is an ongoing goal, especially if there is an interruption in the public health infrastructure. Infectious disease outbreaks can also occur in the recovery phase of disasters, and occasionally disaster workers introduce new organisms into the area.

People in a community will be affected physically and emotionally, depending on the type, cause, and location of the disaster; its magnitude and extent of damage; the duration; and the amount of prewarning provided. Immediate effects may include loss of life and morbidity, but other health effects such as those during and after disaster disease outbreaks may be delayed.

Although the immediate emotional response to a disaster by civilians may be unpredictable, the response is not always a negative one. For example, the terrorist attacks of September 11, 2001, created extreme anger and grief but also led to a marked increase in compassion and patriotism. Thousands of people helped, from donating blood and money to rescuing individuals from the buildings. Four days after the attack, buying an American flag was nearly impossible, as most stores had sold out (Associated Press, 2001). Within 1 month of the attack, an estimated $757 million in cash contributions and hundreds of truckloads of goods had been donated to help the families of victims and rescue workers (Yates, 2001). This was the worst human-made disaster in American history, killing more than 2500 civilians and 460 emergency responders. Yet, the terrorist attacks of September 11 will also be remembered for how they unified the country (Rand Corporation, 2004).

The psychological effects of September 11 were different from those of more contained, single-event disasters. The attack was unexpected and of great magnitude, with much uncertainty and fear about what might happen next. Not knowing when or if a subsequent attack will occur may sustain fear and anger.

Another U.S. disaster raised similar issues. At 7:10 A.M. EDT on August 29, 2005, Hurricane Katrina made landfall in southern Plaquemines Parish, Louisiana, as a category 3 hurricane. Starting as a natural disaster, its consequences were compounded by a human-made disaster caused by flooding from levee failure. Later joined by Hurricane Rita, Hurricane Katrina affected the Gulf Coast and the nation in ways that will be felt for generations to come. It is the costliest U.S. disaster ever, with economic estimates of more than $125 billion (National Oceanic and Atmospheric Administration [NOAA], 2007). The hurricane, floods, and more than 1800 confirmed deaths created traumatic stress that rose to unbearable levels in New Orleans, resulting in a tense and sometimes violent aftermath (Reagan, 2005). New Orleans was typically described as a war zone in the weeks following the disaster, as was the Gulfport-Biloxi coastline in Mississippi, where 90% of the buildings were demolished. Hundreds of thousands of people lost access to their homes and their jobs as a result of Hurricane Katrina. Although the response and recovery efforts eventually superseded any natural recovery efforts in the history of the country, many residents of both Louisiana and Mississippi believed that the help was too little, too late. Despite the enormous efforts of people and the vast amounts of money spent to help the area recover, there is much work to be done and more funds will be needed to restore the area (Institute for Southern Studies [ISS], 2009).

*Stress Reactions in Individuals.* A traumatic event can cause moderate to severe stress reactions. Individuals react to the same disaster in different ways depending on their age, cultural background, health status, social support structure, and general ability to adapt to crisis. Symptoms that may require assistance are listed in Table 23-2.

People who are affected by a disaster often have an exacerbation of an existing chronic disease. For example, the emotional stress of the disaster may make it difficult for people with diabetes to control their blood glucose levels. Grief results in harmful effects on the immune system. It reduces the function of cells that protect against viral infections and tumors. Hormones produced by the body's flight-or-fight mechanism also play a role in mediating the effects of grief. Those with mental health issues may experience increased symptoms (CDC, 2012a).

Older adults' reactions to disaster depend a great deal on their physical health, strength, mobility, independence, and income (Banks, 2013) (Figure 23-6). They can react deeply to the loss of personal possessions because of the high sentimental value attached to the items and their irreplaceable value. Their need for relocation depends on the extent of damage to their home or their compromised health. They may try and conceal the seriousness of their health conditions or losses if they fear loss of independence. Box 23-7 lists other populations at higher risk for serious disruption postdisaster, many of them the same populations at risk for adverse health effects predisaster as well.

The effect of disasters on young children (Figure 23-7) can be especially disruptive (National Institute of Mental Health [NIMH], 2013). Young children may respond with regressive behaviors such as thumb-sucking, bedwetting, crying, and clinging to parents. Older children tend to re-experience images of the traumatic event or have recurring thoughts or sensations, or they may intentionally avoid reminders, thoughts, and feelings related to disaster events. Children may have heightened sensitivity to sights, sounds, or smells and may experience exaggerated responses or difficulty with usual activities. Children not immediately impacted by a disaster can also be affected by it. The constant bombardment of disaster stories on television

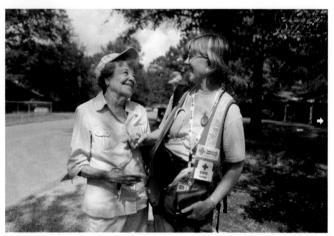

**FIG 23-6** Older adults and disaster. Red Cross nurse Jeanne Pollard chats with Ora White Church, 88, while making door-to-door visits with families in flood-damaged neighborhoods in Picayune, Mississippi, after Hurricane Isaac. (Courtesy of the American Red Cross Photo Library, photo by Talia Frenkel/American Red Cross, Washington, DC. From: http://media.redcross.org/sites/. Retrieved January 2015.)

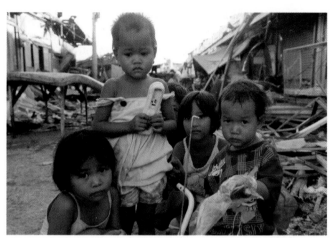

**FIG 23-7** Children and disaster. In 2013, one week after Typhoon Haiyan made landfall, residents of Tanauan, the Philippines, struggle to cope amidst the devastation. Every house in the city of 50,000 was badly damaged or destroyed. The effects of a disaster on young children can be especially disruptive. (Courtesy of the American Red Cross Photo Library, photo by Patrick Fuller/International Federation of Red Cross and Red Crescent Societies, Geneva, Switzerland. From: http://media.redcross.org/sites/. Retrieved January 2015.)

| TABLE 23-2 | Common Responses to a Traumatic Event | | |
|---|---|---|---|
| **COGNITIVE** | **EMOTIONAL** | **PHYSICAL** | **BEHAVIORAL** |
| Poor concentration | Shock | Nausea | Suspicion |
| Confusion | Numbness | Light-headedness | Irritability |
| Disorientation | Feeling overwhelmed | Dizziness | Arguments with friends and loved ones |
| Indecisiveness | Depression | Gastrointestinal problems | Withdrawal |
| Shortened attention span | Feeling lost | Rapid heart rate | Excessive silence |
| Memory loss | Fear of harm to self and/or loved ones | Tremors | Inappropriate humor |
| Unwanted memories | Feeling nothing | Headaches | Increased/decreased eating |
| Difficulty making decisions | Feeling abandoned | Grinding of teeth | Change in sexual desire or functioning |
| | Uncertainty of feelings | Fatigue | Increased smoking |
| | Volatile emotions | Poor sleep | Increased substance use or abuse |
| | | Pain | |
| | | Hyperarousal | |
| | | Jumpiness | |

From Substance Abuse and Mental Health Services Administration (SAMHSA): *Coping with a Traumatic Event: Information for Health Professionals.* 2005. From: http://media.samhsa.gov/MentalHealth/TraumaticEvent.aspx?from=carousel&position=1&date=3112011. Retrieved January 2015.

### BOX 23-7 Populations at Greatest Risk for Disruption after Disaster

- Seniors
- Vision and/or hearing impaired
- Women
- Children
- Individuals with chronic disease
- Individuals with chronic mental illness
- Non–English-speaking
- Low income
- Homeless
- Tourists; persons new to an area
- Persons with disabilities
- Single-parent families
- Substance abusers
- Undocumented residents

From National Institutes of Health, National Library of Medicine: *Special Populations: Emergency and Disaster Preparedness.* 2010. Available at http://sis.nlm.nih.gov/outreach/specialpopulationsanddisasters.html. Accessed January 25, 2011.

can cause fear in children. Parental reaction to a disaster will greatly influence children (NIMH, 2013).

Public health nurses should help those in the affected community talk about their feelings, including anger, sorrow, guilt, and perceived blame for the disaster or the outcomes of the disaster. Community members should be encouraged to engage in healthy eating, exercise, rest, daily routine maintenance, limited demanding responsibilities, and time with family and friends.

***Stress Reactions in the Community.*** Communities reflect the individuals and families living in them, both during and after a disaster incident. Four community phases as seen in Figure 23-8 are commonly recognized: (1) heroic, (2) honeymoon, (3) disillusionment, and (4) reconstruction (Duane's

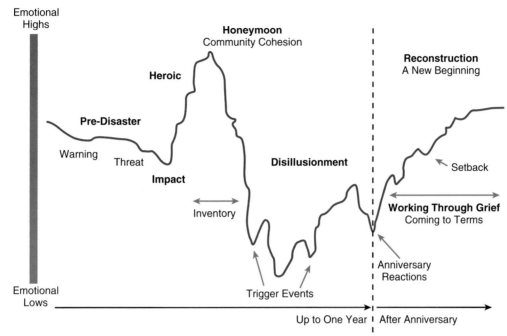

**FIG 23-8** Phases of disaster: Collective reactions. (Courtesy of U.S. Department of Health and Human Services, Substance Abuse and Mental Health Services Administration [SAMHSA]: *Training Manual for Mental Health and Human Services Workers in Major Disasters,* ed 2. Washington, DC, 2000, SAMHSA. From: http://store.samhsa.gov/product/Training-Manual-for-Mental -Health-and-Human-Service-Workers-in-Major-Disasters/SMA96-0538. Retrieved January 2015.)

Dartboard, 2010). The first two phases, the heroic and honeymoon phases, are most often associated with response efforts. The latter two phases, disillusionment and reconstruction, are most often linked with recovery.

During the heroic phase, there is an overwhelming need for people to do whatever they can to help others survive the disaster. First responders, including health and medical personal, will work hours on end with no thought of their own personal or health needs. They may fight needed sleep and refuse rest breaks in their drive to save others. Moreover, deployed responders from outside the disaster area may be unfamiliar with the terrain and inherent dangers. Those with supervisory responsibilities need to take necessary breaks and attend to their health needs. This means back-up plans must be made sooner than later. Exhausted, overworked responders present a danger to themselves and the community served.

In the honeymoon phase, survivors may be rejoicing that their lives and the lives of loved ones have been spared. Survivors will gather to share experiences and stories. The repeated telling to others creates bonds among the survivors. A sense of thankfulness over having survived the disaster is inherent in their stories.

The disillusionment phase occurs as time elapses and people notice that additional help and reinforcement are not coming as quickly as in the initial response. Fatigue and gloom can result and exhaustion starts to takes its toll on volunteers, rescuers, and medical personnel. The community begins to realize that a return to the previous normal is unlikely and that they

must make major changes and adjustments. Nurses in response must consider the psychosocial impact and the resulting emotional, cognitive, and spiritual implications. Public health nurses should identify groups/population segments particularly at risk for burnout and exhaustion, to include volunteers involved in response efforts. They may need breaks and reminders for nourishment. In addition, those in shock and those consumed by grief related to loss of loved ones will need compassionate care, with possible referrals to mental health counseling resources.

The last phase, reconstruction, is the longest. Recovery as a disaster cycle phase is addressed later in this chapter. Homes, schools, churches, and other community elements need to be rebuilt and reestablished. The goal is to return to a new state of normalcy. Community needs may still be extensive; the nurse continues to function as a member of the interprofessional team to provide and assure provision of the best possible coordinated care to the population.

## Role of the Public Health Nurse in Disaster Response

The role of the public health nurse during a disaster depends a great deal on the nurse's experience, professional role in a community disaster plan, and prior disaster knowledge to include personal readiness. Public health nurses bring leadership, policy, planning, and practice expertise to disaster preparedness and response (Association of Public Health Nurses [APHN], 2014). One thing is certain about disasters: continuing change. Public health nursing roles in disaster are generally consistent with the

## KEY POINTS—cont'd

- *Healthy People 2020* objectives are linked in many ways to the disaster management cycle, because a disaster incident affects the health of a community in many areas.
- For effectiveness in disaster prevention, preparedness, response, and recovery, nurses must get involved in their community's disaster plan: as a community member, through their workplace, or with a partnering community organization.
- Nurses must be adequately trained and properly associated with an official response organization to best serve those affected by a disaster.
- Becoming knowledgeable about available community resources before a disaster incident will ensure a better coordinated response and recovery.
- Flexibility is a key attribute in providing nursing care during disaster.
- The Public Health Nursing Intervention Wheel is appropriate for daily operations as well as during disaster chaos.
- With any disaster it is always best to use the resources, personnel, and infrastructure of the community itself to promote self-reliance and resilience.
- Our nation's planning efforts for disaster continue to develop, test, and evaluate the goal of a unified, well-coordinated public and private national response.
- The public health nursing role in the disaster management cycle includes helping clients maintain a safe environment and advocating for environmental safety measures in the community; risk communication and client education; community assessment to include rapid needs assessment; public health triage; and surveillance and field epidemiology.
- Triage in a disaster setting involves both individual and population-based approaches, and everything possible for one individual is provided while determining how to promote the greatest good for the greatest number of those affected.
- People in a community react differently to a disaster depending on the type, cause, and location of the disaster; its magnitude and extent of damage; its duration; and the amount of warning that was provided.
- Individual variables that cause people to react differently include their age, cultural background, health status, social support structure, and general adaptability to crisis.
- The affected community experiences four stages of stress during disaster: heroic, honeymoon, disillusionment, and reconstruction.
- The recovery phase begins almost immediately after a disaster occurs.
- Community organizations and social networks can foster community resiliency across the disaster cycle.
- The nurse assisting in disaster relief efforts must maintain self-health, both physically and mentally, to be of service to his or her family and clients.
- Ongoing community assessment is just as important as initial rapid needs assessment. Surveillance reports indicate the continuing status of the affected population and the effectiveness of ongoing relief efforts.

## CLINICAL DECISION-MAKING ACTIVITIES

1. Select a vulnerable population within your community and determine what needs the group would have in time of disaster. *What community resources are currently available to help this group? Where is the gap in services?*
2. Describe the role of the public health nurse across the disaster management cycle: prevention (mitigation and protection), preparedness, response, and recovery. *How do you practice nursing across these stages? How do you work with other members of the team?*
3. Interview a nurse who has responded to a disaster. *What role did the nurse play? Were his or her interventions provided at the individual, population level or both? Can you describe two specific examples?*
4. Conduct an interview with a leader from the Emergency Management Agency, American Red Cross, Medical Reserve Corps, or other agency involved with disaster management. *What is your community's plan for response to a disaster? What agencies are involved?*
5. Discuss the advantages and disadvantages of serving on a disaster team in your own community. *Are you a good candidate to serve on a disaster team? What about your personal preparedness? Is there a work conflict? How (or does) this differ from day-to-day nursing practice?*
6. Contact your local public health department to determine its role in a local disaster. Describe a specific nurse's role in disaster management. *How does that nurse navigate interprofessional practice?*
7. Determine what the disaster plan is where you work. Get specific details and share them with others who are important to you.

## REFERENCES

American College of Emergency Physicians (ACEP): *America's Emergency Care Environment: A State-by-State Report Card—2014.* 2014. From: http://www.emreportcard.org/uploadedFiles/EMReportCard2014.pdf. Retrieved January 2015.

American Nurses Association (ANA): *Adapting Standards of Care under Extreme Conditions: Guidance for Professionals during Disasters, Pandemics, and Other Extreme Emergencies.* 2008. From: http://www.nursingworld.org/MainMenuCategories/

WorkplaceSafety/Healthy-Work-Environment/DPR/TheLawEthicsofDisasterResponse/AdaptingStandardsofCare.pdf. Retrieved January 2015.

American Nurses Association (ANA): *Code of Ethics for Nurses.* Silver Spring, MD, 2010a, ANA.

American Nurses Association (ANA): *Who Will Be There? Ethics, the Law and a Nurse's Duty to Respond in a Disaster.* 2010b. From: http://www.nursingworld.org/MainMenuCategories/WorkplaceSafety/Healthy-Work-Environment/DPR/

Disaster-Preparedness.pdf. Retrieved January 2015.

American Red Cross: *Disaster Mental Health Handbook*. Washington, DC, 2012, Disaster Services.

American Red Cross: *Disaster Health Services Guidance*. Washington, DC, 2013, Disaster Services.

American Red Cross: *About Us*. 2014. From: http://www.redcross.org/about-us. Retrieved January 2015.

Associated Press: As patriotism soars, flags are hard to come by. *USA Today* 2001. From: http://usatoday30.usatoday.com/news/nation/2001/09/16/flag-shortage.htm. Retrieved January 2015.

Association of Public Health Nurses (APHN): *The Role of the Public Health Nurse in Disaster Preparedness Response, and Recovery: A Position Paper*. 2014. From: http://www.phnurse.org/index.php?option=com_content&view=article&id=120&Itemid=547. Retrieved January 2015.

Association of State and Territorial Directors of Nursing (ASTDN): *Every State Health Department Needs a Public Health Nursing Leader*. 2008. From: http://www.phnurse.org/docs/Every_State_Health_Dept._Needs_a_PHN_Leader_2008.pdf. Retrieved January 2015.

Banks L: Caring for elderly adults during disasters: improving health outcomes and recovery. *Southern Med J* 106:94–98, 2013.

Burkle FM: Population-based triage management in response to surge-capacity requirements during a large-scale bioevent disaster. *Acad Emerg Med* 13:1118–1129, 2006.

Centers for Disease Control and Prevention (CDC): *Disaster Mental Health for Responders: Key Principles, Issues and Questions*. 2012a. From: http://emergency.cdc.gov/mentalhealth/responders.asp. Retrieved January 2015.

Centers for Disease Control and Prevention (CDC): *Preparedness and Response for Public Health Disasters: Community Assessment for Public Health Emergency Response (CASPER)*. 2012b. From: http://www.cdc.gov/nceh/hsb/disaster/casper.htm. Retrieved January 2015.

Centers for Disease Control and Prevention (CDC): *Strategic National Stockpile (SNS)*. 2012c. From: http://www.cdc.gov/phpr/stockpile/stockpile.htm. Retrieved January 2015.

Centers for Disease Control and Prevention (CDC): *About One Health*. 2013. From: http://www.cdc.gov/onehealth/index.html. Retrieved January 2015.

Centers for Disease Control and Prevention (CDC): *Emergency Preparedness and Response: Bioterrorism*. 2014a. From: http://www.bt.cdc.gov/bioterrorism/. Retrieved January 2015.

Centers for Disease Control and Prevention (CDC): *Public Health Information Network (PHIN)*. 2014b. From: http://www.cdc.gov/phin/. Retrieved January 2015.

Chandra A, Acosta J, Sterns S, et al: *Building Community Resilience to Disasters: A Way Forward to Enhance National Health Security*. Santa Monica, CA, 2011, Rand Corporation. From: http://www.rand.org/content/dam/rand/pubs/technical_reports/2011/RAND_TR915.pdf. Retrieved January 2015.

Crippen DW: *Disaster Management: Lessons from September 11, 2001*. Sydney, Australia, 2002. presented at the 8th World Congress of Intensive and Critical Care Medicine.

Department of Homeland Security (DHS): *Homeland Security Act of 2002: Title 1—Department of Homeland Security*. 2002. From: http://www.dhs.gov/homeland-security-act-2002. Retrieved January 2015.

Department of Homeland Security (DHS): *National Preparedness Guidelines*. 2007a. From: http://www.dhs.gov/national-preparedness-guidelines. Retrieved January 2015.

Department of Homeland Security (DHS): *Target Capabilities List: A Companion to the National Preparedness Guidelines* [version 2.0]. 2007b. From: http://www.fema.gov/pdf/government/training/tcl.pdf. Retrieved January 2015.

Department of Homeland Security (DHS): *Presidential Policy Directive / PPD-8: National Preparedness*. 2011. From: http://www.dhs.gov/presidential-policy-directive-8-national-preparedness. Retrieved January 2015.

Department of Homeland Security (DHS): *National Response Framework (NRF)*. 2013. From: http://www.fema.gov/national-response-framework. Retrieved January 2015.

Dilley M, Chen RS, Deichmann U, et al: *Natural Disaster Hotspots: A Global Risk Analysis* [Disaster Risk Management Series No. 5]. Washington, DC, 2005, World Bank. From: https://openknowledge.worldbank.org/handle/10986/737. Retrieved January 2015.

Duane's Dartboard: 2010. Duanehallock.com/2010/01/27phases-of-disaster-recover/. Accessed Febuary 2, 2015.

Federal Emergency Management Agency (FEMA): *Guidance on Planning for Integration of Functional Needs Support Service in General Population Shelters*. 2010. From: http://www.fema.gov/pdf/about/odic/fnss_guidance.pdf. Retrieved January 2015.

Federal Emergency Management Agency (FEMA): *Emergency Management Institute (EMI)*. 2012. From: http://www.training.fema.gov/EMI/emi.asp. Retrieved January 2015.

Federal Emergency Management Agency (FEMA): *Emergency Support Function #8—Public Health and Medical Services Annex*. 2013a. From: http://www.fema.gov/media-library/assets/documents/32198?id=7359. Retrieved January 2015.

Federal Emergency Management Agency (FEMA): *Homeland Security Exercise and Evaluation Program (HSEEP)*. 2013b. From: https://www.llis.dhs.gov/HSEEP. Retrieved January 2015.

Federal Emergency Management Agency (FEMA): *National Incident Management System (NIMS)*. 2013c. From: http://www.fema.gov/national-incident-management-system. Retrieved January 2015.

Federal Emergency Management Agency (FEMA): *2013 National Preparedness Report*. 2013d. From: http://www.fema.gov/media-library/assets/documents/32509?id=7465. Retrieved January 2015.

Federal Emergency Management Agency (FEMA): *Robert T. Stafford Disaster Relief and Emergency Assistance Act as Amended, and Related Authorities as of April 2013*. 2013e. From: https://www.fema.gov/media-library/assets/documents/15271?fromSearch=fromsearch&id=3564. Retrieved January 2015.

Federal Emergency Management Agency (FEMA): *Disaster Declarations for 2013*. 2014a. From: http://www.fema.gov/disasters/grid/year/2013. Retrieved January 2015.

Federal Emergency Management Agency (FEMA): *National Exercise Program (NEP)—Capstone Exercise 2014*. 2014b. From: http://www.fema.gov/national-exercise-program-nep-capstone-exercise-2014. Retrieved January 2015.

Federal Emergency Management Agency (FEMA): *Ready: Caring for Animals*. 2014c. From: http://www.ready.gov/caring-animals. Retrieved January 2015.

Federal Emergency Management Agency (FEMA): *Resource Library*. 2014d. From: http://www.fema.gov/national-preparedness-resource-library. Retrieved January 2015.

Huffington Post: *Superstorm Sandy Deaths, Damage and Magnitude: What We Know One Month Later*. November 29, 2012. From: http://www.huffingtonpost.com/2012/11/29/superstorm-hurricane-sandy-deaths-2012_n_2209217.html. Retrieved January 2015.

Inajima T, Adelman J, Okada Y: *Fukushima disaster was man-made, investigation finds*. Bloomberg Businessweek. July 5, 2012. From: http://www.bloomberg.com/news/2012-07-05/fukushima-nuclear-disaster-was-man-made-investigation-rules.html. Retrieved January 2015.

Institute for Southern Studies (ISS): *Grading the Katrina Recovery: How Gulf Coast Leaders Rate the President and Congress Four Years after the Storm*. August/September 2009. From: http://www.nesri.org/sites/default/files/Grading_Katrina_Year_Report.pdf. Retrieved January 2015.

Institute of Medicine (IOM): *Catastrophic Disaster Response*. Washington, DC, 2012, National Academies Press.

International Council of Nurses (ICN): *Disaster Response Network*. 2013. From: http://www.icn.ch/Disaster-Response-Links/Disaster-Response-Network, http://www.nesri.org/sites/default/files/Grading_Katrina_Year_Report.pdf. Retrieved January 2015.

International Federation of Red Cross and Red Crescent Societies (IFRC): *World Disasters Report 2013: Technology and the Future of Humanitarian Action*. Geneva, Switzerland, 2013, Imprimerie Chirat. From: www.ifrc.org/wdr2013. Retrieved January 2015.

Leonard HB, Howitt AM: Acting in time against disasters: a comprehensive risk-management framework. In Howard K, Michael U, editors: *Learning from Catastrophes: Strategies for Reaction and Response*. Upper Saddle River, NJ, 2010, Wharton School Publishing. From: http://www.hks.harvard.edu/programs/crisisleadership/publications/articles. Retrieved January 2015.

National Aeronautics and Space Administration (NASA): *Natural Disaster Hotspots: A Global Risk Analysis, Earth Observatory*. 2005. From: http://econ.worldbank.org/external/default/main?pagePK=64165259&theSitePK=469372&piPK=64165421&menuPK=64166322&entityID=000160016_20051123111032. Retrieved January 2015.

National Institute of Mental Health (NIMH): *Helping Children and Adolescents Cope with Violence and Disasters: What Parents Can Do*. 2013. From: http://www.nimh.nih.gov/health/publications/helping-children-and-adolescents-cope-with-violence-and-disasters-parents/index.shtml?utm_source=twitterfeed&utm_medium=twitter. Retrieved January 2015.

National Institute of Occupational Health and Safety (NIOSH): *Traumatic Incident Stress*. 2013. From: http://www.cdc.gov/niosh/

topics/traumaticincident/. Retrieved January 2015.

National Oceanic and Atmospheric Administration (NOAA): *Hurricane Katrina*. 2007. From: http://www.nhc.noaa.gov/archive/2005/KATRINA.shtml. Retrieved January 2015.

Naval Postgraduate School (NPS): *Directives, Instructions, Specifications, and Standards*. Monterey, CA, 2014, Dudley Knox Library. From: http://libguides.nps.edu/presidentialdocs. Retrieved January 2015.

Noji EK: *The Public Health Consequences of Disasters*. New York, 1997, Oxford University Press.

Oklahoma City National Memorial & Museum: *Those Who Were killed*. 2010. From: http://www.oklahomacitynationalmemorial.org/secondary.php?ordering=7&view=19&section=1&catid=24. Retrieved January 2015.

Polivka B, Stanley S, Gordon D, et al: Public health nursing competencies for public health surge events. *Public Health Nurs* 25:159–165, 2008.

Powell T, Hanfling D, Gostin LO: Emergency preparedness and public health: the lessons of Hurricane Sandy. *JAMA* 308:2569–2570, 2012. From: http://scholarship.law.georgetown.edu/cgi/viewcontent.cgi?article=2149&context=facpub. Retrieved January 2015.

Powell-Young YM, Baker JR, Hogan JG: Disaster ethics and healthcare personnel: a model case study to facilitate the decision making process. *Online J Health Ethics* 3, 2013. From: http://aquila.usm.edu/ojhe/vol3/iss2/3. Retrieved January 2015.

Rand Corporation: *Compensating the Victims of 9/11*. Santa Monica, CA, 2004, RAND. From: http://www.rand.org/pubs/research_briefs/RB9087/index1.html. Retrieved January 2015.

Reagan M, editor: *CNN Reports: Katrina: State of Emergency*. Kansas City, MO, 2005, Andrews McMeel Publishing.

Shehab N, Anastario MP, Lawry L: Access to care among displaced Mississippi residents in FEMA travel trailer parks two years after Katrina. *Health Aff* 27:w416–w429, 2008.

Stanley S, Bulecza S, Gopalani S: Psychological impact of disasters on communities. In Couig MP, Kelley PW, editors: *Annual Review of Nursing Research: Disasters and Humanitarian Assistance*. New York, 2012, Springer Publishing.

Stanley S, Polivka B, Gordon D, et al: The ExploreSurge Trail Guide and Hiking Workshop: discipline specific education for public health nurses. *Public Health Nurs* 25:166–175, 2008.

United Nations Development Programme: *2011 Global Assessment Report on Disaster Risk Reduction*. 2012. From: http://www.undp.org/content/undp/en/home/librarypage/crisis-prevention-and-recovery/2011-global-assessment-report-on-disaster-risk-reduction/. Retrieved January 2015.

University of Minnesota School of Public Health: *Effectiveness of Simulated Disaster Response Scenarios*. 2014. From: http://sph.umn.edu/research/u-seee/. Retrieved January 2015.

Uscher-Pines L, Chandra A, Acosta J: The promise and pitfalls of community resilience. *Disaster Med Public Health Prep* 7:603–606, 2013.

U.S. Department of Health and Human Services (USDHHS): *Healthy People 2020: A Roadmap to Improve All Americans' Health*. 2010. From: http://www.healthypeople.gov. Retrieved January 2015.

U.S. Department of Health and Human Services (USDHHS): *National Health Security Strategy of the United States of America*. 2013a. From: http://www.phe.gov/Preparedness/planning/authority/nhss/Pages/default.aspx. Retrieved January 2015.

U.S. Department of Health and Human Services (USDHHS): *Public Health Emergency. Pandemic and All-Hazards Preparedness Reauthorization Act (PAHPRA)*. 2014. From: https://www.phe.gov/Preparedness/legal/pahpa/Pages/pahpra.aspx. Retrieved February 2015.

Veenema TG: *Disaster Nursing and Emergency Preparedness for Chemical, Biological, and Radiological Terrorism and Other Hazards*. New York, 2012, Springer Publishing.

Vinter S, Lieberman DA, Levi J: Public health preparedness in a reforming health care system. *Harv Law Policy Rev* 4:339–360, 2010. From: http://healthyamericans.org/assets/files/HLPR_TFAH.pdf. Retrieved January 2015.

World Association for Disaster and Emergency Medicine (WADEM): *Nursing Section Overview*. 2013. From: http://www.wadem.org/nursing.html. Retrieved January 2015.

World Health Organization (WHO): *Disaster Risk Management for Health: Overview*. 2011. From: http://www.who.int/hac/events/drm_fact_sheet_overview.pdf. Retrieved January 2015.

Yates J: Gifts, letters piling up at N.Y. relief centers. *Chicago Tribune* 2001. From: http://articles.chicagotribune.com/2001-10-06/news/0110060083_1_relief-workers-aid-workers-bears. Retrieved January 2015.

# 24

# Public Health Surveillance and Outbreak Investigation

Surveillance is a critical role function for n
in the community. A comprehensive understan
edge of the surveillance systems and how the
nurses improve the quality and the usefulr
collected for making decisions about needed
vices, community actions, and public healt
(Chapter 23 provides additional information).
features indicate it:

- Is organized and planned
- Is the principal means by which a populatic
  is assessed
- Involves ongoing collection of specific data
- Involves analyzing data on a regular basis
- Requires sharing the results with others
- Requires broad and repeated contact with
  personal health issues
- Motivates public health action as a result of
  - Reduce morbidity
  - Reduce mortality
  - Improve health

Surveillance is important because it gene
of a disease or event outbreak patterns (in
geographic distribution, and susceptible pc
knowledge can be used to intervene to reduc
an occurrence at the most appropriate point
the most effective ways. Surveillance is built o
of epidemiologic principles of agent, host, an
relationships and on the natural history of c
tions (see Chapter 12). Surveillance systems
to engage in effective continuous quality imp
ties within organizations and to improve
(Veenema, 2013).

Surveillance focuses on the collection of pro
data. Process data focus on what is done (i.e., :
or protocols for health care delivery). Outcor
changes in health status. The activities generat
these data aim to improve public health resp
example of process data is collection of data a
tion of the eligible population vaccinated aga
any one year. Outcome data in this case are th
(new cases) of influenza among the same p
same year.

Although surveillance was initially devote
and reducing the spread of infectious diseases
monitor and reduce chronic diseases and injui
mental and occupational exposures (Centers fo
and Prevention [CDC], 2014e; Veenema, 201
sonal health behaviors. Surveillance systems
other professionals monitor emerging infectic
ist outbreaks (Pryor and Milligan, 2013). Bic
example of an event creating a critical publi
that involves environmental exposures that mi
This event also requires serious planning in o
respond quickly and effectively. Biological ter
as "the deliberate release of viruses, bacteria
(agents) used to cause illness or death in pe
plants" (http://www.bt.cdc.gov/bioterrorism)

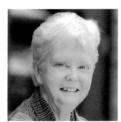

*Marcia Stanhope, PhD, RN, FAAN*
Dr. Marcia Stanhope is currently an Associate of the Tufts and Associates Search Firm, Chicago, Ill. She is also a consultant for the nursing program at Berea College, Kentucky. She has practiced community and home health nursing, has served as an administrator and consultant in home health, and has been involved in the development of two nurse-managed centers. At one time in her career, she held a public policy fellowship and worked in the office of a U.S. Senator. She has taught community health, public health, epidemiology, policy, primary care nursing, and administration courses. Dr. Stanhope formerly directed the Division of Community Health Nursing and Administration and served as Associate Dean of the College of Nursing at the University of Kentucky. She has been responsible for both undergraduate and graduate courses in population-centered nursing. She has also taught at the University of Virginia and the University of Alabama, Birmingham. During her career at the University of Kentucky she appointed to the Good Samaritan Foundation Chair and Professorship in Community Health Nursing, and was honored with the University Provost's Public Scholar award. Her presentations and publications have been in the areas of home health, community health and community-focused nursing practice, as well as primary care nursing.

## ADDITIONAL RESOURCES

Ⓔ **Evolve Website http://evolve.elsevier.com/Stanhope**
- *Healthy People 2020*
- WebLinks—Of special note, see the link for these sites:
  - National Notifiable Disease Surveillance System
  - Enhanced Surveillance Project
- Quiz
- Case Studies

- Glossary
- Answers to Practice Application
- Appendix D.3: Prevention and Control of Pandemic Influenza: Individuals and Families

## OBJECTIVES

*After reading this chapter, the student should be able to do the following:*

1. Define public health surveillance.
2. Analyze types of surveillance systems.
3. Identify steps in planning, analyzing, interviewing, and evaluating surveillance.
4. Recognize sources of data used when investigating a disease/condition outbreak.
5. Relate the role of the nurse in surveillance and outbreak investigation to the national core competencies for public health nurses.

## KEY TERMS

Disease surveillance has been a part of pu
since the 1200s, during the investigations
in Europe. During the 1600s John Grau
damental principles of public health incl
outbreak investigation, and in the 1700s
the first public health laws to provide
health and care of the population of the s
century, William Farr introduced the m
veillance and, along with the United S
Britain, began required reporting syster
eases. In 1901, the United States begar
reporting cases of cholera, smallpox, and
the United States began national reportin
By 1935 the first national health survey
and in 1949 the National Office of Vit
weekly mortality and morbidity statistic
*Health Reports.* This activity was later trar
for Disease Control and Prevention, who
*Morbidity and Mortality Weekly Report* i
tions, reporting mechanisms, and data co
tial to surveillance and disease outbreak in
et al, 2012).

The Constitution of the United State
powers" necessary to preserve health saf
events (see Chapter 8). These powers
surveillance. State and local "police pov
surveillance activities. Health departmer

---

### HOW TO  Develop a Program Plan

A. Define the problem
B. Formulate the plan
  1. Assess population need
    a. Who is the program population?
    b. What is the need to be met?
    c. How large is the client population to be served?
    d. Where are they located?
    e. How does the target population define the need?
    f. Are there other programs addressing the same need? (Describe.)
    g. Why is the need not being met?
  2. Establish program boundaries
    a. Who will be included in the program?
    b. Who will not be included? Why?
    c. What is the program goal?
  3. Program feasibility
    a. Who agrees that the program is needed (stakeholders: administrators, providers, clients, funders)?
    b. Who does not agree?
  4. Resources (general)
    a. What personnel are needed? What personnel are available?
    b. What facilities are needed? What facilities are available?
    c. What equipment is needed? What equipment is available?
    d. Is funding available to support the project? Is additional funding needed?
    e. Are resources being donated (space, printing, paper, medical supplies)?
      (1) Type
      (2) Amount
  5. Tools used to assess need
    a. Census data
    b. Key informants
    c. Focus groups
    d. Community forums
    e. Existing program surveys
    f. Surveys of client population
    g. Statistical indicators (e.g., demographic and morbidity/mortality data)
C. Conceptualize the problem
  1. List the potential solutions to the problem.
  2. What are the risks of each solution?
  3. What are the consequences?
  4. What are the outcomes to be gained from the solutions?
  5. Draw a decision tree to show the problem-solving process used.
D. Detail the plan
  1. What are the objectives for each solution to meet the program goal?
  2. What activities will be done to conduct each of the alternative solutions listed under C1 and based on objectives?
  3. What are the differences in the resources needed for each of the alternative solutions?
  4. Which of the alternative solutions would be chosen if the resources described under B4 were the only resources available?
  5. Who would be responsible or accountable for implementing the plan?
E. Evaluate the plan
  1. Which of the alternative solutions is most acceptable to the following:
    a. The client population
    b. The agency administrator
    c. You
    d. The community
  2. Which of the alternative solutions appears to have the most benefits to the following:
    a. The client population
    b. The agency administrator
    c. You
    d. The community
  3. On the basis of cost, which alternative solution would be chosen by the following:
    a. The client population
    b. The agency administrator
    c. You
    d. The community
F. Implement the program plan
  1. On the basis of data collected, which of the solutions has been chosen?
  2. Why should the agency administrator approve your request? Give a rationale.
  3. Will additional funding be sought?
  4. When can the program begin? Give date.

Developed by M. Stanhope and based on the Basic Program Planning Model (Nutt, 1984: Issel, 2013)

---

 **HEALTHY PEOPLE 2020**

### *Example of* Healthy People 2020 *Goals for Program Planning*

| Focus Area | Overall Goal | Objective | Measuring the Objective |
|---|---|---|---|
| IID-23: Immunization and infectious diseases | Attain high-quality, longer lives free of preventable disease, disability, injury, and premature death. | IID-11: Increase routine vaccination coverage levels for adolescents. | IID: 11-1: Increase (action verb) to one dose of tetanus-diphtheria-acellular pertussis (Tdap) booster vaccine by 13 to 15 years (purpose) for 80% of this age group (operational indicator) by 2020 (time frame). |

USDHHS: *Healthy People 2020: A Roadmap for Health.* Washington, DC, 2010, U.S. Government Printing Office.

Quality assurance programs are prime examples of program evaluation in health care delivery. Evaluation data are used to justify continuing programs in public health. Program evaluation focuses on whether goals were met and the efficiency and effectiveness of program activities. Many methods of program evaluation are described in the literature. One of the primary methods of evaluation used in health care today is Donabedian's (1982; updated in 2003) classic evaluative framework, which examines the structure, process, and outcomes of a program. Other models and frameworks have been developed using this approach (McDonald, 2007). The tracer method and case register are examples of other methods applied to program evaluation. (See Chapter 26 for further discussion.)

Program records and a community index serve as the major source of information for program evaluation. Surveys, interviews, observations, and diagnostic tests are ways to assess client and community responses to health programs. Cost studies help identify program benefits and objectiveness (Refer to chapter 5) (CDC, 2012).

As financial resources become scarce, nursing and the health care system must be able to justify their existence, prove that their services are responsive to client needs, and show their concern for being accountable. Planning and evaluation will assist in meeting these objectives.

## Planning for the Evaluation Process

Planning for the evaluation process is an important part of program planning. When the planning process begins, the plan for evaluating the program should also be developed. All persons to be involved in implementing a program should be a part of the plan for program evaluation. Assessment of need is one component of evaluation. The basic questions to be answered, after carefully considering the data collected from a census, key informants, community forums, surveys, or health statistics indicators, are as follows:

1. Will the objectives and resources of this program meet the identified needs of the client population?
2. Is the program relevant?

Once need has been established and the program is designed, the nurse must continue plans for program evaluation. As a part of the planning process, Posavac (2011) described six steps to use for continuing program evaluation (Figure 25-3):

1. Identify the key people for evaluation. Program personnel, program funders, and the clients of the program should be included in planning for evaluation.
2. Arrange preliminary meetings to discuss the question of how the group wants to evaluate the program and where to start. If the program planners and others agree on an evaluation, the resources needed to do the evaluation must be identified. Evaluation is necessary even though some may not be interested in it. Nurses can help others see that without evaluation, money to support programs will not be available, or the need for a new nurse to help with the work cannot be justified. In health care today, there is great emphasis on outcomes of care. The only way to see outcomes is through evaluation.
3. After the key people have met and considered the questions in the previous steps, they are ready to begin the evaluation

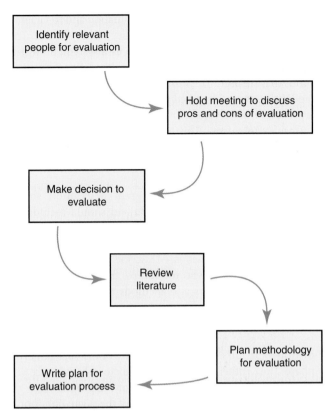

**FIG 25-3** Six steps in planning for program evaluation.

process. Even though evaluation may be desired, the decision to conduct the evaluation may be an administrative one, based on available resources and existing circumstances. For example, if a program evaluation were attempted in a situation in which program personnel wanted it but clients chose to be uncooperative, evaluation efforts would be unsuccessful.

4. Examine the literature for suggestions about the appropriate methods and techniques for evaluation and their usefulness in program evaluation. If an agency has chosen to use an external evaluator, this person may make suggestions about the questions to be answered in the evaluation process. These questions are based on the program goals. Nurses who have reviewed the literature and communicated with others affected by the evaluation can determine whether the evaluation suggestions are appropriate for the situation.
5. Plan the method to be used, including decisions about what goals and objectives will be measured, how they will be measured, and for what population.
6. Write a plan that outlines the mission and goals of the overall program, the type of evaluation to be done, the operational measures to be used to evaluate the program goals, the choice of who will do the evaluation (i.e., internal or external personnel), the available resources for conducting the evaluation, and the readiness of the organization, personnel, and clients for program evaluation. Nurses at all levels of education and preparation can participate in program planning and evaluation.

## Evaluation Process

A framework for evaluation in public health has been developed by the Centers for Disease Control and Prevention (CDC) to guide understanding about program evaluation and to facilitate integration of evaluation in the public health system. This framework defines program evaluation as a systematic way to improve and to account for public health actions by using methods that are useful, feasible, ethical, and accurate. Six interdependent steps are identified that must be part of an evaluation process (USDHHS, 2011):

1. *Engage stakeholders*—This includes those who are involved in planning, funding, and implementing the program, those who are affected by the program, and the intended users of its services.
2. *Describe the program*—The program description should address the need for the program and should include the mission and goals. This sets the standard for judging the results of the evaluation.
3. *Focus the evaluation design*—Describe the purpose for the evaluation, the users who will receive the report, how it will be used, the questions and methods to be used, and any necessary agreements.
4. *Gather credible evidence*—Specify the indicators that will be used, sources of data, quality of the data, quantity of information to be gathered, and the logistics of the data gathering phase. Data gathered should provide credible evidence and should convey a well-rounded view of the program.
5. *Justify conclusions*—The conclusions of the evaluation should be validated by linking them to the evidence gathered and then appraising them against the values or standards set by the stakeholders. Approaches for analyzing, synthesizing, and interpreting the evidence should be agreed on before data collection begins to ensure that all needed information will be available.
6. *Ensure use and share lessons learned*—Use and dissemination of findings require deliberate effort so that the lessons learned can be used in making decisions about the program (CDC, 2012).

## Sources of Program Evaluation

Both quantitative and qualitative methods may be used to conduct an evaluation; however, the strongest evaluation designs combine both qualitative and quantitative methods. Major sources of information for program evaluation are the program clients, program records, and community indexes.

Qualitative methods such as site visits, structured observations of interventions, or open-ended interviews may be used (Trickett et al, 2011). The program participants, or clients of the service, have a unique and valuable role in program evaluation. Whether the clients, for whom the program was designed, accept the services will determine to a large extent whether the program achieves its goal. Thus, their reactions, feelings, and judgments about the program are very important to the evaluation. For example, to garner feedback from participants in a program, an evaluator may use a written survey in the form of a questionnaire or an attitude scale. Interviews and observations are other ways of obtaining feedback about a program. Attitude scales are probably used most often, and they are usually phrased in terms of whether the program met its objectives. The client satisfaction survey is an example of an attitude

scale often used in the health care delivery system to evaluate the program objectives (Finkelstein et al, 2011). Client input into the development of evaluation tools ensures that the questions and approaches are more acceptable to the clients and that the tools effectively elicit the information needed.

The second major source of information for program evaluation is program records, especially clinical records. Clinical records provide the evaluator with information about the care given to the client and the results of that care. To determine whether a program goal has been met, one might summarize the data from a group of records. For example, if one overall goal were to reduce the incidence of low-birth-weight babies through prenatal care, records would be reviewed to obtain the number of mothers who received prenatal care and the number of low-birth-weight babies born to them. Records would be reviewed from the beginning of the program and at the end of a specific time frame, such as at the end of each year. Care must be taken to ensure that any review and use of clinical records complies with HIPAA regulations. (For details about HIPAA compliance, see http://aspe.hhs.gov/admnsimp/index.shtml.)

The third major source of evaluation is epidemiologic data. Mortality and morbidity data measuring health and illness are probably cited more frequently than any other single index for program evaluation. These health and illness indicators are useful in evaluating the effects of health care programs on the total community. Incidence and prevalence data are valuable indexes for measuring program effectiveness and impact, and these data are readily available on the Internet. Useful sites for such data include vital statistics available at state department of health sites, the CDC, and the U.S. Census site. Most counties and communities have their own sites, and many of these contain very useful demographic and health data.

An example of a national program based on a needs assessment of the U.S. population is the national health objectives program *Healthy People 2020* (USDHHS, 2010). *Healthy People* documents have been published every 10 years since 1980. The data gathered from each 10-year period have been used to evaluate the population needs met and the assessment of needs for the next *Healthy People* document.

The Healthy Communities Program (USDHHS, 2010) and named community health status indicators project suggests activities to evaluate national health objectives related to communities. The example shown in the Healthy People 2020 box on p. 559 highlights injury and violence prevention. This box shows that objectives include an action verb, a result, an operational indicator, and a time frame for implementing the objective (10 years, begun in 2010).

The Levels of Prevention box provides examples of applying levels of prevention to program planning and evaluation.

## Aspects of Evaluation

The aspects of program evaluation include the following (USDHHS, 2011):

1. *Relevance*—Need for the program
2. *Adequacy*—Program addresses the extent of the need
3. *Progress*—Tracking of program activities to meet program objectives

## HEALTHY PEOPLE 2020

### Objectives Focus Areas

1. Access to Health Services
2. Adolescent Health
3. Arthritis, Osteoporosis, and Chronic Back Conditions
4. Blood Disorders and Blood Safety
5. Cancer
6. Chronic Kidney Diseases
7. Dementias, including Alzheimer's
8. Diabetes
9. Disability and Health
10. Early and Middle Childhood
11. Educational and Community-Based Programs
12. Environmental Health
13. Family Planning
14. Food Safety
15. Genomics
16. Global Health
17. Healthcare-Associated Infections
18. Health Communication and Health IT
20. Hearing and Other Sensory or Communication Disorders (Ear, Nose, Throat—Voice, Speech, and Language)
21. Heart Disease and Stroke
22. HIV
23. Immunization and Infectious Diseases
24. Injury and Violence Prevention
26. Maternal, Infant, and Child Health
27. Medical Product Safety
28. Mental Health and Mental Disorders
29. Nutrition and Weight Status
30. Occupational Safety and Health
31. Older Adults
32. Oral Health
33. Physical Activity and Fitness
34. Preparedness
35. Public Health Infrastructure
36. Respiratory Diseases
37. Sexually Transmitted Diseases
38. Sleep Health
40. Substance Abuse
41. Tobacco Use
42. Vision

Three other objectives are under development: numbers 19, 25, 39.
USDHHS: *Healthy People 2020: A Roadmap for Health.* Washington, DC, 2010, U.S. Government Printing Office.

## HEALTHY PEOPLE 2020

### Example of a Measurable National Health Objective

In the *Healthy People* focus area of injury and violence prevention, one objective is:

- IPV-5: Increase (action verb) the number of States and the District of Columbia where 90% of deaths of children aged 17 years and under (operational indicator) due to external causes are reviewed by a child fatality review team (purpose), by 2020 (time frame).

USDHHS: *Healthy People 2020: A Roadmap for Health.* Washington, DC, 2010, U.S. Government Printing Office.

## 🗎 LEVELS OF PREVENTION

### Program Planning and Evaluation

**Primary Prevention**
Plan a community-wide program with the local school system and health department to serve healthy meals and snacks in all schools to promote good childhood nutrition.

**Secondary Prevention**
Develop screening programs for all school children to determine the incidence/prevalence of childhood obesity before implementing the program.

**Tertiary Prevention**
Evaluate the incidence/prevalence of obesity among school children after the implementation of the program and provide programs to reduce complications from the condition.

4. *Efficiency*—Relationship between program outcomes and the resources spent
5. *Effectiveness*—Ability to meet program objectives and the results of program efforts
6. *Impact*—Long-term changes in the client population
7. *Sustainability*—Enough resources to continue the program

The How To box suggests questions that may be asked about program evaluation using this process.

The following paragraphs provide an explanation of each step in program evaluation.

*Relevance.* Evaluation of relevance is an important component of the initial planning phase. As money, providers, facilities, and supplies for delivering health care services are more closely monitored, the needs assessment done by the nurse will determine whether the program is needed.

*Adequacy.* Evaluation of adequacy looks at the extent to which the program addresses the entire problem defined in the needs assessment. The magnitude of the problem is determined by vital statistics, incidence, prevalence, and expert opinion.

*Progress.* The monitoring of program activities, such as hours of services, number of providers used, number of referrals made, and amount of money spent to meet program objectives, provides an evaluation of the progress of the program. This type of evaluation is an example of formative or process evaluation, which occurs on an ongoing basis while the program exists. This provides an opportunity to make effective day-to-day management decisions about the operations of the program. Progress evaluation occurs primarily while implementing the program. The nurse who completes a daily or weekly log of clinical activities (e.g., number of clients seen in clinic or visited at home, number of phone contacts, number of referrals made, number of community health promotion activities) is contributing to progress evaluation of the nursing service.

*Efficiency.* If the reason for evaluation is to examine the efficiency of a program, it may occur on an ongoing basis as formative evaluation or at the end of the program as a summative evaluation. The evaluator may be able to determine whether the program provides better benefits at a lower cost than a similar program, or whether the benefits to the clients, or number of clients served, justify the costs of the program.

**HOW TO** Do a Program Evaluation

*To do a program evaluation, first choose the type of evaluation you wish to conduct. Second, identify the goal and objectives for the evaluation. Third, decide who will be involved in the evaluation. Fourth, answer the questions related to the type of evaluation as follows:*

A. *Program relevance: needs assessment (formative)*
 1. *Use answers to all questions listed in section B of How To Develop a Program Plan.*
 2. *On the basis of the needs assessment, was the program necessary?*

B. *Adequacy*
 1. *Is the program large enough to make a positive difference in the problem/need?*
 2. *Are the boundaries of the services defined so that the problem/ need can be addressed for the target population?*

C. *Program progress (formative)*
 1. *Monitor activities (circle which this reflects: daily, weekly, monthly, annually).*
  a. *Name the activities provided.*
  b. *How many hours of service were provided?*
  c. *How many clients have been served?*
  d. *How many providers are there?*
  e. *What types of clients have been served?*
  f. *What types of providers were needed?*
  g. *Where have services been offered (e.g., home, clinic, organization)?*
  h. *How many referrals have been made to community sources?*
  i. *Which sources have been used to provide support services?*
 2. *Budget*
  a. *How much money has been spent to carry out activities?*
  b. *Will more/less money be needed to conduct activities as outlined?*
  c. *Will changes to objectives and activities be needed to sustain the program?*
  d. *What changes do you recommend and why?*

D. *Program efficiency (formative and summative)*
 1. *Costs*
  a. *How do costs of the program compare with those of a similar program to meet the same goal?*
  b. *Do the activities outlined in C1 compare with the activities in a similar program?*

 c. *Although this program costs more/less than expected, is it needed? Why?*
 2. *Productivity (may use national or state averages for comparison)*
  a. *How many clients does each type of staff see per day (e.g., registered nurses, clinical nurse specialists, nurse practitioners)?*
  b. *How does this compare with similar programs?*
  c. *Although the productivity level of this program is low/high, is the program needed? Why?*
 3. *Benefits*
  a. *What are the benefits of the program to the clients served?*
  b. *What are the benefits to the community?*
  c. *Are the benefits important enough to continue the program? Why? (Look at cost, productivity, and outcomes of care.)*

E. *Program effectiveness (summative)*
 1. *Satisfaction*
  a. *Is the client satisfied with the program as designed?*
  b. *Are the providers satisfied with the program outcomes?*
  c. *Is the community satisfied with the program outcomes?*
 2. *Goals*
  a. *Did the program meet its stated goal?*
  b. *Are the client needs being met?*
  c. *Was the problem solved for which the program was designed?*

F. *Impact (summative)*
 1. *Long-term changes in health status (1 year or more)*
  a. *Have there been changes in the community's health?*
  b. *What are the changes seen (e.g., in morbidity or mortality rates, teen pregnancy rates, pregnancy outcomes)?*
  c. *Have there been changes in individuals' health status?*
  d. *What are the changes seen?*
  e. *Has the initial problem been solved or has it returned?*
  f. *Is new or revised programming needed? Why?*
  g. *Should the program be discontinued? Why?*

G. *Sustainability*
 1. *Was the program funded as a demonstration or by an external agency?*
 2. *Can money and resources be found to continue the program after the initial funding is gone?*
 *Depending on the answers to the questions, the program can be found to be successful or unsuccessful.*

*Effectiveness and impact.* An evaluation of program effectiveness may help the nurse evaluator determine both client and provider satisfaction with the program activities, as well as whether the program met its stated objectives. However, if evaluation of impact is the goal, long-term effects such as changes in morbidity and mortality must be investigated. Both effectiveness and impact evaluations are usually summative evaluation functions primarily performed as end-of-program activities.

*Sustainability.* A program can be continued only if there are resources for the program. Ongoing evaluation of sustainability is important!

## ADVANCED PLANNING METHODS AND EVALUATION MODELS

After a need and a client demand for a program have been determined through the needs assessment process, the next step

in the development of the program is to choose a procedural method that will assist the nurse in planning the program to be offered. The following is offered for students who are more advanced in their career and need to consider several methods of program planning plus more extensive evaluation models for program management.

Five planning methods are discussed in this section:
1. Program planning method (PPM)
2. Multi-attribute utility technique (MAUT)
3. Planning Approach to Community Health (PATCH)
4. Assessment Protocol for Excellence in Public Health (APEXPH)
5. Mobilizing for Action through Planning and Partnership (MAPP)

PPM is a more general approach to program planning, whereas MAUT offers guidelines for identifying and tracking specific program activities essential to program success. PATCH,

APEXPH, and MAPP are PPMs that were designed by the CDC and the National Association of County Health Officials with input from local and state health departments. All of these approaches establish the basis for program evaluation.

## Program Planning Method

PPM is a technique using the nominal group technique described by Delbecq and Van de Ven in 1971. The nurse can use this method to involve clients more directly in the planning process. PPM is a five-stage process to identify program needs. It focuses on three levels of planning groups composed of clients, providers, and administrators. The client or consumer group relays a list of problems to the provider group, who in turn aids the client group by presenting the solutions to the problems to the administrative group (Issel, 2013).

The stages of PPM are compared with MAUT's planning process in Table 25-5. The five stages are as follows:
1. *Problem diagnosis.* Each client in the group works with all other members of the group to develop a written problem list, one problem at a time. After all problems have been shared and recorded, they are discussed by the total client group. After the discussion, clients select the problems with the highest priority by voting on the ranking of each problem.
2. *Expert provider group identifies solutions for each of the problems identified by the clients.*
3. *Client and provider groups present their problems and suggested solutions* to the administrative group to determine the possibilities of developing a program to resolve one or more of the problems using one or more of the solutions. In this phase, clients and providers are seeking acceptance from the administrators who control the program resources.
4. *Alternative solutions to the problem are identified,* and the pros and cons of each are analyzed.
5. *Clients, providers, and administrators select the best plan* for program implementation. In this phase, the link between

the planned solutions and the problem is evaluated, pointing out strengths and limitations of the proposed program plan.

A nurse might use this technique for developing school health services within the total community or in one school. A nurse working with a senior citizens group might use this method to identify the priority needs for nursing clinic services at the health department. It is important to note that this method is used to obtain consensus among all persons involved in the program: clients, providers, and administrators. Consensus is most helpful in having a successful program. The process may also be used in a community decision-making activity in which community representatives come together to decide health care service needs for the entire community.

## Multi-Attribute Utility Technique

MAUT is a planning method based on decision theory (Saaty and Vargus, 2013). This method can be adapted for making decisions about the care of a single client or about national health care programs. Recently it has been used to evaluate nursing practice. The purpose of MAUT is to separate all elements of a decision and to evaluate each element separately for its effects on the overall decision, considering available options.

If money is no object, then the option with the highest use value is the best decision. However, if this option exceeds the budget, the next best option may be the alternative to choose. The steps of MAUT (listed in Box 25-2) relate closely to the basic planning process described by Nutt (1984) as shown in Table 25-5.

Steps 1 and 2 of MAUT relate to problem formulating. Step 3 involves conceptualizing the program alternatives, and steps 4 through 9 focus on detailing and the implications of each option. Step 10 involves the evaluating phase of planning or the choice of the best solution as identified in steps 4 through 9. Placing quantitative values on solutions to meet program needs is most helpful in the implementing phase of planning

## TABLE 25-5  Planning Methods Compared with Basic Planning Process

| Basic Planning | PPM | PATCH | APEXPH | MAUT | MAPP |
|---|---|---|---|---|---|
| Formulating | Problems identified by client. | Community members identify health priorities. | Assess community capacity to address health problems. | Identify target populations and program objectives. | Assess community themes and strengths, health status, and strategic issues. |
| Conceptualizing | Provider group identifies solution. | Stakeholders use data to develop program activities. | Assess with community the strengths and health problems. | Identify alternative problem solutions. | Formulate goals and strategies. |
| Detailing | Analyze available solutions. | Design comprehensive program to meet identified health priorities. | Choose plan based on community capacity resources. | Identify criteria for choice; rank and weight; calculate value. | Develop plan for action; engage in visioning. |
| Evaluating | Clients, providers, and administrators select best plan. | Use process evaluation to improve program. | Support recommendations for program change. | Choose best alternatives. | Evaluate the plan. |
| Implementing | Best plan presented to administrators for funding. | | Partners implement the plan. | | Assess community ability to change and implement the plan. |

---

### BOX 25-2   Ten Basic Steps of the Multi-Attribute Utility Technique Method

1. Identify the person or aggregate for whom a problem is to be solved. Who is the client for whom the program is being planned?
2. Identify the issue(s) or decision(s) that is (are) relevant. This step involves the identification of the program objectives.
3. Identify the options to be evaluated. The program planner identifies the available options or action alternatives to accomplish the program goals.
4. Identify the relevant criteria related to the value of each option. The program planner places a value on competing options or alternatives or identifies criteria to be considered in making a choice between them.
5. Rank the criteria in order of importance. The program planner decides which of the criteria are most important and which are least important for meeting program goals.
6. Rate criteria in importance. In this step the program planner assigns an arbitrary rating of 10 to the least important criterion. In considering the next least important criterion, the planner decides how many times more important it is than the least important criterion. If it is considered twice as important, the dimension will be assigned a 20. If it is only considered half as important, it will be assigned a 15. If it is considered four times as important, it will be assigned a 40. The process is continued until all criteria have been rated.
7. Add the importance rate, divide each by the sum, and multiply by 100. This process is called *normalizing* the weights. It is recommended that the number of criteria be kept between 6 and 15. Therefore, in this initial process, the planner can be concerned with only general criteria for choosing action alternatives.
8. Measure the location of the option being evaluated by each criterion. The planner may ask a colleague or expert to estimate on a scale of 0 to 100 the probability that a given option from step 3 will maximize the value of the criterion from step 4.
9. Calculate the use of options. The program planner will obtain the usefulness of each identified action alternative by multiplying the weight for each criterion (step 7) by the rating of an option for each criterion (step 8) and adding the products. The sum of the products for each action is termed the *aggregate utility*.
10. Decide on the best alternative to meet the program objective. The action alternative with the highest aggregate use is considered the best decision for meeting the program objectives.

Kabassi K, Vroom M: MAUT and adaptive techniques for web based educational software. *Instruct Sci* 34(2):313–358, 2006.

(e.g., convincing administrators of the need for such a program). However, caution must be taken in using all planning methods, because the best solution reflects the bias of the planner.

### Planning Approach to Community Health (PATCH)

The PATCH model, which has not been emphasized as much in recent years, was developed in the 1980s by the CDC with input from state and local health departments. The model was developed using as a framework the PRECEDE model developed by Laurence Green in the 1970s. The PRECEDE model was used originally for planning health education programs (Glanz and Bishop, 2010).

Although this model was originally developed to strengthen health promotion activities, the PATCH model is used by communities and agencies to plan, develop, implement, and evaluate both health promotion and disease prevention programs. Application of PATCH emphasizes community participation and ownership by all who are involved. The PATCH process includes the following:

- Mobilizing the community
- Collecting and analyzing data to support local health issues
- Choosing health priorities
- Setting objectives and standards to denote progress and success
- Developing and implementing multiple intervention strategies to meet objectives
- Evaluating the process to detect the need for change
- Securing support of the public health infrastructure within the target community

These elements are essential to the success of any community-based program:

- Participation in the planning process by community members (stakeholders)
- Use of data to help stakeholders select health priorities and develop and evaluate program activities
- Development by stakeholders of a comprehensive approach to design the program to meet the identified health needs
- Use of process (formative) evaluation to improve the program and provide feedback to the stakeholders
- Increase in the capacity of the community to address a variety of health priorities by improving the health program planning skills of the stakeholders

The PATCH model has been useful in developing programs to address *Healthy People 2020* goals (http://www.cdc.gov). PATCH materials are available online at the CDC.

### Assessment Protocol for Excellence in Public Health (APEXPH)

Following the development of the PATCH model in 1987, the CDC, partnering with the National Association of City and County Health Officers (NACCHO) and other organizations, developed its APEXPH model. The model was introduced for use in 1999.

The APEXPH model incorporates the three core functions of public health in assessment, assurance, and policy development. Although the model was developed for use by local health departments, it can be adapted to fit other situations and resources. The model framework includes the following:

- Process for assessing agency organization and management
- Process for working with communities to assess the health of a community as well as a community's strengths and health problems
- Process for integrating plans for resolving health problems based on the capacity, resources, and community members partnering to implement the plan

This model uses the strategic planning process of Nutt (1984) and has three elements:

1. Assessing internal organization capacity to address the community's health problems
2. Assessing and priority setting for the community's health problems
3. Implementing the plan to address these problems

Application of the APEXPH process is useful for the following:
- Supporting recommendations for change in programs/services
- Highlighting the need for improvements in program functions

If APEXPH is applied along with the project budget process, key stakeholders may unite to discuss health and program priorities and options for providing services as well as to make plans for the year (http://www.cdc.gov). Workbooks and other resources are available through NACCHO at their website (http://www.naccho.org).

## Mobilizing for Action through Planning and Partnership (MAPP)

The strategic planning model MAPP can be applied at the community level to improve the community's health. Application of this model helps to identify public health issues and priorities and to identify resources to address the priorities.

As with PATCH and APEXPH, it is important that the community feels ownership of the process. The community's strengths, needs, and wishes are integral to the process.

Two figures (Figures 25-4 and 25-5) show the MAPP process and the community roadmap to a healthier community. The phases of the MAPP process are as follows:

A. Organize for success/partnership development.
　1. Organize agencies.
　2. Recruit partners.
　3. Prepare to implement MAPP.
B. Visioning.
　1. Work toward long-range goals through a shared vision and common values.

C. Engage in four assessment processes.
　1. Assess community themes and strengths.
　　a. Identify issues.
　　b. Identify interest to community.
　　c. Explore quality of life perceptions.
　　d. Identify community assets.

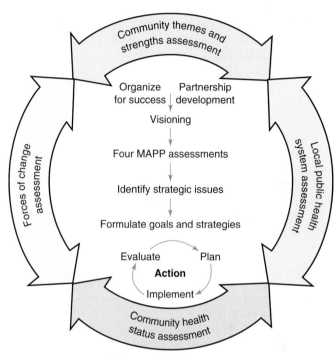

FIG 25-4 MAPP process.

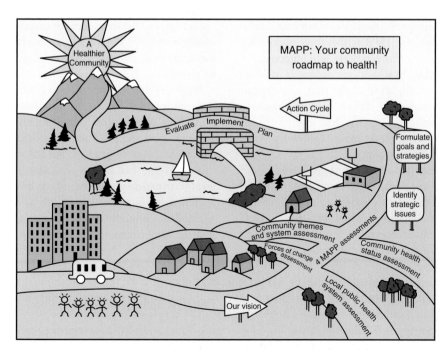

FIG 25-5 MAPP roadmap to community's health.

2. Assess local public health system.
    a. Identify all agencies and other partners who contribute to the public's health.
    b. Measure each partner's capacity to participate; what can each partner contribute?
    c. Measure the performance of each partner; how have they addressed issues in the past?
3. Assess the health status of the community.
    a. Assess available data.
    b. Assess quality of life.
    c. Assess community risk factors.
4. Assess ability of community to change.
    a. Identify forces for change.
    b. Identify forces against change.
D. Identify strategic issues.
    1. What are the health issues that need to be addressed?
    2. Which are the most important?
    3. Where should the community begin?
E. Formulate goals and strategies.
    1. Which goals will be met?
    2. Which strategies will be used to meet the goals?
F. Act.
    1. Participants develop plan for action.
    2. Implement the plan.
    3. Evaluate the implementation.

Two products are available to assist in implementing the MAPP process (Figure 25-4): the NACCHO website (see the WebLinks on this book's Evolve site) and the MAPP toolbox (http://www.naccho.org).

The five models of program planning presented here may be adapted to use with a single program or with a community.

## Evaluation Models and Techniques
### Structure-Process-Outcome Evaluation

The method for evaluation of programs by Donabedian (1982) was initially directed primarily toward medical care but is applicable to the broader area of health care. He describes three approaches to assessment of health care: structure, process, and outcome.

- Structure refers to settings in which care occurs. It includes materials, equipment, qualification of the staff, and organizational structure (Donabedian, 1982). This approach to evaluation is based on the assumption that, given a proper setting with good equipment, good care will follow. However, this assumption is not strongly supported.
- Process refers to whether the care that was given was "good" (Donabedian, 1982), competent, or preferred. Use of process in program evaluation may consist of observing practice but more likely consists of reviewing records. The review could focus on whether documentation of preventive teaching was on the clinical record. Audits using specific criteria are examples of the use of process.
- Outcome refers to results of client care and restoration of function and survival (Donabedian, 1982), but is also used in the sense of changes in health status or changes in health-related knowledge, attitude, and behavior. Thus program outcomes may be expressed in terms of mortality, morbidity, and disability for given populations, such as infants, but they could be expressed in a broader sense through health promotion behaviors such as weight control, exercise, and abstinence from tobacco and alcohol.

Donabedian's model of evaluating program quality is a popular model and is widely used for evaluation in the health care field. It can be useful in evaluating program effectiveness. The Center for Medicare and Medicaid Services and other third-party payers are currently placing more emphasis on outcome evaluation. It is essential that nurses begin to develop outcome criteria for client interventions.

### Tracer Method

The Board of Medicine of the National Academy of Sciences developed a program to evaluate health service delivery called the tracer method (Papanicolas and Smith, 2013). The tracer method of evaluation of programs is based on the premise that health status and care can be evaluated by viewing specific health problems called tracers. Just as radioactive tracers are used to study the thyroid gland, specific health problems are selected to evaluate the delivery of health and nursing services. Examples of conditions selected as tracers are cardiovascular disease, diabetes, obesity, smoking patterns, and breast and cervical cancer. This approach can be used to compare the following:

- Health status among different population groups and in different geographic locations
- Health status in relation to social status, economic level, medical care, nursing care, and behavioral variables
- Various arrangements for health care delivery

The tracer method is a useful technique for looking at the efficiency, effectiveness, and effect of a program.

### Case Register

Systematic registration of a contagious disease has been a practice for many years. Denmark began a national register of tuberculosis in 1921 (Friis and Sellers, 2010). Its contribution to the reduction in the incidence of contagious diseases has been widely recognized. Case registers (Issel, 2013) are also used for acute and chronic diseases (e.g., cancer and myocardial infarction).

Registers collect information from defined groups, and the information may be used for evaluating and planning services, preventing disease, providing care, and monitoring changes in patterns and care. The method is described here because of its use in evaluation of services. The answers to the questions listed in Box 25-3, asked before and after implementing a program, give information about the effects of the program. A tuberculosis register indicates the degree to which infection is being controlled. Cancer registers make state, regional, national, and international comparisons possible, and they provide clues to causes of disease. They are also used to direct the development of programs specific to population needs.

## PROGRAM FUNDING

Providing adequate funding for programs to meet the needs of populations can be a challenge to nurse managers in communities. When money is not available to support endeavors that

## BOX 25-3  Examples of Questions Asked About Cases for Case Register

1. What is the incidence of disease? What is the prevalence? What differences in incidence and prevalence are there between one community and another?
2. What percentage of clients recover? What percentage die?
3. Where does death occur?
4. How long do clients wait before contacting a health care provider?
5. How long is it before they are seen by a health care provider?
6. How many cases are associated with other major risk factors?
7. How many cases are associated with environmental factors such as water hardness or air pollution?
8. What happens after clients leave the hospital and when they return to work? Are there rehabilitation programs?
9. How many clients had been seen by a health care provider shortly before the problem occurred?
10. What prevention measures are taken for persons considered susceptible?

serve the public good, nonprofit organizations may seek funding from outside the organization. Such funding may be in the form of gifts, contracts, or grants.

Gifts are philanthropic contributions from individuals, foundations, businesses, religious or civic organizations, or voluntary associations. Many organizations engage in extensive development efforts to solicit monetary gifts that support the agency's goals. Contracts are awarded for the performance of a specific task or service, usually to meet guidelines specified by the organization making the award. Contracts are frequently used by the government to purchase services of others to perform certain services. Grants are awards to nonprofit organizations to allow recipients to implement activities of their own design that address the interests of the funding agency. Grants are given by the government, foundations, and corporations.

Nurse leaders working in nonprofit agencies may write grants to fund community programs that meet the needs of at-risk populations. Development of a proposal is guided by concepts and principles of program planning and evaluation that have been discussed in this chapter. Successful **grant writing** meshes the plan for the envisioned program of the applying organization with the criteria set forth by the funding agency. A grant proposal is a means of recording plans for establishing, managing, and evaluating a program into a written document. Funding agencies provide guidelines for grant applications, and it is essential to follow those specific guidelines if grant funding is to be acquired. In general, however, most grant proposals include certain essential components.

First, it is important to identify the target population and define the problem(s) that the project intends to address. Specific data, conditions, or circumstances that illustrate the problem and that document the need (e.g., environmental characteristics, economic conditions, population characteristics, and health status indicators) should be included and discussed. Health services should be discussed in relationship to availability, accessibility, and acceptability to the target population

within both the public and private sectors. Identification of duplication or gaps in services that result in unmet needs should be addressed.

The second component is the description of the program that is being proposed. The program description should provide details about what is planned, how it will be done, where it will be done, and by whom. This section should present the reviewer with a clear understanding of the details of the program structure and function. It should be apparent that the program is realistic and can be accomplished. This section includes goals, objectives, action steps, and anticipated outcomes that describe how, when, and by whom each activity will be accomplished to achieve the outcome of the objective for which it was written.

Plans for evaluation address the method that will be used to ensure ongoing and timely review of the specific action steps and objectives involved in achieving the stated goal (formative) and to assess program outcomes (summative).

Applicants for grant funds should develop a realistic operating budget that is appropriate to the requirements of the project. The budget represents the plan for how the program will be implemented and reflects the project's proposed spending plan.

## ⟫ LINKING CONTENT TO PRACTICE

Program planning skills and knowledge are essential for public health nurses. In *Public Health Nursing: Scope and Standards of Practice* (ANA, 2013), the first standard is that of assessment. This addresses the issue of conducting needs assessments and having the ability to collect multiple sources of data, analyze population characteristics, problem solve, and set priorities based on the data collected. Standard 2 speaks to using the assessment data to diagnosis health problems with input from the client population. Standards 3 through 5 address the nurses' roles in identifying health status outcomes, planning and implementing processes to address the health problem, and directing strategies to meet the outcomes. Standard 6 discusses the nurses' role in evaluation including participating in process and outcome evaluation by monitoring activities in programs.

The four professional organizations dedicated to public health nursing—The Association of State and Territorial Directors of Nursing (now APHN), The Association of Community Health Nursing Educators, The Public Health Nursing section of the APHA, and the American Nurses Association—have banned together to form an organization called the Quad Council. This council developed a document identifying the domains of practice for public health nurses. One of the domains is Policy Development and Program Planning Skills. The competencies the nurse needs for this domain of practice related to program management are:

- Manages public health programs consistent with public health laws and regulations.
- Develops a plan to implement policy and programs.
- Develops mechanisms to monitor and evaluate programs for their effectiveness and quality (Quad Council, 2011).

New baccalaureate nurses will want to be knowledgeable and be able to participate in program management; graduate nurses will want to be able to direct programs. Appendix B describes a Program Planning and Design process to use for practicing the content from this chapter. Try out this process on the development of a small program of interest to you and the client population you want to serve and the community level health problem of interest to you.

## PRACTICE APPLICATION

The following is a real-life example of the application of the program management process by an undergraduate nursing student. This activity resulted in the development and implementation of a nurse-managed clinic for the homeless. This example shows how students as well as providers can make a difference in health care delivery. It also illustrates that no mystery surrounds the program management process.

Eva was listening to the radio one Sunday afternoon and heard an announcement about the opening of a soup kitchen within the community for the growing homeless population. She was beginning her public health nursing course and wanted to find a creative clinical experience that would benefit herself as well as others. The announcement gave her an idea. Although it mentioned food, clothing, shelter, and social services, nothing was said about health care.

Eva was interested in finding a way to provide nursing and health care services at the soup kitchen. Which of the following should she do?

A. Talk with key leaders to determine their interest in her idea.
B. Review the literature to find out the magnitude of the problem.
C. Survey the community to determine if others are providing services.
D. Discuss the idea with members of the homeless population.
E. Consider potential solutions to the health care problems.
F. Consider where she would get the resources to open a clinic.
G. Talk with church leaders and nursing faculty members to seek acceptance for her idea.

**Answers can be found on the Evolve site.**

## KEY POINTS

- Planning and evaluation are essential elements of program management and vital to the survival of the nursing discipline in health care delivery.
- The program management process is population focused and is parallel to the nursing process. Both are rational decision-making processes.
- The health care delivery system has grown in the past century, making health planning and evaluation very important.
- Comprehensive health planning grew out of a need to control costs.
- A program is an organized approach to meet the assessed needs of individuals, families, groups, populations, or communities by reducing or eliminating one or more health problems and addressing health disparities.
- Planning is defined as selecting and carrying out a series of actions to achieve a stated goal.
- Evaluation is defined as the methods used to determine if a service is needed and will be used, whether a program to meet that need is carried out as planned, and whether the service actually helps the people it intended to help.
- To develop quality programs, planning should include four essential elements: assessment of need and problem diagnosis, identification of problem solutions, analysis and comparison of alternative methods, and selection of the best plan and planning methods.
- The initial and most critical step in planning a health program is assessment of need. Assessment focuses on the needs of the population who will use the services planned.
- Some of the major tools used in needs assessment are census data, community forums, surveys of existing community agencies, surveys of community residents, and statistical indicators about demographics, morbidity, and mortality of the population.

- The major benefit of program evaluation is to determine whether a program is fulfilling its stated goals. Quality assurance programs are prime examples of program evaluation.
- Plans for implementing and evaluating programs should be developed at the same time.
- Program records and community indexes and health data serve as major sources of information for program evaluation.
- Planning programs and planning for their evaluation are two of the most important ways in which nurses can ensure successful program implementation.
- Cost studies help identify program benefits, effectiveness, and efficiency.
- Program planning helps nurses and agencies focus attention on services that clients need.
- Planning helps everyone involved understand their role in providing services to clients.
- The assessment of need process provides an evaluation of the relevance that a new service may have to clients.
- A decision tree is a useful tool to choose the best alternative for solving a problem.
- Setting goals and writing objectives to meet the goals are necessary to evaluate program outcomes.
- *Healthy People 2020* is an example of a national program based on needs assessment that has stated goals and objectives on which the program can be evaluated.
- Program planning models include PPM, MAUT, PATCH, APEXPH, and MAPP.
- Program evaluation includes assessing structure, process, and outcomes of care.
- Grant writing is a tool used by nurse managers to provide resources for needed services.
- Grant proposals are documents that incorporate principles of program planning and evaluation.

## CLINICAL DECISION-MAKING ACTIVITIES

1. Choose the definitions that best describe your concepts of a program, planning, and evaluation. Explain how each of these definitions can help you in accomplishing planning and evaluation.
2. Apply the program planning process to an identified clinical problem for a client group with whom you are working in the community. Give specific examples.
   A. Assess the client needs and existing resources.
   B. Choose tools appropriate to the assessment of unmet needs.
   C. Analyze the overall planning process of arriving at decisions about implementing a program.
   D. Summarize the benefits for program planning that apply to your situation.
3. Given the situation just described, choose three or four of your classmates to work with you on the following projects:

A. Plan for evaluation of the program in activity 2.
B. Apply the evaluation process to the situation.
C. Identify the measures you will use to gather data for evaluating your program.
D. Identify the sources you will tap to gain information for program evaluation.
E. Analyze the benefits of program evaluation that apply to your situation.
F. Talk with a nurse or an administrator working in the community about the application of program planning and evaluation processes at the local agency. Compare their answers to your research. What are some of the difficulties that your group and the agency had in evaluating a program?

## REFERENCES

American Nurses Association: *ANA's nurses' efforts pay off in historic health care bill signing*, March 2010. Available at www.nurseworld.com/healthcarereform. Accessed February 18, 2011.

American Nurses Association: *Public Health Nursing: Scope and Standards of Practice*, ed 2. Silver Springs, MD, 2013, American Nurses Association.

American Planning Association: *Planning and community health research center 2013 annual report*, National Centers for Planning, 2013. Available at https://www.planning.org/nationalcenters/health/pdf/planningandcommhealthannualreport.pdf. Accessed July 31, 2014.

Brownson RC, Fielding JE, Maylahn CM: Evidence-based public health: a fundamental concept for public health practice. *Annu Rev Public Health* 30:175–201, 2009.

Centers for Disease Control and Prevention: *A framework for program evaluation*, 2012. Available at: www.cdc.gov. Accessed 10/12/2014.

Centers for Disease Control and Prevention: *Measles still threatens health security*, press release, 12/5/2013. Available at: www.cdc.gov. Accessed 10/12/2014.

Centers for Disease Control and Prevention: *A planning model*, 2014. Available at www.cdc.gov. Accessed 10/12/2014.

Centers for Disease Control and Prevention: *Conducting a community needs assessment*, field guidelines, 2014b. Available at www.cdc.gov. Accessed 10/12/2014.

Delbecq A, Van de Ven A: A group process model for problem identification and program planning. *J Appl Behav Sci* 7:466, 1971.

Donabedian A: *Explorations in Quality Assessment and Monitoring*, vol 2. Ann Arbor, MI, 1982, Health Administration Press.

Donabedian A: *An Introduction to Quality Assurance in Health Care*. New York, 2003, Oxford University Press.

Finkelstein SM, Speedie SM, Zhou X, et al: Perception, satisfaction and utilization of the VALUE home telehealth service. *J of Telemedicine and Telehealth* 17(6):288–292, 2011.

Friis RH, Sellers T: *Epidemiology for Public Health Practice*, ed 4. Sudbury, MA, 2010, Jones and Bartlett Publishers.

Glanz K, Bishop DB: The role of behavioral science theory in development and implementation of public health interventions. *Annu Rev Public Health* 31:399–418, 2010.

IHI: *Population health management* 2012. Available at www.ihealthtran.com. Accessed 10/12/2014.

Issel LM: *Health Program Planning and Evaluation: A Practical, Systematic Approach for Community Health*, ed 3. Boston, 2013, Jones and Bartlett.

Jefferson Area Board of Aging: What we do and who we are. *JABA facts*, 2010. Available at http://www.jabacares.org/. Accessed January 31, 2011.

Kabassi K, Vroom M: MAUT and adaptive techniques for web based educational software. *Instruct Sci* 34(2):313–358, 2006.

Kettner PM, Moroney RM, Martin LL: *Designing and Managing Programs: An Effectiveness-Based Approach*. Thousand Oaks, CA, 2012, Sage.

McDonald KM: *Closing the quality gap: a critical analysis of quality improvement strategies* (vol 7 care coordinators), 2007. Available at www.ncbi.nim.nih.gov. Accessed 10/12/2014.

NACCHO: *Definitions of community health assessments and community health improvement plans*, 2014. Avaliable at: www.naccho.org. Accessed 10/12/2-14.

Nutt P: *Planning Methods for Health and Related Organizations*. New York, 1984, Wiley.

Papanicolas I, Smith PC: *Health System Performance Comparison: An Agenda for Policy, Information and Research*. New York, NY, 2013, Open University Press.

Posavac EJ: *Program Evaluation: Methods and Case Studies*, ed 8. Englewood Cliffs, NJ, 2011, Prentice Hall.

Quad Council of Public Health Nursing Organization: *Quad Council competencies for public health nursing*, Summer 2011. Available at http://www.resourcecenter.net/images/ACHNE/Files/QuadCouncil CompetenciesForPublic HealthNurses_Summer2011.pdf. Accessed July 11, 2014.

Royse D, Thyer BA, Padgett DK: *Program Evaluation: An Introduction*, ed 5. Belmont, CA, 2010, Wadsworth.

Ruffolo DC, Andresen PA, Winn KL: Meeting the needs of a community: teaching evidence-based youth violence prevention

initiative to members of strategic communities. *J Trauma Nurs* 20(1):24–30, 2013.

Saaty TL, Vargas LG: *Decision Making with the Analytic Network Process*, ed 2. New York, NY, 2013, Springer.

Sanders G: *Introduction to medical decision making and decision analysis*, Duke University Raleigh, NC, 2009. Available at www.hsrd.research.va.gov. Accessed 10/12/2014.

Shin P, Sharac B, Barber Z, et al: *Community Health Centers: A 2013 Profile and Prospects as ACA Implementation Proceeds Mar 17, 2015*, Accessed at KFF.org. 4/1/2015.

Sparer MS: Health policy and health reform. In Kovner AR, Knickman JR, editors: *Jonas and Kovner's Health Care Delivery in the United States*, ed 10. New York, 2011, Springer.

Trickett EJ, Beehler S, Deutsch C, et al: Advancing the science of community-level interventions. *Am J Publ Health* 101(8):1410–1419, 2011.

University of North Carolina Health Services Library: *Finding information for a community health assessment*, 2014. Available at http://www.hsl.unc.edu/services/guides/communityHealth.cfm. Accessed January 31, 2011.

USDHHS: *Healthy People 2020: A Roadmap for Health*. Washington, DC, 2010, U.S. Government Printing Office.

USDHHS: *Introduction to Program Evaluation for Public Health Programs: A Self-Study Guide*. Atlanta, GA, 2011, Centers for Disease Control and Prevention.

# 26

# Quality Management

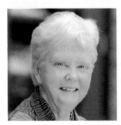

## Marcia Stanhope, PhD, RN, FAAN

Dr. Marcia Stanhope is currently an Associate of the Tufts and Associates Search Firm, Chicago, Ill. She is also a consultant for the nursing program at Berea College, Kentucky. She has practiced community and home health nursing, has served as an administrator and consultant in home health, and has been involved in the development of two nurse-managed centers. At one time in her career, she held a public policy fellowship and worked in the office of a U.S. Senator. She has taught community health, public health, epidemiology, policy, primary care nursing, and administration courses. Dr. Stanhope formerly directed the Division of Community Health Nursing and Administration and served as Associate Dean of the College of Nursing at the University of Kentucky. She has been responsible for both undergraduate and graduate courses in population-centered nursing. She has also taught at the University of Virginia and the University of Alabama, Birmingham. During her career at the University of Kentucky she appointed to the Good Samaritan Foundation Chair and Professorship in Community Health Nursing, and was honored with the University Provost's Public Scholar award. Her presentations and publications have been in the areas of home health, community health and community-focused nursing practice, as well as primary care nursing.

## ADDITIONAL RESOURCES

**ⓔ Evolve Website http://evolve.elsevier.com/Stanhope**
- *Healthy People 2020*
- Quiz
- WebLinks
- Case Studies

- Glossary
- Answers to Practice Application
- Resource Tools
  - Resource Tool 46.A: Core Competencies and Skills Levels for Public Health Nursing

## OBJECTIVES

*After reading this chapter, the student should be able to do the following:*

1. Explain differences in total quality management/continuous quality improvement (TQM/CQI).
2. Evaluate the role of QA/QI in CQI.
3. Analyze the historical development of the quality process in nursing and describe the changes developing under managed care.
4. Evaluate approaches and techniques for implementing CQI and the method of documentation.
5. Plan a model QA/QI program.
6. Identify the purposes for the types of records kept in community and public health agencies.

## KEY TERMS

accountability, p. 572
accreditation, p. 574
audit process, p. 580
certification, p. 575
charter, p. 575
client-centered care, p. 588
concurrent audit, p. 580
continuous quality improvement, p. 569
credentialing, p. 574
evaluative studies, p. 582
evidence-based practice, p. 588
licensure, p. 574
malpractice litigation, p. 584
managed care, p. 571
managed care organizations (MCOs), p. 570
Nurse Licensure Compact Administrators (NLCA), p. 574

outcome, p. 582
partnerships, p. 571
practice guidelines, p. 578
peer review organization (PRO), p. 573
process, p. 582
professional review organizations (PRO), p. 581
Professional Standards Review Organization (PSRO), p. 581
quality assurance/quality improvement (QA/QI), p. 572
quality improvement, p. 570
quality improvement organization (QIO), p. 573
recognition, p. 575
records, p. 587
report cards, p. 570
retrospective audit, p. 580
risk management, p. 581
safety, p. 588

## CHAPTER OUTLINE

**Definitions and Goals**
**Historical Development**
**Approaches to Quality Improvement**
   General Approaches
   Specific Approaches
**TQM/CQI in Community and Public Health Settings**
   Using QA/QI in CQI
   Traditional Quality Assurance
**Client Satisfaction**
   Malpractice Litigation

**Model CQI Program**
   Structure
   Process
   Outcome
   Evaluation, Interpretation, and Action
**Records**
   Community and Public Health Agency Records

Although the concept of quality assurance has been a part of the health care arena for a number of years, it is only in the last few years that major movement to improve health care quality has begun in the United States. The Institute of Medicine (IOM, 2001), not confident of the health care systems' ability to deliver the quality of care expected, set forth a series of recommendations to transform systems to meet Americans' expectations. Very little is known about quality of care in this country for two reasons: (1) a variety of definitions of *quality* are used, and (2) it is difficult to obtain comparable data from all providers and health care agencies.

However, in the Healthcare Research and Quality Act of 1999 (PL 106-129), Congress mandated that the Agency for Healthcare Research and Quality (AHRQ) produce an annual report on health care quality in the United States beginning in fiscal year 2003. This National Healthcare Quality Report (NHQR) is a collaborative effort among the agencies of the U.S. Department of Health and Human Services (USDHHS) and includes a broad set of performance measures that will be used to monitor the nation's progress toward improved health care quality. The NHQR represents the broadest examination of quality of health care, in terms of number of measures and number of dimensions of care, ever undertaken in the United States. The report represents progress toward improving quality as well as recommendations for how to improve quality outcomes (USDHHS, 2014).

The NHQR is intended to serve a number of purposes, such as demonstrating the validity (or lack) of concerns about quality; documenting whether health care quality is stable, improving, or declining over time; and providing national benchmarks against which specific states, health plans, and providers can compare their performance (AHRQ, 2014b; NCQA, 2013a).

In a changing health care market, the demand for quality has become a rallying point for health care consumers. All consumers, including private citizens, insurance companies, industry, and the federal government, are concerned with the highest quality outcomes at the lowest cost (Clancy and Lloyd, 2011). In addition to the demand for higher quality and lower cost, the public wants health care delivered with greater access, and health care that is accountable, efficient, and effective. Moreover, consumers want information about quality. Information is empowering to the consumer. With the expanded use of the Internet, access to information about quality in health care is readily available, ranging from talking to consumers about quality health care (http://www.talkingquality.gov) to clinical practice guidelines that promise to improve care for all (http://www.guideline.gov). **Total quality management** (TQM) is a management philosophy that includes a focus on client, **continuous quality improvement** (CQI), and teamwork (Kelly, 2011). Although relatively new in public health care, the concepts of TQM/CQI have been tried and proven in industry at large. The terms *total quality management, continuous quality improvement, total quality,* and *organization-wide quality improvement* are often used interchangeably. However, they have different meanings. As indicated, TQM refers to a management philosophy that focuses on the statistical processes by which to assess work done with the goal of organization-wide quality effectiveness. TQM is often referred to as TQ, and both acronyms have the same meaning. CQI, while different from the other three terms, can be implemented not only to address system problems, but also to maintain and enhance good performance through the use of differing techniques. Everyone in the public health or community-based organization is involved in CQI—the leaders, the staff, and the client. By obtaining facts about work processes (e.g., all the steps in certifying a child for the women, infants, and children nutritional program [WIC]), it is possible to discover which steps are unnecessary (i.e., non–value adding) and to eliminate those steps to produce better health outcomes for individuals and communities (Oakland,

| BOX 26-1 | **Commonly Used Abbreviations** |
| --- | --- |
| AACN | American Association of Colleges of Nursing |
| ACHNE | Association of Community Health Nursing Educators |
| AHRQ | Agency for Healthcare Research and Quality (formerly AHCPR) |
| ANA | American Nurses Association |
| APHA | American Public Health Association |
| CCNE | Commission on Collegiate Nursing Education |
| CHAP | Community Health Accreditation Program |
| CMS | Centers for Medicare and Medicaid Services (formerly HCFA) |
| CQI | Continuous Quality Improvement |
| HEDIS | Health Plan Employer Data and Information Set |
| IOM | Institute of Medicine |
| JCAHO | Joint Commission on Accreditation of Healthcare Organizations |
| MCO | Managed Care Organization |
| NCQA | National Committee for Quality Assurance |
| NHQR | National Healthcare Quality Report |
| NLN | National League for Nursing |
| NPHPSP | National Public Health Performance Standards Program |
| OCQI | Outcomes-Based Quality Improvement |
| QA | Quality Assurance |
| QI | Quality Improvement |
| QIO | Quality Improvement Organization |
| TQI | Total Quality Improvement |
| TQM | Total Quality Management |

2014). Box 26-1 presents several abbreviations that are commonly used in health care and quality management.

Both consumers and providers have a vested interest in the quality of the health care system to do the following:

1. Improve safety of care to save lives
2. Reduce costs by using effective interventions
3. Increase client confidence in health care delivery regardless of setting (NQF, 2010)

Kovner and Jonas state that in health care there is a direct link between doing a good job and individual and professional survival. Health care providers pride themselves on individual achievement and responsibility for good client outcomes (Kovner and Knickman, 2011). Health care organizations are natural extensions of health care providers and thus can demonstrate their responsibility for optimal outcomes through a rigorous quality improvement process. The application of quality improvement strategies through the following six areas of performance could affect both process and outcomes of health care:

1. Consistently providing appropriate and effective care
2. Reducing unjustified geographic variation in care
3. Eliminating avoidable mistakes
4. Lowering access barriers
5. Improving responsiveness to clients
6. Eliminating racial/ethnic, gender, socioeconomic, and other disparities and inequalities in access and treatment (USDHHS, 2011a)

In the 1990s the United States entered a new era of population-centered, community-controlled delivery of care in which managed care organizations (MCOs) played an integral role. MCOs are agencies such as health maintenance organizations (HMOs) and preferred provider organizations (PPOs)

designed to monitor and deliver health care services within a specific budget. Currently providers, clients, payers, and policy makers all have input into the quality measurement process. The Health Plan Employer Data and Information Set (HEDIS), a data collection arm of the National Committee for Quality Assurance (NCQA), provides performance information, or report cards, for 90 percent of America's health plans. In 2012, 538 health insurance plans, including HMOs and PPOs, reported audited HEDIS data to show the level of quality performance (NCQA, 2013b). In the ACA (KHN, 2014) accountable care organizations (ACO) are being promoted. The ACO may involve a network of physicians.

Although introduced in the 1990s, report cards for public health agencies are currently being developed and promoted to measure quality health care in communities. The term *community health report card* refers to different types of reports, community health profiles, needs assessments, scorecards, quality of life indicators, health status reports, and progress reports. All of these reports are critical components of community-based approaches to improving the health and quality of life of communities (UK, 2014).

An example at the national level is the Community Health Status Indicator (CHSI) Project, which is a collaborative effort between the Health Resources and Services Administration (HRSA), the Association of State and Territorial Health Officials (ASTHO), the National Association of County and City Health Officials (NACCHO), and the Public Health Foundation. In 2000, the project published and disseminated community health status reports for all U.S. counties. These reports provided county-level data, including peer county and national comparisons, for every county in the country. The goal of CHSI is to provide an overview of key health indicators for local communities and to encourage dialogue about actions that can be taken to improve a community's health. The CHSI report was designed not only for public health professionals, but also for members of the community who are interested in the health of their community. They are designed to support health planning by local health departments, local health planners, community residents, and others interested in community health improvement. The CHSI report contains over 200 measures for each of the 3141 U.S. counties. Although CHSI presents indicators like deaths resulting from heart disease and cancer, it is imperative to understand that behavioral factors such as tobacco use, diet, physical activity, alcohol and drug use, and sexual behavior substantially contribute to these deaths (NICHSR, 2012).

These community health improvement initiatives have grown out of three major trends: (1) an increasing recognition of the importance of local community action to solve local problems, (2) an increasing emphasis on outcomes and accountability, and (3) the Healthy Cities/Healthy Communities movement (see Chapter 20). The Healthy Cities/Healthy Communities movement views community health and its determinants broadly, and they use a set of indicators (to track their progress) that reflects this broad definition. These indicators might include the following:

- Physical and mental health status
- Educational achievement
- Economic prosperity

- Public safety
- Adequate housing and transportation
- A clean and safe physical environment
- Recreational and cultural opportunities (Braunstein and Lavizzo-Mourey, 2011)

Community health report cards can be a useful tool in efforts to help identify areas where change is needed, to set priorities for action, and to track changes in population health over time. The report card may be used to track leading causes of morbidity and mortality in a community, looking at trends over time to see if public health interventions have improved health care outcomes. The card may also be used to assess a specific chronic disease, like diabetes, to determine the health status of the community for this particular disease (CDC, 2010). The report card may be used as an internal measure of public health program outcomes and CQI measures within the agency (Gunzenhauser et al, 2010).

In 2014, HEDIS measures of care included several that address public health issues, including BMI reduction and maintenance, smoking or tobacco use quit rates, and physical activity levels (NCQA, 2014).

As a part of a movement to provide quality health care in communities, health departments are increasingly examining their place in promoting quality (CDC, 2014). Sollecito and Johnson (2013) state that public health and CQI are connected because of the use of systems approaches that public health takes in identifying problems and developing interventions. Aspects of planning, implementing, and evaluating by TQM fall under each of the core public health functions of assessment, assurance, and policy development. However, it is with the assurance core function, related to ensuring available access to the health care services essential to sustain and improve the health of the population, that TQM programs must be undertaken. Public health cannot ensure services that improve health if those services lack quality. Public health will want to maintain quality in its workforce and continually evaluate the effectiveness of its services whether service is delivered to the individual, the community, or the population.

At least four documents provide report cards on how well the United States is performing on improving safety of health care delivery, quality of and access to care across population groups, progress and opportunities for improving health care quality, and the state of health care quality. These reports are published regularly by the Agency for Health Care Research and Quality, the National Quality Forum, and the National Committee for Quality Assurance.

Nurses are in a perfect position to implement strategies to improve population-centered health care. Community assessments, identification of high-risk individuals, use of targeted interventions, case management, and management of illnesses across a continuum of care are strategies suggested as part of the focus in improving the health of communities (Quad Council of Public Health Nursing Organizations, 2011). These strategies have long been used by nurses.

The growth of the managed care industry has changed the face of health care in the United States, both in how health care is delivered and in how it is received by consumers. Consumers are forming partnerships in communities to counteract the

power of MCOs by holding them accountable for health outcomes in relation to costs. The ACA's (KHN 2014) emphasis on ACOs is promoting the managed care approach to health care delivery with quality indicators. Partnerships are using data-based community assessments to improve health and to ensure that communities receive quality services. Projects are being funded to meet this goal (Kresge Foundation, 2014).

Because of managed care agencies and consumer demands for quality nursing, objective and systematic evaluation of nursing care is a priority for the nursing profession. Since organized nursing is committed to direct individual accountability, is evolving as a scientific discipline, and is concerned about how costs of health services limit access, it demands delivery and evaluation of quality service aimed at superior client outcomes (ANA, 2009). In the public health arena, the Quad Council of Public Health Nursing Organizations (2011), which includes four nursing organizations—the ANA, the Association of Community Health Nursing Educators, the APHA public health nurses, and the Association of Public Health Nurses—has identified competencies for public health nursing based on the Council on Linkages Between Academia and Public Health Practice document of 2008 with the most recent update on these competencies occurring in 2014 (Council on Linkages). Other states have developed models to document outcomes attributable to nursing interventions and are adding methods for evaluating total quality (Minnesota Department of Health, 2001; Keller et al, 2004a, 2004b; Sakamoto and Avila, 2004; Smith and Bazini-Barakat, 2004; University of Wisconsin-Madison, 2010). Box 26-2 is a list of the areas of nursing interventions that nurses will want to be able to use. (See Chapter 9 for the most recent updates on the Keller et al model of the Intervention Wheel.)

### BOX 26-2   The Areas of Public Health Nursing Interventions for Quality Population-Centered Health Care

| Interventions | Chapter |
|---|---|
| Advocacy | 5, 6, 10, 16, 22, 30, 32, 34, 37, 46 |
| Case finding | 22, 32, 33, 42 |
| Case management | 19, 22, 30, 32, 33, 42, 46 |
| Coalition building | 8, 18, 20 |
| Collaborating | 21, 22, 26, 32, 39, 41, 45 |
| Community organizing | 18, 20 |
| Consulting | 40, 41 |
| Counseling | 9, 14, 30, 32, 36, 39, 42, 45, 46 |
| Delegated functions | 40, 41 |
| Disease and health event investigation | 12, 13, 14, 23, 24 |
| Health teaching | 9, 13, 14, 16, 17, 20, 36, 38, 39, 40, 42, 43, 44, 45 |
| Outreach | 33, 35, 46 |
| Policy development and enforcement | 1, 8, 10, 18, 27, 30, 33 |
| Referral and follow-up | 10, 22, 27, 28, 32, 46 |
| Social marketing | 13, 18, 34, 38 |
| Survey | 18, 24 |

From Minnesota Department of Health, Division of Community Health Services: Public health interventions: applications for public health nursing practice, St Paul, MN, March 2001, p 1, Public Health Nursing Section.

The competencies for public health leadership developed by the Council on Linkages (2001, updated 2014) are crucial to ensure the quality and performance of the public health workforce. See Resource Tool 46.A on the Evolve website for a list of the competencies.

Records are maintained on all health care system clients to provide complete information about the client and to show the quality of care being given to the client within the system. Records are a necessary part of a CQI process, as are the tools and methods for evaluating quality. Electronic health records are becoming more common and are aiding in decreasing errors, increasing quality, and monitoring interventions (Keyser et al, 2009).

## DEFINITIONS AND GOALS

The IOM definition of quality is "the degree to which health services for individuals and populations increase the likelihood of desired health outcomes and are consistent with current professional knowledge" (2001, p. 1000; 2011). The AHRQ defines quality health care as doing the right thing, for the right client, and having the best possible results (2014a). Quality in public health is defined as "the degree to which policies, programs, services, and research for the population increase desired health outcomes and conditions in which the population can be healthy" (IOM, 2013, p. 3).

However, a definition of quality rests largely on the perception of the client, the provider, the care manager, the purchaser, the payer, or the public health official. Whereas the physician views quality in a more technical sense, the client may look at the personal outcome; the manager, purchaser, or payer may consider the cost-effectiveness; and the public health official will look at the appropriate use of health care resources to improve population health (AHRQ, 2012).

According to the AHRQ (2012), problems with quality of care were divided into five groups: variation of service, underuse of service, overuse of service, misuse of service, and disparities in quality. Variation in service refers to the lack of standards of practice continuity. This variation is often seen between regional, state, and local health care services and stems from lack of evolutionary health care practice and not keeping abreast of the constant changes taking place in health care (evidence-based practice) (NCQA, 2013b; IOM, 2011). Underuse of service refers to conservative treatment practices. As an example, there is a lack of immunizations for pneumonia given to Asians 65 years or older as a preventive measure as compared with immunization levels of whites (AHRQ, 2014b). Overuse of service refers to the over-ordering of unnecessary tests, surgeries, and treatments. This overuse drives up the cost of already expensive health care. Misuse of service refers to client safety issues and how disability and mortality can be reduced. With diligent care by health care providers, client injury and death can be avoided (IOM, 2011). Disparities in quality refer to racial, ethnic, and socioeconomic disparities in accessibility and affordability of health care (AHRQ, 2014b).

The term *health services* applies to a wide range of health delivery institutions. Of particular interest to public health is the question of access to appropriate and needed services, a well-prepared workforce, and improvement in the status of the population's health. Client satisfaction and well-being and the processes of client–provider interaction should be considered as well.

TQM is a process-driven, customer-oriented management philosophy that includes leadership, teamwork, employee empowerment, individual responsibility, and continuous improvement of system processes to yield improved outcomes (Oakland, 2014). Under TQM, quality is defined as customer satisfaction. Quality assurance/quality improvement (QA/QI) is the promise or guarantee that certain standards of excellence are being met in the delivery of care. Van den Heuvel, Niemeijer, and Does (2013) discuss what is called the *Juran trilogy*. This consists of quality planning, quality control, and quality improvement. This trilogy combines components of QA as well as CQI to improve client outcomes in health care delivery.

QI is defined as "systematic and continuous actions that lead to measureable improvement in health care services and the health status of targeted patient groups" (USDHHS, 2011b). QI in public health is the use of a deliberate and defined improvement process, such as plan-do-check-act (PDCA), which is focused on activities that are responsive to community needs and improving population health. It refers to a continuous and ongoing effort to achieve measurable improvements in the efficiency, effectiveness, performance, accountability, outcomes, and other indicators of quality in services or processes that achieve equity and improve the health of the community (Bialek et al, 2010).

QA is concerned with the accountability of the provider and is only one tool in achieving the best client outcomes. Accountability means being responsible for care and answerable to the client (Sollecito and Johnson, 2013). Under QA/QI, quality may have a variety of definitions. According to Kaplan and colleagues (2010), QA should consist of peer review leading to QI to improve health care delivery. Client standards of care and safety issues are the core of QA.

The AHRQ has indicated that the assurance of quality is organized around four dimensions (effectiveness, client safety, timeliness, and client centeredness) and is assessed using four stages of care [staying healthy (primary prevention), getting better (secondary prevention), living with illness or disability, and coping with end of life (tertiary prevention)] (AHRQ, 2014b, 2014c).

Quality traditionally has been an important issue in the delivery of health care. QA programs historically have ensured this accountability. The goals of QA and QI are on a continuum of quality, and in public health they are (1) to continuously improve the timeliness, effectiveness, safety, and responsiveness of programs, and (2) to optimize internal resources to improve the health of the community (Riley et al, 2010).

Under a CQI philosophy, QA and QI are but two of the many approaches used to ensure that the health care agency fulfills what the client thinks are the requirements for the service. QA focuses on finding what providers have done wrong in the past (e.g., deviations from a standard of care found through a chart audit). CQI operates at a higher level on the quality continuum but requires the commitment of more organization resources to move in a positive direction. CQI focuses on the sources of differences in the ongoing process of health care delivery and seeks to improve the process (Kelly, 2011; Sullivan, 2013).

The process of health care includes two major components: technical interventions (e.g., how well procedures are accomplished, accurate assessments, and effective interventions) and interpersonal relationships between public health practitioner and client. Both contribute to quality care, and both can be evaluated. Several approaches and techniques are used in quality programs. *Approaches* are methods used to ensure quality, and *techniques* are tools for measuring differences in quality (Kovner and Knickman, 2011).

Traditional approaches to quality focus on assessing or measuring performance, ensuring that performance conforms to standards, and providing remedial work to providers if those standards are not met. Such a definition of quality is too narrow in health care systems that try to meet the needs of many clients, both internal and external to the agency. CQI requires constant attention and should involve surveillance of all records while there is still the opportunity to intervene in both the client's care and the practitioner's actions. Comprehensive data analysis is necessary to detect process failure. Many agencies use some of the TQM/CQI concepts, such as client satisfaction questionnaires, but have not adopted the entire management philosophy. However, because QA/QI methods have traditionally been used and are still in use in many agencies, the QA/QI concepts will be covered.

 **HEALTHY PEOPLE 2020**

Goal of Improving Access to Comprehensive, High-Quality Health Care, and Examples of Objectives to Eliminate Health Disparities
- AHS-1: Increase the proportion of persons with health insurance.
- AHS-5: Increase the proportion of persons who have a specific source of ongoing care.
- AHS-7: Increase the proportion of persons who receive evidence-based clinical preventive services.

From U.S. Department of Health and Human Services: Healthy People 2020, Washington, DC, 2010, U.S. Government Printing Office.

## HISTORICAL DEVELOPMENT

Improving the quality of care has been a part of nursing since the days of Florence Nightingale. In 1860 Nightingale called for the development of a uniform method to collect and present hospital statistics to improve hospital treatment. Nightingale was a pioneer in setting standards for nursing care. The movement to establish nursing schools in the United States came in the late 1800s from a desire to set standards that would upgrade nursing care. In the early 1900s efforts were begun to set similar standards for all nursing schools. From 1912 to 1930 interest in quality nursing education led to the development of nursing organizations involved in accrediting nursing programs. Licensure has been a major issue in nursing since 1892. By 1923 all states had permissive or mandatory laws directing nursing practice.

After World War II, the attention of the emerging nursing profession focused on establishing a scientific method of practice. The nursing process was the chosen method and included evaluation of how nursing activities helped clients (Maibusch, 1984). QA/QI was the evaluative step in the nursing process.

The 1950s brought the development of QA measurement tools. One of the first tools was Phaneuf's nursing audit method (1965), which has been used extensively in population-centered nursing practice.

In 1966, the American Nurses Association (ANA) created the Divisions on Practice. As a result, in 1972, the Congress for Nursing Practice was charged with developing standards to institute QA programs. The Standards for Community Health Nursing Practice were distributed to ANA Community Health Nursing Division members in 1973. In 1986, 1999, and in 2005, with updates in 2007 and 2013, the scope and standards were again revised with a change in focus from community health nursing to public health nursing.

In 1972, the Joint Commission on Accreditation of Hospitals (JCAH) clearly stated the responsibilities of nursing in its description of standards for nursing services. The JCAH called on the nursing industry to clearly plan, document, and evaluate nursing care provided. In the mid-1980s, the JCAH became the Joint Commission on Accreditation of Healthcare Organizations (JCAHO) and began developing quality control standards for hospital and home health nursing. JCAHO is now known as The Joint Commission (TJC) and presently incorporates CQI principles in its standards.

Also in 1972, the Social Security Act (PL 92-603) was amended to establish the Professional Standards Review Organization (PSRO) and to mandate the process review of the delivery of health care to clients of Medicare, Medicaid, and maternal and child health programs. The PSRO program later became the Peer Review Organization (PRO) under the 1983 Social Security amendments. The purpose of the PROs was to monitor the implementation of the prospective reimbursement system for Medicare clients (the diagnosis-related groups [DRGs]). Although PSROs were intended for physicians, PROs made QI a primary issue for all health care professionals. The PRO was renamed the QIO, or the quality improvement organization (QIO), and is mandated to improve the quality and efficiency of Medicare funded services (CMS, 2014a).

In response to increasing charges of malpractice, the government passed the National Health Quality Improvement Act of 1986. Although it was not funded until 1989, its two major goals were to encourage consumers to become informed about their practitioner's practice record and to create a national clearinghouse of information on the malpractice records of providers. The emphasis of this act continued to be on the structure of care rather than the process or outcomes of care (NAHQ, 1993; Zale and Selvan, 2009). (See Chapter 25 for discussion of structure, process, and outcome.)

Efforts to strengthen nursing practice in the community have been carried out by several nursing organizations, including the ANA, the Public Health Nursing Section of the American Public Health Association (APHA), the Association of State and Territorial Directors of Nursing (now APHN), and the Association of Community Health Nursing Educators (ACHNE). The quality of nursing education is a major concern of the ACHNE, which was established in 1978. In 1993, 2000, 2003, and 2007, five reports published by this organization identified the curriculum content required to prepare nursing students for practice in the community (ACHNE, 1993, 2000a/2009, 2000b, 2003, 2007). In 2005, and again in 2007, the Quad Council reviewed scopes and standards of population-focused (public health) and community-based nursing practice and developed new standards to guide the profession in obtaining the best health outcomes for the populations they serve. These standards were updated again in 2013. QA/QI programs remain the enforcers of standards of care for many agencies that have not elected to engage in a program of CQI. These activities are called *assurance activities* because they make certain that those policies and procedures are followed so that appropriate quality services are delivered.

The Council on Linkages between Academia and Public Health Practice (the Council) is a coalition of representatives from 17 national public health organizations. Since 1992, the Council has worked to further academic/practice collaboration to ensure a well-trained, competent workforce and a strong, evidence-based public health infrastructure. The Council is funded by the CDC and staffed by the Public Health Foundation. The most recent core competencies were updated in 2014. These competencies are used in QA/QI as performance measurements of providers to ensure quality of services (Council on Linkages, 2014).

## APPROACHES TO QUALITY IMPROVEMENT

Two basic approaches exist in QI: *general* and *specific*. The general approach involves a large governing or official body's evaluation of a person's or agency's ability to meet criteria or standards. Specific approaches to QI are methods used to manage a specific health care delivery system in an attempt to deliver care with outcomes that are acceptable to the consumer. QA/QI programs that evaluate provider and client interaction through compliance with standards historically have been used alone to monitor quality care. In a TQM approach, CQI with QA/QI methods are an integral, but not the only, tool for ensuring quality or customer satisfaction.

### General Approaches

General approaches to protect the public by ensuring a level of competency among health care professionals are *credentialing, licensure, accreditation, certification, charter, recognition,* and *academic degrees.* Although there has been a long history of public oversight of quality in the United States, this public oversight increasingly involves the private sector. Public oversight for quality emerged when the private market failed to focus on health care quality. Previously mentioned reports about quality are indicators of public sector involvement in public oversight of quality.

**Credentialing** is generally defined as the formal recognition of a person as a professional with technical competence, or of an agency that has met minimum standards of performance.

These mechanisms are used to evaluate the agency structure through which care is provided and the outcomes of care given by the provider. Credentialing can be mandatory or voluntary. Mandatory credentialing requires laws. State nurse practice acts are examples of mandatory credentialing. Voluntary credentialing is performed by an agency or an institution. The certification examinations offered by the ANA through the American Nurses Credentialing Center are examples of voluntary credentialing. Licensing, certification, and accreditation are all examples of credentialing (ANCC, 2014).

**Licensure** is one of the oldest general QA approaches in the United States and Canada. Individual licensure is a contract between the profession and the state. Under this contract, the profession is granted control over entry into, and exit from, the profession and over quality of professional practice (NCSBN, 2014a).

The licensing process requires that written regulations define the scope and limits of the professional's practice. Job descriptions based on these regulations set minimum and maximum limits on the functions and responsibilities of the practitioner. Licensure of nurses has been mandated by law since 1903. Today all 50 states have mandatory nurse licensure, which requires all individuals who practice nursing, whether it be for money or as a volunteer, to be licensed. A new approach to interstate practice requires a pact between states so that nurses can practice across state borders (NCSBN, 2014b). Although reciprocity (which means nurses can have their license accepted through an application process if there is agreement between the states requiring application) exists among states for nursing licensure, interstate practice without approval is an issue for state boards of nursing. The states' compact agreements were to reduce the barriers for interstate practice. The mutual recognition model of nurse licensure allows a nurse to have one license (in his or her state of residency) and to practice in other states (both physically and electronically when giving advice through programs like "ask a nurse"), subject to each state's practice law and regulation. Under mutual recognition, a nurse may practice across state lines unless otherwise restricted. This is referred to as a multistate nurse licensure model, specifically referred to as the Nurse Licensure Compact (NLC). All states that currently belong to the NLC also operate the single-state licensure model for those nurses who do not reside legally in an NLC state or do not qualify for multistate licensure. To achieve mutual recognition, each state must enact legislation or regulation authorizing the NLC. States entering the compact also adopt administrative rules and regulations for implementation of the compact.

Once the compact is enacted, each compact state designates a Nurse Licensure Compact Administrator to facilitate the exchange of information between the states relating to compact nurse licensure and regulation. On January 10, 2000, the **Nurse Licensure Compact Administrators (NLCA)** were organized to protect the public's health and safety by promoting compliance with the laws governing the practice of nursing in each party state through the mutual recognition of party state licenses (NCSBN, 2014b).

**Accreditation**, a voluntary approach to QI, is used for institutions. Since 1954 the National League for Nursing (NLN), a voluntary organization, has had established standards for inspecting nursing education programs. In 1997 the NLN board established an accrediting body as an independent organization: the NLN Accrediting Commission (NLNAC). The name of this organization is now the Accreditation Commission for Nursing Education (ACEN) (NLN, 2014). In 1997 the American Association of Colleges of Nursing (AACN), also a voluntary organization supporting baccalaureate and higher degree programs, established an affiliate—the Commission on Collegiate Nursing Education (CCNE)—to accredit baccalaureate and higher degree nursing programs (CCNE, 2014). In 1966 community health/home health program standards were established by the NLN for the purpose of accrediting these programs through their Community Health Accreditation Program, now an independent organization (CHAP, 2014). In addition, state boards of nursing accredit basic nursing programs so that their graduates are eligible for the licensing examination. In some states, state boards of nursing accredit graduate programs.

The accreditation function is quasi-voluntary. Although accreditation appears to be a voluntary program, it is often linked to government regulation that encourages programs to participate in the accrediting process. Examples include the federal Medicare regulations restricting payments only to accredited public health and home health care agencies (CMS, 2014b).

Accreditation, whether voluntary or required, provides a means for effective peer review and an opportunity for in-depth review of program strengths and limitations. Accreditation applies external pressure and places demands on institutions to improve quality of care. In the past, the accreditation process primarily evaluated an agency's physical structure, organizational structure, and personnel qualifications. However, beginning in 1990, more emphasis was placed on evaluation of the outcomes of care and on the educational qualifications of the person providing the care.

In the past there has not been a mechanism for accrediting public health agencies. In 2007 the Public Health Accreditation Board (PHAB) was incorporated, after public health leaders explored the feasibility of a national accreditation program. The field saw the need for, and value of, public health accreditation, and advocated for the implementation of a national voluntary program. The PHAB was developed in accordance with the recommendations generated by the Exploring Accreditation Steering Committee. The Steering Committee was comprised primarily of state and local public health officials, including boards of health. The committee called on the expertise from other specialty areas engaged in accreditation. The PHAB is a nonprofit organization and is developing and testing national standards and processes that will be used to assess the strengths and areas for improvement in public health (PHAB, 2014).

The PHAB mission is to promote and protect the health of the public by advancing the quality and performance of *all* public health departments in the United States. The PHAB works toward creating a high-performing public health system that will make the United States the healthiest nation. The CDC and the Robert Wood Johnson Foundation are funders, and

partners, of PHAB. The goal is for the accreditation program and the accrediting process, which began in 2011, to be self sustaining.

Certification, another general approach to quality, combines features of licensure and accreditation. Certification is usually a voluntary process within professions. Educational achievements, experience, and performance on an examination determine a person's qualifications for functioning in an identified specialty area. The American Nurses Credentialing Center provides certification in several areas of nursing (ANCC, 2014). Many other professional nursing specialty credentialing organizations also provide for individual certification.

Although usually a voluntary process, certification can also be a quasi-voluntary process. For example, to function as a nurse practitioner in all but three states, one must show proof of educational credentials and take an examination to be certified to practice within the boundaries of the state (Fitzgerald, 2013).

Major concerns exist about certification as a QA mechanism. Data are lacking about the clinical competence of the practitioner at the time of certification because clinical competency is usually not measured by a written test. Although better data exist about the quality of the practitioner's work after the certification process, the American Nurses Credentialing Center conducted a research program to look at how certification is related to the work of the certified nurse (Blegen, 2012; Boltz et al, 2013; Kendall-Gallagher et al, 2011; Martinez, 2011). Except for occupational health nurses and nurse anesthetists, certification has not been universally recognized by employers as an achievement beyond basic preparation, so financial rewards have been few (Keefe, 2010).

Although the nursing profession has accepted the certification process as a mechanism for recognizing competence and excellence, certifying bodies must help nurses communicate the importance of certified nurses to the public.

Charter, recognition, and academic degrees are other general approaches to QA. Charter is the mechanism by which a state government agency, under state laws, grants corporate status to institutions with or without rights to award degrees (e.g., university-based nursing programs).

Recognition is a process whereby one agency accepts the credentialing status of and the credentials conferred by another. For example, most state boards of nursing accept nurse practitioner credentials that are awarded by the American Nurses Credentialing Center or by one of the specialty credentialing agencies. Academic degrees are titles awarded to individuals recognized by degree-granting institutions as having completed a predetermined plan of study in a branch of learning. There are four academic degrees awarded in nursing, with some variety at each degree level: Associate of Arts/Sciences; Bachelor of Science in Nursing; master's degrees, such as Master of Science in Nursing and Master of Nursing; and doctoral degrees, such as Doctor of Philosophy and Doctor of Nursing Practice.

Although these general quality management methods are important and should continue, newer and better approaches must be devised. If performance in the area of quality health care is to advance, better diagnosis of performance problems and corrective strategies that are effective will be necessary (USDHHS, 2011a). The National Network of Public Health Institutes (2010) a toolkit designed to improve quality performance in public health, developed a toolkit.

An approach to recognition is the Magnet nursing services recognition status given by the American Nurses Credentialing Center to agency nursing services that, after an extensive review, are considered excellent. This program began with recognition of excellent hospital nursing services. The Magnet program has expanded to include nursing home and home health agencies, Reapplication for Magnet status must occur every 4 years to ensure that Magnet organizations stay at the top of their games (ANCC, 2014).

## Specific Approaches

Historically, QA programs conducted by health care agencies have measured or assessed the performance of individuals and how they conformed to standards set forth by accrediting agencies. TQM as a management philosophy uses CQI methods that incorporate many tools, including QA, to increase customer satisfaction with quality care. According to the AHRQ, quality health care means doing the right thing, at the right time, in the right way, for the right people—and having the best possible results (AHRQ, 2012, 2014b). To the Institute of Medicine (IOM, 2001, p. 3), quality health care is care that is as follows:

• *Effective*—Providing services based on scientific knowledge to all who could benefit and refraining from providing services to those not likely to benefit
• *Safe*—Avoiding injuries to clients from the care that is intended to help them
• *Timely*—Reducing waits and sometimes harmful delays for both those who receive and those who give care
• *Client-centered*—Providing care that is respectful of and responsive to individual client preferences, needs, and values and ensuring that client values guide all clinical decisions
• *Equitable*—Providing care that does not vary in quality because of personal characteristics such as gender, ethnicity, geographic location, and socioeconomic status
• *Efficient*—Avoiding waste, including waste of equipment, supplies, ideas, and energy

QA seeks to eliminate errors before negative outcomes can occur rather than waiting until after the fact to correct individual performance.

Health care agencies have only recently paid heed to the tenets of TQM. This management philosophy has been used in Japanese industry since the post–World War II era when W. Edwards Deming was invited to Japan to help rebuild its broken economy. In addition to Deming, people associated with the total quality concept are Walter Stewart (who first published on the subject), Joseph M. Juran, Armand F. Feigenbaum, Phillip B. Crosby, Genichi Taguchi, and Kaoru Ishikawa. Unlike traditional QA programs, the focus of CQI is the *process* of delivering health care. This focus on process avoids placing personal blame for less-than-perfect outcomes. Applying TQM in health care allows management to look at the contribution of all systems to outcomes of the organization.

### QSEN FOCUS ON QUALITY AND SAFETY EDUCATION FOR NURSES

**Targeted Competency: Quality Improvement**
Use data to monitor the outcomes of intervention processes, and use improvement methods to design and test changes to continuously improve the quality and safety of health care systems.
Important aspects of quality improvement include:
• **Knowledge:** Recognize that nursing and other health professions students are parts of systems and intervention processes that affect outcomes for clients and families
• **Skills:** Identify gaps between local practices and best practice
• **Attitudes:** Value own and others' contributions to outcomes in local community settings

**Quality Improvement Question**
You are working as a home care nurse and are discovering a trend of frequent readmissions to the hospital of many of your clients with heart failure. Using the quality assurance approach, consider the following questions:
• What is being done now?
• Why is it being done?
• Is it being done well?
• Can it be done better?
• Should it be done at all?
• Are there improved ways to deliver service?
• How much is it costing?
• Should certain activities be abandoned or replaced?
To which aspects of your clients' quality of life and care transitions will you apply these questions?

**Answer**
It would be helpful to look at a group of clients discharged from the hospital. Are they receiving adequate education and preparation to return home? You could also gather data about how clients are being managed by the community. How often are they following up with their primary care clinician? Are clients adequately educated to monitor their own fluid status, weight, and dietary restrictions? Are there community-based cardiovascular care programs that can help clients maintain optimum health and avoid exacerbations?

Prepared by Gail Armstrong, PhD(c), DNP, ACNS-BC, CNE, Associate Professor, University of Colorado Denver College of Nursing.

Deming's (1986, p. 23) guidelines are summarized by his 15-point program:
1. Create, publish, and give to all employees a statement of the aims and purposes of the company or other organization. The management must demonstrate constantly their commitment to this statement.
2. Learn the new philosophy, top management, and everybody.
3. Understand the purpose of inspection, for improvement of processes and reduction of costs.
4. End the practice of awarding business on the basis of price tag alone.
5. Improve constantly and forever the system of production and service.
6. Institute training.
7. Teach and institute leadership.
8. Drive out fear. Create trust. Create a climate for innovation.
9. Optimize toward the aims and purposes of the company the efforts of teams, groups, and staff areas.

10. Eliminate exhortations for the workforce.
11. Eliminate numerical quotes for production. Instead, learn and institute methods for improvement.
12. Eliminate management by objective. Instead, learn the capabilities of processes and how to improve them.
13. Remove barriers that rob people of pride of workmanship.
14. Encourage education and self-improvement for everyone.
15. Take action to accomplish the transformation.

Deming's first point emphasizes that an organization must have purpose and values. Health care providers have a clear idea of their values and have been committed to quality in the past, as demonstrated by codes of ethics and standards of care. However, successful TQM and CQI processes rely on a cultural change within an organization and the full support of management. With respect to providing quality health care, a paradigm shift from individual provider responsibility to team responsibility must occur (Sollecito and Johnson, 2013). A guiding principle is a customer orientation focused on positive health outcomes and perceived satisfaction. Customer (client) satisfaction surveys must be done for both internal and external users of services.

Personnel policies that are motivating as well as continuous training/learning opportunities are crucial to any CQI program. Deming's eighth point addresses driving out fear. Fear in this context means the fear of being fired for being innovative or taking risks. In the CQI process, individuals are not blamed for failures in the system and therefore are motivated through the group to continually look for problems and improve system performance.

TQM works best in a flat organizational structure. This means there are very few supervisors between the staff and the director. This organization operates with an interprofessional team approach and a separate but parallel management quality council that monitors strategy and implementation. Teams are empowered to solve problems and locate opportunities for system improvement. Shewhart's plan-do-check-act cycle serves as a guideline for the team approach to problem solving. This approach is also known as the Demming wheel. Steps include the following (Deming, 1986, p. 88; Deming Institute, 2014):

1. PLAN: Ask questions, such as: What could be the most important accomplishments of this team? What changes might be desirable? What data are available? Are new observations needed? If yes, plan a change or implement a test. Decide how to use the observations.
2. DO: Carry out the change or test decided upon.
3. CHECK: Observe the effects of the change. Study the results. What did we learn? What can we predict?
4. ACT: Repeat the cycle, if the changes worked, or implement a different strategy if the first plan was flawed, or revise the initial strategy based on the changes needed.

A suggested way to start the problem-solving process with a team in step 1 is brainstorming (Simon, n.d.). Brainstorming is getting everyone's input about a possible process situation with no team member criticizing the suggestion. Because TQI organizations are data driven, moving to step 2 requires that ongoing statistics be collected. Differences from the mean (average) or norm are detected through consistent use of tools, such as the flow chart, the Pareto chart (used to compare the importance of differences between groups of data), cause-and-effect diagrams, check sheets (see p. 583 for a client satisfaction check sheet), histograms, control charts, regression, and other statistical analyses (e.g., QA data and techniques, risk management data, risk-adjusted outcome measures, and cost-effectiveness analysis) (Sollecito and Johnson, 2013). Steps 3, 4, and 5 are self-explanatory.

Joseph Juran built on Deming's initial quality work and became a supporter of building quality into all processes. The *Juran trilogy* provides an effective way to compare the tasks of quality planning, QA, and QI. Quality planning involves determining who the clients are, the needs of those clients, the service that fulfills the needs, and the process to produce that service. QA evaluates the performance of that service, compares it with the service goals, and then makes corrections if necessary. QI makes sure the infrastructure exists to enable individuals to identify improvement projects. Management of QI establishes project teams and provides those teams with the resources needed to carry out improvement projects (Van den Heuvel et al, 2013).

## TQM/CQI IN COMMUNITY AND PUBLIC HEALTH SETTINGS

Guidelines provided by the 1991 APHA *Model Standards* linked standards to meeting the health goals for the nation in the year 2000 (Sollecito and Johnson, 2013). *Healthy People 2000* and APHA *Model Standards* (APHA, 1991) provided not only lists of priority health objectives for the nation and a way for public health to implement TQM/CQI, but also the most current statistics and scientific knowledge about health promotion and disease prevention. *Healthy People in Healthy Communities* (USDHHS, 2001) provided the objectives with their stated targets, measurement tools, and reflected intended performance expectations.

*Healthy People 2010* built on *Healthy People 2000* and contained modified and additional objectives for promoting health and preventing disease (USDHHS, 2000). An important part of the framework of *Healthy People 2010* was eliminating health disparities and ensuring access to quality health care for all. After extensive review of the *Healthy People 2010* objectives, new goals and objectives were developed for *Healthy People 2020* (USDHHS, 2010). The goals for *Healthy People 2020* are as follows:

- Attain high-quality, longer lives free of preventable disease, disability, injury, and premature death.
- Achieve health equity, eliminate disparities, and improve the health of all groups.
- Create social and physical environments that promote good health for all.
- Promote quality of life, healthy development, and healthy behaviors across all life stages.

Although all of the goals speak to quality of life and health, goal two specifically addresses issues related to quality of health care delivery.

In addition, the *Planned Approach to Community Health* (PATCH) (CDC, 1995 with update in 2010); the Assessment Protocol for Excellence in Public Health (APEXPH), *APEXPH in Practice* (NACCHO, 1995, 2014); and most recently the *Mobilizing for Action through Planning and Partnerships* (MAPP) process (NACCHO, 2014) provide methods of assessing community needs to see how well health departments are operating to meet existing standards (see Chapter 25).

As health care reform continues, especially with the implementation of the Affordable Care Act, public health agencies face competition and are trying to reform themselves. A promising outcome of reform is how private health care and public health can come together in a community-level effort to monitor performance and improve health (see Chapter 3).

Recognizing the many factors that cause health problems and the fragmenting that continues to exist in the health care system, the public-private collaborative framework supported by the *Healthy People* documents involves many stakeholders, including public health, in monitoring the health of entire communities. Performance monitoring is defined as "a continuing community-based process of selecting indicators that can be used to measure the process and outcomes of an intervention strategy for health improvement (making the results available to the community as a whole) to inform assessments of an effective intervention and the contributions of accountable agencies to this" (*Healthy People*, 2020, 2011). These indicators would measure processes or states that contribute to health, and thus the processes are potentially alterable. As previously noted, there are four documents that monitor the quality and safety of health care, including the contributions of public health. Box 26-3 provides highlights from each of these reports.

Home health care agencies have increasingly adopted QI programs because of the competition that exists. Congruent with the TQM philosophy, meeting customer expectations is essential for home health care agencies. Models for QA/QI in home health care have been developed to improve the quality of care in TQM frameworks emphasizing processes, empowerment, collaboration, consumers, data and measurement, and standards and outcomes (Oakland, 2014). Datasets of clinical information, such as those developed through the Omaha System (see Chapter 40) and the OASIS toolkit from the National Association of Home Care and Hospice (NAHC, 2010), are useful in measuring quality of care. In 2003 the Home Health Care Quality Initiative (HHQI) was developed by the USDHHS to provide consumers with data on the quality of home health services. *Home Health Compare,* posted on the Medicare website, is a home health report card available to consumers nationwide (USDHHS, 2014).

Finally, in the area of standards and guidelines, Honoré and Scott (2010) address six priority areas of performance that need improvement. One of these areas is consistently providing appropriate and effective care. This area is applicable to all health care practitioners, including nurses. Evidence-based practice guidelines are one way to deliver consistent, up-to-date care and to improve outcomes for individuals, communities, and populations. Every year the American Cancer Society (ACS) provides a summary of current cancer screening guidelines for health care professionals and updates the guidelines at least every five years, or sooner if new evidence warrants an

## BOX 26-3 National Quality and Safety Reports

| Name of Report | Most Recent Results |
|---|---|
| The National Health Care Quality Report, Agency for Healthcare Research and Quality, began publication in 2003 and has published for ten years | Assesses four dimensions of quality: effectiveness, client safety, timeliness, and client centeredness. Between 2003-2013:<br>• Health care quality is getting better.<br>• Large variation in quality across states.<br>• 70% of recommended care actually received.<br>• Access is fair and getting worse.<br>• There has been no change in the disparities in health care over time and it is poor. |
| The State of Health Care Quality, 2013; The National Committee for Quality Assurance | Has been published annually for 18 years. Assesses HEDIS to determine quality improvement across third-party payers.<br>• Reports after more than a decade of progress in quality of care<br>• There is stagnant or declining performance in appropriate use of antibiotics.<br>• Childhood obesity measures improving.<br>• Childhood immunization results mixed.<br>• Sustained decline in initiation of alcohol and drug treatment.<br>• Better care in Medicaid HMOs. |
| National Healthcare Disparities Report, 2013; The Agency for Healthcare Research and Quality | Published since 2000 for 13 years. Assesses 11 dimensions of quality including safety:<br>• Findings indicate disparities in quality and access remain common, with blacks, Hispanics, and Asians receiving worse care then whites.<br>• Poor people receive worse care then high income persons.<br>• For some quality measures, persons with limited activity receive poorer care. |
| Safe Practices for Better Healthcare, 2010; The National Quality Forum | Published first in 2003, then in 2006 and 2009. The 2010 update report presents 34 safe practices with descriptions of their safety impact.<br>• Adverse health care events continue to be a leading cause of death and injury.<br>• Evidence indicates that the 34 safe practices identified are effective in improving safety.<br>• Although many of the 34 practices can be adapted to public health, two can be specifically applied in public health: a quality workforce and influenza prevention. |

update (Smith et al, 2014). The use of guidelines helps in gathering data on the effectiveness and outcomes of nurse interventions (Matthew-Maich et al, 2013). The AHRQ, formerly the Agency for Healthcare Policy and Research (AHCPR), has played a major role in developing clinical practice guidelines.

*Guidelines* are protocols or statements of recommended practice developed by governmental and health care agencies, and by professional organizations; they are based on the distilling of scientific evidence and expert opinion that guide a clinician in decision making. Guidelines provide research-based evidence for interventions and promote improved health outcomes. Using research findings as guidelines or frames of reference can improve nurses' awareness of new or better ways to practice, allow for documentation of nurse interventions, and improve outcomes at all levels of public health nursing practice (Matthew-Maich et al, 2013) (see Chapter 9). Keystones of evidence-based practice guidelines arise from client concerns, clinical experience, best practices, and clinical data and research (Malloch and Porter-O'Grady, 2010). Clinical practice guidelines are systematically developed statements to assist practitioner and client decisions about appropriate health care for specific clinical circumstances (as discussed in Chapter 15). An example of criteria for clinical practice guidelines are those set forth by the AHRQ and available on the Internet at the National Guideline Clearinghouse (NGC) website (http://www.guideline.gov/) (NGC, 2010).

- The practice guideline contains systematically developed statements that include recommendations, strategies, or information that assists health care practitioners and clients make decisions about appropriate health care for specific health care circumstances.
- The practice guideline was produced under the auspices of specialty associations; relevant professional societies, public or private organizations, government agencies at the federal, state, or local level; or health care organizations or plans. A practice guideline developed and issued by an individual not officially sponsored or supported by one of the above types of organizations does not meet the inclusion criteria for the NGC.
- Corroborating documentation can be produced and verified that a systematic literature search and review of existing scientific evidence published in peer reviewed journals was performed during the guideline development. A guideline is not excluded from the NGC if corroborating documentation can be produced and verified detailing specific gaps in scientific evidence for some of the guideline's recommendations.
- The full text guideline is available upon request in print or electronic format (for free or for a fee) in English. The guideline is current and the most recent version produced. Documented evidence can be produced or verified that the guideline was developed, reviewed, or revised within the last 5 years (http://www.guideline.gov/contact/coninclusion.aspx).

One of the quality reports published by the clearinghouse each year is the *National Healthcare Disparities Report*, the most recent being 2013. The most recent guideline development and updates are related to cancer control.

Primary care practice guidelines are available in the *Guide to Clinical Preventive Services* (USPSTF, 2014) and the population-based *Guide to Community Preventive Services* available on the CDC website. This guide is an ongoing process of the Taskforce on Community Preventive Services that offers information on changing risk behaviors; reducing specific diseases, injuries and impairments, and environmental concerns; and state-of-the-art public health activities. Nurses need guidelines to reduce differences in care practices, to improve outcomes on the basis of the best research available, and to deliver effective care to individuals, communities, and populations.

## Using QA/QI in CQI

QA/QI methods and tools help agencies conform to standards required by external accrediting agencies. QA/QI provides a way to identify examples of substandard care and to improve that care when standards are not met. QA is focused on problem detection, whereas CQI is focused on problem prevention and continuous improvement. In QA, little attention is paid to preventing errors or problems and finding out who owns the quality issues. Furthermore, the QA process may stop unless another problem is found. Sollecito and Johnson (2013) point out differences in traditional management models that use performance standards versus those that use TQM (Table 26-1). The most important difference is in the emphasis on QA, or simply identifying the problem in the traditional management model versus the emphasis on CQI in the total quality management model. In TQM the problem is identified and measures are implemented to correct the problem. The TQM model is required in health care delivery because of the standards set by the national accrediting agencies such as TJC. Public health, through the public health accrediting process begun in 2011, is required to emphasize TQM.

Positive steps of a known QA program can be integrated into a CQI approach. Strengths of QA include a history of expertise in developing evaluation of structure, identifying high-priority problems, and developing knowledge in QA and information systems (de Jonge et al, 2011). These strengths can be used advantageously in a CQI effort.

## Traditional Quality Assurance

Traditional QA programs can fit well with the CQI process. The overall goal of specific QA approaches is to monitor the process and outcomes of client care. The goals of CQI are as follows:

| TABLE 26-1   **Traditional Management Model Compared with Total Quality Management (TQM) Model** | |
|---|---|
| **Traditional Model** | **TQM Model** |
| Legal or professional authority | Collective or managerial responsibility |
| Specialized accountability | Process accountability |
| Administrative authority | Participation |
| Meeting standards | Meeting process and performance expectations |
| Longer planning horizon | Shorter planning horizon |
| Quality assurance | Continuous improvement |

1. To identify problems between provider and client through QA methods
2. To intervene in problem cases
3. To provide feedback regarding interactions between client and provider
4. To provide documentation of interactions between client and provider

Specific approaches are often implemented voluntarily by agencies and provider groups interested in the quality of interactions in their setting. However, state and federal governments require mandatory programs within public health agencies. For example, periodic utilization review, peer reviews (audits), and other QA measures are required in public health agencies that receive funds from state taxes, Medicaid, Medicare, and other public funding sources. Examples of specific approaches to QA are agency staff review committees for peer review (Banner Health, 2012), utilization review committees for Medicare and Medicaid, research studies, quality improvement organization (QIO) monitoring, client satisfaction surveys, risk management, and malpractice lawsuits.

### Staff Review Committee

Staff review committees are the most common specific approach to QA in the United States. Staff review committees are designed to monitor client-specific aspects of certain levels of care. The audit is the major tool used to evaluate quality of care.

The audit process (Figure 26-1) consists of six steps:
1. Select a topic for study.
2. Select explicit criteria for quality care.
3. Review records to determine whether criteria are met.
4. Do a peer review for all cases that do not meet criteria.
5. Make specific recommendations to correct problems.
6. Follow-up to determine whether problems have been eliminated.

Two types of audits are used in nursing peer review: concurrent and retrospective. The concurrent audit is a process audit that evaluates the quality of ongoing care by looking at the nursing process. Concurrent audit is used by Medicare and Medicaid to evaluate care being received by public health/home health clients. The audit data look at the group, population, or community served. The advantages of this method are as follows:

- Identification of problems at the time care is given
- Provision of a mechanism for identifying and meeting client needs during the intervention
- Implementation of measures to fulfill professional responsibilities
- Provision of a mechanism for communicating on behalf of the client

The disadvantages of the concurrent audit are as follows:
- It is time consuming
- It is more costly to implement than the retrospective audit
- Because the intervention is ongoing, it does not present the total picture of the outcomes of the intervention that the client ultimately will receive

The retrospective audit, or outcome audit, evaluates quality of care through evaluation of the nursing process at the end of

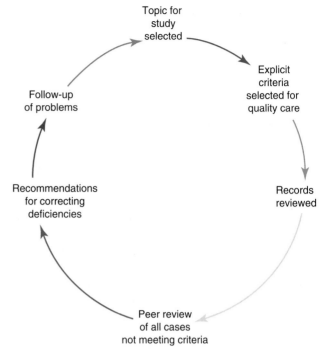

**FIG 26-1** The audit process.

a program or as an audit of the long-term impact of a program within the health care system. The advantages of the retrospective audit are that it provides the following:

- Comparison of actual practice to standards of care
- Analysis of actual practice findings
- A total picture of care given to a population or group of clients
- More accurate data for planning corrective action

Disadvantages of the retrospective audit method are as follows:

- The focus of evaluation is directed away from ongoing care.
- Client problems (group or population or community) are identified after care is offered through the program; thus corrective action can be used only to improve the care of future clients.

Currently in public health, program record audits are done to determine the processes and outcomes of care, such as family planning audits, WIC audits, breast and cervical cancer screening audits, billing coding (to audit costs) and registration audits. Programs regarding physical activity, nutrition, obesity, arthritis, smoking cessation, and others are all designed to address the major causes of morbidity and mortality locally, statewide, and nationwide. The audits assist in determining the progress being made in reducing morbidity and mortality.

### Utilization Review

The purpose of utilization review is to ensure that care is needed and that the cost is appropriate. Utilization review is more likely used in HMOs, other MCOs, and ACOs including Medicaid or Medicare state-level managed care programs. There are three types of utilization review:

1. *Prospective:* An assessment of the necessity of care before giving service

2. *Concurrent:* A review of the necessity of services while care is being given
3. *Retrospective:* An analysis of the necessity of the services received by the client after the care has been given

Each of these reviews assesses the appropriate cost of care. Prospectively, care can be denied and money saved. Concurrently, services can be cut if they are not found to be essential. Retrospectively, payment can be denied to the provider if the care was not necessary.

Utilization review began in the middle part of the twentieth century out of concern for increasing health care costs. The first committees were developed by insurance companies and professional groups. Utilization review committees became mandatory under the 1965 Medicare law as a way to control hospital costs.

The utilization review process includes development of explicit criteria regarding the need for services and the length of service. Utilization review has been used primarily in hospitals to establish the need for client admission and to determine the length of hospital stay. In community and public health, especially home health care, utilization review establishes criteria for admission to agency service, the number of visits a client may receive, the eligibility for client services (e.g., a nursing aide or physical therapist), and discharge.

Utilization review has several advantages:
- It helps clients avoid unnecessary care.
- It may encourage clients to consider alternative care options, such as home health care rather than hospital care.
- It can provide guidelines for staff and program development.
- It provides for agency accountability to the consumer.

The major disadvantage of utilization review is that not all clients fit the classic picture presented by the explicit criteria used to determine approval or denial of care. For example, an older adult client was admitted to a home health care agency for management after hospital discharge. The client was paraplegic as a result of a cerebrovascular accident. After several weeks of physical and speech therapy, the client showed little sign of progress. The utilization review committee considered the client's condition to be stable and did not recognize the continued need for management to prevent future complications; therefore, Medicare payment was denied.

Appeal mechanisms have been built into the utilization review process used by Medicare and Medicaid. The appeal allows providers and clients to present additional data that may help to reverse the original decision to deny payment.

### Risk Management

Risk management committees are often a part of the CQI program of a community agency. Risk management seeks to reduce the agency's liability because of grievances brought against them. The risk management committee reviews all risks to which an agency is exposed. It reviews client and personnel safety policies and procedures and determines whether personnel are following the rules. Examples of problems reviewed by a risk management committee in public health clinics include administering incorrect vaccination dosage, pediatric client injury caused by a fall from an examination table, or injury to the nurse from a needlestick in the sexually transmitted diseases

### EVIDENCE-BASED PRACTICE

This mixed-methods study sought to identify factors that support or hinder the development of a quality improvement culture in public health agencies. The researchers conducted case studies of ten agencies that participated in early quality improvement efforts. Agency staff who participated in National Association of County and City Health Officials (NACCHO)-sponsored quality improvement trainings were invited to complete a survey. Health directors and quality improvement teams from these agencies were also interviewed. The investigators found that agencies that were successful in creating a positive quality improvement culture had the following characteristics: had leadership support; had participated in national quality improvement initiatives; had a greater number of staff trained in quality improvement; had quality improvement teams that met regularly with decision-making authority; reported that accreditation was a major driver to quality improvement work; and had a history of evidence-based decision making and use of quality improvement to address emerging issues. The investigators reported that the role of accreditation preparation as a driving force in quality improvement appears to diminish as an agency develops a quality improvement culture. The researchers noted that common barriers to creating a quality improvement culture included lack of time and resources and relevance of quality improvement to daily work. However, they also reported that staff used quality improvement to overcome these barriers.

**Nurse Use**

Leadership and teamwork within an organization plays a key role in creating a positive quality improvement environment. Community health nurses are in a prime position to be leaders in their organizations in developing a quality improvement environment.

From Davis MV, Mahanna E, Joly B, et al: Creating quality improvement culture in public health agencies. *Am J Public Health* 104(1):e98–e104, 2014.

clinic at the health department or as a result of an accident while making a home visit. Incident reports are reviewed by the risk management committee for appropriate, accurate, and thorough documentation of any problem that occurs relating to clients or personnel. In addition, patterns are identified from looking at program data that may require changes in policy or staff development to correct the problem. As a part of risk management, grievance procedures are established for both clients and personnel.

### Professional Review Organizations/Quality Improvement Organizations

The **Professional Standards Review Organization (PSRO)** was established in 1972 in an amendment to the Social Security Act (PL 92-603) as a publicly mandated utilization and peer review program. This law provided that medical, hospital, and nursing home care under Medicare, Medicaid, and Title V Maternal and Child Health Programs would be reviewed for appropriateness and necessary care to be reimbursed.

In 1983 Congress passed the Peer Review Improvement Act (PL 97-248), creating professional review organizations (PROs). PROs replaced PSROs and are directed by the federal government to reduce hospital admissions for procedures that can be performed safely and effectively in an ambulatory surgical setting on an outpatient basis. The goal was to reduce inappropriate or unnecessary admissions or invasive procedures by specific practitioners or hospitals. Quality measures include reducing unnecessary admissions caused by previous substandard care, avoidable complications and deaths, and unnecessary surgery or invasive procedures (Chassin and Loeb, 2011). The PRO is now known as the Quality Improvement Organization.

Institutions contracting with QIOs for quality reviews are usually state organizations that establish criteria for care on the basis of local patterns of practice, and they are private contractors to CMS and mostly not-for-profit organizations. They may have on their board health care providers who are independent from the QIO and the board must have at least one consumer. QIOs must define their operational objectives, monitor access to care, cost of care, and quality concerns, and protect the Medicare Trust. Professionals working under the regulation of QIOs should develop accurate and complete documenting procedures to ensure compliance with the criteria of the QIO (CMS, 2014a).

Debate has occurred over the limits and benefits of the federally mandated quality review process. Limits include jeopardizing professional autonomy because decision making regarding care includes professionals, consumers, and government representatives. Another limitation of this process is the development of a costly control mechanism whereby client care activities may be determined by cost rather than by professional criteria. The benefit of the QIO system has been the development of standards and the peer review mechanisms to increase accountability for care provided.

TQM provides direction for managing a system of care, whereas CQI using QA/QI focuses on the care a client receives within the system.

## Evaluative Studies

Evaluative studies for quality health care increased during the twentieth century. Studies demonstrate the effect of nursing and health care interventions on client populations. Three key models have been used to evaluate quality: Donabedian's structure-process-outcome model, the tracer method, and the sentinel method.

Donabedian's model (1981, 1985, 2003) introduced three major methods for evaluating quality care:

1. **Structure**: Evaluating the setting and instruments used to provide care; examples of structure are facilities, equipment, characteristics of the administrative organization, client mix, and the qualifications of health providers
2. **Process**: Evaluating activities as they relate to standards and expectations of health providers in the management of client care
3. **Outcome**: The net change or result that occurs as a result of health care

The three methods may be used separately to evaluate a part of care. However, to get an overall picture of quality of care, they should be used together.

The tracer method described by Kessner and Kalk (1973) is a measure of both process and outcome of care and is used today. This method is more effective in evaluating health care of groups than of individual clients. It is also more effective in evaluating care delivered by an institution than care delivered by an individual provider. The following are essential

characteristics for implementing the tracer method (Papanicolas and Smith, 2013; Kelly, 2011):

1. A tracer, or a problem, that has a definite impact on the client's level of functioning
2. Well-defined and easily diagnosed characteristics
3. Population prevalence high enough to permit adequate data collection
4. A known variation resulting from use of effective health care
5. Well-defined management techniques in prevention, diagnosis, treatment, or rehabilitation
6. Understood (documented) effects of nonmedical factors on the tracer

Client groups selected for tracer outcome studies in nursing would have the following:

1. A shared health problem
2. Receiving a similar intervention
3. Sharing similar needs
4. Located in the same community
5. Having a similar lifestyle
6. Being at the same illness stage

The tracer method provides nurses with data to show the differences in outcomes as a result of nursing care standards.

The **sentinel** method of quality evaluation is based on epidemiologic principles. This method is an outcome measure for examining specific instances of client care (Kelly, 2011). Changes in the sentinel indicate potential problems for others. For example, increases in encephalitis in certain communities may result from increases in mosquito populations. Data may be collected at the health department through a state or local required disease reporting system. The health department would be notified and an immediate mosquito control strategy would be put into place. Such an intervention would include, for example, nurses notifying the population to remove standing water around the outside of homes, such as animal water bowls, rain barrels, and gutter downspout water collection pools. Flyers may be sent home with school children or given to clients visiting the public health clinics, and media announcements may be used. In addition, the environmental office at the health department may inspect local swimming pools and may also implement a nighttime mosquito spraying program throughout the community.

---

| HOW TO    **Conduct a Sentinel Evaluation**

- *Identify cases of unnecessary disease, disability, and complications (for example, tuberculosis).*
- *Count the deaths from these causes.*
- *Examine the circumstances surrounding the unnecessary event (or sentinel), in detail.*
- *Review morbidity and mortality rates as an index for comparison; determine the critical increase in the untimely event, which may reflect changes in quality of care. Example: Compare the incidence and prevalence of TB cases before the increased population occurred.*
- *Explore health status indicators, such as changes in social, economic, political, and environmental factors that may have an effect on health outcomes. Example: Overcrowding in the shelter where migrant workers stay (environmental) and the inability to follow-up on testing because of the transient nature of the population (social).*

## CLIENT SATISFACTION

Client satisfaction is another approach to measuring quality of care. Client satisfaction can be assessed using in-person or telephone interviews and mailed questionnaires. Satisfaction surveys are used to assess care received during an admission to a specific agency, to assess a client's personal nursing care, or to assess the total care that the client received from all services.

Satisfaction surveys may measure the interventions used for client care, attitudes about the care received and the providers of care, and perceptions of the situation (environment) in which the care was received. Clients are often more critical of interpersonal and situational components of care than of the interventions of care.

Satisfaction surveys are an essential aspect of QA. Survey data provide clues to reasons for client compliance or noncompliance with plans of care. Although consumers may not view quality in the same light as the health professional, surveys provide data about health-seeking behaviors, the probability of malpractice litigation, and the likelihood of continuing client-provider-agency relationships—always an important measure for community-based and public health agencies (Oakland, 2014) (Figure 26-2).

Please mark the following questions using the scale.

| Domain | Example | Strongly Agree | Somewhat Agree | Agree | Somewhat Disagree | Strongly Disagree |
|---|---|---|---|---|---|---|
| Affective support | 1. The visiting nurse was understanding of my health concerns. | | | | | |
| | 2. The nurse gave me encouragement in regard to my health problems. | | | | | |
| Health information | 3. I got my questions answered in an individual way. | | | | | |
| | 4. The information I received from the nurse helped me to take care of myself at home. | | | | | |
| Decision control | 5. I was included in decision making. | | | | | |
| | 6. I was included in the planning of my care. | | | | | |
| Technical competencies | 7. The care I received was of high quality. | | | | | |
| | 8. Decisions regarding my health care were of high quality. | | | | | |
| Accessibility | 9. The nurse was available when I needed help. | | | | | |
| | 10. The nurse was on time. | | | | | |
| Overall satisfaction | 11. Overall, I was satisfied with my health care. | | | | | |
| | 12. The care I received was of high quality. | | | | | |

**FIG 26-2** Client satisfaction tool domains and examples.

## Malpractice Litigation

Malpractice litigation (i.e., a lawsuit) is a specific approach to QA imposed on the health care delivery system by the legal system. Malpractice litigation typically results from client dissatisfaction with the provider and with the content of the care received. Nursing is not immune from malpractice litigation. Nursing must continue to have a sound QA program that ensures quality care. This will reduce the risk of quality control measures being imposed by an external source, such as the legal system. As a true example, a public health nurse was individually sued by a new family to the community because the nurse repeated an immunization the child had already received prior to moving to the community. The result was Guillain-Barré syndrome. The nurse was found at fault even though the parents did not provide the physician's record of immunizations to the nurse. It was the nurse's responsibility to follow standard guidelines and to obtain the essential records prior to proving the immunization. The public health department was dismissed from the lawsuit because of immunity granted to state agencies.

## MODEL CQI PROGRAM

The primary purpose of a QA/QI program is to ensure that the results of an organized activity are consistent with the expectations. All personnel affected by a QI program should be involved in its development and implementation. Although administration and management are responsible for the quality of services, the key to that quality is in the personnel who deliver the service: their knowledge, skills, and attitudes.

Figure 26-3 shows a model that identifies the basic components of a QI program. QI programs answer the following questions about health care services and nursing care:

1. What is being done now?
2. Why is it being done?
3. Is it being done well?
4. Can it be done better?
5. Should it be done at all?
6. Are there improved ways to deliver the service?
7. How much does it cost?
8. Should certain activities be abandoned or replaced?

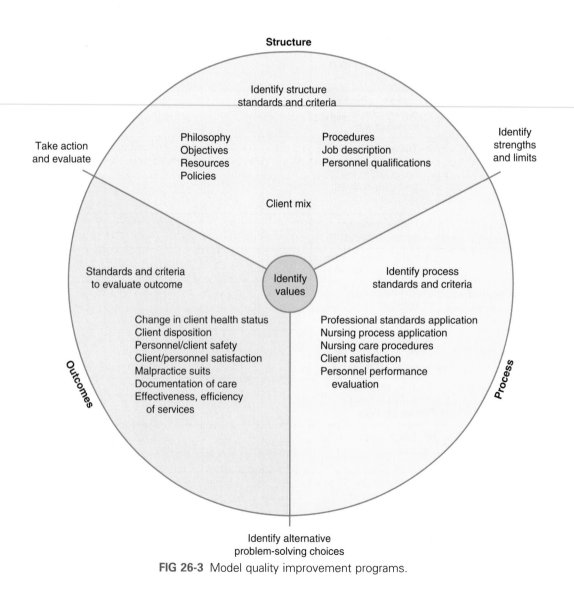

**FIG 26-3** Model quality improvement programs.

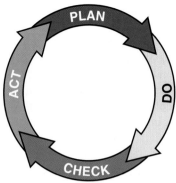

FIG 26-4 The plan-do-check-act (PDCA) model of continuous quality improvement. The concept of the PDCA cycle was originally developed by Walter Shewhart, the pioneering statistician who developed statistical process control in the Bell Laboratories in the United States during the 1930s. It is often referred to as the "Shewhart Cycle." It was adopted in the 1950s by W. Edwards Deming, and is often referred to as the "Deming Wheel."

As a part of answering the questions and determining changes that can improve services, public health can use the PDCA model. The steps of the model are shown in Figure 26-4.

The PDCA is a model for continuous improvement and can be used after an audit of a program, for example to begin a new improvement project or when developing a new or improved design of a process, product, or program. It can also be used to define a repetitive work process or for planning data collection and analysis to verify and prioritize problems or root causes, which are actually the system problems that lead to the problem. It is also used to implement change.

The PDCA procedure involves the following steps:

1. **Plan.** Recognize an opportunity and plan a change.
2. **Do.** Test the change. Carry out a small-scale study.
3. **Check.** Review the data, analyze the results, and identify what has been learned.
4. **Act.** Take action based on what was learned in the check/study step: If the change did not work, go through the cycle again with a different plan. If successful, incorporate what you learned from the test into wider changes. Use what was learned to plan new improvements, and begin the cycle again. Beginning the cycle again defines the continuous program of CQI. This is also referred to as a rapid cycle improvement process in health care.

Donabedian's framework for evaluating health care programs using the components of structure, process, and outcome can be used in developing a QI program. *Outcome* is the most important ingredient of a program because it is the key to evaluating providers and agencies by accrediting bodies, by insurance companies, and by Medicare and Medicaid through QIOs, report cards, and other accrediting agencies.

## LINKING CONTENT TO PRACTICE

The PDCA model is being used in public health to promote CQI. A brief example of how to apply this model is given below.

This approach was designed to improve new mother and baby outcomes by improving nurse/client communication processes. This model for improvement includes four components recommended by the Institute of Healthcare Improvement: (1) aims and goals, (2) performance measures, (3) strategies and ideas for changes, and (4) the use of PDCA cycles.

1. The goal of the project is to improve health outcomes for at-risk new mothers and babies involved in the nurse home visiting program by offering a daily telephone consultation to answer questions and provide support up to 3 months after the baby's birth.

2. The performance measures include:
   A. An assessment of the numbers of nurses on the home visiting team who could successfully answer the questions of the mothers who received the daily consultation.
   B. The second measure is a retrospective record audit at 6 months to assess the progress of the mothers who had access to the daily call as compared with mothers who were involved in the program prior to the daily phone consult.

3. The strategies include:
   A. A work session of the nurses to review their knowledge about parenting and caring for a new baby up to 3 months using a simple pretest.
   B. An update on what new mothers need to know to bond with their babies and to provide for the new babies' needs followed by a post-test of the nurses' knowledge.
   C. The development of the process for the daily phone consultation including a checklist of assessment questions the nurse might ask and time built in to respond to parent's questions.

   **Plan:** Plan a mock "daily consult" call to a public health nurse (or a fellow student) with her first baby. Develop different scenarios for the public health nurse to respond to in order to assess each home visiting nurse's ability to respond to the mother's questions, such as feeding techniques, bathing, crying, and holding the baby.

   **Do:** Engage each of the home visiting nurses in participating in the mock calls.

   **Check:** Assess the abilities of each of the nurses to respond to the questions from the new mother by having the public health nurse use a simple yes/no checklist of prepared questions.

   Assess how efficient the nurse is in completing the consultation. Can answers to the questions be noted immediately, or does help need to be sought from others prior to answering the mother's question? Use a checklist to identify the time on the call, and ability to independently answer the questions.

   **Act:** If the nurses were able to provide the consultation efficiently and without assistance, implement the process with new mothers and babies, use PDCA for the implementation to identify any problems with the process.

   If the nurses were unable to efficiently provide the consult, provide additional education and tools to increase their efficiency. Use the PDCA process until the nurses are able to efficiently provide the consult.

   The PDCA cycle is continuously repeated until the administration, the nurses, and the clients are satisfied that the process is working.

   Data from these small tests will provide realistic estimates of the percentage of the nurses who can successfully engage in consultation via phone. The purpose in the initial assessment and education of the nurses is to ensure faster consults so more mothers and babies can be contacted in a short period without adding to the nurses' workload, while potentially reducing the amount of time for the home visit because the mother may be better prepared to care for the baby's needs with this support. The improvement process may enlist the support of all nursing staff and administration and create a change in the work environment through the development of a planned phone consultation process for all clients who may receive home visits.

   As students develop questions, they also develop a PDCA approach to answering those questions.

From Cronenwett L, Sherwood G, Barnsteiner J, et al: Quality and safety education for nurses, Nurs Outlook 55(3):122-131, 2007.

## Structure

The vision, values, philosophy, and objectives of an agency serve to define the structural standards of the agency. Evaluation of structure is a specific approach to looking at quality. In evaluating the structure of an organization, the evaluator determines whether the agency is adhering to the stated philosophy and objectives and to its vision and stated values. Is the agency providing services to populations across the life span? Are primary, secondary, and/or tertiary preventive services offered? Standards of structure are defined by the licensing or accrediting agency (e.g., the Community Health Accreditation Program's [CHAP's] standards for accrediting home health agencies).

Identifying values, the first step in a QA program, serves to define the beliefs of the agency about humanity, nursing, the community, and health. The beliefs of the community, the population to be served, and the providers of care are equally important to the agency, and all need to be considered to provide quality service.

Identifying standards and criteria for QA begins with writing the philosophy and objectives of the organization. Program objectives define the intended results of nursing care, descriptions of client behaviors, and/or change in health status to be demonstrated on discharge.

Once objectives are formulated, the resources needed to accomplish the objectives should be identified. The personnel, supplies and equipment, facilities, and financial resources that are needed should be described. Once resources are determined, policies, procedures, and job descriptions should be formed to serve as behavioral guides to the employees of the agency. These documents should reflect the essential nursing and other health provider qualifications needed to implement the services of the agency.

Standards of structure are evaluated internally by a committee composed of administrative, management, and staff members for the purpose of doing a self-study. Standards of structure are also evaluated by a utilization review committee, often composed of an external advisory group with community representatives for all services offered through an agency, such as a nurse, a public health physician, an environmental engineer, a sanitation engineer, a health educator, a board member, and an administrator from a similar agency. The data from these committees identify the strengths and weaknesses of the agency structure.

## Process

The evaluation of process standards is a specific look at the quality of care being given by agency providers, such as nurses. Agencies use a variety of methods to determine criteria for evaluating provider activities: conceptual models; the standards of care of the provider's professional organization, such as the ANA's *Scope and Standards of Public Health Nursing Practice* (ANA, 2013) (see Chapter 1); or the nursing process. The activities of the nurse are evaluated to see whether they are the same as the nursing care procedures defined by the public health agency.

The primary approaches used for process evaluation include the peer review committee and the client (often community) satisfaction survey. The techniques used for process evaluation are direct observation, focus groups, questionnaire, interview, written audit, and video or digital recordings of client and provider encounters.

Once data are collected to evaluate nursing process standards, the peer review committee reviews the data to identify strengths and weaknesses in the quality of care delivered. The peer review committee is usually an internal committee composed of representatives of the nursing staff who are trained to administer audit instruments and conduct client interviews.

## Outcome

The evaluation of outcome standards, or the result of nursing care, is one of the more difficult tasks facing nursing today. Identifying changes in the client's health status that result from nursing care provides nursing data that demonstrate the contribution of nursing to the health care delivery system. Research studies using the tracer or sentinel method to identify client outcomes and client satisfaction surveys can be used to measure outcome standards. Measures of outcome standards include client data about the changes in the community in low-birth-weight babies as a result of improved prenatal care and client compliance with care through the WIC program.

From these data, strengths and weaknesses in nursing care delivery can be determined. The most common measurement methods are direct physical observations and interviews. Instruments have also been developed to measure general health status indicators in home health. The Omaha Visiting Nurse Association problem classification system includes nursing diagnosis, protocols of care, and a problem rating scale to measure nursing care outcomes. In addition, the ANA has developed 10 areas for data collection of outcome criteria in community-based, non–acute care settings, including pain management, consistency of communication, staff mix, client satisfaction, prevention of tobacco use, cardiovascular disease prevention, caregiver activity, identification of primary caregiver, activities of daily living, and psychosocial interactions (Rowell, 2001). Nursing has been involved primarily in evaluating program outcomes to justify program expenses rather than in evaluating client outcomes.

Outcome evaluation assumes that health care has a positive effect on client status. The major problem with outcome evaluation is determining which nursing care activities are primarily responsible for causing changes in client status. Recently, studies have been conducted on nurse-sensitive indicators, such as failure to rescue, that show the importance of nurse staffing in adverse client outcomes (Doran, 2011; McCormack et al, 2010). In nursing, many uncontrolled factors in the field, such as environment, community services, and family relationships, have an effect on client status. Often it is difficult to determine whether these factors are the cause of changes in client status or whether nursing interventions have the most effect.

Types of problems studied in a QA program include reasons for the following:

- Client death (population mortality)
- Client injury (population morbidity)
- Personnel and client safety
- Agency liability
- Increased costs

## TABLE 26-2   Quality Assurance Measures

| Structure | Process | Outcome |
|---|---|---|
| Internal agency | Peer review committees | Internal agency committees |
| Self-study | Prospective audit | Evaluative studies |
| Review agency documents | Concurrent audit | Survey health status |
|  | Retrospective audit |  |
| External agency | Client | Client |
| Regulatory audit | Satisfaction survey | Malpractice suits |
|  | Utilization review | Satisfaction survey |

- Denied reimbursement by third-party payers (decreased program funding by government)
- Client complaints
- Inefficient service
- Staff noncompliance with standards of structure
- Lack of resources
- Unnecessary staff work and overtime
- Documenting of care
- Client health status (population health status)
  Table 26-2 summarizes QA measures.

### Evaluation, Interpretation, and Action

Interpreting the findings of a quality care evaluation is an important part of the process. It allows differences between the quality care standards of the agency and the actual practice of the nurse or other health providers to be identified. These patterns reflect the total agency's functioning over time and generate information for decisions to be made about the strengths and limits of the agency. Regular intervals for evaluation should be established within the agency, and periodic reports should be written so that the combined results of structure, process, and outcome efforts can be analyzed and health care delivery patterns and problems can be identified. These reports should be used to establish an ongoing picture of changes that occur within an agency to justify nursing services.

Identifying choices of possible courses of action to correct the weaknesses within the agency should involve both the administration and the staff. The courses of action chosen should be based on their importance, cost, and timeliness. For example, if there is a nursing problem in the recording of client health education, the agency administration and staff may analyze the problem to see why it is occurring. Reasons for lack of record-keeping given by the nurses include a lack of time to do paperwork properly, workloads that reduce the amount of time spent with clients, and lack of available resources for health education. If such reasons are given, it would not be appropriate for management to deal with the problem by providing a staff development program on the importance of doing and recording health education; it would be more important to assess how to provide the time and resources necessary for the nurses to offer health education to the clients. Economically, it may be more beneficial to provide personal data assistants or laptop computers and clerical assistance so that nurses can make notes at the point of implementation, thereby providing more client contact time, or it may be more beneficial economically to employ an additional nurse and reduce workloads.

Taking action is the final step in the QA/QI model. Once the alternative courses of action are chosen to correct problems, actions must be implemented for change to occur in the overall operation of the agency. Follow-up and evaluation of actions taken must occur to improve quality of care. Although health provider evaluation will continue to be included in a QI effort, the focus of a CQI effort emphasizes the process and not the person. The assumption here is that health care professionals and other employees customarily want to do the best job possible for the client, and problems or differences in a process should not be automatically attributed to their behavior. Although frequent feedback should be given to all employees, the hallmark of QI is continuous learning. Staff development must be ongoing for all employees. (The Levels of Prevention box shows prevention levels related to quality management.)

### LEVELS OF PREVENTION

#### Quality Management

**Primary Prevention**

The nurse participates in a parent education program to improve the immunization level of children in the local elementary school and develops a strategy for follow-up.

**Secondary Prevention**

Agency evaluation, using a retrospective audit of records of the immunization program, determines that the vaccine-preventable infectious disease rates have declined in the elementary school after the implementation of the parent education program.

**Tertiary Prevention**

A review of the public health report card indicated that community incidence of complications from vaccine-preventable diseases have declined over a 2-year period after the implementation of the parent education program.

Documentation is essential to evaluating quality care in any organization. The following section focuses on the kinds of documentation that normally occur in a community agency.

## RECORDS

Records are an important part of the communication structure of the health care organization. Accurate and complete records are required by law and must be kept by all government and nongovernment agencies. In most states, the state departments of health stipulate the kinds of records to be kept and their content requirements for community agencies.

Records provide complete information about the client (whether a family, group, population or community), indicate the extent and quality of services being given, resolve legal issues in malpractice suits, and provide information for education and research.

### Community and Public Health Agency Records

Within the community or public health agency, many types of records are kept and used to predict population trends in a community, to identify health needs and problems, to prepare and justify budgets, and to make administrative decisions. The kinds of records kept by the agency may include reports of accidents, births, census, chronic disease, communicable disease, mortality rates, life expectancy, morbidity rates, child and spouse abuse, occupational illness and injury, and environmental health.

Other types of records kept within the agency are those used to maintain administrative contact and control of the organization. Three types of records make up this category: clinical, provider service, and financial. The *clinical record* is the client health record. The *provider service records* include information about the number of clinic clients seen daily, the immunizations given, home visits made daily, transportation and mileage, the provider's time spent with the client, and the amount and kinds of supplies used. The service record is completed on a daily basis by each provider and is summarized monthly and annually to indicate trends in health care activities and costs related to personnel time, transportation, maintenance, and supplies. The provider service records are used to compare with the agency's *financial records* of salaries, overhead, and transportation costs, and they serve as the basis for the cost accounting system. These records are basic to peer review and audit.

Three additional kinds of service records seen in the community agency are the central index system, the annual implementation plan, and the annual summary of agency activities. The *central index system* is a data filing system that indicates the services requested, services offered, active and inactive clients of the agency, and a profile of the agency's clients.

The *annual implementation plan* (often referred to as the strategic plan or tactical plan) is developed at the beginning of each fiscal year to define the short- and long-term goals of the agency. The annual implementation plan serves as the basis for the agency's annual summary. The *annual summary* reflects the success of the agency in meeting the annual objectives, the changes in population trends and health status during the year, the actual versus the projected budget requirements, the number of services offered, the number of clients served, and the plans and changes recommended for the future. This plan serves as the basis for the evaluation of agency structure.

As an outgrowth of QA efforts in the health care system, comprehensive methods are being designed to document and measure client progress and client outcome from agency admission through discharge. An example of such a method is the client classification system developed at the Visiting Nurses Association of Omaha, Nebraska (Martin, 2005; The Omaha System, 2014). This comprehensive method for evaluating client care has several components: a classification system for assessing and categorizing client problems, a database, a nursing problem list, and anticipated outcome criteria for the classified problem. Such schemes are viewed as having the potential to improve the delivery of nursing care, documentation of care, and the descriptions of client care. Briefly, implementing a comprehensive documentation method improves nursing assessment, planning, implementation, and evaluation of client care; it also allows the organization of important client information for more effective and efficient nurse productivity and communication (see Figure 26-2).

## ⟫ LINKING CONTENT TO PRACTICE

The Robert Wood Johnson Foundation (RWJF) funded a project initiative focusing on the development of competencies and resources to enhance the ability of nursing professionals to deliver high-quality and safe nursing care. The Quality Safety Education for Nurses collaboration identified and defined six quality and safety competencies for nursing. In addition, the project allowed for the development of proposed targets for the knowledge, skills, and attitudes of students for each of the six competencies identified by the Institute of Medicine as: client-centered care, teamwork and collaboration, evidence-based practice, quality improvement, safety, and informatics. The overall goal for the Quality and Safety Education for Nurses (QSEN) project is to meet the challenge of preparing future nurses who will have the knowledge, skills, and attitudes (KSAs) necessary to continuously improve the quality and safety of the health care systems within which they work. The following are the definitions for each of the six competencies and examples of the chapters in the text where content can be found and related to the competency:

Client-centered care: Recognize the client or designee as the source of control and full partner in providing compassionate and coordinated care based on respect for client's preferences, values, and needs. (Chapters 4, 6, 7, 9, 12, 14, 15, 19)

Teamwork and Collaboration: Function effectively within nursing and interprofessional teams, fostering open communication, mutual respect, and shared decision making to achieve quality client care. (Chapters 5, 6, 8, 10, 16, 18, 20-22, 26-28, 30, 32-35, 37, 39, 41, 45, 46)

Evidence-Based Practice (EBP): Integrate best current evidence with clinical expertise and client/family preferences and values for delivery of optimal health care. (All chapters, with emphasis in Chapters 15 and 26)

Quality Improvement (QI): Use data to monitor the outcomes of care processes and use improvement methods to design and test changes to continuously improve the quality and safety of health care systems. (Chapters 3, 8, 10, 12, 14, 18, 20, 24, 25, 26)

Safety: Minimizes risk of harm to clients and providers through both system effectiveness and individual performance. (Chapters 12, 13, 14, 23, 24, 28, 39-46)

Informatics: Use information and technology to communicate, manage knowledge, mitigate error, and support decision making. (Chapters 23-26)

All of these competencies are addressed in this text as the competencies relate to public health nursing practice. The knowledge, skills, and attitudes related to QI are addressed in this chapter and one area of the QI competency appears in the following table.

| Knowledge | Skills | Attitudes |
|---|---|---|
| Describe approaches for changing processes of care | Design a small test of change in daily work (using an experiential learning method such as PDCA) | Value local change (in individual practice or team practice on a unit) and its role in creating joy in work |
| | Practice aligning the aims, measures, and changes involved in improving care | Appreciate the value of what individuals and teams can to do to improve care |
| | Use measures to evaluate the effect of change | |

From Institute of Medicine: Health professions education: a bridge to quality, Washington, DC, 2003, National Academies Press.

## PRACTICE APPLICATION

Oscar, a nursing student, has been working in the migrant farm-worker clinic and has noted that each practitioner uses a different educational method for teaching good nutrition practices to newly diagnosed diabetic clients. The clinic has seen a substantial increase in the number of new diabetic clients in the Hispanic farmworker population. Oscar knows that practice guidelines for teaching nutrition practices exist in his clinical facility and that charts have an area to note nutrition education information. He also knows that for nurses to be most effective and ensure quality client outcomes, research-based practice guidelines should be used by all nurses in the health department.

As part of his course, Oscar must prepare a teaching plan and conduct a class on a health care problem. He obtains permission from his instructor and the director of the clinic to conduct an in-service program. The purpose of Oscar's in-service program is to instruct the nursing staff how to teach newly diagnosed diabetic clients good nutrition practices. He obtains and studies the guidelines about teaching good

nutrition practices from the National Guideline Clearinghouse titled Diabetes Type 1 and 2 Evidence-based Nutrition Practice Guideline for Adults (2010), and he researches the methodological background for development of the guidelines. Oscar's native language is Spanish, so this will help him in determining whether brochures for newly diagnosed diabetic clients regarding good nutrition convey the appropriate message.

As part of his in-service program, Oscar keeps demographic records on attendees and conducts before-and-after tests of knowledge, adding questions about the present use of the guidelines. He plans to follow up with the nurses in 6 months with a further test and questions about use of the guidelines. The director will help him determine an outcome measure that can be used with the client population to show effective use of the guidelines.

A. What outcome measure would be useful in this project?
B. How will this help in the overall assessment of quality in the nursing service?

**Answers can be found on the Evolve site.**

## KEY POINTS

- The health care delivery system is the largest employing industry in the United States; society is demanding increased efficiency and effectiveness from the system.
- The actual quality and safety of care in the United States is being assessed regularly and reported in four reports.
- Because of varying definitions, logistics, and data collection methods, quality is difficult to assess accurately.
- Responding to the quality of care question, the federal government has instituted several quality improvement programs. Among these are the National Healthcare Quality Report (NHQR) that is used to monitor the nation's progress toward improved health care quality; the Center for Medicare and Medicaid Services (CMS) Outcomes Based Quality Improvement (OBQI) for home health; and the National Committee for Quality Assurance (NCQA), which provides performance information, or report cards, for health care agencies.
- Quality improvement is the tool used to ensure effective and efficient care.
- The managed care industry is changing the face of the American health care delivery system and how quality is defined and measured.
- Objective and systematic evaluation of nursing care has become a priority within the profession for several reasons, including the effects of cost on health care access, consumer demands for better quality care, and increasing involvement of nurses in formulating public and health agency policy.
- Total quality management is a management philosophy new to the public health care arena. It is prevention oriented and process focused. Its primary focus is to deliver quality health care. One measure of quality is customer satisfaction.

- Public and private sectors are forming partnerships to monitor the performance of all players in health care delivery to improve the health of communities. The different players in the health care system have different perceptions of quality.
- Quality assurance/quality improvement (QA/QI) is the monitoring of client care activities to determine the degree of excellence attained in implementing activities.
- Quality assurance has been a concern of the profession since the 1860s, when Florence Nightingale called for a uniform format to gather and disseminate hospital statistics.
- Licensure has been a major issue in nursing since 1892.
- Two major categories of approaches exist in QA/QI today: general and specific.
- Accreditation is an approach to quality control used for institutions, whereas licensure is used primarily for individuals.
- Certification combines features of both licensing and accreditation.
- Three major models have been used to evaluate quality: Donabedian's structure-process-outcome model, the sentinel model, and the tracer model.
- A fourth model to evaluate quality—the PDCA model—has been adopted by the public health system.
- Seven basic components of a quality improvement program are (1) identifying values, (2) identifying structure, process, and outcome standards and criteria, (3) selecting measurement techniques, (4) interpreting the strengths and weaknesses of the care given, (5) identifying alternative courses of action, (6) choosing specific courses of action, and (7) taking action.

## KEY POINTS—cont'd

- Records are an integral part of the communication structure of a health care organization. Accurate and complete records are by law required of all agencies, whether governmental or nongovernmental.
- QA/QI mechanisms in health care delivery are the mechanisms for controlling the system and requesting accountability from individual providers within the system. Records

help establish a total picture of the contribution of the agency to the client community.
- Delivering quality care to individuals, communities, and populations falls under the 10 essential services of public health.
- Evidence-based practice guidelines can help population-centered nurses document the outcomes and effectiveness of their interventions.

## CLINICAL DECISION-MAKING ACTIVITIES

1. Write your own definition of TQM; compare your definition with the one given in the text. Are they the same or different? Give justification for your answer.
2. How does traditional QA/QI fit with the CQI effort? Explain the relative importance of a continuing QA/QI effort.
3. Interview a nurse who is a coordinator of or is responsible for QA/QI in a local health agency. Ask the following questions and add your own. Do the answers to the questions relate to what you have learned about QA/QI? Explain.
   A. Does the agency subscribe to the TQM approach to management?
   B. If not, is the agency incorporating elements of the TQM process as outlined by Deming (1986) in his 15 points?
   C. Is a traditional method of management used to ensure quality?
   D. Describe the components of the QA/QI program.
   E. How are records used in your QA/QI effort?
   F. Discuss the approaches and techniques that are used to implement the QA/QI program.

   G. How has the QA/QI program changed in the health agency over the past 20 years?
   H. What influence has the QA/QI program had on decreasing problems attributable to process? To provider accountability?
   I. List and describe the types of records usually kept in a community health agency. Explain the purpose of each type of record.
4. Identify partnerships necessary to ensure quality health outcomes for your community from data gathered in a community assessment. Explain why these partners are necessary.
5. Find the *Guide to Community Preventive Services* on the CDC website, and look for the segments on smoking cessation or tuberculosis control. How could you use this information in your practice in health?
6. Explain the nurse's responsibilities and role in the CQI program.

## REFERENCES

Agency for Healthcare Research and Quality: *Disparities in Healthcare Quality Among racial and Ethnic Groups.* Rockville, MD, 2012, USDHHS. AHRQ Pub. No. 12-0006-1-EF.

Agency for Healthcare Research and Quality: *2013 National Healthcare Disparities Report.* Rockville, MD, May 2014a, USDHHS. AHRQ Pub. No. 14-0006.

Agency for Healthcare Research and Quality: *2013 National Healthcare Quality Report.* Rockville, MD, 2014b, USDHHS. AHRQ Pub. No. 14-0005.

Agency for Healthcare Research and Quality: *Your Guide to Choosing Quality Health Care.* Rockville, MD, 2014c, AHRQ.

American Nurses Association: *The Scope and Standards of Public Health Nursing Practice.* Washington, DC, 1999, The Association.

American Nurses Association: *Public Health Nursing: Scope and Standards of Practice.* Silver Springs, MD, 2007, The Association.

American Nurses Association: *Public Health Nursing: Scope and Standards of Practice.* Silver Springs, MD, 2009, The Association.

American Nurses Association: *Public Health Nursing: Scope and Standards of Practice,* ed 2. Silver Springs, MD, 2013, American Nurses Association.

American Nurses Association: *Code of Ethics for Nurses with Interpretive Statements.* Washington, DC, 2013, ANA.

American Nurses Credentialing Center: *Magnet recognition program.* 2014. Accessed 10/14/2014 at www.nursescredentialing.org.

American Nurses Credentialing Center: *Accreditation.* 2014. Accessed 10/14/2014 at www.nursescredentialing.org.

American Public Health Association: *Healthy Communities 2000: Model Standards, Guidelines for Community Attainment of the Year 2000 National Health Objectives,* ed 3. Washington, DC, 1991, APHA.

Association of Community Health Nursing Educators: *Perspectives on Doctoral Education in Community Health Nursing.* Lexington, KY, 1993, ACHNE.

Association of Community Health Nursing Educators: *Essentials of Baccalaureate Nursing Education for Entry Level Community Health Nursing Practice.* Chapel Hill, NC, 2000a, updated 2009, ACHNE.

Association of Community Health Nursing Educators: *Graduate Education for Advanced Practice Education in Community/Public Health Nursing.* Chapel Hill, NC, 2000b, ACHNE.

Association of Community Health Nursing Educators: *Graduate Education for Advanced Practice in Community Public Health Nursing.* New York, 2003, ACHNE.

Association of Community Health Nursing Educators: *Graduate Education for Advanced Practice Public Health Nursing: at the Crossroads.* Chapel Hill, NC, 2007, ACHNE.

Banner Health: *The quality improvement committee peer review.* 2012. Available at: www.bannerhealth.com. Accessed 10/14/2014.

Bialek R, Carden J: Supporting public health departments' quality improvement initiatives: lessons learned from the Public Health Foundation. *J Public Health Manag Pract* 16(1):14–18, 2010.

Blegen MA: Does certification of staff nurses improve patient outcomes? *Evid Based Nurs* 15:54–55, 2012.

Boltz M, Capezuti E, Wagner L, et al: Patient safety in medical-surgical units: can nurse certification make a difference? *Medsurg Nurs* 22(1):26–37, 2013.

Braunstein S, Lavizzo-Mourey R: How the health and community development sectors are combining forces to improve health and well-being. *Health Aff* 30(11):2042–2051, 2011.

Centers for Disease Control and Prevention: *Planned Approach to Community Health: Guide for Local Coordinators.* Atlanta, 1995, CDC, National Center for Chronic Disease Prevention and Health Promotion, and updated 2010.

Centers for Disease Control and Prevention: *National Public Health Performance Standards (NPHPS)*. 2014. Available at http://www.cdc.gov/nphpsp/. Accessed August 1, 2014.

Centers for Medicare and Medicaid: *Quality improvement organizations*. 2014a. Available at www.cms.gov. Accessed 10/14/2014.

Centers for Medicare and Medicaid: *Accreditation*. 2014b. Available at www.cms.gov. Accessed 10/14/2014.

Chassin MR, Loeb JM: The ongoing quality improvement journey: next stop, high reliability. *Health Aff* 30(4):559–568, 2011.

Clancy C, Lloyd R: High quality health care. In Kovner AR, Knickman JR, editors: *Jonas and Kovner's Health Care Delivery in the United States*, ed 10. New York, NY, 2011, Springer.

Commision on Collegiate Nursing Education. *Accreditation standards for nursing*. 2014. Available at www.ccne.nihc.edu. Accessed 10/14/2014.

Community Health Accreditation Partners: *Home health accreditation*. 2014. Available at www.chapinc.org. Accessed 10/14/2014.

Council on Linkages Between Academia and Public Health Practice: *The Core Competencies for Public Health Professionals*. Washington, DC, 2014, The Public Health Foundation.

Davis MV, Mahanna E, Joly B, et al: Creating quality improvement culture in public health agencies. *Am J Public Health* 104(1):e98–e104, 2014.

de Jonge V, Nicolaas JS, van Leerdam ME, et al: Overview of the quality assurance movement in health care. *Best Pract Res Clin Gastroenterol* 25(3):337–347, 2011.

The Deming Institute: *Plan, do, check, act model*. 2014. Available at www.deming.org. Accessed 10/14/2014.

Deming WE: *Out of the Crisis*. Cambridge, MA, 1986, Massachusetts Institute of Technology, Center for Advanced Engineering Study.

Donabedian A: *Explorations in Quality Assessment and Monitoring*, vol 2. Ann Arbor, MI, 1981, Health Administration Press.

Donabedian A: *Explorations in Quality Assessment and Monitoring*, vol 3. Ann Arbor, MI, 1985, Health Administration Press.

Donabedian A: *An Introduction to Quality Assurance in Health Care*. New York, 2003, Oxford University Press.

Doran DM: *Nursing Outcomes: The State of the Science*, ed 2. Sudbury, MA, 2011, Jones & Bartlett.

Fitzgerald M: *State Licensure and Certification: Myths and Realities*. 2013, Fitzgerald Health Education Association. Available at: www.fhea.com.

Gunzenhauser JD, Eggena ZP, Fielding JE, et al: The quality improvement experience in a high-performing local health department: Los Angeles County. *J Public Health Manag Pract* 16(1):39–48, 2010.

Healthy People 2020: *Implementing Healthy People 2020 MAP-IT: A guide to using Healthy People 2020 in your community*. 2011. Available at www.healthy people2002.gov. Accessed June 17, 2011.

Honoré PA, Scott W: *Priority Areas for Improvement of Quality in Public Health*. Washington, DC, November 2010, USDHHS.

Institute of Medicine: *Crossing the Quality Chasm*. Washington, DC, 2001, National Academy Press.

Institute of Medicine: *Health Matters*. Washington, DC, 2011, National Academy Press.

Institute of Medicine: *Toward Quality Measures for Population Health and the Leading Health Indicators*. Washington, DC, 2013, The National Academies Press.

Kaiser Health News: *Accountable Care Organizations Explained*. 2014, Kaiser Family Foundation. Available at: www.khn.org.

Kaplan HC, Brady PW, Dritz MC, et al: The influence of context on quality improvement success in health care: a systematic review of the literature. *Milbank Q* 88(4):500–559, 2010.

Keefe S: *Advance: nurses salary survey: results in! Many hospitals don't need to increase salaries to be competitive—for now*, March 1, 2010. Available at www.advanceweb.com.

Keller LO, Strohschein S, Lia-Hoagberg B, et al: Population-based public health interventions: practice-based and evidence-supported, Part I. *Public Health Nurs* 21:453–468, 2004a.

Keller LO, Strohschein S, Schaffer MA, et al: Population-based public health interventions: innovations in practice, teaching and management, Part II. *Public Health Nurs* 21:469–487, 2004b.

Kelly D: *Applying Quality Management in Health Care: A Systems Approach*, ed 3. Washington, DC, 2011, Health Administration Press.

Kendall-Gallagher D, Aiken LH, Sloane DM, et al: Nurse specialty certification, inpatient mortality, and failure to rescue. *J Nurs Scholarsh* 43(2):188–194, 2011.

Kessner DM, Kalk CE: Assessing health quality—the case for tracers. *N Engl J Med* 288:189, 1973.

Keyser DJ, Dembosky JW, Kmetik K, et al: Using health information technology–related performance measures and tools to improve chronic care. *Jt Comm J Qual Patient Saf* 35(5):248–255, 2009.

Kovner AR, Knickman JR, editors: *Jonas and Kovner's Health Care Delivery in the United States*, ed 10. New York, NY, 2011, Springer.

The Kresge Foundation: *Community health partnerships*. 2014. Available at www.kresge.org. Accessed 10/14/2014.

Maibusch RM: Evolution of quality assurance for nursing in hospitals. In Schroder PS, Maibusch RM, editors: *Nursing Quality Assurance*. Rockville, MD, 1984, Aspen.

Malloch K, Porter-O'Grady T: *Introduction to Evidence-Based Practice in Nursing and Health Care*, ed 2. Sudbury, MA, 2010, Jones and Bartlett.

Matthew-Maich N, Ploeg J, Dobbins M, et al: Supporting the uptake of nursing guidelines: what you really need to know to move nursing guidelines into practice. *Worldviews Evid Based Nurs* 10(2):104–115, 2013.

Martin S: *The Omaha System: A Key to Practice, Documentation, and Information Management*, ed 2. St. Louis, 2005, Mosby.

Martinez JM: Hospice and palliative nursing certification: the journey to defining a new nursing specialty. *J Hosp Palliat Nurs* 13(6):S29–S34, 2011.

McCormack B, Dewing J, Breslin L, et al: Developing person-centered practice: nursing outcomes arising from changes to the care environment in residential settings for older people. *Int J Older People Nurs* 5(2):93–107, 2010.

Minnesota Department of Health, Division of Community Health Services: *Public Health Interventions: Applications for Public Health Nursing Practice*. St Paul, MN, March 2001, Public Health Nursing Section.

National Association of City and County Health Officials: *APEXPH in Practice*. Washington, DC, 1995, NACCHO.

National Association of City and County Health Officials: *Mobilizing for Action Through Planning and Partnerships: Web-Based Tool*. Washington, DC, 2014, NACCHO. Available at: http://mapp.naccho.org. Accessed 10/14/2014.

National Association for Healthcare Quality: *Risk Management: NAHQ Guide to Quality Management*. Skokie, Ill, 1993, NAHQ Press.

National Association of Home Care: *Uniform data set for home care and hospice*. 2010. Available at http://www.nahc.org/NAHC/Research/unidata.html. Accessed February 5, 2011.

National Committee for Quality Assurance: *HEDIS: Health Plan for Employee and Data Information set*. Washington, DC, 2013a, NCQA.

National Committee on Quality Assurance: *National Healthcare Quality Report*. Rockville, MD, 2013b, Agency for Healthcare Quality and Research, USDHHS.

National Committee on Quality Assurance: *State of Health Care*. Rockville, MD, 2014c, Agency for Healthcare Quality and Research, USDHHS.

National Council of State Boards of Nursing: *Nurse licensure*. 2014. Available at www.ncsbn.org. Accessed 10/14/2014.

National Council of State Boards of Nursing: *Nurse licensure compact*, 2014. Available at www.nlca.ncsbn.org. Accessed 10/14/2014.

National Guideline Clearinghouse: *Fact Sheet*. Rockville, MD, 2010, Agency for Healthcare Research and Quality, USDHHS.

National Information Center on Health Services Research and Health Care Technology (NICHSR): *Community Health Status Indicators (CHSI): Questions and Answers*. Bethesda, MD, 2012, National Institute of Health, U.S. National Library of Medicine. Available at: http://www.nlm.nih.gov/nichsr/healthindicators/CHSI_Q_and_A.html. Accessed July 31, 2014.

National League for Nursing: *Accreditation Commission for Education in Nursing*. 2014. Avaliable at www.acenursing.org. Accessed 10/14/2014.

National Network of Public Health Institutes: *Public health performance improvement toolkit*. 2013c. Available at www.nnphi.org. Accessed 10/14/2014.

National Quality Forum: *Safe practices for better healthcare*. 2010. Available at http://www.ahrq.gov/qual/nqfpract.htm. Accessed 10/14/2014.

Oakland JS: *Total Quality Management and Operational Excellence: Text with Cases*, ed 4. New York, NY, 2014, Routledge.

The Omaha System: *Omaha system overview 2014*, 2014. Available at http://www.omahasystem.org/overview.html. Accessed September 15, 2014.

Papanicolas I, Smith PC: *Health System Performance Comparison: An Agenda for Policy, Information and Research*. New York, NY, 2013, Open University Press.

Phaneuf M: A nursing audit method. *Nurs Outlook* 5:42, 1965.

Public Health Accreditation Board: *National Voluntary Accreditation Program for Public Health Agencies*. Washington, DC, 2014, PHAB.

Quad Council of Public Health Nursing Organization: *Quad Council competencies for public health nursing,* Summer 2011. Available at http://www.resourcenter.net/images/ACHNE/Files/QuadCouncilCompetenciesForPublicHealthNurses_Summer2011.pdf. Accessed July 11, 2014.

Riley WJ, Moran JW, Corso LC, et al: Defining quality improvement in public health. *J Public Health Manag Pract* 16(1):5–7, 2010.

Rowell PA: Beyond the acute care setting: community-based non-acute care nursing-sensitive indicators. *Outcomes Manag Nurs Pract* 5:24, 2001.

Sakamoto SD, Avila M: The public health nursing practice manual: a tool for public health nurses. *Public Health Nurs* 21:179–182, 2004.

Simon K: *Effective brainstorming in SixSigma,* n.d. Available at http://www.isixsigma.com/library/content/c010401a.asp. Accessed April 12, 2007.

Smith K, Bazini-Barakat N: A public health nursing practice model: melding public health practice with the nursing process. *Public Health Nurs* 20:42–48, 2004.

Smith RA, Manassaram-Baptiste D, Brooks D, et al: Cancer screening in the United States, 2014: a review of current American Cancer Society guidelines and current issues in cancer screening. *CA Cancer J Clin* 64(1):30–51, 2014.

Sollecito WA, Johnson JK: *McLaughlin and Kaluzny's Continuous Quality Improvement in Health Care,* ed 4. Burlington, MA, 2013, Jones & Bartlett.

Sullivan DT: Healthcare quality. In DeNisco SM, Barker AM, editors: *Advance Practice Nursing: Evolving Roles for the Transformation of the Profession,* ed 2. Burlington, MA, 2013, Jones & Barlett.

University of Kansas: *The community toolbox.* 2014. Avaliable at www.ctb.ku.edu. Accessed 10/14/2014.

University of Wisconsin-Madison, School of Nursing: *Wisconsin Public Health Nursing Practice Model, Companion Notes.* 2010, Linking Education and Practice for Excellence in Public Health Nursing (LEAP). Available at: http://www.son.wisc.edu/LEAP/pdfs/WPHN_companion_2010_07.pdf. Accessed February 5, 2011.

U.S. Department of Health and Human Services: *Healthy People 2010: Understanding and Improving Health,* ed 2. Washington, DC, 2000, U.S. Government Printing Office.

U.S. Department of Health and Human Services: *Healthy People in Healthy Communities.* Washington, DC, February 2001, U.S. Government Printing Office.

U.S. Department of Health and Human Services: *Healthy People 2020.* Washington, DC, 2010, U.S. Government Printing Office.

U.S. Department of Health and Human Services: *HHS Action Plan to Reduce Racial and Ethnic Health Disparities.* Washington, DC, April 2011a, USDHHS.

U.S. Department of Health and Human Services: *Quality Improvement.* Rockville, MD, 2011b, Health Resources and Services Administration (HRSA).

U.S. Department of Health and Human Services: *Home health compare: Medicare* 2014: Available at http://www.hhs.gov. Accessed 10/14/2014.

U.S. Department of Health and Human Services: *2013 National Health Care Quality Report.* Rockville MD, May 2014, Agency for Health Care Quality and Research. AHRQ Pub. No. 14-0005.

United States Preventive Services Task Force: *US clinical preventive services,* 2014. Avaliable at www.uspstf.gov.

Van den Heuvel J, Niemeijer GC, Does RJMM: Measuring healthcare quality: the challenges. *Int J Health Care Qual Assur* 26(3):269–278, 2013.

Zale JM, Selvan MS: Interfaces between quality improvement, law, and medical ethics. In Varkey P, editor: *Medical Quality Management: Theory and Practice.* Sudbury, PA, 2009, Jones and Barlett.

# PART 5

# Health Promotion with Target Populations Across the Life Span

The family is a major influence on the individual's concept of health and illness. It is within the family that a person's sense of self-esteem and personal competence is developed. The action taken by or for the person with a health problem depends on this sense of self-worth and the family's definitions of health and illness. Environmental, social, cultural, and economic factors, as well as the resources of the community to meet health needs, influence the family's health risks and reaction to health. The goals of the nation for the year 2020 focus on changing the overall health of the nation, with emphasis on the specific health and health care issues of populations. Through family support the individual may develop the responsibility to participate in activities that will lead to a healthier lifestyle.

Major health problems of individuals can be identified and related to their developmental phase. This factor becomes evident when age-specific morbidity data are reviewed. Nurses can influence the actions and reactions to health of all individuals in the community from birth through senescence. The nurse can influence the health of children by introducing healthy parenting behaviors, risk factor appraisal, and age-appropriate interventions.

Women and men are faced with many life changes and challenges, some of which are gender specific. Previous lifestyles and increases in stress from social, environmental, and economic constraints often result in risk for major health problems during adulthood.

The nurse's primary function with persons of all ages should be to promote quality as well as a long and healthy life. As the elderly segment of the population continues to grow, the health care delivery system and nurses must address and plan strategies to cope with increasing longevity and chronic health problems.

Attention is also focused on the needs of compromised populations. *Healthy People 2020* has a specific goal to promote the health and well-being of compromised populations. Over 15% of the United States population has some type of long-lasting condition. Nursing interventions must be refined to assist this group in meeting their health care needs. As the nurse studies and gathers evidence about the health issues of populations such as children, women, men, and the elderly, he/she can better understand how to assess and plan for care of individuals who are members of these compromised populations. Community-oriented nurses assess the risk of age-related issues in populations, promote the development of programs and policies that will promote initiatives to enhance population health status, and ensure that such programs are available to address the health risks of these target populations.

# 27

# Working with Families in the Community for Healthy Outcomes

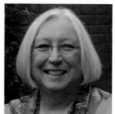

### *Joanna Rowe Kaakinen, PhD, RN*

Dr. Joanna Rowe Kaakinen has been a family nurse scholar for the last 25 years. She has written extensively about family nursing. She is a reviewer for the *Journal of Family Nursing,* the *Journal of Family Relations,* a member of the International Association of Family Nurses, and a member of the National Council of Family Relations. She has presented nationally and internationally on family nursing. Dr. Kaakinen is a Professor in the School of Nursing at the Linfield College School of Nursing in Portland, Oregon.

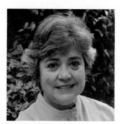

### *Jackie F. Webb, FNP-BC, MS, RN*

Jackie Webb has been a practicing family nurse practitioner for over 25 years, working primarily with underserved populations. She was also director for student health services for a small New England college for almost 10 years, serving young adults. She has taught nursing students both at the undergraduate and graduate levels for the past 15 years. Currently she is a professor at Linfield College School of Nursing in Portland, Oregon. She is currently a doctoral student at Oregon Health Sciences University in Portland, Oregon. Her research focus is looking at innovations in health care delivery.

## ADDITIONAL RESOURCES

## OBJECTIVES

*After reading this chapter, the student should be able to do the following:*

1. Explain the multiple ways public health nurses work with families and communities.
2. Identify challenges to working with families in the community.
3. Describe family function and structure.
4. Describe family demographic trends and demographic changes that affect the health of families.
5. Compare and contrast three social science theoretical frameworks nurses use when working with the family in the community.
6. Work with families using a strength-based approach to assess, develop, and evaluate family action plans.

## KEY TERMS

The health of communities is directly related to the health of its families (ANA, 2007; APHA, 2010; Eddy, Bailey, and Doutrich, 2015). The importance of establishing collaborative relationships with families for providing care has been well documented in public health nursing literature (Wald, 1915; Paavilainen and Astedt-Kurki, 1997; Jonsdottir, Litchfield, and Pharris, 2003; Porr, Drummond, and Olson, 2012). Public health nurses must have skills to move competently between working with individual families, bridge relationships between families and the community, advocate for family and community legislation, and influence policies that promote and protect the health of populations. Therefore, public health nurses must integrate knowledge and practice of family nursing and community health nursing (APHA, 2014) in meeting the needs of families.

Family nursing is a philosophy and a science that is based on the following assumptions: health and illness are family events; what affects one family member affects the whole family; and health care practices, decisions, and behaviors are made within the context of the family (Kaakinen and Hanson, 2015a).

*Public health nursing practice* has a secondary focus: the "synthesis of nursing theory and public health theory applied to promoting, preserving and maintaining the health of populations through the delivery of personal health care services to individuals, families, and groups. The focus of practice is the health of individuals, families and groups and the effect of their health status on the health of the community as a whole" (p. 596) Refer to the inside cover of this text for a table about distinctions in practice.

Nurses practicing in the community use the core competencies for public health professionals (PHF, 2011 and the core public health functions of assessment, assurance, and policy development to promote the interconnectedness of individual health with the health of families and communities (Eddy et al, 2015). The Linking Content to Practice box shows the applications of public health nursing practice from a family perspective. The Healthy People 2020 box highlights four new objectives that have been identified as leading health issues that address ways to improve the health of families and the nation. Nurses who practice with a family nursing philosophy and theory base will improve the health of families, their members, and the community.

## LINKING CONTENT TO PRACTICE

In this chapter the public health core functions with the essential services below are applied to family nursing.

**Assessment**
- Monitor health status of families to identify community health problems.
- Diagnose and investigate health problems and health hazards in the community that affect families.
- Evaluate effectiveness, accessibility, and quality of personal and population-based health services.

**Policy Development**
- Develop policies and plans that support family and community health efforts.
- Enforce laws and regulations that protect health and ensure safety of families in the community.
- Research for new insights and innovative solutions to health problems.

**Assurance**
- Link people to needed personal health services and assure the provision of health care when otherwise unavailable.
- Assure a competent public health and personal health care workforce.
- Mobilize community partnerships to identify and solve health problems.

## HEALTHY PEOPLE 2020

New objectives specific to families and family nursing that relate to a leading health issue.
- AHS 1: Increase the proportion of persons with health insurance
- AH-5-1: Increase the proportion of students who graduate with a regular diploma 4 years after starting the 9th grade
- D-5: Improve glycemic control among persons with diabetes, especially those with A1C greater than 9%
- NWS-9 & 10: Reduce the proportion of adults and children who are obese

From: US Department of Health and Human Services: *Healthy People 2020*, Washington DC, 2010, US Government Printing Office.

## CHALLENGES FOR NURSES WORKING WITH FAMILIES IN THE COMMUNITY

Numerous challenges exist that affect the practice of family nursing in a community setting. Many of the following challenges have been recognized in the family nursing literature for a long time, yet they persist in the current health care system. One role for the nurse would be to advocate that the following challenges be addressed in federal and state health care policies and programs.

### Definition of Family

Now more than ever, the traditional definition of family is being challenged with the legalization of same-sex marriages. There is still no universally agreed on definition of family (Kaakinen and Hanson, 2015a).

Public health nurses and family nurses struggle on a daily basis with the conflict between the narrow traditional legal definition of family used in the health care system and by social policy makers and the broader term used by the family. Family, as defined and implemented in the health care system, continues to be based on the legal notions of relationships such as biological/genetic blood ties and contractual relationships such as adoption, guardianship, or marriage. However, the family system and family nurses use the following broader definition of family: "Family refers to two or more individuals who depend on one another for emotional, physical, and/or financial support. The members of the family are self-defined" (Hanson, 2005).

Given the current social and political climate, nurses need to adopt the open definition described above because the families they work with have a wide variety of family structures. Nurses who work with the people in the individual's everyday world have a higher likelihood of helping them to achieve better health outcomes.

### Transitions of Care

Nurses have a pivotal role relative to communication of information in transitions of care between agencies that frequently result in hospital admission or readmission. Nationally, the number of home health care clients who were admitted to the hospital between 2002 and 2006 was 28.3% (AHCRQ, 2008). The majority of these hospital admissions in home health care clients occurred within 7 days of admission to the home health agency (Vasquez, 2008). It is estimated that about 20% of individuals discharged from a hospital in the United States are readmitted within 30 days (Cloonan, Wood, and Riley, 2013). Of the estimated $17.5 billion in Medicare spending on readmissions, approximately $12 billion is potentially preventable (Centers for Medicare and Medicaid Services, 2013). Individuals most at risk for readmissions are males over 75 years of age, African American, hospitalized with a medical diagnosis, and without insurance other than Medicare (Cloonan et al, 2013).

There are communication issues between health care providers within the community agencies, such as incomplete or missing documentation, that result from rushed assessments. Rushed procedures and failure to follow the plan of action and standards of care are known causes of hospital readmissions (Vasquez, 2008). Persons at high risk for readmission rates parallel those of the population with low health literacy rates (Cloonan et al, 2013; Berkman et al, 2011). Approximately 35% of adults in the United States have limited literacy skills, with an additional 30 million adults who have below basic literacy skills (Berkman et al, 2011). A systematic review of the literature indicated that low health literacy was associated with increased health care use, inappropriate drug use, low use of preventive services, and overall poorer health (Berkman et al, 2011).

It is crucial that home health care staff have current updates on evidence-based practice, standards of care, and interventions to ensure quality health outcomes. Nurses practicing in the community have a significant role in working with multiple health care systems to improve communication and evidence-based design protocols to improve the quality of care and the health of the home health population (Ventura et al, 2010).

Nurses must develop and hone excellent negotiation skills because they spend a significant amount of time arranging for limited services for their under-insured and uninsured clients and families. In working with families, communication and teaching will be more effective if hours of service match the times of day when family members, specifically the family care provider, can attend appointments. Bringing a companion to office visits benefits communication (Wolff et al, 2009; Wolff and Roter, 2008), especially for those with low health literacy (Rosland et al, 2011); enhances shared decision making (Clayman et al, 2005); and improves the sharing of information (Eggly et al, 2006). Involving family in the care of the client improves self-management of health care, results in fewer medication errors (Kinnersley et al, 2007; Wolff et al, 2009), and improves health outcomes (Weinberg et al, 2007). Based on this information about companion participation, it is crucial that nurses involve family as much as possible in their interactions and decisions with clients.

## Uninsured, Underinsured, and Limited Services

Nursing practice in the community presents various challenges such as knowing how to access health care resources for clients and understanding how recent health care reforms are transforming the landscape of our current health care system. Uninsured clients are those who do not have health insurance for any family member. Underserved are individuals who have minimal insurance coverage and usually have a high deductible. Individuals with limited services are people who may have trouble accessing health care and/or experience barriers to health care. For example, a family with insurance coverage may live in a rural area that does not have a primary health care provider or services near them. The main goals of the Affordable Care Act (ACA) of 2010 were to provide U.S. citizens with patient protection and affordable health care, and decrease the overall cost of health care (see Chapter 3 for more discussion). The ACA is designed to offer premium subsidies to help eligible individuals and their families purchase insurance coverage when affordable employer sponsored insurance is not available. Questions remain about how this affordability protection will be applied in situations where self-only coverage offered by an employer is affordable but family coverage is not.

The U.S. Supreme Court ruled that the ACA Medicaid expansion is a voluntary program for states. As a result, not all states have expanded Medicaid coverage. What this means for persons living in states that have expanded Medicaid coverage is that they qualify for either Medicaid or reduced costs on a private insurance plan if they earn up to $16,104 a year for one person or $32,913 for a family of four (CMS, 2013). For persons living in states that have not expanded Medicaid coverage it means if their income is more than 100% of the federal poverty level (about $11,490 a year as a single person or about $23,550 for a family of four) they qualify to buy a private health insurance plan in the Marketplace and may get lower costs based on their household size and income (CMS, 2013).

The ACA is estimated to insure at least half of the United States population that is currently uninsured (USDHHS, 2012). The individuals that make up the uninsured are predominantly undocumented immigrants, citizens who choose not to enroll in Medicaid, residents of states that opt out of the Medicaid expansion provision, and citizens whose cost of health care is 8% or more of their total income (USDHHS, 2012). Undocumented immigrants, who are prohibited from enrolling in Medicaid and purchasing coverage through the new health insurance exchanges, are projected to constitute 25% of the uninsured after the major provisions of the ACA are fully implemented (USDHHS, 2012). Providing health care to the uninsured is already a challenge and will continue to require creative solutions even after the ACA is fully implemented.

Nurses must be adept at working among health care systems to find resources and services for the large population of uninsured clients and families. The number of uninsured Americans in 2010 was 49 million or roughly 16.3% of the total population (DHHS, 2011). A 2014 survey by the Commonwealth Fund suggests that the number of uninsured has dropped significantly since the beginning of the enrollment period in 2013 (Commonwealth Fund, 2014). The percentage of children under the age of 18 without health insurance in 2010 was 9.8%, which significantly decreased from 12% in 1999 due to the expansion of coverage to the Children's Health Insurance Program (CHIP). Since the enactment of the 2010 Affordable Care Act, children can now remain on their parents' insurance plans until the age of 26.

Employer-sponsored insurance continues to be the largest source of health insurance coverage, with 55.3% of the U.S. population covered. However, it is important to note the differences in insurance coverage among minority populations. Hispanics have the highest uninsured rates at 30.7% and blacks are at 20.8%; only 11.7% of non-Hispanic whites are uninsured (USDHHS, 2011).

The demand for primary care will be driven over the next decade and a half not only by the ACA mandates, but also by an aging population and an overall growth in the size of the U.S. population. This growth in demand also accompanies a shift from acute care services to more chronic care management as the nation's disease patterns change as the population ages (Dower & O'Neil, 2011). Various studies projecting current or imminent shortages in primary care providers are shifting attention away from the traditional physician model of care to nurse practitioners, who now account for about 19% of the U.S. primary care workforce, and physician assistants, who account for 7% of the U.S. workforce (Green, Savin & Lu, 2013). Nurse practitioners and physician assistants not only provide effective care but they can also meet the growing demands for primary care providers (Green et al, 2013).

The lack of insurance makes finding adequate services for clients and families difficult. In some areas federal and state funding for care in health clinics is free or available for a minimal fee. However, because the number of primary health care clinics is limited, care is often provided based on the number of volunteer health care providers working that day in the clinic. Many clinics are program based, such as family planning clinics, sexually transmitted disease (STD) clinics, and immunizations clinics. Thus, it is difficult to meet the needs of the uninsured or underinsured populations.

*Practice & Research*, ed 5. Philadelphia, 2015, FA Davis.

Kim-Godwin YS, Bomar PJ: Family health promotion. In Kaakinen JR, Coehlo DP, Steele R, et al, editors: *Family Health Nursing: Theory, Practice & Research*, ed 5. Philadelphia, 2015, FA Davis.

King V, Scott ME: A comparison of cohabiting relationships among older and younger adults. *J Marriage Family* 67:271–285, 2005.

Kinnersley P, Edwards A, Hood K, et al: Interventions before consultations for helping patients, address their information needs. *Cochrane Database Systematic Review* (3):CD004565, 2007. PMID: 17636767.

Kreider RM, Ellis R: *Living arrangements of children: 2009: Household economic studies*, 2011a. Available from http://www.census.gove/prod/2011pubs/p70-126.pdf. Accessed March 23, 2014.

Kreider RM, Ellis R: *Number, timing and duration of marriage and divorces: 2009. Household economic studies*, 2011b. Available at http://www.census.gov/prod/2011pubs/p70-125.pdf. Accessed March 23, 2014.

Kreider RM, Elliot DB: *American's Families and Living Arrangements: 2007, Current Population Reports, P 20-561*. Washington, DC, 2007, U.S. Census Bureau.

Leahey M, Svavarsdottir EK: Implementing family nursing: how do we translate knowledge into clinical practice? *J Fam Nurs* 15(4):445–460, 2009.

Lofquist D, Lugaila T, O'Connell M, et al: *Households and families:2010*. 2010 Census briefs No. C23010BR-14, U.S. Census Bureau, Department of Commerce Economics and Statistics Administration, 2012. Available at http://www.census.gov/prod/cen2010/briefs/c2010br-14.pdf. Accessed March 23, 2014.

Marco CA, Moskop JC, Schears RM, et al: The ethics of health care reform: impact on emergency medicine. *Academic Emergency Med* 19(4):461–468, 2012.

Martin JA, Hamilton BE, Ventura SJ, et al: Births, Final data for 2010. *National Vital Statistics Reports* 61:1–100, 2012. Available at http://www.cdc.gov/nchs/data/nvsr/nvsr51_01.edf. Accessed March 23, 2014.

McGoldrick M, Gerson R, Petry SS: *Genograms: Assessment and Interventions*, ed 3. New York, 2008, W.W. Norton.

National Alliance for Family Caregiving: *Caregiving in the U.S*, 2009. Available at http://assets.aarp.org/rgcenter/il/caregiving_09_es.pdf. Accessed March 23, 2014.

National Alliance for Family Caregiving: *Young Caregivers in the United States*, 2005. Available at http://www.caregiving.org/data/youngcaregivers.pdf. Accessed March 23, 2014.

National Bureau of Economic Research: *The effect of Medicare on medical expenditures, mortality, and spending risk*, 2013. Retrieved from http://www.nber.org/aginghealth/fall05/w11619.html. Accessed April 4th, 2014.

National health interview survey: *Summary health statistics for the US population*, 2012. Available at www.cdc.gov/nchs/data/series/sr_10/sr10_259.pdf. Accessed March 23, 2014.

Olson DH, Gorall DM: Circumplex model of marital and family systems. In Walsh F, editor: *Normal Family Processes*, ed 3. New York, 2003, Guilford, pp 514–517.

Osborne C, McLanahan S: Partnership instability and child well-being. *J Marriage Family* 69:1065–1083, 2007.

Paavilainen E, Astedt-Kurki P: The nurse-client relationship as experienced by public health nurses: Toward a better collaboration. *Public Health Nurs* 14:135–188, 1997.

Peters DJ, Dieckann N, Dixon A, et al: Less is more in presenting quality information to consumers. *Med Care Res Rev* 64(2):169–190, 2007.

PEW: *Family caregivers online*, 2012. Available at http://www.pewinternet.org/files/old-media/Files/Reports/2012/PIP_Family_Caregivers_Online.pdf. Accessed March 23, 2014.

Phillips JA, Sweeney MM: Premarital cohabitation and marital disruption among white, black and Mexican American women. *J Marriage Family* 67:296–314, 2005.

Porr C, Drummond J, Olsen K: Establishing therapeutic relationships with vulnerable and potentially stigmatized clients. *Quality Health Research* 22:384–396, 2012.

Public Health Foundation: *Core competencies for public health professionals*, 2011. Available at http://www.phf.org/resourcestools/Documents/Core_Competencies_for_Public_Health_Professionals_2010May.pdf. Accessed March 22, 2014.

Ray S: Cohabitation effects on kids. *Psychol Today*, March 2013. Available at http://www.psychologytoday.com/blog/adulthood-whats-the-rush/201303/cohabitations-effect-kids. Accessed March 23, 2014.

Region X: *IPP Committee: Infertility prevention project: program guidelines and data collection*, 2000. Available at http://www.oregon.gov/DHS/ph/std/ipp/

overview.shtml. Accessed February 10, 2011.

Rosland AM, Piette JD, Choi HJ, et al: Family and friend participation in primary care visits of patients with diabetes or heart failure: patient and physician determinants and experiences. *Med Care* 49:37–45, 2011.

Salmond S: Who is family? Family and decision making. In Lewenson SB, Truglio-Londrigan M, editors: *Decision-Making in Nursing: Thoughtful Approaches for Practice*. Sudbury, MA, 2008, Jones and Bartlett, pp 89–104.

Schoen R, Canudas-Romo V: Timing effects on divorce: 20th century experience in the United States. *J Marriage Family* 68:749–758, 2006.

Shin HB, Kominski RA: *Language use in the United States: 2007. American Community Survey Reports, ACS-12*, 2010. Available at www.census.gov/prod/2010pubs/acs-12.pdf. Accessed March 23, 2014.

Siskowski C: Young caregivers: effect of family health situations on school performance. *J School Nursing* 22:163–169, 2006.

Smith CM: Home visit: opening the doors for family health. In Maurer FA, Smith CM, editors: *Community public Health Nursing Practice: Health for Families and Populations*, ed 4. St Louis, 2009, Saunders, pp 302–326.

Speros C: Health literacy: concept analysis. *J Adv Nurs* 50(6):633–640, 2005.

Tabacco A: Nursing assessment of the family. In Votroubek W, Tabacco A, editors: *Pediatric Home Care for Nurses: A Family-Centered Approach*, ed 3. Boston, 2010, Jones & Bartlett, pp 59–80.

Touliatos J, Perlmutter B, Straus M: *Handbook of family measurement techniques*. Newbury Park, CA, 2001, Sage.

U.S. Census Bureau: *Employment status of women, by marital status and presence and age of children: 1960 to 2005*, 2008. Available at http://www/census/gov/compendia. Accessed April 8, 2010.

U.S. Census Bureau: *Completed fertility for women 40 to 44 years old by single race in combination with other races and selected characteristics: June 2010* (Detailed Table 7), 2010a. Available at http://www.census.gov/hhes/fertility/data/cps/2010.html. Accessed March 23, 2014.

U.S. Census Bureau: *Women who had a child in the last year per 1,000 women, by race, Hispanic origin, nativity status, and selected characteristics: June 2010. Detailed fertility tables* (Table 4), 2010b. Available at http://www.census.gov/hhes/fertility/data/cps/2010.html. Accessed March 23, 2014.

U.S. Census Bureau: *Family groups: 2011* (Table FG10), 2011a. Available at http://www.census.gov/hhes/families/data/cps2011.html. Accessed March 22, 2014.

U.S. Census Bureau: *Population 65 years and over in the United States: 2011. American community survey*, 2011b. Available from Retrieved from http://factfinder2.census.gov/faces/tableservices/jsf/pages/productview.xhtml?pid=ACS_11_1YR_S0103&prodType=table. Accessed March 23, 2014.

U.S. Census Bureau: *Marital status of people 15 years and over, by age, sex, personal earnings, race, and Hispanic origin/1, 2011* (Table A1), 2011c. Available at http://www.census.gov/hhes/families/data/cps2011.html. Accessed March 23, 2014.

U.S. Census Bureau: *Unmarried partners of the opposite sex, by presence of children: 1960 to present* (Table UC-1), 2011d. Available at www.census.gov/population/socdemo/hh-fam/uc1.xls. Accessed March 23, 2014.

U.S. Census Bureau: *All parent/child situations, by type, race, and Hispanic origin of householder or reference person: 1970 to present* (Table FM-2), 2011e. Available at http://www.census.gov/hhes/families/data/families.html. Accessed March 23, 2014.

U.S. Census Bureau: *Living arrangements of children under 18 years/1 and marital status of parents, by age, sex, race, and Hispanic origin/2 and selected characteristics of the child for all children* (Table C3), 2011f. Available at http://www.census.gov/hhes/families/data/cps2011.html. Accessed March 23, 2014.

U.S. Census Bureau: *Families, by presence of own children under 18: 1950 to present* (Table FM-1), 2011g. Available at http://www.census.gov/hhes/families/data/families.html. Accessed March 23, 2014.

U.S. Census Bureau: *Households, families, subfamilies and married couples:1080-2010*, 2012a. Available at http://www.census.gov/compendia/statab/2012/tables/12s0059.pdf. Accessed March 22, 2014.

US Department of Health and Human Services: *Overview of the Uninsured in the United States: Summary of the 2011 Population Survey*. Washington DC, 2011. from: www.aspe.hhs.gov. Accessed July 2012.

US Department of Health and Human Services: *Overview of the Uninsured in the United States: Summary of the 2012 Population Survey*. Washington DC, 2012. from: www.aspe.hhs.gov. Accessed March 22, 2014.

Vasquez MS: Preventing rehospitalization through effective home health nursing care. *Home Health Nurse* 26(2):75–81, 2008.

Ventura MS, Brown D, Archibald T, et al: *Improving care transitions and reducing hospital readmissions: establishing the evidence for community-based implementation strategies through the care transitions theme, The Remington Report*, 2010. Available at http://www.cfmc.org/caretransitions/files/Care_Transition_Article_Remington_Report_Jan_2010.pdf. Accessed February 10, 2011.

Wald L: *The House on Henry Street*. New York, 1915, Holt.

Weinberg DB, Lusenhop RW, Gittell JH, et al: Coordination between formal providers and informal caregivers. *Health Care Manag Rev* 32(2):140–149, 2007.

White JM, Klein DN: *Family Theories: An Introduction*, ed 3. Thousand Oaks, CA, 2008, Sage.

Wolff J, Roter D: Hidden in plain sight: medical visit companions as a resource for vulnerable older adults. *Arch Int Med* 168(13):1409–1415, 2008.

Wolff JL, Roter DL, Given B, et al: Optimizing patient and family involvement in geriatric home care. *J Healthcare Qual* 31(2):24–33, 2009.

# Family Health Risks

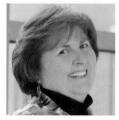

### Debra Gay Anderson, PhD, PHCNS-BC

Dr. Debra Gay Anderson is a faculty member at the University of Kentucky's College of Nursing. She is certified as a clinical specialist in public/community health nursing and has provided health care for the homeless and other vulnerable populations. Dr. Anderson has taught public health, epidemiology, leadership, and research courses at both the graduate and undergraduate levels. The focus of her program of research, publications, and presentations is vulnerable populations, primarily women who have experienced homelessness, domestic violence or workplace violence. Dr. Anderson completed her doctoral studies and a family nursing postdoctoral fellowship at Oregon Health Sciences University in Portland, Oregon. Dr. Anderson is an active member of the American Public Health Association (APHA) and has served in various leadership capacities, including Chair of the Public Health Nursing Section of APHA.

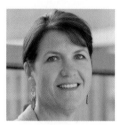

### Hartley Feld, RN, MSN, PHCNS-BC

Hartley Feld received her Masters of Science in Nursing, Community and Public Health nursing specialty, in 2006 from the University of Kentucky. She is board certified as a Public Health Clinical Nurse Specialist. Ms. Feld is a lecturer and clinical instructor in Community and Public Health Nursing. Her clinical interests include global health, health care economics, determinants of health, and vulnerable populations.

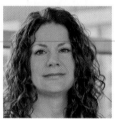

### Mollie Aleshire, DNP, FNP-BC, PPCNP-BC

Dr. Mollie E. Aleshire is a faculty member at the University of Kentucky College of Nursing and is certified as a family nurse practitioner and pediatric primary care nurse practitioner. Dr. Aleshire has taught interprofessional health systems, health promotion, and primary care prevention in both undergraduate and graduate courses. She received a Master of Science in Nursing and a Doctor of Nursing Practice from the University of Kentucky. Dr. Aleshire's clinical and scholarship interests include prevention strategies in primary care settings and health issues of young women and female adolescents.

## ADDITIONAL RESOURCES

ⓔ **Evolve Website http://evolve.elsevier.com/Stanhope**
- *Healthy People 2020*
- Quiz
- Case Studies
- WebLinks
- Glossary
- Answers to Practice Application
- Resource Tools
  - Resource Tool 5.A: Schedule of Clinical Preventive Services

- Resource Tool 27.A: Family Systems Stressor-Strength Inventory
- Resource Tool 27.B: Case Example of Family Assessment

**Appendix**
- Appendix E: Friedman Family Assessment Model (Short Form)

## OBJECTIVES

*After reading this chapter, the student should be able to do the following:*

1. Evaluate the various approaches to defining and conceptualizing family health.
2. Analyze the major risks to family health.
3. Analyze the interrelationships among individual health, family health, and community health.
4. Explain the relevance of knowledge about family structures, roles, and functions for family-focused nursing in the community.
5. Discuss the implications of policy and policy decisions, at all governmental levels, on families.
6. Explain the application of the nursing process (assessment, planning, implementation, evaluation) to reducing family health risks and promoting family health.

What is a "family?" Is there one definition that fits all families? Is there a new normal? Was there ever a true "normal" family? In 2011, Lisa Belkin wrote an opinion piece for *The New York Times*, "A 'Normal' Family." In her article, she discussed seven trends identified by the Pew Research Center. The trends were "more unmarried couples raising children; more gay and lesbian couples raising children; more single women having children without a male partner to help raise them; more people living together without getting married; more mothers of young children working outside the home; more people of different races marrying each other; and more women not ever having children" (Belkin, 2011).

Although Belkin is referring to current family incarnations, history demonstrates that the makeup of families is in constant flux, depending on the current socioeconomic pragmatism. We are reminded of Abraham Lincoln's father leaving his two children following the death of their mother for the purpose of bringing back a new mother. Was that a "normal" family? Sarah Bush Johnston Lincoln, with three children, married Thomas Lincoln, following the deaths of both of their spouses and, in addition to their combined five children, raised a cousin of Nancy Hank Lincoln. Today, we might call that a "blended" family. We refer to Lincoln's family simply to demonstrate that the "traditional" family was never the "normal" family. As family

makeup transitions, those families are often the ones that are the most vulnerable because they do not conform to traditional societal expectations.

Regardless of makeup, the family as a client unit is basic to the practice of population-centered nursing, and nurses are responsible for promoting healthy families in society. As such, families are described as a unique population in public health. The purpose of this chapter is to make the reader aware of influences, both individual and societal, that place families at risk for poor health outcomes, and to discuss how positive outcomes for diverse families can be accomplished through appropriate nursing interventions.

The expanding definition of the family unit presents today's nurse with an array of challenges and opportunities to address the health needs of families. First, it is essential to place the family in the context of the twenty-first century. Many Americans tend to idealize *family* and wish for a return to family values of the past and a golden time for families. However, historical demographic statistics reveal that this prevalence of the idealized family that has often been portrayed in the media never actually existed. Rather than arguing for a return to the "traditional family" (male breadwinner and woman at home), serious discussions are needed about how to help today's diverse families succeed. A focus on all family structures is a moral and ethical imperative in the promotion of the health of individuals as well as the health of the community (Nightingale et al, 1978; Wright and Leahey, 2013).

The varying family structures of today need to be recognized and examined to better understand both the strengths and weaknesses associated with each. Only by doing this will we be able to help all families live healthy and productive lives. Nurses can play an active role in leading and facilitating this learning process. This facilitation can enable better-informed health care policy decisions that have a positive effect on single-parent families, remarried and stepfamilies, gay and lesbian families, grandparent-headed families, and ethnically diverse families, as well as "traditional" families.

A nation's family health care **policy** is a primary determinant of **family health**. Family policy means anything that is done by the government that directly or indirectly affects families. Family health policy and its relative effectiveness demonstrates a government's understanding of families and its role in promoting their health, with an important desired outcome being that families derive a sense of empowerment and are able to take responsibility for their own health (Chinn, 2012). The responsibility for family health programs is shared by the federal government with state and local governments. Each state, as well as regions within states, has programs and laws related to family services. The United States is one of the richest and most technologically advanced countries in the world today and yet, despite the profusion of technological advances and the continually growing proportion of the national budget spent on health care, the disparities in health status between different populations of families has continued to grow (FAMILIES USA, 2014). These disparities have resulted, at least in part, from previous attempts to develop and implement "family policies" that either directly or indirectly affect specific issues related to family health but which have failed to take a comprehensive system-wide approach.

Although many disparities and inequities continue in the United States, the health care disparities related to insurance coverage should begin to change as the **Affordable Care Act** (ACA) expands. At the 2014 Health Action Conference, FAMILIES USA, Vice President Joe Biden spoke of the importance of the Affordable Care Act (discussed throughout this text) and the importance of the ACA for families in the United States. The specific benefits he highlighted were the coverage of pre-existing conditions, mental health coverage, the disparity in the cost of insurance for women and men, the more than three million young adults on their parents' insurance policies, and not receiving medical care simply because one does not have insurance (Biden, 2014). Nursing has a rich history in social activism and social justice which should be continued, emphasizing advocacy and policy work to help families and communities become healthier for all populations.

Evidence to date suggests that the United States could benefit from a cohesive family policy designed to enhance the well-being of all families. Such a policy would go a long way toward preventing future crises in vulnerable family populations, such as those in or on the verge of poverty or families overwhelmed with abuse and neglect, by providing a structural safety net to help families to maintain their health in times of disaster, economic downturns, unemployment, health crises, and other situations. An effective family health policy may consider as its foundational element an infrastructure of programs designed to provide access to primary and preventive health care. The building of this foundation requires a multiprofessional process in which nurses can be actively involved. Nurses are educated in community assessment, planning, development, and evaluation activities that emphasize and address issues crucial to promoting and sustaining primary family health. Nurses looking to positively influence family health will want to be aware of and actively participate in the ongoing national debate and dialogue on family health policy that embraces their role as principal constituents in building healthy families.

In establishing health objectives for the nation, an emphasis has been placed on both health promotion and risk reduction. Reducing the risks to segments of the population is a direct way to improve the health of the general population. Specific objectives have been identified related to specific health risks for families. The family is an important environmental factor that affects the health of individuals as well as a social unit whose health is basic to that of the community and the larger population. It is within the family that health values, health habits, and health risk perceptions are developed, organized, and carried out. Individuals' health behaviors are affected by and acted out within the family environment, the larger community, and society.

Family health habits are developed in the same manner in the context of community norms and values, and on the basis of availability and accessibility. For example, in a television commercial for an over-the-counter stimulant, a man is featured who is able to coach his child's basketball team, work at a rehabilitation center, and work as a borough inspector for the city, all while pursuing a college degree at night. The commercial credits the drug for providing the man with the energy needed to be successful in all of these areas. The message is clear: you can, and must, do it all, and taking drugs to succeed is a viable option. The health risks to individual and family health are affected by the societal norms—in this example, the norm is increasing productivity through drugs.

To intervene effectively and appropriately with families to reduce their health risk and thereby promote their health, nurses need to understand not only family structure and functioning, but also family theory, nursing theory, and models of health risk (see Chapters 9, 17, and 27). In addition, the effective nurse needs to look beyond the individual and the family in order to understand the complex environment in which the family exists. Increasing evidence of the effects of social, biological, economic, and life events on health requires a broader approach to addressing health risks for families. Nurses and the communities they serve have a vital interest in exploring new and appropriate options for structuring nursing interventions with families to decrease health risks and to promote health and well-being for all families. It is important for the nurse to focus on families who share similar health risks as a population. Working and planning interventions to reduce health risks in family populations provides a mechanism for shared communication and support among families as well as efficient and effective health care interventions that will not only make the families, but the community as a whole, healthier.

## EARLY APPROACHES TO FAMILY HEALTH RISKS

### Health of Families

Historically, the study of the family relative to health and illness focused on three major areas: (1) the effect of illness on families, (2) the role of the family in the cause of disease, and (3) the role of the family in its use of services. In his classic review of the family as an important unit, Litman (1974) pointed out the important role that the family (as a primary unit of health care) plays in health and illness and emphasized that the relationship between health, health behavior, and family "is a highly dynamic one in which each may have a dramatic effect on the other" (p. 495). At about this same time, Mauksch (1974) proposed the idea of distinguishing between family health and individual health. Pratt's (1976) examination of the role of the family in health and illness included the role of family health in the promotion of healthy or unhealthy behavior. Pratt proposed and described the *energized family* as being an ideal family type that was most effective in meeting health needs. The energized family is characterized as promoting freedom and change, active contact with a variety of other groups and organizations, flexible role relationships, equal power structure, and a high degree of autonomy in family members. Doherty and McCubbin (1985) proposed a family health and illness cycle consisting of six phases, beginning with family health promotion and risk reduction and continuing through the family's vulnerability to illness, their illness response, their interaction with the health care system, and finally their ways of adapting to illness.

### Health of the Nation

In recent years, increased attention has been given to improving the health of everyone in the United States. As a result of major public health and scientific advances, the leading causes of morbidity and mortality have shifted from infectious diseases to chronic diseases, accidents, and violence, all of which have strong lifestyle and environmental components. A classic population-focused study in Alameda County, California (Belloc and Breslow, 1972) demonstrated the relationships between seven lifestyle habits and decreased morbidity and mortality. These habits were (1) sleeping 7 to 8 hours daily, (2) eating breakfast almost every day, (3) never or rarely eating between meals, (4) being at or near recommended height-adjusted weight, (5) never smoking cigarettes, (6) moderate or no use of alcohol, and (7) regular physical activity. These same lifestyle health habits are still important for improved health in the twenty-first century.

The Alameda study has been supported by Dan Buettner's (2009) work with The National Geographic Society and their examination of communities around the world who have not only longevity, but quality of life. Public health nurses will want to read *The Blue Zones: 9 Lessons for Living Longer* for in-depth case studies. The nine lessons include the following:

1. Move naturally: Be active without thinking about it;
2. Hara Hachi Bu: Painlessly cut calories by 20 percent;
3. Plant slant: Avoid meat and processed foods;
4. Grapes of life: Drink red wine in moderation;
5. Purpose now: Take time to see the big picture;
6. Downshift: Take time to relieve stress;
7. Belong: Participate in a spiritual community;
8. Loved ones first: Make family a priority; and
9. Right tribe: Be surrounded by those who share Blue Zone values.

A growing body of literature supports the notion that lifestyle and the environment interact with heredity to cause disease. In response to these findings and to the limited effect of medical interventions on the growing incidence and prevalence of injuries and chronic disease, the government launched a major effort to address the health status of the population. Part of this effort was a report by the Division of Health Promotion and Disease Prevention of the Institute of Medicine that examined the critical components of the physical, socioeconomic, and family environments related to decreasing risk and promoting health (Nightingale et al, 1978). *The Surgeon General's Report on Health Promotion and Disease Prevention* (Califano, 1979) described the risks to good health in the United States at that time. As a result of these reports, health objectives for the nation were established and then evaluated and restated for the year 2000 and again for 2010 (USDHHS, 2000). The *Healthy People 2020* objectives extend the work of the three past documents. An innovative part of this latest *Healthy People* (USDHHS, 2010) update has been a move to become more creative and inclusive. The focus challenges health care providers with a national goal of improving health and will provide the necessary background for future policy initiatives to reduce risk in all populations. Of the four goals, three are particularly important to families:

- Achieve health equity, eliminate disparities, and improve the health of all groups.
- Create social and physical environments that promote good health for all.
- Promote quality of life, healthy development, and healthy behaviors across all life stages.

With the notion of **risk**, any factor resulting in a predisposition toward or an increased likelihood of ill health takes on increased importance. Specific attention is being paid to those environmental and behavioral factors that lead to ill health with or without the influence of heredity. Reducing health risks is a major step toward improving the health of the nation. Although the family is considered an important environment related to achieving important health objectives, limited attention and research have been directed at family health risks and the role of society in promoting healthy families.

## CONCEPTS IN FAMILY HEALTH RISK

Pender's Health Promotion Model (2010), described in the latest edition of her textbook, continues to be useful in research

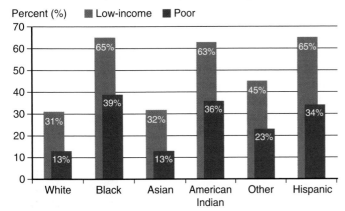

**Percentage of children in low-income and poor families by race/ethnicity, 2011**

©National Center for Children in Poverty (www.nocp.org)
Basic Facts About Low-income Children Under 18 Years, 2011

**FIG 29-1** Percentage of children living in poverty and low income by ethnicity in 2011. (From National Center for Children in Poverty: Basic facts about low income children, 2013. Available at www.nccp.org. Accessed February 19, 2015.)

income of half of the federal poverty level (Federal Interagency Forum on Child and Family Statistics, 2013; Jiang et al, 2014). About 30% of children born to immigrant parents live below the federal poverty level compared with 19% of children of native-born parents (AAP, 2013). The federal poverty level for 2012 was defined as a family income of less than $23,364 for a family of four whereas low income (the amount of income necessary to provide for the family's basic needs) is two times the federal poverty level, or $46,728.

Minority children, most notably black and Hispanic children, have higher proportions of living at poverty or low-income levels (Figure 29-1). Characteristics that put children at risk for living in low-income families are parents without a high school degree, having a lack of parental employment, and living in a single-parent household. Children's ability to learn in school and reach their full cognitive ability is affected by low-income status. Children living in poverty experience a higher incidence of behavioral, social, and emotional problems (Jiang et al, 2014).

In addition, U.S. children face other challenges. More than 10% of American households with children experience low food security (Wight & Thampi, 2010). Low food security, a lack of available food and access to food on a regular basis, affects children's physical health, development, and school performance. Homelessness is increasing for American children and is highly correlated to poverty status and the lack of affordable housing. It is estimated that over 200,000 children have no place to live on any given day with 1.6 million U.S. children experiencing homelessness each year (National Center on Family Homelessness, 2011).

## Immigrant Children

Children of immigrant families represent the largest growing portion of the U.S. population with approximately 18 million immigrant children (1 in every 4 U.S. children). Of those, 89% are born in the U.S. and have citizenship (Child Trends Data Base, 2012). "Immigrant children" are defined as those who were born in a foreign country or children born in the U.S. who live with a parent(s) who was born in a foreign country. When compared to nonimmigrant children, immigrant children are more likely to have poor to fair health.

Immigrant children face many challenges to good health, including lack of health insurance, poverty, language barriers, and substandard housing. These families often experience or fear discrimination related to anti-immigration sentiment and this impacts access to health care and child health outcomes. Nurses should advocate for culturally and linguistically effective comprehensive health care, provide preventive screenings and referrals as appropriate, and encourage early education services for the support of optimal development in immigrant children (AAP, 2013).

## Access to Care

Access to quality health services is one of the focus areas of *Healthy People 2020* (USDHHS, 2010). Children with health care coverage are more likely to have a regular and accessible source of health care. In 2012, 8.9% of all children had no health insurance. For children living in poverty, the uninsured rate for children was 13% (U.S. Census Bureau, 2013). With the implementation of the Affordable Care Act (ACA), the number of children covered by government health insurance programs has been increasing.

The Medicaid program, established by the Social Security Act in 1965, is a state-administered health insurance program financed jointly by the federal and state governments. Children under 18 years of age living in a household with an income level at or below 133% of the federal poverty level or children meeting disability requirements qualify for this program. The program provides health services at no cost to participants and includes outpatient visits, hospitalization, laboratory testing, immunizations, well care/preventive services, and dental care (CMMS, 2014a).

The Children's Health Insurance Plan (CHIP) was the result of federally mandated legislation passed in 1997 to expand health insurance to the nation's uninsured children. The Children's Health Insurance Program Reauthorization Act of 2009 has continued to provide insurance to over 5 million American children. CHIP is a federal and state partnership directed toward uninsured children and pregnant women in families with incomes too high to qualify for state Medicaid programs but usually too low to afford private coverage. Following federal guidelines, each state determines the model of its particular CHIP program, which includes the eligibility parameters, benefit package, payment levels for coverage, and administrative process. The program is jointly financed by the federal and state governments, and administered by the states (CMMS, 2014b). CHIP enrollment eligibility requirements are:

- Family income too high for Medicaid qualification (up to $44,100 for family of 4)
- Uninsured children under 19 years of age in the home

CHIP coverage includes:
- Primary care provider/specialist visits
- Immunizations
- Hospitalizations and ED visits

Under the ACA, 21 states are mandated to expand their Medicaid coverage to fully provide comprehensive coverage to children of families at 133% of the federal poverty level. This eliminates the "stairstep" eligibility rules that were previously in place in these states and limited enrollment of children in Medicaid. Currently, Medicaid and CHIP combined provide health coverage to over 43 million children (Kaiser Family Foundation, 2013). This remains an area of outreach opportunity for nurses to identify potential families eligible for Medicaid and CHIP and provide appropriate referrals to state agencies. It is expected that as the ACA is fully implemented, health insurance coverage for children will continue to increase, improving access and health outcomes for this population.

## Infant Mortality

Promotion of healthy pregnancies is a focus of *Healthy People 2020*. The *Healthy People 2020* target goal for the U.S. infant mortality rate is 4.5 infant deaths per 1000 live births. The U.S. infant mortality rate dropped to a record low of 6.15 infant deaths per 1,000 live births in 2010 (down 3.8% from 2009), although the infant mortality rate for the black population was 2.2 times greater when compared to the white population (Murphy et al, 2013). Although infant death rates have decreased, the United States has a higher infant mortality rate than 50 other nations (Central Intelligence Agency, 2014) and its position in a global ranking has consistently fallen over past years.

Infant mortality rates are critical indicators of a country's overall health. Infant mortality rates are associated with a variety of factors such as maternal health, socioeconomic circumstances, quality and access to medical care, and community health practices.

## Risk-Taking Behaviors

Risk behaviors are any behaviors that place early and middle adolescents at risk for physical, emotional, or psychological harm. Much progress has been made through health promotion and education to decrease risk factors in adolescents. The Youth Risk Behavior Surveillance System (YRBSS) indicates that many teens continue to engage in risk behaviors with smoking tobacco (15.7%), using marijuana (23.4%), and drinking alcohol (34.5%). Increasingly, drugs of abuse are inhalants. Nationally, 8.9% of high school students have breathed the contents of aerosol spray cans, sniffed glue, or inhaled any paints or sprays to get high one or more times (Kann et al, 2014). In regards to motor vehicle safety, 7.6% of adolescents reported never wearing a seat belt while 21.9% rode in the car with an intoxicated driver. Nationwide, 41.4% of teens shared that they texted or e-mailed while driving, an increase of 7% from 2011. The overall prevalence of risk behaviors indicates the continued emphasis on primary and secondary prevention and education with the adolescent population.

Despite extensive education campaigns, adolescents continue to engage in sexual activity (34%) with only 59.1% using condoms during intercourse and 15% of teens reporting that they had sexual intercourse with four or more partners (Kann et al, 2014). These risk behaviors increase the risk for unintended pregnancies and sexually transmitted infections. Yet the birth rate for teenagers (15-19 years) did drop 6% to an all-time low rate of 29.4 per 1000 in 2010 (USDHHS, 2013a). This number remains a significant concern for public health nurses because teen pregnancy creates a significant socioeconomic burden on society and the family.

Nurses should be aware of the factors associated with increased adolescent risk-taking behaviors: poor academic performance, poor parental role models, low self-esteem, lack of a supportive social environment, and poverty. Individual assessment of an adolescent's risk-taking behavior can provide the direction to focus education and interventions. Providing after-school extracurricular activities, identifying a positive adult role model, and engaging teens in support systems to build self-esteem can reduce risk-taking behaviors in at-risk adolescents.

The misuse and abuse of prescription stimulant medication to treat attention-deficit hyperactivity disorder (ADHD) has risen in past years. Misuse of these drugs occurs in 2% to 8% of children and adolescents. Misuse ranges from selling or trading the prescription stimulant, taking a prescription stimulant with no ADHD symptoms, taking more than the recommended dose, or taking it by a route other than the prescribed route (i.e., inhaling an oral medication) (Lakhan & Kirchgessner, 2012). It is vital to promote community and family awareness of this problem and educate children and adolescents on the dangers of taking others' prescription medications.

# CHILD DEVELOPMENT

## Growth and Development

Growth is the measurable aspect of the individual's size and follows a predictable pace that is evaluated at regular intervals to determine if a child is growing based on standard parameters. Development involves the observable changes in the individual and relates to physical, psychosocial, and cognitive achievements. Growth and development in children is an ongoing, dynamic process that results in physical, cognitive, and emotional changes (Figure 29-2). Health visits or well-child checkups are scheduled at key ages to monitor these processes and provide anticipatory guidance to families. Nursing assessments include growth and health status, developmental level, and the quality of the parent–child relationship. (See Tables 29-2, 29-3, 29-4, and 29-5 for considerations and issues to address at each stage.) The recommendations for preventive pediatric health care (see Resource Tool 5.A on the Evolve site) list components of well-child assessments. Further tools and specific interventions are included in Appendixes D and E.

## Developmental Theories

Many developmental theories provide perspectives on children's growth and development. The work of Erik Erikson on psychosocial development emphasizes that personality development culminates in the achievement of ego identity, which involves accepting oneself and having the skills for healthy

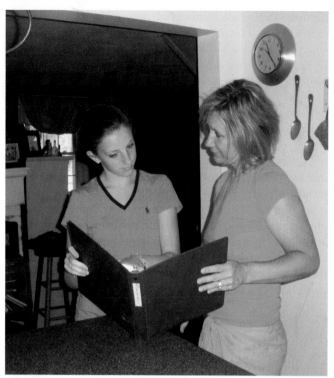

**FIG 29-2** Conflict between parents and teenagers is normal as teenagers experience physical and emotional growth processes.

| TABLE 29-1 | Developmental Screening Tools |
|---|---|
| **Tool** | **Purpose** |
| Denver II | Domain specific development (gross and fine motor, social, language) |
| Ages and Stages Questionnaire | Social and emotional development |
| Parents' Evaluation of Developmental Status (PEDS) | General developmental and behavioral screening |
| Modified Checklist for Autism in Toddlers (M-CHAT) | Autism spectrum disorder |
| Pediatric Symptom Checklist | Coping and mental health concerns |

functioning in society. According to Erickson, development is a continual process that occurs in distinct stages with a developmental crisis needing resolution at each stage and some degree of mastery being achieved before proceeding successfully to the next stage. All new development is rooted in prior experiences, and difficulty resolving the crisis will cause problems progressing through the subsequent stages.

The work of Jean Piaget is widely used to understand the process of cognitive development. According to Piaget, learning results from actively manipulating objects and information followed by a mental processing of the event. As the child interacts with the environment, new objects and problems are discovered. The child creates mental schemes or thought patterns to understand the encounter. This permits the child to receive information from the world, make sense of it, and predict future events. Development occurs as the schemes increase in scope and complexity. Piaget identified four stages of cognitive development that represent increasing problem-solving ability. As one will remember from pediatric courses, these stages are sensorimotor, preoperational, concrete, and formal operations (Shaffer & Kipp, 2013).

Bronfenbrenner's human ecology theory emphasizes the complex relationship between the growing child and his/her immediate environment. Children are greatly influenced by the environments in which they spend time and one of the most important environments in affecting growth is the family environment. Educational programs, communities, and other environmental factors also influence the child's development. Children learn to accommodate to their environment and alter themselves based on environmental interactions. This theory explains that individuals do not develop in isolation but in relation to their home and family, school, community, and society (Shaffer & Kipp, 2013).

## Developmental Screening

Developmental screening is a process designed to identify children who should receive more intensive assessment or diagnosis of potential developmental delays. These delays may be in any of the developmental domains—gross motor, fine motor, language, or social skills. Developmental screening promotes early detection of delays and improves child health and well-being for identified children. In the United States, 15% of children have a developmental disability such as autism, attention-deficit disorder, hearing loss or a language delay (AAP, 2011a). Nurses are critical to early screening and identification of developmental delays in young children and appropriately initiating referrals to maximize school readiness and maximum achievement. Multiple screening tools are available and are selected based on the nurse's role in the community (Table 29-1).

Children with delayed skills or other disabilities may qualify for special services that provide individualized education programs in public schools that are free of charge to families. Nurses can be effective health advocates for these children within educational settings. The passage of the updated version of the Individuals with Disabilities Education Act 2004 (IDEA) promotes a collaborative focus on meeting the needs of children with disabilities (Department of Education, 2006). Parents, educators, administrators, nurses, and other team members collaboratively develop a plan—the individualized education plan (IEP)—to help children succeed in school. The IEP explains the goals the team sets for a child during the school year as well as any special support needed to help achieve these goals.

## IMMUNIZATIONS

Increasing immunization coverage for children remains a significant focus of the *Healthy People 2020* objectives. Currently, 92% of the nation's 19- to 35-month-old children have received all of the polio vaccinations as well as 87% of hepatitis B vaccinations in the recommended series but only 53% have received the complete hepatitis A series (CDC, 2013a). For adolescents, vaccination rates continue to rise steadily for this age group. For those aged 13 to 17 years, 84% received the recommended tetanus-diphtheria-acellular pertussis vaccine (Tdap) and 74% received the meningococcal conjugate vaccine (MCV4). Lowest immunization rates are noted for the human papillomavirus vaccine (HPV4) series, with 53% of girls receiving one dose and only 34% receiving the full three-dose series by 17 years of age (CDC, 2013b). Routine immunization of children is very successful in the prevention of selected diseases. The ultimate challenge is making sure that children receive immunizations.

## Barriers

There are several barriers to successful immunizations. These include vaccine cost, vaccine refusal by parents, vaccine shortages, and changes in vaccine scheduling and recommendations. Health disparities in vaccinations continue to exist. Children living in poverty have lower immunization rates than their peers, and African American adolescents have lower immunization rates compared with white adolescents (Burns et al, 2010). It is important to educate parents to obtain immunizations for their children and to focus on the issue at every encounter with families.

Parental fears about vaccines prevent children from getting immunized. Parents readily access the Internet for information about vaccines, and disreputable sites provide parents with incorrect vaccine information. It is critical for nurses to educate families on the safety and efficacy of vaccinations. Scientific studies have not found a relationship between immunizations and autism, sudden infant death syndrome, diabetes, neurologic disabilities, deafness, or cancer. Parents question the need to vaccinate because the incidence of vaccine-preventable diseases is low. However, Japan, Great Britain, and Sweden stopped the use of the pertussis vaccine, and within 5 years there were epidemic levels of the disease and rising death rates (CDC, 2011a). When a parent chooses not to vaccinate their child, this puts the child and others at risk.

Shortages of vaccines have periodically occurred as a result of manufacturing problems, and the U.S. Department of Health and Human Services (USDHHS) has focused on maintaining adequate manufactured supplies of vaccines. When a shortage does occur, the CDC provides priority administration guidelines for highest-risk clients. When the immunization schedule is revised, there can be delays in practitioners implementing the new recommended vaccination schedules. Nurses must continually review the CDC recommendations for any changes to implement within the public health and community settings.

Vaccines and vaccine administration costs are high and those families without health insurance often find following the vaccination recommendations financially prohibitive. A federal program established in 1995, Vaccines for Children (VFC), provides free vaccines to eligible children, including those without health insurance coverage, children enrolled in Medicaid, American Indians and Alaskan Natives, and children whose health insurance does not cover vaccines. Identifying children who qualify for VFC is a primary prevention strategy of population-focused nurses.

## Immunization Theory

The goal of immunization is to protect by using immunizing agents to stimulate antibody formation (see Chapter 13 for types of immunity). Immunizing agents for active immunity are in the form of toxoids and vaccines. A toxoid is a bacterial toxin (e.g., from the bacteria that cause tetanus and diphtheria) that has been heated or chemically treated to decrease virulence but not antibody-producing ability. Vaccines are suspensions of attenuated (live) or inactivated (killed) microorganisms. Examples include pertussis (inactivated bacteria); measles, mumps, and rubella (live attenuated viruses); and hepatitis B (inactivated virus) (see Chapter 13) (CDC, 2012a).

The neonate receives placental transfer of maternal antibodies. This natural passive immunity lasts for about 2 months. Protection is temporary and is only to diseases to which the mother has adequate antibodies. The immune system of both term and preterm infants is capable of adequate antibody response to immunizations by 2 months of age. Generally, this is the recommended age to start immunizations; the exception is the hepatitis B series which begins at birth (CDC, 2012a).

The interval between immunizations is important to the immune response. After the first injection, antibodies are produced slowly and in small concentrations (the primary response). When subsequent injections of the same antigen are given, the body recognizes the antigen and antibodies are produced much faster and in higher concentration (the secondary response). Because of this secondary response, once an initial immunization series has been started, it does not need to be restarted if interrupted, regardless of the length of time elapsed. Once the initial series is completed, boosters are required at appropriate intervals to maintain an adequate concentration of antibodies. (Further information about immunizing agents is available on the Evolve website).

## Recommendations

Immunization recommendations rapidly change as new information and products are available. The recommended immunization schedule guidelines for children from birth through 18 years and the catch-up immunization schedule have been approved by the U.S. Public Health Services Advisory Committee on Immunization Practices (ACIP), the American Academy of Pediatrics (AAP), the American Academy of Family Physicians (AAFP), and the American College of Obstetricians and Gynecologists (ACOG) (CDC, 2014a). Current recommendations for children and adolescents can be found on the Evolve website. The main goal of the guidelines is to provide flexibility to ensure that the largest number of children will be immunized. All health care providers are urged to assess immunization status at every encounter with children and to update immunizations whenever possible.

## Contraindications

There are relatively few contraindications to giving immunizations. Minor acute illness is not a contraindication. Immunizations should be deferred with moderate or acute febrile illnesses because the reactions may mask the symptoms of the illness.

The side effects of the immunization may be accentuated by the illness (CDC, 2012a).

People with the following conditions are not routinely immunized and require medical consultation: pregnancy, generalized malignancy, immunosuppressive therapy or immunodeficiency disease, sensitivity to components of the agent, or recent administration of immune serum globulin, plasma or blood (CDC, 2012a).

## Legislation

The National Childhood Vaccine Injury Act became effective in 1988. It requires providers to counsel parents and clients about the risks and benefits of the immunizing agent as well as possible side effects. Informed consent is recommended. Vaccine information statements (VIS) are used for this purpose. The VIS is an information sheet produced by the CDC that explains both the benefits and risks of a vaccine. Federal law requires that a VIS be given to parents or legal guardians before each vaccine dose is given (CDC, 2012a).

The Vaccine Adverse Event Reporting System (VAERS) is a national safety surveillance program. It requires providers and vaccine manufacturers to report any adverse effects following the administration of routinely recommended vaccinations. The program has been effective in tracking and identifying adverse effects associated with vaccinations. In 1999, VAERS detected reports of intussusception above what would be expected to occur by chance alone after the administration of the RotaShield rotavirus vaccine. Subsequently, this vaccine was pulled from manufacturing and the vaccine formulation was redeveloped (CDC, 2012a).

---

### QSEN FOCUS ON QUALITY AND SAFETY EDUCATION FOR NURSES

**Targeted Competency**

Teamwork and collaboration: Refers to the ability to function effectively with nursing and interprofessional teams and to foster open communication, mutual respect, and shared decision making to provide quality client care

- **Knowledge:** Recognize the contributions of other individuals and groups in helping clients achieve health goals
- **Skill:** Integrate contributions of others who play a role in helping clients achieve health goals
- **Attitude:** Respect the unique attributes and contributions of others

**Question**

Teamwork and Collaboration Question: The PHN Quad Council defines one competency for PHNs as analytic and assessment skills. The PHN uses available data and resources related to social determinants of health when planning care for clients. From this chapter you know that the built environment includes the physical environment where the child client lives, plays, goes to school, shops, and seeks safety. This environment assists the child in managing health risks. Many persons and groups assist the child in this endeavor. To determine the potential or real health risks of a child client, what information would you gather and from whom? How would you use the data from your assessment? Name a health risk and discuss the interventions you might plan and the health education you would offer to promote the child's health. What would you see as the role of other individuals and groups in the community to assist you or to take the lead in assisting the child and family? Be specific.

---

## THE BUILT ENVIRONMENT

A **built environment** is simply defined as the person's human-made or modified surroundings in which they live, work, and partake in recreation (Renalds et al, 2010). This is the actual physical environment in which children live and includes neighborhood access to recreation opportunities, grocery stores, the home environment, and the consideration of general safety for children in their physical environments. A child's built environment is influential in the managing of risk factors for obesity, amount and type of physical activity, risk for injuries, and exposure to environmental toxins. Therefore, as nurses, assessing a child's built environment provides a foundation for identifying interventions and education to promote health and prevent injuries and diseases. (See Evidence-Based Practice box.)

---

### EVIDENCE-BASED PRACTICE

California has a large Hmong population. Despite having health insurance, community providers noted that the Hmong children consistently had lower than national and state levels for immunizations. The authors conducted a study to determine the primary barriers for this cultural group related to immunizing their children. The study identified two primary barriers to immunization: lower socioeconomic status and greater use of traditional Hmong health care (shamans and herbalists) (Baker et al, 2010).

**Nurse Use**

We often make assumptions about the barriers to positive health decisions or behaviors. This study demonstrates that cultural differences can be influential in making health care decisions. By targeting the specific population of concern, nurses can identify the specific barriers that prevent parents from obtaining preventive health care. Public health nurses can then develop interventions and education to address those specific barriers and improve pediatric health.

Baker D, Dang M, Diaz R: Perception of barriers to immunization among parents of Hmong origin in California. *AJPH* 100:839–845, 2010.

---

### Obesity

Obesity rates in American children have risen to epidemic levels over the past few decades. These increases are noted for all children aged 2 to 18 years regardless of gender or ethnicity. The CDC defines **overweight** as a body mass index (BMI) at or above the 85th percentile and lower than the 95th percentile, and **obesity** is defined as a BMI at or above the 95th percentile for children of the same age and sex when plotted on the CDC growth charts (Table 29-2) (CDC, 2012b). Recently, it has been recommended to monitor the World Health Organization (WHO) growth standards for children younger than 2 years. Those infants and toddlers who measure above the 97.7th percentile of WHO weight for recumbent length growth standards are considered high risk for obesity (Ogden et al, 2014).

The 2011-2012 prevalence of the overweight and the obese combined is 23% in children ages 2 to 5 years, 35% for children ages 6 to 11 years, and 35% for adolescents 12 to 19 years. The prevalence of obesity in children is approximately 8% for ages 2 to 5 years, 18% for ages 6 to 11 years, and 21% for ages 12 to

## TABLE 29-2  Centers for Disease Control and Prevention Classification of Body Mass Index (BMI) for Children Age 2 Years and Above

| Plotted Percentile for Age and Gender | BMI Interpretation |
| --- | --- |
| <5th percentile | Underweight |
| 5th-85th percentile | Normal |
| 85th-95th percentile | Overweight |
| >95th percentile | Obese |

From Centers for Disease Control and Prevention: Classification of body mass index, 2015. Available at http://www.cdc.gov/.

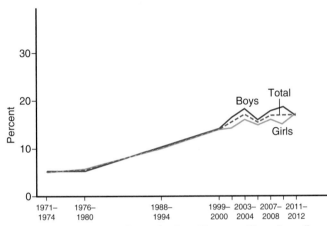

**FIG 29-3** Obesity prevalence for 2 to 19 years. (Data from Fryer C, Carroll M, et al: Health E-Stat: Prevalence of obesity among children and adolescents: United States, trends 1963-1965 through 2011-2012, 2013. Centers for Disease Control and Prevention, National Center of Health Statistics. Available at www.cdc.gov. Accessed March 15, 2015.)

19 years (Ogden et al, 2014) (Figure 29-3). Comparing these 2012 National Health and Nutrition Examination Survey (NHANES) findings with 2004 NHANES results demonstrates that prevalence rates for obesity have remained stable with a decrease (5.5%) for the 2 to 5 year age range (Ogden et al, 2014). In addition, 8.1% of infants and toddlers had high weight for recumbent length, indicating a substantial risk for obesity in childhood.

The physiological consequences of childhood obesity are extensive and significantly impact the health status of American children. Research has clearly identified strong relationships between being obese as a child and increased disease risk and disease burden in the cardiovascular, metabolic, musculoskeletal, respiratory, and renal systems (May et al, 2012; Papandreou et al, 2012; Papoutsakis et al, 2013; Paulis et al, 2014; Morandi & Maffeis, 2013). Another critical consequence for children is the negative psychological and social impact of obesity with decreased self-esteem; higher incidence of depression, sadness, and anxiety; problems with social relationships; and higher reports of being the victim of bullying (Puhl et al, 2012; Ting et al, 2012; Griffiths et al, 2010).

Multiple factors contribute to the likelihood that a child will become overweight or obese. Genetics and genetic susceptibility are certainly contributing components, although the genetic composition of the population has been stable over time, thereby failing to account for a sudden rise in obesity in recent years (Garver et al, 2013). Within the literature, three modifiable risk factors for the development of childhood obesity have been identified. These risk factors are screen time (including television, computer/tablet, phone, and video games), physical activity engagement, and dietary intake/eating behaviors (Hoelscher et al, 2013; Vollmer & Mobley, 2013; Fakhouri et al, 2013).

A rising comorbidity for childhood obesity is type 2 diabetes mellitus (T2DM). Currently, about 151,000 U.S. children and adolescents have T2DM (CDC, 2013c). Children and adolescents diagnosed with type 2 diabetes are usually between 10 and 19 years old, are obese with a strong family history for T2DM, and have insulin resistance (Springer et al, 2013). Most children and adolescents with T2DM have poor glycemic control with hemoglobin A1C levels between 10% and 12%. T2DM affects all ethnic groups but occurs more frequently in non-white groups with the highest prevalence in American Indian youth (CDC, 2013c).

Screening for T2DM is recommended for children with a BMI of 85th to 95th percentile with two risk factors of family history of diabetes, belonging to a racial minority group, or with signs of insulin resistance; all children with a BMI above the 95th percentile; and at age 10 years or onset of puberty. In addition, these children should be screened for hypercholesterolemia and hypertension, which are also associated with childhood obesity (Springer et al, 2013). Nurses can be instrumental in the management of T2DM in children by educating and counseling.

### Built Food Environments

A discussion on the risk factors for childhood obesity should be considered within the context of a child's environment. The emerging research on the relationship of built environments and obesity evaluates the factors within an individual's environment that may contribute on a macro- or micro-level to the development of obesity. The current literature focuses on the role of the built environment in increasing energy consumption while decreasing energy expenditure and looks at the interaction of the individual with his or her environment that influences health (Gose et al, 2013).

For children, the built environment as it relates to nutrition includes both macro- and micro-level considerations. On the community, or macro level, the factors of the built environment that influence nutrition and risk factors for obesity include a greater reliance on convenience foods and fast foods, increasing portion sizes, and the **food landscape** (He et al, 2012). The food landscape evaluates the accessibility and availability of healthy foods, and it is clear that low-income neighborhoods have limited access to stores offering fruits and vegetables (Dutko et al, 2012).

Close proximity to fast food restaurants and convenience stores are negatively correlated with daily fruit and vegetable consumption for school age children (He et al, 2012). Many urban and rural Americans live in areas termed as food deserts, which are defined as having limited access to affordable and nutritious foods. The inability to easily obtain nutritious foods has been identified as a contributing factor to the development of obesity and obesity-related diseases. More than 23.5 million American households live in low-income areas more than 1 mile from a supermarket (Dutko et al, 2012).

The factors on the macro level interact closely with those factors on the micro level. For children, the micro-level factors of the built environment that influence nutrition include the home food environment. The home food environment factors include home availability and accessibility of fruits and vegetables, parent role modeling, child feeding practices, and general parenting style (Osei-Assibey et al, 2012).

## Obesity Prevention

A united national movement is underway to reduce risk factors for developing obesity in children. The current White House administration is promoting the "Let's Move!" campaign as a comprehensive and coordinated initiative to prevent childhood obesity. The initiative emphasizes four primary components: healthy schools, access to affordable and healthy food, raising children's physical activity levels, and empowering families to make healthy choices (White House, 2014).

### ♥ HEALTHY PEOPLE 2020

The *Healthy People 2020* priority focus areas of prevention include a direct focus on achieving the goals of reducing the proportion of children who are overweight or obese, increasing the proportion of daily servings of fruits for children, and increasing the proportion of daily servings of vegetables for children.

From: US Department of Health and Human Services: Healthy People 2020, Wash DC, 2010, US Government Printing Office.

Promoting good nutrition and dietary habits is a key to maintaining child health. The first six years are the most important for developing sound lifetime eating habits. Parents as primary caregivers are most influential in teaching children specific eating behaviors through their own child feeding practices. Child feeding practices are a primary factor in the development of eating behaviors for children and include the level of control the parent or caregiver exerts over the type and amount of food the child eats, the role modeling of eating behaviors, the feeding cues given to the child, and the actual

mealtime environment and routine. The resulting learned eating behaviors then follow an individual through adolescence and into adulthood (Anzman et al, 2010).

*Collaboration between agencies is critical to implementing community based interventions to reduce childhood obesity. Shape NC is an innovative partnership that provides grant funding and training resources to improve obesity risk factors for young children. The resources extend to 100 North Carolina counties and improve policies, practices and outdoor environments in child care centers and communities so that more children are entering kindergarten at a healthy weight. Within 18 months of implementation, Shape NC has shown an increase from 49% to 65% of daycares meeting best practices for obesity prevention. The program is well on its way to reaching the goal of 75% of all daycares meeting best practices and supporting young children in maintaining a healthy weight (National Institute for Health Care Management, 2012).*

## Nutrition Assessment

Physical growth serves as an excellent measure of adequacy of the diet. Measurements of height and weight, plotted on appropriate growth curves at regular intervals, allow assessment of growth patterns. Head circumference is followed until age 3. For children less than 2 years, the weight for recumbent length is assessed at regular intervals. Those infants and toddlers who measure above the 97.7th percentile of WHO growth standards are considered high risk for obesity. For children 2 years and older, the body mass index (BMI) should be calculated (kilograms/[meters]$^2$) based on the weight and height measurements. BMI for age and gender is plotted on the standardized BMI-for-age charts available through the CDC. Children falling outside the expected growth patterns can then be identified and interventions implemented (ADA, 2008).

A 24-hour diet recall by the parent is a helpful screening tool to assess the amount and variety of food intake. If the recall is fairly typical for the child or adolescent, the nurse can compare the intake with basic recommendations for the child's or adolescent's age. It is important to ask about parent's concerns regarding diet. It is also helpful to look at the family's meal patterns. Other important parts of the nutrition assessment include amount of physical activity and any behavior problems that occur during meals. Table 29-3 offers guidelines to daily requirements for all ages.

## TABLE 29-3  Daily Dietary Recommendations: Childhood and Adolescence

| Food Group* | 2-3 Years | 4-8 Years | 9-13 Years | 14-18 Years |
|---|---|---|---|---|
| Milk: Try to select low-fat sources of milk, cheese, yogurt | 2 cups | 2-2½ cups | 3 cups | 3 cups |
| Meat and Beans: Lean meats, beans, eggs, seafood | 2 oz | 4 oz | 5 oz | 5-6½ oz |
| Vegetables: Fresh vegetables best choice | 1 cup | 1-1½ cups | 2-2½ cups | 2½-3 cups |
| Fruits: Limit fruit juices | 1 cup | 1-1½ cups | 1½ cups | 2 cups |
| Grains: Half of grains should be whole grains Cooked pasta or rice, bread, cereals | 3 oz | 5 oz | 5-6 oz | 6-8 oz |

*Recommendations are per day for each group.
Adapted from U.S. Department of Agriculture: Choose my plate, 2015. www.USDA.gov.

## Physical Activity

Physical activity levels contribute significantly to the overall health of children, particularly related to their risk for obesity. Fewer children are meeting the recommended physical activities levels today compared with previous generations. There are several contributing factors including the physical built environment, changes in school practices for physical education, and increased screen time.

Some children are at higher risk for not getting enough physical activity, particularly those children living in poverty in urban neighborhoods that are unsafe for outdoor playtime and with limited access to playgrounds and parks (CDC, 2010a). Even in suburban areas, parents are wary of allowing their children to play unsupervised outdoors. Few families live in locations where they can regularly walk or bike to school or for errands. As a society, Americans have become increasingly sedentary, which contributes greatly to obesity and the development of many chronic diseases.

The CDC recommends that every child and adolescent gets 60 minutes of physical activity daily. This should primarily consist of moderate-intensity aerobic activity and it is recommended that vigorous-intensity aerobic, muscle strengthening, and bone strengthening activities be incorporated at least three times a week (CDC, 2011b). This can be accumulated throughout the day with smaller increments of activity, those obtained during school, at home, and while engaged in leisure or sports activities. It is important to encourage families to be active together since this promotes greater physical activity levels in children. It also provides family time for promoting family engagement, connection, and communication. Table 29-4 shows developmental guidelines for physical activity promotion.

According to the most recent NHANES data, all age groups are failing to meet recommended daily activity levels. For children 6 to 11 years of age, 41.8% get 60 minutes of moderate activity daily; this drops to 7.6% for 12- to 15-year-olds and just 7.7% for 16- to 19-year-old adolescents (Tudor-Locke et al, 2012). Of significant note, girls are much more sedentary than boys, with the disparity increasing with age.

## Schools

Children and adolescents spend much of each weekday in school. Based on the results of a recent study, there is strong evidence that physical activity improves academic achievement with grades and standardized tests (CDC, 2010b). Currently, 48% of high school students attend physical education classes one or more days a week with only 29.4% attending physical education classes five days per week (Kann et al, 2014). In addition, 54% of adolescents in the United States play on at least one sports team, with more males participating in sports than females.

Schools have a vital ability to influence student health and academic achievement through federal and state school policies. Quality physical education requires adequate time (at least 150 minutes for elementary schools and 225 minutes for secondary

| TABLE 29-4 | Physical Activity Recommendations by Age Group |
|---|---|
| **Age Group** | **Recommendations** |
| Infants and toddlers (0-2 years) | Safe, minimally structured play environment<br>　Promote outdoor activities and exploration under supervision of a responsible adult<br>　No television viewing<br>　Organized exercise classes are not recommended |
| Preschoolers (2-6 years) | Encourage free play and exploration under proper supervision<br>　Provide unorganized play with opportunity for running, swimming, tumbling, throwing, catching with supervision<br>　Take short walks with family member; limit use of strollers for transportation<br>　Limit television viewing to <2 hours/day |
| Elementary school age (6-9 years) | Encourage free play with emphasis on basic skills acquisition<br>　Promote walking, dancing, jumping rope<br>　Organized sports (soccer, baseball) can be started but should be flexible with rules, allowing free time in practice<br>　Take walks, short bike rides together as a family<br>　Limit television viewing, video games to <2 hours/day |
| Middle school age (10-12 years) | Encourage physical activities enjoyed with families and friends<br>　Emphasize skills acquisition with increased focus on strategies<br>　Participation in complex sports (football, basketball) is appropriate<br>　Weight training can begin with good supervision and small weights<br>　Limit television viewing, video games to <2 hours/day |
| Adolescents | Encourage physical activities that are enjoyed with friends and considered fun to the teen<br>　Promote personal fitness—running, yoga, dance, swimming<br>　Encourage active transportation—biking and walking<br>　Weight training is safe for this age<br>　Limit television viewing, video games to <2 hours/day |

Data from American Academy of Pediatrics: Policy statement: active healthy living: prevention of childhood obesity through increased physical activity. *Pediatrics* 117(5):1834–1842, 2006. Reaffirmed by the American Academy of Pediatrics, as a continuing policy May 2009.

schools per week), teacher preparation and professional support, and adequate facilities and class size. Recommendations to meet high levels of physical activity in schools include strategies that integrate physical activity into structured classroom activities, encouraging more unstructured play, expanding extracurricular activities promoting physical activity, and guiding adolescents in developing their own personal fitness goals and plans (CDC, 2013d).

The *Healthy People 2020* objectives include a focus on increasing the proportion of adolescents and children who engage in moderate to vigorous activity on a daily basis, increasing the proportion of adolescents who spend at least 50% of school physical education class time being physically active, and increasing the proportion of adolescents who participate in daily school physical education. Nurses will want to be active in educating school administrators and school boards on the benefits of physical activity in improving children's and adolescents' physical health, cognitive performance, and behavior. Nurses should be engaged in policy revisions in the school systems to restore compulsory, quality, daily physical education classes; retain school recess; and expand extracurricular activities that promote physical activity before and after schools.

## Media

The concept of "media" has changed significantly over the past decade. In addition to television and movies, media now includes the Internet, video games, computers/tablets, and cell or smartphones. Social media is another avenue in which Americans interact with peers, family, and friends. With the extensive incorporation of media and social media into our society, its impact on children and adolescents is significant. Children and adolescents now spend more time engaged with media than any other activity except for sleeping; on average over 7 hours each day. Currently, 20.8% of 6- to 11-year-olds and 26.1% of teens have excessive screen time (Wethington et al, 2013). With video viewing alone, adolescents spend an average of 5 hours online, 8 hours on a mobile device, and 99 hours per month watching videos of some type (Office of Adolescent Health, 2013).

Research has strongly correlated increased use of media with an increased sedentary lifestyle, obesity, hypercholesterolemia, and hypertension. In addition to the negative physiological effects, exposure to such extensive media has been correlated to desensitization to violence and increased aggression, greater sexual content exposure and increased sexual activity, and lower academic performance if the child or adolescent has a television in the bedroom (AAP, 2009a).

Interventions need to be based on the goal of lifestyle changes for the entire family. The AAP recommends that children and adolescents over the age of 2 years be limited to 2 hours per day of media screen time and that children under 2 years do not have any screen time (Strasburger et al, 2010). Televisions, video game systems, tablets, phones, and computers should be kept out of the child's or adolescent's bedroom and in open spaces in the home (Wethington et al, 2013). Parents should engage in media and social media viewing with their children to discuss appropriate content, avoid exposing young children to PG-13 or R-rated movies, and role model limited media usage.

Nurses are uniquely positioned within the community to effect change in the childhood obesity rates. With the knowledge and skills to identify children as at risk or obese, nurses can develop interventions for healthy change for these families and refer to providers appropriately. Education on healthy eating, child feeding practices, and physical activity levels are necessary for individuals, families, and groups within the community. Nurses have the abilities and knowledge to develop creative programs to provide families with the skills to grow their own gardens and cook healthy meals. Advocating for exercise trails and physical activity programs within the community will improve the health of families living in the vicinity. It is clear from obesity research that a community-based approach is most effective at reducing obesity rates and improving health. The following list highlights some guidelines on nutrition education for families:

- Breastfeeding is the recommended exclusive feeding choice for infants from birth to 6 months and should be continued until 1 year of age. Breastfeeding is associated with a lower risk for developing childhood obesity.
- Parents' responsibilities are to provide healthy meals and snacks for their children. It is their child's responsibility to decide how much to eat.
- Limit 100% fruit juices and avoid all other sugary beverages. These are empty calories and fill children up so they are not hungry at meals. Appropriate beverages are milk and water.
- For toddlers and preschoolers, it sometimes takes 10 to 15 tastes of a new food before they learn to like that food. Be persistent!
- Parents should role model good eating behaviors—lots of fruits and vegetables, no sugary beverages, and little to no "junk" food or "fast" food.
- Family meals are important for teaching manners, listening to hunger cues, and having quality family time together.
- Encourage children to help with food selection and preparation as appropriate to developmental skills. Allow them to select new foods to try in the produce section of the grocery store.
- Avoid using food as a punishment or reward. Do not expect your child to "clean their plate." These feeding techniques have been associated with increased risk for obesity.
- Turn off the television during meals and do not let your child eat in front of the television. Children do not listen to their cues of satiety when distracted.
- Cook meals at home. Broil, bake, stir-fry, or poach foods rather than frying.
- Modify family eating habits to include low-fat food choices. Serve calorically dense foods that incorporate the food guide pyramid: whole grains, fruits, vegetables, lean protein foods, and low-fat dairy products.
- Encourage family members to stop eating when they are satisfied. Encourage recognizing hunger and satiation cues.
- Schedule regular times for meals and snacks. Include breakfast and do not skip meals.

- Have low-calorie, nutritious snacks ready and available. Avoid having empty-calorie junk foods in the home. Plan for healthy snacks when eating "on the run," such as granola, fruits, and nuts.
- Decrease salt, sugar, and fat. Increase complex carbohydrates—whole grains.
- Maintain regular activity (e.g., exercise, sports) and limit television viewing.
- Select family activities and vacations that include or focus on physical activity (hiking, bicycling, swimming).

## Injuries and Accidents

Unintentional injuries are the leading cause of morbidity and mortality in the United States for young people ages 1 to 19 years. Unintentional injuries are any injuries sustained by accident such as falls, drowning or motor vehicle accidents. It is one of the most under-recognized public health problems facing the United States today, with more than 9,000 children dying from a preventable injury in 2009. Reducing injuries from unintentional causes, as well as from violence and abuse, is a goal of *Healthy People 2020*. More than 8.4 million children were seen in emergency departments in 2009 for treatment from an unintentional injury (MMWR, 2012).

Motor vehicle crashes remain the leading cause of death for unintentional injuries in children and teens. One research study found that 72% of almost 3500 observed car and booster seats were mishandled in a way that could possibly increase a child's risk of injury during a crash. It is recommended by the National Highway Traffic Safety Administration for children to remain in booster seats until they are at least 8 years of age or 4 feet, 9 inches tall (Figure 29-4). A study found that booster seats reduced injury risk by 59% compared with seat belts alone for children ages 4 to 7 years. National standards recommend that all children ages 12 years and younger ride in the back seat because they are at significant risk of injury from airbag deployment, and the back seat is known as the safest part of the vehicle if a crash occurs. Even for adolescents to age 16 years, sitting in the back seat is associated with a 40% decrease in the risk of serious injury (Borse et al, 2008; CDC 2014b).

Drowning, poisonings, and burns account for most of the other deaths. For infants, the leading cause of death

is suffocation (Table 29-5). From 2000 to 2009, the rates of unintentional infant suffocation deaths increased by 54% leading to an overall increase in newborn and infant death rates (MMWR, 2012). To effectively implement prevention strategies, nurses need to understand the developmental factors that place this population at risk.

### Developmental Considerations

*Infants.* Infants have the second highest injury rate of all groups of children; their small size contributes to some types of injury. The small airway may be easily occluded. The small body fits through places where the head may be entrapped. In motor vehicle crashes, small size is a great disadvantage and increases the risk for crushing or being propelled into surfaces.

The second half of infancy brings major accomplishments in gross motor activities. Rolling, sitting, pulling up, and walking bring safety concerns. Their developing motor skills remain immature, which limits their ability to escape from injury and places them at risk for drowning, suffocating, and burns (CDC, 2012c).

*Toddlers and Preschoolers.* This population experiences a large number of nonfatal falls and being struck by or against an

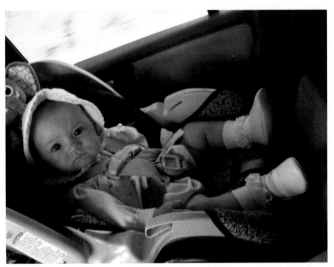

FIG 29-4 Children should always be restrained while riding in a vehicle.

| TABLE 29-5 | Leading Causes of Unintentional Injury Death Among U.S. Children 0 to 19 Years, 2000-2009 | | | | |
|---|---|---|---|---|---|
| Rank | 0-1 Years | 1-4 Years | 5-9 Years | 10-14 Years | 15-19 Years |
| 1 | Suffocation (77%) | Drowning (31%) | MVT-related* (49%) | MVT-related* (68%) | MVT-related* (67%) |
| 2 | MVT-related* (8%) | MVT related* (25%) | Drowning (15%) | Transportation Other (15%) | Poisoning (9%) |
| 3 | Drowning (4%) | Fire burns (12%) | Burns/fire (11%) | Drowning (10%) | Drowning (6%) |
| 4 | Fire burns (2%) | Transportation Other (10%) | Transportation Other (9%) | Burns/fire (6%) | Transportation Other (4%) |
| 5 | Poisoning (2%) | Suffocation (9%) | Suffocation (3%) | Suffocation (5%) | Falls (1%) |

*MVT-related: Motor vehicle traffic–related includes motor vehicle injuries, pedestrian injuries.
Centers for Disease Control and Prevention, National Center for Injury Prevention and Control: National Action Plan for Child Injury Prevention, Atlanta (GA), 2012C, CDC, NCIPC.

object. They are active and lack an understanding of cause and effect, and their increasing motor skills make supervision difficult (CDC, 2012c). They are inquisitive and have relatively immature logic abilities.

*School-Age Children.* The school-age group has the lowest injury death rate. At this age, it is difficult to judge speed and distance, placing them at risk for pedestrian and bicycle accidents. Boys are twice as likely as girls to sustain a nonfatal bicycle injury, and the highest injury rate is at 10 to 14 years of age. Universal use of bicycle helmets would prevent most deaths. Peer pressure and lack of parental role modeling often inhibits the use of protective devices such as helmets and limb pads (CDC, 2012c).

*Adolescents.* Motor vehicle–related injuries and violence are the leading causes of morbidity and mortality for adolescents. Risk-taking becomes more conscious at this time, especially among boys. The injury death rates for boys are twice as high as those for girls. Adolescents are at the highest risk of any age group for motor vehicle deaths and fatal poisonings. Use of weapons and drug and alcohol abuse play an important role in injuries in this age group. Homicides are the second leading cause of death for U.S. adolescents (Borse et al, 2008; CDC, 2012c).

In a survey of adolescents, 24.7% reported being in a physical fight at least one time in the previous 12 months, and 7.1% reported missing school at least one day in the previous month because they felt unsafe at school or on their way to school. Suicide is the third leading cause of death among youths between the ages of 15 and 24 years. Poor social adjustment, psychiatric problems, and family disorganization increase the risk for suicide (Kann et al, 2014; Federal Interagency Forum on Child & Family Statistics, 2013).

For all ages, families should be given anticipatory guidance in the high-risk areas for each age group to promote safety and injury prevention. Nurses can use community centers, schools, workplaces, and health centers to provide teaching to families on how to prevent injuries in their children.

## Sports Injuries

Encouraging participation in team sports and individual sports and active leisure activities can increase the physical activity of children and adolescents. Children who are active in sports should have annual sports physicals, and guidelines for sports safety should be discussed as follows:

- Children should be grouped according to weight, size, maturation, and skill level.
- Qualified and competent persons should be available for supervision during games and practices.
- Adequate and appropriate-size equipment should be available.
- Goals should be developmentally and physically appropriate for the child.

Approximately 2.6 million children a year are seen in the emergency department for sports and recreational injuries (CDC, 2012c).

To protect children and adolescents during sports, families require education on selecting age and physically appropriate

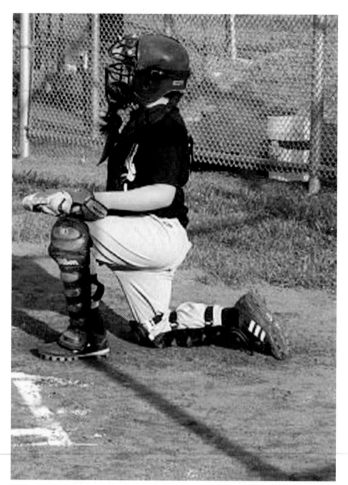

**FIG 29-5** Involvement in developmentally appropriate sports promotes physical activity and skills acquisition.

activities, using the correct safety gear, maintaining the safety gear in good condition, and practicing good body mechanics (Figure 29-5). Management of acute injuries sustained during sports should be monitored closely by coaches and primary care providers. The incidence of concussions, or brain injuries, is 3.8 million per year in the United States (USDHHS, 2013b).

The state of Washington passed the first law on concussion in sports in 2009, the Zackery Lystedt Law. Between 2009 and 2012, 43 states (as well as the District of Columbia) passed laws on concussions in sports for youth and/or high school athletes. Many of these laws are known as "Return to Play" laws. The CDC's *Heads Up* program provides recommendations and educational materials to health professionals, coaches, and parents to increase knowledge related to sports-related concussions in youth. Recognition of concussions and proper treatment is critical to prevent repeat concussions, which can cause long-term problems (USDHHS, 2013b) (Table 29-6).

## Child Maltreatment

In 2011, 3.7 million children were reported abused or neglected with about 681,000 cases confirmed by Child Protective Services. For the same year, about 1750 U.S. children (2.1 deaths per 100,000 children) died as a result of maltreatment (CDC, 2013e). In 2011, 35% of victims of child maltreatment

## TABLE 29-6   Recognizing a Concussion in an Athlete

| Signs Observed by Coaches/Parents | Symptoms Reported by Athlete |
|---|---|
| • Appears dazed, stunned, confused | • Headache or "pressure" in head |
| • Forgets sports plays | • Nausea or vomiting |
| • Moves clumsily | • Balance problems, dizziness, double/blurred vision |
| • Answers questions slowly | • Sensitivity to light and/or noise |
| • Loses consciousness (even briefly) | • Feeling sluggish, foggy, or groggy |
| • Shows behavior or personality changes | • Concentration or memory problems |
| • Cannot recall events prior to or after hit or fall | • Confusion or does not "feel right" |

From U.S. Department of Health and Human Services: Heads up, concussion in youth sports: a fact sheet for coaches, 2013b. Available at www.cdc.gov.

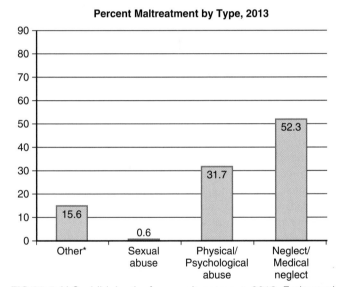

**Percent Maltreatment by Type, 2013**

FIG 29-6 U.S. child deaths from maltreatment, 2013. Estimated 1,217 deaths in 2013. (U.S. Department of Health and Human Services, Administration for Children and Families, Administration on Children, Youth and Families, Children's Bureau: Child Maltreatment 2138, 2013. Available from http://www.acf.hhs.gov/programs/cb/stats_research/index.htm#can.)

were less than 3 years of age and infants less than 1 year of age had the highest incidence of abuse.

Child maltreatment is defined as any act or series of acts of commission or omission by an adult that results in harm, potential for harm, or threat of harm to a child. Acts of commission (abuse) include physical abuse, sexual abuse, and psychological abuse; acts of omission (neglect) include failure to provide (physical neglect, emotional neglect, medical/dental neglect, educational neglect) and failure to supervise (inadequate supervision, exposure to violent environments) (Figure 29-6) (Leeb et al, 2008).

Child maltreatment occurs in all socioeconomic, racial, and ethnic groups. Yet African American, American Indian/Native American, and multiracial children experienced higher rates of victimization. Children under the age of 4 years and those children with special needs are at highest risk. Children are most likely to be maltreated by their parents, and common parental characteristics include a poor understanding of child development and children's needs, history of abuse in the family of origin, substance abuse in the household, and nonbiological transient caregivers in the home (e.g., mother's boyfriend). Families at highest risk for maltreatment are those families experiencing social isolation, family violence, parenting stress, and poor parent–child relationships (Zimmerman & Mercy, 2010).

The consequences of child maltreatment are often devastating. Children experience long-term physical consequences as well as negative psychological and behavioral consequences. Abusive head trauma (AHT), also known as shaken baby syndrome, results from violent shaking or shaking and impacting of the head of an infant or young child. Intracranial injury, subdural bleeding, retinal hemorrhages, and skull fractures can result, leading to death or survival with associated motor impairments, visual deficits, and cognitive deficits (AAP, 2012a).

Preventive strategies are necessary to reduce the incidence of child maltreatment. Parental education should be started prenatally to prevent AHT. Nurses can use home visiting programs, peer mentoring programs, preschool and Head Start programs, and public health centers to identify at-risk families and provide support and education to prevent child maltreatment. Nurses can provide education to those individuals in the community who work with children on recognizing signs of abuse and how to report suspected maltreatment. Increased awareness within the community and early intervention can prevent maltreatment from occurring and rescue children from violent and unsafe abuse situations.

### Injury Prevention

Health care provider offices, schools, community centers, public health centers, and daycare/preschool facilities provide opportunities to teach children, adolescents, and their families about prevention of injuries. Safety and health promotion can be incorporated into required health education courses within the school systems. Community-sponsored car seat and seat belt safety checks and safety fairs are another way to educate families (CDC, 2012c). Early home visitation programs to high-risk families resulted in a reduction of 48% in child abuse. Injury prevention is a topic that should be addressed at all health visits (Zimmerman & Mercy, 2010).

*Reducing Gun Violence.* Although rates have fallen, deaths of children and adolescents from firearm-related injuries were 11.4 per 100,000 in 2009. The NYRBSS survey of adolescents found that 5.1% had carried a gun on at least one day during the previous month. Witnessing gun violence or knowing the victims affects children indirectly (AAP, 2012b).

A recent study compared firearm-related mortality rates in urban and rural settings. The study found no significant differences in the death rates between the settings but noted a difference in the firearm intent that resulted in deaths for children and adolescents. The urban victims died from high rates of firearm homicide while the rural victims experienced high rates of firearm suicide and unintentional firearm-related accidental deaths. This study provides evidence that to reduce firearm mortality effectively, prevention strategies should be geared for the specific type of firearm injury issue within the community of interest (Nance et al, 2010).

Characteristics associated with gun violence include history of aggressive behaviors, poverty, school problems, substance abuse, and cultural acceptance of violent behavior. Young children are inquisitive and often imitate in play what they see in the media and on television. A significant number of accidental firearm injuries and deaths in children occur in the homes of friends and family members (AAP, 2012b). Interventions must begin early and address each of these factors.

The *Healthy People 2020* objectives seek to reduce the number of high school students who carry weapons. Nurses can actively participate in efforts to reduce gun violence among young people in the following ways (AAP, 2012c):
- Urge legislators to support gun control legislation, assault weapons bans, and eliminate gun show loopholes.
- Collaborate with schools to develop programs to discourage violence among children.
- Encourage families to remove guns from their homes. If unable to do this, educate families to:
  - Store all firearms unloaded and uncocked in a securely locked container. Only the parents should know where the container is located.
  - Store the guns and ammunition in separate locked locations.
  - When handling or cleaning a gun, never leave it unattended, even for a moment; it should be in the parent's view at all times.
- Initiate community programs focusing on gun storage and safety at school.
- Educate parents on communicating with the homeowners of the homes their children visit regarding gun access and safety.
- Children and adolescents learning to hunt in rural areas should take gun safety courses.
- Identify populations at risk for violence and target aggression or anger management.
- Discourage mixing alcohol or drugs with guns.
- Encourage families to avoid gun violence in media sources at home.

*Promoting Safe Playgrounds and Recreation Areas.* Schools, daycare centers, families, and community groups often need guidance toward developing safe places for children to play. Each year, more than 200,000 children are treated in emergency departments for injuries sustained on playgrounds and play sets. Approximately 45% of playground-related injuries are severe injuries and include fractures, internal injuries, concussions, dislocations, and amputations. Between 1990 and 2000, 147 children under the age of 14 died from playground-related injuries. These deaths were attributable to

strangulation (56%) and falls (20%) to the playground surface, with most of these deaths (70%) occurring on home playgrounds (CDC, 2012d).

The U.S. Consumer Product Safety Commission has published guidelines for public and home playground safety. Guidelines cover structure, materials, surfaces, and maintenance of equipment:
- Playgrounds should be surrounded by a barrier to protect children from traffic.
- Activity centers should be distributed to avoid crowding in one area.
- Surfaces should be finished with substances that meet Consumer Product Safety Commission (CPSC) regulations for lead.
- Durable materials should be used.
- Sand, gravel, wood chips, and wood mulch (not CCA treated) are acceptable surfaces for limiting the shock of falls.
- Equipment should be inspected regularly for protrusions that could puncture skin or entangle clothes.
- Inspect equipment for openings/angles that allow for possible head entrapment.
- Multiple-occupancy swings, animal swings, rope swings, and trampolines are not recommended.

The developmental skills of specific ages are incorporated, as well as recommendations for physically challenged children. Nurses can use these guidelines to help the community establish standards for play areas (Figure 29-7).

Nurses share responsibility in the prevention of intentional and unintentional injuries in the pediatric population. Assessment of the characteristics of the child, family, and environment identifies risk factors. Interventions include anticipatory guidance, modification of the environment, and safety education. Education focuses on age-appropriate interventions based on knowledge of leading causes of death and risk factors. Topics to consider are listed in Box 29-1.

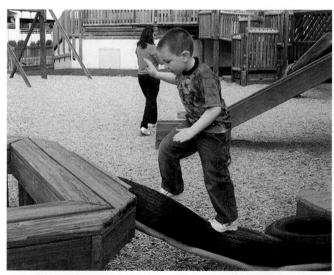

**FIG 29-7** Playground injuries are frequent among young children.

## BOX 29-1  Injury Prevention Topics

- Car restraints, seat belts, air-bag safety
- Preventing fires, burns
- Poison prevention
- Preventing falls
- Preventing drowning, water safety
- Bicycle safety
- Safe driving practices
- Sports safety
- Pedestrian safety
- Gun control
- Decreasing gang activities
- Substance abuse prevention

(See also the Evolve website)

## HEALTH PROBLEMS OF CHILDHOOD

### Acute Illnesses

Acute illnesses are those illnesses with an abrupt onset and are usually of a short duration. For children, it is common for viruses to spread easily through daycares, preschools, and school systems. Nurses use developmental factors at each age to plan assessment and intervention strategies to prevent the spread of illnesses between children. Community-focused interventions, education, and programs can prevent many childhood illnesses.

Hand washing is a simple and reliable strategy to reduce the incidence of acute illnesses in children. The How To box below provides guidelines for the nurse to teach families about hand washing. Infants and young children are particularly at risk for contracting viral and bacterial illnesses spread by contact because their immune systems are not yet fully developed. Focusing community education on preschools, daycare centers, and other programs that serve the families of infants and young children can reduce the occurrence of acute illnesses (Aronson & Shope, 2013).

Several strategies can be used to reduce the occurrence of acute illnesses as follows: sanitizing objects such as toys that are handled by multiple children each day to prevent the spread of diseases; practicing good hand hygiene and diaper disposal techniques in daycares to prevent the spread of illnesses; and educating parents, daycares, and schools on when to keep children home to prevent putting others at risk for illness (Aronson & Shope, 2013).

Influenza is a common viral illness that affects children and adolescents primarily during the winter months. It is a highly contagious acute febrile illness of the nose, throat, and lungs that leads to missed school days and can result in complications including pneumonia and infrequently death. The best prevention strategy is vaccinations for all children ages 6 months and above. It is important to educate families about the need for vaccination and home management of symptoms (Aronson & Shope, 2013).

Nurses can focus on preventive measures and promote high vaccination rates, good hand washing hygiene and early identification to prevent the spread of illness. If a child or adolescent

### HOW TO  Teach Families About Hand Washing

*Use the guidelines below when counseling families about hand washing.*

*Always wash your hands before:*
- *Preparing foods*
- *Eating*
- *Touching someone who is sick*
- *Inserting or removing contact lenses*

*Always wash your hands after:*
- *Preparing foods, particularly raw meats or poultry*
- *Using the toilet*
- *Changing a diaper*
- *Touching animals, animal toys, leashes, or animal waste*
- *Blowing your nose, coughing, or sneezing into your hands*
- *Touching someone who is sick*
  *Or anytime you feel that your hands need washing!*

*How to wash your hands:*
- *Wet your hands with warm running water*
- *Apply soap (liquid, bar, or powder)*
- *Lather your hands well*
- *Rub your hands vigorously for at least 20 seconds (sing the "Happy Birthday" song)—scrub all surfaces including between your fingers, under your nails, backs of your hands, and your wrist*
- *Rinse your hands well*
- *Dry your hands with a clean towel, disposable towel, or air dryer*
- *Use your towel to turn off the faucet if possible*

is diagnosed with influenza, parents can be instructed to keep children at home until symptoms have improved and fever has been gone for 24 hours. Nurses can be actively involved in developing community-based policies in the event of a pandemic, and this may include plans for mass immunizations, specific flu clinics, and protocols for school closures (Aronson & Shope, 2013).

### SIDS/SUIDS

Sudden infant death syndrome (SIDS) is defined as the sudden death of an infant under 1 year of age that remains unexplained after a thorough case investigation, including performance of a complete autopsy, examination of the death scene, and review of the clinical history (AAP, 2011b). Sudden unexpected infant death (SUID) is a term that describes any sudden and unexpected death that occurs in infancy; this includes both explained (i.e., suffocation, infection, trauma) and unexplained cases (SIDS). The peak age for SIDS deaths occurs between 2 and 3 months of age, although SIDS may occur up to 1 year of age. There are specific independent risk factors for SIDS (AAP, 2011b):

- Prone or side-lying sleep position
- Sleeping on a soft surface
- Maternal smoking during pregnancy
- Overheating
- Late or no prenatal care
- Young maternal age
- Preterm birth and/or low birth weight
- Male gender
- Lack of immunizations

There are consistently higher rates of SIDS in non-Hispanic black and American Indian/Alaska Native infants—two to three times the national average. The incidence has decreased more than 50% since the "Back to Sleep" campaign was promoted in 1994. There is no test to identify infants who may die, making this a frustrating clinical problem. Nurses should teach the preventive measures that follow:

- Supine position only for infants—no side lying or prone
- No smoking during pregnancy or in home after birth
- Use a firm sleep surface—no soft bedding, no pillows, no stuffed animals, no sleeping on chairs or sofas, no sleeping with adults or in a waterbed
- Offer a pacifier at naptime and bedtime—reduces risk
- Avoid overheating and overbundling—room temperature should be between 68° and 72° F
- Continue "Back to Sleep" campaign (AAP, 2011b)

When an infant dies from SIDS, the family requires tremendous support. The nurse provides empathetic support and assists the family as they progress through the grief process and provides guidance for siblings and other family members. Referral to support groups may be helpful.

## Oral Health

Oral health is recognized as an integral component of overall health for children and adolescents. Dental caries in early childhood has been identified by the CDC as one of the most prevalent infectious diseases and the incidence is more common in children living in poverty or low socioeconomic status. Access to pediatric dental care is a barrier to meeting the oral health care needs of children in the United States (Hallas & Shelley, 2009).

Nurses are well positioned to provide oral health screenings and to educate families on preventive oral health topics. Children should be referred to a qualified dentist by 1 year of age. Families should receive anticipatory guidance on optimal use of fluorides, proper nutrition and dietary practices, prevention of poor oral health habits and tooth decay, age-appropriate dental injury prevention, and proper care of teeth and gingival tissue (AAP, 2008).

## Chronic Health Conditions

Improved medical technology has increased the number of children surviving with chronic health problems. In addition, environmental factors are leading to an increase in certain chronic health conditions. At present, it is estimated that about 26% of American children have a chronic health condition (Van Cleave et al, 2010). Some examples of common chronic conditions in children are Down syndrome, spina bifida, cerebral palsy, asthma, ADHD, diabetes, congenital heart disease, cancer, hemophilia, bronchopulmonary dysplasia, and AIDS.

Despite the differences in the specific diagnoses, all of these families have complex needs and face similar problems. Several variables exist to assess for each child and family:

- What is the actual health status? Is the condition stable or life threatening?
- What is the degree of impairment to the child's ability to develop?

- What types of treatments and therapy are required and with what frequency?
- How often are health care visits and hospitalizations required?
- To what degree are the family routines disrupted?

The common issues nurses will want to evaluate for these families include the following:

- All children and adolescents with chronic health problems need routine health care. The same issues of pediatric health promotion and acute health care need to be addressed with this group. The use of the medical home (discussed later in the chapter) is very important for this population.
- Ongoing medical care specific to the health problem needs to be provided. Examples include monitoring for complications of the health problem, medications management, dietary adjustments, and coordination of therapies. Evaluation of the effectiveness of the treatment plan is critical.
- Care is often provided by multiple specialists. There is a need for coordinating the scheduling of visits, tests or procedures and the treatment regimen.
- Skilled care procedures are often required and may include suctioning, positioning, medications, feeding techniques, breathing treatments, physical therapy, and use of appliances.
- Equipment needs are often complex and may include monitors, oxygen, ventilators, positioning or ambulation devices, infusion pumps, and suction machines.
- Educational needs are often complex. Communication between the family, the team of health care providers, school administrators, and teachers is essential to meet the child's health and educational needs.
- Safe transportation to health care services and school must be available. Several barriers may exist, including family resources, location, and the burden of supportive equipment.
- Financial resources may not be adequate to meet the needs.
- Behavioral issues include the effect of the condition on the child's behavior as well as on other family members.

The ultimate goal is for children with chronic health conditions to achieve optimal health and functioning. Identifying barriers for individual families and overall community barriers is a focus for nurses. Developing support groups, advocating for improved community access to resources, and educating those working with these children on their conditions and needs will promote the family's functioning. The How To box below details a community nursing approach to supporting a child with ADHD.

## Mental Health

Psychosocial stressors have increased over the years for children and mental health issues are a priority health concern for children and adolescents. There are many underlying causes for mental health problems in children, ranging from lead poisoning to exposure to violence in the home. Approximately 1 in 5 children and adolescents in the United States has a diagnosable mental health disorder. Children who live in poverty, live with

**HOW TO** Implement a Community Nursing Approach to a Chronic Illness: ADHD

*The following describes the steps the nurse in the community will follow to support a child with ADHD:*

- *Assessment: Obtaining history, physical, parent/family assessment, environmental assessment, learning, and psychoeducational evaluations*
- *Behavioral modifications: (home and school) Teaching families techniques to support clear expectations, consistent routines, positive reinforcement for appropriate behavior, and consequences for negative behaviors*
- *Classroom modifications: Consulting with family and teachers to meet individual needs for remediation or alternative instruction methods if necessary; structuring activities to respond to the child's needs*
- *Support: Referring family to family therapy/counseling, support groups, or mental health services to assist development of positive coping behaviors*
- *Medications: Consulting with physician to monitor and evaluate therapeutic and adverse effects*
- *Follow-up: Assessing at 3- to 6-month intervals when stable; dynamic process affected by relationships with others; behaviors will change with age; problem may persist through adulthood*

a single parent, or are exposed to violence are at higher risk for developing a mental health condition. Only 21% of children with a mental health or substance abuse problem are currently receiving treatment (AACAP, 2009).

Some of the common mental health problems diagnosed in children and adolescents are anxiety disorders, autism spectrum disorders, depression, bipolar disorder, conduct disorder, oppositional defiant disorder, and substance abuse (AACAP, 2009). Each of these mental health diagnoses has a specific set of criteria for diagnosis found in the DSM-V. Early recognition and coordinated management of pediatric mental health issues is critical to a child's functioning in school, home, and the community.

More than 2 million U.S. children during the past 10 years have experienced the stress and emotions associated with being separated from a parent deployed for active duty. These children experience symptoms of depression (25%), excess worry (50%), and sleep problems (50%). By understanding the stressors of military deployment, nurses can identify and provide the support (and referrals) needed to help these children (Siegle & Davis, 2013).

Many families can be at a loss for the behaviors or symptoms they observe in their child. A sense of embarrassment may prohibit parents from seeking help. Nurses can be instrumental in promoting community awareness about common mental health problems in children and identifying resources for families. The use of the medical home to coordinate management of mental health problems is important in the ability to provide oversight of subspecialties, medications, and therapies. A challenge for treating pediatric mental health disorders is an inadequate number of practitioners specializing in pediatric mental health, which may leave some families without adequate support and resources (AAP, 2009b).

## Bullying

Bullying has always been an issue for children and adolescents. With the extensive use of texting, e-mails, social networking, and other means of electronic communication among tweens and adolescents, cyber bullying has become a significant problem within communities. Girls are more likely to be victims of cyber bullying, and victims report thinking about self-harm and/or suicide as a result of bullying. Cyber bullying includes sending hurtful messages, starting rumors and uploading and sharing unflattering or altered photographs of the victims via an electronic means. Many cyber bullies use avatars or other ways of disguising their true identity, which makes it difficult for the victim to know who the bully is. The victims often do not report cyber bullying for fear of retaliation from the bully and experience emotional and behavioral symptoms along with school-related problems (Suzuki et al, 2012).

## Environmental Health

The built environment that children and adolescents live in directly affects their health. Growth, size, and behaviors place the pediatric population at greater risk for damage from various toxins. Lead poisoning is one of the most common environmental health hazards. Pesticides, mercury exposure, plasticizers, and poor air quality also pose serious risks (National Institute of Environmental Health Science, 2014). Common toxins and sources of pediatric exposure are listed in Table 29-7.

Growing tissues absorb toxins readily. Developing organ systems are more susceptible to damage. Smaller size means increased concentration of toxins per pound of body weight. The fact that children are short exposes them to lower air spaces, where heavy chemicals tend to concentrate. Outdoor play, especially during summer months, increases the opportunity for exposure to air pollutants. Chewing and mouthing behaviors offer contact to toxins such as lead. Playing on the floor increases exposure to chemicals in rugs and flooring. Rolling and playing in grass can result in pesticide exposure and playground materials that are treated with chemicals put children at risk. Exposure risks for adolescents are similar to those for adults and are primarily through work, school, and hobbies (NIEHS, 2014).

It is critical to assess for these environmental health hazards during health care visits. Referral for treatment may be necessary. Counseling families on risk reduction is important to children's health. Population-focused nurses identify environmental problems within the community and target at-risk populations with community interventions (see Table 29-8 for examples). Bringing screening programs into neighborhoods at risk may facilitate early identification and prevent complications. Lobbying efforts and education can effect public policy changes to make the environment healthier. The following case presentation gives an example of how a school environment can lead to health problems.

A child's built environment includes exposure to media and the resulting influence on behavior and choices. Food and beverage corporations spend over $1.6 billion each year on advertising that specifically targets children. Much of this advertising uses licensed cartoon characters to promote food products, and

| TABLE 29-7 | Common Environmental Agents Hazardous to Children |
|---|---|
| **Toxins** | **Sources** |
| Arsenic | Food, water |
| Asbestos | Building materials: insulation, ceilings, floor tiles |
| Carbon monoxide | Space heaters, woodstoves, fireplaces, engine exhaust, tobacco smoke |
| Dioxins | Contaminated foods, water, and soil |
| Lead | Paint, dust, soil, water, occupational exposure (e.g., battery plant), hobbies (e.g., stained glass) |
| Mercury | Water contamination, fish, thermometer/sphygmomanometer breakage |
| Molds | Food, ubiquitous to moist outdoor and indoor environment |
| Nitrites, nitrates | Water, food |
| Nicotine, benzene, tars | Environmental tobacco smoke |
| Particulate matter-nanomaterials | Outdoor air pollution, dust mites, animal dander, roach parts |
| Pesticides | Food, soil, plants, water, air, topical application for lice treatment, home and school insect management |
| Phthalates and bisphenol (BPA) | Linings of canned foods, children's toys, vinyl flooring, hard plastics made of polycarbonate (many sports water bottles and baby bottles) |
| Radon | Soil and rock, the air, ground water, surface water |
| Solvents/volatile organic compounds | Furniture, carpet, building materials, solvents and degreasers, cleaning products, acetone, formaldehyde |
| Styrene | vapors from building materials, photocopiers, tobacco smoke |
| Ultraviolet light | Outdoor sun exposure, tanning beds |

From: National Institutes of Environmental Health: Your Environment your health, 2015, Triangle Park, North Carolina, Accessed at www.NIEHS. Nih.gov. March 24, 2015.

| TABLE 29-8 | Prevention Strategies Applied to Environmental Hazards |
|---|---|
| **Prevention Strategies** | **Examples** |
| **Primary** | |
| Identification of at-risk populations | Substandard housing communities |
| | Pregnant women |
| | Children with asthma |
| Health education about environmental risks | Poison prevention |
| | Responses to poor air quality alerts |
| | Discontinue use of plasticizers |
| Formation of public health policies | Air/water quality standards |
| | Safety inspections: playgrounds, schools, daycare centers |
| | Standards for lead levels in imported products intended for children |
| Research to assess impact of environmental hazards on the pediatric population | Developing reference ranges/biological markers to assess toxic levels in children |
| | Identify long-term physiological and cognitive consequences of exposure to environmental toxins |
| **Secondary** | |
| Early detection, treatment, and referral for management of environmental toxins | Removal of at-risk persons when lead hazards are detected |
| | Assessment of lead levels of populations of at-risk children with treatment of individuals as indicated |
| **Tertiary** | |
| Restoration of environment and occupants to healthier state | Asbestos/lead abatement of buildings |
| | Radon remediation of homes |
| | Replacement of heating, ventilation, air conditioning, systems contaminated with mold |
| | Chelating agents for individuals with lead toxic levels |

Modified from Burns C, Dunn A, Sattler B: Resources for environmental health problems. *J Pediatr Health Care* 16:3, 2002.

the majority of those products are of poor nutritional value. The heart of the question is whether this advertising is effective in influencing children's food choices. A study by Roberto et al (2010) looked at the preferences of preschool children for food packaged with a licensed cartoon character. The study found that preschoolers rated the taste of the foods packaged with the licensed character over the identical food without the character packaging. The children also selected the high-density character-packaged foods more often. Nurses in the community can use this information to provide guidance to parents to limit exposure to television and media, make healthy food choices for their children, and avoid unhealthy foods packaged with licensed cartoon characters. Nurses can also advocate for stricter advertising laws for those unhealthy foods targeted to children.

## Lead Poisoning

Lead is a heavy metal that is absorbed into the body primarily through ingestion. Lead poisoning is defined as a serum lead

## BOX 29-2  Steps to Minimize Lead Exposure in Contaminated Toys and Products

- Read recall notices from the CPSC (www.cpsc.gov) and do not buy recalled toys.
- Check old toys at home to make sure they have not been recalled.
- Avoid purchasing toys secondhand from yard sales and flea markets.
- Check labels and recommended ages on all toy labels and follow recommendations.
- Do not purchase children's costume jewelry or allow children to play with adult costume jewelry.

level above 10 µg/dL and it causes significant neurologic, cardiovascular, and renal disease. A *Healthy People 2020* goal is to eliminate elevated blood lead levels in all children. More than 310,000 children younger than 5 years have elevated lead levels, and the most common exposure is through lead-based paints and lead-contaminated soil and dust in houses built before 1987 (Warniment et al, 2010).

Another exposure risk is through imported toys and costume jewelry that are painted with a lead-based paint. Young children are exposed through their mouthing behaviors. If a piece of contaminated costume jewelry is accidentally swallowed, the high lead concentration can result in death. In 2007, the U.S. Consumer Products Safety Commission (CPSC) issued numerous recalls for these toys and passed the Consumer Product Safety Improvement Act in 2008 which requires third-party testing and certification of all imported toys and products marketed to children (Galvez et al, 2009).

Universal screening for lead poisoning of all children at ages 1 and 2 years is recommended. This screening is recommended when children receive well-child or EPSDT screening at regular intervals. In addition, families should be assessed for environmental risk factors to determine the need for screening at other ages. Specific guidelines for minimizing lead exposure through contaminated toys are included in Box 29-2.

## LEVELS OF PREVENTION

| Lead Poisoning | Obesity |
| --- | --- |
| **Primary Prevention** | **Primary Prevention** |
| Community education about lead exposure, lead sources in the community, and the adverse health consequences for children. | Offer healthy cooking classes for families in the community. |
| **Secondary Prevention** | **Secondary Prevention** |
| Implement universal screening for all children ages 1 and 2 years that present to the community health centers and primary care practices. | Conduct child body mass index screenings in community daycares and preschools. |
| **Tertiary Prevention** | **Tertiary Prevention** |
| Provide families with guidance and resources for lead abatement and to eliminate lead exposure for children with blood lead levels >10 µg/dL. | Develop individualized weight loss plans and counsel children identified as obese on lifestyle changes. |

## Mercury

Mercury is another heavy metal that is highly toxic. The most common exposure for humans is the ingestion of contaminated fish. Mercury poisoning is determined with a blood mercury level of 5.8 µg/L or above. Mercury poisoning can result in significant developmental deficits with the fetuses of pregnant women at particular risk. Screening for dietary intake and other possible exposures is critical to identification of risk factors (Bose-O'Reilly et al, 2010). The nurses' responsibility is to educate families on how to minimize mercury exposure risks. It is recommended that families eat commercially caught fish that are low in mercury (tilapia, Alaskan salmon, herring). For pregnant women, women of child-bearing age, breastfeeding mothers, and young children, these steps are recommended:

- Avoid ingesting shark, tilefish, and king mackerel because of the high mercury levels
- Limit intake of tuna to 4 to 6 ounces each week and all other fishes to 12 ounces each week

## Plasticizers

Phthalates and bisphenol (BPA) are chemicals that are commonly added to plastics to create flexibility and durability. Exposure to these products has caused significant adverse health effects in animal studies. Human studies have noted a link between BPA and cardiovascular and liver disease. The possible exposures for children are many and include the linings of canned foods (ready-to-feed formulas), children's toys, and hard plastics made of polycarbonate (many sports water bottles and baby bottles). Increased exposure occurs when these products are exposed to high heat, which occurs with the sterilization of baby bottles. The half-life of these plasticizers is very short, which makes it difficult to thoroughly screen for exposure (Galvez et al, 2009).

The Consumer Products Safety Improvement Act of 2008 provided guidelines for eliminating these plasticizers nationally from children's products. Continued education of families is needed until all of these plasticizers are no longer available for purchase; recommendations on avoiding second-hand children's products should be promoted (Consumer Product Safety Commission, 2013).

## Environmental Tobacco Smoke

Environmental tobacco smoke (ETS) is exhaled smoke, smoke from burning tobacco or smoke from the mouthpiece or filter end of a cigarette, cigar or pipe. Cigarettes have many known poisons, and both cigarettes and ETS were classified as Class A known human carcinogens in 1992 by the Environmental Protection Agency (EPA). Parents often do not understand or believe the effects of smoking on children. Children, particularly those under age 5 years and those living in poverty, have higher levels of exposure to ETS. The recent introduction of electronic cigarettes is also considered to be a risk for ETS. An initial study found cancer-causing substances in all of the e-cigarette samples that were tested (Goniewicz et al, 2013).

Children exposed to ETS experience increased episodes of middle ear infections, asthma, upper respiratory tract infections, and more missed school days. Prenatal exposure to ETS is linked to preterm births, low birth weight, and increased risk for several childhood cancers. Prenatal exposure is also linked to the fetal brain becoming sensitized to nicotine, leading to greater addiction when exposed at an older age. Children living in smoking households with a parent role modeling smoking are more likely to start smoking (AAP, 2009c).

Interventions to discourage smoking focus on the parent, the child or adolescent, and public policy. Nurses in public health should offer educational programs for parents dealing with the negative effects of smoking on children, specific interventions to stop smoking, and ways to create a smoke-free environment. Anti-smoking programs directed toward children and teenagers are more successful if the focus is on short-term effects rather than on long-term effects. Developmentally, children and teenagers cannot visualize the future to imagine the consequences of smoking. Teaching social skills to resist peer pressure is critical (CDC, 2014c).

Nurses should become politically active in the area of smoking. Policies to ban tobacco advertising, enforce restrictions of sale to minors, increase funds for anti-smoking education, and restriction of public smoking may reduce the incidence of smoking. Community-based interventions to reduce smoking and ETS exposure are included here.

- Collaborate with schools to provide tobacco-free environments (for all school facilities, vehicles, and events).
- Work with schools to provide prevention curricula in elementary, middle, and high schools.
- Develop or identify smoking cessation programs and provide information to health care providers and workplaces in the community.
- Provide education to families on the dangers of ETS exposure for children and adolescents.
- Partnership with community merchants to enforce minors' access laws
- Advocate for local policy change to limit smoking in public and private enterprises (CDC, 2014c).

## MODELS FOR HEALTH CARE DELIVERY TO CHILDREN AND ADOLESCENTS

Nurses are in a position to work with specific populations through programs targeting the health care needs of children and particularly those at risk. In the following section, strategies for promoting the health care of children and adolescents are described.

### Family-Centered Medical Home

A family-centered medical home is a partnership between a child or adolescent, the child or adolescent's family, and the pediatric team who oversees the child or adolescent's health and well-being within a community-based system that provides uninterrupted care to promote optimal health outcomes. The medical home incorporates preventive, acute, and chronic care from birth through transition to adulthood. The medical home emphasizes an integrated health system with collaboration of care from an interprofessional team of primary care physicians, specialists and subspecialists, other health professionals, hospitals and health care facilities, public health, and the community working with children and families (Malouin, 2013).

Approximately 58% of all children have a medical home compared with 47% of children with special health care needs. It is imperative to increase the use of medical homes for all children, particularly children with special health care needs (Homer et al, 2008). A child with Down syndrome will greatly benefit from collaborative care from the primary care provider, subspecialty physicians, school system, community therapists, family support groups, and other community resources to achieve optimal health.

A successful medical home relies on the multitude of supports that are brought to the service delivery system that surrounds the family and community. Families can trust that there is a place where their child or adolescent is provided holistic care that addresses all aspects of physical, mental, and emotional health. The medical home is not a specific building, but it is a system of care that is accessible, continuous, comprehensive, coordinated, compassionate, and culturally effective. Nurses in the community play an active role as a team member of the medical home by identifying resources for families, referring families to a medical home, and participating in the health care of children in medical homes.

### Motivational Interviewing

Motivational interviewing is a focused communication strategy in which the parents are encouraged to set goals, identify personal barriers, and identify potential mechanisms to overcome the barriers to make safety and health promotion changes for their child. This can be an effective intervention to promote healthy changes within the family environment (Barnes, 2012). It can be easily implemented by nurses in primary care settings and public health clinics under limited time constraints and is readily incorporated into the medical home model.

Motivational interviewing emphasizes a collaborative approach to behavior change instead of a prescriptive approach (Figure 29-8). Nurses use open-ended questioning and reflection to encourage the parent or adolescent to share their identified barriers to change. When individuals demonstrate positive comments toward change, the nurse expands upon those

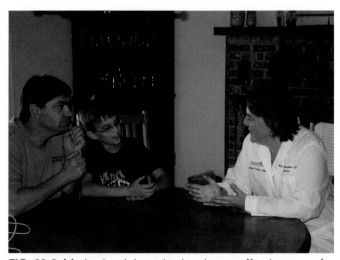

**FIG 29-8** Motivational interviewing is an effective way for nurses to intervene with families and promote positive behavioral change in the home.

comments and provides further support for that change. This strategy is very effective with positive health behavior changes such as smoking cessation, healthy eating, and safety behaviors. (See Appendix F.1 in the back of the book.)

## ROLE OF THE POPULATION-FOCUSED NURSE IN CHILD AND ADOLESCENT HEALTH

Population-focused nurses have the opportunity to work with families to achieve growth toward many of the *Healthy People 2020* objectives. They practice in a variety of settings, including community health centers, school-based clinics, and home health programs. They provide care through well-child clinics, immunization programs, federally mandated programs (such as the nutrition program Women, Infants, and Children [WIC]) or specific state-funded programs, such as Head Start.

With passage of the ACA, strategies to implement improved access include expanding the role of nurses and the settings for practice. The nursing process and a knowledge base of the factors unique to the pediatric population provide a framework of care. Nursing, through developing and coordinating community services and through formation of public policies, promotes the well-being of children and families within the community. Assessments are made to identify the needs and target populations at risk. Programs based on the needs of specific at-risk populations are developed for the delivery of health care.

The nursing plan of care includes three major components. The first is the management of actual or potential health problems. The second involves both education and anticipatory guidance. This enables families to understand what to expect in the areas of growth and development as well as social,

emotional, and cognitive changes. Nurses offer information to promote healthy lifestyles and to prevent acute and chronic health problems as well as unintentional injuries. A third role is case management or coordination of care. For example, the nurse coordinates referrals to community agencies, other health care services or providers or assistance programs. Box 29-3 lists community resources.

---

### BOX 29-3 Community Resources for Pediatric Health Care

- Children's service clinics
- Well-child clinics
- Immunization clinics
- Infectious disease clinics
- Children's specialty services
- Family violence/child abuse centers
- Homeless shelters
- School health programs
- Head Start
- Parents Anonymous
- Crisis hotlines
- Community education classes
- Early intervention/developmental services
- Childbirth education classes
- Breastfeeding support groups
- Parent support groups
- Family planning clinics
- Women, Infants, and Children (WIC) programs
- Medicaid and CHIP
- Youth employment/training programs

---

### ⫸ LINKING CONTENT TO PRACTICE

In this chapter, emphasis is placed on the community health needs of children and adolescents within the context of the family. The public health core functions of disease prevention, health promotion, and the three levels of health services are directly related to the pediatric population and their specific population needs. To meet the core public health competencies, nurses must learn how to assess children and adolescents using developmental principles to determine safety risks for injury and environmental health exposures. Policy and program development for the pediatric population is geared toward improving the built environment in which a child grows and providing parents with education on health promotion strategies like smoking cessation to improve their child's

health. Nurses develop competencies in communication strategies with children of varying developmental levels and recognize the various locations in the community that need education on promoting the health of children (e.g., daycare centers, schools). Basic health services such as well-child care and immunizations are critical to the health of the pediatric population, and the nurse is poised as a leader within the medical home model of health care delivery for children and adolescents. This chapter prepares the community health nurse to provide comprehensive, developmentally appropriate education to families; deliver basic health care services in a holistic approach; and develop community programming to improve safety and environmental wellness for children and adolescents.

## ♥ HEALTHY PEOPLE 2020

### *Objectives Focused on Children and Adolescents*

**Education and Community-Based Programs**
- ECB-4: Increase the proportion of elementary, middle, and senior high schools that provide school health education to promote personal health and wellness in the following areas: hand washing or hand hygiene; oral health; growth and development; sun safety and skin cancer prevention; benefits of rest and sleep; ways to prevent vision and hearing loss; and the importance of health screenings and checkups.
- ECB-7: Increase the proportion of middle, junior high, and senior high schools that provide comprehensive school health education to prevent health problems in the following areas: unintentional injury; violence; suicide; tobacco use and addiction; alcohol or other drug use; unintended pregnancy; HIV/AIDS and STD infection; unhealthy dietary patterns; inadequate physical activity; and environmental health.

**Environmental Health**
- EH-8: Eliminate elevated blood lead levels in children.

**Immunizations and Infectious Disease**
- IID-7: Achieve and maintain effective vaccination coverage levels for universally recommended vaccines among young children.

**Injury/Violence Prevention**
- IVP-16: Increase use of age appropriate child restraints in cars.

**Nutrition and Weight Status**
- NWS-10: Reduce the proportion of children and adolescents who are overweight or obese.

**Physical Activity and Fitness**
- PA-4: Increase the proportion of the nation's public and private schools that require daily physical education for all students.

**Tobacco Use**
- TU-15: Tobacco-free environments in schools, including all school facilities, property, vehicles, and school events.

From: US Department of Health and Human Services: Healthy People 2020, Wash DC, 2010, US Government Printing Office.

## ▍ PRACTICE APPLICATION

Sam is a 4-year-old boy brought to the clinic by his mother for his 4-year well-child check and immunizations. Sam will be attending the local Head Start program in the fall. He is the oldest of three children and his siblings are 9 months and 35 months. His mother is a single parent who works at a local restaurant as a waitress. Sam and his siblings are insured by Medicaid. Sam's mother is 24 years old and the family lives with the maternal grandparents. Sam's mother is in good health and does not smoke or abuse drugs. Sam has been watched by his grandmother since birth and is exposed to cigarette smoke in the home by both grandparents.

On the developmental exam, Sam is very cooperative, eager to please, and speaks clearly. His development is significant for failure to identify three colors, count to 5, or recognize any letters. His gross motor skills are appropriate but he only scribbles when given a crayon. Sam reports watching television shows with his family for fun. On physical examination, Sam has a >95th percentile BMI for age/gender but no other abnormal exam findings are noted. Hearing and vision are within normal limits for age.

Based on the previous scenario, answer the following questions:

A. What additional history and assessment information should you collect based on the child's home environment?
B. What immunizations and lab tests are indicated based on his age and risk factors?
C. What education should you give this mother on changes in the home to promote development? To reduce ETS exposure? To ensure safety?
D. Based on the BMI percentile, what additional nutrition and dietary practices information should you obtain?
E. What interventions and education should you provide to this mother regarding Sam's obesity and associated risk factors?
F. In an analysis of the Medicaid child population in Sam's medical home, the population-focused nurse found that a number of children had similar risk factors. Is there a population-level intervention the nurse may want to use to reduce the risk in the future child population?
**Answers can be found on the Evolve site.**

## ▍ KEY POINTS

- Physical growth and development is an ongoing process resulting in physical, cognitive, and emotional changes that affect health status.
- Good nutrition is essential for healthy growth and development, and it influences disease prevention in later life.

- Childhood obesity is increasing in prevalence. Modifiable risk factors include dietary intake, physical activity, and screen viewing time.
- Immunizations are successful in prevention of selected diseases. Barriers to immunizing children are parental concerns,

## KEY POINTS—cont'd

cost, vaccine shortages, and changes in recommended vaccine scheduling.

- The built environment is influential on a child's physical, emotional, and psychosocial health. Nurses can design interventions for families and communities to improve a child's environment if improvement is indicated.

- The family is critical to the growth and development of the child. Social support has a powerful influence on successful parenting.

- Unintentional injuries are the major cause of morbidity and mortality in the child and adolescent population. Most are preventable. Nurses have a major role in anticipatory guidance and prevention.

- Population-focused nurses have a strong role in the prevention of, identification of, and education about child maltreatment. Child advocacy is critical to reduce the incidence of abuse and neglect in childhood.

- Minimizing complications of the major health risks to the pediatric and adolescent population follows the goals of *Healthy People 2020* initiatives.

- The pediatric population is vulnerable to environmental hazards. Decreasing exposure and identifying problems early are important areas for interventions by population-focused nurses.

- Nurses are involved in strategies to meet the needs of the pediatric population and their families in the community.

- The family-centered medical home is a successful system for coordinating health care for children and for facilitating continuous family support and health management.

- Children who are low income or live in poverty are at increased risk for violence, injuries, and environmental hazards.

- The use of motivational interviewing can facilitate positive health behavior changes for families with children.

## CLINICAL DECISION-MAKING ACTIVITIES

1. Develop a plan of immunization for a 5½-year-old who has had one DTaP, Hib, and IPV. Be specific about due dates for immunizations.

2. Develop a screening program for children and adolescents who live in a low-income older neighborhood with a large percentage of Hispanic residents. What risk factors would you consider in the process? Have you examined the thoughts of others in the community that might affect the success of the screening program? Be specific.

3. Plan a survey of a school district to determine its "friendliness" to children with chronic health problems. How would you implement changes?

4. Develop a community program for smoking cessation. Identify how you will target parents and caregivers of children.

Discuss how you will incorporate the concept of ETS exposure in your program.

5. Develop nutrition education programs for (1) mothers who are breastfeeding their infants, (2) a group of 5-year-olds in a kindergarten class, and (3) a group of high school sophomores. What factors do these programs have in common? How do they differ?

6. Administer a safety survey (e.g., the Injury Prevention Program [TIPP] from the American Academy of Pediatrics, or develop your own) to assess the home environment of a 6-month-old and a 5-year-old. Develop a plan of education and anticipatory guidance for the family. How would you apply this information to a larger population?

## REFERENCES

American Academy of Child and Adolescent Psychiatry: Committee on health care access and economics task force on mental health: improving mental health services in primary care: reducing administrative and financial barriers to access and collaboration. *Pediatrics* 123(4):1248–1251, 2009.

American Academy of Pediatrics: Policy statement: preventive oral health intervention for pediatricians. *Pediatrics* 122(6):1387–1394, 2008. doi: 10.1542/peds.2008.2577.

American Academy of Pediatrics: Policy statement: media violence. *Pediatrics* 124(5):1495–1503, 2009a. doi: 10.1542/peds.2009-2146.

American Academy of Pediatrics: Policy statement: the future of

pediatrics: mental health competencies for pediatric primary care. *Pediatrics* 124:410–421, 2009b.

American Academy of Pediatrics: Technical report: secondhand and prenatal tobacco smoke exposure. *Pediatrics* 124:e1017–e1044, 2009c.

American Academy of Pediatrics: Trends in the prevalence of developmental disabilities in US children 1997-2008. *Pediatrics* 127(6):1034–1042, 2011a.

American Academy of Pediatrics: Task force on sudden infant death syndrome: SIDS and other sleep-related infant deaths: expansion of recommendations for a safe infant sleeping environment. *Pediatrics* 128:1030,

2011b. doi: 10.1542/peds.2011-2284.

American Academy of Pediatrics: Abusive head trauma (shaken baby syndrome), 2012a. Available at http://www.aap.org/en-us/about-the-aap/aap-press-room/aap-press-room-media-center/Pages/Abusive-Head-Trauma-Fact-Sheet.aspx. Accessed on September 24, 2014.

American Academy of Pediatrics: Firearm-related injuries affecting the pediatric population. *Pediatrics* 130(5):e1416–e1423, 2012b. doi: 10.1542/peds.2012-2481.

American Academy of Pediatrics: Gun violence policy recommendations, 2012c. Available at http://www.aap.org/en-us/advocacy-and-policy/federal-advocacy/Documents/

AAPGunViolencePrevention PolicyRecommendations_Jan2013.pdf. Accessed on September 20, 2014.

American Academy of Pediatrics: Policy statement: providing care for immigrant, migrant, and border children. *Pediatrics* 131(6):e2028–e2034, 2013.

American Dietetic Association: Position of the American Dietetic Association: Nutrition guidance for healthy children ages 2 to 11 years. *J Am Dietetic Assoc* 108(6):1038–1047, 2008. doi: 10.1016/j.jada.2008.04.005.

Anzman SL, Rollins BY, Birch LL: Parental influence on children's early eating environments and obesity risk: implications for prevention. *Int J Obes*

34(7):1116–1124, 2010. doi: 10.1038/ijo.2010.43.

Aronson SS, Shope TR: *Managing Infectious Diseases in Child Care and Schools*, ed 3. Elk Grove Village III, 2013, American Academy of Pediatrics.

Baker DL, Dang MT, Ly MY, et al: Perception of barriers to immunization among parents of Hmong origin in California. *Am J Public Health* 100(5):839–845, 2010. doi: 10.2105/AJPH .2009.175935.

Barnes AJ: Promoting health behaviors in pediatrics: motivational interviewing. *Pediatric Rev* 33:e33–e57, 2012.

Borse NN, Gilchrist J, Dellinger AM, et al: *CDC Childhood Injury Report: Patterns of Unintentional Injuries Among 0-19 Year Olds in the United States, 2000-2006*. Atlanta, 2008, CDC, National Center for Injury Prevention and Control.

Bose-O'Reilly S, McCarty KM, Steckling N, et al: Mercury exposure and children's health. *Curr Problems Pediatric Adolesc Health Care* 40(8):186–215, 2010. doi: 10.1016/j.cppeds.2010.07.002.

Burns J, Walsh L, Popovich J: Practical pediatric and adolescent immunization update. *J Nurse Practitioners* 6(4):254–266, 2010.

Centers for Disease Control and Prevention: *State Indicator Report on Physical Activity*. Atlanta, 2010a, U.S. Department of Health and Human Services.

Centers for Disease Control and Prevention: *The Association Between School Based Physical Activity, Including Physical Education, and Academic Performance*. Atlanta, 2010b, Department of Health and Human Services.

Centers for Disease Control and Prevention: Some common misconceptions about vaccination and how to respond to them, 2011a. Available at http:// www.cdc.gov/vaccines/vac-gen/6mishome.htm. Accessed September 24, 2014.

Centers for Disease Control and Prevention: How much physical activity do children need? 2011b. Available at http://www.cdc.gov/ physicalactivity/everyone/guidelines/ children.html. Accessed September 19, 2014.

Centers for Disease Control and Prevention: *The Pink Book: Epidemiology and Prevention of Vaccine-Preventable Diseases*, ed 12, 2012a. Available at http:// www.cdc.gov/vaccines/pubs/ pinkbook/downloads/prinvac.pdf. Accessed September 19, 2014.

Centers for Disease Control and Prevention: Basic Facts about Childhood Obesity, 2012b. Available at http://www.cdc.gov/

obesity/childhood/basics.html. Accessed April 14, 2014.

Centers for Disease Control and Prevention: National Center for Injury Prevention and Control: National Action Plan for Child Injury Prevention, 2012c. Available at http://www.cdc.gov/safechild/nap. Accessed September 22, 2014.

Centers for Disease Control and Prevention: Playground injuries: fact sheet, 2012d. Available at http://www.cdc.gov/Homeand RecreationalSafety/Playground -Injuries/playgroundinjuries -factsheet.htm. Accessed September 24, 2014.

Centers for Disease Control and Prevention MMWR: National, state, and local area vaccination coverage among children aged 19-35 months—US 2012. *MMWR* 62(36):733–743, 2013a.

Centers for Disease Control and Prevention: MMWR: National and state vaccination coverage among adolescents aged 13-17 years—US 2012. *MMWR* 62(34):685–693, 2013b.

Centers for Disease Control and Prevention: Children and diabetes, 2013c. Available at http:// www.cdc.gov/diabetes/projects/ cda2.htm. Accessed on September 20, 2014.

Centers for Disease Control and Prevention: High quality physical education, 2013d. Available at http://www.cdc.gov/healthyyouth/ pecat/highquality.htm. Accessed on September 24, 2014.

Centers for Disease Control and Prevention: Child Maltreatment, Facts at a Glance, 2013e. National Center for Injury Prevention and Control, Division of Violence Prevention. Available at http:// www.cdc.gov/ViolencePrevention/ childmaltreatment/index.html. Accessed September 28, 2014.

Centers for Disease Control and Prevention: Birth-18 years & catch-up immunization schedules, 2014a. Available at http:// www.cdc.gov/vaccines/schedules/ hcp/child-adolescent.html. Accessed on September 20, 2014.

Centers for Disease Control and Prevention: Child passenger safety, 2014b. Available at http:// www.cdc.gov/Motorvehiclesafety/ Child_Passenger_Safety/. Accessed April 14, 2014.

Centers for Disease Control and Prevention: Youth tobacco prevention, 2014c. Available at http://www.cdc.gov/tobacco/youth/ index.htm. Accessed September 20, 2014.

Centers for Disease Control and Prevention: Classification of body mass index, 2015. Available at http://www.cdc.gov/.

Centers for Medicare & Medicaid Services (CMMS): Medicaid benefits, 2014a. Available at

http://www.medicaid.gov/Medicaid -CHIP-Program-Information/By -Topics/Benefits/Medicaid-Benefits .html. Accessed on April 14, 2014.

Centers for Medicare & Medicaid Services (CMMS): Children's Health Insurance Plan (CHIP), 2014b. Available at http:// www.medicaid.gov/Medicaid-CHIP- Program-Information/By-Topics/ Childrens-Health-Insurance- Program-CHIP/Childrens-Health- Insurance-Program-CHIP.html. Accessed April 14, 2014.

Central Intelligence Agency: The World Factbook: Infant Mortality Rate, 2014. Available at https:// www.cia.gov/library/publications/ the-world-factbook/ rankorder/2091rank.html. Acccessed April 14, 2014.

Child Trends Data Base: Immigrant Children—Indicators On Children and Youth, 2012. Available at http:// www.childtrends.org/wp-content/ uploads/2012/07/110_Immigrant_ Children.pdf.

Consumer Product Safety Commission: Phthalates, 2013. Available at http://www.cpsc.gov/ Business–Manufacturing/ Business-Education/Business- Guidance/Phthalates-Information/. Accessed September 24, 2014.

Department of Education: Assistance to states for education of children with disabilities and preschool grants for children with disabilities. *Fed Regist* 71(156):46541–46845, 2006. Available at: www.idea.ed .gov/download/finalregulations .pdf. Accessed September 20, 2014.

Dutko P, Ver Ploeg M, Farrigan T: USDA characteristics and influential factors of food deserts. Economic Research Service, Economic Research Report Number 140, August 2012.

Fakhouri TH, Hughes JP, Brody DJ, et al: Physical activity and screen-time viewing among elementary school-aged children in the US from 2009-2010. *JAMA Pediatrics* 167(3):223–229, 2013. doi: 10.1001/2013.jamapedia trics.122.

Federal Interagency Forum on Child and Family Statistics: America's Children: Key Indicators for Well-being, 2013. Available at http://www.childstats.gov/pdf/ ac2013/ac_13.pdf.

Fryer C, Carroll M, et al: Health E-Stat: Prevalence of obesity among children and adolescents: United States, trends 1963-1965 through 2011-2012, 2013. Centers for Disease Control and Prevention, National Center of Health Statistics. Available at www.CDC.gov. Accessed March 15, 2015.

Galvez M, Graber N, Sheffield P, et al: Hot topics in environmental health. *Contemp Pediatr* 26(7):34–47, 2009.

Garver W, Newman S, Gonzales- Pacheco D, et al: The genetics of childhood obesity and interaction with dietary macronutrients. *Genes in Nutrition* 8:271–287, 2013.

Goniewicz ML, Knysak J, Gawron M, et al: Levels of selected carcinogens and toxicants in vapour from electronic cigarettes. *Tob Control* 2013. doi: 10.1136/ tobaccocontrol-2012-050859. [published online 6 March 2013].

Gose M, Plachta-Danielzik S, Willie B, et al: Longitudinal influences of neighbourhood built and social environment on children's weight status. *Int J Environ Res Public Health* 10:5083–5096, 2013. doi: 10.3390/ijerph10105083.

Griffiths LJ, Parsons TJ, Hill AJ: Self-esteem and quality of life in obese children and adolescents: a systematic review. *Int J Pediatric Obesity* 5:282–304, 2010. doi: 10.3109/17477160903473697.

Hallas D, Shelley D: Role of pediatric nurse practitioners in oral health care. *Acad Pediatr* 9(6):462–466, 2009.

He M, Tucker P, Irwin JD, et al: Obesogenic neighbourhoods: the impact of neighbourhood restaurants and convenience stores on adolescents' food consumption behaviors. *Public Health Nutr* 15(12):2331–2339, 2012. doi: 10.1017/S1368980012000584.

Hoelscher JM, Kirk S, Ritchie L, et al: Position of the Academy of Nutrition and Dietetics: Interventions for the prevention and treatment of pediatric overweight and obesity. *J Acad Nutrit Dietetics* 113(10):1375–1394, 2013. doi: 10.1016/j.jand.2013 .08.004.

Homer C, Perrin J, Romm D, et al: A review of the evidence for the medical home for children with special health care needs. *Pediatrics* 122:e922–e937, 2008.

Jiang Y, Ekono M, Skinner C: Basic facts about low-income children, children under 18 years 2012, 2014: National Center for Children in Poverty. Available at http:// www.nccp.org/publications/ pub_1089.html. Accessed April 15, 2014.

Kaiser Family Foundation: Aligning eligibility for children: moving the stairstep kids to Medicaid, 2013. Available at http://kff.org/medicaid/ issue-brief/aligning-eligibility-for- children-moving-the-stairstep-kids- to-medicaid/. Accessed on April 14, 2014.

Kann L, Kinchen S, Shanklin SL, et al: Youth risk behavior surveillance Federal register, United States, 2013. *MMWR* 63(4):1–168, 2014.

Lakhan SE, Kirchgessner A: Prescription stimulants in individuals with and without attention deficit hyperactivity disorder: misuse, cognitive impact, and adverse effects. *Brain Behav* 2(5):661–677, 2012. doi: 10.1002/brb3.78.

Leeb RT, Paulozzi L, Melanson C, et al: *Child Maltreatment Surveillance: Uniform Definitions for Public Health and Recommended Data Elements*, Version 1.0. Atlanta (GA), 2008, Centers for Disease Control and Prevention, National Center for Injury Prevention and Control.

Malouin RA: *Positioning the Family and Patient at the Center: A Guide to Family and Patient Partnership in the Medical Home*. American Academy of Pediatrics, Elk Grove Village, IL, 2013, National Center for Medical Home Implementation.

May AL, Kuklina EV, Yoon PW: Prevalence of cardiovascular disease risk factors among US adolescents 1999-2008. *Pediatrics* 129(6):1035–1041, 2012. doi: 10.1542/peds.2011-1082.

MMWR: Vital signs: unintentional injury deaths among persons aged 0-19 years-United States, 2000-2009, 2012. Available at http://www.cdc.gov/mmwr/preview/mmwrhtml/mm61e0416a1.htm.

Morandi A, Maffeis C: Urogenital complications of obesity. *Best Pract Res Clin Endocrinol Metabolism* 27:209–218, 2013.

Murphy SL, Xu J, Kochanek KD: Deaths: Final data for 2010. *Natl Vital Stat Rep* 61(4):1–117, 2013.

Nance M, Carr B, Kallan M, et al: Variation in pediatric and adolescent firearm mortality rate in rural and urban U.S. counties. *Pediatrics* 125(6):1112–1118, 2010. doi: 10.1542/peds.2009-3219.

National Center for Children in Poverty: Basic facts about low income children, children under 18 years, 2012, 2013, 2014. Available at http://www.nccp.org/publications/pub_1089.html. Accessed September 28, 2014.

National Center on Family Homelessness: *The Characteristics and Needs of Families Experiencing Homelessness*. Needham, Ma, 2011, National Center on Family Homelessness.

National Institute for Environmental Health Science: Children's health, 2014: Available at http://www.niehs.nih.gov/health/topics/population/children/index.cfm. Accessed September 24, 2014.

National Institute for Health Care Management: Preventing early childhood obesity in North Carolina, 2012: Available at http://www.nihcm.org/pdf/Shape_NC_FINAL_electronic_091012.pdf. Accessed September 19, 2014.

National Institutes of Environmental Health: Your Environment your health, 2015, Triangle Park, North Carolina, Accessed at www.NIEHS.Nih.gov. March 24, 2015.

Office on Adolescent Health: Teen media use part 1—increasing and on the move, 2013. Available at http://www.hhs.gov/ash/oah/news/e-updates/eupdate-nov-2013.html. Accessed September 30, 2014.

Ogden CL, Carroll MD, Kit BK, et al: Prevalence of childhood and adult obesity in the United States, 2011-2012. *J Am Med Assoc* 311(8):806–814, 2014. doi: 10.1001/jama.2014.732.

Osei-Assibey G, Dick S, Macdiarmid J, et al: The influence of the food environment on overweight and obesity in young children: a systematic review. *BMJ Open* 2:e001538, 2012. doi: 10.1136/bmjopen-2012-001538.

Papandreou D, Karabouta Z, Pantoleon A, et al: Investigation of anthropometric, biochemical and dietary parameters of obese children with and without non-alcoholic fatty liver disease. *Appetite* 59:939–944, 2012.

Papoutsakis C, Priftis KN, Drakouli M, et al: Childhood overweight/obesity and asthma: is there a link? A systematic review of recent epidemiologic evidence. *J Acad Nutrition Dietetics* 113(1):77–105, 2013. doi: 10.1016/j.jand.2012.08.025.

Paulis WD, Silba S, Koes BW, et al: Overweight and obesity are associated with musculoskeletal complaints as early as childhood: a systematic review. *Obes Rev* 15:52–67, 2014. doi: 10.1111/obr.12067.

Puhl RM, Peterson JL, Luedicke J: Weight-based victimization: Bullying experiences of weight loss treatment-seeking youth. *Pediatrics* 131(e1):1–9, 2012. doi: 10.1542/peds.2012-1106.

Renalds A, Smith TH, Hale PJ: A systematic review of built environment and health. *Fam Community Health* 33(1):68–78, 2010.

Roberto CA, Baik J, Harris JL, et al: Influence of licensed characters on children's taste and snack preferences. *Pediatrics* 126:88–93, 2010.

Shaffer D, Kipp K: *Developmental Psychology: Childhood and Adolescents*, ed 9. Independence Ky, 2013, Cengage Learning.

Siegle BS, Davis BE: Health and mental health needs of children in U.S. military families. *Pediatrics* 131(6):e2002–e2015, 2013. doi: 10.1542/peds.2013-0940.

Springer SC, Silverstein J, Copeland K, et al: Management of type 2 diabetes mellitus in children and adolescents. *Pediatrics* 131:e648, 2013. doi: 10.1542/peds/2012-3496.

Strasburger V, Jordan A, Donnerstein E: Health effects of media on children and adolescents. *Pediatrics* 125:756–767, 2010.

Suzuki K, Asaga R, Sourander A, et al: Cyberbullying and adolescent mental health. *Int J Medical Health* 24(1):27–35, 2012. doi: 10.1515/IJAMH.2012.005.

Ting W, Huang C, Tu Y, et al: Association between weight status and depressive symptoms in adolescents: role of weight perception, weight concern, and dietary restraint. *Europ J Ped* 171:1247–1255, 2012.

Tudor-Locke C, Camhi SM, Troiano RP: A catalog of rules, variables, and definitions applied to accelerometer data in the National Health and Nutrition Examination Survey, 2003-2006. *Prev Chronic Dis* 9:110332, 2012.

U.S. Census Bureau: Current population survey 2012, 2013. Available at http://www.census.gov/. Accessed September 20, 2014.

U.S. child deaths from maltreatment, 2013. Estimated 1,217 deaths in 2013. (*U.S. Department of Health and Human Services, Administration for Children and Families, Administration on Children, Youth and Families, Children's Bureau (2013). Child Maltreatment 2138.* Available from http://www.acf.hhs.gov/programs/cb/stats_research/index.htm#can.).

U.S. Department of Agriculture: Choose my plate, 2015. www.USDA.gov.

U.S. Department of Health and Human Services: *Healthy People 2020*, Washington, D.C., 2010, U.S. Government Printing Office.

U.S. Department of Health and Human Services: Birth rates for US teenagers reach historic lows for all age and ethnic groups, 2013a. Available at http://www.cdc.gov/nchs/data/nvsr/nvsr62/nvsr62_09.pdf#table02. Accessed April 12, 2014.

U.S. Department of Health and Human Services: Heads up, concussion in youth sports, 2013b. Available at http://www.cdc.gov/concussion/HeadsUp/youth.html. Accessed April 12, 2014.

Van Cleave J, Gortmaker S, Perrin J: Dynamics of obesity and chronic health conditions among children and youth. *J Am Med Assoc* 303(7):623–630, 2010.

Vollmer RL, Mobley AR: Parenting styles, feeding styles, and their influence on child obesogenic behaviors and body weight—a review. *Appetite* 71:232–241, 2013.

Warniment C, Tsang K, Galazka SS: Lead poisoning in children. *Am Fam Physician* 81(6):751–760, 2010.

Wethington H, Pan L, Sherry B: The association of screen time, television in the bedroom and obesity among school-aged youth: 2007 national survey of children's health. *J School Health* 83(8):573–581, 2013.

White House: Let's Move! 2014 Available at http://www.letsmove.gov/. Accessed April 12, 2014.

Wight V, Thampi K: Basic facts about food insecurity among children in the US 2008, 2010, National Center for Children in Poverty. Available at http://www.nccp.org/publications/pub_956.html. Accessed April 14, 2014.

Zimmerman F, Mercy JA: A better start: child maltreatment prevention as a public health priority, Zero to Three, 2010. Available at http://www.zerotothree.org/maltreatment/child-abuse-neglect/30-5-zimmerman.pdf. Accessed on April 14, 2014.

# Major Health Issues and Chronic Disease Management of Adults Across the Life Span

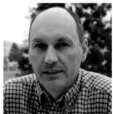

### Monty Gross, PhD, RN, CNE, CNL

Dr. Monty Gross is Clinical Nurse Educator for the Veterans Health Administration in Las Vegas, Nevada. He received his BS in Communications from Clarion University of Pennsylvania and his BSN and MSN from the University of Virginia. In 2006 he completed his PhD from Virginia Tech. He has practiced nursing in acute care, critical care, and underserved communities in Latin America. He has taught nursing as an Associate Professor at the undergraduate and graduate levels. Staying engaged in academia, he teaches as an adjunct faculty.

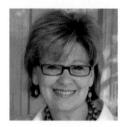

### Linda Hulton, PhD, RN

Dr. Linda Hulton is Professor of Nursing at James Madison University (JMU) and Coordinator of the Doctor of Nursing Practice (DNP) program. She received her BSN in nursing from Roberts Wesleyan College and her Masters and PhD in nursing from the University of Virginia. Her areas of research interest and practice are adolescent health promotion, unintended pregnancy, and health care for the homeless. In 2012, she received the James Madison University CISAT Distinguished Teaching Award. She has had her scholarly work published in *Issues in Comprehensive Pediatric Nursing, Sigma Theta Tau's Online Journal of Knowledge Synthesis in Nursing,* the *Journal of Gynecological and Neonatal Nursing, The Journal of School Nursing,* and the *Journal for Specialists in Pediatric Nursing.* At JMU, she teaches graduate courses in research, community health, and analytic methods.

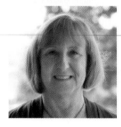

### Sharon Strang, RN, DNP, APRN, FNP-BC

Dr. Sharon Strang is an Associate Professor of Nursing and faculty in the Graduate School at James Madison University. She is a Board Certified Family Nurse Practitioner who practices at a free clinic. She received her BSN from Duquesne University in Pittsburgh, PA, and her Masters of Science in Nursing from the University of Pennsylvania at Edinboro. Sharon completed a Post Masters Nurse Practitioner Certificate Program at Old Dominion University and received her DNP from the University of Virginia. The focus of her doctoral studies and grant writing is chronic disease. She has presented at national nursing and education conferences and published in nursing education and nurse practitioner journals. In 2005 she received the Virginia Council of Nurse Practitioner's nurse practitioner in education award and in 2011 she received the Virginia Council of Nurse Practitioner's Distinguished Nurse Practitioner award. She is licensed as a Chronic Disease and Diabetes Self-Management Master Trainer by Stanford University.

## ADDITIONAL RESOURCES

(e) **Evolve Website http://evolve.elsevier.com/Stanhope**
- Healthy People 2020
- Quiz
- Case Studies
- WebLinks—Of special note see the links for these sites:
  - American Cancer Society
  - American Diabetes Association
  - American Heart Association
  - American Stroke Association
  - CDC Men's Health
  - Food and Drug Administration
  - Men's Health Network
  - National Cancer Institute
- National Center for Complementary and Alternative Medicine
- National Institute of Mental Health
- National Women's Health Information Center
- United States Department of Health and Human Services
- Glossary
- Answers to Practice Applications
- Resource Tools
  - Resource Tool 30.A: Lifestyle Assessment Questionnaire
  - Resource Tool 30.B: Health Risk Appraisal for Older Adults

## OBJECTIVES

*After reading this chapter, the student should be able to:*
1. Define terms commonly used in the care of adults.
2. Describe historical and current perspectives of adult health and health policy.

3. Discuss sources of population-based public health data and health status indicators about adults to be used to align community resources to support adults with chronic illnesses.

## OBJECTIVES—cont'd

4. Use appropriate assessment tools and development strategies to care for adults across the life span.
5. Discuss the concepts of self-management and the implementation of the Chronic Care Model to support adults with chronic illness.

6. Explain the dynamic forces that contribute to shared and gender specific diseases, health disparities, cultural diversity, and the role of social and behavioral factors that contribute to culturally competent care of adults in their communities.

## KEY TERMS

abuse, p. 673
adult day health, p. 688
advanced medical directives, p. 674
Americans with Disabilities Act (ADA), p. 673
anorexia, p. 681
assisted living, p. 688
bisexual, p. 686
body mass index, p. 680
bulimia, p. 681
cancer, p. 679
cardiovascular disease, p. 677
caregiver, p. 673
caregiver burden, p. 673
Chronic Care Model (CCM), p. 676
chronic disease, p. 672
community-based model, p. 687
diabetes, p. 678
do-not-resuscitate order, p. 674
durable medical power of attorney, p. 674
erectile dysfunction, p. 685
Family and Medical Leave Act (FMLA), p. 673
financial exploitation, p. 674
frail elderly, p. 687
gay, p. 686
gestational diabetes mellitus (GDM), p. 681
health, p. 672
health screenings, p. 683
health status indicators, p. 674
heart disease, p. 677
home health, p. 688
hospice, p. 688
hypertension, p. 678
injury, p. 687
impoverished, p. 686

lesbian, p. 686
life expectancy, p. 675
living will, p. 674
long-term care, p. 688
menopause, p. 682
men's health, p. 683
mental health, p. 678
neglect, p. 674
obesity, p. 680
Office on Women's Health, p. 681
Older Americans Act (OAA), p. 673
osteoporosis, p. 682
palliative care, p. 688
patient-centered medical home, p. 687
Patient Self-Determination Act, p. 674
Personal Responsibility and Work Opportunity
    Reconciliation Act, p. 673
physical activity, p. 678
preconceptual counseling, p. 681
prostate cancer, p. 684
rehabilitation, p. 689
reproductive health, p. 681
respite care, p. 688
self-management, p. 677
sexually transmitted disease, p. 679
sexually transmitted infection, p. 679
stroke, p. 678
Temporary Assistance for Needy Families
    (TANF), p. 673
testicular cancer, p. 684
unintended pregnancy, p. 681
weight control, p. 680
women's health, p. 672
—*See Glossary for definitions*

## CHAPTER OUTLINE

**Historical Perspectives on Adult Men and Women's Health**
**Health Policy and Legislation**
    Ethical and Legal Issues and Legislation for Older Adults
    Environmental Impact
**Health Status Indicators**
    Mortality
    Morbidity
**Adult Health Concerns**
    Chronic Disease
    Cardiovascular Disease

Hypertension
Stroke
Diabetes
Mental Health
Cancer
STDs/HIV/AIDS
Weight Control
**Women's Health Concerns**
    Reproductive Health
    Gestational Diabetes

This chapter provides an overview of major health issues of adults that occur at various stages of life. Nurses struggle with these numerous and complex topics. Changes in population demographics signal challenges of limited resources and increased prevalence of persons living with multiple chronic conditions. Unhealthy lifestyles, environmental pollution, and politics are a sample of factors a nurse will need to consider in population-centered health care. Descriptive statistics are frequently provided to help illustrate the significance of a disease or condition. Despite many pressing issues and political debates, there are abundant opportunities to improve the health of the population. There is strong evidence that community interventions, such as those designed for disadvantaged populations to improve diabetes care, can improve health through political involvement and strategies such as implementing well-planned programs (Brownson et al, 2009). Significant changes are rapidly occurring in health care and in the communities through policy changes and research. Nurses will be better prepared to practice by having a better understanding of these major health issues.

# HISTORICAL PERSPECTIVES ON ADULT MEN AND WOMEN'S HEALTH

Men and women have always faced a wide array of health issues that transition over time to impact their lives and the community. Gender is a major social determinant of health. Gender equity positively impacts a variety of factors, such as decision making, income allocation, and application and observance of norms, which affect health. Gender inequalities span throughout time and all societies, damaging the health of both genders, but in the majority of societies throughout the world women lose out to men (Fernández-Sáez et al, 2013). Social and political climates influence research and funding agendas that ultimately affect how health care is delivered in the community. A gender gap has existed where the emphasis on health issues and community focus has given priority to one gender over the other through research, policies, and funding. This has resulted in the focus of prevention and treatment being on one or the other gender, depending on social and political time period.

Historically men have dominated the medical and research professions because of cultural and societal norms. At the

beginning of the twentieth century, discussions of women's health focused primarily on reproduction and women's roles as mothers. In the 1920s, with the birth control movement in its initial stages, women's health expanded to address family planning and reproductive health. Women began to be empowered by the suffragette movement, winning the right to vote in 1920. As the women's rights movement gained momentum, women's health issues and the research of those issues displaced many issues of men. In the 1980s recommendations were made by the U.S. Public Health Services Task Force on Women's Health Issues to increase gender equity in biomedical research and the establishment of guidelines for including women in federally sponsored studies (Alexander et al, 2007; Public Health Reports, 1985). In 1990 the Society for Women's Research was founded. Through political action of the National Institute of Health (NIH), legislation once again included women and other minorities in research studies (NIH Revitalization Act of 1993).

During the nineteenth and twentieth centuries, illness and death rates from infectious diseases decreased and those of chronic diseases increased for men and women in western countries. Due to refinement and understanding of germ theory and the use of medical and public health strategies such as immunizations, pasteurization, and antibiotics, primary infections declined (Egger, 2012). Health policies and programs were implemented to reduce the spread of infections and increase life span. These activities began the shift in focus to chronic illnesses, such as cardiovascular disease and cancers.

# HEALTH POLICY AND LEGISLATION

Health policy is action taken by public and private agencies to promote health. It is a reflection of the values held in society and can greatly influence the health of the citizens overall. Legislation consists of laws that regulate health care and promote health. Nursing practice and the care provided is impacted by policy and legislation. Nurses can serve as change agents to improve health care through engaging in health policy. To be fully engaged in improving health care from the bedside to the community level, nurses must understand how policy and legislation, along with other system factors such as social, cultural, and economic forces, can be incorporated into planning care for clients and use their skills as collaborators and communicators to improve health policy (Ressler and Glazer, 2010).

The following are five examples of important federal legislation that has influenced the health of adults and their lives in communities: The Older Americans Act of 1965, the Americans with Disabilities Act of 1990, the Family and Medical Leave Act of 1993, the Personal Responsibility and Work Opportunity Reconciliation Act of 1996, and the Patient Protection and Affordable Care Act of 2010.

The Older Americans Act (OAA), originally passed in 1965, established the Administration on Aging (AOA) and state agencies to provide for the social service needs of older people. The mission of the AOA is to help older adults maintain dignity and live independently in their communities through a comprehensive and coordinated network across the United States (AOA, 2010). In 2008, of the $1.9 billion funding allotted to the AOA, two thirds supported state and community grants for multiple social and nutritional service programs. Title III of the OAA authorizes funding for nonprofit area agencies on aging to coordinate social services that provide supportive and nutritional services, family caregiver support, and disease prevention and health promotion activities. The services are available to all people age 60 or over, specifically targeted to those with the greatest economic or social need.

In 1990, the Americans with Disabilities Act (ADA) was passed, providing protection against discrimination to millions of Americans with disabilities. A disability is generally defined by the ADA as a physical or mental impairment that substantially limits one or more major life activities, a person who has a history or record of such an impairment, or a person who is perceived by others as having such an impairment (Americans with Disabilities Act of 1990, as amended with ADA Act of 2008, n.d.). The ADA legislation requires government and businesses to provide disabled individuals with equal opportunities for jobs, education, access to transportation and public buildings, and other accommodations for both physical and mental limitations.

The Family and Medical Leave Act (FMLA), initially passed in 1993, provides job protection and continuous health benefits where applicable for eligible employees who need extended leave for their own illness or to care for a family member. Gender equality was expanded with FMLA to offer women the ability to better manage both a career and a family (Guy, 2013). However, FMLA is limited. It only permits eligible employees to take 12 weeks of unpaid leave during a 12-month period for limited situations such as birth, adoption, or care for a serious illness of self or family members. It also only applies to employees who worked for at least 12 months in companies that have 50 or more employees (U.S. Department of Labor Wage and Hour Division [WHD] The Family and Medical Leave Act of 1993). Frequently caregivers provide unpaid care for their family members, including aging parents, children, grandchildren, and partners. Often adults find themselves struggling to balance work and caring for a family member. More families find themselves in this struggle as more women enter the workforce and work full time. Caregivers' multiple roles and responsibilities are frequently coupled with financial strain, which can lead them to experience caregiver burden.

In 1996 Congress passed the Personal Responsibility and Work Opportunity Reconciliation Act, commonly known as "welfare reform." This law targeted women who received public assistance and changed the previous Aid to Families with Dependent Children (AFDC) to Temporary Assistance for Needy Families (TANF)—a work program that mandates that women heads-of-household find employment to retain their benefits. The Administration for Children and Families (ACF), within the Department of Health and Human Services (USDHHS) is responsible for federal programs such as TANF that promote the economic and social well-being of families, children, individuals, and communities (ACF, n.d.).

The Patient Protection and Affordable Care Act (2010), also known as the Affordable Care Act (ACA) was passed by Congress and signed into law by President Obama in March 2010. The ACA has been considered the most significant reform law passed since Medicare and Medicaid were enacted in 1965. Some of the key features of the ACA include an end to health plans limiting or denying benefits to children under 19 years of age due to a pre-existing condition. Children under the age of 26 can be covered under their parent's health plan, lifetime coverage limits were stopped, no copayment is needed for preventive care, and access to insurance is provided for uninsured individuals (Kominski, 2014). The law is complex and expensive. As such, ACA is a continuing source of debate.

The nurse serves in a unique position for advocacy and support of health legislation and policy that supports the physical, mental, and social well-being of adults. Advocacy can be accomplished in a variety of ways such as lobbying, public speaking, participating in grassroots activities, and staying abreast of proposed legislation that influences the health of men and women, their families, and communities.

## Ethical and Legal Issues and Legislation for Older Adults

Ethical issues regarding the care and treatment of older adults arise regularly. As the population continues to age and technological advances continue to be developed, complex ethical and legal questions will continue to increase. The most common of these issues involve decision making—assessment of the ability of the client to make decisions, the appropriate surrogate decision-maker, disclosure of information to make informed decisions, level of care needed on the basis of function, and termination of treatment at the end of life. One often-overlooked concern of older persons is abuse. The National Center on Elder Abuse (NCEA), within the Administration on Aging, notes that abuse encompasses physical, emotional, and sexual abuse, as well as exploitation, neglect, and abandonment. Identification of abuse consists of recognizing the following: (a) The willful infliction of physical pain or injury, (b) infliction of debilitating mental anguish and fear, (c) theft or mismanagement of money or resources, and (d) unreasonable confinement or the depriving of services.

It is estimated that every year one out of 10 older adults experiences abuse or neglect by a caregiver, with only a fraction of cases being reported (Hoover and Polson, 2014). Although legal definitions vary from state to state, the NCEA defines neglect as "the refusal or failure to fulfill any part of a person's obligations or duties to an elder. Neglect may also occur if the person who has fiduciary responsibilities fails to pay for items or necessary home care services or, on the part of the in-home service provider, to provide the necessary care (NCEA, n.d., p. 2). Older persons can make independent choices with which others may disagree. Their right to self-determination can be taken from them if they are declared incompetent. According to the Older Americans Act, financial exploitation is the "illegal or improper act or process of an individual, including a caregiver, using the resources of an older individual for monetary or personal benefit, profit or gain" (Administration on Aging, n.d., p. 1).

During the assessment process, nurses will want to be aware of contradictions between injuries and the explanation of their cause, codependency issues between client and caregiver, and substance abuse by the caregiver. Hoover and Polson (2014) suggest asking open-ended questions to patients presenting with signs of injuries or abuse, such as, "Can you tell me what happened? and "What do you remember about how this injury occurred?" The local social services agency or area agency on aging can help with information on reporting requirements. Nurses can play a key role in reducing elder abuse.

The Patient Self-Determination Act of 1991 requires those providers receiving Medicare and Medicaid funds to give clients written information regarding their legal options for treatment choices if they become incapacitated. A routine discussion of advanced medical directives can help ease the difficult discussions faced by health care professionals, families, and clients. The nurse can help an individual complete a values history instrument. These instruments ask questions about specific wishes regarding different medical situations. "Your Life Your Choices: Planning for Future Medical Decisions: How to Prepare a Personalized Living Will" (Pearlman et al, 2010) is a valuable resource to help people by using scenarios and information to guide people through the process of developing advanced medical directives. There are two parts to the advanced directives. The living will allows the client to express wishes regarding the use of medical treatments in the event of a terminal illness. A durable medical power of attorney is the legal way for the client to designate someone else to make health care decisions when he or she is unable to do so. A do-not-resuscitate order (DNR) is a specific order from a physician not to use cardiopulmonary resuscitation. Physician Orders for Life-Sustaining Treatment (POLST) are becoming common to specify end-of-life care or resuscitation orders for patients not in cardiopulmonary arrest. The POLST document is brightly colored and signed by the physician and the patient, depending on the state, and specifies medical orders to be carried out by health care workers when the patient is unable to speak. The difference between a POLST form and an advance directive is that the POLST is usable throughout the community (Buck and Fahlberg, 2014). State laws vary widely regarding the implementation of these tools, so it is important to consult a knowledgeable source for information. It is also important to involve the family,

and especially the designated decision-maker or agent, in these discussions so that everyone is clear about the client's choices.

## Environmental Impact

The impact of an unhealthy environment adds significantly to the burden of disease for men and women. Men and women are often exposed to different environmental factors because of upbringing, employment, cultural, or tradition variations.

It is important to understand that the hosts (men and women) may respond differently to environmental factors. For example, Clougherty (2010) reports that women and girls are affected more than men and boys by air pollution. Both gender (a social construct) and sex (a biological construct) are factors that make identification of the impact of environmental hazards on men and women more complex. Social and environmental factors influence adults' choices of health behaviors. Understanding how these factors impact health outcomes will require additional research and policy analysis (USDHHS, 2010). Conducting gender analysis as part of research would help clarify influences of environment on social and biological differences between men and women.

Governmental programs are in place to improve environmental health. The Centers for Disease Control and Prevention (CDC) Environmental Hazards and Effects Program (EHEP) is designed to prevent and control disease or death and to promote health and quality of life that result from interactions between people and their environments. The program uses indicators to assess and monitor progress on goals to improve the environmental health (CDC, National Center for Environmental Health, 2009). It is incumbent on community health nurses to decrease the burden of disease resulting from an unhealthy environment.

## HEALTH STATUS INDICATORS

Health status indicators are the quantitative or qualitative measures used to describe the level of well-being or illness present in a defined population or to describe related attributes or risk factors. They can be represented in the form of rates, such as mortality and morbidity, or proportions, such as percentages of a given population that receive immunizations (Community Health Status Indicators, 2009). Data on local communities are available through the Community Health Status Indicators Reports. This report is a collection of nationally available data for localities, including vital statistics, census, infectious disease, environmental health, health care indicators, employment indicators, and many of the vulnerable populations estimates (Community Health Status Indicators Working Group, 2009).

While health status indicators in the United States show persistent health disparities among ethnic and racial groups, the awareness of these disparities remains low among the general public (Benz et al, 2011). Persons with low socioeconomic status are more likely to be affected by chronic illness such as diabetes, hypertension, and human immunodeficiency virus (HIV). They are also less likely to be screened for colorectal cancer or vaccinated against influenza (Meyer et al, 2013).

Over the past decade, efforts to reduce chronic disease risk factors in adults have resulted in less-than-expected improvements. The CDC developed the *Futures Initiative* (2005) as part of a major strategic planning process and developed a set of Health Protection Goals to track measures of mortality and morbidity by life stages (CDC, 2005). The goals were categorized by four themes, each with an overarching goal: Healthy People in Every Stage of Life, Healthy People in Healthy Places, People Prepared for Emerging Health Threats, and Healthy People in a Healthy World. Improvements were noted among all life stages with the exception of adults. Adults reported continued declining trends in perceived health status and dramatic declines in healthy weight indicators (Roy et al, 2009).

## EVIDENCE-BASED PRACTICE

Health assessment and early detection are foundations for health promotion. Finding essential health indicators for older adults can better reflect the health status of the older adult population and efficiently detect their health problems in a timely and economical manner. This study aimed to explore the pertinent health indicators and to form a model of health for older adults. This study had two phases. Phase I began with sending evaluation surveys to a panel of ten professional experts to generate health indicators for older adults. Phase II was a preliminary determination of the extent of health predictions using these indicators by conducting a descriptive study involving a stratified random sample of 55 community-dwelling older adults. Results demonstrated three domains (physical health, psychological health, and social-economic health) and four constructs (activities of daily living, physical status, emotional health, and social engagement).

### Nurse Use

Results of this study can be used for making health policy and/or setting goals for interventions. In addition, nurses who care for older adults may use the health indicators to plan and control the given quality of care.

From Chen K, Hung H, Lin H, et al: Development of the model of health for older adults. *Journal of Advanced Nursing* 67(9):2015–2025, 2011. Doi: 10.1111/j.1365-2648.2011.05643.x

## Mortality

Life expectancy is a measure that is often used to gauge the overall health of a population. Although the United States spends more money per capita on health than any other country, other developed countries have a longer life expectancy for both genders. As illustrated in Figure 30-1, in the United States, life expectancy ranked 25th out of 37 countries and territories for men (75.2 years) and 23rd for women (80.4 years) (MMWR, 2008). However, these ranking methods did not reflect changes in health outcomes over time. A recent study (Kindig and Cheng, 2013) found that female mortality rates increased in 42.8% of U.S. counties, while male mortality rates increased in only 3.4%. Several factors were associated with lower mortality rates, including higher educational levels, not living in the South or West, and low smoking rates.

A comparative study of U.S. population health used data from the massive Global Burden of Disease (GBD) effort (U.S. Burden of Disease Collaborators, 2013). Significant improvements in U.S. health included an increase in overall life expectancy from age 75.2 to 78.2. Age-standardized years of life lost (YLL) rates increased for Alzheimer disease, drug use disorders, chronic kidney disease, and falls. Ischemic heart disease, lung cancer, stroke, chronic obstructive pulmonary disease, and road injury were diseases and injuries with the largest number of YLLs in 2010 (U.S. Burden of Disease Collaborators, 2013).

Life expectancy and mortality rates also vary among ethnic/racial groups in the United States. Health disparities are strikingly apparent in life expectancy, death rates, and other measures of health status (CDC Health Disparities and Inequalities Report, 2013). For instance, African Americans in 2009 had the highest death rates from heart disease and stroke compared with other racial and ethnic populations. They also had the highest death rates from homicide, with rates among African American males highest across all age groups (CDC Health Disparities and Inequalities Report, 2013). The gap in life expectancy between white adults and African American adults persists but has narrowed since 1990 (National Center for Health Statistics, 2009). The age-adjusted death rate was 1.3 times greater, infant mortality rate 2.4 times greater, and maternal mortality rate 3.4 times greater for the African American population than for the white population. Life expectancy for the white population exceeded that for the African American population by 5.0 years (Heron et al, 2009).

## Morbidity

When healthy years of life are increased, longer life spans are generally considered desirable. However, increasing prevalence of chronic diseases and other conditions associated with aging can increase functional limitations and affect quality of life. Moreover, being male or female leads to different socialization, expectations, and lifestyles that affect and interact with health in complex ways. Of particular concern is the high prevalence of adults with risk factors such as tobacco use, high cholesterol, obesity, and insufficient exercise habits, which are associated with chronic disease. Cholesterol levels have been dropping, in particular for the older adults, because of a large increase of drug therapies (NCHS, 2009). The leading risk factors related to disability-adjusted life-years (DALYs) in the United States are dietary risks, tobacco smoking, high body mass index, hypertension, high fasting plasma glucose, physical inactivity, and alcohol use (U.S. Burden of Disease Collaborators, 2013).

The prevalence of diabetes, serious heart conditions, and hypertension among adults 45 to 64 years of age is strongly associated with poverty status. In lower-income populations, modifiable risk factors for these diseases are more common. The number of poor adults 45 to 64 with hypertension was similar to the percentage of higher-income persons who were 65 to 74 years of age (NCHS, 2009).

Although women live longer than men, by about 5 years, they do not necessarily live those extra years in good physical and mental health. Women are more likely to use health services and report greater rates of disability. For instance, men have higher blood pressure levels than women through middle age. However, after menopause, women may be more affected by increased blood pressure. Women also present with different risk factors and symptoms for cardiac-related conditions.

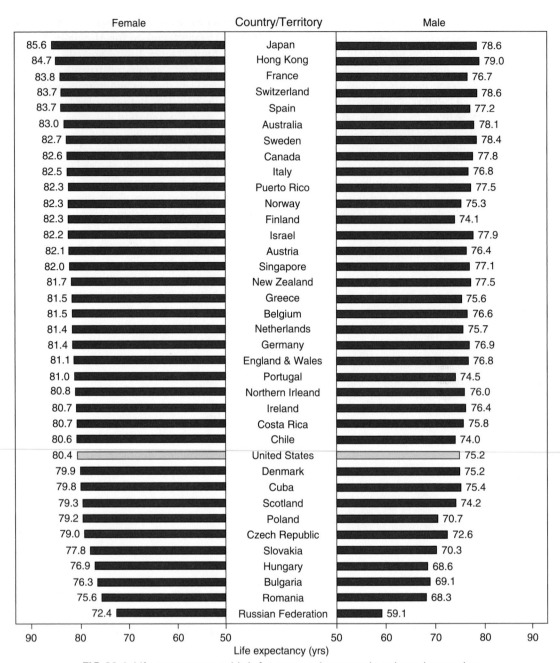

FIG 30-1 Life expectancy at birth for men and women in selected countries.

Women often report more jaw/neck pain, dyspnea, back pain, fatigue, paroxysmal nocturnal dyspnea, and palpitations. Men and women were equally likely to report midsternal chest pain or pressure (Shin et al, 2009).

## ADULT HEALTH CONCERNS

### Chronic Disease

In 1988 the CDC created the National Center for Chronic Disease Prevention and Health Promotion (NCCDPHP). Chronic illness has become a public health problem of great proportions. The most common and costly chronic diseases are heart disease, diabetes, stroke, cancer, and arthritis. Eighty-four

percent of all health care spending in 2006 was for the 50% of the population who have one or more chronic medical conditions (Robert Wood Johnson Foundation, 2010). Chronic disease is the leading cause of preventable deaths, disability, and decreased quality of life. The CDC has identified four modifiable health risk behaviors for the prevention of chronic disease. These are lack of physical activity, poor nutrition, tobacco use, and excessive alcohol use (NCCDPHP, 2014). Many models have been developed to guide the delivery of care to people with chronic illness. A complex health care system and community model was developed with the funding of the Robert Wood Johnson Foundation. This model is Wagner's Chronic Care Model (CCM).

## ❤ HEALTHY PEOPLE 2020

### *Selected Objectives Relevant to Major Health Issues and Chronic Disease of Adults*

**Arthritis, Osteoporosis, and Chronic Back Conditions**
- AOCBC-7: Increase the proportion of adults with doctor-diagnosed arthritis who receive health care provider counseling.
- AOCBC-10: Reduce the proportion of adults with osteoporosis.

**Cancer**
- C-1: Reduce the overall cancer death rate.

**Diabetes**
- D-3: Reduce the diabetes death rate.

**Educational and Community-Based Programs**
- ECBP-9: (Developmental) Increase the proportion of employees who participate in employer-sponsored health promotion activities.

**Environmental Health**
- EH-3: Reduce air toxic emissions to decrease the risk of adverse health effects caused by airborne toxics.

**Genomics**
- G-1: Increase the proportion of women with a family history of breast and/or ovarian cancer who receive genetic counseling.
- G-2: (Developmental) Increase the proportion of persons with newly diagnosed colorectal cancer who receive genetic testing to identify Lynch syndrome (or familial colorectal cancer syndromes).

**Heart Disease and Stroke**
- HDS-2: Reduce coronary heart disease deaths.
- HDS-3: Reduce stroke deaths.

**Older Adults**
- OA-1: Increase the proportion of older adults who are up to date on a core set of clinical preventive services.

**Physical Activity and Fitness**
- PAF-2: Increase the proportion of adults that meet current Federal physical activity guidelines for aerobic physical activity and for muscle strength training.

U.S. Department of Health and Human Services: *Healthy People 2020*, 2010. Retrieved from http://www.healthypeople.gov/2020/default .aspx 9/11/2014

The CCM identifies the essential elements of a health care system that encourages high-quality chronic disease care. These elements are the community, the health system, self-management support, delivery system design, decision support, and clinical information systems. Evidence-based change concepts under each element, in combination, foster productive interactions between informed clients who take an active part in their care and providers with resources and expertise (Model Elements, 2014). The CCM continues to be implemented and evaluated today. Using electronic health records, provider reminders for key evidence-based care components, interprofessional teams communicating regularly, and community health classes to educate people with chronic diseases are ways the CCM is being implemented. A modification of the CCM to include health literacy was suggested by Koh et al (2013).

Chronic disease self-management (CDSMP) is one intervention that has shown positive outcomes for people with chronic diseases. The U.S. Administration on Aging initiated CDSMP in 2009. Within two years 9305 workshops were offered to more than 100,000 middle-aged and older adults (Ory et al, 2013). Studies have shown improvement in health behaviors, health outcomes, and reduced health care utilization. A recent study showed significant reductions in emergency room visits and hospitalizations. Potential savings of $364 per participant and a national savings of $3.3 billion could result if only 5% of the U.S. population participated (Ahn et al, 2013). Opportunities exist for additional studies to identify effective models and strategies. Nurses should consider using models and strategies that have shown improvements in health behaviors or outcomes when planning community interventions.

Family remains an important source of support for people with chronic disease. A recent review of programs to increase effective family support showed that programs that train families in supportive communication techniques have improved both health behaviors and client symptom management (Rosland and Piette, 2010).

## Cardiovascular Disease

About 83.6 million American adults have one or more types of cardiovascular disease (CVD). The leading cause of death for African Americans, American Indians or Alaska Natives, Hispanics, and whites in the United States is heart disease. It is the leading cause of death for both men and women. Heart disease was responsible for 31.9% of deaths in 2010 (Go et al, 2014). The annual cost of heart disease for 2010 to the United States was estimated to be $315.4 billion. In response to the high incidence and mortality rates of heart disease, the American Heart Association (AHA) has the following goal: "By 2020, to improve the cardiovascular health of all Americans by 20 percent while reducing deaths from cardiovascular diseases and stroke by 20 percent" (American Heart Association, 2010). Progress is being made in this area as from 2000 to 2010 death rates attributable to CVD declined by 31% (Go et al, 2014). However, with the increased rates of obesity and diabetes in children, future prevalence may increase.

Approximately 23 of the *Healthy People 2020* objectives focus on cardiovascular disease. Reaching these objectives means intervening with all ethnicities in the United States. However, there continue to be gaps in knowledge and awareness for heart disease, particularly in women. In a 2009 survey of 2300 women age 25 or older, 60% of white women were aware that heart disease was the leading cause of death for women. However, only 43% of African American women, 44% of Hispanic women, and 34% of Asian women knew the major cause of death for their gender. Knowledge of heart attack signs and symptoms has not increased since 1997 among all women surveyed, and only 53% of the women surveyed said they would call 911 if they thought they were having a heart attack (Mosca et al, 2010). Improvement in this area has also been noted. Mosca et al (2013) found that "Between 1997 and 2012, the rate of awareness of CVD as the leading cause of death nearly doubled (56% versus 30%; P < 0.001). The rate of awareness among black and Hispanic women in 2012 (36% and 34%, respectively) was similar to that of white women in 1997 (33%). In 1997, women were more likely to cite cancer than CVD as the leading killer (35% versus 30%), but in 2012, the trend reversed (24% versus 56%)." The trend of the data is encouraging but the overall knowledge of women and minority women remains low.

## Hypertension

High blood pressure, or hypertension, is estimated to occur in one in three, or approximately 78 million Americans. Uncontrolled hypertension leads to heart attack, stroke, kidney damage, and a host of other complications. Only 82% of people with hypertension are aware that they have the disease. Hypertension is controlled in 53% of people with the disease, 75% are under current treatment, and 47% do not have it controlled (AHA, 2014). Although these numbers are not optimal, blood pressure control has improved significantly over time; however, racial, ethnic, and socioeconomic differences have not shown significant improvement. There is no significant difference in prevalence between men and women, but there are racial and ethnic differences in hypertension rates among both men and women. Forty-four percent of African Americans have hypertension; this is the highest ethnic prevalence (AHA, 2007). A recent discovery is the connection between obstructive sleep apnea and hypertension. Konecny et al (2014) examined the evidence on sleep apnea and hypertension and noted that sleep apnea is a modifiable and highly prevalent factor in the development of hypertension. Once hypertension is present, CPAP averages only a modest 2 mm Hg drop in blood pressure (p. 208).

## Stroke

Strokes have decreased in the United States since the 1950s. The actual number of stroke deaths declined by 22.8% from 2000 to 2010 (Go, 2014). However, the estimated prevalence of stroke in 2010 was 6.8 million for people equal to or greater than 20 years of age. Approximately 795,000 people each year experience a new or recurrent stroke. The lifetime risk for stroke is higher in women ($\approx$1 in 5) than in men ($\approx$1 in 6), and since women live longer than men and strokes increase with age, more women than men are likely to die from stroke. African Americans have almost twice the risk of first-time strokes as whites. Mexican Americans also have an increased incidence of stroke over non-Hispanic whites. The prevalence of strokes is projected to increase 21.9% by 2030 (Go, 2014).

One *Healthy People 2020* objective is to reduce stroke deaths to 48 in 100,000. Community-based programs and policies regarding stroke care from initial signs and symptoms to after-treatment have been developed by the AHA and other organizations. The CDC's Division for Heart Disease and Stroke Prevention (DHDSP) is promoting the use of community health workers (CHWs) to support healthy living strategies that would reduce the prevalence of stroke as well as other chronic conditions (Brownstein et al, (2013). Collaboration between

health care institutions, community leaders, emergency medical services, CHWs, and support groups within the community is needed for programs to be effective. Nurses can direct efforts toward smoking reduction, since the incidence of ischemic stroke is twice as high in smokers as in adults who do not smoke (AHA, 2010).

## Diabetes

Diabetes is a serious public health challenge for the United States. Between 1980 and 1990 the number of new cases remained stable, but from 1990 to 2010 the annual number of new cases almost tripled. Increases in obesity, decreases in leisure-time physical activity, and the aging population are associated with this dramatic increase in the incidence of type 2 diabetes (CDC, 2012a). An estimated 19.7 million Americans were dianosed with diabetes mellitus in 2010 (Go, 2014). Diabetes is an epidemic, with 1 in 12 to 13 adults reportedly having diabetes, costing the nation approximately $174 billion each year. It is also estimated that for every three people who have diabetes, there is another who does not know he or she has it. Age-adjusted diabetes was diagnosed in 16.1% of American Indian and Alaska Natives, 8.4% of Asian Americans, 11.8% of Hispanics, 12.6% of non-Hispanic African Americans, and 7.1% of non-Hispanic whites. The many complications associated with diabetes include heart disease, stroke, hypertension, retinopathy, kidney disease, neuropathies, amputations, and dental disease (CDC, 2012a).

At least 18 of the goals of *Healthy People 2020* are related to diabetes. There is a tremendous need in the community to strive to limit the toll this disease takes on the person and the community. Social and economic factors related to health and well-being need to be addressed.

Primary prevention includes educating adults about nutrition and the risks of obesity, smoking, and physical inactivity. Community interventions addressing healthy eating, exercise, and weight reduction can also benefit adults at risk for diabetes. Secondary prevention includes screening for diabetes with finger-stick blood glucose tests or glucose tolerance tests. Screening is also accomplished by thorough history and physical examination. Tertiary prevention targets activities aimed at reducing the complications of the disease (see Levels of Prevention box).

## Mental Health

Mental disorders are a common cause of disability. According to the 2012 National Survey on Drug Use and Health: Mental Health Findings, there were an estimated 43.7 million (18.6%) adults in the United States with any mental illness in the prior year and 9.6 million (4.1%) of those were categorized as serious mental illness (U.S. Department of Health and Human Services, 2013). As described previously, gender makes a difference regarding environmental impact on health. Similarly, gender influences how a person responds to stress, presents with symptoms, experiences the course of illness, and accesses and uses mental health services (Forchuk et al, 2009). Although both men and women suffer from the burden of mental illness, women experience certain conditions such as anxiety and

## LEVELS OF PREVENTION

### Cardiovascular Disease in Women and Prevention of HIV in Men

**Primary Prevention**

*Collaborating with a variety of organizations such as the American Heart Association to design and implement interventions aimed at reducing women's risk for cardiovascular disease.*

The nurse advises men who have sex with other men to use a new latex condom during oral or anal sex. In group and individual counseling about HIV, the nurse indicates to clients that they should not share needles, syringes, razors, or toothbrushes.

**Secondary Prevention**

*Establishing screening clinics in community settings for cholesterol and hypertension.*

The nurse advises an infected man to swallow all of his highly active antiretroviral therapy (HAART) medication on schedule. The nurse advises a man who had unprotected sex to be tested with a standard enzyme-linked immunosorbent assay (ELISA), followed by a confirmatory Western blot test.

**Tertiary Prevention**

*Developing a community-based exercise program for a group of women who have cardiovascular disease.*

The nurse teaches men newly diagnosed with HIV to exercise regularly, eat a balanced nutritious diet, sleep at least 8 hours a day, and stop or limit alcohol. The nurse advises clients not to donate blood, plasma, or organs.

| TABLE 30-1 | Deaths Caused by Cancers* | |
|---|---|---|
| **Population** | **Men** | **Women** |
| White | 218.7 | 153.4 |
| African American | 278.8 | 176.9 |
| Hispanic | 145.4 | 101.4 |
| Native American | 137.0 | 108.9 |
| Asian/Pacific Islander | 128.2 | 93.3 |

*Rates are per 100,000.
From Centers for Disease Control and Prevention: Rates for new cancer cases and deaths by race/ethnicity and sex, n.d. Available at www.cdc.gov.

depression more often than men, yet men have a higher suicide rate (Riska, 2009). It is important to consider sex and gender when generating meaningful knowledge and interventions to promote the health of both men and women.

Researchers are exploring how biological factors, including genetics and sex hormones, affect women's increased risk for depression. Other scientists are focusing on how psychosocial factors such as life stress, trauma, and interpersonal relationships contribute to women's depression (Danielsson et al, 2009). Although the roles men and women traditionally fulfill in society continue to be the framework of much mental health research, additional focus is addressing cultural or other factors to explain differences (Riska, 2009).

Mental illness is generally viewed by society in a negative manner (Bos et al, 2009). This social stigma leads to guilt, low self-esteem, social isolation, and ultimately to poorer health (Stuenkel and Wong, 2009). Community education programs will want to focus on speakers who address audiences to educate them and dispel the stereotypes and fears often applied by society to individuals with mental illness. Local and mass media outlets can be incorporated to broadcast positive aspects of those living with mental disabilities and functioning as a productive part of society.

## Cancer

Cancers of all types are a serious public health concern (Table 30-1). Cancer is the second leading cause of death in the United States, surpassed only by heart disease. As of January 1, 2012, approximately 13.7 million Americans with a history of cancer

were alive, some of whom were cancer free. The American Cancer Society's (ACS) 2014 Cancer Facts and Figures reports an estimated 585,720 cancer deaths in 2014, 176,000 of which resulted from tobacco use. In the same year, about 1,665,540 new cancer cases are projected to be diagnosed. The report also gave estimates by the National Institutes of Health that place the overall costs of cancer in 2009 at $216.6 billion. Of this total, $86.6 billion is for direct medical costs and $130 billion for indirect costs or those resulting from lost productivity related to illness or premature death. These costs could be reduced by removing barriers to care such as lack of health insurance and improving the health literacy of Americans.

Early screening and detection, promotion of healthy lifestyles, expansion of access to services, and improvement in cancer treatments will help reduce the burden of cancer and disparities. For example, the declining death rates from colorectal cancer are largely attributed to screening and risk factor reduction (Edwards et al, 2009). Finding cancer lesions in a precancerous state, such as those found in cervical, colorectal, and breast cancer, allows for treatment while in a highly treatable stage. Obesity, physical inactivity, smoking, heavy alcohol consumption, a diet high in red or processed meats, and insufficient intake of fruits and vegetables are risk factors for colorectal cancer. Reducing these risk factors will reduce the incidence of the disease.

Public health agencies, health care providers, and communities must work together to reduce the burden of cancer on society. The *Healthy People 2020* goal is to reduce the number of overall cancer cases as well as the illness, disability, and death caused by cancer. Education on the hazards of tobacco use and second-hand smoke, eating a healthy diet and limiting daily consumption of alcohol, and exposure to ultraviolet rays are examples of topics for education programs that will reduce the burden of cancer on society.

## STDs/HIV/AIDS

Sexually transmitted diseases (STDs) refer to more than 25 infectious organisms, such as viruses, bacteria, or parasites, transmitted primarily through sexual activity. Some other means of transmission include lice, mother-to-child transmission during pregnancy or breastfeeding, or contaminated needles used in drug use or surgery. The term sexually transmitted infections (STIs) is also used synonymously, although there are distinctions. Shuford (2008) explained that *STI* is a broader term meaning that the body has had an invasion and multiplication of microorganisms, whereas *STD* signifies that pathology or damage has occurred with or without symptoms. STDs continue to be a major burden to society and have tremendous health and economic consequences in the United States despite their relatively preventable nature. The costs to the U.S. health care system related to STDs are as much as $15.3 billion annually (CDC, 2008).

The CDC (2008) estimates there are approximately 19 million new STD infections each year, with almost half occurring in people from 15 to 24 years of age. Many cases go undiagnosed, so the true burden is not fully known. In 2008, more than 1.5 million cases of chlamydia and gonorrhea occurred, making them the two most reported infectious diseases. Females are at greater risk for STDs as a result of biological differences and other factors. Syphilis, once close to elimination, has reemerged, primarily related to men who have sex with men (MSM), but not in all cases (CDC, 2008). People with an STD are more susceptible to and two to five times more likely to acquire an HIV infection (CDC, 2013).

In the United States approximately 1.1 million people were diagnosed or undiagnosed with HIV infection (CDC, 2013). The HIV incidence is about 50,000 new infections per year, which appears stable. Seventy-eight percent of new HIV infections and 63% of all of these new infections occurred in MSMs. African Americans accounted for 44% of the HIV/AIDS cases whereas Hispanics/Latinos accounted for 21% of new cases in 2010.

The *Healthy People 2020* goal is to promote responsible sexual behaviors, strengthen community capacity, and increase access to quality services to prevent STDs and their complications (USDHHS, 2010b). Nurses have a role in this goal and can serve as advocates by focusing on the high-risk behaviors of men and women, as well as on the factors in their communities that lead to STDs. High-risk populations should be considered when assessing for clients' risk for STDs, including pregnant women, adolescents, MSM, women who have sex with women (WSW), and older clients (Waski and Kachlic, 2009). Interventions to improve education, employment opportunities, and adequate housing—as well as those to decrease drug use, isolation, and poverty—can have a critical impact on this epidemic. The CDC/HRSA Advisory Committee on HIV/AIDS and STD Prevention (CHAC) recommend the following: (1) early detection and treatment of curable STDs should become a major, explicit component of comprehensive HIV prevention programs at national, state, and local levels; (2) in areas where STDs that facilitate HIV transmission are prevalent, screening and treatment programs should be expanded; (3) HIV testing should always be recommended for individuals who are diagnosed with or suspected to have an STD; and (4) HIV and STD prevention programs in the United States, together with private and public sector partners, should take joint responsibility for implementing these strategies (see How To box).

## Weight Control

Americans spend a great deal of time, energy, and money in the never-ending pursuit of the beautiful body. One study indicated

---

**HOW TO**

*To reduce the prevalence of STDs, the CDC/HRSA Advisory Committee on HIV/AIDS and STD Prevention (CHAC) recommend the following:*

- *Early detection and treatment of curable STDs should be a major, explicit component of comprehensive HIV prevention programs at national, state, and local levels.*
- *In areas where STDs that facilitate HIV transmission are prevalent, screening and treatment programs should be expanded.*
- *HIV testing should always be recommended for individuals who are diagnosed with or suspected to have an STD.*
- *HIV and STD prevention programs in the U.S., together with private and public sector partners, should take joint responsibility for implementing these strategies.*
- *Social, behavioral, and biomedical interventions should also be included in a comprehensive HIV prevention program.*

Centers for Disease Control and Prevention: *CDC fact sheet: the role of STD prevention and treatment in HIV prevention*, 2010. Available at http://www.cdc.gov/std/hiv/stds-and-hiv-fact-sheet-press.pdf. Accessed April 15, 2014.

---

that spending on overweight and obesity could be as much as 10%, or $147 billion, of U.S. health care costs (Finkelstein et al, 2009). In 1998 the National Institutes of Health (NIH) began using the calculation of **body mass index** (BMI) to define overweight and obesity in individuals. BMI is the relationship of body weight and height. A BMI of 25 to 29.9 is defined as overweight, whereas a BMI of 30 and above is considered obese (WIN, 2008) (Table 30-2).

Overweight and obesity are topics addressed numerous times in *Healthy People 2020*. According to the AHA (2009), 145 million Americans age 20 and older are overweight or obese (BMI ≥ 25.0 kg/m²). This number is composed of 76.9 million men and 68.1 million women. Of the total 145 million, 74.1 million are obese (BMI ≥ 30.0).

**Obesity** has many effects on health and is linked to a number of major health problems. Nurses can provide education regarding obesity's risks to health. The educational offerings can be fashioned after a community health model using the levels of prevention to establish effective interventions for adults at risk for **weight control** issues. For example, only about one third of all adults meet the 2008 Physical Activity Guidelines (CDC, 2008). Therefore, a community prevention project aimed at

**TABLE 30-2  BMI Determination and Interpretation**

| BMI* | Category |
|---|---|
| ≤18.5-24.9 | Normal weight |
| 25.0-29.9 | Overweight |
| 30.0-39.9 | Obesity |
| ≥40 | Extreme obesity |

*Body mass index is a method used to determine optimal weight for height and is an indicator for obesity or malnutrition.
From National Institutes of Health: Do you know the health risks of being overweight? Rockville, MD, 2004, USDHHS.

increasing activity levels would help in prevention of obesity and subsequent illnesses of diabetes and heart disease.

In addition to obesity, other eating disorders have increased among U.S. women. Common eating disorders seen in women include anorexia nervosa and bulimia. **Anorexia** is defined as a fear of gaining weight coupled with disturbances in perceptions of the body. Excessive weight loss is the most noticeable clue to this disorder. Individuals with anorexia rarely complain of weight loss because they view themselves as normal or overweight. Many of these women also struggle with psychological problems, including depression, obsessive symptoms, and social phobias. **Bulimia** is characterized by a persistent concern with the shape of the body along with body weight, recurrent episodes of binge eating, a loss of control during these binges, and use of extreme methods to prevent weight gain, such as purging, strict dieting, fasting, use of laxatives or diuretics, or vigorous exercise (NIMH, 2014).

Through comprehensive physical and psychosocial assessments, as well as histories of dietary practice, nurses identify women with eating disorders and provide appropriate referrals. Weight control strategies include promoting healthy eating habits and regular physical activity. At a population level, nurses advocate against advertising that promotes exceptionally thin bodies for women. They also promote community-wide exercise and healthy eating programs.

## WOMEN'S HEALTH CONCERNS

It is preferable to emphasize prevention in adult health care. Screening, immunizations, and a healthy lifestyle are important for women of all ages. The **Office on Women's Health** (USDHHS, 2014) works through policy, education, and model programs to improve the health of women and girls. This agency has guidelines that include screening tests and disease-specific information for women. The Agency for Research and Health Quality (ARHQ) was mandated by Congress to provide annual reports on health care quality and disparities. Women are one of the populations addressed in this report.

### Reproductive Health

Women often use health care services for **reproductive health** concerns. A number of *Healthy People 2020* objectives address areas related to women's reproductive health (see the Maternal Infant and Child Health section of the *Healthy People 2020*.

Nurses are in a unique position to advocate for policies that increase women's access to services for reproductive health. In addition, many nurses discuss contraception with women of child-bearing age. Contraceptive counseling requires accurate knowledge of current contraceptive choices and a nonjudgmental approach. The goal of contraceptive counseling is to ensure that women have appropriate instruction to make informed choices about reproduction. The choice of contraceptive method depends on many factors, including the woman's health, frequency of sexual activity, number of partners, and plans to have future children. Except for abstinence, no method provides a 100% guarantee against **unintended pregnancy** or disease (USDHHS, 2014).

**Preconceptual counseling** addresses risks before conception and includes education, assessment, diagnosis, and intervention. The purpose is to reduce and/or eliminate health risks for women and infants. One major health problem that could be significantly impacted by preconceptual counseling is the problem of neural tube defects. More than 300,000 babies annually are born with neural tube defects (anacephaly and spina bifida). In the United States, it is estimated that the annual health care costs for people with spina bifida exceed $200 million. The United States is part of a global initiative to reduce these numbers. Research has shown that intake of folic acid can significantly reduce the occurrence of these very serious and often fatal neural tube defects by 50% to 70%. The goal of one *Healthy People 2020* objective is to increase the proportion of pregnancies begun with the recommended folic acid level; a recommendation was made that women capable of or planning a pregnancy take 400 mcg of folic acid daily (CDC, 2012b). Supplementation of cereal and masa flour, surveillance, and detection of levels are part of the initiatives currently being conducted with worldwide partners (NCBDDD, 2014).

Another concern critical to preconception awareness is exposure to substances such as alcohol. A major preventable cause of birth defects, mental retardation, and neurodevelopmental disorders is fetal exposure to alcohol during pregnancy. Although fetal alcohol syndrome disorders (FASD) are declining in the United States, they remain a preventable public health problem. According to the Substance Abuse and Mental Health Services Administration (SAMSHA) in 2010, FASD affects 40,000 babies born in the United States each year. The rate is higher (15 to 25 per 10,000) among some Native American tribes (SAMSHA, 2009). The CDC and the American Academy of Pediatrics recommend no alcohol during pregnancy. Cannon et al (2012) sought to prevent FAS by studying the characteristics of birth mothers. They discovered that predictors were older age, American Indian/Alaska Native or African American ethnicity, unmarried, unemployed, and without prenatal care. In addition they were more likely to be smokers, Medicaid recipients, have a history of treatment for alcohol abuse or confirmed alcoholism, and to have used marijuana or cocaine during their pregnancy. Community interventions have been shown to help decrease the consumption of alcohol during pregnancy. Studies are needed with interventions that target this risk group for children with FAS.

Nurses will want to be involved in community-based interventions for women. They can conduct motivational classes and participate in campaigns that print and broadcast advertisements informing women of child-bearing age that drinking during pregnancy can cause birth defects. Nurses can serve as advocates not only to encourage their clients to use prenatal care services, but also to work toward the establishment of services that are accessible, affordable, and available to all pregnant women.

### Gestational Diabetes

**Gestational diabetes mellitus** (GDM) is a condition characterized by carbohydrate intolerance that is first identified or develops during pregnancy. The incidence of gestational diabetes is increasing in the United States. Gestational diabetes has a higher incidence among African Americans, American Indians, and Hispanic/Latino Americans. According to the CDC (2011), after the pregnancy ends 5% to 10% of women will continue with diabetes or have a 35% to 60% chance of developing diabetes within the next 10 to 20 years.

Clearly, interventions are needed to prevent gestational diabetes and its consequences for both mother and baby. A meta-analysis of studies regarding physical activity and gestational diabetes was conducted by Tobias et al (2011). Higher levels of physical activity were significantly associated with a lower risk of developing gestational diabetes mellitus. This association occurred with physical activity that occurred before pregnancy or in early pregnancy (p. 223). Nursing interventions related to activity levels are imperative in reproductive women and their unborn children.

## Menopause

During menopause the levels of the hormones estrogen and progesterone change in a woman's body. This change leads to the cessation of menstruation. Decline in these hormone levels can affect the vaginal and urinary tract, cardiovascular system, bone density, libido, sleep patterns, memory, and emotions (NIA, 2014).

Women's attitudes toward menopause vary greatly and are influenced by culture, age, support, and the recounted experiences of other women. For decades, however, the prevailing medical view of menopause was a state of deficiency that required hormone replacement to reduce heart disease and osteoporosis. A more positive outlook on menopause encourages women to view it as a transitional and natural stage in the life of a woman.

For decades, many U.S. women used hormone replacement therapy (HRT), although HRT remained untested by rigorous scientific study. A clinical trial launched in 1991, the Women's Health Initiative, set out to test specific effects HRT had on women's health, especially its effects on heart disease and osteoporosis. Researchers concluded that HRT did not prevent heart disease and that to prevent heart disease women should avoid smoking, reduce fat and cholesterol intake, limit salt and alcohol intake, maintain a healthy weight, and be physically active. Scientists also concluded that HRT should be used to prevent osteoporosis only among women who are unable to take non-estrogen medications (NOF, 2014).

### Complementary and Alternative Therapies

The change in the recommendations regarding HRT led many women to seek alternative approaches for the management of menopausal symptoms. Women experiencing menopause frequently report symptoms including hot flashes, vaginal dryness, and irregular menses. Examples of alternative therapies are those actions that are taken by women instead of HRT. Complementary therapies are those taken to augment (or as a complement to) HRT. The listing of alternative/complementary therapies for menopausal symptoms can be an endless task, but Box 30-1 provides common examples. The National Center for Complementary and Alternative Medicine at the National

---

**BOX 30-1  Examples of Alternative/Complementary Therapies for Menopausal Symptoms**

- Acupuncture
- Acupressure
- Massage therapy
- Healing touch
- Aromatherapy
- Guided imagery
- Chiropractic healing
- Yoga
- Tai Chi
- Qi gong
- St. John's wort
- Black cohosh
- Soy and isoflavones
- Ginseng
- Kava
- Red clover
- Dong quai

---

Institutes of Health (2012) notes that alternative therapies may or may not be helpful in reducing menopausal symptoms and that more research should be done to determine the scientific benefits and risks of these therapies. A systematic review of the literature on mind-body therapies for menopausal symptoms was conducted by Innes et al in 2010. They noted that yoga-based and certain other mind-body therapies may be beneficial, but recommended further study.

### Breast Cancer

In 2014 an estimated 232,670 U.S. women will be diagnosed with breast cancer. Of that number, an estimated 40,000 women will die. The breast cancer death rate in the United States has been declining since 1989-1990. The death rate has been declining an average of 1.9% per year over the last 10 years. In 2010, there were an estimated 2,829,041 women living with breast cancer (ACS, 2014b). Although the incidence of breast cancer is higher in white women than in African American women, the death rate for African American women is higher. Secondary prevention that includes screening activities, such as mammography and clinical breast examination, makes a difference in death rates. Early detection can promote a cure whereas late detection typically ensures a poor prognosis (NCI, 2014b).

### Osteoporosis

Osteoporosis, or *porous bone*, is a disease "marked by reduced bone strength leading to an increased risk of fractures, or broken bones" (NIAMSD, 2014). This is the most common bone disease, affecting 40 million people in the United States, and is most common in white and Asian women. Among women more than 50 years of age, approximately one out of every two women will have an osteoporosis-related fracture—that is 2 million fractures annually that are attributed to osteoporosis. Hip fractures have the most impact on quality of life and one in 5 people who suffer hip fractures over the age of 50 will die in the year following their fracture (NIAMSD, 2014). According to the National Osteoporosis Foundation's Clinician's Guide to Prevention and Treatment (2014, Version 1), the cost of care for hip fractures is projected to be $25.3 billion by 2025.

Prevention includes diets rich in calcium and vitamin D and avoiding medications that cause bone loss. Exercise also improves bone density, especially weight-bearing activities such as walking, running, stair climbing, and weight lifting. Limiting alcohol consumption and avoiding smoking are also important. Home assessment and correction of risk factors for falls, bone density testing, and annual height measurements help with fracture prevention. Finally, several medications are approved for the prevention of osteoporosis in the United States (NOF, 2014).

## MEN'S HEALTH CONCERNS

The health status of one gender impacts the health status of the other gender, the children, and ultimately society. For example, when a male is ill and cannot work, the family and society are impacted economically and work productivity is reduced. The family can suffer from lack of income. If the male dies, the widow generally experiences the loss of companionship and assumes the responsibilities of the lost spouse. Resources to promote and sustain health outcomes of both genders must be balanced for the overall health of the community. However, although a vital aspect of community health, men's health is often overlooked and factors exist that prevent men from reaching their full health potential. Factors such as "socioeconomic status, access to health care, male acculturation to health issues, harmful perceptions about masculinity, and lack of understanding of male health behaviors contribute to poor health outcomes for men" (Giorgianni et al 2013, p. 343). There are a wide range of poorer overall health status and health outcomes for men in the United States that result in an approximately 5-year shorter life span for men than women. Giorgianni et al (2013) provide examples of these different outcomes; for example, more men than women smoke (21.5% versus 17.3%), more men are overweight (72.3% versus 64.1), and men are less likely to receive routine care or seek out care early in the disease process than women. Changing these health behaviors could significantly improve the health outcomes of men.

Although health policies, campaigns, and community health organizations offer services for men, there are disparities that emphasize women's health and other barriers that negatively impact men's health (Broom and Tovey, 2009). Several barriers to men reaching their full health potential have been identified. Men do not participate in health care to the same level as women, apparently because of the traditional masculine gender role learned through socialization (Giorgianni et al, 2013). Only 57% of U.S. men see a doctor, nurse practitioner, or physician assistant compared with 74% of women (AHRQ, 2010). Even fewer Hispanic (35.5%) and African American (43.5%) men compared with white (63%) men made appointments for routine medical care. Men are socialized to ignore pain, be self-reliant, and be achievement oriented. Large numbers of men do not receive the health screenings intended to prevent and identify disease. Men are more often employed in dangerous jobs and incur more work-related injuries than women (Berdahl and Zodet, 2010). Not only do these behaviors limit the opportunity to prevent disease through screening, health education, and counseling, but also once they are diagnosed, management and treatment will be more difficult.

Disparities and barriers such as these provide opportunities and challenges for nurses. By being aware of disparities and barriers in the health care system and recognizing that something should be done, nurses can help reduce the bias and remove barriers to health for both genders. Nurses will want to develop strategies to get men involved in lifestyle changes that prevent illness. All health care providers can do a better job at reaching out to men and offer the guidance and knowledge to improve men's health. Nurses can take an active role in public policy development and implementation. The role also includes encouraging men to identify primary care providers and obtain a physical examination and the appropriate recommended screening tests.

Men who can establish a working relationship with their health care provider and participate in the recommended screening tests may live healthier, happier, and longer lives. Refer to Box 30-2 for a variety of screening tests with suggested frequencies. Health screenings as well as other prevention strategies for adults are regularly updated by AHRQ. Some health screenings are clearly beneficial while health care providers and researchers debate the benefit of other screening procedures. As

### BOX 30-2 Prevention Strategies for Adults

**Dental Health**
- Regular dental examinations
- Floss; brush with fluoride toothpaste

**Health Screening**
- Blood pressure
- Height and weight
- Nutritional screening (obesity)
- Lipid disorders (men 35 and older; women 45 and older)
- Papanicolaou (Pap) test (all women sexually active with a cervix)
- Colorectal cancer (adults 50 and older)
- Mammogram (women 40 and older)
- Osteoporosis (postmenopausal women 60 and older)
- Problem drinking
- Depression screening
- Tobacco use/tobacco-causing diseases
- Rubella serology or vaccination (women of child-bearing age)
- Chlamydia (sexually active women age 25 and younger; women older than 25 with new/multiple sexual partners)
- Testicular cancer (symptomatic males)
- Coronary heart disease screening (EEG; exercise treadmill)
- Syphilis screening (for at-risk population only)
- Diabetes mellitus (adults with hypertension or hyperlipidemia)

**Chemoprophylaxis**
- Multivitamin/folic acid (women planning or capable of pregnancy)
- Aspirin prevention (CAD at-risk adults)

**Immunizations**
- Tetanus-diphtheria (TD) boosters
- Rubella (women of child-bearing age)
- Pneumococcal vaccine (adults 65 and older)
- Influenza vaccine (adults 65 and older/at risk/annually)

From: Agency for health care quality and research, US preventive services taskforce: The guide to clinical preventive services, 2009, Rockville Md, AHRQ a health care professional, it is important to keep up to date on current research and literature to identify the appropriate screenings for the specific population served.

Nurses can assume many roles to fulfill responsibilities to improve the health of men in the community. As an educator, the nurse provides the knowledge and skill for replacing unhealthy behaviors with a healthy lifestyle. As a client advocate, the nurse supports and interacts with those agencies to obtain the needed resources. The nurse acts as a change agent to assess needs and system influences, identify and set priorities, plan and implement programs for men, and evaluate results. Working within groups and communities, nurses can identify needs and priorities and develop interventions to reduce health risks and improve the health status not only of men, but also of their wives, mothers, daughters, and sisters and the communities in which they live.

## Cancers Unique to Men
### Prostate Cancer

In 2011, 209,292 men in the United States were diagnosed with prostate cancer and 27,970 died from the disease (U.S. Cancer Statistics Working Group, 2014). According to the National Cancer Institute (NCI, 2014a), approximately 15% of men will be diagnosed with prostate cancer in their lifetime. The NCI estimates that 233,000 new cases will be diagnosed in 2014. It is the most common non-skin cancer and the second leading cause of cancer deaths in the United States (NCI, 2014a). African American men have higher rates (223.9/100,000) of prostate cancer compared to all races (147.8/100,000. Prostate cancer is linked to changes in the DNA of a prostate cancer cell and high levels of male hormones, but the exact cause of prostate cancer is unknown (ACS, 2014a).

The ACS recommends men be informed about risks and possible benefits of prostate cancer screening. The information should be provided at age 50 for men of average risk for prostate cancer and age 45 for men at high risk, such as African American men and men who have had a father, brother, or son diagnosed with prostate cancer before age 65. Men who have had several of these family members diagnosed with prostate cancer at an early age should be informed about prostate screening at age 40 (ACS, 2014a).

Two screening tests include the prostate-specific antigen (PSA) and the digital rectal examination (DRE). The PSA test is not accurate in terms of sensitivity or specificity. This blood test produces many false-positive results because many factors can elevate the PSA, such as infections, ejaculation, exercise such as bike riding, and benign prostatic hyperplasia (BPH). The DRE is a procedure where the physician inserts a well-lubricated, gloved index finger into the rectum to palpate the prostate gland and examine the rectum for masses. The examiner is unable to palpate the anterior aspects of the prostate, reducing the accuracy of this examination. Men find this examination unpleasant and another reason for avoiding health care (ACS, 2014a).

### Testicular Cancer

Testicular cancer is the most common solid tumor diagnosed in males between the ages of 15 and 40 years, with the peak incidence between the ages of 18 and 40 years. The ACS predicted 8480 new cases of testicular cancer and 350 deaths in 2010 (ACS, 2013. Age-adjusted incidence showed 6.4 of 100,000 white men and 1.2 of 100,000 African American men were diagnosed with testicular cancer, with a mortality rate of 0.3 of 100,000 and 0.2 of 100,000, respectively. Unfortunately, the cause of testicular cancer is unknown. The only established relationship to testicular cancer is cryptorchidism. The good news is that testicular cancer is rare, and the 5-year survival rate by race was reported as 95.7% for white men and 88.4% for African American men.

The American Cancer Society (ACS) recommends a testicular exam by a doctor as part of a routine cancer-related check-up (ACS, 2013). Because painless testicular enlargement is commonly the first sign of testicular cancer, the testicular self-examination has traditionally been recommended for men. Some testicular cancers might not cause symptoms until they have grown and/or metastasized. However, in 2004 the U.S. Preventive Services Task Force (USPSTF) updated previously published guidelines that significantly altered that tradition for asymptomatic adolescent and adult males (USPSTF, 2004). The new guidelines state:

*The USPSTF found no new evidence that screening with clinical examination or testicular self-examination was effective in reducing mortality from testicular cancer. Even in the absence of screening, the current treatment interventions provided very favorable health outcomes. Given the low prevalence of testicular cancer, limited accuracy of screening tests, and no evidence for the incremental benefits of screening, the USPSTF concluded that the harms of screening exceeded any potential benefits.*

## Depression

More women than men are classified as having depression (6.6% and 4.4%, respectively) for all ages (Pratt and Brody, 2010). Wilhelm (2009) reported that the rates of depression vary between genders based on the type of depression. Of particular concern for men is that higher rates of depression can be found in the unemployed, socially disadvantaged, those who abuse substances, and those with more than one medical condition. There are reasons to believe that men with depression often go unrecognized and underreported. Men tend to be stoic and do not verbalize how they feel and are reluctant to talk about health issues, and men often do not have positive relationships with their health care provider.

The suicide rate is four times greater for men, although women are diagnosed twice as often with major depression. It has been suggested that this difference is due to gender bias in the criteria used to diagnose depression and suggests that men may have more difficulty recognizing or acknowledging depression "because of socially reinforced masculinity norms, including self-reliance, restrictions of emotions and toughness" (Rochlen et al, 2010, p167). Much of how gender is manifested in individuals is learned through socialization. How men manifest signs and symptoms of depression may result in low numbers of men diagnosed with depression because men are socialized to hide their feelings. Ultimately, men are seen with more incidences of avoidance behavior, anger, violence, and finally suicide. Nurses should recognize how men can manifest depression and be aware of the importance of developing a therapeutic relationship. Through the therapeutic relationship the experience of depression can be normalized, the biological and social factors in depression can be explained, and the positive outcome of depression treatment can be communicated.

## Erectile Dysfunction

Erectile dysfunction (ED), also known as impotence, is the consistent inability to achieve or maintain an erection sufficient for satisfactory sexual performance. Up to 52% of men between the ages of 40 and 70 are affected by ED and it is associated with decreased quality of life. ED can lead to withdrawal from intimacy, emotional stress, lower self-esteem, and avoidance of physical contact. The incidence of ED significantly increases with age, and 55% to 70% of men aged 77 to 79 years are sexually active (McMahon, 2014). It can occur in association with cardiovascular disease, diabetes, hypertension, hypercholesterolemia, smoking, spinal cord injury, prostate cancer, genitourinary surgery, psychiatric disorders, and the use of alcohol and drugs (Douglass and Lin, 2010).

It is now known that ED is an independent marker for increased cardiovascular disease with vascular disease of the penile arteries (Jackson and Kirby, 2014). Men with ED and no cardiac symptoms should have a thorough cardiac assessment. Lifestyle changes to reduce weight, manage hypertension and diabetes, stop smoking, reduce alcohol consumption and stress, and start exercising regularly will reduce risk.

Although ED may be discussed more openly with health care providers since the increased publicity generated from the marketing of the medications for ED, many men will still be embarrassed and reluctant to discuss the subject. A variety of treatments are available and can be discussed with the health care provider. Men who respond positively to treatment for ED report significantly better quality of life. With this evidence of positive response, health care providers should be proactive in discussing ED with men.

In summary, regardless of the prevalence differences in the health problems described in this section between men and women, appropriate health care services must be provided. Men and women need to be encouraged equally to take advantage of these services.

## HEALTH DISPARITIES AMONG SPECIAL GROUPS OF ADULTS

Health disparities present political implications and influence government actions, including the commitment of resources to address them. In the United States, the government describes health disparities as a continuing and persistent gap in health status between genders, ethnicities, economic statuses, and those who represent the majority populations (NPA, 2010). The causes are complex, but there are two major factors including inadequate access to care and substandard quality of care (NPA, 2010).

Certain groups have been recognized as experiencing health disparities and have become a priority for policy efforts. Many factors contribute to disparities in health and health care for special groups of adult men and women, including education, insurance status, segregation, immigration status, health behaviors and lifestyle choices, health care provider behavior, employment, and the nature and operation of the health system in communities (Kosoko-Lasaki et al, 2009). In particular, poverty is a strong underlying current throughout all of the special groups.

### Adults of Color

In 2000, about 33% of the U.S. population identified themselves as members of racial or ethnic minority groups. By 2050, these groups are projected to account for almost half of the U.S. population (NHDR, 2008). Improvements in preventive care, chronic care, and access to care have led to improvements to the health of some populations in areas such as mammograms and smoking cessation counseling. However, the complete picture of disparities is different for each population. For instance, non-Asian racial/ethnic minorities continue to experience higher rates of HIV diagnoses than whites. When compared with whites, a lower percentage of blacks diagnosed with HIV were prescribed antiretroviral therapy and a lower percentage of both blacks and Hispanics had suppressed viral loads (CDC Health Disparities & Inequalities Report, 2013). Diabetes prevalence is highest among non-Hispanic blacks, Hispanics, and those of mixed races (CDC Health Disparities & Inequalities Report, 2013). Although addressing these disparities appears daunting, the intent is to close the gap with regard to the health disparities in adults of color while at the same time preserving and respecting the richness and unique influences of various cultures. Population-focused nurses are positioned to advocate for culturally sensitive and gender-sensitive programs necessary in communities where adults of color may reside.

### Incarcerated Adults

Since 2000 the U.S. prison population grew at the slowest rate (0.8%) in 2008, reaching 1,610,446 sentenced prisoners (U.S. Department of Justice, Bureau of Justice Statistics, 2009). However, while this appears to be positive, it does create a challenge to nurses who will be caring for this special population in other community settings. An increase in the number of prison releases has led to offenders being released to the community without supervision. African American males were incarcerated at a rate six and one half times higher than white males. The proportion of prisoners under state or federal jurisdiction was 93% men and 7% women (Sabol et al, 2009). Women are more likely to be serving time for property and drug offenses rather than violent crimes.

Inmates have been shown to have more chronic diseases such as hypertension, diabetes, asthma, chronic liver disease, and HIV than the general population (Kulkarni et al, 2010). Upon release from correctional institutions, ex-offenders face interruptions in their medical care stemming from limited resources, limited ability to access health care, and a lack of adequate discharge planning (Wang et al, 2008; Kulkarni et al, 2010).

Over the past 40 years, legal, social, and political factors have led to the current epidemic of psychiatric disorders in the U.S. prison system. Incarcerated populations with major psychiatric disorders (major depressive disorder, bipolar disorders, schizophrenia, and non-schizophrenic psychotic disorders) have a substantially increased risk of multiple incarcerations. The greatest increase may be among inmates with bipolar disorders (Baillargeon et al, 2009). Nurses can support and deliver beneficial continuity of care reentry programs to help those who are mentally ill connect with community-based mental health programs at the time of release from prison to decrease recidivism rates (Baillargeon et al, 2009).

## Lesbian/Gay/Bisexual Adults

Lesbian/gay/bisexual (LGB) adults represent a sometimes hidden special population, in part because of the social stigma associated with homosexuality coupled with the fear of discrimination. Several studies have documented health disparities by sexual orientation in population-based data and have revealed differences in health between LGB adults and their heterosexual counterparts, including higher risks of poor mental health, smoking, higher risk of disability, and excessive drinking (Dilley et al, 2010; Conron et al, 2010; Fredriksen-Goldsen et al, 2013) To improve the health of lesbian/gay/bisexual adults, services that address their unique needs are warranted. Safe places where this special population can voice their concerns and receive effective health promotion, disease prevention, and treatment are critical. Clarification of ways in which sexual orientation is associated with health outcomes will be critical to developing appropriate health interventions (Bostwick et al, 2010).

## Adults with Physical and Mental Disabilities

Many issues confront adults with disabilities. Concerns associated with health, aging, civil rights, abuse, and independent living are but a few examples of the types of problems facing this population. In 2007, 69 million adults 18 years of age and over had either basic actions difficulty (including movement or emotional difficulty or trouble seeing or hearing) or complex activity limitation (such as work or self-care limitations). This was an increase by 8 million over the past 10 years. One quarter of adults 18 to 64 years of age had at least one basic actions difficulty or complex activity limitation in 2007, compared with 62% of adults 65 years of age and over (NCHS, 2009).

Adults with lifelong disabilities are more likely to have chronic conditions and multiple comorbidities than adults with no limitations (Dixon-Ibarra and Horner-Johnson, 2014). For instance, adults with developmental disabilities may be at a high risk for obesity and its sequelae (Bazzano et al, 2009). This may be due to individual and community factors including physical challenges, cognitive limitations, medications, lack of accessible adaptive fitness facilities, and segregation from the community in general. A community-based health intervention program called "The Healthy Lifestyle Change Program" targeted adults with developmental disabilities. This program used a twice-weekly education and exercise program to increase knowledge, skills, and self-efficacy regarding health, nutrition, and fitness with peer mentors serving as participatory leaders and motivators. Outcomes were improved lifestyles, weight loss success, and increased life satisfaction (Bazzano et al, 2009).

Nurses can develop an awareness of the many health-related issues facing adults with disabilities. In particular, care should be taken to recognize the physical barriers that prevent disabled adults from accessing health care, such as structures that are not accessible despite the ADA recommendations. Developing health promotion programs targeted at this vulnerable, high-risk group can assist in overall well-being.

## Impoverished and Uninsured Adults

According to the Stanford Center on Poverty and Inequity's *National Report Card*, the official poverty rate increased from 12.5 in 2007 to 15.0 percent in 2012 and the child poverty rate increased from 18.0 percent in 2007 to 21.8 percent in 2012 (Danziger and Wimer, 2014). Poverty affects acute and chronic conditions, accumulates over the life course, and is transmitted across generations. It limits education and employment opportunities, leaving individuals susceptible to weaker social integration, low control, depressive symptoms, and often a fatalistic outlook (Sanders et al, 2008). Often the stress of poverty may lead to poor dietary habits, tobacco use, and inconsistent personal hygiene. Health disparities, including chronic illness and health care services, are consistently associated with socioeconomic differences. The vulnerable homeless, impoverished rural, migrant, and public housing communities suffer from an increased burden of disease and greater morbidity and mortality than the general population (Custodio et al, 2009).

Adults who are insured will access health care services more often, including obtaining recommended screening and care for chronic conditions, thus reducing the overall costs of potential catastrophic illness (Wilper et al, 2009). Although President Obama signed the Patient Protection and Affordable Care Act along with the Health Care and Education Reconciliation Act in March 2010 (United States Congress, Public Law 111-148, 2010), many changes such as health insurance mandates did not begin until 2014. The Rand Corporation reported that by March 2014:

> *Overall, we estimate that 9.3 million more people had health care coverage in March 2014, lowering the uninsured rate from 20.5 percent to 15.8 percent. This increase in coverage is driven not only by enrollment in health insurance marketplace plans, but also by gains in employer-sponsored insurance and Medicaid. Enrollment in employer-sponsored insurance plans increased by 8.2 million and Medicaid enrollment increased by 5.9 million, although some individuals did lose coverage during this period. The authors also found that 3.9 million people are now covered through the state and federal marketplaces and less than 1 million people who previously had individual-market insurance became uninsured during the period in question. While the survey cannot tell if this latter group lost their insurance due to cancellation or because they simply felt the cost was too high, the overall number is very small, representing less than 1 percent of people between the ages of 18 and 64 (Carman and Eibner, 2014).*

Under the Affordable Care Act (ACA), states can extend Medicaid eligibility to nearly all adults with income no more than 138% of the federal poverty level. However, compared with adults who were already enrolled in Medicaid prior to the ACA, a substantial proportion of uninsured adults with chronic conditions do not have good disease control and may require intensive medical care following Medicare enrollment (Decker et al, 2013).

Nurses can be uniquely involved in community assessments to document pockets of poverty within their communities. For example, housing is a fundamental determinant of health and provides shelter and privacy. Exposure to cracks in ceilings and walls, inadequate heat, mold, poor ventilation, pesticide residue, excessive moisture, leaky pipes, and lead paint are all health hazards that can be addressed by nurses. Recent research has also found that health resilience to poverty was supported by protective factors in built and social environments. (See Chapter 29 for discussion of the built environment.) When poverty itself cannot be eliminated, improving the quality of the built and social environments can foster resilience to the harmful effects of poverty (Sanders et al, 2008).

## Frail Elderly

In the past decade, the United States experienced a 15% increase in the population 65 years of age and older. By 2020, this group is expected to increase another 36% (A Profile of Older Americans, 2009). In addition, the population of those 85 years and older is projected to increase another 15% by 2020. Most older persons have at least one chronic condition and many have multiple conditions, putting them at risk of experiencing frailty while living in a community setting.

Frailty is a geriatric syndrome that places older adults at risk for adverse health outcomes, including falls, worsening disability, institutionalization, and death (Espinoza and Hazuda, 2008). It is a complex state of impairment that signifies loss in areas of physical functioning, physiological resiliency, metabolism, and immune response (Hackstaff, 2009).

The prevalence of frail elderly in the population poses a major public health dilemma since the majority of this group will reside in a community setting, placing new demands on health care systems, family caregivers, and community resources. To improve the health of frail elderly, community-based nursing programs will need to address racial/ethnic and socioeconomic disparities.

The elder-friendly community model identifies four domains needed by the elderly, including having basic needs met, social and civic engagement, physical and mental health and well-being, and independence for the frail and disabled (Feldman and Oberlink, 2003). This model identifies independence for the frail elderly as the ability to "age in place" with specific indicators that focus on activities of daily living, transportation, and caregivers' ability to complement formal services. Community-level characteristics, including security issues, accessible shopping, and adequate transportation services are important community resources (Weierbach and Glick, 2009). Nurses can use this model to incorporate both individual and community factors that are necessary for elderly to live and thrive in community settings.

## COMMUNITY-BASED MODELS FOR CARE OF ADULTS
### Nursing Roles

Communities are where people live, work, and socialize. Community health settings include public health departments, nurse-managed health centers, ambulatory care clinics, and home health agencies. Nurses are involved in direct care, providing self-care information, contributing to the supervision of paraprofessionals, or collaborating with other disciplines to provide the most appropriate, high-quality, cost-effective care at the most appropriate level and location.

Knowledge of community resources is a fundamental part of caring for the adult with special needs in any community. The nurse assesses the need for and helps develop the resources. Every community has an area agency on aging that coordinates planning and delivery of needed services, and it can be a good resource for the nurse. Most communities have information and referral systems as well as a public directory of services available.

The complex nature of chronic illness with care focused primarily on maximizing functional status and well-being is particularly suited to nursing's holistic focus (Lupari et al, 2011). The Doctor of Nursing Practice (DNP) role brings specific competencies and nursing backgrounds to the role of primary care provider. A recent community-based model to provide care for frail elders highlights three areas of expertise that advanced practice nurses in the DNP role can provide: management of complex chronic illness, illness and injury prevention, and promotion of quality of life (Auer and Nirenberg, 2008).

### Community Care Settings
#### Patient-Centered Medical Homes

A traditional part of community care for adults with chronic illness is the use of primary care practices. Health care systems with a primary care focus have better outcomes, including better quality, lower costs, less inequality in health care and health, and better population health when compared with systems based on other approaches to health care. The patient-centered medical home (PCMH) moves beyond primary care to include new approaches to organizing practice to enhance its responsiveness to individual patient needs (Stange et al, 2010). The following are established basic tenets for the concept of PCMH:

1. A relationship between the patient and medical provider
2. A provider who takes charge of total patient care, including arrangements for specialty care
3. Open access to health care
4. Ongoing care managed by the same provider to assure coordination and collaboration
5. Quality and safety as key aspects of the system
6. Transparent and fair payment (Rittenhouse and Shortell, 2009)

For patients with chronic illnesses, one approach to PCMH is to include physician assistants (PAs) and nurse practitioners (NPs) on primary care teams. This approach has demonstrated positive outcomes in the measure of quality of diabetes care and use of health care services (Everett et al, 2013).

## Senior Centers

Senior centers were developed in the early 1940s to provide social and recreational activities. Now many centers are multipurpose, offering recreation, education, counseling, therapies, hot meals, and case management, as well as health screening and education. Some even offer primary care services. Nurses have a unique opportunity to provide services to a group of older persons who wish to remain independent in the community (Weierbach and Glick, 2009; Truncali et al, 2010).

## Adult Day Health

Adult day health is for individuals whose mental or physical function requires them to obtain more health care and supervision. It serves as more of a medical model than the senior center, and often individuals return home to their caregivers at night. Some settings offer respite care for short-term overnight relief for caregivers. This provides caregivers the opportunity to work or have personal time during the day. Support groups for caregivers may be offered by nurses.

## Home Health, Palliative Care, and Hospice

Home health can be provided by multidisciplinary teams. Nurses provide individual and environmental assessments, direct skilled care and treatment, and provide short-term guidance and instruction. Nurses often function independently in the home and must rely on their own resources and knowledge to improvise and adapt care to meet the client's unique physical and social circumstances. They work closely with the family and other caregivers to provide necessary communication and continuity of care. (See Chapter 41 for more details.)

Palliative care is the broad term used to describe the care provided by an interdisciplinary team consisting of physicians, nurses, social workers, chaplains, and other health care professionals. Coyle (2010) describes the distinctive features of palliative care nursing as "a whole person" philosophy of care. This care is provided across a continuum of different settings, including the life span, the illness trajectory, the patient's death, and the family's bereavement. Often, the terms *hospice* and *palliative care* are used interchangeably. Palliative care is a broader concept and includes the entire continuum of care. Hospice care is always palliative care, but not all palliative care is hospice care (Coyle, 2010).

Hospice represents a philosophy of caring for and supporting life to its fullest until death occurs. The hospice team encourages the client and family to jointly make decisions to meet physical, emotional, spiritual, and comfort needs (see palliative care in the Content Resources section of the Evolve website).

## Assisted Living

Assisted living covers a wide variety of choices, from a single shared room to opulent independent living accommodations in a full-service, life-care community. The differences are related to the type and extent of the amenities provided and the contract signed for them. The role of the nurse varies depending on the philosophy and leadership of the management of the facility. The nurse generally provides assessment and interventions, medication review, education, and advocacy (Counsell et al, 2006; Auer and Nirenberg, 2008).

## Long-Term Care and Rehabilitation

Nursing homes, or long-term care facilities, house only about 5% of the older population at a given time; however, 25% of those adults older than 65 will spend some time in a nursing home. Nursing homes provide a safe environment, special diets and activities, routine personal care, and the treatment and management of health care needs for those needing rehabilitation, as well as for those needing a permanent supportive residence. Rehabilitation is a combination of physical, occupational, psychological, and speech therapy to help debilitated persons maintain or recover their physical capacities. **Rehabilitation** is typically needed for older adults after a hip fracture, stroke, or prolonged illness that results in serious deconditioning (Olsson et al, 2009).

Like hospitals, nursing homes are paid using the prospective payment model based on the nursing assessment. A recent new model developed by nurse practitioners used collaborative practice techniques to change care management for frail and elderly nursing home residents, which reduced hospitalizations by 45%, reduced emergency room visits by 50%, and effectively reduced the incidence of acute episodes in the nursing home setting (Kappas-Larson, 2008).

 **LINKING CONTENT TO PRACTICE**

The information in this chapter focuses on the health issues of adult and older adult men and women from a population perspective as opposed to the individual or family. In practice, the knowledge, skills, and attitudes, such as those identified by the Quad Council for Public Health Nursing, transcend other public health disciplines. Therefore, nurses practicing in community health need to foster the ability to work effectively with interprofessional teams across a variety of organizations to accomplish goals to improve community health. Working in interprofessional teams is a core competency identified by the Institute of Medicine (IOM) and involves essential features such as "sections related to self, team, team communication and conflict resolution, effect of team on safety and quality, and the impact of systems on team functioning" (Cronenwett et al, 2007, p. 123).

## PRACTICE APPLICATION

During her community clinical time in nursing education, Laura had the opportunity to accompany Marie, her preceptor, on an initial home visit to a young woman named Josie. Josie was a 20-year-old single woman who had come to the public health center last week for a gynecological examination because she thought she might have some sort of infection. During the visit, Josie mentioned to the clinic nurse that she did not have any food in her house. After the examination the clinic nurse made a referral to the women's resource service center for a home visit and for inclusion of Josie into their case management program.

When Marie and Laura arrived at Josie's apartment, they immediately noted that the living areas were devoid of furniture; however, there was a soiled mattress on the floor of the living room. Dirty clothing was on the floor; empty take-out food sacks and trash littered the area. The kitchen area was also dirty, with evidence of cockroach infestation.

Marie and Laura noticed that Josie appeared to be uncomfortable and had difficulty interacting with either of them. Marie explained that they were there because the nurse at the clinic had asked them to stop by and see if there was any way that they might help Josie with her health care needs and living situation. Immediately Josie began to cry. She had been with her abusive boyfriend until about 3 weeks ago when she asked him to leave. Marie and Laura learned that since that time, Josie had been prostituting as a way to survive. She was frightened and thought that her boyfriend was going to return and harm her. She also feared that she was pregnant.

Based on this situation, what would be potential actions that Laura and her preceptor Marie might take?

A. Make an appointment for Josie to return to the women's clinic for pregnancy testing.

B. Suggest to Josie that she focus on cleaning up her apartment, reminding her of the hazards of spoiled food.

C. Refer Josie to a safe-house shelter as a victim of domestic violence.

D. Make a referral for food delivery from a local church.

**Answers are in the back of the book.**

The nurse in a local public health department talks with the director of the department, who needs to determine what major public health issues exist in the community and prioritize them to better allocate resources. The director formed a committee to assist in this process. The director asks the nurse to participate on the committee because of the nurse's interest in men's health. The director asks the nurse to identify up to 10 major health issues in the community, prioritize them, and recommend strategies to improve men's health in the community. The director wants a report supporting conclusions and strategies that the department could implement.

Based on the previous scenario, answer the following questions:

A. What information do you want to collect?

B. How would you identify priorities in your area?

C. What positive and negative factors may be influencing these issues?

D. How would you select strategies to improve health issues?

  1. What interventions, if any, are currently being used, and are they effective?

  2. Who are the key participants that would need to be involved in improving the issues?

  3. Have these issues been addressed effectively in other communities? If they have, what have they done?

**Answers can be found on the Evolve site.**

## KEY POINTS

- The health of adults is embedded in their communities.
- Societal factors influence the distribution of health and disease.

- Women's health advocates have widened the framework of women's health by focusing on social, psychological, cultural, political, and economic as well as biological factors.

## KEY POINTS—cont'd

- The complexities of women's lives—their educational levels, income, culture, ethnicity/race, and a host of other identities and experiences—shape their health.
- The Office on Women's Health (OWH) works to address inequities in research, health services, and education that have traditionally placed women at risk for health problems.
- The problem of unintended pregnancy exists among adolescents as well as adult women.
- Women's attitudes toward menopause vary greatly and are influenced by culture, age, support, and the shared experiences of other women.
- Cardiovascular disease (CVD) is the leading cause of death among U.S. adults.
- Diabetes has increased dramatically in the United States during the last decade.
- Women in the United States experience depression at higher rates than do men.
- Overall, white women have a higher incidence rate for all cancers while African American women have higher mortality rates.
- Most U.S. women contract HIV/AIDS by heterosexual transmission.
- The Bureau of Justice reports a dramatic rise in the number of women in state and federal prisons.
- Research findings indicate that lesbians and bisexual women have higher prevalence rates of several risk factors than their heterosexual counterparts with regard to smoking, alcohol use, and lack of preventative cancer screening.
- Poverty among female heads of household reflects the disparities that exist in the United States among various ethnic/racial groups because female-headed African American and Hispanic families suffer disproportionately higher rates of poverty than do other families.
- Research shows that older women, especially women of color from lower socioeconomic groups, experience higher rates of chronic illness and disability than their white and more affluent counterparts.
- One out of every two American women more than 50 years of age will experience an osteoporosis-related fracture in her lifetime.
- Men are reluctant to seek health care and are not well connected to the health care system.
- Large numbers of men do not receive the health screenings intended to prevent and identify disease.
- To improve health outcomes for men, chronic disease prevention and control programs should combine individual and population-based strategies developed in collaboration with community members and developing infrastructure to address environmental and policy change.
- Although adverse working conditions and numerous pathological conditions clearly are detrimental to men's health, there is a great need to focus on the mental health of men.
- The nurse acts as a change agent to assess needs and system influences, identify and set priorities, plan and implement programs, and evaluate results.

## CLINICAL DECISION-MAKING ACTIVITIES

1. Interview three women, each from a different culture, about their experiences accessing health care. Are there differences in their stories about how they meet their health care needs? Do variances in ethnicity and culture present barriers to accessing health care?
2. Review current legislation that deals with women's health. Note patterns or trends in the issues that are being considered by the Senate or the House of Representatives. Are there obvious gaps in legislation that adversely affect women's health?
3. Considering breast cancer, apply the levels of prevention to women in underserved areas. Describe approaches to meeting their health care, social needs, and psychological needs. What barriers might prevent an effective program addressing breast cancer?
4. Contact your local public health office to determine what services are available for women. Identify community resources and agencies targeted for women. How do these organizations communicate their services to women in the community?
5. Propose a community-based intervention for women with HIV. Describe various program components such as goals and objectives, evaluation methods, and program outcomes.
6. Identify a men's health issue in your community. Contact local health agencies in your area to determine what strategies are currently in place to address the issue.
7. Based on the issue identified in question 6, search the Internet for evidence-based practices related to the issue.
8. Think about television, movie, or magazine portrayals of men and identify both positive and negative influences the media may have on men's health.
9. Locate several websites focusing on men's health topics. Using criteria for credible websites from Health on the Net Foundation (www.hon.ch), evaluate those sites for credible health information.

# REFERENCES

"Administration on Aging" long term care ombudsman program complaint codes, nd, Retrieved from: WWW.aoa.gov. 9/11/2014.

Administration on Aging: About AoA, 2010. Retrieved from: WWW.aoa.gov. 9/11/2014.

Agency for Healthcare Research and Quality: Men shy away from routine medical appointments, AHRQ News and Numbers, 2010. Retrieved from: http://www.ahrq.gov. 9/11/2014.

Ahn S, Basu R, Smith ML, et al: The impact of chronic disease self-management programs: healthcare savings through a community-based intervention. *BMC Public Health* 13:1141, 2013. doi: 10.1186/1471-2458-13-1141.

Alexander LL, LaRosa JH, Bader H, et al: *New Dimensions in Women's Health*, ed 4. Boston, 2007, Jones and Bartlett.

American Cancer Society: Do I have Testicular Cancer? 2013. Retrieved from: http://www.cancer.org/cancer/testicularcancer/moreinformation/doihavetesticularcancer/do-i-have-testicular-cancer-self-exam.9/11/2014.

American Cancer Society: *Cancer Facts and Figures 2014*, Atlanta, 2014a, ACS. Retrieved from: http://www.cancer.org. 9/11/2014.

American Cancer Society: Prostate Cancer Overview, 2014b. Retrieved from: http://www.cancer.org/Cancer/ProstateCancer/OverviewGuide/prostate-cancer-overview-what-causes. 9/11/2014.

American Heart Association: Overweight and Obesity Statistics, 2007. Retrieved from: http://grfw.org/presenter.jhtml?identifier=30009479/11/2014.

American Heart Association: Women, Heart Disease, and Stroke, 2010. Retrieved from: www.americanheart.org. 9/11/2014.

Aministration for Children and Families: About ACF, nd, Retrieved from: www.acf.hhs.gov. on 9/11/2014.

Americans with Disabilities Act of 1990, as amended with ADA Amendments Act of 2008, (n.d.). Retrieved from: http://www.ada.gov/pubs/adastatute08.htm. 9/11/2014.

Auer P, Nirenberg A: Nurse practitioner home-based primary care: a model for the care of frail elders. *Clin Schol Rev* 1(1):33–39, 2008.

Baillargeon J, Binswanger I, Penn J, et al: Psychiatric disorders and repeat incarcerations: the revolving prison door. *Am J Psychiatry* 166(1):103–109, 2009.

Bazzano A, Zeldin A, Diab I, et al: The Healthy Lifestyle Change Program: a pilot of a community-based health promotion intervention for adults with developmental disabilities. *Am J Prev Med* 37(6S1):S201-S208, 2009.

Benz J, Espinosa O, Welsh V, et al: Awareness of racial and ethnic health disparities has improved only modestly over a decade. *Health Aff* 30:1860–1867, 2011.

Berdahl T, Zodet M: Medical care utilization for work-related injuries in the United States 2002-2006. *Med Care* 48(7):645–651, 2010.

Bos A, Kanner D, Muris P, et al: Mental illness stigma and disclosure: consequences of coming out of the closet. *Issues Ment Health Nurs* 30:509–513, 2009.

Bostwick W, Boyd C, Hughes T, et al: Dimensions of sexual orientation and the prevalence of mood and anxiety disorders in the United States. *Am J Public Health* 100(3):468–475, 2010.

Broom A, Tovey P: *Men's Health: Body, Identity and Social Context*, West Sussex, England, 2009, Wiley-Blackwell.

Brownson R, Chriqui J, Stamatakis K: Policy, politics, and collective action. *Am J Public Health* 99(9):1576–1582, 2009.

Brownstein J, Mirambeau A, Roland K: News from the CDC: Using web-based training to translate evidence on the value of community health workers into public action. *Transl Behav Med* 3(3):229–230, 2013. doi: 10.1007/s13142-013-0204-5.

Buck H, Fahlberg B: Using POLST to ensure patient's treatment preferences. *Nursing* 44(3):16–17, 2014.

Cannon M, Dominique Y, O'Leary L, et al: Characteristics and behaviors of mothers who have a child with fetal alcohol syndrome. *Neurotoxicol Teratol* 34(1):90–95, 2012.

Carman K, Eibner C: Changes in Health Insurance Enrollment Since 2013: Evidence from the RAND Health Reform Opinion Study, Rand Corporation Research Reports, 2014. Retrieved from: http://www.rand.org/content/dam/rand/pubs/research_reports/RR600/RR656/RAND_RR656.pdf9/11/2014.

Centers for Disease Control and Prevention: The Futures Initiatives, 2005. Retrieved from: http://www.cdc.gov/futures/9/11/2014.

Centers for Disease Control and Prevention: Chronic Disease Prevention and Health Promotion, 2007. Retrieved from: http://www.cdc.gov/chronicdisease/overview/index.htm9/11/2014.

Centers for Disease Control and Prevention: Sexually Transmitted Disease in the United States, 2008. Retrieved from: http://www.cdc.gov/std/stats08/trends.htm. 9/11/2014.

Centers for Disease Control and Prevention: National Center for Environmental Health, 2009. Retrieved from: http://www.cdc.gov/nceh/ehhe/about.htm. 9/11/2014.

Centers for Disease Control and Prevention: CDC Fact Sheet: The Role of STD Prevention and Treatment in HIV Prevention, 2010. Retrieved from: http://www.cdc.gov/std/hiv/stds-and-hiv-fact-sheet-press.pdf. 9/11/2014.

Centers for Disease Control and Prevention: *National Diabetes Fact Sheet: National Estimates and General Information on Diabetes in the United States, 2011*, Atlanta, GA, 2011, USDHHS, CDC. Retrieved from: http://www.cdc.gov/diabetes/pubs/factsheet11.htm. 9/11/2014.

Centers for Disease Control and Prevention: *Diabetes Report Card 2012*, Atlanta, GA, 2012a, Centers for Disease Control and Prevention, U.S. Department of Health and Human Services. Retrieved from: http://www.cdc.gov/diabetes/pubs/pdf/diabetesreportcard.pdf. 9/11/2014.

Centers for Disease Control and Prevention: National Center on Birth Defects and Developmental Disabilities Annual Report, 2012b, USDHHS, CDC. Retrieved from: http://www.cdc.gov/ncbddd/aboutus/annualreport2012/index.html9/11/2014.

Centers for Disease Control and Prevention: Health Disparities and Inequalities Report, 2013, USDHHS, CDC. Retrieved from: http://www.cdc.gov/mmwr/preview/ind2013_su.html#HealthDisparities2013. 9/11/2014.

Centers for Disease Control and Prevention: HIV in the United States: At a Glance, 2013. Retrieved from: http://www.cdc.gov/hiv/pdf/statistics_basics_factsheet.pdf. 9/11/2014.

Clougherty JE: A growing role for gender analysis in air pollution epidemiology. *Environ Health Perspect* 118(2):167–175, 2010.

Community Health Status Indicators Report, 2009, USDHHS. Retrieved from: http://www.cdc.gov/CommunityHealth/homepage.aspx?j=1. 9/11/2014.

Conron K, Mimiaga M, Landers S: A population-based study of sexual orientation identity and gender differences in adult health. *Am J Public Health* 100(1):1953–1960, 2010.

Counsell S, Callahan C, Buttar A, et al: Geriatric Resources for Assessment and Care of Elders (GRACE): a new model of primary care for low income senior. *J Am Geriatr Soc* 54(7):1136–1141, 2006.

Coyle N: Introduction to palliative nursing care. In Ferrel BR, Coyle N, editors: *Textbook of Palliative Nursing*, ed 3. Oxford, UK, 2010, Oxford University Press, pp 3–11.

Cronenwett L, Sherwood G, Barnsteiner J, et al: Quality and safety education for nurses. *Nurs Outlook* 55:122–131, 2007.

Custodio R, Gard A, Graham G: Health information technology: addressing health disparity by improving quality, increasing access, and developing workforce. *J Health Care Poor Underserved* 20:301–307, 2009.

Danielsson U, Bengs C, Lehti A, et al: Struck by lightning or slowly suffocating-gender trajectories into depression. *BMC Fam Pract* 10:56, 2009. doi: 10.1186/1471-2296-10-56.

Danziger S, Wimer C: Poverty. The Stanford Center on Poverty and Inequality: National Report Card, 2014. Retrieved from: http://web.stanford.edu/group/scspi/sotu/SOTU_2014_CPI.pdf. 9/11/2014.

Decker S, Kostova D, Kenney G, et al: Health status, risk factors, and medical conditions among persons enrolled in Medicaid vs. uninsured low-income adults potentially eligible for Medicaid under the Affordable Care Act. *JAMA* 309(24):2579–2586, 2013. doi: 10.1001/jama.2013.7106.

Dilley J, Simmons K, Boysun M, et al: Demonstrating the importance and feasibility of including sexual orientation in public health surveys: health disparities in the Pacific Northwest. *Am J Public Health* 100(3):460–467, 2010.

Dixon-Ibarra A, Horner-Johnson W: Disability status as an antecedent to chronic conditions: National Health Interview Survey, 2006-2012. *Prev Chronic Dis* 11:130251, 2014. doi: 10.5888/pcd11.130251.

Douglass M, Lin J: Erectile dysfunction and premature ejaculation: underlying causes and available treatments. *Formul J* 45:17–45, 2010.

Edwards BK, Ward E, Kohler BA, et al: Annual report to the nation on the status of cancer, 1975-2006, featuring colorectal cancer trends and impact of interventions (risk factors, screening, and treatment) to reduce stress. *Cancer* 16(3):544–573, 2009. Retrieved from: http://www3.interscience

.wiley.com/cgi-bin/fulltext/12320 6036/HTMLSTART. 9/11/2014.

Egger G: In search of germ theory equivalent for chronic disease. *Prev Chronic Dis* 9:110301, 2012. doi: http://dx.doi.org/10.5888/pcd9.110301.

Espinoza S, Hazuda H: Frailty in older Mexican-American and European-American Adults: is there an ethnic disparity?. *J Am Geriatr Soc* 56:1744–1749, 2008.

Everett C, Thorpe C, Palta M, et al: Physician assistants and nurse practitioners perform effectives roles on team caring for medicare patients with diabetes. *Health Aff* 32(11):1942–1948, 2013. doi: 10.1377/hlthaff.2013.0506.

Feldman P, Oberlink M: The advantage initiative: developing community indicators to promote the health and well-being of older people. *Fam Community Health* 26:268–274, 2003.

Fernández-Sáez J, Ruiz-Cantero MT, Guijarro-Garí M, et al: Looking twice at the gender equity index for public health impact. *BMC Public Health* 13(1):1–10, 2013. doi: 10.1186/1471-2458-13-659.

Finkelstein EA, Trogdon JG, Cohen JW, et al: Annual medical spending attributable to obesity: payer- and service-specific estimates. *Health Aff* 28(5):s822–s831, 2009.

Forchuk C, Jensen E, Csiernik R, et al: Exploring differences between community-based women and men with a history of mental illness. *Issues Ment Health Nurs* 30:495–502, 2009.

Fredriksen-Goldsen K, Kim H, Barkan S, et al: Health disparities among lesbian, gay, and bisexual older adults: Results from a population-based study. *Am J Public Health* 103(10):1802–1809, 2013. doi: 10.2105/AJPH.2012.301110.

Giorgianni S, Porche D, Williams S, et al: Developing the discipline and practice of comprehensive men's health. *Am J Mens Health* 7(4):342–349, 2013. doi: 10.1177/1557988313478649.

Go AS, Mozaffarian D, Roger VL, et al: Heart disease and stroke statistics—2014 update: a report from the American Heart Association. *Circulation* 129:399–410, 2014. doi: 10.1161/01. cir.0000442015.53336.12.

Guy M: American Political Science Association 2013 annual meeting. Retrieved April 13, 2014, from: http://ssrn.com/abstract= 2300429.

Hackstaff L: Factors associated with frailty in chronically ill older adults. *Soc Work Health Care* 48:798–811, 2009.

Heron M, Hoyert D, Murphy S, et al: Deaths: final data for 2006. *Natl Vital Stat Rep* 57(14), 2009. Retrieved from: http://www.cdc

.gov/nchs/data/nvsr/nvsr57/ nvsr57_14.pdf. 9/11/2014.

Hoover R, Polson M: Detecting elder abuse and neglect: Assessment and intervention. *Am Fam Physician* 89(6):453–460, 2014.

Innes KE, Selfe TK, Vishnu A: Mind-body therapies for menopausal symptoms: a systematic review. *Maturitas* 66(2):135–149, 2010.

Jackson G, Kirby M: Erectile dysfunction increases cardiovascular risk: time to reduce it. *Trends Urol Men's Health* 5(1):28–30, 2014.

Kappas-Larson P: The evercare story: reshaping the health care model, revolutionizing long-term care. *J Nurs Pract* 4(2):132–136, 2008.

Kindig D, Cheng E: Even as mortality fell in most US counties, female mortality nonetheless rose in 42.8 percent of counties from 1992 to 2006. *Health Aff* 32(3):451–458, 2013.

Koh HK, Brach C, Harris LM, et al: A proposed 'Health Literate Care Model' would constitute a systems approach to improving patients' engagement in care. *Health Aff* 32(2):357–367, 2013.

Kominski G, editor: *Changing the U.S. Health Care System: Key Issues in Health Services Policy and Management*, San Francisco, CA, 2014, Jossey-Bass.

Konecny T, Kara T, Somers K: Obstructive sleep apnea and hypertension: An update. *Hypertension* (63):203–209, 2014.

Kosoko-Lasaki S, Cook C, O'Brien R: *Cultural Proficiency in Addressing Health Disparities*, Sudbury, MA, 2009, Jones and Bartlett.

Kulkarni S, Baldwin S, Lightstone A, et al: Is incarceration a contributor to health disparities? Access to care of formerly incarcerated adults. *J Community Health* 35:268–274, 2010. doi: 10.1007/ s10900-010-9234-9.

Lupari M, Coates V, Adamson G, et al: "We're just not getting it right": How should we provide care to the older person with multi-morbid chronic conditions. *J Clin Nurs* 20:1225–1235, 2011.

McMahon C: Erectile dysfunction. *Intern Med J* 44(1):18–26, 2014. doi: 10.1111/imj.12325.

Meyer P, Penman-Aguilar A, Campbell V, et al: Conclusion and future directions: CDC Health Disparities and Inequalities Report. *MMWR Surveill Summ* 62(03):184–186, 2013.

NIMH: What are eating disorders? USDHHS, National Institutes of Health, 2014. Rockville, MD.

Model Elements: Improving Chronic Illness Care, 2014. Available at: http://www.improvingchroniccare .org/index.php?p=Model_Elements &s=18. Accessed October 2, 2014.

Morbidity and Mortality Weekly Report: Center for Disease Control and Prevention. Life expectancy ranking at birth, by sex: selected countries and territories, 2008. Retrieved from: http:// www.cdc.gov/mmwr/preview/ mmwrhtml/mm5713a8.htm. 9/11/2014.

Mosca L, Hammond G, Mochari-Greenberger H, et al: Fifteen-year trends in awareness of heart disease in women: results of a 2012 American Heart Association national survey. *Circulation* 127:1254–1263, 2013.

Mosca L, Mochari-Greenberger H, Dolar R, et al: Twelve-year follow-up of American women's awareness of cardiovascular disease risk and barriers to heart health. *Circ Cardiovasc Qual Outcomes* 3(2):120–127, 2010.

National Cancer Institute: 2014a. Prostate cancer. Available at: http:// seer.cancer.gov/statfacts/html/prost .html. Accessed October 01, 2014.

National Cancer Institute: 2014b. Breast cancer. Available at: http://www .cancer.gov/cancertopics/types/ breast. Accessed October 2, 2014.

National Center for Chronic Disease Prevention and Health Promotion (NCCDPHP): Health Risk Factors That Cause Chronic Disease, 2014. Retrieved from: http:// www.cdc.gov/chronicdisease/ overview/. 9/11/2014.

National Center for Complementary and Alternative Medicine: Get the Facts, Menopausal Symptoms and Complimentary Health Practices, 2012. Available at: http:// nccam.nih.gov/health/menopause/ menopausesymptoms. Accessed October 2, 2014.

National Center for Elder Abuse: Why should I care about elder abuse? Nd Retrieved from: www.ncea.aoa.gov.9/11/2014.

National Center for Health Statistics (NCHS): *Health, United States, 2009: With Special Feature on Medical Technology*, Hyattsville, MD, 2009, us govt printing office Wash DC.

National Healthcare Disparities Report: AHRQ Publication No. 09-0002, 2008, USDHHS. Retrieved from: www.ahrq.gov/qual/qrdr08.htm.

National Institute on Aging: Hormones and Menopause, 2014. Available at: http://www.nia.nih.gov/health/ publication/hormones-and-menopause#what. Accessed October 2, 2014.

National Institute of Arthritis and Musculoskeletal and Skin Diseases: *Osteoporosis*, 2014. Available at: http://www.niams.nih.gov/Health _Info/Osteoporosis/default.asp#10. Accessed October 2, 2014.

National Institutes of Health: Overweight and obesity statistics, *National Institutes of Health* WIN: 2008. Available at: http://win.niddk.

nih.gov/Publications/tools.htm#body massindex. Accessed February 22, 2011.

National Osteoporosis Foundation: *Clinician's Guide to Prevention and Treatment of Osteoporosis*, Washington, DC, 2014. National osteoprosis foundation. Retrieved from: http://www.nof.org/ professionals/pdfs/NOF_ ClinicianGuide2009_v7.pdf. 9/11/2014.

National Institute of Mental Health: What Are Eating Disorders? USDHHS. *National Institutes of Health*, 2014. Rockville, MD.

National Partnership for Action (NPA): Office of Minority Health, Health Disparities, 2010. Retrieved from: http://minorityhealth.hhs.gov/. 9/11/2014.

Olsson L, Hansson E, Ekman I, et al: A cost-effective study of a patient-centered integrated care pathway. *J Adv Nurs* 65(8):1626–1635, 2009.

Ory MG, Smith ML, Kulinski KP, et al: Self-management at the tipping point: Reaching 1000,000 Americans with evidence-based programs. *J Am Geriatr Soc* 61(5):821–823, 2013.

Pearlman R, Starks H, Cain K, et al: Your Life Your Choices: Planning for Future Medical Decisions: How To Prepare a Personalized Living Will, 2010. Retrieved from: http:// books.google.com/books?id=ECKSr 69RNuEC&lpg=PP1&dq=inauthor% 3A%22Robert%20Pearlman%22&p g=PP2#v=onepage&q&f=false. 9/11/2014.

Pratt LA, Brody DJ: Depression and smoking in the US Household population, Aged 20 and over 2005-2008, 2010. Retrieved from: www.cdc.gov. 9/11/2014.

A Profile of Older Americans: Administration on Aging, 2009, USDHHS. Retrieved from: http:// www.aoa.gov/AoARoot/Aging_ Statistics/Profile/2009/docs/2009 profile_508.pdf. 9/11/2014.

Women's health. Report of the Public Health Services task for on women's health issues. *Public Health Rep* 100(1):73–106 , 1985.

Ressler P, Glazer G: Legislative: Nursing's engagement in health policy and healthcare through social media. *Online J Issues Nurs* 16(1):2010. Retrieved from: http:// www.nursingworld.org/MainMenu Categories/ANAMarketplace/ ANAPeriodicals/OJIN/Tableof Contents/Vol-16-2011/No1-Jan -2011/Health-Policy-and-Healthcare -Through-Social-Media.html or doi: 10.3912/OJIN.Vol16No01LegCol01. 9/11/2014.

Riska E: Men's mental health. In Broom A, Tovey P, editors: *Men's Health: Body, Identity and Social Context*, West Sussex,

UK, 2009, Wiley-Blackwell, pp 145–162.

Rittenhouse D, Shortell S: The patient-centered medical home. *JAMA* 301(19):2038–2040, 2009.

Robert Wood Johnson Foundation: *Chronic Care: Making the Case for Ongoing Care*, Princeton, NJ, 2010, Robert Wood Johnston Foundation. Retrieved from: http://www.rwjf.org/content/dam/farm/reports/reports/2010/rwjf54583. 9/11/2014.

Rochlen A, Paterniti D, Epstein R, et al: Barriers in diagnosing and treating men with depression: A focus group report. *Am J Mens Health* 4(2):167–175, 2010. doi: 10.1177/1557988309335823.

Rosland A, Piette J: Emerging models for mobilizing family support for chronic disease management: a structured review. *Chronic Illn* 6(7):17–21, 2010. doi: 10.1177/1742395309352254.

Roy K, Haddix A, Ikeda R, et al: Monitoring progress toward CDC's health protection goals: health outcome measures by life stage. *Public Health Rep* 124:304–316, 2009.

Sabol WJ, West HC, Cooper M: Prisoners in 2008. Bureau of Justice Statistics Bulletin, 2009, U.S. Department of Justice. Retrieved from: www.ojp.usdoj.gov/bjs/. 9/11/2014.

Sanders A, Lim S, Sohn W: Resilience to urban poverty: theoretical and empirical considerations for population health. *Am J Public Health* 98(6):1101–1106, 2008.

Shin J, Martin R, Howren M: Influence of assessment methods n reports of gender differences in AMI symptoms. *West J Nurs Res* 31(5):553–568, 2009.

Shuford JA: What Is the Difference Between Sexually Transmitted Infection (STI) and Sexually Transmitted Disease (STD)? 2008. Retrieved from: http://www.medinstitute.org/public/132.cfm. 9/11/2014.

Stange K, Nutting P, Gill J: Defining and measuring the Patient-Center Medical Home. *J Gen Intern Med* 25(6):601–612, 2010. doi: 10.1007/s11606-010-1291-3.

Stuenkel D, Wong V: Stigma. In Larsen PD, Lubkin IM, editors: *Chronic Illness: Impact and Intervention*, Sudbury, MA, 2009, Jones and Bartlett.

Substance Abuse and Mental Health Services Administration: Fetal Alcohol Syndrome Thru the Lifespan, 2009. Retrieved from: www.samhsa.gov. 9/11/2014.

Tobias DK, Zhang C, Van Dam RM, et al: Physical activity before and during pregnancy and risk of gestational diabetes mellitus: a meta-analysis. *Diabetes Care* 34(1):223–229, 2011.

Truncali A, Dumanosvsky T, Stollman H, et al: Keep on Track: a volunteer-run community-based intervention to lower blood pressure in older adults. *J Am Geriatr Soc* 58(6):1177–1183, 2010.

United States Congress: *Public Law 111-148*, Washington, D.C, 2010, United States Government Printing Office. Retrieved from: https://democrats.senate.gov/pdfs/reform/patient-protection-affordable-care-act-as-passed.pdf. 9/11/2014.

US Burden of Disease Collaborators: The state of US health, 1990-2010: burden of diseases, injuries, and risk factors. *JAMA* 310(6):591–608, 2013. doi: 10.1001/jama.2013.13805.

U.S. Cancer Statistics Working Group: *United States Cancer Statistics: 1999–2011 Incidence and Mortality Web-Based Report*, Atlanta, GA, 2014, Department of Health and Human Services, Centers for Disease Control and Prevention, and National Cancer Institute. 2014.

U.S. Department of Health and Human Services, National Women's Health Information Center: Teen Talk II, 2010. Retrieved from: http://www.womenshealth.gov/index.cfm. 9/11/2014.

U.S. Department of Health and Human Services: Healthy People 2020, 2010. Retrieved from: http://www.healthypeople.gov/2020/default.aspx. 9/11/2014.

U.S. Department of Health and Human Services: Results from the 2012 National Survey on Drug Use and Health: Mental health findings, 2013. Retrieved from: http://store.samhsa.gov/product/Results-from-the-2012-National-Survey-on-Drug-Use-and-Health-NSDUH-H-47-Mental-Health-Findings/SMA13-4805. 9/11/2014.

U.S. Department of Health and Human Services: Office of Women's Health, 2014. Retrieved from: www.hrsa.gov. 9/11/2014.

U.S. Department of Justice, Bureau of Justice Studies: Prisoners in 2008, 2009. Retrieved from: http://bjs.ojp.usdoj.gov/index.cfm?ty=pbdetail&iid=1763. 9/11/2014.

U.S. Department of Labor Wage and Hour Division (WHD): The Family and Medical Leave Act of 1993, n.d. Retrieved from: http://www.dol.gov/whd/regs/statutes/fmla.htm. 9/11/2014.

U.S. Preventive Services Task Force: Folic acid for the prevention of neural tube defects: U.S. Preventive Services Task Force recommendation statement. *Ann Intern Med* 150:626–631, 2009.

U.S. Preventive Services Task Force: Screening for testicular cancer: U.S. Preventive Services Task Force recommendation statement, 2004. *Ann Intern Med* 154:483–486, 2004.

Wang E, White M, Jamison R, et al: Discharge planning and continuity of health care: Findings from the San Francisco County jail. *Am J Public Health* 98(12):2182–2184, 2008.

Waski M, Kachlic M: A review of common sexually transmitted diseases. *Formulary* 44:78–85, 2009.

Weierbach F, Glick D: Community resources for older adults with chronic illness. *Holist Nurs Pract* 23(6):355–360, 2009.

Wilhelm K: Men and depression. *Aust Fam Physician* 38(3):102–105, 2009.

Wilper AP, Woolhandler S, Lasser KE, et al: Health insurance and mortality in U.S. adults. *Am J Public Health* 99(12):2289–2295, 2009.

# 31

# Disability Health Care Across the Life Span

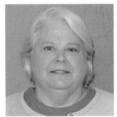

## *Lynn Wasserbauer, RN, FNP, PhD\**

Lynn Wasserbauer earned an undergraduate degree in Zoology from The State University of New York, Oswego, the BS and MS in nursing from the University of Rochester, and the PhD and FNP certificate from the University of Virginia. She is a nurse practitioner at The University of Rochester Medical Center. Her current practice is in psychiatric nursing.

## ADDITIONAL RESOURCES

**Ⓔ Evolve Website http://evolve.elsevier.com/Stanhope**
- Healthy People 2020
- WebLinks
- Quiz
- Case Studies
- Glossary
- Answers to Practice Application
- Resource Tools
  - Resource Tool 5.A: Schedule of Clinical Preventive Services

- Resource Tool 31.A: The Living Will Directive
- Resource Tool 31.B: Assessment Tools for Communities with Physically Compromised Members
- Resource Tool 31.C: Assessment Tools for Families with Physically Compromised Members
- Resource Tool 31.D: Assessment Tools for Physically Compromised Individuals
- Appendix
  - Appendix F.1: Instrumental Activities of Daily Living (IADLs) Scale

## OBJECTIVES

*After reading this chapter, the student should be able to do the following:*
1. Define terms related to disability.
2. Discuss implications of developmental disability, physical disability, or chronic illness.
3. Identify the conditions that may contribute to disability.
4. Discuss the effects of being disabled on the individual, the family, and the community.

5. Describe the implications of being disabled for selected (low-income) populations.
6. Discuss selected issues for those who are disabled (abuse, health promotion).
7. Discuss the objectives of *Healthy People 2020* as they relate to disability.
8. Examine the nurse's role in caring for people who are disabled.

## KEY TERMS

Americans with Disabilities Act, p. 695
burden of chronic disease, p. 698
children with special health care needs (CSHCN), p. 697
chronic disease, p. 697
disability, p. 695
developmental disability, p. 697

dual diagnosis, p. 699
functional limitations, p. 696
medical model of disability, p. 695
social model of disability, p. 695
—*See Glossary for definitions*

---

*Special thanks to Susan Kennel, PhD, RN, CPNP and Carol Lynn Maxwell-Thompson, MSN, RN, FNP-C, who authored this chapter in the seventh edition of the text.

Foundational to the American system of government is the belief that all citizens are entitled to protection of individual civil rights. Unfortunately, individuals with disabilities were among the last groups in the United States to receive civil rights protection. Until the late twentieth century, widespread discrimination against the disabled made it difficult for them to feel fully integrated into society. As a result of this discrimination, the disabled often were literally shut in and shut out of much of American society. The Americans with Disabilities Act (ADA) of 1990 was the first comprehensive civil rights legislation for individuals with disabilities. One effect of this legislation is a greater emphasis on community care for the disabled, rather than institutionalization, and there is a growing emphasis on providing that care in as "home-like" an environment as possible.

One of the many challenges for the disabled is access to appropriate health care. Although not all care can be delivered at home, public health nurses are uniquely positioned to serve as care providers and managers for community-dwelling disabled individuals. Having an understanding of disabilities, disability rights, and the legislation specifically enacted to decrease discrimination will assist nurses in intervening and advocating for the disabled.

This chapter provides an overview of disabilities, defines key terms, and reviews the effects of disabilities on individuals, families and communities. The relationships between disabling conditions and *Healthy People 2020* are discussed. Also reviewed is the nurse's role in planning and providing or securing appropriate interventions for individuals, families, and communities to manage or prevent these health problems.

## UNDERSTANDING DISABILITIES

### Models of Disability

There is no single accepted definition for disability. The definition of disability varies depending on common use of the word or the specific agency defining the term. With regard to health care, the medical model of disability is generally used to conceptualize disability. In this model, disability is considered to be a function of physical characteristics or conditions that place an individual at a disadvantage compared with those who do not have the characteristic or condition. This model places emphasis on the disabled person and the need to modify the course of illness, or as much as possible to give the disabled person a "normal" life. The Social Security Administration uses this model for determination of disability. In the social model of disability, emphasis is placed on systemic barriers as well as societal attitudes and stigmas that contribute to the perception that those with limitations or physical illnesses are disabled. In this model the focus is on the need to change society and not the individual with a disability. This model has led to a focus on civil rights for the disabled and the need for legislation addressing discrimination (Scullion, 2010).

### Disability Defined

Disability is defined by *Webster's* as "A condition (such as an illness or injury) that damages or limits a person's physical or mental abilities; the condition of being disabled; limitation in the ability to pursue an occupation because of a physical or mental impairment; a program providing financial support to one affected by a disability; lack of legal qualification to do something or a disqualification, restriction, or disadvantage" (Merriam-Webster, 2014).

### Census Determination of Disability

The last time that disability data were collected using the standard long-form for the decennial census was in 2000 and the population was assessed to determine and define disability based on functional limitations. The Census Bureau collected data on the number of individuals with disabilities. Six specific subpopulations of disability were identified and included employment disability, sensory disability, mental disability, physical disability, self-care disability, and go-outside-the-home disability (American Community Survey, 2012).

Beginning with the 2010 Census, disability data were obtained using the American Community Survey (ACS), a yearly supplement to the decennial census, and the Survey of Income and Program Participation (SIPP), a continuous survey of a national panel of households with each panel lasting approximately four years. The definition of disability was also changed in an attempt to improve the response rate and gather more reliable information. For the ACS the current definition of disability includes the following: hearing difficulty/vision difficulty, cognitive difficulty, ambulatory difficulty, self-care difficulty, and independent living difficulty data (ACS, 2012).

The SIPP survey categorizes types of disabilities into communicative (difficulty seeing, hearing, or having their speech understood); physical (used an assistive device, had difficulty with a specific task such as climbing a flight of stairs, or had a specific illness such as arthritis); and mental (had a cognitive disability or had a mental or emotional problem that interfered with everyday activities) domains. These changes may appear subtle; however, by reclassifying disabilities it became easier to obtain more detailed disability data (Brault, 2012).

Box 31-1 lists the top ten causes of disability in the United States.

## Social Security Disability

The Social Security Administration (SSA), who ultimately determines the individual's status for disability benefits, defines disability as the inability "to engage in any substantial gainful activity (SGA) because of a medically-determinable physical or mental impairment(s): That is expected to result in death, or That has lasted or is expected to last for a continuous period of at least 12 months" (SSA, 2014, p. 5). An individual's inability to perform any SGA is the criteria used by the Social Security Administration to determine disability. A gainful work activity is: "Work performed for pay or profit; or Work of a nature generally performed for pay or profit; or Work intended for profit, whether or not a profit is realized" (SSA, 2014, p. 5).

The Social Security Administration and Workman's Compensation Systems determine the patient's disability based on

clinical evidence. The health care provider should consult the office of Disability Determination Services in the Social Security Administration or the Workman's Compensation Department for guidelines from individual states since requirements may vary.

## Americans with Disabilities Act

According to the ADA, the term *disability* means, with respect to an individual, (1) a physical or mental impairment that substantially limits one or more of the major life activities of such an individual, (2) a record of such an impairment, or (3) being regarded as having such an impairment (ADA, 1990, Section 3 [2]).

Thus, individuals who are clearly diagnosed with an illness that limits functioning in one or more major life activities are covered. According to ADA guidelines disability status is based on a person's ability to complete major life activities independently. Major life activities refer to self-care, receptive and expressive language, learning, mobility, self-direction, capacity for independent living, and financial sufficiency.

Also covered by the ADA are individuals who have a history of an illness, those who have been considered (possibly erroneously) to have had an illness, or those who have been treated as if they had a disabling illness. The intent of the ADA is to reduce "discrimination based not only on simple prejudice, but also on stereotypical attitudes and ignorance about individuals with disabilities" (Jones, 1991, p. 34). This means that individuals may have been misdiagnosed or inappropriately treated as if they had an illness or disability. Because of this, these individuals may not have had the same opportunities as do nondisabled individuals. An example of this is intelligence testing or assessment of cognitive ability. If there was an underestimate of intelligence or functioning, an individual may not have been allowed full access in education. This then may have limited his or her ability to be prepared for higher education.

## Functional Disability

In 2001 the World Health Organization (WHO) redefined The International Classification of Impairments, Disabilities and Handicaps from 1980. This new classification, called the International Classification of Functioning, Disability and Health (ICF), provides standardized language for measuring, classifying, and defining disability. The new definition of disability considers not only medical problems, but also physical, social, attitudinal, and personal factors (WHO, 2014). In the new classification, functioning and disability are determined by the complex interaction between the health condition of the individual and environmental and personal factors. It recognizes that external factors beyond body structures and functions contribute to the disability. The emphasis is on function rather than the condition or the disease. It is relevant across cultures, age groups, and genders and is a useful way to measure health outcomes (WHO, 2014).

Functional limitations occur when individuals experience difficulty performing basic activities of daily living because of their disability. Examples of functional limitations include difficulty standing, walking, climbing, grasping, and reading.

Emphasis is placed on the level of function rather than on the purpose of the activity, so that functional limitation can be associated with the disability. For example, impairment in the strength or range of motion of the arm could lead to functional limitations in grasping or reaching. Affected individuals may have difficulty performing basic self-care activities such as bathing and dressing.

## Additional Definitions

The term children with special health care needs (CSHCN) is defined by the Maternal and Child Health Bureau (MCHB) of the U.S. Department of Health and Human Services as "those who have or are at increased risk for a chronic, physical, developmental, behavioral or emotional condition and who also require health and related service of a type or amount beyond that required by children generally" (MCHB, 2013, p. 1). This definition is broad and includes children with many conditions and risk factors. The prevalence of special health care needs increases with age and varies with race and ethnicity. The children with the highest prevalence of special health care needs are Native American/Alaska Native children, multiracial zchildren, and non-Hispanic white children. The lowest rates are in Hispanic children and non-Hispanic Asian children (MCHB, 2013).

The term developmental disability, as defined by the National Center on Birth Defects and Developmental Disabilities of the Centers for Disease Control and Prevention (CDC), is a chronic impairment that occurs during development and up to age 22 and lasts throughout the person's lifetime. The disability limits the functioning of an individual in at least three of the following areas: self-help, language, learning, mobility, self-direction, independent living, and economic self-sufficiency (CDC, 2014b).

Chronic disease, or illness, refers to any long-lasting condition or illness. Disease processes (e.g., diabetes mellitus, cancer, heart disease) and congenital or acquired conditions (e.g., Down syndrome, severe burns, amputation of a limb) are examples of chronic diseases. Therefore, concepts related to disabilities and functional limitations may apply to individuals with a chronic disease or other conditions. For nurses working with these clients, the onset, course, outcome, and degree of limitation are important factors to consider when determining the meaning of the disease to individuals and the families.

Persons with disabilities have often been defined by their illness or disability. Defining someone by their disease or disability is devaluing and disrespectful. It can also place artificial limitations on an individual's potential and value. Language is powerful. The word *handicapped* symbolized the person with a disability begging with a "cap in his hand." The term *disabled* is often used to describe cars that are disabled, indicating they are broken, not functioning, or defective. Whereas we may refer to *things* that are broken or defective, people with disabilities are not broken. Rather than saying a baby has a birth defect, a better term would be to say a child has a congenital disability. The Person First Movement was initiated in an effort to promote acceptable language for people with disabilities. The Person First Movement advocates for political correctness in defining persons with disabilities. In other words, refer to a "woman who is blind" rather than a "blind woman" or a "person with diabetes" rather than a "diabetic" (Disability is Natural, 2014).

Definitions of disability need to take into account the degree of disability, the limitations it imposes, and the degree of dependence that occurs as a result of the disability. These definitions can range from minor to severe. Situational factors also affect the disability experience and influence the individual's ability to cope and function in society. Nurses and the interdisciplinary team need to be included, informed, and involved in the science of disability and rehabilitation to be influential in the decision making related to practice, policy, training, research, and funding.

---

### ⟫ LINKING CONTENT TO PRACTICE

Within public health nursing, there has been a commitment to caring for people in their communities and working to build the health of communities. The Council on Linkages (2012) has identified several core competencies for public health professionals, including public health nurses.

**Tier 1 Core Competencies** apply to public health professionals, including nurses, who are not in management. Responsibilities of these public health professionals may include basic data collection and analysis, fieldwork, program planning, outreach activities, programmatic support, and other organizational tasks.

**Tier 2 Core Competencies** apply to individuals with program management and/or supervisory responsibilities. Responsibilities may include program development, program implementation, program evaluation, establishing and maintaining community relations, managing timelines and work plans, presenting arguments, and recommendations on policy issues.

**Tier 3 Core Competencies** apply to individuals at a senior/management level and leaders of public health organizations. In general, an individual who is responsible for the major programs or functions of an organization, setting a strategy and vision for the organization, and/or building the organization's culture can be considered to be a Tier 3 public health professional.

Public health nurses working in any tier are needed to ensure that disabled individuals are properly cared for in the community. This may involve providing or directing care, or understanding disability legislation and programs for which individual/families are eligible. Public health nurses may also be involved in developing and implementing programs for the disabled or being the chief executive officer of an agency that advocates for the disabled.

---

## SCOPE OF THE PROBLEM

### Number of Disabled Americans

According to the most recent data from the Survey of Income and Program Participation collected in 2010, approximately 18.7%, or 56.7 million civilian, noninstitutionalized men, women, and children in the United States reported a disability. Prevalence rates by type of disability are as follows: vision 3.3%; hearing 3.1%; lower body limitations 12.6%; upper body limitations 8.2%; difficulty with at least one ADL 2.1%; difficulty with one or more IADL 6.4%; and cognitive, mental, or emotional 6.3% (Brault, 2012).

### Number of Disabled Worldwide

According to data obtained from the World Health Survey, approximately 785 million (15%) of the world's population 15 years of age and older have some type of disability and 110 million people (2.2%) have significant difficulty functioning. This number is increasing annually in part because of the increase in chronic diseases, injuries, automobile crashes, violence, an aging population, and improvements in the methodologies used to measure disability. Minorities, including women, and the poor are disproportionately affected by being disabled. Worldwide, most of the people with disabilities have limited access to basic public health services and rehabilitation (WHO, 2011).

## Burden of Chronic Disease

Another way to consider disability data is to look at the burden of chronic disease. According to 2010 worldwide data obtained from The Global Burden of Disease Study, the prevalence of chronic diseases such as depression and diabetes is increasing faster than public health concerns such as malnutrition and infectious disease (Currie, 2013).

Although not all individuals with chronic diseases are disabled, the following data from the CDC provide convincing evidence that chronic diseases contribute significantly to the development of disability. Chronic diseases such as heart disease, stroke, cancer, diabetes, and arthritis are some of the most common, costly, and preventable of all health problems in the United States. Approximately 7 out of 10 deaths among

Americans each year are from chronic diseases. Heart disease, cancer, and stroke account for more than 50% of all deaths each year. In 2005 nearly 50% of the adult population, or almost 133 million Americans, had at least one chronic illness (CDC, 2010a).

## Additional Causes of Disability

Disabilities among the chronically ill are common, and the CDC reports that about one fourth of people with chronic conditions have one or more daily activity limitations. For example, arthritis is the most common cause of disability, with nearly 19 million Americans reporting activity limitations. Diabetes continues to be the leading cause of kidney failure, nontraumatic lower-extremity amputations, and blindness among adults ages 20 to 74 (CDC, 2010a).

There is an obesity epidemic in the United States and according to the CDC (2014c), more than one third of adults, or 72 million Americans, are obese. People who are obese are more likely to develop chronic medical problems and have higher medical costs than people of normal weight. Moreover, older adults who are obese are more likely to have disabilities related to functional impairment.

Several other conditions and inherited problems can cause disability as seen in (Figure 31-1). These include genetic disorders, acute and chronic illnesses, violence, tobacco use, lack of access to health care, as well as failure to eat correctly, exercise

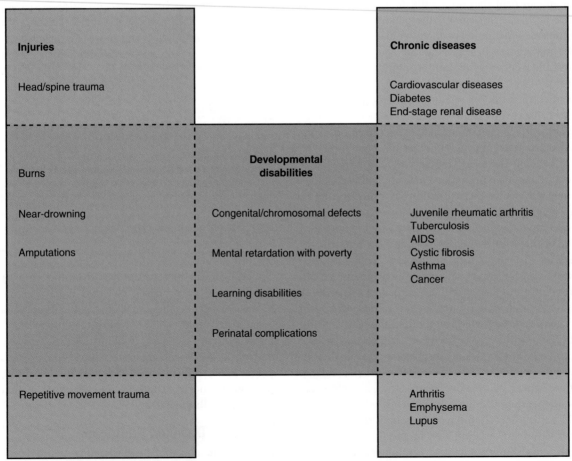

**FIG 31-1** Examples of conditions related to being physically compromised.

regularly, or manage stress effectively. In addition, substance abuse, environmental problems, and unsanitary living conditions can cause disability. The people reporting these causes identified difficulty with functional limitations, difficulty with activities of daily living (ADLs)/instrumental activities of daily living (IADLs), or inability to do housework, or to work at a job or business (CDC, 2014a).

Falls among the elderly, especially the frail elderly, are common and one third of adults over the age of 65 fall every year. Of these falls approximately 20% to 30% result in moderate to severe injury and can cause temporary or permanent disability. This places the elderly at greater risk for loss of independence and physical mobility that can in turn cause additional medical problems. This loss of independence places additional burdens on family members and caregivers to provide assistance with ADLs and IADLs (CDC, 2013). A thorough nursing assessment can identify factors placing a community-dwelling elder at risk for falls. The assessment should include functional impairments, medications, and environmental factors that increase fall risk. Early assessment and intervention can prevent a fall and decrease development of additional medical problems and disability.

## Childhood Disability

An estimated 15.1% of children in the United States have special needs, which may be developmental, behavioral, or emotional in nature. Moreover, 23.0% of households with children have at least one child with a special health need. Children with special health care needs require such things as prescription medication (86%), specialty medical care (48%), vision care (35%), mental health care (28%), specialized therapies (27%), and medical equipment (11%). Many families with children with special needs have difficulty obtaining services due to waiting lists and difficulty getting to appointments (17.8%), child not eligible for the service (10.8%), trouble getting the needed information (9.0%), the cost of the service (14.9%), and the service not being available in the area (11.2%) (MCHB, 2013).

Of the children with special health care needs, 20.8% are under the age of 5; 38.7% are between the ages of 6 and 11; and 40.5% are age 12 through 17. Moreover, children with special health care needs are more likely to be boys (59.3%) than girls (40.7%) (MCHB, 2013). Childhood disability may be developmental or acquired and may be a result of prenatal damage, perinatal factors, acquired neonatal factors, or early childhood factors. These may include genetic factors, prematurity, infections, traumatic or toxic exposure, or nutritional factors. Although the etiology of many childhood disabilities remains unknown, preventive screening for genetic disorders including developmental disabilities is critical for early detection and medical intervention. Newborn screening, immunization programs, and genetic counseling prevent disabilities. Neonatal screening for phenylketonuria (PKU), hypothyroidism, thalassemias, and other disorders has greatly reduced childhood disabilities.

## Mental Illness

Often an overlooked source of disability is that related to mental disorders. According to the WHO (2013), mental health problems, including depression, are among the 20 leading causes of disability worldwide. In the United States, the National Institute of Mental Health (2010) estimates that each year approximately 57.5 million Americans over the age of 18 (26.2%) have a diagnosable mental disorder. Major depressive disorder is the leading cause of disability in the United States for individuals ages 15 to 44. For individuals with one diagnosable mental illness, almost 45% meet criteria for a second or third mental illness. Multiple diagnoses, including individuals with a dual diagnosis, increase the severity of disability and functional impairment.

## THE EFFECTS OF DISABILITIES

The costs of chronic disability to the injured persons, family, employers, and society are significant. In 2010 the SIPP estimated that of the noninstitutionalized population ages 21 to 64 who had any type of disability, only 41.1% were employed as compared to the nondisabled population (79.1%). Moreover, employment rates varied by type of disability: 73.4% of individuals with a disability related to communication were employed, while 40.8% of those with physical disabilities and 51.9% of people with mental disabilities were employed (Brault, 2012).

Disability status also affects annual household income, as can be seen in a 2010 survey of the median monthly household income among households with or without a disabled individual age 21 to 64. The monthly household income for households with a disabled member was $1,961 whereas the monthly income for households without a disabled member was $2,724. Perhaps of more significance are the number of individuals with disabilities who live in poverty. Moreover, the number of individuals living in poverty increases with the severity of disability. Twenty-eight percent of people with severe disability, 17.9% of people with nonsevere disability, and 14.3% of people with no disability live in poverty (Brault, 2012).

Nurses provide care for persons who are disabled, for their families, for the populations and subpopulations they comprise, and for the communities in which they live. Remember that some clients prefer to be regarded as being physically or mentally challenged or compromised, whereas others may think such terms minimize the importance of the needs and problems of people who are disabled. The extent to which the disabled person may need extra support, care, and services from the family unit and the community is shown in Box 31-2. These relationships are best understood by looking at the stress placed on the individual.

### Effects on the Individual

According to the U.S. Department of Health and Human Services, disabilities are characteristics of the body, mind, or senses that affect a person's ability to engage independently in some or all aspects of day-to-day life. Many types of disabilities exist, and they affect people in various ways. People may be born with a disability, develop a disability from being sick or injured, or acquire a disability with the aging process. Most men, women, and children of all ages, races, and ethnicities will

## BOX 31-2   Potential Effects of Being Physically Compromised

### Individuals, Families, and Communities

**Individuals**
- Related health problems (e.g., nutrition, oral health, hygiene, limited activity/stamina)
- Self-concept/self-esteem
- Life expectancy and risk for infection and secondary injury
- Developmental tasks; change in role expectations

**Families**
- Stress on family unit
- Need for use of external resources to help family meet role expectations
- Options limited in use of any discretionary income
- Social stigma

**Communities**
- Need/demand to reallocate resources
- Discomfort or fear from lack of knowledge of disability
- Need to comply with legislation
- Services provided by health department, health care providers
- Need for other services beyond medical diagnosis (e.g., transportation)

experience disability at some time during their lives (Erickson et al, 2012).

As the population ages, the likelihood of developing a disability increases. For example, 10.1% of individuals 18 to 64 years old have a disability, 25.0% of those 65 to 74 have a disability, and 75% of those over 75 have a disability. Disability is not a sickness, and most people with disabilities are healthy and without a documented chronic illness. However, persons with disabilities may be at greater risk for developing illnesses as a result of their condition. For example, someone with decreased mobility can suffer from the problems of immobility such as obesity, skin breakdown, osteoporosis, pneumonia, malnutrition, or loneliness. Most persons with disabilities can and do work, play, learn, and enjoy healthy lives (Erickson et al, 2012).

Many disabled people try to discourage the image that they are helpless and pitiful. For example, *Murderball* is a documentary film about several quadriplegic rugby players who play competitive rugby in wheelchairs. Their motto is "Smashing stereotypes one hit at a time!" These individuals promote the idea of living and working independently (U.S. Quad Rugby Association, 2010).

### Children: Infancy Through Adolescence

Children who live with a disability are affected in many ways. In an effort to decrease childhood obesity, greater emphasis has been placed on increasing children's physical activity. In spite of this goal, children with any type of disability continue to be less physically active and at greater risk of obesity than their healthy peers. This is in part due to the relative lack of available opportunities for disabled children to participate in organized and spontaneous play. Moreover, nondisabled children and parents have also had negative attitudes about interacting or playing with disabled children (Obrusnikova et al, 2010; Reinehr et al, 2010).

Children and adolescents with special health care needs are also at higher risk to experience psychological maladjustment compared with their healthy peers. The risk of psychological problems such as depression and anxiety is correlated with the degree of physical impairment, not with the level of disease activity. For some, the inability to participate in certain physical activities affects their feelings of belonging and self-worth (Wilson and Clayton, 2010; WHO, 2012).

A particular problem for children with cognitive disabilities is difficulty with accurately interpreting social cues. These children are less likely to understand a social interaction that differs from usual and predictable interactions. As a result of misinterpreting social cues, children with cognitive disabilities are at a disadvantage in developing age-appropriate friendships. This can contribute to increased social isolation for many disabled children (Leffert et al, 2010).

For other children, managing the effects of their disability may cause embarrassment and they may choose to isolate themselves from others. For example, students who have spina bifida or renal disease might need to leave classrooms or other school settings quickly to use the bathroom. Having to explain this need to their classmates could call unwanted attention to these children and their diseases. However, disabled children can overcome some of these obstacles if they have families who are able to provide the support necessary for the development of more positive self-images and a feeling of inclusiveness. The use of assistive technology such as computers can enhance learning and decrease obstacles related to inadequate education (Heywood, 2010; Murchland and Parkyn, 2010; WHO, 2012).

The unique issues and challenges experienced by adolescents with disabilities have not been studied as well as those that affect younger children and adults. This population is often overlooked by advocacy groups for the disabled and by most of the new initiatives developed for disabled persons. However, the years between 10 and 18 are difficult ones for most adolescents, and the needs of those who are disabled are similar to those of their healthy peers (i.e., education, peer relationships, recreation, and planning for the future). In addition to the expected challenges experienced by adolescents, those who are disabled must also deal with prejudice, discrimination, and social isolation because of their disability (Redmon, 2010; WHO, 2012).

Disabled adolescents are often viewed as asexual by their healthy peers. However, they are as sexually active as healthy adolescents. They view themselves as "normal" even though they realize that others perceive them differently. Moreover, disabled adolescents are just as likely as their nondisabled peers to engage in risky sexual activity. This places them at risk for unplanned pregnancy and sexually transmitted diseases. Therefore, they should receive the same amount of sexual education as their unaffected peers (Maart, Jelsma, 2010; WHO, 2012).

### Adults

According to The Center for an Accessible Society (CAS) (2014), more than 3 million people in the United States require help from another person to live independently. Many adults receive some, but not enough, help to meet their needs. With inadequate community support, an individual may experience

Researchers studied the effect of psychosocial education given to mothers who had an intellectually disabled child. The researchers wanted to know if providing education to mothers would decrease the mothers' risk of depression, as well as increase their perception of how well their family functioned. The study was a randomized controlled study of 75 women with intellectually disabled children; 40 in the intervention group and 35 in the control group. The intervention group received once weekly educational sessions over four weeks. At the conclusion of the study the researchers found there was a statistically significant difference between the two groups. The mothers who received education were less likely to be depressed and they perceived that their family functioned better.

**Nurse Use**

This study provides additional evidence that psychosocial education can contribute to the overall health and wellness of mothers with a disabled child. Nurses are often in a position to develop educational programs after assessing what information is needed. It's important for nurses working with families of children with disabilities to have psychosocial educational material available. Moreover, public health nurses should also maintain a database of community services and supports to make appropriate referrals for additional education and support.

Yildirim A, Hacihasanoglu R, Karakurt P: Effects of a nursing intervention program on the depression and perception of family functioning of mothers with intellectually disabled children. *J Clin Nurs* 22(1-2):251–261, 2013.

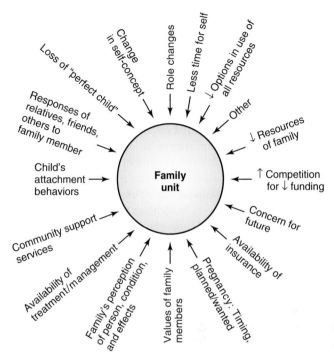

**FIG 31-2** Factors influencing a family unit when a member is physically compromised.

hunger, injuries, falls, or other problems that contribute to the development of secondary health problems, disabilities, and possibly early death. Becoming disabled increases the risk of placement in a nursing home or other long-term care facility, contributing to both decreased community participation and limited social integration for the disabled.

It is estimated that those persons who live by themselves receive only 56% of the help they need, while those living with family members or friends receive 80% of what they need. Informal supports such as family members and friends frequently have multiple work, family, and community responsibilities. This makes it difficult for them to consistently meet the needs of the disabled. Those without informal supports must rely on formal supports, which are increasingly limited in difficult financial times (CAS, 2014).

In addition, millions of Americans depend on Medicaid to finance their long-term services (CAS, 2014). For example, 80% of all Medicaid long-term care funds go to nursing homes or other institutional service providers, even though many of these people could receive services in their own homes. A personal assistant could make it possible for a disabled person to live at home instead of in an institution. Many Americans think that nursing homes are the only alternative for long-term care. However, the elderly often prefer the freedom and control of living at home. Many states offer community-based services such as home health care services and senior services. In home supportive services (IHSS) provide home health services to the aged, blind, or disabled. In addition, adult protective services exist to receive reports of abuse of elders or dependent adults.

Computer technology and use of the Internet can increase the independence of people with disabilities. Homebound persons can access a computer and order groceries, shop for needed items, research issues, participate in online discussions, and communicate with friends and family. With newer technologies, blind persons can access the computer as well as sighted persons. Even persons who cannot hold a pen or who lack fine-motor skills can use speech recognition and other technologies to write letters, pay bills, and perform other tasks using the computer and Internet (CAS, 2014). However, only one fourth of persons with disabilities own computers, and only one tenth use the Internet. The elderly and African Americans with disabilities, especially low-income or low-education-level elders, rarely take advantage of these new technologies. Fortunately, computers and associated equipment for the disabled has become less expensive. Moreover, there are organizations that provide low-cost or free computer equipment for qualified disabled individuals (CAS, 2014).

## Effects on the Family

Most people who are physically disabled are cared for at home by one or more family members. Figure 31-2 lists some of the issues and concerns that occur when a family member is disabled and shows the effect of the disability on the family unit. As this figure shows, the entire family system is affected when one member is disabled.

A report conducted by AARP found that the number of individuals providing care to family members is increasing and the care provided is more complex. Family members provide a wide range of services including coordinating care, transportation to medical care, providing direct medical care, and using medical equipment. This caregiver burden can result in stress, depression, financial problems, as well as physical and social isolation (Diament, 2011; WHO, 2011).

## Children: Infancy Through Adolescence

A child's disability may have long-term effects on the family, primary caregiver, and the marital relationship. Providing care for these children places additional demands on the family, particularly the mother. Mothers of children with special health care needs report higher levels of stress, anxiety, depression, and feelings of isolation compared with mothers of unaffected children. In addition, employment is difficult and sometimes impossible to secure for the parents of children who require extensive care. This is especially true for mothers, single parents, and low-income families who may be unable to afford child care for their disabled children. In addition to the day-to-day physical care these children require, the caregiver must also access and coordinate physical, occupational, and speech therapy as well as specialty care and additional educational services (Bilgin and Gozum, 2009; Wei and Yu, 2012).

The cost of caring for a child with a disability often affects the family's financial well-being. Children with special health care needs are more likely than the general population of children to have health insurance. However, one third of the children with disabilities who have insurance have inadequate coverage to meet their needs. Moreover, 21.6% of CSHCN have conditions that create financial problems for their families. This is due to high out-of-pocket expenses, the services required not being covered, or the child not having access to appropriate providers (Laskar et al, 2010; MCHB, 2013).

Although children with special health care needs are more likely to have health insurance through Medicaid, children from low-income families who lack medical insurance are at a particular disadvantage because their families may be unable to afford the care they need. Siblings of children with special health care needs are at higher risk for developing emotional and psychological problems compared with their unaffected peers. For example, they tend to express more psychosomatic illnesses, anxiety disorders, and aggressive behaviors compared with siblings of nondisabled children (O'Brien et al, 2009; Dauz et al, 2010).

Conversely, these siblings are often found to be more mature, altruistic, responsible, and independent when compared with siblings of nondisabled children. Whether a child suffers or benefits from having a disabled brother or sister depends on the attitude of the parents toward the disability and their coping methods, the economic circumstances of the family, the communication among family members, and the degree of parental affection and attention received by the nondisabled child (Dyke et al, 2009; MCHB, 2013).

## Adults

Having a physically disabled adult in a family causes enormous stress on the rest of the members. There may be a significant loss of income when a parent is unable to work because of a disability, and disability prevents people from earning a living. Another effect on multigenerational families is caregiver burden. Well children in the family may have unmet needs due to the disability of a parent. Moreover, the children may have to assume the role of caregiver if other supports are not available.

Adults who are responsible for caring for their own children as well as one or both of their parents have been termed the "sandwich generation." These adults often struggle with burnout as well as increased marital stress when faced with caring for an elderly parent with a disability (Roth et al, 2009; Council for Disability Awareness, 2013).

## Effects on the Community

The presence of physically disabled people and their families in the community has far-reaching effects on all aspects of community life. The prevention of disability and providing community support for caretakers need to be priorities. The community may be called on to respond in new ways to these citizens as a result of federal laws affecting those who are disabled.

## Children: Infancy Through Adolescence

Families of children with disabilities need the support of their communities as they care for their disabled children at home. Children with disabilities have rights, including the right to remain at home rather than become institutionalized. The concept of providing mainstream inclusive health care is essential. Moreover, family services should also include education regarding available services and how to access them (WHO, 2012).

Children who are chronically ill or disabled and who enter school for mainstream education require educational support from the public school system as mandated in the Individuals with Disabilities Education Act (IDEA). IDEA is outlined in Box 31-3. In addition, IDEA requires states to provide appropriate services to infants and children from birth to age 5 who have or are at risk for disability. Examples of such services include speech therapy, occupational therapy, physical therapy, play therapy, and behavioral therapy (U.S. Department of Education, 2010). As seen in Figure 31-5 preterm infants have many health care needs if they are to grow and develop to their highest potential.

Although the provision of appropriate services for disabled infants and children is mandated by IDEA, states vary in the nature and quantity of services they provide for eligible children. In addition, public schools must evaluate their effectiveness with students who are disabled. This can add to the cost of

---

> **BOX 31-3** **Individuals with Disabilities Education Act (IDEA)**
>
> The Individuals with Disabilities Education Act federal law was developed:
> - To ensure that all children with disabilities have available to them a free, appropriate public education that emphasizes special education and related services designed to meet their unique needs and prepare them for employment and independent living
> - To ensure that the rights of children with disabilities and their parents are protected
> - To assist states, localities, educational service agencies, and federal agencies to provide for the education of all children with disabilities
> - To assess and ensure the effectiveness of efforts to educate children with disabilities

U.S. Department of Education: *Building the legacy: IDEA 2004*, 2010: author. Available at www.idea.ed.gov. Accessed April 8, 2014.

educating children. Increased education for pediatricians and nurses can increase supportive and knowledgeable collaboration for the development of early intervention programs in the schools (National Dissemination Center for Children with Disabilities, 2012). As seen in Figure 31-6 having a disabled family member requires many adjustments and may cause enormous stress on the rest of the family.

## Adults

Former Surgeon General Richard H. Carmona sought to improve the health and wellness of persons with disabilities. To achieve this goal, in 2005 he published a call to action which encouraged (1) health care providers to see and treat the whole person, not just the disability, (2) educators to teach about disability, (3) the public to focus on a person's abilities, not just the disability, and (4) the community to ensure accessible health care and wellness services to persons with disabilities (Carmona, 2005).

These goals have been only partially achieved as evidenced by the WHO (2011) World Report on Disability that again calls for action to address barriers and inequities for people with disabilities. The recommendations are as follows: enable access to all mainstream systems and services; invest in specific programs and services for people with disabilities; adopt a national disability strategy and plan of action; involve people with disabilities; improve human resource capacity; provide adequate funding and improve affordability; increase public awareness and understanding; improve disability data collection; and strengthen and support research on disability.

Persons with disabilities that affect mobility are at risk for health problems of the multiple body systems related to mobility/immobility. Persons with mobility-associated problems can suffer damage to any system. Some of the problems that develop with the musculoskeletal system include foot drop, muscular atrophy, contractures, or fractures. Respiratory and circulatory function can be compromised by pneumonia or deep vein thrombosis. Renal problems such as infection, incontinence, or renal calculi are common problems related to immobility. Decubiti and skin breakdown and rashes can develop from immobility and/or incontinence of bowel and bladder. Malnutrition or obesity could also be related to effects of immobility.

## SPECIAL POPULATIONS

### Low-Income Populations

Physically compromised individuals often experience poverty, as do other special population groups including single parents and their children, the aged, the unemployed, and members of racial and ethnic minorities. Persons with low income have less access to health care throughout their lives and are less likely to participate in all levels of prevention. Therefore, they are at greater risk for the onset of disabling conditions and for more rapid progression of disease processes. Those in poverty could also be at greater risk for disabling conditions resulting from lifestyle choices (e.g., injuries; tobacco, alcohol, or drug abuse; and inadequate nutrition).

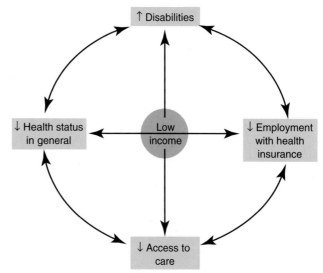

**FIG 31-3** Relationships of poverty and disability.

People who are disabled and live in poverty are less likely to have the resources to provide for their own special needs. Those who are disabled are often unemployed, even though they may be able to work and are seeking jobs. Employers may be reluctant to hire people whose conditions may increase employer-provided health insurance costs. This is another barrier to adequate insurance and access to health care for the disabled. Other factors that affect low-income, physically compromised clients' access to needed services are inadequate transportation, lack of coordination of care, and limited locally available services for those who cannot pay for them. Figure 31-3 illustrates the relationship between poverty and disabilities.

## SELECTED ISSUES

### Abuse and Neglect

Individuals with disabilities are more likely to experience some form of abuse or neglect during their lifetime compared with individuals without disabilities. Examples of abuse and neglect include physical harm, inappropriate sexual contact, emotional or verbal threats, withholding care, not providing adequate supervision, and not providing needed medical care. Abuse and neglect also include withholding medical information, denying the opportunity to participate in decision making, including decisions about medical care and the right to refuse care, and financial exploitation (Missouri Department of Health & Senior Services (MDHSS), 2014). (Figure 31-4 illustrates the relationships among the family member with a disability, the caregiver, the environment and the intersection with abuse).

While all individuals with disabilities are at risk for abuse and neglect, children, the elderly, and women are at particular risk. Children are dependent on adults and require care, supervision, guidance, and financial support to achieve normal growth and development. The responsibility for and care of healthy, nondisabled children poses many challenges for parents. When a child is born with or develops a disability the developmental, physical, and financial needs can become

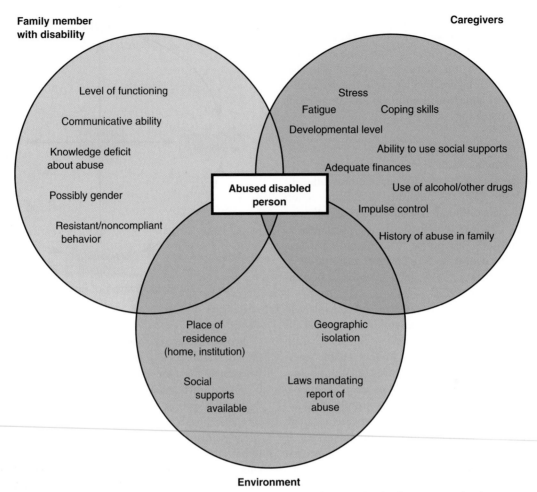

**Family member with disability**

Level of functioning

Communicative ability

Knowledge deficit about abuse

Possibly gender

Resistant/noncompliant behavior

**Caregivers**

Stress

Fatigue    Coping skills

Developmental level

Ability to use social supports

Adequate finances

Use of alcohol/other drugs

Impulse control

History of abuse in family

**Abused disabled person**

Place of residence (home, institution)

Geographic isolation

Social supports available

Laws mandating report of abuse

**Environment**

FIG 31-4 Factors influencing the abuse of those who are physically compromised.

overwhelming. According to the U.S. Department of Health and Human Services (2012) risk factors for the abuse/neglect of disabled children can be stratified to societal factors, such as believing disabled children are asexual or do not feel pain; family or parental factors, which include the child being viewed as different, parents who are embarrassed by their disabled child, or families with inadequate social support or resources; and child-related factors, which include being male, having challenging/difficult behaviors, or requiring extensive physical care.

An interesting study conducted by researchers with the Interactive Autism Network found that children with autistic spectrum disorders (ASD) were three times more likely to be bullied than children without ASD. One form of bullying is intentionally provoking a child with ASD to the point of emotional breakdown or physical violence. According to this study children with ASD are also more likely to be bullies, due to aggressive outbursts or poorly developed social skills. Many children with ASD are unable to make socially appropriate comments and may inappropriately comment on another child's physical characteristics, such as telling other children they are ugly or fat (Anderson, 2012).

In general, the elderly are at increased risk for abuse and neglect. The elderly who also have disabilities are at additional

risk due to their increased dependency needs. The most common type of abuse reported by disabled individuals is care related. Because many disabled individuals are dependent on others for basic care, they are at risk for experiencing neglect and at times cruel physical care from their care providers. Financial abuse is another common way elderly disabled persons are mistreated. Community-dwelling elderly living with family may be threatened with institutionalization in a nursing home if they report the abuse or complain (Missouri Department of Health and Senior Services, 2014).

Women and girls with disabilities face many challenges and often have to face "double discrimination." There is worldwide gender discrimination in such areas as access to housing, education, training, employment, and salary equity. Being female also places one at risk for sexual exploitation, abuse, neglect, and violence. Women with disabilities are at increased risk of this type of abuse because of the powerlessness of women in many parts of the world, the lack of resources, and women being undervalued (United Nations, 2010).

## Health Promotion

Health promotion usually focuses on the primary prevention of conditions that may lead to disability (e.g., smoking cessation to prevent lung cancer). Actually all three levels of prevention

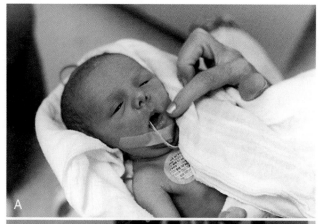

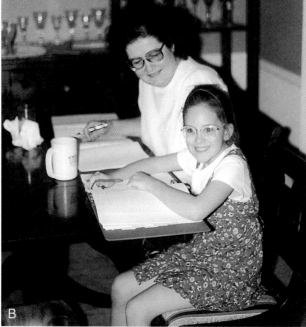

FIG 31-5 **A,** An at-risk infant girl who was 1 month premature and delivered by cesarean section because of abruption. This child's Apgar scores were 1 at 1 minute of age and 3 at 5 minutes of age. **B,** The same child at 10 years of age. She is profoundly hearing impaired. Her parents' commitment has helped her to be mainstreamed successfully and she is able to do her own homework.

apply to physically compromised clients (see the Levels of Prevention box). They need information and counseling for health-promoting behaviors and for prevention of the progression of a condition or pathology.

Health promotion is a multidimensional concept that applies to all individuals regardless of disability. Strategies are needed to expand the knowledge base of health promotion for those who are disabled. Persons with chronic disabilities have frequently defined themselves in terms of their physical problems and sick role. However, they need all the prevention activities of the nondisabled. This includes immunizations, exercise, weight control, use of safety precautions, safe sex practices, stress reduction, as well as screening and treatment of disease not related to their disability.

In addition, health promotion and prevention programs for persons with disabilities should focus on preventing complications from the effects of immobility and the disease process. The complications of immobility and the disease process need to be prevented to ensure optimal independent and healthy living, thus allowing the individual with disabilities the opportunity to have a productive and happy life.

Many health promotion and disease prevention needs are similar across the life span (e.g., exercise, diet, avoidance of excess substance use, and injury prevention). However, specific problems and interventions to deal with these needs vary according to age, specific disabling condition, and developmental status. For example, nutritional needs of premature infants are related to obtaining adequate energy, protein, fat, vitamins, and minerals. An older adult with type 2 diabetes mellitus may be concerned primarily with reducing the risk of experiencing a myocardial infarction.

Persons with disabilities need appropriate nutrition. Therefore, nurses may consult with dietitians or refer clients to them for assistance. Speech therapists may also be needed for persons with chewing or swallowing difficulties. Occupational health professionals focus on the activities of daily living and often use adaptive equipment to promote success and independence with ADLs. Families and professionals can work together to meet the nutritional needs of persons with disabilities and chronic health care problems.

Health promotion and disease prevention for those who are physically compromised have not been emphasized in primary care or in rehabilitation. It is especially important to establish

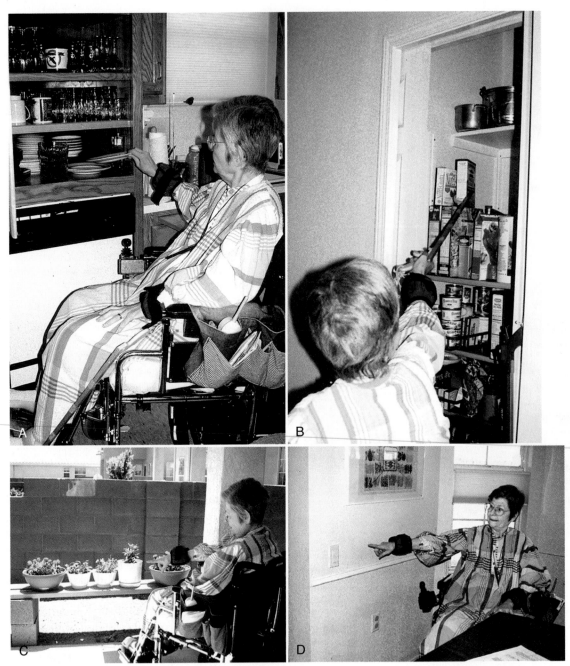

**FIG 31-6** This disabled woman is able to live in and maintain her own home, including growing plants and flowers, with the help of easy-access devices and lower light fixtures and cabinets.

lifelong health-promoting behaviors in children who are disabled. Unfortunately, parents may be so overwhelmed by caring for such children that this aspect of care is not considered.

## *Healthy People 2020* Objectives

Selected objectives from *Healthy People 2020* for persons with disabilities are highlighted in the Healthy People 2020 box. Many of the objectives address concerns discussed in this chapter regarding increasing health promotion and wellness activities for individuals with disabilities. In addition, there is greater emphasis on increasing access to services, which can increase independence and foster community living.

The *Healthy People 2020* objectives are a useful tool available to nurses to evaluate if individuals with disabilities are receiving adequate services. Moreover, these objectives can serve as national benchmarks for individuals with disabilities with regard to their health, use of community services, leisure activities, and overall quality of life. Nurses can use the *Healthy People 2020* objectives to advocate for increased physical activity and wellness programs for the disabled. This can be done by working with community and disability organizations to ensure compliance with the ADA and by educating others about the *Healthy People 2020* objectives. (U.S. Department of Health and Human Services, 2013).

Selected objectives are listed here that pertain to persons with disabilities.

**Systems and DH-1 Policies**
- DH-1: Increase the number of population-based data systems used to monitor *Healthy People 2020* objectives that include in their core a standardized set of questions that identify people with disabilities.
- DH-2: Increase the number of tribes, states, and the District of Columbia that have public health surveillance and health promotion programs for people with disabilities and caregivers.

**Barriers to Health Care**
- DH-5: Increase the proportion of youth with special health care needs whose health care provider has discussed transition planning from pediatric to adult health care.
- DH-7: Reduce the proportion of older adults with disabilities who use inappropriate medications.

**Environment**
- DH-8: Reduce the proportion of people with disabilities who report having physical or program barriers to local health and wellness programs.
- DH-9: Reduce the proportion of people with disabilities who encounter barriers to participating in home, school, work or community activities.

**Activities and Participation**
- DH-13: Increase the proportion of people with disabilities who participate in social, spiritual, recreational, community, and civic activities to the degree that they wish.
- DSC-14: Reduce the proportion of people with disabilities reporting delays in receiving primary and periodic preventive care due to specific barriers.

U.S. Department of Health and Human Services: *Healthy People 2020: Disability and Health,* 2013: author. Available at www.healthypeople.gov. Accessed April 11, 2014.

# ROLE OF THE NURSE

Many factors influence the role of nurses who work with individuals with disabilities. These factors include the community's awareness of these persons and the commitment to their health needs. Also, the missions of the agencies where nurses work influence the type of services they provide to special groups. For example, the structure and priorities of a community-based agency determine whether a nurse will care for the general population or focus on service to a specific population. If funding sources are dedicated to particular programs (e.g., tuberculosis control, maternal–child health services), care for those who are disabled may be dispersed throughout several program areas and may be difficult to identify.

In dealing with those who are disabled, a nurse's role may also change as the focus varies among the levels of individuals, families, groups, or entire communities. For example, at the level of the individual, nurses may provide nursing care for ventilated patients at home. Nurses also serve as educators who provide clients at any level with sufficient knowledge to enable them to care for their own needs. At the community level, nurses may provide information about certain causes of disability and aim to reduce the behaviors that precede the development of disability, such as spinal cord injury. The closely

| **HOW TO** **Promote Appropriate Use of Asthma Medications by Children** |

A. Collaborate/coordinate efforts with health care provider managing child's asthma.
  1. Personnel in all areas in which a child uses drugs need to be informed of regimen.
  2. Be aware of factors that could affect adherence to regimen:
    - Prolonged therapy
    - Medications used prophylactically
    - Delayed consequences of nonadherence
    - Drugs expensive, hard to use
    - Family concerns about side effects
    - Adherence less likely with mild or severe asthma; most likely with moderate asthma
    - Child with cognitive or emotional problems
    - Poorly functioning family
    - Strong alternative health beliefs
    - Multiple caregivers
B. Assess child's adherence to regimen.
  1. Count pills; use float test for remaining amount in inhalers (gross estimate).
  2. Ask child, "In an average week, how many puffs of your inhaler do you actually get?"
  3. Obtain refill history from pharmacist (information can be obtained from child's health care provider).
C. Interventions
  1. Educate child, parents, and other caregivers.
  2. Encourage adaptation of regimen to family's needs.
    - Health care provider may need additional information about family situation.
    - Signed, dated, written permission to exchange information with such a provider is needed.
  3. Encourage consideration of acceptability of medication to child, family.
  4. Be encouraging, caring, supportive, and willing to work with family.
  5. Follow-up and monitor progress closely, including school attendance, when appropriate.
  6. Consider home visits (e.g., to assess/manage environmental triggers).
  7. Identify an "asthma partner" (i.e., another adult besides parents when they do not reliably monitor child).
  8. Use a contract for adherence.
  9. In extreme cases, especially with young and/or ill children, consider reporting family to child protective services for medical neglect.

related counseling role is of value because clients learn to improve their problem-solving skills with guidance from the nurse. The How To box that follows discusses ways to promote the appropriate use of asthma medications by children.

Nurses serve as advocates for individuals and families or groups. An advocate is a person who speaks on behalf of those who are unable to speak for themselves. One of the potential problems with this role is that nurses may unintentionally foster excessive dependence by individuals, families, or other groups. Nurses should focus on using advocacy to support those who need this service. Moreover, having an opportunity to observe nurses using their advocacy skills may assist clients to feel more comfortable in being advocates for themselves or for family members. For example, nurses might advocate for a school environment that is adapted to the specific needs of children who require wheelchairs but who do not necessarily have to be limited to their chairs, without explicitly telling the children when they should use their wheelchairs. In addition, nurses may help family caregivers of disabled individuals by validating that the caregiver may have unmet needs and by helping them to identify ways their needs can be met.

As referral agents, nurses maintain current information about agencies with services that are of potential use to those who are disabled. Referral, a common practice for nurses, is the process of directing clients to the resources that can meet their needs. For self-directed clients and families, information about an agency's services, phone number, and address may be adequate. For families with little understanding of how systems work, more specific guidance and case conferences may be necessary to coordinate clients' health-related and educational needs.

As health care providers with a goal of making basic care universally accessible, nurses are positioned well to ensure that the full range of prevention and information about health promotion is made available to individuals with disabilities. On a more individualized basis, the nurse in a case manager role works to meet the needs of clients by developing a plan of care for them to help them reach individual goals. Although nurses may direct others to carry out the plan, they are responsible for evaluating the plan's effectiveness. For example, clients who have been disabled because of complications from diabetes mellitus may have several immediate problems. They may need to adjust to the amputation of one or more limbs, as well as learn new skills to improve management of their diabetes in an effort to prevent additional complications. Nurses (as case managers) will develop plans with clients and families to meet these needs and establish time frames to evaluate specific outcomes.

In the coordinator role, nurses are not responsible for developing overall plans of client care. Instead, responsibilities include assisting clients and families by organizing and integrating the resources of other agencies or care providers to meet clients' needs most efficiently. For example, with the family's agreement, a nurse may arrange for the family to see a social worker on the same day they bring their children to an appointment in a pediatric cardiology clinic.

Nurses are collaborators when they take part in joint decision making with clients, families, groups, and communities. Collaboration with other care providers is of particular importance in coordinating care and assisting a disabled person to understand the full range of services available. For example, nurses may work with agencies or groups who make decisions about community housing for those who are physically disabled.

In the nursing as case finder role, nurses identify individuals with disabilities who have unmet service needs. For example, nurses may arrange developmental, vision, and hearing screenings for young children. Although a nurse's efforts are for particular clients, the focus of case finding is on monitoring the health status of entire groups or communities. Nurses may also identify those who are members of vulnerable populations and who, although not presently affected by an illness, are at high risk for acquiring the disease. Such people may have limited or no access to health promotion or disease prevention services, or they may be unaware of those for which they are eligible.

Nurses may function as change agents at all levels, including the health care delivery system. A change agent is one who originates and creates change. This process includes identifying a need for change, enlightening and motivating others as to this need, as well as starting and directing the proposed change. Nurses may function in the role by helping to obtain more appropriate health care services for those who are disabled. The most up-to-date information on national and local resources for individuals with disabilities can be found on the Internet. Two excellent resources are Connecting the Disability Community to Information and Opportunities (www.disability.gov) and Disability Resource (www.disabilityresources.org). The following Quality and Safety in Nursing Education box provides useful information regarding teamwork and collaboration in caring for a person who is part of a special needs population.

---

**QSEN** FOCUS ON QUALITY AND SAFETY EDUCATION FOR NURSES

*Quality and Safety Focus*

**Targeted Competency: Teamwork and Collaboration**
Function effectively within nursing and interprofessional teams, fostering open communication, mutual respect, and shared decision making to achieve quality patient care.
Important aspects of teamwork and collaboration include:

- **Knowledge:** Recognize contributions of other individuals and groups in helping patient/family achieve health goals
- **Skills:** Integrate the contributions of others who play a role in helping patient/family achieve health goals
- **Attitudes:** Respect the unique attributes that members bring to a team, including variations in professional orientations and accountabilities

**Teamwork and Collaboration Question**
You are a VA home care nurse who has extensive experience in caring for returned veterans who are recovering from spinal cord injuries. You have been approached by the VA Hospital to help develop a program to reduce recurring admissions to the acute care setting for this population. Specifically, there are models from leading rehabilitation hospitals that a Spinal Cord Injury Nurse Advice Line can effectively help clients and families address commonly recurring complications like neurogenic bladder and skin breakdown. Employing an "Ask-A-Nurse" model, a Spinal Cord Injury Nurse Advice Line is a call-in resource. The development team is asking your input on which team members should be involved in development of this local initiative. If successful, the model may be implemented nationally across the VA Medical System.

What contributions will the following team members make to a Spinal Cord Injury Nurse Advice Line?

- Patients with spinal cord injuries
- Families of patients with spinal cord injuries
- Primary care providers
- Neurologists
- Urologists
- Wound care nurses
- Emergency room physicians
- Case managers

Prepared by Gail Armstrong, PhD(c), DNP, ACNS-BC, CNE, Associate Professor, University of Colorado Denver College of Nursing

## BOX 31-4   Categories of Federal Legislation for Those With Disabilities

**Education**
- Early childhood special education
- Elementary and Secondary Education Act and amendments
- Vocational education for those who are disabled

**Rehabilitation**
- Vocational
- Medical, including Medicare and Medicaid
- Rehabilitation

**Services**
- Economic assistance
- Facility construction and architectural design
- Deinstitutionalization and independent living
- Civil rights and advocacy

The International Center for Disability Resources on the Internet: *Legal, Advocacy, Policy, and Political Issues,* 2010: author. Available at www.icdri.org/legal. Accessed April 11, 2014.

## BOX 31-5   Summary of Legislation

- Communications Act of 1934 and Telecommunications Act of 1996
- Elementary and Secondary Education Act of 1965
- Architectural Barriers Act of 1968
- Rehabilitation Act of 1973
- Individuals with Disabilities Education Act (IDEA) of 1975
- Civil Rights of Institutionalized Persons Act of 1980
- Voting Accessibility for the Elderly and the Handicapped Act of 1984
- The Air Carrier Access Act of 1986
- The Fair Housing Act of 1988
- Americans with Disabilities Act (ADA) of 1990
- National Voter Registration Act of 1993
- The Developmental Disabilities Act and Bill of Rights Act of 2000
- No Child Left Behind Act of 2001
- The Individuals with Disabilities Education Improvement Act of 2004

U.S. Department of Justice: *A guide to disability rights laws,* 2012: author. Available at www.ada.gov/cguide.pdf. Accessed April 11, 2014.

## LEGISLATION

A nurse who works with physically disabled clients may have a caseload of clients of all ages, while another nurse, such as a school nurse, may see clients in a specific age group. Nurses need to be knowledgeable about the legislation that relates to populations for whom they provide nursing care. Box 31-4 summarizes categories of historically significant federal legislation designed to benefit those who are disabled, and Box 31-5 summarizes key disability rights legislation.

The U.S. Department of Justice (USDOJ, 2012) provides *A Guide to Disability Rights Law*. This publication provides an overview of federal civil rights laws designed to ensure equal opportunity for people with disabilities. This guide is an excellent reference about legislation and disability rights information. The document is available in multiple formats including large print, Braille, and audio.

Rehabilitation services were originally developed through legislation for veterans of World War I. In time, others who were physically disabled were regarded less as sources of embarrassment to their families and more as citizens who should participate as fully as possible in all aspects of society. This change in attitude was reflected in changing laws affecting the disabled.

The Rehabilitation Act of 1973 was the first legislation designed specifically to eliminate discrimination against the disabled. This act required all federal agencies and programs receiving federal funds to hire disabled workers. The Rehabilitation Act was an important piece of legislation that defined disability clearly and increased opportunities for some disabled Americans. However, additional legislation was needed to provide more inclusive protection for individuals with disabilities and to extend the benefits of the Rehabilitation Act to encompass more than federal programs. The ADA of 1990 was designed to decrease discrimination and increase opportunities for all disabled Americans by providing more comprehensive protection for them (Allarie, 2005; Lair and Kale, 2005).

The ADA was signed into law July 26, 1990. The act makes it illegal for state and local governments, private employers, employment agencies, labor organizations, and labor-management committees to discriminate against the disabled in employment, public accommodations, transportation, state and local government operations, and telecommunications (ADA, 1990). Cutting across the specific policy provisions of the ADA are four global goals that clarify the intent of the legislation. For persons with a disability, the ADA is designed to promote (1) equality of opportunity, (2) full participation in society and social integration, (3) independent living, and (4) economic self-sufficiency (ADA, 1990). "The ADA provides comprehensive civil rights protection for qualified individuals with disabilities" (Walk et al, 1993, p. 92). The ADA addresses four areas as shown in Box 31-6.

According to the ADA (1990), a qualified employee or applicant with a disability is a person who, with or without reasonable accommodation, can perform the essential functions of the job in question. Reasonable accommodations may include but are not limited to the following:
- Making existing facilities that are used by employees readily accessible to and usable by persons with disabilities
- Job restructuring, modifying work schedules, reassignment to a vacant position
- Acquiring or modifying equipment or devices; adjusting or modifying examinations, training materials, or policies; and providing qualified readers or interpreters

Employers may not ask qualified job applicants questions about the existence, nature, or severity of a disability. Qualified applicants may be asked about their ability to perform job functions. A job offer may be made conditional based on the results of a medical examination, but only if that examination is required for all applicants for the same job. In addition, the examination must be job related and consistent with the employer's business needs. Individuals who use illegal drugs or who are intoxicated at work are not covered under the ADA. Tests for illegal drugs are not subject to the ADA's restrictions on examinations. Employers may hold illegal drug users and alcoholics to the same performance standards as other employees.

Service animals are defined and protected under the ADA. Service animals are working animals that are individually trained to perform tasks for persons with disabilities. These tasks may include guiding someone who is blind, alerting persons who are deaf, pulling wheelchairs, and other special tasks. Under the ADA, businesses and other organizations who serve the public, including restaurants, hotels, taxis, stores, medical offices and hospitals, theaters, and parks, are required to allow service animals to accompany a disabled person into all areas open to the general public.

The Fair Housing Act of 1988 prohibits housing discrimination based on race, color, religion, sex, disability, familial status, and national origin. This includes private as well as public housing. The Act also requires new multifamily housing with four or more units to be accessible for persons with disabilities.

The Civil Rights of Institutionalized Persons Act of 1980 authorizes the attorney general to investigate conditions of confinement in state and local institutions such as prisons, detention centers, jails, nursing homes, and institutions for persons with psychiatric or developmental disabilities. Civil lawsuits

may be initiated on the behalf of the person if harmful or neglectful conditions are found (Guiding Light Foundation (GLF), 2010).

According to the Department of Justice, the Voting Accessibility for the Elderly and the Handicapped Act of 1984 requires polling places across the United States to be accessible for persons with disabilities during federal elections. In addition, states are responsible for ensuring available registration and voting aids for disabled and elderly voters, including telecommunication devices for the deaf (GLF, 2010).

The National Voter Registration Act of 1993, also known as the Motor Voter Act, makes it easier for all Americans to vote. Because of the low registration turnout of minorities and persons with disabilities, this act requires all offices of state-funded programs to provide program applicants with voter registration forms, to assist them in completing the forms, and to transmit the forms to the appropriate office (GLF, 2010).

The Air Carrier Access Act of 1986 prohibits discrimination by airlines. Persons with disabilities do not have to give advance notice before they fly. Moreover, unless there is a safety concern, they cannot be discriminated against with regard to seat assignment (GLF, 2010).

IDEA of 1975 is federal legislation that guarantees all children with disabilities ages 3 through 21 years the right to a free and appropriate public school education that will meet their individual needs. This law protects the rights of parents, guardians, and surrogate parents to fully participate in educational decisions. Special education including physical education is defined in this law, and special instruction is to be provided at no cost to parents. Special education was created to meet the special needs of children with disabilities.

According to IDEA, children with disabilities are those who have one or a combination of the following conditions and therefore would benefit from special education: autism, blindness, deafness, hearing impairment, mental retardation, multiple disabilities, orthopedic impairment, serious emotional disturbance, specific learning disabilities, traumatic brain injury, visual impairment, and other health impairments (U.S. Department of Education (USDE), 2010).

## Basic Rights Under IDEA

*Free and appropriate public education (FAPE)*—The child's education must be designed to meet the child's special needs.

*Appropriate evaluation/assessment*—Each child with a disability must receive a complete educational assessment before being placed in a special education program.

*Individualized education plan (IEP)*—This plan must be focused and modified on a set of goals and objectives to meet the child's individual needs.

*Education in the least restrictive environment (LRE)*—Children with disabilities should be educated as much as possible with their peers who do not have disabilities.

*Parent and student participation in decision making*—Parent and student participation and communication are encouraged. Parents are members of the IEP team and are included in evaluation, eligibility, and placement.

*Early intervention services for children and their families*—Funds are allocated to infants who have disabling conditions and/or developmental delays. An individualized family service plan (IFSP) is developed that details the early intervention services to enhance the child's development and strengthen the family (National Dissemination Center for Children with Disabilities, 2012).

The No Child Left Behind Act of 2001 expands parental roles in their child's education. This law reauthorized the Elementary and Secondary Education Act of 1965, the principal federal law governing elementary and secondary education. According to the USDE, it is built on four concepts: accountability, doing what works according to the scientific research, expanding parental options, and expanding local control and flexibility. This bill does the following:

- Supports learning in the early years, hopefully preventing learning disabilities
- Provides more information for parents about their child's programs
- Alerts parents to important information about their child's performance
- Gives more resources to schools
- Gives children and parents a lifeline
- Improves teaching and learning by providing better information to teachers
- Ensures that teacher quality is a high priority
- Allows more flexibility

The Individuals with Disabilities Education Improvement Act of 2004 is the nation's special education law and serves 6.8 million children and youth with disabilities (USDE, 2010).

The Developmental Disabilities Act and Bill of Rights Act of 2000 requires the Administration of Developmental Disabilities (ADD) under the USDHHS to ensure that people with developmental disabilities and their families receive the services and support they need. The disabled and their families must also be given the opportunity to participate in the planning and implementation of these services. The ADD is a federal agency within the USDHHS and is responsible for implementation and administration of The Developmental Disabilities Act and Bill of Rights Act of 2000 and the disability provisions of the Help Americans Vote Act. There are eight areas of emphasis for ADD: employment, education, child care, health, housing, transportation, recreation, and quality assurance. The ADD meets these requirements through four programs:

1. *State Councils on Developmental Disabilities (SCDD):* Each state has a council whose function is to increase the independence, productivity, inclusion, and community integration of persons with developmental disabilities.
2. *Protection and Advocacy Agencies (P&As):* Every state has a system to empower, protect, and advocate on the behalf of persons with developmental disabilities. The system investigates incidents of abuse, neglect, or discrimination based on disability.
3. *University Centers for Excellence in Developmental Disabilities—Education, Research, and Services (UCEDD):*

This program provides support to a national network of university centers to carry out interdisciplinary training, services, technical assistance, and information dissemination activities. Its purpose is to increase independence, productivity, and integration into communities.

4. *Projects of National Significance:* The purpose of this program is to focus on emerging issues, provide technical assistance, conduct research regarding disability issues, and develop state and federal policy (www.acf.hhs.gov). In addition, most states and many large cities and counties have their own laws prohibiting discrimination on the basis of disability. Such laws offer greater protection to employees by extending coverage to smaller employers, by using more expansive definitions of disability than those used under the ADA, and by expanding the duty of employers to assist employees with disabilities to move to new positions for which they are qualified. Box 31-7 lists federal agencies with developmental disability activities.

---

**BOX 31-7   Federal Agencies with Developmental Disability Activities**

- Administration on Developmental Disabilities (ADD)
- Center for Medicaid and Medicare Services—Medicaid and the State Children's Health Insurance Program can help children and adults obtain health care coverage
- DisabilityInfo.gov—provides information about disability resources in the federal government
- Maternal and Child Health Bureau (MCHB)—promotes the health of mothers and children; provides newborn hearing screening, information on child health and safety and information on genetics
- Medline plus Health Information, National Library of Medicine—online resource for information
- National Council on Disability (NCD)—ensures that persons with disabilities have the same opportunities as others; promotes policies and programs that assist people with disabilities
- National Institutes of Health (NIH)—conducts and funds research on developmental disabilities
- National Institute on Disability and Rehabilitation Research (NIDRR)—promotes the participation of persons with disabilities in their communities
- Office of Disability Employment—focus is to increase job opportunities for people with disabilities; this office is within the U.S. Department of Labor
- Office of Special Education Programs (OSEP)—improves the lives of children and youth with disabilities from birth to adulthood through education and support services; this office is within the U.S. Department of Education
- Office on Disability—oversees the implementation of federal disability policies and programs; fosters interactions between the U.S. Department of Health and Human Services, other federal and state agencies, and private-sector groups
- Rehabilitative Services Administration (RSA)—helps persons with disabilities get jobs and live more independently; RSA is part of the U.S. Department of Education

Centers for Disease Control and Prevention: *Federal agencies with developmental disability activities*, 2010b: author. Available at www.cdc.gov. Accessed April 11, 2014.

## PRACTICE APPLICATION

A referral was made to a public health department from a nearby regional level III neonatal intensive care unit (NICU) regarding discharge plans for a developmentally delayed infant. The infant, Joel, was born at 27 weeks gestation and had remained in intensive care for 7 months. His hospital course was complicated by respiratory distress syndrome, bronchopulmonary dysplasia, and intraventricular hemorrhage. At the time of discharge, Joel was receiving neither supplemental oxygen nor medications and was taking all of his feedings orally. There were strong indications of spastic diplegia and he was diagnosed as having severe retinopathy of prematurity with the expectation of eventual blindness.

Family financial resources were extremely limited. Although Medicaid coverage was available for subsequent needs, the family owed more than $100,000 to the hospital. Joel's grandmother agreed to care for him while his 17-year-old mother Mary finished high school. Joel's father, who is also 17 years old and unemployed, had not been active with Mary and her mother in the hospital discharge-planning program. His involvement with Mary and Joel was expected to be minimal. The hospital was seeking a home evaluation before discharge.

What would you consider to be the first step in completing the home evaluation?

**Answers can be found on the Evolve site.**

## KEY POINTS

- Nurses have many opportunities to influence the care of individuals with disabilities through health promotion activities. Health education is important for parents who might be at high risk for having a disabled child, for children at risk for accidents and injuries, and for adults with chronic illnesses who might prevent disability through careful health practices.
- Many of the *Healthy People 2020* objectives apply to physically compromised individuals, their families, and communities.
- Physically compromised individuals need to participate in health promotion to prevent the onset of a new health disruption, to strengthen their well-functioning aspects, and to prevent further deterioration of their health.
- Nursing interventions for physically compromised clients require attention to their health as well as to the environment in which they live.
- Nurses influence policy decisions that affect the health and well-being of compromised individuals.
- Nurses must know both federal and state laws pertaining to disabilities to most effectively assist clients and their families.

## CLINICAL DECISION-MAKING ACTIVITIES

1. Divide the class or the clinical group into two teams and debate the following: Children with developmental disabilities should or should not be mainstreamed into classrooms with nondisabled children.
2. During a home visit first to an adult and then to a child who have a chronic illness that leaves them physically compromised, answer the following questions:
   A. Could this disability have been prevented? If so, what steps could a nurse have taken to provide health promotion activities that would have prevented the occurrence of the disabling condition?
   B. What role, if any, does the environment play in the onset of this compromising health condition?
   C. What preventive activities are currently needed to ensure the highest possible quality of life for this person?
3. For the next week, look at each building you enter and consider the following:
   A. What accommodations have been made to allow physically compromised people to enter this building?
   B. What accommodations should still be made?
   C. Who should pay for these architectural accommodations?
4. Spend one day following your usual schedule using either crutches or a wheelchair, so that you can understand better what it means to be physically compromised and have special needs.
5. Using a telephone book, community resource directory, or the web pages for your town, identify all agencies whose scope of work is devoted to assisting special needs individuals and their families.

## REFERENCES

Allarie SH: Employment and satisfaction outcomes from a job retention intervention delivered to persons with chronic diseases. *Rehabil Couns Bull* 48:100–109, 2005.

American Community Survey: *Disability*, 2012. author. Available at: www.census.gov/people/ disability/methodology/acs. Accessed April 1, 2014.

Americans with Disabilities Act of 1990, PL 101–336, 1990.

Anderson C: *IAN research report: Bullying and Children with ASD*, 2012. author. Available at: www.iancommunity.org/cs/ ian_research_reports/ ian_research_report_bullying. Accessed April 9, 2014.

Bilgin S, Gozum S: Reducing burnout in mothers with an intellectually disabled child: an education programme. *J Adv Nurs* 65:2552–2561, 2009.

Brault M: *Americans with Disabilities: 2010: Current Population Reports*, 2012. author. Available at: www.census.gov/prod/2012pubs/ p70-131.pdf. Accessed March 1, 2014.

Carmona R: *The Surgeon General's Call to Action to Improve the Health and Wellness of Persons with Disabilities*, 2005. author. Available at:

www.surgeongeneral.gov/about. Accessed April 8, 2014.

Center for an Accessible Society: *Independent Living for a Million Adults Jeopardized by a Shortfall of a Few Hours of Help*, 2014. author. Available at: www.accessiblesociety.org/topics. Accessed April 8, 2014.

Centers for Disease Control and Prevention: *Chronic Diseases and Health Promotion*, 2010a. author. Available at: www.cdc.gov/ chronicdisease/overview/index. Accessed April 5, 2014.

Centers for Disease Control and Prevention: *Federal Agencies with Developmental Disability Activities*, 2010b: author. Available at www.cdc.gov. Accessed April 11, 2014.

Centers for Disease Control and Prevention: *Falls among Older Adults: An Overview*, 2013. author. Available at: www.cdc.gov/ homeandrecreationalsafety/falls/ adultfalls.html. Accessed April 8, 2014.

Centers for Disease Control and Prevention: *Causes of Disability*, 2014a. author. Available at: www.cdc.gov/Features/ dsAdultDisabilityCauses. Accessed April 5,2014.

Centers for Disease Control and Prevention: *Classifications of Diseases Functioning, and Disability*, 2014b. author. Available at: www.cdc.gov/nchs/icd. Accessed April 5, 2014.

Centers for Disease Control and Prevention: *Disability and Obesity*, 2014c. author. Available at: www.cdc.gov/ncbddd/ disabilityandhealth/obesity.html. Accessed April 8, 2014.

The Council for Disability Awareness: *Disability Statistics*, 2013. author. Available at: www .disabilitycanhappen.org. Accessed April 8, 2014.

Council on Linkages Between Academia and Public Health Practice: *Core Competencies for Public Health Professionals*: Tiers, 2012. author. Available at: www.phf.org/programs/ corecompetencies. Accessed February 26, 2014.

Currie D: Major causes of disability, death shift around the globe: Chronic diseases now taking the lead. *The Nation's Health*, 2013. Available at: www.thenationshealth.apha publications.org. Accessed April 6. 2014.

Dauz WP, Piamjariyakul U, Graff JC, et al: Developmental disabilities: effects on well siblings. *Issues Compr Pediatr Nurs* 33:39–55, 2010.

Diament M: *Families Increasingly Shoulder Caregiving Burden*, 2011. author. Available at: www.disabilityscoop.com. Accessed April 8, 2014.

Disability is Natural: *People First Language*, 2014. author. Available at: www.disabilityisnatural.com/ explore/people-first-language. Accessed April 5, 2014.

Dyke P, Mulroy S, Leonard H: Siblings of children with disabilities: challenges and opportunities. *Acta Paediatr* 98:23–24, 2009.

Erickson W, Lee C, von Schrader S: *Disability Statistics from the 2012 American Community Survey (ACS)*, 2014. Cornell University Employment and Disability Institute (EDI). Available at: www.disabilitystatistics.org. Accessed April 8, 2014.

Gallaudet University National Deaf Education Center: *Americans with Disabilities Act*, 2014. author. Available at: www.gallaudet.edu/ clerc_center/information_and_ resources/info_to_go/laws/ada.html. Accessed April 11, 2014.

Guiding Light Foundation: *Disability Laws*, 2010. author. Available at: www.guidinglightfoundation.org. Accessed April 11.2014.

Heywood J: Childhood disability: ordinary lives for extraordinary families. *Community Pract* 83:19–22, 2010.

International Center for Disability Resources on the Internet: *Legal, Advocacy, Policy, and Political Issues*, 2010. author. Available at: www.icdri.org/legal. Accessed April 11, 2014.

Jones NL: Essential requirements of the act: A short history and overview. *Milbank Q* 69(Suppl 1–2):25–54, 1991.

Lair PL, Kale KD: Post-offer medical exam was premature. *HR Magazine* 50:163, 2005.

Laskar AR, Gupta VK, Kumar D, et al: Psychosocial effect and economic burden on parents of children with locomotor disability. *Indian J Pediatr [serial online]* 2010. Available at: www.ncbi.nlm.nih.gov/ pubmed. Accessed April 8. 2014.

Leffert JS, Siperstein GN, Widaman KF: Social perceptions in children with intellectual disabilities: the interpretation of benign and hostile intentions. *J Intellect Disabil Res* 54:168–180, 2010.

Maart S, Jelsma J: The sexual behavior of physically disabled adolescents. *Disabil Rehabil* 32:438–443, 2010.

Maternal and Child Health Bureau: *The National Survey of Children with Special Health Care Needs Chartbook 2009-2010*, 2013. author. Available at:

www.mchb.hrsa.gov. Accessed April 5, 1014.

Merriam-Webster On-Line Dictionary: *Disability*, 2014. author. Available at: www.merriam-webster.com. Accessed March 26, 2014.

Missouri Department of Health & Senior Services: *Abuse, Neglect, and Exploitation of the Elderly and Disabled*, 2014. author. Available at: www.health.mo.gov/safety/ abuse. Accessed April 9, 2014.

Murchland S, Parkyn H: Using assistive technology for schoolwork: the experience of children with physical disabilities. *Disabil Rehabil Assist Technol* 5(6):438–447, 2010.

National Dissemination Center for Children with Disabilities: *IDEA—the Individuals with Disabilities Education Act*, 2012. author. Available at: www.nichcy.org. Accessed April 11, 2014.

National Institute of Mental Health: *The Numbers Count: Mental Disorders in America*, 2010. author. Available at: www.nimh.gov/health/ publications. Accessed April 8. 2014.

O'Brien I, Duffy A, Nicholl H: Impact of childhood chronic illness on siblings: a literature review. *Br J Nurs* 18(1358):1360–1365, 2009.

Obrusnikova I, Block M, Dillon S: Children's beliefs toward cooperative playing with peers with disabilities in physical education. *Adapt Phys Activ Q* 27:127–142, 2010.

Redmon SJ: Healthcare transitions for adolescents and young adults with special healthcare needs and/or disabilities. *Prof Case Manag* 15:170, 2010.

Reinehr T, Dobe M, Winkel K, et al: Obesity in disabled children and adolescents: an overlooked group of patients. *Dtsch Arztebl Int* 107:268–275, 2010.

Roth DL, Perkins M, Wadley VG, et al: Family caregiving and emotional strain: associations with quality of life in a large national sample of middle-aged and older adults. *Qual Life Res* 18:679–688, 2009.

Scullion PA: Models of disability: their influence in nursing and potential role in challenging discrimination. *J Adv Nurs* 66:697–707, 2010.

Social Security Administration: *Red Book*, 2014. author. Available at: www.ssa.gov/redbook/eng/ definedisability. Accessed April 5, 2014.

United Nations: *Women and Girls with Disabilities*, 2010. author. Available at: www.un.org/ disabilities. Accessed April 9, 2014.

United States Quad Rugby Association: *Murderball*, 2010. author. Available at: www.quadrugby.com/murderball/ faqs.html. Accessed April 8, 2014.

U.S. Department of Education (USDE): *Building the Legacy: IDEA 2004*, 2010. author. Available at: www.idea.ed.gov. Accessed April 8, 2014.

U.S. Department of Health and Human Services, Children's Bureau: *The Risk and Prevention of Maltreatment of Children with Disabilities*, 2012. author. Available at: www.childwelfare.gov/pubs/ prevenres/focus. Accessed April 11, 2014.

U.S. Department of Health and Human Services: *Healthy People 2020: Disability and Health*, 2013. author. Available at: www.healthypeople.gov. Accessed April 11, 2014.

U.S. Department of Justice: *A Guide to Disability Rights Laws*, 2012. author. Available at: www.ada.gov/ cguide.pdf. Accessed April 11, 2014.

Walk EE, Ahn HC, Lampkin PM, et al: Americans with Disabilities Act. *J Burn Care Rehabil* 14:92–98, 1993.

Wei X, Yu JW: The concurrent and longitudinal effects of child disability types and health on family experiences. *Maternal Child Health J [serial online]*, 2012. Available at: www.ncbi.nlm.nih.gov/pubmed. Accessed April 8, 2014.

Wilson PE, Clayton GH: Sports and disability. *Phys Med Rehabil Clin N Am* 2:S46–S54, 2010.

World Health Organization: *World Report on Disability*, 2011. author. Available at: www.who.int/ disabilities/world_report/2011. Accessed April 5, 2014.

World health Organization: *Early Childhood Development and Disability: A Discussion Paper*, 2012. author. Available at: www.who.int/disabilities/ publications/other/ECDD_final word.doc. Accessed April 8, 2014.

World Health Organization: *10 Facts on the State of Global Health*, 2013. author. Available at: www.who.int/features/factfiles/ disability. Accessed April 8, 2014.

World Health Organization: *Towards a Common Language for Functioning, Disability and Health*, 2011. author. *Available* at: www.who.int/ classifications/icf/en. Accessed April 5, 2014.

Yildirim A, Hacihasanoglu R, Karakurt P: Effects of a nursing intervention program on the depression and perception of family functioning of mothers with intellectually disabled children. *J Clin Nurs* 22(1–2):251–261, 2013.

# Promoting and Protecting the Health of Vulnerable Populations

The chapters in this section of the text describe the myriad ways in which the social determinants of health affect people. There is a growing body of information that tells us that one of the most powerful ways to improve the health of the community is to consider and hopefully improve the social determinants of health. The World Health Organization (2012) defines social determinants of health as "conditions in which people are born, grow, live, work, and age, including the health system" and which are "shaped by the distribution of money, power, and resources at global, national and local levels" (para 1). Social determinants of health include social, political, and economic factors, and include living environments and conditions, geographic location, and social class. Populations that lack adequate socioeconomic and psychosocial resources have a greater exposure to violence, alcohol, tobacco and other drugs, mental health issues, and poverty. Migrant workers are often included in a population that is high risk for health disruptions due to their work and transitory lifestyle. Homeless persons and pregnant teens are also high-risk populations due to the circumstances that they face. Solutions to the many problems described in the chapters in this part of the text require an integrated behavioral, social, and health care approach. This approach must begin with a commitment to primary health care. Primary health care involves a partnership between public health and primary care to address the problems of society as well as of individuals and families. The chapters in Part 6 discuss some of the most common problems seen in communities. There is hope that health care reform will positively intervene in the social determinants that affect the groups described in this part of the text.

---

World Health Organization: *Social determinants of health.* Retrieved from http://www.who.int/social_determinants/en/. March 20, 2015.

# 32

# Vulnerability and Vulnerable Populations: An Overview

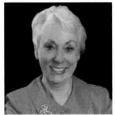

*Jeanette Lancaster, PhD, RN, FAAN\**

Dr. Lancaster is Professor and Dean Emerita of Nursing at the University of Virginia. She has edited this book with Dr. Marcia Stanhope through its previous eight editions.

## ADDITIONAL RESOURCES

ⓔ**Evolve Website http://evolve.elsevier.com/Stanhope**
- NCLEX® Review Questions
- Case Study, with Questions and Answers

- Glossary
- Clinical Application Answers

## OBJECTIVES

*After reading this chapter, the student should be able to do the following:*

1. Describe population groups who might be considered vulnerable.
2. Identify the ways in which these populations often have health disparities compared with the general population.
3. Analyze trends that have influenced both the development of vulnerability among certain population groups and social attitudes toward vulnerability.

4. Analyze the effects of public policies on vulnerable populations and on reducing health disparities experienced by these populations.
5. Examine the multiple individual and social factors that contribute to vulnerability.
6. Evaluate strategies that nurses can use to improve the health status, and eliminate health disparities, of vulnerable populations including governmental, community, and private programs.

## KEY TERMS

advocacy, p. 722
barriers to access, p. 719
case management, p. 728
comprehensive services, p. 722
cumulative risks, p. 716
determinants of health, p. 718
disadvantaged, p. 717
disenfranchisement, p. 717
federal poverty guideline, p. 719
health disparities, p. 717
human capital, p. 717

linguistically appropriate health care, p. 722
poverty, p. 719
resilience, p. 716
risk, p. 716
social determinants of health, p. 718
social justice, p. 722
vulnerability, p. 716
vulnerable population group, p. 716
wrap-around services, p. 721
—*See Glossary for definitions*

---

*In previous editions of this textbook, Chapter 32 was skillfully authored by Juliann G. Sebastian. Dr. Sebastian is Professor and Dean of the College of Nursing at the University of Nebraska. Her contributions to the development of this chapter have been enormous over the years and in several editions.

This chapter discusses the concept of *vulnerability* and the nursing roles for meeting the health needs of vulnerable population groups. Selected population groups that are at greater risk than others of poor health outcomes are described briefly in this chapter and in depth in other chapters in this book. The relationship between health disparities, health equity, and vulnerability is described. Public policies that have influenced vulnerable groups and the effects of these policies are explored. The nature of vulnerability is analyzed and factors that predispose people to vulnerability, outcomes of vulnerability, and the cycle of vulnerability are described. Two of the overarching goals of *Healthy People 2020* are to achieve equity, eliminate disparities, and improve the health of all groups; and to create social and physical environments that promote good health for all (U.S. Department of Health and Human Services [USDHHS], 2010). Nursing interventions to break the cycle of vulnerability and to eliminate health disparities are possible at the individual, family, group, community, and population levels, and examples of interventions are discussed. This chapter also describes how nurses use the nursing process with vulnerable population groups and presents case examples to illustrate nursing actions.

## VULNERABILITY: DEFINITION, RISK FACTORS, AND HEALTH DISPARITIES

Vulnerability is defined as susceptibility to actual or potential stressors that may lead to an adverse effect. Vulnerable populations are typically considered to be those that are at greater risk for poor health status and that have poor access to health care. As discussed in Chapter 12, risk is an epidemiologic term indicating that some people have a higher probability of illness than others. In the epidemiologic triangle, the agent, host, and environment interact to produce illness or poor health. The natural history of disease model explains how certain aspects of physiology and the environment, including personal habits, social environment, and physical environment, make it more likely that a person will develop particular health problems (Friis, 2010). For example, a smoker is at risk for developing lung cancer because cellular changes occur with smoking. However, not everyone who is at risk develops health problems. Some individuals are more likely than others to develop the health problems for which they are at risk. These people are more vulnerable than other people.

The web of causation model helps to explain what happens in these situations. A vulnerable population group is a subgroup of the population that is more likely to develop health problems as a result of exposure to risk and to have worse outcomes from these health problems than the rest of the population. That is, the interaction among many variables creates a more powerful combination of factors that predispose the persons in that group to illness. Vulnerable populations often experience multiple cumulative risks, and they are particularly sensitive to the effects of those risks. Risks come from environmental hazards (e.g., lead exposure from lead-based paint from peeling walls or paint used in toy manufacturing, melamine added to milk supplies), social hazards (e.g., crime, violence), personal behavior (e.g., diet, exercise habits, smoking), or biological or genetic makeup (e.g., congenital addiction, compromised immune status). Members of vulnerable populations often have multiple illnesses, with each affecting the other. Some members of vulnerable populations do not succumb to the health risks that impinge on them. It is important to learn what factors help these people to resist, or have resilience to, the effects of vulnerability. Vulnerability is a global concern, with different populations being more vulnerable in different countries. Several vulnerable population groups are discussed in Chapters 33 through 38 and in Chapters 11, 13, 14, and 31.

Examples of vulnerable populations of concern to nurses are persons who are poor and homeless, persons with special needs, pregnant teens, migrant workers and immigrants, individuals with mental health problems, people who abuse addictive substances, persons who have been incarcerated, persons who have or who are at risk for communicable and infectious diseases including persons who are HIV positive or have hepatitis B virus (HBV) or sexually transmitted diseases (STDs). Genetics also plays a role in vulnerability and influences a person's resilience to socioeconomic adverse conditions (Braveman and Gottlieb, 2014).

Benatar (2013) cites potentially avoidable factors that are often ignored by what he calls privileged societies and that could be alleviated by appropriate approaches. These are as follows: a bad start in life, such as in utero factors including material deprivation, abuse, substance abuse, or poor care; physical and emotional deprivation during childhood and adolescence; inadequate education and lack of exposure to social and environmental factors needed to promote adolescent development; inadequate access to the basic living conditions for a healthy life; lack of training for work that will allow the person to develop independently; and a lack of a sense of belonging and as a valued citizen (Benatar, 2013, p. 43).

Vulnerable populations are more likely than the general population to suffer from health disparities. Health disparities refer to the wide variations in health services and health status among certain population groups. For more than two decades, *Healthy People* has had an overarching goal that focused on intervening in disparities. The goal in *Healthy People 2000* was to reduce health disparities, and the goal moved to remove health disparities in *Healthy People 2010*. *Healthy People 2020* has expanded the goal to aim to achieve health equity, eliminate disparities, and improve the health of all groups. *Healthy People 2020* describes health equity as attaining the highest possible level of health for all people and includes eliminating health disparities (USDHHS, 2010). Thirty-eight topic areas in *Healthy People 2020* emphasize access, chronic health problems, injury and violence prevention, environmental health, food safety, education and community-based programs, health communication, health information technologies, immunization and infectious diseases, and public health infrastructure, among others. These topic areas are discussed in chapters throughout the text.

 **HEALTHY PEOPLE 2020**

### *Objectives for Vulnerable Populations*

Following are examples of objectives that nurses who work with vulnerable populations might want to note:

- AHS-1: Increase the proportion of persons with health insurance.
- AHS-6: Reduce the proportion of individuals who are unable to obtain or delay obtaining necessary medical care, dental care, or prescription medicines.
- HIV-4: Reduce the number of new HIV cases among adolescents and adults.
- EMC-2.5: Increase the proportion of parents with children under the age of 3 years whose doctors or other health care professionals talk with them about positive parenting practices.

*AHS*, Access to Health Services; *EMC*, Early and Middle Childhood. From U.S. Department of Health and Human Services (USDHHS): *Healthy People 2020*. Washington, DC, 2010, USDHHS. Retrieved February 2015 from http://www.healthypeople.gov/.

As discussed in other chapters, *Healthy People 2020* is an implementation guide for all federal and most state health initiatives. It is especially relevant to a discussion of vulnerable populations because these underserved and disadvantaged populations have fewer resources for promoting health and treating illness than does the average person in the United States. For example, a family or individual below the federal poverty line is considered disadvantaged in terms of access to economic resources. These groups are thought to be vulnerable because of the combination of risk factors, health status, and lack of resources needed to access health care and reduce risk factors.

Areas that show health disparities across population groups include infant mortality, mortality among children under 5 years of age, and age-adjusted mortality rates. In 2010, the mortality rate for black infants was 2.2 times the rate for white infants, with black infant deaths being 11.6 per 1000 live births in contrast to 5.19 infant deaths per 1000 live births for white infants (Murphy et al, 2013). Life expectancy at birth for white

males and females in 2010 was 76.4 and 81.1 years of age, respectively, and for black males and females, 71.4 and 77.7 years, respectively; the life expectancy for Hispanic males was 78.8 years, and Hispanic females had the highest life expectancy of 83.8 years (Murphy et al, 2012).

African Americans have significantly higher death rates from prostate and breast cancer and from heart disease than non-Hispanic whites living in the United States. Hispanics have higher mortality rates from diabetes than non-Hispanic whites living in the United States. Race and ethnicity are not thought to be the causes of these disparities, although research is underway to determine biological susceptibilities by race, ethnicity, and gender. Rather, poverty and low educational levels are more likely to contribute to social conditions in which disparities develop. People who are poor often live in unsafe areas, work in stressful environments, have less access to healthful foods and opportunities for exercise, and are more likely to be uninsured or underinsured.

## FACTORS CONTRIBUTING TO VULNERABILITY

Vulnerability results from the combined effects of limited resources. Limitations in physical resources, environmental resources, personal resources (or human capital), and biopsychosocial resources (e.g., the presence of illness, genetic predispositions) combine to cause vulnerability (Aday, 2001). Poverty, limited social support, and working in a hazardous environment are examples of limitations in physical and environmental resources. People with pre-existing illnesses, such as those with communicable or infectious diseases or chronic illnesses such as cancer, heart disease, or chronic airway disease, have less physical ability to cope with stress than those without such physical problems. Human capital refers to all of the strengths, knowledge, and skills that enable a person to live a productive, happy life. People with little education have less human capital because their choices are more limited than those of people with higher levels of education.

Vulnerability has many aspects. It often comes from a feeling of lack of power, limited control, victimization, disadvantaged status, disenfranchisement, and health risks. Vulnerability can be reversed by obtaining resources to increase resilience. Useful nursing interventions to increase resilience include case finding, health education, care coordination, and policy making related to improving health for vulnerable populations.

One aspect of vulnerability, disenfranchisement, refers to a feeling of separation from mainstream society. The person does not seem to have an emotional connection with any group in particular or with the larger society. Some groups such as the poor, the homeless, and migrant workers are "invisible" to society as a whole and tend to be forgotten in health and social planning. Vulnerable populations are at risk for disenfranchisement because their social supports are often weak, as are their linkages to formal community organizations such as churches, schools, and other types of social organizations. They also may have few informal sources of support, such as family, friends, and neighbors. In many ways, vulnerable groups have limited control over potential and actual health needs. In many communities, these groups are in the minority and disadvantaged because typical health planning focuses on the majority. Disadvantage also results from lack of resources that others may take for granted. Vulnerable population groups have limited social and economic resources with which to manage their health care. For example, women may endure domestic violence rather than risk losing a place for them and their children to live. Women who are among the working poor are more likely to become homeless when they leave an abusive partner. They may not be able to pay for a place to live when they lose their partner's income.

## Social Determinants of Health

Social and economic factors contribute heavily to vulnerability. Social determinants of health include a range of social, political and economic factors that include socioeconomic status, living conditions, geographic location, social class, education, environmental factors, nutrition, stress, and prejudice that lead to resource constraints, poor health, and health risk (Wilensky and Satcher, 2009; Lathrop, 2013). From an international perspective, the World Health Organization (WHO, 2015) states that many factors in combination affect the health of individuals and communities. Specifically, "whether people are healthy or not is determined by their circumstances and environment." The WHO, consistent with *Healthy People 2020*, describes three overall determinants of health to be (1) the social and economic environment, (2) the physical environment, and (3) the person's individual characteristics and behaviors. The WHO also notes that individuals are unlikely to be able to directly control many of the determinants of health, and this is directly related to vulnerability. That is, when people experience adverse determinants of health that they cannot control, they are predisposed to becoming vulnerable. The WHO, 2015 cites seven examples of factors that affect health. There are many more factors that affect health, as noted later in the *Healthy People 2020* document. The seven WHO factors are as follows (WHO, 2015, pp. 1-2):

1. Income and social status: Higher income and social status are associated with better health.
2. Education: Low education is linked with poor health, more stress, and lower self-confidence.
3. Physical environment: Safe water and clean air; healthy workplaces; safer homes, communities, and roads; and good employment and working conditions, especially when the person has more control, all contribute to good health.
4. Social support networks: Family, friends, and community as well as culture, customs, traditions, and beliefs affect health.
5. Genetics, as well as personal behavior and coping skills, affect health.
6. Health services: Access and use of services affect health.
7. Gender: Men and women suffer from different types of diseases at different ages. See Figure 32-1 for a street scene that depicts factors that could influence the determinants of health.

*Healthy People 2020* (USDHHS, 2010) discusses the importance of social determinants of health by including "Create social and physical environments that promote good health for

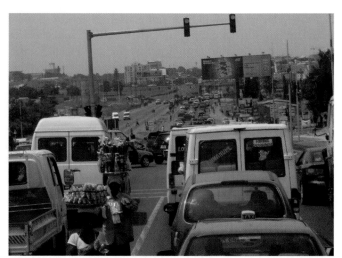

**FIG 32-1** Example of a street scene that could influence the determinants of health.

all" as one of the four overarching goals. This document explains that it is important to understand the relationship between how population groups experience "place" and the effect that "place" has on the social determinants of health. This concept is consistent with an ecologic framework that examines the effect that people have on the environment and vice versa. *Healthy People 2020* lists 15 examples of social determinants of health: (1) availability of resources to meet daily needs; (2) access to educational, economic, and job opportunities; (3) access to health services; (4) quality of education and job training; (5) availability of community-based resources in support of community living and opportunities for recreation; (6) transportation options; (7) public safety; (8) social support; (9) social norms and attitudes; (10) exposure to crime, violence, and social disorder; (11) socioeconomic conditions; (12) residential segregation; (13) language/literacy; (14) access to mass media and emerging technologies; and (15) culture. This document also lists seven examples of physical determinants of health: (1) natural environment, such as green space and weather; (2) built environment, such as buildings, sidewalks, bike lanes, and roads; (3) worksites, schools, and recreational settings; (4) housing and community design; (5) exposure to toxic substances and other physical hazards; (6) physical barriers, especially for people with disabilities; and (7) aesthetic elements (USDHHS, 2010, pp. 3-4). A useful diagram is also provided that depicts how the five key areas (determinants) of economic stability, education, social and community context, health and health care, and neighborhoods and the built environment serve as a framework for an approach to understanding the social determinants of health (USDHHS, 2010, p. 4) (Figure 32-2).

As mentioned, social status influences health in a variety of ways. First, the more wealth the person has, the more likely the person is to have access to better foods, more education, a safer community, recreation, and health care. These resources serve as protective barriers again chronic disease, injury, and premature mortality (Lathrop, 2013). Nursing interventions are designed to help vulnerable populations gain the resources needed for better health and reduction of risk factors.

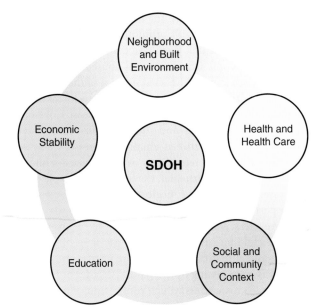

**FIG 32-2** Five key areas of social determinants of health as found in *Healthy People 2020*. (Retrieved February 2015 from http://www.healthypeople.gov/2020/topics-objectives/topic/social-determinants-health?topicid=39.)

Poverty is a primary cause of vulnerability, and it is a growing problem in the United States. The chronic stress of factors such as poverty, unemployment, and poor education can lead to maladaptive physical responses and disease (Lathrop, 2013). Poverty is a relative state. The federal definition of poverty is used to develop eligibility criteria for programs such as Medicaid and welfare assistance. In 2014 the federal poverty guideline for a family of four was $23,850 for all states except Hawaii and Alaska. Both Alaska and Hawaii have higher poverty guideline levels (USDHHS, 2010). However, many people who earn just a little more than the federal poverty guideline are unable to pay for their living expenses but are ineligible for assistance programs. See Chapter 3 for a discussion of the Patient Protection and Affordable Care Act of 2010, and its implementation and effect on individuals and families. The implementation of this Act is bringing substantial changes to the U.S. health care system including a new emphasis on prevention (Lathrop, 2013).

As discussed in Chapter 10, people who are poor are more likely to live in hazardous environments that are overcrowded and have inadequate sanitation, work in high-risk jobs, have less nutritious diets, and have multiple stressors, because they do not have the extra resources to manage unexpected crises and may not even have adequate resources to manage daily life. Poverty often reduces an individual's access to health care. In the developed countries of the world, this is more likely to be a problem for those just above the poverty line, who are not eligible for public support, whereas in developing countries poverty is correlated with decreased access to health care. Chapter 33 provides a more thorough discussion of poverty and also discusses how poverty can lead to homelessness.

Education plays an important role in health status. Although education is related to income, educational level seems to influence health separately. Higher levels of education may provide people with more information for making healthy lifestyle choices. More highly educated people are better able to make informed choices about health insurance and providers. Education also may influence perceptions of stressors and problem situations and give people more alternatives (Shi and Stevens, 2010). Finally, education and language skills affect health literacy. Chapter 16 discusses health literacy and its effect on health.

Access to health care may be more limited for low socioeconomic groups. Barriers to access are policies and financial, geographic, or cultural features of health care that make services difficult to obtain or so unappealing that people do not seek care. Examples include offering services only on weekdays without providing evening or weekend hours for working adults, being uninsured or underinsured, not having reasonably convenient or economical transportation, or providing services only in English and not in the population's primary language. Also, services for families may be offered in locations that make it difficult for people who do not have reliable forms of transportation. Removing these barriers by providing extended clinic hours, low-cost or free health services for people who are uninsured or underinsured, transportation, mobile vans, and professional interpreters helps improve access to care (Shi and Stevens, 2005). The interactions among multiple socioeconomic stressors make people more susceptible to risks than others with more financial resources, who may cope more effectively.

As discussed in Chapter 33, extreme poverty, in the form of homelessness or marginal housing, is related to risk for physical, dental, and mental health problems; food insecurity; and limited access to health care (Baggett et al, 2010). Those who are homeless or marginally housed have even fewer resources than poor people who have adequate housing. Homeless and marginally housed people must struggle with heavy demands as they try to manage daily life. These individuals and families do not have the advantage of consistent housing and must cope with finding a place to sleep at night and a place to stay during the day or must move frequently from one residence to another, as well as find food, before even thinking about health care. Lack of access to nutritious food on a regular basis poses serious health problems (Borre et al, 2010).

### Health Status

Age is related to vulnerability, because people at both ends of the age continuum are often less able physiologically to adapt to stressors. For example, infants of substance-abusing mothers risk being born addicted and having severe physiological problems and developmental delays. Because mental and physical problems in adulthood are often associated with childhood stressors such as poverty and emotional deprivation it is important to reduce or eliminate early health disparities (Hillemeier et al, 2013). See Figure 32-3. *Healthy People 2020* includes objectives related to equity for young children for prenatal and early childhood health promotion, decrease in preterm birth and low birth weight, optimal intake of nutrition, and weight and healthy development for school readiness (USDHHS, 2010). Elderly individuals are more likely to develop active infections

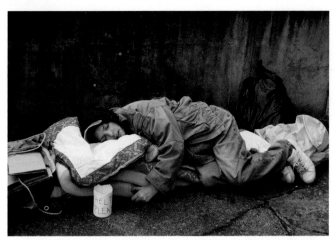

**FIG 32-3** People who become homeless often once had a home and a family. (© 2012 Photos.com, a division of Getty Images. All rights reserved. Image #135090280.)

from communicable diseases such as the flu or pneumonia and generally have more difficulty recovering from infectious processes than younger people because of their less effective immune systems. Older people also may be more vulnerable to safety threats and loss of independence because of their age, multiple chronic illnesses, and impaired mobility. Chapter 37 discusses substance abuse, and Chapter 13 describes communicable disease risk.

Also, changes in normal physiology can predispose people to vulnerability. This may result from disease processes, such as in someone with single or multiple chronic diseases. As discussed in Chapter 14, infection with HIV is a pathophysiological situation that increases vulnerability to opportunistic infections.

A person's life experiences, especially those early in life, influence vulnerability or resilience. For example, children who survive disasters may experience difficulties in later life if they do not receive adequate counseling. Examples of protective social factors include social support, self-esteem, and self-efficacy (thinking you can handle situations and cope) (Braveman and Gottlieb, 2014). Specifically, higher levels of confidence in one's ability or internal locus of control appears to protect children (particularly adolescents) from the negative effects of disaster and trauma. Persons with an internal locus of control believe that they control their behavior and do not depend entirely on external people, events, or forces to control behavior. It is the person's perception of his or her level of personal control that influences the person's decisions. Persons with a high level of internal locus of control are more likely to participate in health screenings and take responsibility for their health. That is, they believe they can control to some extent their health outcomes. For example, a woman with a high internal locus of control would participate regularly in yoga and exercise classes to increase flexibility and build strength to preserve her bone and muscle tone. Vulnerable population groups often develop an external locus of control. They may believe that events are outside their control and result from bad luck or fate. People with an external locus of control have more difficulty

taking action or seeking care for health problems. They may minimize the value of health promotion or illness prevention because they do not think they have control over their health destinies. Also, people who have been abused or have experienced chronic stress may have used up a lot of the reserves that others would normally have for coping with new forms of stress. A study by investigators at the Centers for Disease Control and Prevention (Middlebrooks and Audage, 2008) looked retrospectively at the link between childhood stressors and adult health. This study was referred to as the Adverse Childhood Experiences Study. In particular, the investigators looked at the stress caused by child abuse, neglect, and repeated exposure to intimate partner violence. They discussed three kinds of stress: (1) positive stress, which comes from short-lived adverse events and which children can manage with the help of supportive adults; (2) tolerable stress, which is more intense but still short-lived, such as stress arising from a natural disaster or frightening accident; or (3) toxic stress, which results from intense adverse experiences sustained over time. Children cannot handle toxic stress alone. Stress response activated for an extended length of time can lead to permanent developmental changes in the brain. The support of helping adults can enable the child's stress response to return to normal. As is discussed in Chapter 38, child maltreatment can be a source of toxic stress.

## OUTCOMES OF VULNERABILITY

Outcomes of vulnerability may be negative, such as a lower health status than the rest of the population, or they may be positive with effective interventions. Vulnerable populations often have worse health outcomes than other people in terms of morbidity and mortality. These groups have a high prevalence of chronic illnesses, such as hypertension, and high levels of communicable diseases, including tuberculosis (TB), hepatitis B, and sexually transmitted diseases (STDs), as well as upper respiratory tract infections, including influenza. They also have higher mortality rates than the general population because of factors such as poor living conditions, diet, and health status, as well as crime and violence, including domestic violence.

There is often a cycle to vulnerability. That is, poor health creates stress as individuals and families try to manage health problems with inadequate resources. For example, if someone with acquired immunodeficiency syndrome (AIDS) develops one or more opportunistic infections and is either uninsured or underinsured, that person and the family and caregivers will have more difficulty managing than if the person had adequate insurance. Vulnerable populations often suffer many forms of stress. Sometimes when one problem is solved, another quickly emerges. This can lead to feelings of hopelessness, which result from an overwhelming sense of powerlessness and social isolation. For example, substance abusers who feel powerless over their addiction and who have isolated themselves from the people they care about may see no way to change their situation. Nursing interventions should include strategies that will increase resources or reduce health risks to decrease health disparities between vulnerable populations and populations with more advantages (Flaskerud and Winslow, 2010).

## PUBLIC POLICIES AFFECTING VULNERABLE POPULATIONS

Three pieces of legislation have provided direct and indirect financial subsidies to certain vulnerable groups. The Social Security Act of 1935 created the largest federal support program in history for elderly and poor Americans. This act was intended to ensure a minimal level of support for people at risk for problems resulting from inadequate financial resources. This was accomplished by direct payments to eligible individuals. Later, the Social Security Act Amendments of 1965, Medicare and Medicaid, provided for the health care needs of older adults, the poor, and disabled people who might be vulnerable to impoverishment resulting from high medical bills or poor health status from inadequate access to health care. These acts created federal and state third-party health care payers. Title XXI of the Social Security Act, enacted in 1998, created the State Children's Health Insurance Program (SCHIP), which provides funds to insure currently uninsured children. The SCHIP is jointly funded by the federal and state governments and administered by the states. Using broad federal guidelines, each state designs its own program, determines who is eligible for benefits, sets the payment levels, and decides on the administrative and operating procedures. President Obama signed the Children's Health Insurance Program Reauthorization Act of 2009 (CHIPRA). This legislation provided states with new funding, new program options, and a range of new incentives for covering children through Medicaid and the Children's Health Insurance Program (CHIP) (Centers for Medicare and Medicaid Services, 2009).

The Balanced Budget Act of 1997 also influenced the use of resources for providing health services. In an attempt to curb the rapid growth in spending on home health and financial fraud in that industry, the Health Care Financing Administration (HCFA) moved toward prospective payment for home health services. HCFA also set more stringent regulations about which services were reimbursed and for how long and limited access to care for certain vulnerable groups, such as frail elders, chronically ill individuals whose care is largely home based, and people who are HIV positive. The goal is to ensure that care is appropriate, rather than to limit access. Nurses and other health care providers must work closely with families to determine the kinds of services needed to foster self-care and the optimal timing of these services. The Balanced Budget Act of 1997 also reduced payments for services for Medicare beneficiaries, resulting in some providers choosing not to treat them. This means that people with major health needs (i.e., some chronically ill and the elderly) may have limited access to care. There are a variety of Medicare supplemental insurance plans, including those for prescription drugs, and the costs of the plans vary considerably depending on the level of coverage provided. Choosing the right supplemental plan is complex. Two useful sources of information about supplemental plans are the American Association of Retired Persons (http://www.aarp.org) and the U.S. government website for Medicare (http://www.Medicare.gov).

Finally, one law focuses on the privacy and security of personal health information. The Health Insurance Portability and Accountability Act of 1996 (HIPAA) was intended to help people keep their health insurance when moving from one place to another. Ensuring the privacy and security of personal health information means that electronic and paper health records, case management, referrals, and physical space layouts (such as computer screen visibility and clinic registration sheets) must be managed to protect the client's privacy and safeguard the privacy of personal health information. In certain cases, health information for public health uses may be shared with appropriate public health agencies, such as in cases of suspected abuse or when investigating a communicable disease outbreak. As electronic health networks become more widely used, some provisions of this law may need to be updated (Greenberg et al, 2009).

The Balanced Budget Act of 1997 had some shifts in payment with the stipulations related to home health care. In an attempt to curb the rapid growth in spending on home health care and financial fraud in that industry, the Health Care Financing Administration (now the Centers for Medicare and Medicaid Services [CMS]) instituted prospective payment for home health services. The goal was to ensure that care was needed, rather than to limit access. Nurses and other health care providers work closely with families to determine the kinds of services needed to foster self-care, and the optimal timing of these services. The Patient Protection and Affordable Care Act of 2010 has provisions for reducing the growth of future Medicare expenditures (Newhouse, 2010). See Chapters 3, 5, and 8 for more detail on health care financing and the economics of health care. See also http://www.healthcare.gov/law/index.html and http://healthlawguide.aarp.org/.

## NURSING APPROACHES TO CARE IN THE COMMUNITY

As discussed in Chapter 2, the history of public health nursing, nurses beginning with Florence Nightingale, have known that the physical and social environments influenced the health of patients. Later Lillian Wald, when she established the Henry Street Settlement, provided nursing care and education to the community through health promotion including education, modification of the environment, and disease control (Lathrop, 2013). There is a trend toward providing more comprehensive, family-centered services when treating vulnerable population groups. It is important to provide comprehensive, family-centered, "one-stop" services. Providing multiple services during a single clinic visit is an example of one-stop services. If social assistance and economic assistance are provided and included in interdisciplinary treatment plans, services can be more responsive to the combined effects of social and economic stressors on the health of special population groups. This situation is sometimes referred to as providing wrap-around services, in which comprehensive health services are available and social and economic services are "wrapped around" these services. Although this is an excellent approach to care, it is not available in all or even most areas in the United States.

It is helpful to provide comprehensive services in locations where people live and work, including schools, churches, neighborhoods, and workplaces. Comprehensive services are health services that focus on more than one health problem or concern. For example, some nurses use stationary or mobile outreach clinics to provide a wide array of health promotion, illness prevention, and illness management services in migrant camps, schools, and local communities. A single client visit may focus on an acute health problem such as influenza, but it also may include health education about diet and exercise, counseling for smoking cessation, and a follow-up appointment for immunizations once the influenza is over. The shift away from hospital-based care includes a renewed commitment to the public health services that vulnerable populations need to prevent illness and promote health, such as reductions of environmental hazards and violence and assurance of safe food and water.

Referring clients to community agencies involves much more than simply making a phone call or completing a form. Nurses should make certain that the agency to which they refer a client is the right one to meet that client's needs. Nurses can do more harm than good by referring a stressed, discouraged client to an agency from which the client is not really eligible to receive services. Nurses should help the client learn how to get the most from the referral. As discussed in the chapter related to nurse managed health centers (see Chapter 21), nurses are critical safety net providers to vulnerable populations. Nurses in these centers aim to provide comprehensive care that includes referrals, follow-up, and advocacy. They often serve populations that have low incomes, may be members of minority groups, may be homeless, or may lack adequate insurance coverage, as well as other groups of vulnerable people.

Nurses also focus on advocacy and social justice concerns. Advocacy refers to actions taken on behalf of another. Nurses may function as advocates for vulnerable populations by working for the passage and implementation of policies that lead to improved public health services for these populations. For example, a nurse may serve on a local coalition for uninsured people and another may work to develop a plan for sharing the provision of free or low-cost health care by local health care organizations and providers.

Social justice includes the concepts of egalitarianism and equality. Braveman (2014, p. 129) says that at the heart of social justice is "justice with respect to the treatment of more advantaged vs. less advantaged socioeconomic groups when it comes to health and health care." A society that subscribes to the concept of social justice would be one that values equality and recognizes the worth of all members of that society. Such a society would provide humane care and social supports for all people. Nurses who function in advocacy roles and facilitate change in public policy are intervening to promote social justice. Nurses can be advocates for policy changes to improve social, economic, and environmental factors that predispose vulnerable populations to poor health. The overriding nursing goal for care of all people, including those who come from vulnerable populations, is to provide safe and quality care. See the Quality and Safety Education for Nurses (QSEN) box for information on quality care.

It is important for nurses to provide culturally and linguistically appropriate health care. Linguistically appropriate health care means communicating health-related information in the recipient's primary language when possible and always in a language the recipient can understand. It also means using words that the recipient can understand. The factors that predispose people to vulnerability and the outcomes of vulnerability create a cycle in which the outcomes reinforce the predisposing factors, leading to more negative outcomes. Unless the cycle is broken, it is difficult for vulnerable populations to improve their health. Nurses can identify areas in which they can work with vulnerable populations to break the cycle. The nursing process guides nurses in assessing vulnerable individuals, families, groups, and communities; developing nursing diagnoses of their strengths and needs; planning and implementing appropriate therapeutic nursing interventions in partnership with vulnerable clients; and evaluating the effectiveness of interventions.

## QSEN FOCUS ON QUALITY AND SAFETY EDUCATION FOR NURSES

Targeted Competency: Quality Improvement—Use data to monitor the outcomes of care processes and use improvement methods to design and test changes to continuously improve the quality and safety of health care systems.

Important aspects of quality improvement include:
- **Knowledge:** Explain the importance of variation and measurement in assessing quality of care.
- **Skills:** Use quality measures to understand performance.
- **Attitudes:** Value measurement and its role in good client care.

### Quality Improvement Question

Examine health statistics and demographic data in your geographic area to determine which vulnerable groups are predominant. Look on the web for examples of agencies you think provide services to these vulnerable groups. If the agency has a web page, read about the target population they serve, the types of services they provide, and how they are reimbursed for services. Learn about different agencies and share results during class. On the basis of your findings, identify gaps or overlaps in services provided to vulnerable groups in your community. Which data do these agencies collect to demonstrate the efficacy of their services? How could you deal with these gaps and overlaps to help clients receive needed services?

Prepared by Gail Armstrong, PhD(c), DNP, ACNS-BC, CNE, Associate Professor, University of Colorado Denver College of Nursing.

It is also important to consider that there can be ethical dilemmas associated with working with vulnerable populations. The Evidence-Based Practice box describes ethical dilemmas that arose in an academic-community partnership designed to learn about the experiences of undocumented immigrants who sought health care in Toronto, Canada.

In some situations, the nurse works with individual clients. The nurse also develops programs and policies for populations of vulnerable persons. In both examples, planning and implementing care for members of vulnerable populations involve partnerships between the nurse and client and build on careful assessment. Nurses need to avoid directing and controlling clients' care because this might interfere with their being able to establish a trusting relationship and may inadvertently foster a cycle of dependency and lack of personal health control. The

## EVIDENCE-BASED PRACTICE

Using an academic-community partnership, a study was conducted to understand the experiences of undocumented immigrants seeking health care in Toronto, Canada. A team composed of the principal investigator, three researchers, and a group of nine undocumented immigrants used a community-based participatory research process to examine the experiences of the immigrants. Representatives from the community-based organization (CBO) had a pre-existing, strong and trusting relationship with the study participants. Two ethical dilemmas arose. Two of the participants thought that the researcher who was asking them questions was a spy for the Canadian Border Services Agency (CBSA). These two participants had not attended the orientation session. They were concerned when asked about their immigration status during the informed consent process. To solve this dilemma, the team decided that the CBO worker should ask for the informed consent because trust was present in that relationship. A second ethical dilemma arose when one participant told the principal investigator (PI) that she was suicidal. The PI was unprepared to deal with this information, and the team decided that in future interviews the PI would tell the participants that she was not a mental health professional. They also determined that the team needed to have access to a mental health professional in the event they learned information that needed follow-up.

### Nurse Use

When ethical dilemmas arise in either research or client care, it is essential to identify them and immediately try to seek a solution. This study is a good example of how the team learned a great deal from their project. They put the project on hold in order to reflect, analyze, synthesize, and evaluate the facts.

Source: Campbell-Page RM, Shaw-Ridley MS: Managing ethical dilemmas in community-based participatory research with vulnerable populations. *Health Promot Pract* 17:485–490, 2013.

most important initial step is for nurses to demonstrate they are trustworthy and dependable. For example, nurses who work in a community clinic for substance abusers must overcome any suspicion that clients may have of them and eliminate any fears clients may have of being manipulated.

Nurses working with vulnerable populations may fill numerous roles, including those listed in Box 32-1. They identify vulnerable individuals and families through outreach and case finding. They encourage vulnerable groups to obtain health services, and they develop programs that respond to their needs. Nurses teach vulnerable individuals, families, and groups

strategies to prevent illness and promote health. They counsel clients about ways to increase their sense of personal power and help them identify strengths and resources. They provide direct care to clients and families in a variety of settings, including storefront clinics, mobile clinics, shelters, homes, neighborhoods, worksites, churches, and schools.

The following are some examples of care to clients, families, and groups: (1) a nurse in a mobile migrant clinic might administer a tetanus booster to a client who has been injured by a piece of farm machinery and may also check that client's blood pressure and cholesterol level during the same visit; (2) a home health nurse seeing a family referred by the courts for child abuse may weigh the child, conduct a nutritional assessment, and help the family learn how to manage anger and disciplinary problems; (3) a nurse working in a school-based clinic may lead a support group for pregnant adolescents and conduct a birthing class; and (4) a nurse may work with people being treated for TB to monitor drug treatment compliance and ensure that they complete their full course of therapy.

## ⟫ LINKING CONTENT TO PRACTICE

Generalist and staff public health nurses should have competencies in eight domains as defined by the Quad Council of Public Health Nursing Organizations (2011). Each of the eight competencies is important in working with vulnerable populations. Public health nurses working with vulnerable populations should be able to analyze data and determine when a problem exists with an individual and within a vulnerable population group. They should be able to identify options for programs or policies that could be helpful to these populations and communicate their ideas and recommendations clearly. Public health nurses should be able to provide culturally competent interventions for individuals or for vulnerable populations. As an example, a public health nurse should be able to collect and analyze data related to the prevalence of violence among women in the community; identify key stakeholders; evaluate the cultural preferences of the population; work with others to develop a program to meet a defined need within this population, including preparation of a basic budget for the program; and ensure that the program is culturally appropriate for the population. The Council on Linkages between Academia and Public Health Practice (2010) published a similar list for public health professionals, including but not limited to public health nurses. This list includes an emphasis on evaluation and ongoing improvement of programs. In this example, the nurse would evaluate the program developed for women who are victims of violence and work with others to develop and implement quality improvements on a regular basis.

Public health nurses also serve as population health advocates and work with local, state, or national groups to develop and implement healthy public policy. They also collaborate with community members and serve as community assessors and developers, and they monitor and evaluate care and health programs. Nurses often function as case managers for vulnerable clients, making referrals and linking them to community services. Case management services are especially important for vulnerable persons because they often do not have the ability or resources to make their own arrangements. They may not be able to speak the language, or they may be unable to navigate the complex telephone systems that many agencies establish. They also serve as advocates when they refer clients to other

## BOX 32-1   Nursing Roles When Working with Vulnerable Population Groups

- Case manager
- Health educator
- Counselor
- Direct care provider
- Population health advocate
- Community assessor and developer
- Monitor and evaluate of care
- Case manager
- Advocate
- Health program planner and implementer
- Participant in developing health policies

agencies, work with others to develop health programs, and influence legislation and health policies that affect vulnerable populations.

The nature of nurses' roles varies depending on whether the client is a single person, a family, or a group. For example, a nurse might teach an HIV-positive client about the need for prevention of opportunistic infections, may help a family with an HIV-positive member understand myths about transmission of HIV, or may work with a community group concerned about HIV transmission among students. In each case, the nurse teaches individuals how to prevent infectious and communicable diseases. The size of the group and the teaching method for each group differ.

Health education is often used in working with vulnerable populations. The nurse should teach members of populations with low educational levels what they need to do to promote health and prevent illness rather than directing health education to groups that the nurse thinks might be at high risk even though there is no evidence to support the perception.

## Levels of Prevention

*Healthy People 2020* (USDHHS, 2010) objectives emphasize improving health by modifying the individual, social, and environmental determinants of health. One way to do this is for vulnerable individuals to have a primary care provider who both coordinates health services for them and provides their preventive services. This primary care provider may be an advanced practice nurse or a primary care physician. Another approach is for a nurse to serve as a case manager for vulnerable clients and, again, coordinate services and provide illness prevention and health promotion services.

One example of primary prevention is to give influenza vaccinations to vulnerable populations that are immunocompromised (unless contraindicated). Secondary prevention is seen in conducting screening clinics for vulnerable populations. For example, nurses who work in homeless shelters, prisons, migrant camps, and substance abuse treatment facilities should know that these groups are at high risk for acquiring communicable diseases. Both clients and staff need routine screening for TB. Screening homeless adults and providing isoniazid to those who test positive for TB are examples of secondary prevention. An example of tertiary prevention is conducting a therapy group with the residents of a group home for severely mentally ill adults. Nurses who work with abused women to help them enhance their levels of self-esteem are also providing tertiary preventive activities.

## Assessment Issues

Nurses who work with vulnerable populations need good assessment skills, current knowledge of available resources, and the ability to plan care based on client needs and receptivity to help. They also need to be able to show respect for the client. The How To box entitled "Assess Members of Vulnerable Population Groups" lists guidelines for assessing members of vulnerable population groups.

Because members of vulnerable populations often experience multiple stressors, assessment must balance the need to be

---

📄 **LEVELS OF PREVENTION**

### *Related to Vulnerable Populations*

**Primary Prevention**
- Provide culturally and economically sensitive health teaching about balanced diet and exercise.
- Develop a portable immunization chart, such as a wallet card, that mobile population groups such as the homeless and migrant workers can carry with them.

**Secondary Prevention**
- Conduct screening clinics to assess for things such as obesity, diabetes, heart disease, or tuberculosis (TB).
- Develop a way for homeless individuals to read their TB skin test, if necessary, and to transfer the results back to the facility at which the skin test was administered.

**Tertiary Prevention**
- Develop community-based exercise programs for people identified as obese or who have increased blood pressure or increased blood sugar.
- Provide directly observed medication therapy for people with active TB.

---

**HOW TO** Assess Members of Vulnerable Population Groups

**Setting the Stage**
- *Create a comfortable, nonthreatening environment.*
- *Learn as much as you can about the culture of the clients you work with so that you will understand cultural practices and values that may influence their health care practices.*
- *Provide a culturally competent assessment by understanding the meaning of language and nonverbal behavior in the client's culture.*
- *Be sensitive to the fact that the individual or family you are assessing may have other priorities that are more important to them. These might include financial or legal problems. You may need to give them some tangible help with their most pressing priority before you will be able to address issues that are more traditionally thought of as health concerns.*
- *Collaborate with others as appropriate; you should not provide financial or legal advice. However, you should make sure to connect your client with someone who can and will help them.*

**Nursing History of an Individual or Family**
- *You may have only one opportunity to work with a vulnerable person or family. Try to complete a history that will provide all the essential information you need to help the individual or family on that day. This means that you will have to organize in your mind exactly what you need to ask. You should also understand why you need any information that you gather.*
- *It will help to use a comprehensive assessment form that has been modified to focus on the special needs of the vulnerable population group with whom you work. However, be flexible. With some clients, it will be both impractical and unethical to cover all questions on a comprehensive form. If you know that you are likely to see the client again, ask the less pressing questions at the next visit.*
- *Be sure to include questions about social support, economic status, resources for health care, developmental issues, current health problems, medications, and how the person or family manages their health status. Your goal is to obtain information that will enable you to provide family-centered care.*
- *Determine whether the individual has any condition that compromises his or her immune status, such as AIDS, or if the individual*

*is undergoing therapy that would result in immunodeficiency, such as cancer chemotherapy.*

**Physical Examination or Home Assessment**

- *Again, complete as thorough a physical examination (on an individual) or home assessment as you can. Keep in mind that you should collect only data for which you have a use.*
- *Be alert for indications of physical abuse, substance use (e.g., needle marks, nasal abnormalities), or neglect (e.g., underweight, inadequate clothing).*
- *You can assess a family's living environment using good observational skills. Does the family live in an insect- or rat-infested environment? Do they have running water, functioning plumbing, electricity, and a telephone?*
- *Is perishable food left sitting out on tables and countertops? Are bed linens reasonably clean? Is paint peeling on the walls and ceilings? Is ventilation adequate? Is the temperature of the home adequate? Is the family exposed to raw sewage or animal waste? Is the home adjacent to a busy highway, possibly exposing the family to high noise levels and automobile exhaust?*

comprehensive while focusing only on information that the nurse needs and the client is willing to provide. Remember to ask questions about the client's perceptions of his or her socioeconomic resources, including identifying people who can provide support and financial resources. Support from other people may include information, caregiving, emotional support, and help with instrumental activities of daily living, such as transportation, shopping, and babysitting. Financial resources may include the extent to which the client can pay for health services and medications, as well as questions about eligibility for third-party payment. The nurse should ask the client about the perceived adequacy of both formal and informal support networks.

When possible, assessment should include an evaluation of clients' preventive health needs, including age-appropriate screening tests such as immunization status, blood pressure, weight, serum cholesterol, Papanicolaou (Pap) smears, breast examinations, mammograms, prostate examinations, glaucoma screening, and dental evaluations. It may be necessary to make referrals for some of these tests. Assessment should also include preventive screening for physical health problems, for which certain vulnerable groups are at particularly high risk. For example, people who are HIV positive should be evaluated regularly for CD4 cell counts and common opportunistic infections, including TB and pneumonia. Intravenous drug users should be evaluated for HBV, including liver palpation and serum antigen tests as necessary. Alcoholic clients should also be asked about symptoms of liver disease and should be evaluated for jaundice and liver enlargement. Severely mentally ill clients should be assessed for the presence of tardive dyskinesia, indicating possible toxicity from their antipsychotic medications.

Vulnerable populations should be assessed for congenital and genetic predisposition to illness and either receive education and counseling as appropriate or be referred to other health professionals as necessary. For example, pregnant adolescents who are substance abusers should be referred to programs to help them quit using addictive substances during their pregnancies and, ideally, after delivery of their infants. Pregnant women

older than 35 years should receive amniocentesis testing to determine whether genetic abnormalities exist in the fetus.

The nurse should also assess the amount of stress the person or family is having. Does the family have healthy coping skills and healthy family interaction? Are some family members able and willing to care for others? What is the level of mental health in each member? Also, are diet, exercise, and rest and sleep patterns conducive to good health?

The nurse should assess the living environment and neighborhood surroundings of vulnerable families and groups for environmental hazards such as lead-based paint, asbestos, water and air quality, industrial wastes, and the incidence of crime.

# PLANNING AND IMPLEMENTING CARE FOR VULNERABLE POPULATIONS

Nurses who work in community settings may have considerable involvement with vulnerable populations. The relationship with the client will depend on the nature of the contact. Some will be seen in clinics and others in homes, schools, and at work. Regardless of the setting, the following key nursing actions should be used:

- **Create a trusting environment:** Trust is essential, because many of these individuals have previously been disappointed in their interactions with health care and social systems. It is important to follow through and do what you say you are going to do. If you do not know the answer to a question, the best reply is "I do not know, but I will try to find out."
- **Show respect, compassion, and concern:** Vulnerable people have been defeated again and again by life's circumstances. They may have reached a point at which they question whether they even deserve to get care. Listen carefully, because listening is a form of respect, as well as a way to gather information to plan care.
- **Do not make assumptions:** Assess each person and family. No two people or groups are alike.
- **Coordinate services and providers:** Getting health and social services is not always easy. Often people feel like they are traveling through a maze. In most communities a large number of useful services exist. People who need them simply may not know how to find them. For example, people may need help finding a food bank or a free clinic or obtaining low-cost or free clothing through churches or in secondhand stores. Clients often need help in determining whether they meet the eligibility requirements. If gaps in service are found, nurses can work with others to try to get the needed services established. Care for vulnerable populations requires interprofessional collaboration to meet their multiple needs. For example, nurses can work with business and public health leaders to reduce hazardous exposures, develop accessible services, and improve working conditions for low-income employees (Lathrop, 2013). Nurses may need to work with lawmakers, union leaders, urban developers, business leaders, and a range of public health and other health care workers. The following Case Study describes a situation in which a mother faced many obstacles in getting care for her two children (Box 32-2).

## BOX 32-2 Case Study

Felicia is a 22-year-old single mother of three children whose primary source of income is Temporary Assistance to Needy Families (TANF). She is worried about the future because she will no longer be eligible for welfare by the end of the year. She has been unable to find a job that will pay enough for her to afford childcare. Her friend Maria said that Felicia and her children can stay in Maria's trailer for a short time, but Felicia is afraid that her only choice after that will be a shelter.

Felicia recently took all three children with her to the health department because 15-month-old Hector needed immunizations. Felicia was also concerned about 5-year-old Martina, who had had a fever of 100 to 101° F on and off for the past month. Felicia and her friends in the trailer park think that some type of hazardous waste from the chemical plant next door to the park is making their children sick. Now that Martina was not feeling well, Felicia was particularly concerned. However, the health department nurse told her that no appointments were available that day and that she would need to bring Martina back to the clinic on the next day. Felicia left discouraged because it was so difficult for her to get all three children ready and on the bus to go to the health department, not to mention the expense. She thought maybe Martina just had a cold and she would wait a little longer before bringing her back. However, she wanted to take care of Martina's problem before losing her medical card. Felicia is desperate to find a way to manage her money problems and take care of her children.

**Advocate for accessible health care services:** Vulnerable people have trouble getting access to services. Neighborhood clinics, mobile vans, and home visits can be valuable for them. Also, coordinating services at a central location is helpful. These multiservice centers can provide health care, social services, daycare, drug and alcohol recovery programs, and case management. When working with vulnerable populations, it is a good idea to arrange to have as many services as possible available in a single location and at convenient times. This "one-stop shopping" approach to care delivery is very helpful for populations experiencing multiple social, economic, and health-related stresses. Although it may seem difficult and costly to provide comprehensive services in one location, it may save money in the long run by preventing illness.

**Focus on prevention:** Use every opportunity to teach about preventive health care. Primary prevention may include child and adult immunizations and education about nutrition, foot care, safe sex, contraception, and the prevention of injuries or chronic illness. It also includes providing prophylactic antituberculosis drug therapy for HIV-positive people who live in homeless shelters or giving flu vaccine to people who are immune-compromised or older than 65 years of age. Secondary prevention would include screening for health problems such as TB, diabetes, hypertension, foot problems, anemia, or drug use or abuse. People who spend time in homeless shelters, substance abuse treatment facilities, and prisons often get communicable diseases such as influenza, TB, and methicillin-resistant *Staphylococcus aureus* (MRSA). Nurses who work in these facilities should plan regular influenza vaccination clinics and TB screening clinics. When planning these clinics, nurses should work with local physicians to develop signed protocols and should

plan ahead for problems related to the transient nature of the population. For example, nurses should develop a way for homeless individuals to read their TB skin test if necessary and transfer the results back to the facility where the skin test was administered. It is helpful to develop a portable immunization chart, such as a wallet card, that mobile population groups such as the homeless and migrant workers can carry with them.

**Know when to "walk beside" the client and when to encourage the client to "walk ahead":** At times it is difficult to know when to do something for people and when to teach or encourage them to do for themselves. Nursing actions range from providing encouragement and support to providing information and active intervention. It is important to assess for the presence of strength and the ability to problem solve, cope, and access services. For example, a local hospital might provide free mammograms for women who cannot pay. The nurse would need to decide whether to schedule the appointments for clients or to give them the information and encourage them to do the scheduling.

**Know what resources are available:** Be familiar with community agencies that offer health and social services to vulnerable populations. Also follow up after you make a referral to make sure the client was able to obtain the needed help. Examples of agencies found in most communities are health departments, community mental health centers, voluntary organizations such as the American Red Cross, missions, shelters, soup kitchens, food banks, nurse-managed or free clinics, social service agencies such as the Salvation Army or Travelers Aid, and church-sponsored health and social services.

**Develop your own support network:** Working with vulnerable populations can be challenging, rewarding, and at times exhausting. Nurses need to find sources of support and strength. This can come from friends, colleagues, hobbies, exercise, poetry, music, and other sources.

In addition to the nursing actions described, the How To box entitled "Intervene with Vulnerable Populations" summarizes goals and interventions and evaluates outcomes with vulnerable populations.

### HOW TO Intervene with Vulnerable Populations
Goals
- *Set reasonable goals based on the baseline data you collected. Focus on reducing disparities in health status among vulnerable populations.*
- *Work toward setting manageable goals with the client. Goals that seem unattainable may be discouraging.*
- *Set goals collaboratively with the client as a first step toward client empowerment.*
- *Set family-centered, culturally sensitive goals.*

Interventions
- *Set up outreach and case-finding programs to help increase access to health services by vulnerable populations.*
- *Do everything you can to minimize the "hassle factor" connected with the interventions you plan. Vulnerable groups do not have the extra energy, money, or time to cope with unnecessary waits, complicated treatment plans, or confusion. As your*

*client's advocate, you should identify possible hassles and develop ways to avoid them. For example, this may include providing comprehensive services during a single encounter, rather than asking the client to return for multiple visits. Multiple visits for more specialized aspects of the client's needs, whether individual or family group, reinforce a perception that health care is fragmented and organized for the professional's convenience rather than that of the client.*

- *Work with clients to ensure that interventions are culturally sensitive and competent.*
- *Focus on teaching skills in health promotion and disease prevention. Also, teach clients how to be effective health care consumers. For example, role-play asking questions in a physician's office with a client.*
- *Help clients learn what to do if they cannot keep an appointment with a health care or social service professional.*

**Evaluating Outcomes**

- *It is often difficult for vulnerable clients to return for follow-up care. Help your client develop self-care strategies for evaluating outcomes. For example, teach homeless individuals how to read their own tuberculosis (TB) skin test, and give them a self-addressed, stamped card they can return by mail with the results.*
- *Remember to evaluate outcomes in terms of the goals you have mutually agreed on with the client. For example, one outcome for a homeless person receiving isoniazid therapy for TB might be that the person returns to the clinic daily for direct observation of compliance with the drug therapy.*

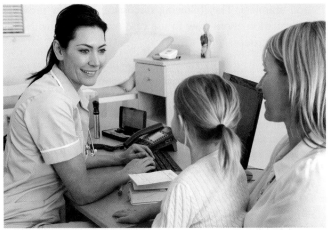

**FIG 32-4** Nurse-managed clinics provide many services to individuals and families. (© 2012 Photos.com, a division of Getty Images. All rights reserved.)

In general, more agencies are needed that provide comprehensive services with nonrestrictive eligibility requirements. Communities often have many agencies that restrict eligibility to make it possible for more people to receive services. For example, shelters may prohibit people who have been drinking alcohol from staying overnight and limit the number of sequential nights a person can stay. Food banks usually limit the number of times a person can receive free food. Agencies are often very specialized as well. For vulnerable individuals and families, this means that they must go to several agencies to obtain services for which they qualify and that meet their health needs. This is tiring and discouraging, and people may forgo help because of these difficulties.

Nurses need to know about community agencies that offer various health and social services. It is important to follow-up with the client after a referral to ensure that the desired outcomes were achieved. Sometimes excellent community resources may be available but impractical because of transportation or reimbursement issues. Nurses can identify these potential problems by following through with referrals, and they can also work with other team members to make referrals as convenient and realistic as possible. Although clients with social problems such as financial needs should be referred to social workers, it is useful for nurses to understand the close connections between health and social problems and know how to work effectively with other professionals. A list of community resources can often be found in the telephone directory or online. The following are examples of agency resources found in most communities:

- Health departments
- Community mental health centers

- American Red Cross and other voluntary organizations
- Food and clothing banks
- Missions and shelters
- Nurse-managed clinics
- Social service agencies such as Travelers Aid and the Salvation Army
- Church-sponsored health and service assistance
- Free clinics and other community services

As seen in Figure 32-4 nurses who work with vulnerable populations often need to coordinate services across multiple agencies for members of these groups. It is helpful to have a strong professional network of people who work in other agencies. Effective professional networks make it easier to coordinate care smoothly and in ways that do not add to clients' stress. Nurses can develop strong networks by participating in community coalitions and attending professional meetings. When making referrals to other agencies, a phone call can be a helpful way to obtain information that the client will need for the visit. When possible, having an interdisciplinary, interagency team plan care for clients at high risk for health problems is effective. Obtain the clients' written and informed consent before engaging in this kind of planning because of confidentiality issues. The following list of tips can be helpful:

- Involve clients in making decisions about the kinds of services they are willing and able to use.
- Work with community coalitions to coordinate services for targeted vulnerable populations.
- Collaborate with legal counsel from the agencies involved in the coalitions to ensure that legal and ethical issues related to care coordination have been properly addressed. Examples of issues to address include privacy and security of clinical data and ensuring compliance with HIPAA, contractual provisions for coordinating care across agencies, and consent to treatment from multiple agencies.
- Develop policies and protocols for making referrals, following up on referrals, and ensuring that clients receiving care from multiple agencies experience the process as smooth

and seamless. The following discussion and box provides information about how to use case management with vulnerable groups.

> **HOW TO  Use Case Management in Working with Vulnerable Populations**
> - *Know available services and resources.*
> - *Find out what is missing; look for creative solutions.*
> - *Use your clinical skills.*
> - *Develop long-term relationships with the families you serve.*
> - *Strengthen the family's coping and survival skills and resourcefulness.*
> - *Be the roadmap that guides the family to services, and help them get the services.*
> - *Communicate with the family and the agencies that can help them.*
> - *Work to change the environment and the policies that affect your clients.*

Two other important categories of resources for vulnerable people are their own personal coping skills and social supports (Aday, 2001). These groups often are resourceful and creative in managing multiple stressors. Nurses can work with clients to help them identify their strengths and draw on those strengths when managing their health needs. Also, clients may be able to depend on informal support networks. Even though social isolation is a problem for many vulnerable clients, nurses should not assume they have no one who can or will help them. Case management involves linking clients with services and providing direct nursing services to them, including teaching, counseling, screening, and immunizing. Lillian Wald was the first case manager. She linked vulnerable families with various services to help them stay healthy (Buhler-Wilkerson, 1993). Nurses are often the link between personal health services and population-based health care. Linking, or brokering, health services is accomplished by making appropriate referrals and following up with clients to ensure that the desired outcomes from the referral were achieved. Nurses are effective case managers in community nursing clinics, health departments, hospitals, and various other health care agencies. Nurse case managers emphasize health promotion and illness prevention with vulnerable clients and focus on helping them avoid unnecessary hospitalization. Figure 32-2 illustrates the coordination and brokering aspect of the nurse's role as case manager for vulnerable populations.

As can be seen, many of these nursing actions are in the realm of case management, in which the nurse makes referrals and links clients with other community services. In the case manager role, the nurse often is an advocate for the client or family. The nurse serves as an advocate when referring clients to other agencies, when working with others to develop health programs, and when trying to influence legislation and health policies that affect vulnerable population groups.

## PRACTICE APPLICATION

Ms. Green, a 46-year-old farm worker pregnant with her fifth child, has come to the clinic requesting treatment for swollen ankles. During your assessment, you learned that she had seen the nurse practitioner at the local health department 2 months ago. The nurse practitioner gave her some sample vitamins, but Ms. Green lost them. She has not received regular prenatal care and has no plans to do so. Her previous pregnancies were essentially normal, although she said she was "toxic" with her last child. She also said that her middle child was "not quite right." He is in the seventh grade at age 15. Ms. Green is 5 feet 2 inches tall, weighs 180 pounds, and has a blood pressure of 160/90. She has pitting edema of the ankles and a mild headache.

Ms. Green says that she usually takes chlorpromazine hydrochloride (Thorazine) but has run out of it and cannot afford to have her prescription refilled. She says that she has been in several mental hospitals in the past and that she has been more agitated lately and now has problems managing her daily activities. As her agitation grows, she says that she usually hears voices and this really makes her aggressive.

None of her children lives with her, and she has no plans for taking care of the infant. She thinks she will ask the child's father, a race track worker, to help her, because she usually travels around the country with him.

A. What additional information do you need to help you adequately assess Ms. Green's health status and current needs?

B. What nursing activities are suggested by her history, physical, and psychological descriptions?

**Answers can be found on the Evolve website.**

## KEY POINTS

- All countries have population subgroups that are more vulnerable to health threats than the general population.
- Vulnerable populations are more likely to develop health problems as a result of exposure to risk or to have worse outcomes from those health problems than the population as a whole.
- Vulnerable populations are more sensitive to risk factors than those who are more resilient, because they are often exposed to cumulative risk factors. These populations include poor or homeless persons, pregnant adolescents, migrant workers, severely mentally ill individuals, substance abusers, abused individuals, people with communicable diseases, and people with sexually transmitted diseases.
- Factors leading to the growing number of poor people in the United States include reduced earnings, decreased availability of low-cost housing, more households headed by women,

## KEY POINTS—cont'd

inadequate education, lack of marketable skills, welfare reform, and reduced Social Security payments to children.

- Poverty has a direct effect on health and well-being across the life span. Poor people have higher rates of chronic illness and infant morbidity and mortality, shorter life expectancy, and more complex health problems.
- Child poverty rates are twice as high as those for adults. Children who live in single-parent homes are twice as likely to be poor than those who live with both parents.
- The complex health problems of homeless people include the inability to obtain adequate rest, sleep, exercise, nutrition, and medication; exposure; infectious diseases; acute and chronic illness; infestations; and trauma and mental health problems.
- Health care is increasingly moving into the community. This began with deinstitutionalization of the severely mentally ill population and is continuing today as hospitals reduce inpatient stays. Vulnerable populations need a wide variety of services, and because these are often provided by multiple community agencies, nurses coordinate and manage the service needs of vulnerable groups.
- Socioeconomic problems, including poverty and social isolation, physiological and developmental aspects of age, poor health status, and highly stressful life experiences, predispose people to vulnerability. Vulnerability can become a cycle, with the predisposing factors leading to poor health outcomes, chronic stress, and hopelessness. These outcomes increase vulnerability.
- Nurses assess vulnerable individuals, families, and groups to determine which socioeconomic, physical, biological, psychological, and environmental factors are problematic for clients. They work as partners with vulnerable clients to identify client strengths and needs and develop intervention strategies designed to break the cycle of vulnerability.

## CLINICAL DECISION-MAKING ACTIVITIES

1. Examine health statistics and demographic data in your geographic area to determine which vulnerable groups are predominant. Look through your phone book or on the Internet for examples of agencies you think provide services to these vulnerable groups. If the agency has a web page, read about the target populations they serve, the types of services they provide, and how they are reimbursed for services. Learn about different agencies and share results during class. On the basis of your findings, identify gaps or overlaps in services provided to vulnerable groups in your community. How could you deal with these gaps and overlaps to help clients receive needed services?

2. Identify nurses in your community who work with vulnerable groups. Invite these nurses to come to class and talk about their experiences. What is their typical day? What are the rewards? What are the challenges? How do they deal with frustration, competing demands, and stress?

3. Discuss welfare reform with your classmates. How does the U.S. welfare system work? Who gets welfare? What should be done to improve the system? Is your state a leader in welfare reform?

4. Suppose you are making a home visit to a person whose home is not clean. Food is everywhere, and roaches are crawling around the house. What do you do if the person asks you to sit down? What if you are offered food?

## REFERENCES

Aday LA: *At Risk in America: The Health and Health Care Needs of Vulnerable Populations in the United States.* San Francisco, 2001, Jossey-Bass.

Baggett TP, O'Connell JJ, Singer DE, et al: The unmet health care needs of homeless adults: a national study. *Am J Public Health* 100:1326–1333, 2010.

Benatar RS: Global health, vulnerable populations, and law. *J Law Med Ethics* 41:42–47, 2013.

Borre K, Ertle L, Graff M: Working to eat: vulnerability, food insecurity, and obesity among migrant and seasonal farmworker families. *Am J Ind Med* 53:443–462, 2010.

Braveman P: What are health disparities and health equity? We need to be clear. *Public Health Rep* 129(Suppl 2):5–8, 2014.

Braveman P, Gottlieb L: The social determinants of health: it's time to consider the causes of the causes. *Public Health Rep* 129(Suppl 2):19–31, 2014.

Buhler-Wilkerson K: Bringing care to the people: Lillian Wald's legacy to public health nursing. *Am J Publ Health* 83:1778–1786, 1993.

Campbell-Page RM, Shaw-Ridley MS: Managing ethical dilemmas in community-based participatory research with vulnerable populations. *Health Promot Pract* 14:485–490, 2013.

Centers for Medicare and Medicaid Services (CMS): *Children's Health Insurance Program Reauthorization (CHPRA)*. Washington, DC, 2009, CMS. From: http://www.medicaid.gov/CHIP/CHIP-Program

-information.html. Retrieved January 2015.

Council on Linkages between Academia and Public Health Practice: *Core Competencies for Public Health Professionals.* Washington, DC, 2010. From: http://www.phf.org/resourcestools/Pages/core_public_health_competencies.aspx. Retrieved February 2015.

Flaskerud JH, Winslow BW: Vulnerable populations and ultimate responsibility. *Issues Ment Health Nurs* 31:298–299, 2010.

Friis RH: *Epidemiology 101* [Essential Public Health series]. Sudbury, MA, 2010, Jones & Bartlett Learning.

Greenberg MD, Ridgely MS, Hillestad RJ: Crossed wires: how yesterday's privacy rules might undercut tomorrow's nationwide

health information network. *Health Aff* 28:450–452, 2009.

Hillemeier MM, Lanza ST, Landate NS, et al: Measuring early childhood health and health disparities: a new approach. *Matern Child Health J* 17:1852–1861, 2013.

Lathrop B: Nursing leadership in addressing the social determinants of health. *Policy Polit Nurs Pract* 14:41–47, 2013.

Middlebrooks JS, Audage NC: *The Effects of Childhood Stress on Health across the Lifespan.* Atlanta, GA, 2008, Centers for Disease Control and Prevention, National Center for Injury Prevention and Control.

Murphy SL, Xu J, Kochanek KD: Deaths: final data for 2010. *Natl Vital Stat Rep* 61:1–117, 2013.

Newhouse JP: Assessing health reform's impact on four key groups of Americans. *Health Aff* 29:1–11, 2010.

Quad Council of Public Health Nursing Organizations: *Core Competencies for Public Health Professionals: A Project of the Council on Linkages between Academia and Public Health Practice Funded by the Health Resources and Services Administration*. 2011. From: http://www.achne.org/quadcouncil. Retrieved January 2015.

Shi L, Stevens GD: Vulnerability and unmet health care needs: the influence of multiple risk factors. *J Gen Intern Med* 20:148–154, 2005.

Shi L, Stevens GD: *Vulnerable Populations in the United States*. San Francisco, 2010, Jossey-Bass.

U.S. Department of Health and Human Services (USDHHS): *Healthy People 2020*. Washington, DC, 2010, USDHHS. From: www.healthypeople.gov/. Retrieved January 2015.

U.S. Department of Health and Human Services (USDHHS): *2014 Poverty Guidelines*, 2010. From: http://aspe.hhs.gov/poverty/14poverty.cfm. Retrieved January 2015.

Wilensky GR, Satcher D: Don't forget about the social determinants of health. *Health Aff* 28:w194–w198, 2009.

World Health Organization (WHO): *Health Impact Assessment (HIA): The Determinants of Health*, 2015. From: http://www.who.int/hia/evidence/doh/en/. Retrieved January 2015.

# 33

# Poverty and Homelessness

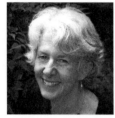

## Ann Connor, DNP, MSN, RN, FNP-BC

Ann Connor holds the BSN, MSN, DNP, and the FNP certificate from the University of Alabama in Birmingham. She is an Assistant Professor-Clinical at the Nell Hodgson Woodruff School of Nursing at Emory University. Her research focuses on *Health literacy and self-management of prescription medications among persons who are homeless.* Dr. Connor has worked with persons who are homeless for 30+ years, for 12 of those years she and her family shared their home, The Community of Hospitality, with persons who were homeless. In 1988, she helped establish Café 458, a restaurant for persons who are homeless, serving as the Chair of the Board of Directors. Since its beginning, Café 458 has served as an interdisciplinary clinical learning site. In the early 1980's Dr. Connor began offering foot care and intentional comfort touch to persons who were living on the streets. Her work served as a catalyst to increase health care access for persons who were homeless. She served as a Family Nurse Practitioner with the Georgia Nurses Foundations Clinics for the Homeless, one of the earliest health care clinics for the homeless. She continues to work with many vulnerable populations including migrant farm worker families in South Georgia.

## ADDITIONAL RESOURCES

ⓔ **Evolve website http://evolve.elsevier.com/Stanhope**
- Healthy People 2020
- WebLinks
- Quiz
- Case Studies
- Glossary
- Answers to Practice Application

## OBJECTIVES

*After reading this chapter, the student should be able to do the following:*

1. Analyze the concept of poverty.
2. Discuss how nurses view and understand poverty, homelessness, and health.
3. Describe the social, political, cultural, and environmental factors that influence poverty and homelessness.
4. Discuss the effects of poverty on the health and well-being of individuals, families, and communities.
5. Analyze the concept of homelessness.
6. Discuss the effects of homelessness on the health and well-being of individuals, families, and communities.
7. Discuss nursing interventions for poor and homeless individuals.

## KEY TERMS

consumer price index, p. 734
crisis poverty, p. 739
cultural attitudes, p. 733
deinstitutionalization, p. 741
Elizabethan poor laws, p. 732
emergency shelters, p. 744
homeless children, p. 743
homelessness, p. 738
homeless persons, p. 744
Interagency Council on the Homeless, p. 743
low-income housing, p. 744
media discourses, p. 733

near poor, p. 734
neighborhood poverty, p. 734
persistent poverty, p. 734
personal beliefs, p. 732
poverty, p. 734
Poverty Threshold Guidelines, p. 734
Stewart B. McKinney Homeless Assistance Act of 1987, p. 743
supportive housing, p. 744
Temporary Assistance to Needy Families, p. 734
Women, Infants, and Children Program, p. 734
—*See Glossary for definitions*

American society values self-reliance, individual responsibility, and personal accountability. Although these cultural expectations are important, our beliefs about personal autonomy can work against the needs of persons who are unable to live independent, successful lives. Discussions about those who are poor and homeless arouse feelings in many Americans. The spectrum of feelings includes those who think people should work hard, save some money, plan for the future, and be able to take care of themselves to others who believe there is a need for society to care for and assist those who are vulnerable and poor. Changes in economic conditions affect many people. In an economic downturn, people often lose their jobs and are no longer able to keep their homes. Some become homeless.

Nurses encounter poor persons, families, and populations in a variety of settings, such as private homes, congregate living situations, schools, churches, clinics, and meal sites. To provide effective care and to advocate for individuals, families, and populations living in poverty, nurses need to understand poverty as a concept with historical, social, political, economic, biological, psychological, and spiritual dimensions. Understanding the concepts of poverty and homelessness begins with an examination of one's beliefs, values, and personal experience. It is also important to develop an appreciation for the history of public responses to poor and homeless persons, and the relationship of this history to contemporary public and personal debates. Nurses must be able to identify health care needs, barriers to care, and essential health care services for poor and homeless individuals, families, and populations. Providing effective nursing interventions requires an understanding of the epidemiology, health problems, and risk factors associated with poverty as well as sources of support and existing programs for these vulnerable populations.

This chapter describes the many ways that poverty and homelessness affect the health status of individuals, families, and communities, and it suggests effective nursing interventions for poor and homeless people. The concepts of poverty and homelessness are examined in historical, economic, political, and spiritual contexts.

## CONCEPT OF POVERTY

Individual perceptions of poverty and poor persons are rooted in social, political, cultural, and environmental factors. Personal beliefs, social values, personal experience, cultural attitudes, media portrayals, and historical factors influence our understanding of poverty. It is important for each of us to be aware of our values and beliefs about poor and homeless persons.

To be effective, nurses must recognize and acknowledge the beliefs, values, and knowledge that form their worldviews and influence the way they practice. Personal beliefs are ideas about the world that a person believes to be true; these beliefs are rooted in societal values. Our attitudes toward poor persons are influenced by societal/cultural values of personal responsibility, individual autonomy, and personal accountability. Although these societal and cultural values have changed little throughout history, there is some evidence that they may be changing because of the magnitude of people affected by the current economic situation.

## Historical Views of Poverty

Public perceptions about poor persons and individual attitudes about what should be done for the poor go back to the Elizabethan Poor Laws. In seventeenth-century England, being poor was no disgrace because nearly everyone lived in poverty. Therefore, people often shared what they had with one another and frequently banded together to help those whose luck had taken a downturn. People become more mobile when the Industrial Revolution began. Increased migration, from rural areas to urban industrial townships, brought with it questions of whom among the downtrodden should be helped. In short, how could society distinguish poor persons deserving assistance from those who did not (Katz, 1989). According to Elizabethan Poor Laws, established in the seventeenth century, persons born within the boundaries of the community should be given assistance by that community. Needy travelers from another community would not be helped and were sent back to their original community, where they would be helped by their own folk.

Society changed to adapt to the Industrial Revolution. It became more difficult to differentiate between the deserving and the undeserving poor. Persons who were down-and-out were classified as deserving of assistance if their poverty was considered to be beyond their control. Widowed women, orphaned children, laborers who were injured on the job, and persons with chronic illness not caused by personal failure were considered deserving of public assistance. Alcoholics, prostitutes, mentally ill persons, and those considered to be lazy were the undeserving poor, and they were denied any type of aid (Katz, 1989).

Societal responses to poverty and homeless persons are deeply rooted in history. This history has helped to shape our cultural attitudes. Our cultural attitudes affect, and are affected by, the media. Therefore, it is important to consider the effects of cultural attitudes and the media on societal responses to poverty and homelessness. As is seen in the next sections, there is no one definition of poverty. The definitions vary depending on the person or agency that is using the definition.

## Cultural Attitudes and the Media's Influence

Cultural attitudes are the beliefs and perspectives that a society values. Perspectives about individual responsibility for health and well-being are influenced by prevailing cultural attitudes. Media discourses, or views, are a way to communicate thoughts and attitudes through literature, film, art, television, newspapers, and the Internet. Media images of persons who are poor influence and are influenced by cultural attitudes and values. Poor persons may be cast in negative ways by the media, which influence what we believe to be true about poor persons.

You can examine your own beliefs, values, and knowledge about vulnerable groups by thinking about the following clinical situations and questions:

- You are conducting health screening at a homeless shelter and one of the clients asks you for money for bus fare. Do you give it to her?
- You are in the home of an older person, and there are many roaches on the kitchen floor. What are your obligations in terms of the client's home environment? Where do you sit if he offers you a chair?
- What is your opinion of individual versus societal responsibility for health and well-being? In other words, who is responsible for helping poor and/or homeless persons? Is it society's responsibility? Is it up to poor or homeless persons to help themselves?
- What interventions would you initiate for a population of poor or homeless families in a local shelter? Would you begin with health screening or elsewhere?
- How do you help people who are homeless adhere to their medication regimen?
- How could you effectively advocate for a group of medically indigent men?
- What do you think about your community conducting a town meeting to consider building a homeless shelter?

There are no easy answers to these questions. However, nurses' behaviors in these situations influence, and are influenced by, their relationships with clients who are poor. It is important to evaluate clients and populations in the context of the environment to develop effective nursing interventions. Treating medical problems alone is inadequate. Instead, care must be multidimensional and include biological, psychological, social, political, cultural, environmental, economic, and spiritual factors.

## DEFINING AND UNDERSTANDING POVERTY

The official poverty measure in the United States is a specific dollar amount that varies by family size but is consistent across the country with the exception of Alaska and Hawaii. It does take into account a family's assets and debt and other factors such as cost of living (which varies in different areas of the country). The 2014 poverty level for a family of four was $23,850 ($1,987/month) and $19,790 ($1,649/month) for a family of three (in the 48 contiguous states and the District of Columbia). The higher levels in both Alaska and Hawaii are adjusted for cost of living in these areas (U.S. Department of Health and Human Services [USDHHS], 2014). The poverty guidelines are used to determine whether a family is eligible for public programs (and in some instances private program eligibility). It is thought that across the nation, families actually need about twice the amount of the official poverty level to meet their basic needs (National Center for Children in Poverty [NCCP], 2014a). There are a number of calculators available to determine basic budget needs. The NCCP (2014b) has a calculator to differentiate between basic needs for families of four living in urban (north vs. south), suburban, and rural areas (see the NCCP's Basic Needs Budget Calculator at http://www.nccp.org/tools/frs/budget.php).

In making their calculations, the NCCP assumes that a family is composed of two parents with one child in school and a preschool child. The calculation below assumes that both parents work full-time. The items included in the basic needs budgets are as follows: rent and utilities, food, child care, health insurance premiums, out-of-pocket medical costs, transportation, other necessities, payroll taxes, and income taxes. To compare the need versus the poverty level, in 2008 (most current figures available using the calculator), a family of four in Houston, Texas, would need $50,624 compared with the same family in rural Decatur County, Iowa, who would need $42,749 per year.

In 2013, the official poverty rate was 154.5%, with 45.3 million people living below the federal poverty level; 19.9% of those 18 years of age or less were living in poverty. This does not include the millions more living near poverty (U.S. Census Bureau, 2014). As mentioned earlier, the number of people living in poverty increases during times of economic stress and when unemployment rates rise.

Because people who live in poverty are not all alike, be sure to listen in order to individualize care and avoid making inappropriate assumptions about their needs. It is important to take the time to know clients by name and to listen to the stories of their lives. Getting to know your clients can begin to break down barriers caused by their fears and isolation as well as barriers caused by your fears as a nurse, which can lead to misunderstandings. It is also helpful to examine social and cultural definitions and considerations related to poverty. Table 33-1 lists the 2014 poverty guidelines for the United States.

## Social and Cultural Definitions of Poverty

As mentioned, income level is used as the key criterion that determines whether someone is poor. Although income

WIC, TANF

**TABLE 33-1 2014 Poverty Guidelines for the 48 Contiguous States and the District of Columbia**

| Persons in Family/Household | Poverty Guideline |
| --- | --- |
| 1 | $11,670 |
| 2 | $15,730 |
| 3 | $19,790 |
| 4 | $23,850 |
| 5 | $27,910 |
| 6 | $31,970 |
| 7 | $36,030 |
| 8* | $40,090 |

*For families/households with more than eight persons, add $4060 for each additional person.
From U.S. Department of Health and Human Services (2014).

continues to be the measurement of choice, poverty is not adequately defined solely by income level. Understanding the social and cultural dimensions of poverty helps to broaden our view of the concept. Poverty refers to having insufficient financial resources to meet basic living expenses. These expenses include costs of food, shelter, clothing, transportation, and medical care. In addition to its economic outcomes, however, poverty has important physical, psychological, and spiritual consequences. People who are poor are more likely to live in dangerous environments, work at high-risk jobs, eat less nutritious foods, and have multiple and unrelenting stressors, such as unemployment, inadequate housing, lack of affordable daycare, and lack of access to regular health care.

Meanings and perceptions of poverty differ across cultures. Most Western cultures view poverty negatively, whereas other cultures often respect the poor. Religious and political differences affect the perceptions people hold of poor and underserved groups. Meanings of lower socioeconomic status can also vary among various groups within a culture.

## Political Dimensions and Causes of Poverty

It is important to examine poverty in terms of its political dimensions. Poverty involves a lack of control over critical resources needed to function effectively in society. The federal government uses two types of guidelines to define poverty: (1) The Poverty Threshold Guidelines are issued by the U.S. Bureau of the Census and are used primarily for statistical purposes; and (2) the Federal Income Poverty Guidelines are issued by the USDHHS and are used to determine whether a person or family is financially eligible for assistance or services from various federal and state programs. The programs include Temporary Assistance to Needy Families (TANF [formerly called Aid to Families with Dependent Children, or AFDC]); Medicaid; the Supplemental Nutritional Assistance Program (SNAP [formerly Food Stamps]); Women, Infants, and Children Program (WIC); and Head Start. Federal poverty guidelines are updated annually to be consistent with the consumer price index (CPI), also called the cost-of-living index. The CPI is a measure of the average change over time in the prices paid by households for a fixed market basket of consumer goods and

services, including housing; electricity; food; clothing; fuels; doctor, dentist, and drug charges; transportation; and other goods and services that people buy for day-to-day living (Bureau of Labor Statistics, 2014).

Many people who earn slightly more than the government-defined income levels (see Table 33-1) are unable to meet living expenses but are not eligible for government assistance programs. Persons whose income is above the federal poverty guidelines but still inadequate are called the near poor. An example would be a family of four with an income of $24,000 (poverty level, $23,850); they are near poor and may not qualify for Medicaid. Although the federal government funds part of Medicaid, each individual state determines eligibility criteria.

The terms persistent poverty and neighborhood poverty are often used to describe social aspects of poverty. Persistent poverty refers to individuals and families who remain poor for long periods and whose poverty is multigenerational. Neighborhood poverty refers to geographically defined areas of high poverty, characterized by run-down housing, high unemployment rates, and poorer health outcomes (Raphael, 2011). It is important for nurses who work with poor populations to know these definitions and to respect poor clients as human beings whose life situations influence their health and well-being.

Poverty in the United States was not recognized as a social problem before the Civil War (Katz, 1989). The prevalent attitude during that time was that poverty was an individual's problem, and poor individuals had only themselves to blame. In general, society did not assume responsibility for alleviating the plight of the poor. However, during the post–Civil War industrialized era, this attitude changed significantly. Widespread unemployment, undesirable working conditions, insufficient wages, and substandard housing forced a rethinking of public responsibility for the poor (Wilson, 1990). Many laws concerning public health and housing were passed. Social reform movements after the Civil War led to an interest in urban poverty research (Bremner, 1956; Miller, 1966). Despite influences of the Depression of the 1930s and national discussion of New Deal legislation, such as the Social Security Act of 1935, the public's interest in the plight of the poor declined (Wilson, 1990).

A resurgence of political activity on behalf of disadvantaged groups occurred during the late 1950s and early 1960s. In 1959 the Kerr-Mills Act increased funds for health care for aged persons (Fine, 1998). In 1961 President Kennedy approved a pilot food program in response to the hunger he observed on the campaign trail (Price, 1994); in 1963 he instructed his administration to develop a major policy effort to combat poverty. After Kennedy's assassination, President Johnson sustained the interest in the antipoverty campaign. Johnson established the War on Poverty in 1964, which emphasized job-training programs and community organization and involvement (Pilisuk and Pilisuk, 1973; Wilson, 1990). In 1964 the Social Security Administration established the income level of the official poverty line. Individuals and families with incomes below the federal poverty line were considered to be living in poverty. In 1965 the Medicare amendments to the Social Security Act were passed. After 1965 considerable research focused on poverty as it related to education, health, housing, the law, and public welfare (Wilson, 1990).

Policy changes during the 1980s led to an emphasis on defense spending rather than on social programs. The visibility of the homeless and the media attention on an underclass of individuals seemed to blame the poor for being poor. However, being poor is often the result of a complex web including the economic environment, income levels, and race. The poverty rate for blacks and Hispanics exceeds the average. In 2011, the rate was 25% to 27% whereas the rate for whites (non-Hispanic) was about 10% (U.S. Census Bureau, 2012).

During the 1990s, record numbers of people received welfare benefits, and this stimulated enthusiasm for reform of the health and welfare systems (Zedlewski, 2002). In 1996 a bill creating the TANF program was enacted. This welfare reform legislation replaced the Aid to Families with Dependent Children program with a program of temporary welfare benefits. Under TANF, eligible persons are provided with benefits for a limited time, and are required to find jobs and/or to enroll in job-training programs. Low-income working families often do not bring home enough money to cover the costs of everyday living. Although there are governmental programs such as tax credits, SNAP (food stamps), WIC, and childcare subsidies, often these supports are not sufficient or not available to all who need them or meet eligibility. Low-income working families are at great risk during times of a weak economy. The loss of a job or a cut in hours of work can disrupt their precarious financial situation. Most of these persons cannot save for a time when times get rough because they barely earn enough to cover regular expenses. Also, many of these workers do not have employee-sponsored health insurance, and an illness can therefore be a devastating financial crisis. Although these employees may be eligible for health insurance through the Affordable Care Act, they may not have enrolled because of reluctance, uncertainty about eligibility or how to enroll, lack of health navigators, etc.

Opinions and beliefs about how to assist those who are poor differ among recipients, taxpayers, politicians, economists, health care providers, and others. Some people believe that welfare benefits for the poor are inadequate, whereas others argue that welfare breeds dependency and illegitimacy. Families receiving welfare benefits also have differing views. There are ongoing political debate about whether to abolish or to reform the benefits available through the TANF, SNAP, and other programs.

The causes of poverty are complex and interrelated. In recent decades the number of adult and older adult Americans living in poverty has decreased in part because of the support provided through Social Security and Medicare benefits, as discussed later. In contrast, the number of women and children living in poverty has increased. The following factors affect the growing number of poor persons in the United States:

- Decreased earnings
- Increased unemployment rates
- Changes in the labor force
- Increase in female-headed households
- Inadequate education and job skills
- Inadequate antipoverty programs

- Inadequate welfare benefits
- Weak enforcement of child support statutes
- Dwindling Social Security payments to children
- Increased numbers of children born to single women
- Trade deficits, debt, involvement in wars
- Outsourcing of American jobs

As most industrialized nations have moved from being industrial economies to service economies, job opportunities have increasingly excluded workers who do not have at least a high school education. Many manufacturing and other jobs at the lower end of the pay scale do not pay sufficient salary to support a family. Lack of adequate health care compounds the effects of poverty on health.

## POVERTY AND HEALTH: EFFECTS ACROSS THE LIFE SPAN

Poverty directly affects health and well-being, leading to the following:

- Higher rates of chronic illness
- Higher infant morbidity and mortality
- Shorter life expectancy
- More complex health problems
- More significant complications and physical limitation from chronic diseases such as asthma, diabetes, and hypertension
- Hospitalization rates greater than those for persons with higher incomes

Poor health outcomes are related to decreased access to health care. Lack of access to health care can be related to inability to pay for care, lack of or inadequate insurance, geographic location, language, provider shortage areas, transportation difficulties, immigration status, inconvenient clinic hours, and negative attitudes of health care providers toward poor clients. These access issues tend to disproportionately impact those who are poor. The first topic area in *Healthy People 2020* deals with access to health services. This area and its objectives are relevant to meeting the needs of poor and homeless people. See the *Healthy People 2020* box for specific objectives.

---

### ♥ HEALTHY PEOPLE 2020

The following are a sampling of health access goals that affect poor and homeless people:

- AHS-1: Increase the proportion of persons with health insurance.
- AHS-2: Increase the proportion of insured persons with coverage for clinical preventive services.
- AHS-3: Increase the proportion of persons with a usual primary care provider.
- AHS-5: Increase the proportion of persons who have a specific source of ongoing care.
- AHS-6: Reduce the proportion of individuals who experience difficulties or delays in obtaining necessary medical care, dental care, or prescription medicines.

From U.S. Department of Health and Human Services (USDHHS): *HealthyPeople.gov: Access to Health Services.* Washington, DC, 2010, USDHHS. Retrieved February 2015 from http://www .healthypeople.gov/2020/topics-objectives/topic/Access-to-Health -Services/objectives

The Affordable Care Act (ACA) is designed to help meet *Healthy People 2020* goals by providing increased health care access through affordable health insurance. The ACA focuses on access to clinical preventive services, increased access to health care providers, and establishing a medical home. At this time the ACA's mechanism for enrolling those who are poor is through Medicaid expansion in each state. This process has been slowed by states that have not expanded their Medicaid enrollment. This delay in the implementation of the ACA presents a significant barrier to assisting the very poorest in accessing health care.

## Poverty among Women

In 2012, just over half (50.3%) of poor families were headed by women (Pew Research Center, 2014). Approximately 14% of the adult female population lives in poverty compared with 10.5% of adult men. Minority women are also disproportionally affected by diabetes, hypertension, overweight and obesity, asthma, HIV/AIDS, and sexually transmitted infections (STIs). Two thirds of newly diagnosed cases of HIV and the highest rates of chlamydia and gonorrhea occur in African American females. Women living in rural areas face additional barriers. They have less income, education, and socioeconomic status and live in areas with fewer providers. These issues contribute to increased rates of chronic disease, injury, and mortality for rural women (USDHHS, 2012).

The relationship between poverty and health is significant. Poverty presents a formidable obstacle to positive health across the life span. Those in lower income groups have poorer health status, and those with poor health have decreased ability to work and improve their socioeconomic status. Many health risks and conditions are linked to education and income. For example, among women aged 25 years and older, 31.0% of those without a high school diploma were living in poverty compared with 4.3% of those with a bachelor's degree. Education is also a strong predictor of health; the more years of schooling, the stronger one's health (National Coalition for the Homeless, 2014; USDHHS, 2012; NCCP, 2014a; Zlotnick et al, 2013).

As discussed earlier, there have been significant changes to welfare support. These reforms affect the health and well-being of childbearing women and their families. When changes in the benefit levels are made, women and their children are often affected. TANF requires that more families work to receive assistance. Funds are targeted to provide childcare subsidies so that women can work. When governmental funds are targeted for a specific area it typically means they are taken from other areas. In this instance there is less funding available to assist those women and children living in poverty who have needs unrelated to child care subsidies. More changes are expected as financial and health care reform in the United States continues and as state and federal budgets continue to be challenged to meet many needs.

## Children and Poverty

Poverty among children in the United States has risen in all racial and ethnic groups and in all geographic settings—urban, suburban, and rural. The poverty rate for children in 2012 was 21.8% higher than for any other age group (U.S. Census Bureau, 2012). Poverty is highest among the youngest children: whereas children represent 24% of the population they comprise 34% of those in poverty. Forty-five percent of all children live in low-income families. Poverty among young African American and Hispanic children is more than three times that of white, non-Hispanic children. Since data were first collected, African American children have experienced significantly high rates of poverty (Children's Defense Fund, 2014; NCCP, 2014a).

Any decrease in social support services increases the number of children living in poverty or near poverty. The decrease in support affects income and access to services, and produces added stress in families. These changes affect the health and well-being of poor children. Young children are at highest risk for the most harmful effects of poverty, especially lack of adequate nutrition, and brain development (Children's Defense Fund, 2014). Children in poverty are more likely to be hungry, sicker, miss more school, and have poorer academic success. Other risk factors for children in poverty include maternal substance abuse or depression, exposure to environmental toxins, trauma, abuse, and lower quality daily care (Children's Defense Fund, 2014; NCCP, 2014a). Poor health in early childhood negatively affects a child's future health. Some of the effects of poverty on children include higher rates of prematurity, low birth weight, birth defects, and infant mortality; an increased incidence of chronic disease, traumatic injuries, or death, nutritional deficits, growth retardation or developmental delays, iron deficiency anemia, and infections; and an increased risk of homelessness and decreased chances for education (Morrell-Bellai et al, 2000). See Box 33-1 for a list of ways in which poverty affects the health of children.

Adolescents are sometimes included in statistics related to childhood poverty. Teens in lower socioeconomic groups have poorer academic achievement, more risky sexual behavior, and higher rates of pregnancy. Teen moms are more likely to drop out of school, be unemployed, and be dependent on welfare programs. African American teens have higher birth rates than white teens and are less likely to graduate from high school (Basch, 2011; Lacour and Tissington, 2011; NCCP, 2014a. See Table 33-2 for the percent of children under 18 years of age who live in low-income families.

---

### BOX 33-1   Effects of Poverty on the Health of Children

- Higher rates of prematurity, low birth weight, and birth defects
- Higher infant mortality rates
- Increased incidence of:
  - Chronic disease
  - Traumatic death and injuries
  - Nutritional deficits
  - Growth retardation and developmental delays
  - Iron deficiency anemia
  - Elevated blood lead levels
  - Infections
- Increased risk for homelessness
- Decreased opportunities for education, income, and occupation

From Morrell-Bellai T, Goering PN, Boydell KM: Becoming and remaining homeless: a qualitative investigation, Issues Ment Health Nurs 21:581-604, 2000.

## TABLE 33-2 Percentage of Children under 18 Years of Age in Low-Income Families, by Race/Ethnicity

| Race/Ethnicity | Percentage in Low-Income Families |
|---|---|
| White children | 32% |
| Black children | 66% |
| Asian children | 32% |
| American Indian children | 64% |
| Children of some other race | 44% |
| Hispanic children | 64% |

National Center for Children in Poverty (2014a).

## Noncustodial Parents

Under current federal law, noncustodial parents are required to provide financial support to their children. Current child support policies are designed to provide financial security to children, prevent single-parent families from entering the welfare system, help single-parent families get off welfare as quickly as possible, and decrease welfare expenditures. Individual states are responsible for locating nonsupporting custodial parents, establishing paternity, and enforcing financial responsibility. In most states, government involvement in locating noncustodial parents begins when the custodial parent applies for TANF.

The current system is criticized because public expectations of financial responsibility for noncustodial parents are based on an assumption that the noncustodial parent is working full time. However, many low-income parents were never married, and many have intermittent work histories. Current policy requires the custodial parent to assign all financial support from the noncustodial parent to the state to equal the amount that the family receives from the welfare (TANF) system. In response to these regulations, many low-income parents often make private, informal arrangements for child support payments. Under these verbal arrangements, the noncustodial parent pays the custodial parent directly. The pejorative term "deadbeat dad" refers to fathers who do not contribute to the financial support of their children. As the number of custodial single fathers increases there may be greater attention to noncustodial mothers who do not contribute to the financial support of their children, because noncustodial mothers are equally responsible under the law to provide for the economic well-being of their children.

## Older Adults and Poverty

An estimated 9.5% of older adults (65 years and older) live in poverty (U.S. Census Bureau, 2014). Poverty rates for this age group are lower, largely because of improvements in Social Security and the Supplemental Security Income (SSI) program. SSI is a federal income supplement program funded by general tax revenues (not Social Security taxes). The SSI program is designed to help older people, those who are blind or disabled, and those who have little or no income. SSI provides cash to meet basic needs for food, clothing, and shelter. The Social Security website (http://www.ssa.gov/) has vast information about eligibility for SSI for children, survivors, retirees, and those with a disability. The site also discusses the benefits available through Medicare and SSI via SNAP (food stamps) and other nutrition programs (Social Security Administration, 2014). Despite the federal benefits available to older persons, certain groups of older adults remain vulnerable to the effects of poverty. Approximately 20% of all black and Hispanic adults (65 years and older) live in poverty compared with only 7.6% whites. Across all groups more than 25% of unmarried older women live at or just above the poverty level (AARP, 2014).

Older adults living at or near poverty are disproportionately more likely to report poor health outcomes compared with those living at higher incomes. They are more likely to have a disability (physical, vision, hearing, or cognitive). Older adults who live in poverty are particularly at risk because they may be alone, unable to manage their personal affairs, and have greater limitations in their functional abilities (bathing, preparing meals, and other daily activities). More than half of those who are poor and old spend greater than 50% of their income on housing costs. This is particularly worrisome because housing costs that exceed 30% are typically considered unaffordable. Food insecurity is another issue affecting this group. Low-income elderly often are unable to access adequate and safe food. Those who are elderly and poor are more likely to seek acute crisis care rather than preventive health care. Many older adults are eligible for benefits and yet do not know how to access them (AARP, 2014).

One client gave the following advice to nurses who care for poor people: (1) treat the poor like everyone else; (2) do not be condescending and do not prejudge; instead ask whether the person can pay his bill, although not everyone can pay for his medications; (3) recommend programs such as food banks, churches, and clothing centers. Remember that poor people have complex needs and they need strong advocates to help them find needed services.

## The Community and Poverty

Conditions in neighborhoods influence health. Poverty is a strong and powerful determinant of health (Zlotnick et al, 2013). Lower socioeconomic neighborhoods have been linked with poorer general health status, chronic conditions, higher mortality and morbidity, poorer birth outcomes, disability, and higher levels of injury and violence. They are more likely to have environmental hazards, rodent and pest infestations, and higher crime rates. They lack safe areas for exercise such as parks, good sidewalks, safe playgrounds, after-school programs, and other options that promote healthy behaviors. The concentration of substandard housing in poorer neighborhoods adds to socioeconomic health disparities. Poorer neighborhoods tend to be targets for drug and alcohol advertising and the presence of liquor stores, where paychecks may be cashed (Robert Wood Johnson Foundation, 2014).

Neighborhood conditions affect whether residents have access to healthy affordable food choices. Access to health care continues to be difficult for those who live in poorer

**CLINICAL DECISION-MAKING ACTIVITIES—cont'd**

community and how could state senators and representatives support such programs?

3. Examine the specific programs identified in the preceding assessment. How do those who need services access them? Working with other students, make appointments with key persons in the agencies identified to find out what each agency offers, which particular aggregate is served, how clients access the services, who is eligible, how the agency receives funding, and what methods are used to evaluate the agency's ability to meet the needs of its targeted aggregates. Give some examples.

4. Identify nurses in your community who work with the homeless or with other vulnerable groups. Invite these nurses to come to a class meeting to share their experiences. What constitutes a typical workday? What are the rewards and challenges of working with vulnerable populations? How do they deal with the frustrations and challenges of their work? What advice might they offer to students working with vulnerable populations? What programs do they recommend? How would you advocate for vulnerable populations in your practice?

5. Imagine yourself as a nurse working in a homeless shelter or making a home visit to a family in an impoverished neighborhood. How have your life experiences and education prepared you (or not) for these situations?

# REFERENCES

AARP: *Older Americans in Poverty: A Snapshot*, 2014. Retrieved February 2015 from http://assets.aarp.org/rgcenter/ppi/econ-sec/2010-03-poverty.pdf. Retrieved February 2015 from http://www.acog.org/~/media/Departments/Adolescent%20Health%20Care/Teen%20Care%20Tool%20Kit/ACOGPreventCare.pdf?dmc=1&ts=20140316T1247342980.

American Nurses Association (ANA): *Scope and Standards of Practice: Public Health Nursing*, ed 2. Silver Spring, MD, 2013, ANA.

Basch C: Teen pregnancy and the acheivement gap among urban minority youth. *J School Health* 81:614–618, 2011.

Bharel M, Lin WC, Zhang J, et al: Health care utilization patterns of homeless individuals in Boston: preparing for Medicaid expansion under the Affordable Care Act. *Am J Public Health* 103(Suppl 2):S311–S317, 2013.

Bremner RH: *From the Depths: The Discovery of Poverty in the United States*. New York, 1956, New York University Press.

Bureau of Labor Statistics: *Consumer Price Index*. Washington, DC, 2014, U.S. Department of Labor. Retrieved February 2015 from http://www.bls.gov/cpi/cpiovrvw.htm.

Cheshire WP: Disorders of thermal regulation. In *Cecil Essentials of Medicine*. Philadelphia, PA, 2010, Saunders Elsevier, pp 1083–1085.

Children's Defense Fund: *The State of America's Children 2014 Report*, 2014. Retrieved February 2015 from http://www.childrensdefense.org/library/state-of-americas-children/2014-soac.html.

Connor A, Donohue ML: Integrating faith and health with persons who are homeless using a parish nursing practice model. *Fam Community Health* 33:123–132, 2010.

Doran KM, Vashi AA, Platis S, et al: Navigating the boundaries of emergency department care: addressing the medical and social needs of patients who are homeless. *Am J Public Health* 103(Suppl 2):S355–S360, 2013.

Dworsky A, Napolitano L, Courtney M: Homelessness during the transition from foster care to adulthood. *Am J Public Health* 103(Suppl 2):S318–S323, 2013.

Fine S: The Kerr-Mills Act: medical care for the indigent in Michigan, 1960-1965. *J Hist Med Allied Sci* 53:285–316, 1998.

Gerber L: Bringing home effective nursing care for the homeless. *Nursing* 43:32–38, 2013.

Goodman S, Messeri P, O'Flaherty B: How effective homelessness prevention impacts the length of shelter spells. *J Hous Econ* 23:55–62, 2014.

Grant R, Gracy D, Goldsmith G, et al: Twenty-five years of child and family homelessness: where are we now? *Am J Public Health* 103(Suppl 2):e1–e10, 2013.

Holtrop K, McNeil S, McWey LM: It's a struggle but I can do it. I'm doing it for me and my kids": the psychosocial characteristics and life experiences of at-risk homeless parents in transitional housing. *J Marital Fam Ther* 2013 (in press). DOI: 10.1111/jmft.12050.

Howett M, Connor A, Downes E: Nightingale theory and intentional comfort touch in management of tinea pedis in vulnerable populations. *J Holist Nurs* 28:244–250, 2010.

Katz MB: *The Undeserving Poor: From the War on Poverty to the War on Welfare*. New York, 1989, Pantheon Books.

Kertesz SG, Holt CL, Steward JL, et al: Comparing homeless persons' care experiences in tailored versus nontailored primary care programs. *Am J Public Health* 103(Suppl 2):S331–S339, 2013.

Kidd SA, Karabanow J, Hughes J, et al: Brief report: youth pathways out of homelessness—preliminary findings. *J Adolesc* 36:1035–1037, 2013.

Lacour M, Tissington LD: The effects of poverty on academic achievement. *Educ Res Rev* 6:522–527, 2011.

Linton KF, Shafer MS: Factors associated with the health service utilization of unsheltered, chronically homeless adults. *Soc Work Public Health* 29:73–80, 2014.

Mental Illness Recovery Center (MIRCI): Home page, 2014. Retrieved February 2015 from http://www.mirci.org/.

Miller HP: *Poverty American Style*. Belmont, CA, 1966, Wadsworth.

Morrell-Bellai T, Goering PN, Boydell K: Becoming and remaining homeless: a qualitative investigation. *Issues Mental Health Nurs* 21:581–604, 2000.

National AIDS Housing Coalition: *Fact Sheet*, 2014. Retrieved February 2015 from http://nationalaidshousing.org/PDF/FactSheet.pdf.

National Alliance to End Homelessness: *Snapshot of Homelessness*, 2014. Retrieved February 2015 from http://www.endhomelessness.org/pages/snapshot_of_homelessness.

National Center for Children in Poverty (NCCP): *Basic Facts about Low-Income Children: Children under 18 Years* [Fact Sheet], 2014a. Retrieved from http://www.nccp.org/publications/pub_1089.html.

National Center for Children in Poverty (NCCP): *Basic Needs Budget Calculator*, 2014b. Retrieved February 2014 from http://www.nccp.org/tools/frs/budget.php.

National Center for Homeless Education: *Homelessness: General Awareness*, 2014. Retrieved February 2015 from http://center.serve.org/nche/ibt/aw_homeless.php.

National Coalition for the Homeless: *Homelessness in America*, 2014. Retrieved February 2015 from http://nationalhomeless.org/about-homelessness/.

New York City Department of Homeless Services: Home page, 2014. Retrieved February 2015 from http://www.nyc.gov/html/dhs/html/home/home.shtml.

Paulson A: Record number of homeless children enrolled in US public schools (++vidoe). CSmonitor http://www.csmonitor.com?USA/Education?2014/0923/Record-number-of-homeless-children-enrolled-in-US-public-schools-video. Retrieved April 3, 2015.

Pew Research Center: *Who's Poor in America? 50 Years into the "War on Poverty," a Data Portrait*, Retrieved February 2015 from http://www.pewresearch.org/fact-tank/2014/01/13/whos-poor-in-america-50-years-into-the-war-on-poverty-a-data-portrait/.

Pilisuk M, Pilusuk P, editors: *Poor Americans: How We Lost the War on Poverty*. New Brunswick, NJ, 1973, Transaction Publishers.

Price J: More mouths, more money. *Washington Times*, April 19, 1994.

Public Health Foundation: *Council on Linkages between Academia and Public Health Practice*, 2014.

Retrieved February 2015 from http://www.phf.org/programs/council/Pages/default.aspx/competenciesinformation.htm.

Raphael D: Poverty in childhood and adverse health outcomes in adulthood. *Maturitas* 69:22–26, 2011.

Robert Wood Johnson Foundation: *Neighborhoods and Health: Exploring the Social Determinants of Health* [Issue Brief #8], 2014. Retrieved February 2015 from http://www.rwjf.org/content/dam/farm/reports/issue_briefs/2011/rwjf70450.

Social Security Administration (SSA): *Official Social Security Website, 2014.* Washington, DC, 2014, SSA. Retrieved February 2015 from http://www.ssa.gov/.

Teruya C, Anderson RM, Arangua L, et al: Health and health care disparities among homeless women. *Women Health* 50:719–736, 2010.

U.S. Census Bureau: *Poverty: 2013 Highlights.* Washington, DC, 2014,

U.S. Department of Commerce. Retrieved February 2015 from http://www.census.gov/hhes/www/poverty/about/overview/index.html.

U.S. Conference of Mayors: *2013 Hunger and Homelessness Survey: a Status Report on Hunger and Homelessness in America's Cities: 31st Survey of Hunger and Homelessness.* Retrieved February 2015 from http://www.usmayors.org/pressreleases/uploads/2013/1210-report-HH.pdf.

U.S. Department of Health and Human Services (USDHHS): *HealthyPeople.gov.* Washington, DC, 2010, U.S. Government Printing Office. Retrieved February 2015 from http://www.healthypeople.gov/2020/topicsobjectives2020/default.aspx.

U.S. Department of Health and Human Services (USDHHS), Health Resources and Services Administration: *Women's Health USA 2012.* Washington, DC, 2012, U.S. Government Printing Office. Retrieved February 2015 from

http://www.mchb.hrsa.gov/whusa12/more/downloads/pdf/whusa12.pdf.

U.S. Department of Health and Human Services (USDHHS): *2014 Poverty Guidelines.* Washington, DC, 2014, U.S. Government Printing Office. Retrieved February 2015 from http://aspe.hhs.gov/poverty/14poverty.cfm.

U.S. Department of Housing and Urban Development: *ASPE Research Brief: Approaches to Low-Income Energy Assistance Funding in Selected States*, 2014. Retrieved February 2015 from http://aspe.hhs.gov/hsp/14/LIHEAP/rb_LIHEAP.cfm.

van den Berk-Clark C, McGuire J: Elderly homeless veterans in Los Angeles: chronicity and precipitants of homelessness. *Am J Public Health* 103(Suppl 2):S232–S238, 2013.

Weber M, Thompson L, Schmiege SJ, et al: Perception of access to health care by homeless individuals seeking services at a day shelter.

*Arch Psychiatric Nurs* 27:179–184, 2013.

Wilson WK: *The Truly Disadvantaged: The Inner City, the Underclass, and Public Policy.* Chicago, 1990, University of Chicago Press.

Yoder JR, Bender K, Thompson SJ, et al: Explaining homeless youths' criminal justice interactions: childhood trauma or surviving life on the streets? *Community Ment Health J* 50:135–144, 2014.

Zazworsky D, Johnson N: It takes a village: a community partnership model in caring for the homeless. *Nurs Admin Q* 38:179–185, 2014.

Zedlewski SR: Family economic resources in the post-reform era. *Future Child* 12:120–145, 2002.

Zlotnick C, Zerger S, Wolfe PB: Health care for the homeless: what we have learned in the past 30 years and what's next. *Am J Public Health* 103(Suppl 2):S199–S205, 2013.

# 34

# Migrant Health Issues

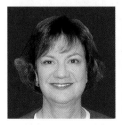

## Marie Napolitano, PhD, RN, FNP

Dr. Marie Napolitano is an associate professor and the Director of the Doctor of Nursing Practice/Family Nurse Practitioner Program at the University of Portland. She earned the BA in nursing from Louisiana State University, the MA in Nursing from the University of Washington, and the PhD from the Oregon Health and Sciences University. She has extensive clinical practice with migrant farmworkers and their families and has been a co-investigator on NIH pesticide exposure studies. Her areas of expertise include nurse practitioner education in the United States and internationally, doctor of nursing practice education, and the integration into practice of cultural considerations regarding immigrant and Latino populations. Her clinical interests include chronic illness self-care management for Latino individuals and families. She is a board member of Project Access Now and a member of the advisory committee of the Migrant Head Start Program in Oregon.

## ADDITIONAL RESOURCES

**Evolve Website http://evolve.elsevier.com/Stanhope**
- *Healthy People 2020*
- WebLinks
- Quiz
- Case Studies

- Glossary
- Answers to Practice Application
- Resource Tool 34.A: Resources for the Nurse Who Is Working with Migrant Farm Workers

## OBJECTIVES

*After reading this chapter, the student should be able to do the following:*

1. Define the terms *migrant farmworker* and *seasonal farmworker* and discuss the lifestyle and work environments that contribute to their health status.
2. Discuss the difficulties with obtaining epidemiologic and health data on this population.
3. Describe occupational and common health problems of migrant farmworkers and their families and the barriers in securing health care.

4. Evaluate programs to determine effectiveness with encouraging health-seeking and health-promoting behaviors among migrant farmworkers and their families.
5. Analyze the role of the nurse in planning and providing culturally appropriate care to migrant farmworkers and their families.
6. Advocate for legislation and policy that would improve the lives and working conditions of migrant farmworkers and their access to health care services.

## KEY TERMS

food insecurity, p. 757
health disparities, p. 756
migrant farmworker, p. 751
Migrant Health Act, p. 753
migrant health centers, p. 753
migrant lifestyle, p. 752

occupational health risks, p. 755
pesticide exposure, p. 755
political advocates, p. 762
seasonal farmworker, p. 751
traditional beliefs and practices, p. 760
—*See Glossary for definitions*

## CHAPTER OUTLINE

**Migrant Lifestyle**
  Housing
**Health and Health Care**
  Access to Health Care
**Occupational and Environmental Health Problems**
  Pesticide Exposure
**Common Health Problems**
  Specific Health Problems

**Children and Youth**
**Cultural Considerations in Migrant Health Care**
  Nurse-Client Relationship
  Health Values
  Health Beliefs and Practices
**Health Promotion and Illness Prevention**
**Role of the Nurse**

Imagine yourself attempting to deliver treatment in a migrant camp to a toddler whose pertussis culture returned positive. The camp is located in an isolated rural community. The toddler lives in a trailer with her parents and siblings and extended family members (13 individuals). The family must also be treated as contacts. No one speaks English, so you have an interpreter with you. The family has just returned from picking strawberries all day in the fields, and they are tired and hungry. The family is willing to give medicine to the toddler because she is sick; however, they do not understand why they must take the medicine also, because they are not sick. The family tells you that they will not be able to take the noon dose because they have no water with them at work. Walking to the drinking barrel will take too long and they will lose income. As a nurse, what would you do? As a starting point, nurses need to be informed about the cultures, lifestyle, and health picture of the migrant and seasonal farmworkers and families that they serve.

Migrant and seasonal farmworkers (MSFWs) are essential to the agricultural industry in the United States, especially with the decrease in family farms and the increase in labor-intensive crop production such as vegetables, fruit, nuts, and ornamental plants. Although the availability and affordability of food in the United States depend on these individuals, their economic status and social acceptance have not reflected the importance of their work. Estimates of the numbers of MSFWs in the United States vary, with sources identifying approximately 1.0 to 1.8 million hired farmworkers. Five states account for 65% of all farmworkers: California, Florida, Washington, Oregon, and North Carolina (U.S. Department of Agriculture, 2007). Numbers vary because of divergent methodologies for estimating numbers and difficulties in counting mobile populations. Large data sources each have unique limitations prohibiting a clear picture of the MSFW population.

According to the U.S. Department of Labor (2013), a **migrant farmworker** is a seasonal farmworker who must travel to do farm work and is unable to return to a permanent residence within the same day. A **seasonal farmworker** returns to his permanent residence, works in agriculture for at least is 25 days or parts of days, and does not work year round only in agriculture. The term *MSFW* also includes migrant food-processing workers, who are defined in the same way as seasonal farmworkers but work in food processing and are unable to return to a permanent residence on the same day. Numbers of migrant crop farmworkers (about 26%) are decreasing whereas those of seasonal farmworkers are increasing (Carroll et al, 2011). Migrant and seasonal farmworkers share many demographic, cultural, and occupational characteristics. Much of the available information on agricultural farmworkers does not distinguish between migrant and seasonal farmworkers.

The majority of MSFWs are foreign-born (72%) and predominantly Mexican (68%) (Carroll et al, 2011). Traditionally, Mexican MSFWs have come from the west central states of Guanajuato, Jalisco, and Michoacán; however, in 2009, 20% of MSFWs came from the nontraditional sending states of southern Mexico including Oaxaca, Guerrero, Chiapas, Puebla, Morelos, and Veracruz (Carroll et al, 2011). The numbers of newly arrived indigenous migrant workers from southern

Mexico and Central America are increasing. These individuals are at higher risk for exploitation due to language difficulties, poverty, and fear. Other workers include African Americans, Jamaicans, Haitians, Laotians, and Thais. The composition of the migrant and seasonal population can vary from region to region in the United States. Of the MSFWs, 52% have legal authorization to work in the United States. Less than 5% of farmworkers are in the United States as a H-2A guest worker (Villarejo, 2012). Foreign-born farmworkers have spent an average of 13 years working in the United States, with more than 50% for 10 to 20 years. Approximately 29% have been in the United States for at least 20 years whereas 26% have been in the country 4 years or less (Carroll et al, 2011). The average number of farm workdays by farmworkers in 2009 was 190 per year, not necessarily on one farm only.

According to the latest analyzed National Agricultural Workers Survey (NAWS) data from 2007 to 2009 (Carroll et al, 2011), MSFWs are young, with an average age of 36 years; 24% are less than 25 years of age. Interestingly, considering the nature of the work, 18% of MSFWs are older than 45 years of age. The majority of MSFWs are male (79%); more than 50% are married with an average of two children. Approximately 59% live with their spouses during their agricultural work. Thirty percent speak English well and 35% cannot speak English at all. The average school grade completed is eighth grade. Up to 40% have completed up to the sixth grade and 28% completed up to the tenth to twelfth grades.

In comparison, the Migrant and Seasonal Farmworker Descriptive Profiles Project (Migrant Clinicians Network [MCN], 2010b) found more single men; fewer women and children (except on the West Coast); an increase in seasonal workers who no longer migrate; greater representation from Central America, the Caribbean, and Pacific; and shifting industry reducing traditional labor crops with less processing. Some regional results were that housing varied in terms of availability and quality, more indigenous individuals were found in the West with corresponding language challenges, and greater labor shortages existed in the West.

## MIGRANT LIFESTYLE

Migrant farmworkers traditionally have followed one of three migratory streams: Eastern, originating in Florida; Midwestern, originating in Texas; and Western, originating in California. However, as workers increasingly travel throughout the country seeking employment, these streams are becoming less distinct. Migrant farmworkers are employed in fruit and nut (35%), vegetable (23%), horticultural (20%), field (16%), and miscellaneous (5%) agricultural venues (Carroll et al, 2011). Eighty-eight percent of farmworkers are hired directly and 12% are labor contracted; however, this method is increasing. The cyclic nature of agricultural work along with its dependence on weather and economic conditions results in considerable uncertainty for migrant farmworkers. These individuals and families leave their homes with the expectation of work at certain sites. Word of mouth from friends or family, newspaper announcements, or previous employment most often determines their destinations. However, on arrival migrant farmworkers may find that other workers have arrived first or that the crops are late, leaving the farmworkers unemployed.

Migrant farmworkers are vulnerable to forced labor (labor trafficking). Labor trafficking is defined as "the recruitment, harboring, transporting, providing, or obtaining of people for forced or coerced labor" (Polaris Project, 2013). Trafficked individuals, especially undocumented, need to work but can find themselves in appalling work conditions and housing without means to leave or report, fearful of retaliation. They may owe debt to their employers or the recruiters from their home countries. Federal and state legislation exist against human trafficking, but in isolated agricultural areas enforcement is difficult. Although exact numbers are not available, it is estimated that the agricultural sector comprises 10% of all foreign nationals trafficked in the United States annually, which is approximately 1450 to 1750 individuals per year (Human Rights Center, 2004) or 5% of all farmworkers (Polaris Project, 2013). The psychological stress can result in physical and mental health problems. Certain questions can be asked to possibly identify a victim of forced labor and should be asked as part of a nursing assessment in an attempt not to frighten the individual. These include:

- What type of work do you do? Are you paid for your work? Are you able to leave your work at any time for another job? Do you owe money to your employer or someone else here? Are you able to leave your living space? Are you required to ask permission to obtain food and medical care?

If a minor is identified, then child-protective services and law enforcement should be notified (Clawson et al, 2009). Richards (2014) recommended involving social workers and others in the plan to assist. The minor should not be left alone until services arrive. For an adult, obtain permission to contact authorities and get a social worker or agency involved. The National Human Trafficking Resource Center hotline (888-373-7888) should be contacted.

The way of life for any migrant farmworker is stressful. Some of the challenges of the migrant lifestyle include leaving one's home every year, traveling, and experiencing uncertainty regarding work and housing, isolation in new communities, and a lack of resources. Farmworkers usually are paid an hourly rate (83%) followed by piece rate pay (11%). The specifics for payment differ depending on the location and type of work. Reports of average income for farmworkers have varied. According to the NAWS 2007-2009 statistics, farmworker families averaged $17,500 to $19,999 per year. Almost 25% of families live below federal poverty limits; however, the numbers of families with incomes below poverty has decreased. Although many farmworker families meet the income tests for federal and state assistance programs, less than 1% of farmworker families receive any assistance (Villarejo, 2012). Undocumented workers are not eligible for these programs; for others, changing residence from state to state, lack of knowledge and lack of access to programs impede use of program assistance. See Figure 34-1 for an example of a group of migrant farmworkers.

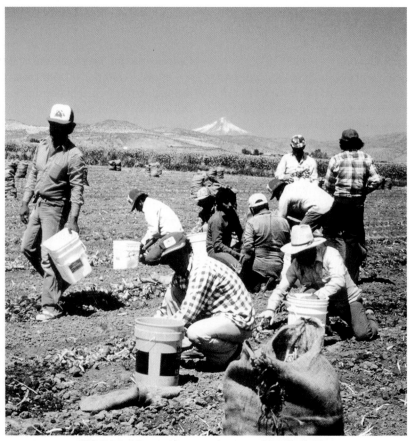

**FIG 34-1** Migrant farmworkers working in fields.

Laws have been enacted that should protect farmworkers. These include the Fair Labor Standards that addresses minimum wage, overtime pay, record keeping, and child labor standards. Farms with fewer than seven workers in a calendar quarter are exempt from minimum wage requirements and farmworkers are not included in overtime pay. The Migrant and Seasonal Agricultural Worker Protection Act mandates that farm contractors, employers, and agricultural associations must disclose employment terms, post information about worker protection at the worksite, pay workers what is due and provide itemized statements, and ensure that housing complies with federal and state safety and health standards. Employers and agricultural associations continuously attempt to weaken or void the law (Farmworker Justice, 2014). The Occupational Safety and Health Act's Field Sanitation Standards (http://www.dol.gov/whd/regs/compliance/whdfs51.htm) ensure drinkable water and accessible sanitation facilities. One section of the Immigration and Nationality Act protects H-2A workers who have permission to work in the United States. As of February 2015, the U.S. Environmental Protection Agency (EPA) has accepted comments and is proposing a stronger Worker Protection Standard (WPS) to safeguard farmworkers from harmful exposures to pesticides. Migrant and seasonal workers often are exempt from the protection of these laws as well as from some Occupational Safety and Health Administration (OSHA) protective provisions due to such allowances as small farm exemptions. Where laws do exist to protect agricultural workers, they may be minimally enforced because of lack of staff and resources. Only three states enforce workplace safety standards regardless of size of farm and numbers of employees: Washington, Oregon, and California.

Migrant and seasonal agricultural workers are considered a unique vulnerable population because of their mobility, the physical demands of the work, social and often geographic isolation, language differences, and high rates of financial impoverishment (National Center for Farmworker Health [NCFH], 2012b). Although MSFW problems are numerous and creating solutions is difficult, some progress has been made in improving the condition of the farmworker population. For example, the latest analyzed NAWS data showed improvement in field sanitation conditions such as the provision of drinking water, field toilets, and hand-washing facilities.

## Housing

Migrant farmworkers often have trouble finding available, decent, and affordable housing. Housing conditions vary between states and localities, and housing arrangements and locations and types of housing differ for migrant and seasonal farmworkers. Housing for migrant farmworkers varies by region; it can be located in camps with cabins, trailers, or houses and be near farms. The author has seen migrant farmworker families living in cars and tents when housing was not available. A recent trend shows that fewer employers provide on-farm housing or labor camps, and farmworkers must rely on private market housing such as apartments. The Housing Assistance Council (HAC), a nonprofit organization whose mission is to improve affordable housing in rural areas, surveyed 4600

farmworker housing units across the country and found 52% of these units to be crowded by federal standards. More than half of the units lacked showers, a laundry machine, or both (Culp and Umbarger, 2004). This prevented farmworkers from removing pesticides from themselves and their clothing in a timely manner. In North Carolina, a study found that substandard housing conditions worsened as the agricultural season progressed (Vallejos et al, 2011). In addition to crowded conditions, housing may lack individual sanitation, bathing or laundry facilities, screens on windows, or fans or heaters. Housing may be located next to fields that have been sprayed with pesticides or where farming machinery poses a danger to children.

Because housing may be expensive, 50 men may live in one house or three families may share one trailer. The health risks of overcrowded housing range from spread of infectious disease to psychosocial effects. While paying for housing during the agricultural season, many farmworker families also support a home-base household. More federal and state programs are seeking to provide private sector housing to farmworker families such as by providing grants to nonprofit agencies serving farmworkers. However, insufficient funds have been provided to meet the demand for farmworker housing.

## HEALTH AND HEALTH CARE

The literature provides only a glimpse into the health status of migrant farmworkers. National data needed to present a clear picture of their health status are unavailable because of such factors as high annual turnover, language, mobility, and concern for immigration status. Regional and local cross-sectional health status studies allow some insights. In the past, the most inclusive health data came from two reports from California: *Suffering in Silence: A Report on the Health of California's Agricultural Workers* (Villarejo et al, 2000) and the California Institute for Rural Studies (CIRS) Agricultural Workers Health Study (Ayala et al, 2001). These reports showed a population at high risk for chronic disease, poor dental health, and mental health problems; higher rates of certain diseases such as tuberculosis (TB), anemia, diabetes, and hypertension; high levels of work injuries and chemical exposures; and detrimental physical and social environments for the children. Accurate morbidity and mortality data are difficult to obtain because of such factors as Mexican-born farmworkers returning to Mexico when no longer working, farmworkers going back to Mexico to receive health services, and easy-to-record infectious diseases decreasing (Villarejo, 2003).

### Access to Health Care

The Migrant Health Act, signed in 1962, provides funds for primary and supplemental health services to migrant workers and their families. These funds are dispersed to 156 migrant health centers in 42 states that serve as models for delivery of services to a difficult-to-reach migrant population. Migrant health centers serve more than 903,089 individuals across the country (Health Resources and Services Administration [HRSA], 2012). However, estimates show that these clinics serve less than 15% of the entire migrant farmworker population. The others will seek medical care from a private physician or an emergency department, or they will not seek help at all. Approximately 55% of farmworkers received health care services of some type over a 2-year period in 2007 to 2008, mainly dental and well-child examinations, including immunizations (Carroll et al, 2011).

Migrant farmworkers have limited access to health care. NAWS findings from 2008 showed that gender, immigration status, migrant status, English proficiency, access to transportation, health status, and access to health care services outside of the United States were associated with health care use. Other nonindependent factors were proximity to the United States–Mexican border, health insurance status, and workplace payment structure (Hoerster et al, 2011).

Factors that limit adequate provision of health care services include the following:

- *Lack of knowledge about services:* Because of their isolation, migrant farmworkers lack the usual sources for information regarding available services, especially if they are not receiving public benefits.
- *Inability to afford care:* According to Villarejo (2012), 75% of hired farmworkers lack health insurance. The Medicaid program, which is intended to serve the poor, often is not available to migrant farmworkers. Workers may not remain in a geographic area long enough to be considered for benefits, or they may lose benefits when they relocate to a state with different eligibility standards. Their salaries may fluctuate each month, making them ineligible during the times

their salaries rise. Employers may not offer health insurance. Undocumented farmworkers are not eligible for Medicaid coverage. Therefore, migrant farmworkers lack health insurance and state program assistance, which further hinders their access to care. Box 34-1 provides information about what migrant farmworkers have said about several factors in their lives. Also, 16 states do not require employers to provide any workers' compensation insurance for migrant or seasonal farmworkers.

- *Affordable Care Act or health insurance subsidies:* Although it is difficult to determine numbers, many farmworkers will not receive employer-mandated health coverage or subsidies because of the small farm exemption and the exclusion of seasonal workers who are employed less than 120 days in the employer's tax year. Undocumented workers are excluded from any employer and individual insurance mandates.
- *Availability of services:* Immigrants are treated differently, depending on whether they were in the United States before the welfare reform legislation of 1996, and depending on the category of their immigration status. Each state determines whether to fill any or part of the services' gap to immigrants. As a result, many legal immigrants and unauthorized immigrants are ineligible for services such as Supplemental Security Income (SSI) and the Supplemental Nutrition Assistance Program (SNAP; food stamps).
- *Transportation:* Health care services may be located a great distance from work or home, and transportation may not be available or may be too costly.

---

## BOX 34-1   What Migrants Say About...

**Health and Health Care**
"What we have to do is re-educate our people and let them know that we have many rights to live and work and to educate and to have health care. And without health care, we cannot have the other three." Unidentified male farmworker, California

**Work Conditions**
"We're used to working. We don't want to be given things. We just want to be respected and to be paid the salaries." Teresa, California

"Right now, because I'm here today [testifying at hearing on work conditions], I may not have my job. Possibly I may not have my job tomorrow." José, California

"We have to get up at 4:00 in the morning so we can pick the strawberries until late—like 7 or 9—before they are too ripe." Unidentified male farmworker, Hillsboro, Oregon

**Pesticide Exposure**
"You go to the fields and you think that it's a foggy day because it's so pretty and it's white, but it's actually the chemicals that have been sprayed." Adelaide, California

"Pesticides presently occupy us tremendously during our work. We wear rubber gloves and that in itself creates a problem because it takes flesh, pieces of flesh from our hands." Guadalupe, California

"Pesticides only cause problems for people who are new to the work or have some physical problem or are weak." Unidentified male farmworker, Parksdale, Oregon

**Housing**
"My slogan is there must be a way to build houses. I believe we have the right to live in a decent way. We are the labor force. It's like we are foreigners—I am a U.S. citizen. Farmworkers come here with hope, but go home worse off than before." Unidentified male farmworker, Colorado

"We have no coolers in the summer and no heaters in the winter. Temperatures range up to 100 degrees in the summer and 30 degrees in the winter. We work out in the open for 12 or more hours and after working there for more than 12 hours, we have no place to rest. This creates a tremendous amount of frustration, not being able to provide the children with the minimum for comfort." Margarita, California

"The foremen even charged (the farmworkers) for sleeping under the trees." Teresa, California

**Women**
"...Another thing I would like to mention is the way we are treated as women. As women we are discriminated with our co-workers because they see us as insignificant beings. The men think that they are superior." Maria, California

"I come with my uncle and cousin and I cook and clean for them—after I come home from the fields." Unidentified female farmworker, Cornelius, Oregon

**Children and Youth**
"...[The children] go out to the fields. They lay under the trees and there is a residue falling on the children. They are picking grapes, what happens? The sprayers are there with the residue falling on the children." Irma, Oregon

"We have worked in the fields! Well, I'm not very young but I've left some of my youth in the work." Juliana, Washington

From Galarneau C, editor: *Under the Weather: Farm Worker Health.* Austin, TX, 1993, National Advisory Council on Migrant Health, Bureau of Primary Health Care, USDHHS.

- *Hours of services:* Many health services are available only during work hours; therefore, seeking health care during work hours leads to loss of earnings and potential loss of employment.
- *Mobility and tracking:* Migrant families move from job to job, but their health care records do not typically travel with them, leading to fragmented services in such areas as TB treatment, chronic illness management, and immunizations. For example, health departments are known to dispense TB medications on a monthly basis. Adequate treatment for TB requires 6 to 12 months of medication. The migrant farmworker who relocates must independently seek out new health services in order to continue medications. The Migrant Clinicians Network (MCN) TB tracking program makes available to a farmworker's current provider any previous provider information that was entered into the tracking program. This tracking helps maintain continuity of TB care for a mobile population (MCN, 2010a).
- *Discrimination:* Although migrant farmworkers and their families bring revenue into the community, they are often perceived as poor, uneducated, transient, and ethnically different. These perceptions foster attitudes and acts of discrimination against them.
- *Documentation:* Unauthorized individuals fear that securing services in a federally funded or state-funded clinic may lead to discovery and deportation.
- *Language:* The majority of migrant farmworkers speak another language as their first language, mostly Spanish, with a growing number speaking dialects. Although migrant health centers may hire bilingual Spanish-speaking staff, interpreters may be difficult to locate for farmworkers speaking local dialects.
- *Cultural aspects of health care:* See the section "Cultural Considerations in Migrant Health Care" (following).

## OCCUPATIONAL AND ENVIRONMENTAL HEALTH PROBLEMS

Agricultural work ranks as one of the most dangerous industries in the United States (Bureau of Labor Statistics, 2012). Hired farmworkers have a five times higher occupational mortality rate than other workers combined (Villarejo, 2012). Heat illness fatalities were identified as especially significant. Heat-related deaths for crop workers exceed those among other types of workers (Centers for Disease Control and Prevention [CDC], 2008). Working conditions, such as standing on ladders, being exposed to chemicals, and using machinery, produce occupational health risks for the migrant farmworkers who may be inadequately protected or educated. Lack of a comprehensive surveillance system makes it difficult to know the extent of all injuries within the farmworker population. Because small farms are excluded from governmental annual injury surveys and maintenance of written injury reports, injury statistics for farmworkers are incomplete (Villarejo, 2012). Injuries are unreported by farmworkers themselves for fear of loss of work and deportation. Injuries such as sprains and strains, fractures, and lacerations are the most common (Cooper et al, 2006). Other injuries include amputations; crush injuries from tractors,

trucks, or other machinery; acute pesticide poisoning; electrical injuries; and drowning in ditches. Safety practices help prevent injuries; however, one study in North Carolina found that safety regulations are not consistently met, especially during the middle of the season, and that farmworkers, especially undocumented farmworkers, tend not to practice safety behaviors (Whalley et al, 2009). This may be due to lack of knowledge, fear of losing time to work, or beliefs regarding who may be harmed. MSFWs rarely have access to workers' compensation or disability benefits (NCFH, 2012a). Farmworkers tend to self-treat with over-the-counter remedies for injuries (Anthony et al, 2010).

The physical demands of harvesting crops 12 to 14 hours a day take their toll on the musculoskeletal system. Stooping to pick strawberries, reaching overhead while on a ladder to pick pears, or lifting heavy crates with straight legs all cause musculoskeletal pain. In one study, prevalence of chronic back pain among farmworkers and family members was 33% during the last migrant season (Shipp et al, 2009).

Naturally occurring plant substances or applied chemicals can cause irritation to the skin (contact dermatitis) or to the eyes (allergic or chemical conjunctivitis). Farmworkers also spend considerable time in the sun, which is dangerous to the skin. Although skin diseases and skin exposure are common, farmworkers seldom seek care from health centers and mostly use self-treatments (Feldman et al, 2009). Infectious diseases caused by poor sanitary conditions at work and home, poor-quality drinking water, and contaminated foods take the form of acute gastroenteritis and parasites. Farmworkers are at higher risk for eye injuries because of the lack of eye protection devices; lack of knowledge about prevention of eye injuries; taking risks to save time (Verma et al, 2011); and exposure to chemicals, pollen, and dust. Chronic eye irritation and sun exposure leads to cataracts, pterygium, and cloudy lens.

### Pesticide Exposure

The majority of the North American food supply is treated with pesticides. Organophosphate pesticides make up the largest group of pesticides in current use. These pesticides are known to be potential hazards. Farmworkers are exposed not only to the immediate effects of working in fields that are foggy or wet with pesticides, but also to the unknown long-term effects of chronic exposure to pesticides. The location of the migrant farmworker's dwelling near fields or orchards can also be a major source of contamination for the worker and his family. Chemicals on clothes worn at work come into contact with farmworker children as parents embrace or carry their children (NCFH, 2009). Organophosphate pesticide metabolites have been confirmed in farmworkers and their children. Studies have found that farmworkers including pregnant women eat fruits and vegetables directly from the fields without washing them (Goldman et al, 2004; Flocks et al, 2007). The U.S. Environmental Protection Agency (EPA) and the Occupational Safety and Health Administration (OSHA) require that farmworkers be given information about pesticide exposure safety. However, migrant farmworkers may not receive this information, they may receive ineffectual training, or they may not understand the information (Napolitano et al, 2002; Whalley et al, 2009).

Also, migrant farmworkers may have preconceived beliefs about pesticides, such as that only weak workers are harmed by them.

The use of personal protection equipment is not prevalent but the provision of gloves, hats, and so forth by employers has been associated with greater use (Levesque et al, 2012). Farmworkers may not have access to protective clothing or they may be unable to afford its purchase; alternatively, they may choose to disregard precautionary procedures and behaviors (such as wearing gloves) that affect their productivity (Arcury and Quandt, 2009; Napolitano et al, 2002). Some workers do not shower when they return from the fields because of their cultural beliefs about being exposed to cooler water while feeling hot from working. Although the worker protection standards are in effect to minimize pesticide risk, migrant farmworker families remain at high risk for exposure. Lack of resources for monitoring pesticide exposure, culturally inappropriate educational methods, migrants' fear of reporting violations and being fired, and language differences are just a few barriers that hinder a safer pesticide environment for migrant farmworkers. The How To box lists ways to recognize the signs and symptoms of pesticide exposure.

> **HOW TO Recognize the Signs and Symptoms of Pesticide Exposure**
> *Signs and symptoms of pesticide exposure vary according to the amount and length of time of exposure. The majority of body systems can be affected by pesticide exposure.*
> - *Acute health effects of pesticide exposure include neuromuscular symptoms (headache, dizziness, confusion, irritability, twitching muscles, muscle weakness, and seizures), respiratory symptoms (shortness of breath, difficulty breathing, and nasal and pharyngeal irritation), gastrointestinal symptoms (nausea, vomiting, diarrhea, and stomach cramps), skin rashes, eye irritation, memory loss, difficulty with concentration, mood changes, and unconsciousness. Symptoms vary depending on whether the pesticide poisoning is mild or severe.*
> - *Effects of chronic exposure are not entirely known but have been related to such illnesses as cancer, Parkinson disease, infertility or sterility, liver damage, and polyneuropathy and neurobehavioral problems.*
> - *Migrant workers may not understand exposure and may relate any symptom to pesticide exposure when the symptom cannot otherwise be explained.*
> - *If symptoms of pesticide exposure are suspected, the nurse should develop a pesticide exposure history. A good example of an exposure form can be found at http://pesticide.umd.edu.*

Not all health professionals are educated to recognize and treat pesticide illness and therefore might attribute the farmworkers' symptoms and physical findings to other causes.

Cancer is an identified but not well-documented health problem for migrant farmworkers associated with their exposure to chemicals. A high prevalence of breast cancer, brain tumors, non-Hodgkin's lymphoma, and leukemia has been found in agricultural communities (Larson, 2001; Ray and Richards, 2001). Farmworkers in California were found to have a higher risk for certain cancers such as lymphomas, prostate

cancer, brain cancer, leukemia, cervical cancer, and stomach cancer (Mills et al, 2009). A registry-based case-control study of breast cancer in farm labor union members in California found that one crop (mushroom) and three chemicals (an organophosphate, malathion, and an organochlorine) were associated with breast cancer risk (Mills and Yang, 2005).

Pesticides also lead to adverse reproductive and developmental outcomes (Arcury and Quandt, 2009); however, study findings differ regarding pesticides and reproductive health. In California, the rate of pesticide poisoning for females is twice that for males (Calvert et al, 2008) while the California Agricultural Workers Health Survey (CAWHS) found that fewer females received training in pesticide safety (Villarejo and McCurdy, 2008). Goldman and colleagues (2004) found that pregnant women were not taking precautions against pesticide exposure; for example, they did not wash their hands before eating, wear protective clothing, or wash their clothes separately from other family members' clothing; they wore clothing and shoes from work into the home and ate fruits and vegetables directly from the fields.

## COMMON HEALTH PROBLEMS

Migrant and seasonal farmworkers suffer from the same acute and chronic health problems as other populations in the United States. However, their lifestyle and racial or ethnic group membership place them at risk for certain health disparities compared with the general population and to have more frequent and more severe health problems than the general population. Health Center Program data (NCFH, 2014), collected in 2010 from 155 Health Resources and Services Administration health centers serving this population, showed that hypertension, diabetes, otitis media, asthma, contact dermatitis and other eczema, depression, and anxiety affected the greater number of patients seen. All dental needs were numerous.

MSFWs may not know that symptoms such as diarrhea or fever might indicate a more serious health problem, and they often do not seek early treatment. The CAWHS found many undiagnosed health problems during physical examinations. These included sexually transmitted infections (STIs), cervical cancer, high blood glucose, high blood pressure, high serum cholesterol, anemia, and untreated dental problems. In addition, there was a high prevalence of obesity (29% male, 38% female). All of these findings left untreated lead to serious health problems such as heart disease, diabetes, and periodontal disease. For children, the most frequently seen minor problems were "rashes, strains, sprains, upper respiratory infections, otitis media, abdominal discomfort, diarrhea, urinary tract infections, anemia, lacerations, headaches, and dizziness" (MCN, 2008, p. 2). Lack of continuity of care and good record keeping often leads the children to being both over- and underimmunized.

Because of the lack of access to health care and health care information, migrant women may not receive prenatal care. One study found that only 42% of farmworker women reported accessing prenatal services early in their pregnancy (first 3 months) compared with 76% nationally (Rosenbaum and Shin,

2005). The Pregnancy Nutrition Surveillance System found that more than 50% of migrant women had less than the recommended weight gain throughout their pregnancies and almost 25% had undesirable birth outcomes, such as low-birth-weight, preterm births, and small-for-gestational-age babies (CDC, 1998). Unfortunately, current data on migrant women are not available from updated reports from the Pregnancy Nutrition Surveillance. Loss of Medicaid coverage for prenatal care for migrant women and lack of state coverage through the Children's Health Insurance Program (CHIP) in Nebraska has resulted in late entry to prenatal care and an increase in pregnancy complications such as fetal abnormalities (Hopewell, 2011). Study findings related to pesticide exposures and pregnancy outcomes have been inconsistent. One study in North Carolina found that if pregnant women were exposed to pesticides, their newborns' risks for various severe physical and neurological developmental abnormalities were increased (Chelminski et al, 2004).

Food insecurity is a more prevalent problem for farmworkers than for the general U.S. population (Cason et al, 2004; Quandt et al, 2004). In Texas and New Mexico, 82% of farmworker families were found to have experienced food insecurity, of which 49% experienced hunger (Weigel et al, 2007). In Georgia, 63% of migrant farmworkers surveyed were found to be food insecure, with 58% of those being hungry (Hill et al, 2011). The risk for workers with children was three times higher than those without children. Lack of transportation, and lack of access to a refrigerator and stove also were risk factors for food insecurity. Quandt and colleagues (2004) found that households with children had a higher prevalence of food hunger and used strategies such as borrowing money, reducing food variety, giving food to children first, and consuming less to cope with not having enough food.

## Specific Health Problems

Among the Latino population in the United States, the prevalence of diabetes is estimated to be three to five times greater than that of the general population, with higher rates of end-stage complications. In 2000, 2 million people, or 10% of Latinos (including farmworkers), were diagnosed with diabetes (Heuer et al, 2004). Data from the NCFH report from the Health Center Program (2014) showed that migrant and seasonal farmworkers had a slightly higher rate of diabetes than nonagricultural patients. The lifestyle of migrant farmworkers makes it difficult to obtain proper nutrition, adhere to weight control measures, and procure continuity of health care and medication administration necessary for good diabetes control. Migrant health centers participating in the Bureau of Primary Health Care's Diabetes Collaborative provide comprehensive and continuous diabetes care and monitoring for their clients. The MCN Health Net allows providers to access information from any of the farmworkers' previous providers who participated in the tracking program, thereby allowing for better continuity of care for diabetes (Box 34-2 provides a brief example of an assessment with migrant farmworkers).

Dental disease is one of the most common health problems for farmworkers of all ages. According to the Centers for Disease

> **BOX 34-2 Example of Assessment with Migrant Farmworkers**
>
> The nurse, working with community partners and migrant camp gatekeepers, visits migrant camps to screen for diabetes (secondary prevention). If a high glucose level is obtained, the nurse refers the individual to a migrant health center or county health department clinic for a complete assessment. For those individuals in a given camp diagnosed with diabetes, the nurse plans and executes a culturally appropriate educational program on self-care for diabetes (tertiary prevention).

Control and Prevention (2013b), Mexican Americans experience higher rates of tooth decay and periodontal disease than do non-Hispanic whites. Disparities in oral health have been documented with the migrant farmworker population (Finlayson et al, 2010). Migrant children also have significantly higher rates of tooth decay and lower rates of treatment (Quandt et al, 2007). Quandt and colleagues (2007) found that 80% of farmworkers in North Carolina had not received dental care in the last year, and that the few who did receive care returned to Mexico for dental care. Many of the people surveyed had inadequate knowledge of oral health and lack of access to care (and the resources to pay). Funding for increasing access to dental care has been insufficient to meet the needs of this population. Without insurance or personal resources and low Medicaid reimbursement, private dentistry is usually not an option for the farmworker. Those migrant health centers with dental care have a high rate of use (NCFH, 2013a), with visits for dental services accounting for one-third of all visits to migrant health centers.

Depression and stress are areas of concern for adult migrants, and this may be related to isolation, economic hardship, their legal status, poor living conditions, and weather conditions that interrupt their work (MCN, 2008). Hiott and colleagues (2008) found that 38% of farmworkers report significant stress. MSFWs identify themselves as highly stressed even though they rate their physical health as good or excellent (Kim-Godwin and Bechtel, 2004). Weigel and colleagues (2007) found that 41% of farmworkers along the United States–Mexico border reported *nervios* (a term used by some Western Hemisphere Hispanics to refer to increased susceptibility to mental stress and symptoms of nervousness), 37% reported depression, and 17% reported heart palpitations that were attributed to anxiety. In North Carolina, 28% of farmworkers surveyed reported higher levels of depressive symptoms (Sandberg et al, 2012). Hovey and Magana (2002) found that migrant women reported significantly more anxiety than migrant men and were at greater risk for anxiety from working all day, cooking, cleaning, taking care of children, experiencing sexual harassment, and seldom receiving maternity leave and prenatal care. Farmworkers, especially males, are reluctant to seek mental health care.

Female farmworkers, especially the undocumented, are a vulnerable population suffering harassment and sexual abuse. According to a report by Human Rights Watch (2012), harassment and sexual abuse are so common that female farmworkers see no escape from its occurrence and believe it is part of the job. The report identified sexually charged language, unwanted touching, stalking, and rape as common occurrences. Most victims do not report these abuses, often feeling powerless; however, many who have reported have not seen their perpetrators prosecuted (Yeung and Rubenstein, 2013). Recently, the U.S. Equal Employment Opportunity Commission filed lawsuits against employers in the Northwest as a means to address sexual harassment.

Drug and alcohol use in migrant communities also has been identified as a significant source of stress (Kim-Godwin and Bechtel, 2004), without a clear picture of the scope of the problem in migrant farmworker communities. One study in North Carolina showed variation in drinking pattern, with 26% of the farmworkers surveyed abstaining from drinking and 27% reporting heavy drinking (Grzywacz et al, 2007). Drinking alcohol poses safety hazards for farmworkers, such as accidents while driving and workplace injuries. Alcohol can also contribute to health problems, greater risk for HIV infection, violence in camps/home sites, domestic violence, and decreased funds for personal and family needs.

The incidence rate for tuberculosis is not known for migrant farmworkers; however, foreign-born immigrants had a rate of 15.8 per 100,000 in 2012, or 11.5 times higher than among native-born individuals (CDC, 2013a). Hispanics of any race had a 6.6 times higher incidence. The majority of migrant farmworkers are foreign-born and Hispanic. MSFWs are at increased risk for TB because of higher rates in their countries of origin (Latin America, Haiti, and Southeast Asia), crowded housing, and malnutrition (NCFH, 2013b). Indigenous farmworkers from southern Mexico and Central America are especially at higher risk (Lowther et al, 2011). Malnutrition and diabetes may affect tuberculosis status. Required long-term treatment is difficult to complete because of mobility, fear of deportation, language barriers, and lack of access to services. Incomplete treatment contributes to resistant TB. The MCN's Health Net TB tracking program fosters continuity and monitoring of TB treatment as migrant farmworkers move to different work and home sites.

Accurate HIV data for migrant farmworkers is difficult to obtain; however, results from relevant studies show that HIV is a health concern for migrant farmworkers. HIV rates increased by almost 8% along the United States–Mexico border from 2003 to 2006 (Espinoza et al, 2009). According to the NCFH report on data from Health Center Programs (2014), migrant/seasonal farmworkers had a slightly lower diagnosis rate of HIV than did nonagricultural workers. Risk factors for this population include lack of accurate knowledge, barriers to health care services, limited education, poverty, sharing needles for common medications such as vitamins and antibiotics, unprotected sexual activity, isolation and separation from families, available prostitution, migration across borders that results in the spread of HIV (NCFH, 2011), and needle-sharing through amateur tattooing (Smith et al, 2009). Beliefs regarding AIDS/HIV also play a role in lack of preventive behaviors. Sanchez and colleagues (2004) found that misconceptions existed, such as HIV no longer being a serious problem in the United States, that it only affects homosexuals, that one does not need to be tested if the person looks healthy, and that HIV is curable. Farmworkers

reported that sexual issues are taboo and not discussed and that married men can have multiple partners (Washington Association of Community and Migrant Health Centers, 2003). Apostolopoulos and colleagues (2006) stated that successful prevention efforts should include reducing migrants' social isolation and using their social networks while educating on condom use and increasing HIV awareness and testing.

Although there is no clear picture on the health status of the migrant farmworker population, available data indicate that this population suffers from challenging health problems that are difficult to address. Nurses can play a vital role in changing this situation.

## CHILDREN AND YOUTH

Migrant farmworker parents want a better future for their children. In fact, this strong desire was the catalyst for many farmworkers to leave their country of origin. These children often appear to the outsider as happy, outgoing, and inquisitive. However, these children suffer from health problems including malnutrition (vitamin A and iron deficiencies), infectious diseases (upper respiratory tract infection, gastroenteritis), dental caries (from prolonged bottle-feeding, bottle-propping, and limited access to fluoride and dental care), inadequate immunization status, pesticide exposure, injuries, overcrowding and poor housing conditions, and disruption of their social and school life, which, not surprisingly, lead to anxiety-related problems. A study of migrant farmworker children in Georgia from 2003 to 2011 found elevated prevalences of obesity, high blood pressure, stunting, and anemia in older children (Nichols et al, 2014). Children living with at least one undocumented parent experience worse health and less access to care and use of public assistance programs (Yoshikawa and Kalil, 2011). See Figure 34-2.

Children may be separated from their farmworker parents for periods of time when parents leave for work away from the home site. Children experiencing their parents' stress with work, housing, and income when they accompany their parents can result in physical, behavioral, and emotional problems. A clear understanding of these children's health and social status is lacking because of their absence in research and epidemiologic studies.

Ziol-Guest and Kalil (2012) found that being uninsured is more likely in families that are undocumented and permanent resident immigrants. Because of this limited health insurance, it is no surprise that many farmworker children have unmet health needs, those children who sought health care did not have a consistent provider, and children were not on a well-child schedule (Gentry et al, 2007). Moving between states and/or being undocumented can affect migrant children's eligibility for Medicaid and the state Children's Health Insurance Program (CHIP).

Migrant adolescents who work in agriculture warrant attention. Although the exact number of youth who work in the fields is not known, the Centers for Disease Control and Prevention estimated that 230,000 youth were employed on U.S. farms in 2008. It is estimated that about 6% of all farmworkers are

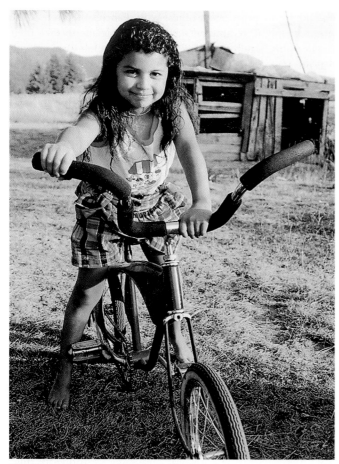

FIG 34-2 Children of migrant farmworkers experience many hardships. They may have to help with the agricultural work while trying to maintain their schoolwork and to fit into two different cultures. These can be difficult efforts, especially if the children have to move a lot or are frequently sick.

between the ages of 14 and 17 years and that many of those children work "off the books" and cannot be documented as workers (NCFH, 2012c). Some adolescents accompany their parents to work or come with others such as an uncle; however, many adolescents come alone. These youth are the most vulnerable to low wages, lack of health insurance or disability insurance, lack of education, social isolation, occupational hazards, and substance abuse and HIV exposure. Cooper and colleagues (2005) found that migrant youth were more likely to have been injured while working. Migrant adolescents have reported increasing substance use (Cooper et al, 2005). Salazar and colleagues (2004) found that migrant adolescents believe that "weak" individuals were the most vulnerable to health problems and that being sick is an inevitable outcome of migrant lifestyle. Health care providers may believe that they are prohibited from caring for minor unaccompanied youth; however, they should be aware of their state's laws on minors' consent to care that could increase access to care for these youth. The 1938 Child Labor Act does not protect farmworker children. Children as young as 12 can work in the fields if they have parental permission. Children ages 16 and older may work in any farm job at any time, including performing hazardous work.

Children of migrant farmworkers may need to work for the family's economic survival. The number of migrant farmworker children under age 14 is unknown. According to the Fair Labor Standards Act, the minimum age at which a child can work in agriculture is 14 years, whereas the age is 16 in other industries. Children 12 to 13 years of age can work on a farm with the parents' consent or if the parent works on the same farm. Children younger than 12 years can work on a farm with fewer than seven full-time workers. Some additional protection is provided to children by the majority of states, such as limiting the number of hours per day and week a child can work.

Federal law does not protect children from overworking or from the time of day they work outside of school. Therefore, children may work until late in the evenings or very early in the mornings every day of the week if not protected by state law or if inadequately monitored. Personal communication with Marie Napolitano and adolescent farmworkers in Oregon revealed that they were frequently too tired after working to do homework and to attend classes. They leave school before the term ends to travel with their families and they arrive late to start school in the fall. Child farmworkers often attend three to five different schools each year as they migrate from one farm to another farm, and these frequent changes in schools and constant fatigue set these children up for failure.

Some children of migrant farmworkers stay home to care for younger children. Girls 8 to 10 years old may remain at the camp site to care for their siblings and other children. The Migrant Head Start Program is a safe, healthy, and educative option for children 6 weeks to 5 years old. However, inadequate funding means there are not enough services for all migrant children. The Migrant Education Program is a state and nationally sponsored summer school program for farmworkers' children more than 5 years of age. However, this program is not available to all eligible migrant youth, especially those living in isolated rural areas.

Nurses can play an important role in the lives of migrant children, as portrayed by migrant children in southern Georgia. During focus groups, these children talked about the importance of nurses in their health and health care (Wilson et al, 2000). For example, one child said, "The nurses teach you how to stay healthy, like good things to eat, how to stay safe, and how to learn in school" (Wilson et al, 2000, p. 143). Another child said, "The nurse also told us how to stay safe in our neighborhood, like staying away from people who drink and take drugs" (Wilson et al, 2000, p. 143).

## CULTURAL CONSIDERATIONS IN MIGRANT HEALTH CARE

To provide culturally effective care to migrant farmworkers, nurses need to be knowledgeable about the cultural backgrounds of these individuals. Because the majority of migrant farmworkers are of Mexican descent, this section focuses on Mexican culture. Although certain health beliefs and practices have been identified with the Mexican culture, the nurse must remember that beliefs and practices differ between regions and localities of a country, and among individuals. Mexico is a multicultural country; therefore, the cultural backgrounds of Mexican immigrants vary depending on their place of origin. There are many indigenous groups in Mexico that speak their own group dialect. Mexican immigrants may or may not understand or speak Spanish. Mexican immigrants who are less educated, have fewer economic resources, and are from rural areas tend to possess more traditional beliefs and practices.

## Nurse-Client Relationship

The nurse is considered an authority figure who should respect *(respeto)* the individual, be able to relate to the individual *(personalismo)*, and maintain the individual's dignity *(dignidad)*. Mexican individuals prefer polite, nonconfrontational relationships with others *(simpatia)*. At times, because of *simpatia*, individuals and families may appear to understand what is being said to them (by nodding their heads) when in actuality they do not understand. The nurse should take measures to validate the understanding of these individuals. The Mexican individual expects to converse about personal matters (chit-chat) for the first few minutes of an encounter. They expect the nurse not to appear rushed and to be a good listener. Humor is appreciated and touching as a caring gesture is seen as a positive behavior.

Mexican clients may not seek care with health professionals first. Instead they may consult with knowledgeable individuals in their family or community (the popular arena of care) or with folk healers (the traditional arena of care). Examples of the members of the popular arena include the "senora," or wise, older woman living in the community; one's grandmother *(la abuela)*; and the local parish priest. If you work with Latino migrant workers, you may relate better with them if you learn some key Spanish words and phrases.

## Health Values

Family, in general, is a significant component of a Mexican individual's health care and social support system. The female in the household is considered to be the caretaker whereas the male is considered to be the major decision-maker. However, Mexican females in certain families have significant influence over most matters including health decisions. Grandmothers and sisters are highly significant to the wife (female) in the immediate family. They provide advice, care, and support. Not all Mexican immigrants have extended families in the United States. If not present, communication may be maintained with family in Mexico, but a support system for these individuals may be lacking.

Love of their children, rather than concern for their own health, may encourage migrant parents to adopt healthier lifestyles. One example is when the parents of a child with asthma choose to stop smoking. In Oregon, when asked if they protected themselves from pesticide exposure, Mexican migrant parents responded negatively in general. However, they were willing to change their behaviors if, as a result, their children would be protected from pesticides (Napolitano et al, 2002).

The Mexican client may be more willing to follow the advice of another Mexican individual with a similar health problem rather than the advice of the health professional. I found that Mexican women with type 2 diabetes were more willing to ask

and adopt the practices of others with diabetes than follow the nonmeaningful, redundant advice of physicians to take their medications, watch their diet, and exercise. One woman, who was unable to differentiate the symptoms of hyperglycemia and hypoglycemia, would drink a bottle of grape juice when she felt her "sugar high," as was recommended by her neighbor.

Although the majority of Mexican immigrants may identify themselves as Catholics, many Mexican individuals belong to other religious groups. The individual's religion may influence his or her health practices such as birth control; however, the nurse cannot assume that a Catholic, for example, will not use some method of birth control. The Quality and Safety in Nursing Education box provides ways to provide client-centered care.

---

**QSEN FOCUS ON QUALITY AND SAFETY EDUCATION FOR NURSES**

**Targeted Competency: Client-Centered Care**
Recognize the client or designee as the source of control and full partner in providing compassionate and coordinated care (interventions) based on respect for the client's preferences, values, and needs.

Important aspects of client-centered interventions include the following:
**Knowledge:** Discuss principles of effective communication.
**Skills:** Assess own level of communication skill in encounters with clients and families.
**Attitudes:** Value continuous improvement of own communication and conflict resolution skills.

**Client-Centered Care Question**
To provide client-centered care, it is important not only to be able to communicate with the person(s) but also to understand their cultural perspectives that influence their health care practices. If you are caring for clients who live in migrant farmworker camps and you observe that they are allowing their children to work several hours both before and after they go to school, how would you approach the situation?
- Would you begin by speaking with the parents?
- Would you speak with the person who owns or manages the farm?
- What would your approach be to those with whom you speak?
- At what point would you consider involving community resources? If you choose this route, what resources would you consider?

Prepared by Gail Armstrong, PhD(c), DNP, ACNS-BC, CNE, Associate Professor, University of Colorado Denver College of Nursing.

---

## Health Beliefs and Practices

In the Mexican culture, health may be considered a gift from God. Another common perception of health is that a healthy person is one who can continue to work and maintain one's daily activities independent of symptoms or diagnosed diseases. The nurse should understand that a Mexican individual may not return for a clinic appointment because the client was capable of working that day. Mexican immigrants may think illness is a punishment from God and may cite this belief as a rationale for why therapies have not cured them. This more commonly occurs with chronic illnesses. There are four more common folk illnesses that a nurse may encounter with the Mexican client. These are *mal de ojo* (evil eye), *susto* (fright), *empacho* (indigestion), and *caida de mollera* (fallen fontanelle).

Symptoms and treatments may vary depending on the individual's or family's origin in Mexico. Other cultural beliefs related to hot-cold balance, pregnancy, and postpartum behaviors *(cuarentena)* have been documented. When experiencing a folk illness, the traditional Mexican individual would prefer to seek care with a folk healer. The more common healers are the *curanderos, herbalistas,* and *espiritualistas.* The most commonly used herbs are chamomile *(manzanilla)*, peppermint *(yerba buena),* aloe vera, cactus *(nopales),* and epazote.

---

### EVIDENCE-BASED PRACTICE

Guidelines recommend that human papillomavirus (HPV) vaccination be routinely administered to girls aged 11 to 12 years old, with catch-up vaccinations being administered between the ages of 13 and 26 years. There are few studies that have included Latina women, especially those from rural areas in low-income families, which includes migrant farmworkers and their children. Luque and colleagues (2012) conducted a study with Latina farmworkers in Central Florida to identify the barriers and benefits to HPV vaccination for this population. Study results showed barriers included lack of transportation and health insurance, language and cultural practices accessing health care, and lack of knowledge regarding the vaccine's purpose. Misperceptions were identified. The perceived benefits included the worthiness of vaccines in general, improving the health of their children, and enhancing communication with their children.

#### Nurse Use

Nurses have the opportunity to provide education regarding the HPV vaccine to migrant farmworkers as individuals in a health care setting or to groups in community settings. Nurses can design their educational programs to include the farmworkers' beliefs about the benefits of vaccine and the prevention of illness in their children's future lives.

---

## HEALTH PROMOTION AND ILLNESS PREVENTION

The same principles of health promotion and illness prevention apply to migrant farmworkers as to other U.S. populations. However, health promotion and disease prevention may be difficult concepts for migrant workers to embrace because of their beliefs regarding disease causality, their irregular and episodic contact with the health care system, and their lower educational level.

Health promotion begins by asking farmworker families which health topics would be of interest to them and whether they are familiar with the available resources to improve their health. Several migrant health programs have recruited migrant workers to serve as outreach workers and lay camp aides to assist in outreach and health education of the workers. Nurses can be part of the planning and education of health workers for outreach educational programs. Evaluation to determine successful outreach educational methods can be undertaken by nurses. These activities demonstrate the core competencies related to the domain of community dimensions of practice skills for public health nursing (Quad Council, 2011). The skills include recognizing community relationships affecting health, collaborating with community partners to promote the health of the population, using group processes to advance community involvement, identifying community assets and resources, and promoting public health programs.

## ROLE OF THE NURSE

As described next, nurses can use primary, secondary, and tertiary prevention actions to help improve the health of migrant farmworkers. Primary prevention activities include education for the prevention of infectious diseases such as HIV, measures to reduce pesticide exposure, and immunizations in childhood and adulthood. Secondary prevention activities include screening for pesticide exposure, TB skin testing, diabetes screening and monitoring activities, and diagnostic testing done for prenatal care. Tertiary prevention includes rehabilitation for musculoskeletal injury, especially low back pain, and treatments for lead poisoning and anemia.

---

### LEVELS OF PREVENTION

#### *Migrant and Farmworker Health Issues*

**Primary Prevention**
Teach migrant workers how to reduce exposure to pesticides.

**Secondary Prevention**
Conduct screening for diabetes in adult farmworkers and for anemia in children in camps.

**Tertiary Prevention**
Educate migrant families regarding appropriate nutrition for an adult with diabetes or a child with anemia.

---

The health status of all people is a function of their ecology, or all that "touches" them. The nurse keeps a finger on the pulse of the community by remaining active with political and social issues that involve the client. The nurse can be a catalyst for change to assess farmworker needs continually, to direct efforts to obtain needed health care services, and to evaluate the success of those efforts. Acting as a community educator knowledgeable about how to obtain the latest information and resources, the nurse can work to assess the infrastructure and needs of the community. Follow-up on assessments by the nurse is critical. For example, the needs assessment might indicate inadequate child and adult immunizations in the migrant population, which may best be provided in the fields, camps, and schools. The nurse may instigate and lead in the creation of an immunization tracking system to share information with other counties and states as the farmworkers migrate.

Nurses can screen and monitor migrant farmworkers' health. Diseases such as TB, diabetes, and hypertension are often missed in a mobile population without regular access to care. Nurses can create screening programs in migrant camps and other farmworker housing. When problems are identified and treated, nurses can monitor the success of medication regimens, preventive measures, and follow-up with the health care system. The nurse can provide culturally specific health promotion and disease prevention programs and materials, as well as information about any further referral sources. The nurse can teach health promotion strategies to lay health promoters who then will educate the migrant community. Box 34-3 lists selected resources for the nurse working with migrant farmworkers. The Clinical Decision-Making Activities at the end of the chapter explore nurses' roles in various health care delivery settings.

**LINKING CONTENT TO PRACTICE**

In this chapter, an overview of the lifestyle and health status of the migrant farmworker population is presented. The public health nurse plays an important role in improving the health of this population. Core competencies within five of the Quad Council Domains of Public Health Nursing guide the nurse in working with migrant farmworkers. These domains are as follows: (1) Analytic/Assessment Skills, which include identifying, describing and using data obtained from working with migrant individuals, families and groups; (2) Policy Development/Program Planning Skills, which are directed toward knowing and applying policies, laws, and regulations toward the delivery of health programs and the protection of the migrant population; (3) Communication Skills, which

are used to identify health literacy of the migrant farmworker and to communicate in a linguistic and culturally appropriate style; (4) Cultural Competency Skills, which allow the nurse to function in a culturally appropriate manner and to assist the public health organization to become more culturally competent when serving migrant farmworker families; and (5) Community Dimension of Practice Skills, which include use of community resources, establishing linkages between community partners to eliminate redundancy and better serve the migrant population, and maintaining partnerships with migrant leaders and agencies serving this population (Quad Council, 2011).

From Quad Council of Public Health Nursing Competencies, 2003. Available at http://www.sphtc.org/phn_competencies_final_comb.pdf. Accessed March 2010.

---

### BOX 34-3   Resources for the Nurse Working with Migrant Farmworkers

**Films and Videos**
- Edward R. Murrow's *Harvest of Shame:* Access at http://billmoyers.com/2013/07/19/watch-edward-r-murrows-harvest-of-shame/
- Migrant Clinicians Network (MCN) resource database: This comprehensive online database (http://www.migrantclinician.org/resources_intro.html) includes downloadable resources as well as links on a wide variety of primary care issues related to migrant farmworkers. Resources include links to other organizations, client education tools, clinical guidelines, MCN program materials, research guidelines, and others.
- *Un Lugar Seguro para Sus Niños:* Video developed as part of a research project with the Center for Research on Occupational and Environmental Health and Oregon Child Development Coalition (Oregon Migrant Head Start), 1999. (Contact the Oregon Child Development Coalition [phone: 503-570-1110] about availability.)

**Written Materials**
- National Center for Farmworker Health: Monograph Series, Migrant Health Issues
- National Center for Farmworker Health: Factsheets on Migrant Farmworkers
- Fields of Tears: Access at www.economist.com/node/17722932/print

**Organizations**
- Migrant Clinicians Network, Inc.
  1515 Capital of Texas Highway South, Suite 220
  Austin, TX 78746
  (512) 328-7682
  http://www.migrantclinician.org
- National Center for Farmworker Health
  1770 FM 967
  Buda, TX 78610
  http://www.ncfh.org
- Farmworker Justice, Inc
  1010 Vermont Ave NW, Suite 915
  Washington, DC 20005
  (202) 783-2628
  http://www.fwjustice.org

Nurses can be social and **political advocates** for the migrant population. Educating communities about these individuals, collecting necessary data on their lives and health, and communicating with legislators and other policy makers at local, state, and national levels are needed actions that nurses are prepared to undertake.

The health of the MSFW population warrants a variety of actions by nurses. Working with this population can be challenging. Insufficient resources, short-term stays in a community, barriers placed by growers, discrimination, and nonenforced legislation are just some of the obstacles that confront the nurse. However, nurses can make a difference in the health of migrant farmworkers and their families.

 **HEALTHY PEOPLE 2020**

### Selected Objectives for Migrant Farmworker Populations

This box lists selected *Healthy People 2020* objectives that relate to health promotion and disease prevention in migrant farmworkers. They were selected on the basis of occupational, lifestyle, and socioeconomic factors that place migrant farmworkers and their families at unique risk for suboptimal health.

**Environmental Health**
- EH-10: Reduce pesticide exposures that result in visits to a health care facility.
- EH-19: Reduce the proportion of occupied housing units that have moderate or severe physical problems.

**Immunization and Infectious Diseases**
- IID-29: Reduce tuberculosis.
- IID-30: Increase treatment completion rate for all tuberculosis patients who are eligible to complete therapy.

**Maternal, Infant, and Child Health**
- MICH-10: Increase the proportion of pregnant women who receive early and adequate prenatal care.

**Occupational Safety and Health**
- OSH-2: Reduce nonfatal work-related injuries.
- OSH-8: Reduce occupational skin diseases or disorders among full-time workers.

From U.S. Department of Health and Human Services: *Healthy People 2020*. Washington, DC, 2010, Office of Disease Prevention and Health Promotion, U.S. Department of Health and Human Services.

The effectiveness of many existing programs dedicated to all levels of prevention and treatment for farmworkers has not been evaluated (Arcury and Quandt, 2007); therefore, opportunities exist for nurses to lead or participate in evaluation of these programs.

## PRACTICE APPLICATION

Maricela is 15 years old and has accompanied her uncle and male cousin to the camp to cook and clean the cabin for them. She also works in the fields picking crops in season. Maricela traveled the East Coast for 6 months with her uncle and cousin. Maricela is originally from Mexico, and Florida is her home base. One evening after finishing her work, Maricela asks to speak with Joan Lewis, the nurse practitioner whose medical van is parked outside the migrant camp where Maricela lives. She tells the nurse that her stomach has been hurting for a while and asks Ms. Lewis for something to stop the pain. While assessing the complaint, Ms. Lewis asks Maricela what she believes has caused the pain. Maricela is very quiet and barely responds to the nurse. She does not make eye contact with Ms. Lewis. Maricela states that she probably ate something hot that upset her stomach. She seems to be in a great hurry and says she does not want her uncle to know she stopped by the van because he would be angry. Ms. Lewis, who speaks fluent Spanish, completes her history but Maricela does not permit the nurse to examine her abdomen. Maricela also would not talk about her last menstrual period. She asks for medicine again and gets up to leave.

A. What do you see as the important points regarding Maricela's situation?

B. What are cultural considerations that may impact the assessment of Maricela's complaint?

C. What could be the possible causes for Maricela's stomach pain? What is your rationale for each cause?

**Answers can be found on the Evolve website.**

## KEY POINTS

- A migrant farmworker is a laborer whose principal employment involves moving from a home base to another location to plant or harvest agricultural products and lives in temporary housing.
- An estimated 1 to 3 million migrant farmworkers are in the United States. These numbers are controversial because of the inconsistency in defining farmworkers and limitations in obtaining data.
- Migrant farmworkers are considered a vulnerable population because of their lifestyle and lack of resources.
- Health problems of migrant farmworkers are linked to their work and housing environments, limited access to health services and education, and lack of economic opportunities.

- Migrant farmworkers are faced with uncertainty regarding work and housing, inadequate wages, unsafe working conditions, and lack of enforcement regarding legislation for field sanitation and safety regulations.
- Farmworkers are exposed not only to the immediate effects in the fields (foggy or wet with pesticides), but also to unknown long-term effects of chronic exposure to pesticides.
- When harvesting is completed, the farmworker becomes simultaneously homeless and unemployed. Forced migration to find employment leaves little time or energy to seek out and improve living standards.
- Children of migrant farmworkers may need to work for the family's economic survival. They are most affected by the disruptive and challenging lifestyle.

## CLINICAL DECISION-MAKING ACTIVITIES

1. Interview rural community leaders regarding migrant farmworkers in your area. What do business owners, teachers, clergy, politicians, and other health professionals say about this population? Can you identify misinformation or lack of information on their parts?

2. Outreach workers are personnel generally hired by an agency, such as a health department, to provide services such as education to migrant persons. Lay health promoters, often past migrants themselves, also provide community-based education. Find out if these roles exist in your community. Interview these individuals or accompany them in their work. Compare and contrast their roles. How are they complementary? How do they overlap? How can they work together to maximize health? How are their approaches to education different (e.g., does one use a protocol or template, whereas the other uses popular education techniques)? How does the outreach worker role and the lay health promoter role compare with the nursing role? How can the nurse work with the outreach worker and the lay health promoter?

3. Find an agency that visits migrant farmworkers in their housing. Ask to accompany them on subsequent visits. What is the condition of the housing? Are there deficits that could impact the health of the inhabitants?

4. Determine eligibility for Medicaid and Aid to Families with Dependent Children services in your state. You may consult the county health department and the state health department. Do migrant workers in your state qualify?

5. Design a temporary clinic to provide health care to migrant workers in your area during crop season. What services would you provide? What hours would you operate? How would you staff the clinic? Where would you get funds?

6. Below are a few settings and RN-delivered services for migrant clients. Can you propose others?
   a. Health department (generally state and county funded)—Nurses monitor communicable diseases and provide treatments for communicable outbreaks such as TB and pertussis.

## CLINICAL DECISION-MAKING ACTIVITIES—cont'd

b. Migrant camps (generally funded through migrant clinics or health departments)—Nurses assess and triage, screen for disease, dispense medications under protocol, provide education, interview families, and coordinate care in conjunction with health department nurses.

c. Migrant clinics (federally funded)—Nurses work with clinics' primary care providers, lead prenatal (both classes and home visits) and diabetes programs, educate regarding illnesses, and visit migrant camps to provide services or follow-up on clinic care.

## REFERENCES

Anthony M, Martin E, Avery A, et al: Self care and health-seeking behavior of migrant farm workers. *J Immigr Minor Health* 12:634–639, 2010.

Apostolopoulos Y, Sonmez S, Kronefeld J, et al: STI/HIV risks for Mexican migrant laborers: exploratory ethnographies. *J Immigr Minor Health* 8:291–302, 2006.

Arcury TA, Quandt SA: Delivery of health services to migrant and seasonal farmworkers. *Annu Rev Public Health* 28:345–363, 2007.

Arcury TA, Quandt SA: Pesticide exposure among farmworkers and their families in the Eastern United States: matters of social and environmental justice. In Arcury TA, Quandt SA, editors: *Latino Farmworkers in the Eastern United States: Health, Safety and Justice.* New York, 2009, Springer.

Ayala M, Clarke M, Kambara K, et al: *In Their Own Words: Farmworker Access to Health Care in Four California Regions.* Davis, CA, 2001, California Institute for Rural Studies.

Bureau of Labor Statistics: *U.S. Department of Labor news release*, October 25, 2012, Retrieved February 2015 from www.bls.gov/news.release/pdf/osh.pdf.

Calvert GM, Karnik J, Mekler LN, et al: Acute pesticide poisoning among agricultural workers in the United States 1998-2005. *Am J Ind Med* 51:883–898, 2008.

Carroll D, Georges A, Saltz R: *Changing Characteristics of U.S. Farm Workers: 21 Years of Findings from the National Agricultural Workers Survey* [presentation to the Immigration Reform and Agriculture Conference: Implications for Farmers, Farm Workers, and Communities. University of California Washington Center, Washington, D.C., May 12, 2011]. Retrieved February 2015 from: http://migrationfiles.ucdavis.edu/uploads/cf/files/2011-may/carroll-changing-characteristics.pdf.

Cason K, Snyder A, Jensen L: *The Health and Nutrition of Hispanic Migrant and Seasonal Farm Workers.* Harrisburg, PA, 2004, Center for Rural Pennsylvania.

Centers for Disease Control and Prevention (CDC): *Pregnancy-Related Behaviors among Migrant Farm Workers—Four States, 1989-1993.* 1998. Retrieved February 2015 from http://www.cdc.gov/mmwr/preview/mmwrhtml/00047114.htm.

Centers for Disease Control and Prevention (CDC): Heat-related deaths among crop workers—United States, 1992-2006. *MMWR Morb Mortal Wkly Rep* 57:649–653, 2008.

Centers for Disease Control and Prevention (CDC): Trends in tuberculosis—United States, 2012. *MMWR Morb Mortal Wkly Rep* 62:201–205, 2013a.

Centers for Disease Control and Prevention (CDC): *Disparities in Oral Health.* 2013b. Retrieved February 2015 from http://www.cdc.gov/OralHealth/oral_health_disparities/.

Chelminski AN, Higgins S, Meyer R, et al: *Assessment of Material Occupational Pesticide Exposures during Pregnancy and Three Children with Birth Defects: North Carolina.* Raleigh, NC, 2004, North Carolina Health and Human Services Department.

Clawson H, Dutch N, Williamson E: *National Symposium on the Health Needs of Human Trafficking Victims* [background brief]. Washington, DC, 2009, U.S. Department of Health and Human Services, Office of the Assistant Secretary for Planning and Evaluation.

Cooper SP, Weller NF, Fox EE, et al: Comparative description of migrant farmworkers versus other students attending rural south Texas schools: substance use, work and injuries. *J Rural Health* 21:362–366, 2005.

Cooper SP, Burau K, Frankowski R, et al: A cohort study of injuries in migrant farm worker families in south Texas. *Ann Epidemiol* 16:313–320, 2006.

Culp K, Umbarger M: Seasonal and migrant agricultural workers: a neglected work force. *AAOHN J* 52:383–390, 2004.

Espinoza H, Hall H, Hu X: *Increases in HIV Diagnosis at U.S.-Mexico Border, 2003-2006,* Official Publication of The International Society for AIDS Education: 21(5 Suppl):19–33, 2009.

Farmworker Justice: *U.S. Labor Law for Farmworkers.* 2014. Retrieved February 2015 from www.farmworkerjustice.org/advocacy-and-programs/US-labor-law-farmworkers.

Feldman SR, Vallejos QM, Quandt SA, et al: Health care utilization among migrant Latino farmworkers: the case of skin disease. *J Rural Health* 25:98–103, 2009.

Finlayson T, Gansky S, Shain S, et al: Dental utilization among Hispanic adults in agricultural worker families in California's Central Valley. *J Public Health Dent* 70:292–299, 2010.

Flocks J, Monaghan P, Albrecht S, et al: Florida farmworkers perceptions and lay knowledge of occupational pesticides. *J Community Health* 32:181–194, 2007.

Gentry K, Quandt SA, Davis SW, et al: Child healthcare in two farmworker populations. *J Community Health* 32:419–431, 2007.

Goldman L, Eskenazi B, Bradman A, et al: Risk behaviors for pesticide exposure among pregnant women living in farm worker households in Salinas, California. *Am J Ind Med* 45:491–499, 2004.

Grzywacz J, Quandt S, Isom S, et al: Alcohol use among immigrant Latino farmworkers in North Carolina. *Am J Ind Med* 50:617–625, 2007.

Health Resources and Services Administration (HRSA): *2012 Health Center Data* [Primary Care: The Health Center Program], 2012. Retrieved February 2015 from http://bphc.hrsa.gov/uds/datacenter.aspx?year=2012.

Heuer L, Hess C, Klug M: Meeting the health care needs of a rural Hispanic migrant population with diabetes. *J Rural Health* 20:265–270, 2004.

Hill B, Moloney A, Mize T, et al: Prevalence and predictors of food insecurity in migrant farmworkers in Georgia. *Am J Public Health* 101:831–833, 2011.

Hiott AE, Grzywacz JG, Davis SW, et al: Migrant farmworker stress: mental health implications. *J Rural Health* 24:32–39, 2008.

Hoerster K, Mayr J, Gabbard S, et al: Impact of individual-, environmental-, and policy-level factors on health care utilization among U.S. farmworkers. *Am J Public Health* 101:685–692, 2011.

Hopewell J: Access to prenatal care: the case of Nebraska. *MCN Streamline* 17:2–5, 2011.

Hovey J, Magana C: Cognitive, affective, and psychological expressions of anxiety symptomatology among Mexican migrant farmworkers: predictors and generational differences. *Community Ment Health J* 38:223–237, 2002.

Human Rights Center, Free the Slaves: *Hidden Slaves—Forced Labor in the United States.* Berkeley, CA, 2004, Human Rights Center, University of California, and Washington, D.C., Free the Slaves. From: https://www.law.berkeley.edu/files/hiddenslaves_report.pdf. Retrieved February 2015.

Human Rights Watch: *Cultivating Fear: The Vulnerability of Immigrant Farmworkers in the U.S. to Sexual Violence and Sexual Harassment.* 2012. Retrieved February 2015 from http://www.hrw.org/sites/default/files/reports/us0512ForUpload_1.pdf.

Kim-Godwin Y, Bechtel G: Stress among migrant and seasonal farmworkers in rural southeast North Carolina. *J Rural Health* 20:271–278, 2004.

Larson A: *Environmental/Occupational Safety and Health, Migrant Health Issues—Monograph Series.* 2001. National Center for Farmworker Health. From: http://www.ncfh.org/docs/02%20-%20environment.pdf. Retrieved February 2015.

Levesque DL, Arif A, Shen J, et al: Effectiveness of pesticide safety training and knowledge about pesticide exposure among Hispanic farmworkers. *J Occup Environ Med* 54:1550–1556, 2012.

Lowther S, Miramontes R, Navara B, et al: *Outbreak of Tuberculosis among Guatemalan Immigrants in Rural Minnesota in 2008* [Public Health Reports], 2011. Retrieved February 2015 from

www.ncbi.nlm.nih.gov/
pubmed/21886333.

Luque J, Castañeda H, Tyson D, et al:
Formative research on HPV vaccine
acceptability among Latina
farmworkers. *Health Promot Pract*
13:617–625, 2012.

Migrant Clinicians Network (MCN):
*Migrant Health Issues: High Risk
General Problems.* 2008. Retrieved
February 2015 from http://
www.migrantclinician.org/
migrant_info/health_problems.html.

Migrant Clinicians Network (MCN):
*TBNet: Ensuring Continuity of Care
through Global Trans-border Patient
Navigation.* 2010a. Retrieved
February 2015 from http://
www.migrantclinician.org/files/
TBNet2010.pdf.

Migrant Clinicians Network (MCN):
*The Migrant/Seasonal Farmworker.*
2010b. Retrieved February 2015
from http://www.migrantclinician
.org/issues/migrant-info/migrant
.html

Mills P, Yang R: Breast cancer risk
in Hispanic agricultural workers
in California. *Int J Occup
Environ Health* 11:123–131,
2005.

Mills P, Dodge J, Yang R: Cancer in
migrant and seasonal hired farm
workers. *J Agromedicine*
14:185–191, 2009.

Napolitano M, Philips J, Beltran M: Un
lugar seguro para sus ninos:
development and evaluation of a
pesticide education video. *J Immigr
Health* 4:35–45, 2002.

National Center for Farmworker
Health (NCFH): *Maternal and Child
Health Fact Sheet.* 2009. Retrieved
February 2015 from http://
www.ncfh.org/pdfs/1387.pdf.

National Center for Farmworker
Health (NCFH): *HIV/AIDS
Farmworker Fact Sheet.* 2011.
Retrieved February 2015 from
http://www.ncfh.org/pdfs/2601.pdf.

National Center for Farmworker
Health (NCFH): *Facts about
Farmworkers.* 2012a. Retrieved
February 2015 from http://
www.ncfh.org/pdfs/2k9/8139.pdf.

National Center for Farmworker
Health (NCFH): *Migrant and
Seasonal Farmworker
Demographics Fact Sheet.* 2012b.
Retrieved February 2015 from
http://www.ncfh.org/pdfs/1389.pdf.

National Center for Farmworker
Health (NCFH): *Child Labor.* 2012c.
Retrieved February 2015 from
http://www.ncfh.org/pdfs/4538.pdf.

National Center for Farmworker
Health (NCFH): *Oral Health.* 2013a.
Retrieved February 2015 from
http://www.ncfh.org/pdfs/2822.pdf.

National Center for Farmworker
Health (NCFH): *Tuberculosis.*
2013b. Retrieved February 2015
from http://www.ncfh.org/
pdfs/2654.pdf.

National Center for Farmworker
Health (NCFH): *A Profile of Migrant
Health: An Analysis of the Uniform
Data System, 2010.* 2014.
Retrieved February 2015 from
http://www.ncfh.org/docs/A%20
Profile%20of%20Migrant%20
Health.pdf.

Nichols M, Stein A, Wold J: Health
status of children of migrant
farmworkers: Farm Worker Family
Health Program, Moultrie, Georgia.
*Am J Public Health* 104:365–370,
2014.

Polaris Project for a World without
Slavery: *Human Trafficking
Legislative Issue Brief: Combating
Labor Trafficking.* 2013. Retrieved
February 2015 from http://
www.polarisproject.org/storage/
documents/policy_documents/
Issue_Briefs/Issue_Brief_Labor_
Trafficking_August_2013.pdf.

Quad Council of Public Health Nursing
Organizations: *Competencies for
Public Health Nursing Practice.*
Washington, DC, 2011, ASTDN.

Quandt S, Arcury T, Early J, et al:
Household food security among
migrant and seasonal Latino
farmworkers in North Carolina.
*Public Health Rep* 119:568–576,
2004.

Quandt SA, Hiott AE, Grzywacz JG,
et al: Oral health and quality
of life of migrant and seasonal
farmworkers in the US community/
migrant health centers. *J Agric Saf
Health* 13:45–55, 2007.

Ray D, Richards P: The potential for
toxic effects of chronic, low dose
exposure to organophosphates.
*Toxicol Lett* 120:343–351, 2001.

Richards T: Health implications of
human trafficking. *Nurs Womens
Health* 18:155–162, 2014.

Rosenbaum S, Shin P: *Migrant and
Seasonal Farmworkers: Health
Insurance Coverage and Access to
Care* [issue paper no. 7314].
Washington, DC, 2005, Kaiser
Commission on Medicaid and the
Uninsured. From: http://
hsrc.himmelfarb.gwu.edu/cgi/
viewcontent.cgi?article=1274&
context=sphhs_policy_facpubs.
Retrieved February 2015.

Salazar M, Napolitano M, Scherer J,
et al: Hispanic adolescent
farmworkers' perceptions
associated with pesticide exposure.
*West J Nurs Res* 26:146–166,
2004.

Sanchez M, Lemp G, Magis-Rodriguez
C, et al: The epidemiology of HIV
among Mexican migrants and
recent immigrants in California and
Mexico. *J Acquir Immune Defic
Syndr* S37:S204–S214, 2004.

Sandberg J, Grzywacz J, Talton J,
et al: A cross sectional exploration
of excessive daytime sleepiness,
depression, and musculo skeletal
pain among migrant farmworkers.
*J Agromedicine* 17:70–80, 2012.

Shipp EM, Cooper SP, del Junco DJ,
et al: Chronic back pain and
associated work and non-work
variables among farmworkers from
Starr County, Texas. *J
Agromedicine* 14:22–32, 2009.

Smith S, Acuna J, Feldman S, et al:
Tattooing practices in the migrant
Latino population: risk for blood
borne disease. *Int J Dermatol*
48:1400–1402, 2009.

U.S. Department of Agriculture (USDA):
*Agricultural Statistics: Annual.*
Washington, DC, 2007, USDA.

U.S. Department of Labor: *Who Are
Migrant and Seasonal
Farmworkers.* 2013. Retrieved
February 2015 from http://
www.doleta.gov/programs/
who_msfw.cfm.

Vallejos Q, Quendt S, Grzywacz J,
et al: Migrant farm workers'
housing conditions across an
agricultural season in North
Carolina. *Am J Ind Med* 54:533–
544, 2011.

Verma A, Schulz MR, Quandt SA,
et al: Eye health and safety
among Latino farmworkers.
*J Agromedicine* 16:143–152,
2011.

Villarejo D: The health of U.S. hired
farm workers. *Annu Rev Public
Health* 24:175–193, 2003.

Villarejo D: *Health Related Inequities
among Hired Farm Workers and
the Resurgence of Labor-Intensive
Agriculture.* Troy, MI, 2012, Kresge
Foundation.

Villarejo D, McCurdy SA: The
California Agricultural Workers
Survey. *J Agric Saf Health*
14:135–146, 2008.

Villarejo D, Lighthall D, Williams D III,
et al: *Suffering in Silence: A Report
on the Health of California's
Agricultural Workers.* Davis, CA,
2000, California Institute for Rural
Studies.

Washington Association of
Community and Migrant Health
Centers: *HIV/AIDS Knowledge and
Prevention Needs Assessment of
Migrant Seasonal Farm Workers.*
2003, p. 11. Retrieved February
2015 from http:www.ncfh.org/?
plugin=ecomm+content=item&
sku=4996.

Weigel MM, Armijos RX, Hall YP,
et al: The household food
insecurity and health outcomes
of U.S.-Mexico border migrant
and seasonal farmworkers.
*J Immigr Minor Health* 9:157–169,
2007.

Whalley LE, Grzywacz JG, Quandt SA,
et al: Migrant farmworker field and
camp safety and sanitation in
eastern North Carolina. *J
Agromedicine* 14:421–436,
2009.

Wilson A, Pittman K, Wold J:
Listening to the quiet voices of
Hispanic migrant children about
health. *J Pediatr Nurs* 15:137–147,
2000.

Yeung B, Rubenstein G; Center for
Investigative Reporting: *Female
Workers Face Rape, Harassment in
U.S. Agricultural Industry.* 2013.
Retrieved February 2015 from
http://cironline.org/reports/
female-workers-face-rape-
harassment-us-agriculture-
industry-4798.

Yoshikawa H, Kalil A: The effects of
parental undocumented states in
the development centers of young
children in immigrant families.
*Child Dev Perspect* 5:291–297,
2011.

Ziol-Guest K, Kalil A: Health and
medical care among the children
of immigrants. *Child Dev* 83:
1494–1500, 2012.

# 35

# Teen Pregnancy

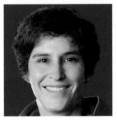

## *Dyan A. Aretakis, RN, FNP, MSN*

Dyan A. Aretakis earned her BSN from the University of Connecticut and the MSN, PNP, and FNP from the University of Virginia. She began her nursing practice in pediatrics at the University of Connecticut and at a regional residential facility for individuals with intellectual developmental disorders. She went on to co-develop a model teen health center at the University of Virginia Health System in 1990 and currently practices in and directs its daily and long-term programs. This unique program provides a range of adolescent and young adult primary health care services as well as community and professional outreach programs.

## ADDITIONAL RESOURCES

ⓔ **Evolve Website http://evolve.elsevier.com/Stanhope**
- *Healthy People 2020*
- WebLinks
- Quiz
- Case Studies
- Glossary
- Answers to Practice Application

## OBJECTIVES

*After reading this chapter, the student should be able to do the following:*

1. Discuss approaches that could be used in providing care to the adolescent client.
2. Identify trends in adolescent pregnancy, births, abortions, and adoption in the United States.
3. Discuss reasons that may affect whether a teenager becomes pregnant.
4. Explain some of the deterrents to the establishment of paternity among young fathers.
5. Develop nursing interventions for the prevention of pregnancy problems that adolescents are at risk for experiencing.
6. Identify nursing activities that may contribute to the prevention of adolescent pregnancy.

## KEY TERMS

abortion services, p. 768
adoption, p. 771
birth control, p. 767
coercive sex, p. 771
dual protection, p. 770
gynecological age, p. 775
intimate partner violence, p. 774
long-acting reversible contraception, p. 770
low birth weight, p. 776
paternity, p. 772

peer pressure, p. 770
prematurity, p. 776
prenatal care, p. 774
repeat pregnancy, p. 776
sexual debut, p. 770
sexual victimization, p. 771
statutory rape, p. 771
weight gain, p. 775
*—See Glossary for definitions*

## CHAPTER OUTLINE

**Adolescent Health Care in the United States**
**The Adolescent Client**
**Trends in Adolescent Sexual Behavior, Pregnancy, and Childbearing**
**Background Factors**
 Sexual Activity and Use of Birth Control

 Peer Pressure and Partner Pressure
 Other Factors
**Young Men and Paternity**
**Early Identification of the Pregnant Teen**
**Special Issues in Caring for the Pregnant Teen**
 Violence

Teen pregnancy is an area of public concern because of its significant effect on communities. Resources to support the special needs of pregnant teenagers are decreasing, and the costs of sustaining young families are prohibitive. Many teenagers who become pregnant are caught in a cycle of poverty, school failure, and limited life options. Even under the ideal circumstances of adequate finances, loving and supportive families, and good birth outcomes, a teen mother must circumvent her own necessary developmental tasks to raise her child.

There is neither a uniform reason that teens become pregnant nor a universally acceptable solution. The causes of teen pregnancy are diverse and affected by changing moral attitudes, sexual codes, and economic circumstances. Teen pregnancy places an enormous strain on the health care and social service systems. Social concern is also raised about the lost potential for young parents when pregnancy occurs, and the academic and economic disadvantages that their children will experience. Nurses are in a key position to understand how teen pregnancy affects both the individual and the community. This chapter presents a variety of issues associated with teen pregnancy and proposes nursing interventions to promote healthy outcomes for individuals and communities.

## ADOLESCENT HEALTH CARE IN THE UNITED STATES

Adolescents are generally healthy, and when they seek health care it is for reasons different from those of adults or young children. The main causes of teen mortality are high-risk behaviors: motor vehicle accidents (usually including alcohol), homicide, suicide, and accidental injuries (such as falls, fires, or drowning). Teens often engage in behaviors that put them at risk for life-threatening diseases. For example, each year, one fourth of both new human immunodeficiency virus (HIV) infections and newly identified sexually transmitted diseases (STDs) occur among adolescents. During the teen years, other behaviors are initiated (e.g., smoking, decreased activity, and poor nutrition) that can ultimately lead to poor health as well as influence behavior change that can significantly alter a young person's life.

National surveys highlight the health issues facing adolescents. There have been some improvements in risk behaviors as well as a worsening of others. Among ninth to twelfth graders participating in the 2013 Youth Risk Behavior Surveillance System, fewer teens reported binge drinking or riding in a car with a driver who had been drinking (Kann et al, 2014).

However, these and other significant risk behaviors continued at high rates. Of ninth to twelfth graders, 38.7% reported current alcohol use (20.8% reported binge drinking); 22.4% of teens were current cigarette smokers; and 40.7% had tried marijuana (23.4% were current users). Mental health issues are also strongly associated with the adolescent years: 29.9% of students reported feeling sad or hopeless for more than 2 weeks; 39.1% of females and 20.8% of males reported these symptoms. Suicidal thoughts with a plan existed for 13.6% of students nationwide, and 10.6% of girls and 5.4% of boys attempted suicide. In addition, 30.3% of students were either obese or overweight, 21% had been told they had asthma, and 10.1% used sunscreen when they were in the sun for more than an hour. It is the collective impact of these behaviors that not only put adolescents at risk during the teenage years but set the stage for adult morbidity and mortality from heart disease, cancer, and diabetes (Centers for Disease Control and Prevention [CDC], 2014.

Adolescents may not seek care for these problems for the following reasons: (1) access to health care may be hindered due to a limited number of professionals with expertise in dealing with teenagers; (2) costs of care or availability of insurance may limit services; (3) adolescents need to believe that their visits are confidential before they will honestly reveal information; and (4) health care professionals must be able to discuss sensitive topics in a nonjudgmental and supportive manner and demonstrate a desire to work with youths. Nurses who want to promote the health of adolescents by providing anticipatory guidance about peer pressure, assertiveness, and future planning need to understand adolescent behaviors, health risks, and the social context in which they live. Involvement and education of the parents about youth culture and development can promote positive and supportive parenting of teens.

## THE ADOLESCENT CLIENT

Adolescents have limited experience in independently seeking health care. When they do seek care, it is often to discuss concerns about a possible pregnancy or to find a birth control method. These teens may also need assistance negotiating complex health care systems. Special approaches in both client interview and subsequent client education are often warranted. The behavior of adolescents toward the nurse can range from mature and competent during one visit to hostile, rude, or distant at other times because behavior often reflects intense anxiety over what the teen is experiencing.

Because client interviews usually begin with evaluation of a chief complaint, teens need to know that their concerns are heard. Health care providers may have their own opinions about what teenagers need and may fail to take the chief complaint seriously. For example, when a teen expresses ambivalence about or a desire to become pregnant, this should be discussed in depth even though the nurse may feel uncomfortable when asked to provide information to a teen about how to conceive. During this interview, the nurse can provide preconception counseling and emphasize the need to achieve good health and to establish a health-promoting lifestyle before pregnancy. Health risks to the mother, as well as to fetal development, can be discussed. The nurse can encourage a young person to consider lifetime goals and discuss how parenthood might affect them. Not only does information presented this way demonstrate that the nurse has heard what the teen is saying, but it also allows the nurse to provide useful health information that may encourage the teen to examine her plans carefully, seriously, and maturely.

It is also important to pay attention to what the teen *fails* to verbalize. Knowledge of adolescent health care issues is valuable so that the nurse can anticipate other health concerns and provide an environment in which the adolescent feels safe about discussing other issues. By creating a caring and understanding atmosphere, the nurse can encourage the young person to discuss concerns about family violence, drugs, alcohol, or dating.

Discussing reproductive health care is a sensitive matter for both teens and many adults. Teens may have difficulty expressing themselves because of a limited sexual vocabulary or embarrassment resulting from their lack of knowledge. The nurse must recognize this potential deficit and embarrassment and assist teens by anticipating concerns. It is also important to allow teens to express themselves in their own language, which may include crude or offensive words. Nurses must learn about common slang expressions and common misconceptions so they do not miss important concerns that a teenager might have. The nurse can offer more appropriate terms once trust is established.

Teens may have difficulty discussing topics that provoke a judgmental reaction, such as discussing STDs (See Box 35-1). The nurse can choose neutral words to evaluate symptoms (e.g., "Has there been a change in your typical vaginal discharge?"). This approach also gives the nurse a chance to educate the young client about normal anatomy and physiology.

Considerable debate exists over whether adolescents should make reproductive health care decisions without their parents' knowledge. As seen in Box 35-2, federal law establishes the adolescent's right for access to contraceptive treatment. Obstacles to services do exist, however, and this may result in a teen not receiving contraceptive information and treatment. Obstacles can include lack of transportation to a health care facility, insufficient money to pay for services, or permission to leave school early to attend an appointment.

Although most minor teens can consent to birth control services in the United States, there is great variability in who may access and release their medical records. In recognition of the importance of confidentiality in reproductive health care, federal

---

> **BOX 35-1    Sexually Transmitted Diseases and Teen Pregnancy**
>
> Sexually transmitted diseases (STDs) affect 25% of sexually experienced teenagers each year. STDs are more easily transmitted to women than men. STD infections among women can contribute to infertility, cancer, and ectopic pregnancy. When a young woman is pregnant, these infections can cause premature rupture of membranes, premature labor, and postpartum infection. Also, the baby can be affected by all STDs in several ways: prematurity and low birth weight, febrile infection after delivery, long-term infection, and even death (e.g., exposure to viral infections such as human papillomavirus and herpes simplex virus).
>
> The pregnant adolescent is at high risk for acquiring an STD because she may not be using barrier protection (e.g., condoms). During the pregnancy, she will require periodic STD screening. STD education and counseling should accompany this screening. Information given should include ways to reduce risk, such as maintaining a mutually monogamous relationship and using latex condoms.

---

> **BOX 35-2    Reproductive Health Care and Adolescents' Rights**
>
> No federal regulation requires a young person to have parents involved in decisions on contraception services provided by federal programs. States cannot prohibit an adolescent access to contraception. Several Supreme Court decisions protect this access:
>
> - 1965: *Griswold v. Connecticut*—the right to prevent pregnancy through the use of contraceptives is protected by the right to privacy.
> - 1972: *Eisenstadt v. Baird*—the right to privacy in contraceptive use is extended to unmarried individuals.
> - 1977: *Carey v. Population Services International*—the right to privacy is specifically extended to minors.

Data from National Abortion and Reproductive Rights Action League Foundation (NARAL): *U.S. Supreme Court Decisions concerning Reproductive Rights: 1927–2012.* Washington, DC, 2014a, NARAL. Retrieved February 2015 from http://www.prochoiceamerica.org/media/fact-sheets/government-federal-courts-scotus-choice-cases.pdf

---

privacy rules were established in 2002 as follow-up to the Health Insurance Portability and Accountability Act of 1996 (HIPAA). This rule, the HIPAA Privacy Rule (or more correctly, the Standards for Privacy of Individually Identifiable Health Information), established that if a minor consented to care, then only that individual could access and release those medical records. However, the Privacy Rule also deferred to existing state law. In many states the laws specify that parents can legally access all the medical records of their minor children (English and Kenney, 2010), which limits the confidentiality assurances offered to a teen seeking reproductive health care. It is incumbent on nurses working with teens to be knowledgeable about state and federal laws so they can accurately inform teenagers of their rights and limitations in seeking reproductive health care.

**Abortion services** for adolescents are not clearly defined. No federal protection is extended to adolescents requesting abortion services, and the adolescent's right to privacy and ability to give consent varies by state (See Box 35-3, which describes abortion and adolescent rights). Confidential care to teenagers may mean the difference in preventing an unwanted pregnancy, an

## BOX 35-3   Abortion and Adolescent Rights

- *Parental consent laws:* One or both parents of a young woman who is under 18 years of age seeking an abortion must give permission to the abortion provider before the abortion is performed. These 25 states have enforceable mandatory consent and notice laws: Alabama, Arkansas, Arizona, California, Idaho, Indiana, Kansas, Kentucky, Louisiana, Maine, Massachusetts, Michigan, Mississippi, Missouri, Montana, Nebraska, New Mexico, North Carolina, North Dakota, Ohio, Pennsylvania, Rhode Island, South Carolina, Tennessee, and Wisconsin.
- *Parental notification laws:* One or both parents of a young woman seeking an abortion must be notified by the abortion provider before the abortion is performed. These laws are in 14 states: Alaska, Colorado, Delaware, Florida, Georgia, Illinois, Iowa, Maryland, Minnesota, Nevada, New Hampshire, New Jersey, South Dakota, and West Virginia.
- *Parental notification and consent laws:* One or both parents of a young woman seeking an abortion must be notified and provide consent before the abortion is performed. These laws are enforced in five states: Oklahoma, Texas, Utah, Virginia, and Wyoming.
- *The following states (11) with parental notification or consent laws permit other trusted adults to stand in for a parent:* Arizona, Colorado, Delaware, Illinois, Iowa, Maine, North Carolina, Pennsylvania, South Carolina, Virginia, and Wisconsin.
- *The following states (four) have laws that have been found unconstitutional and unenforceable:* California, Nevada, New Jersey, and New Mexico.
- *Judicial bypass:* In a 1979 Supreme Court decision, it was ruled that any mandatory parental consent law must allow the young woman an opportunity to be granted an exception or waiver to the law. A young woman could appeal directly to a judge, who would decide either that she was mature enough to make this decision or that the abortion would be in her best interest.

Data from National Abortion and Reproductive Rights Action League Foundation (NARAL): *Who Decides? The Status of Women's Reproductive Rights in the United States,* ed 23. Washington, DC, 2014b, NARAL. Retrieved February 2015 from http://www.prochoice america.org/government-and-you/who-decides/

abortion, and a birth. This care can influence whether prenatal visits begin in the first trimester or in the second or third trimester. Teens have various reasons for pursuing confidential care, including seeking independence as well as serious and well-founded concerns about a parent's potential reaction (e.g., abuse of the teen). Once nurses recognize the reason for confidential care, they can work with teens to discuss reproductive health care needs with the family. To do so, first clarify family values about sexuality and family communication styles with the teen. In a nonhealthy family, referral to community agencies (e.g., child protective services, Al-Anon) may be necessary. However, the nurse may need to honor the adolescent's need for confidentiality for an unknown period and proceed with the usual interventions, such as pregnancy testing, options counseling, and referral for clinical care.

## TRENDS IN ADOLESCENT SEXUAL BEHAVIOR, PREGNANCY, AND CHILDBEARING

In 2012, there were 305,388 births to women under age 20. There was an overall 7% decline from 2011 (8% decline in teens ages 15 to 17; 5% decline in 18- to 19-year-olds). These were the lowest rates since 1945. Of these births, 18.3% were a repeat birth (CDC, 2013). The birth rate in the United States still remains higher than in any other developed nation (Ikramullah et al, 2011). The numbers of teens who become pregnant are generally identified in the following way: by age group (e.g., younger than 15, ages 15-17, ages 18-19, and under age 20), by states, by marital status, by rates (e.g., number of pregnancies, births, and abortions per 1000 young women), and by race/ethnicity (e.g., African American, white, Hispanic/Latino). Births to teenagers make up 11% of all births in the United States (Ikramullah et al, 2011). Teen birth rates increase by age, with the highest rates occurring among 19-year-olds. Pregnancy and birthrates increased steadily among teens of all ages from 1986 to 1991 and declined among teens of all ages and ethnicities from 1991 to 2005. Decreases from 25% to 17% were also noted in the teen repeat birth rate from 1991 to 2012 (CDC, 2013; Ikramullah et al, 2011). Decreases in pregnancy among teens ages 15 to 17 have been attributed to reduced sexual activity (one fourth of the reduction) and the rest result from improved contraceptive use. For teens ages 18 to 19 the reduction is entirely attributed to increased contraceptive use, with evidence showing that the use of long-acting reversible contraceptives tripled among this age group from 2007 to 2009 (Kost and Henshaw, 2014).

Decline in the teen birth rate varies by race, with the highest birth rates among Hispanic teens (46.3 births per 1000), then black teens (43.9 births per 1000) and white teens (20.5 births per 1000) (Office of Adolescent Health, U.S. Department of Health and Human Services [USDHHS], 2015).

In 2010, there were 615,000 pregnancies to American teens between the ages of 15 and 19 years. In this same age group, there were 157,450 abortions. About 5% of all abortions are obtained by minors (Guttmacher Institute, 2014). The reasons most teens give for having an abortion is that they are concerned about how a baby would change their lives. They also say that they do not think they could afford to care for a baby, and they do not feel that they are mature enough to raise a child. A sexually active teen who does not use contraceptives has a 90% chance of becoming pregnant within one year (Guttmacher Institute 2015). Elective abortion rates for teenagers increased from the time of legalization in 1973 until 1988 and then began to decline. This decrease was caused in part by decreases in the pregnancy rate, but may also have resulted from laws that required parental notification or consent for minors requesting abortion services in some states. As of May 2014, laws in 38 states required that minors seeking abortions must have parental involvement in the decision (Guttmacher Institute, 2014).

## BACKGROUND FACTORS

Many adults have difficulty understanding why young people would jeopardize their careers and personal potential by becoming pregnant during the teen years. Adolescents, however, do not view the world in the same way as adults. Teens often feel invincible and therefore do not recognize any risk related to their behaviors or anticipate the consequences. That is, they

their teens may find them more at risk for sexual permissiveness and pregnancy (Bersamin et al, 2008).

## YOUNG MEN AND PATERNITY

Although declines among pregnant female teenagers have been seen over the past 23 years, there are no published data showing the same decline among teen males. About 9% have become fathers before the age of 20. Of this group, two thirds were ages 18 or 19 when they fathered their first child and one third were less than 18 years old. These are conservative numbers because not all teen males are aware that a partner became pregnant nor are they always aware of the outcome of the pregnancy. A review of birth certificate information may not be helpful as many unmarried couples fail to complete the steps required for a father's name to appear. Adolescent males who become fathers are often reported to be second-generation teen parents. Studies demonstrate that they came from poor families, did poorly in school, and engaged in many high-risk behaviors such as gang membership, drugs, and early sexual involvement. These young fathers face special challenges because of concomitant social problems and limited future plans or ability to provide support. There may also be an overlap between young fatherhood and delinquency. Adolescent males who demonstrate law-breaking behaviors, alcohol or substance use, school problems, and aggressive behaviors may have difficulty developing a positive fathering role, yet they are the highest-risk group to become young fathers. Almost half of these teen fathers will go on to father at least one additional child by the age of 22 to 24, sometimes with another mother (9% of the time) (Paschal et al, 2011; Savio Beers and Hollo, 2009).

Paternity, or fatherhood, is legally established at the time of the birth for a teen who is married. However, it is more difficult to establish paternity among nonmarried couples. Some of the difficulty lies in the complexity of the specific state system for young men to acknowledge paternity. In some states, a young man may have to work with the judicial system outside of the hospital after the birth; if he is under age 18, he may need to involve his parents.

Some young couples do not attempt to establish paternity and prefer a verbal promise of assistance for the teen mother and child. Although a verbal commitment may be acceptable when the child is born, the mother may become more inclined to pursue the establishment of paternity later when the relationship ends or for reasons related to financial, social, or emotional needs of the child. Young women who receive state or federal assistance (e.g., Temporary Assistance for Needy Families [TANF], Medicaid) may be asked to name the child's father so the judicial process can be used to establish paternity.

Young men react differently when they learn that their partner is pregnant. The reaction often depends on the nature of the relationship before the pregnancy. Many young men will accompany the young woman to a health care center for pregnancy diagnosis and counseling. A large percentage of young men will continue to accompany the young woman to some prenatal visits and may even attend the delivery. These young men may also want, and need, to be involved with their children

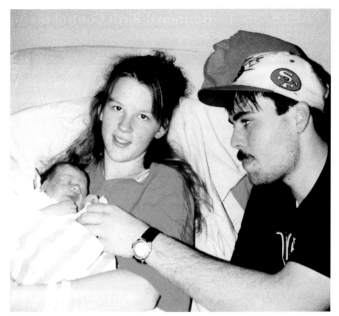

FIG 35-1 It is important to include both the teen mother and the father in teaching about child development.

regardless of changes in their relationships with the teen mother. It is not unusual for a young man to be excluded or even rejected by the young woman's family (usually her mother). He may then begin to act as though he is disinterested when he may really feel that he cannot provide resources for his child or know how to take care of him or her (Savio Beers and Hollo, 2009) (See Figure 35-1).

Nurses can acknowledge and support the young man as he develops in the role of father. His involvement can positively affect his child's development and provide greater personal satisfaction for him and greater role satisfaction for the young mother. Young mothers who report less social support from their baby's father are more apt to be unhappy and distressed in the parenting role and consequently more at risk for abuse of their child (Savio Beers and Hollo, 2009). The immediate concerns revolve around his financial responsibility, living arrangements, relationship issues, school, and work. Establishing an opportunity to meet with the young man and both families is helpful to clarify these issues and identify roles and responsibilities.

Life experiences for a young man will influence behaviors that can lead to a teen pregnancy or prevent a teen pregnancy. Adverse childhood experiences including a history of abuse (especially physical and sexual abuse and domestic violence), mental illness and/or substance abuse in the childhood home, criminal behaviors in the home, and separated parents have been linked to negative behaviors such as early sexual intercourse, multiple partners, and substance use. These behaviors are possible antecedents to male involvement in teen pregnancy (Sipsma et al, 2010).

Age discrepancy between the pregnant teen and her male partner is an important consideration, even when it is 2 years. It raises concern about coercion, potential or actual violence, increased risk for STI, and exposure to greater substance and alcohol use (Volpe et al, 2013). The greatest age discrepancies are seen with the youngest pregnant teens. Although these numbers have decreased, the risk is present with more than half of all females ages 15 and younger reporting first sexual intercourse with a male partner who is more than 3 years older. Protective factors that can reduce the risk of a young teen becoming sexually involved with an older partner include living with both biological parents, greater parental education, and not being born to a teen mother (Child Trends Data Bank, 2013).

## EARLY IDENTIFICATION OF THE PREGNANT TEEN

Some teens delay seeking pregnancy services because they fail to recognize signs such as breast tenderness and a late period, because they are experiencing a variety of other pubertal changes. Most young women, however, suspect pregnancy as soon as a period is late. These young women may still delay seeking care because they falsely hope that the pregnancy will just go away. A teen may also delay seeking care to keep the pregnancy a secret from family members, fearing either an angry or disappointed response or expecting to be forced into a decision that may not be hers.

Nurses must be sensitive to subtle cues that a teenager may offer about sexuality and pregnancy concerns. Such cues include questions about one's fertile period or requests for confirmation that one need not miss a period to be pregnant. Once the nurse identifies the specific concern, information can be provided about how and when to obtain pregnancy testing. The nurse should determine how a teenager would react to the possible pregnancy before completing the test. If the test is negative, the nurse should take the opportunity to assess whether the young woman would consider counseling to prevent pregnancy. A follow-up visit is important after a negative test to determine if retesting is necessary or if another problem exists.

In looking at teen pregnancy from the perspective of levels of prevention, several steps could be taken. These are shown in the Levels of Prevention box.

### LEVELS OF PREVENTION

#### Teen Pregnancy

**Primary Prevention**
Teach young people about sexual practices that will prevent untimely pregnancy.

**Secondary Prevention**
Provide services for early detection of teen pregnancy.

**Tertiary Prevention**
Counsel the young person or young couple about available options, including keeping the baby (and making appropriate plans to care for the child), abortion, and adoption.

A young woman with a positive pregnancy test requires a physical examination and pregnancy counseling. It is advantageous to offer these at the same time so that the counseling is consistent with the findings of the examination. The purpose of the examination is to assess the duration and well-being of the pregnancy, as well as to test for sexually transmitted infection. The pregnancy counseling should include the following: information on adoption, abortion, and child-rearing; an opportunity for assessment of support systems for the young woman; and identification of the immediate concerns she might have (Aruda et al, 2010).

The availability of affordable abortion services up to 13 weeks of gestation varies from community to community. Similarly, second-trimester services may be available locally or involve extensive travel and cost. The nurse should know about abortion services and provide information or refer the pregnant teenager to a pregnancy counseling service that can assist.

The pregnant teenager needs information about adoption, such as current policies among agencies that allow continued contact with the adopting family. Also, church organizations, private attorneys, and social service agencies provide a variety of adoption services with which the nurse should be familiar. Box 35-4 lists guidelines for adoption counseling.

Pregnancy counseling requires that the nurse and young woman explore strengths and weaknesses for personal care and responsibility during pregnancy and parenting. Young women vary in their interest in including the partner or their parents in this discussion. Issues to discuss include education and career plans, family finances and qualifications for outside assistance, and personal values about pregnancy and parenting at this time

### BOX 35-4   Guidelines for Adoption Counseling

1. Assess your own thoughts and feelings on adoption. Do not impose your opinion on the decision-making process of teen mothers.
2. Know about state laws, local resources, and various types of adoption services.
3. Choose language sensitively. Examples follow:
   a. Avoid saying "giving away a child" or "putting up for adoption." It is more appropriate and positive to say "releasing a child for adoption," "placing for adoption," or "making an adoption plan."
   b. Avoid saying "unwanted child" or "unwanted pregnancy." A more appropriate term may be *unplanned pregnancy*.
   c. Avoid saying "natural parents" or "natural child," because the adopted parents would then seem to be "unnatural." The terms *biological parents* and *adoptive parents* are more appropriate.
4. Assess when a discussion of adoption is appropriate. It can be helpful to begin with information on adoption and then explore feelings and concerns over time. Individuals will vary in how much they may have already considered adoption, and this will influence the counseling session.
5. Assess the relationship between the pregnant teen and her partner and what role she expects him to play. Discuss the reality of this.
6. It may be helpful for a pregnant teen to talk with other teens who have been pregnant, are raising a child, have released a child for adoption, or have been adopted themselves.
7. A young woman can be encouraged to begin writing letters to her baby. These can be saved or given to the child when released to the adoptive family.

Modified from Brandsen CK: *A case for adoption*, Grand Rapids, MI, 1991, Bethany.

in their life. Often it is difficult to focus on counseling in any depth at the time of the initial pregnancy testing results. A follow-up visit is usually more productive and should be arranged as soon as possible.

As decisions are made about the course of the pregnancy, the nurse can make referrals to appropriate programs such as WIC (a supplemental food program for women, infants, and children), Medicaid, and prenatal services. The young woman and her family also need to know about expected costs of care and, if there is a family insurance policy, whether it will cover the pregnancy-related expenses of a dependent child. For those without insurance, the family can apply for Medicaid or determine whether local facilities offer indigent care programs (e.g., Hill-Burton programs for assistance with hospital expenses). The nurse can also begin prenatal education and counseling on nutrition, substance abuse and use, exercise, and special medical concerns.

## SPECIAL ISSUES IN CARING FOR THE PREGNANT TEEN

Pregnant teenagers are considered high-risk obstetric clients. Many of the complications of their pregnancy result from poverty, late entry into prenatal care, and limited knowledge about self-care during pregnancy. Nursing interventions through education and early identification of problems may dramatically alter the course of the pregnancy and the birth outcome.

### Violence

Teens are more likely to experience violence during their pregnancies than adult women. Age may be a factor in their greater vulnerability to potential perpetrators that include partners, family members, and other acquaintances. Violence in pregnancy has been associated with an increased risk for substance abuse, poor compliance with prenatal care, and poor birth outcome. In the case of partner violence, young women may be protective of their partners because of fear or helplessness. Eliciting this history from an adolescent is not easy. Be sure to inquire about violence at every visit. Frequent routine assessments are more revealing than a single inquiry at the first prenatal visit. Research has demonstrated that 6% to 55% of pregnant or parenting adolescents reported violence, a rate greater than that reported by adult women (Herrman, 2013). Violence that began during the pregnancy may continue for several years after, with increasing severity. Variations by ethnicity have also been observed during this postpartum period; intimate partner violence may peak at 3 months postpartum among African American and Hispanic/Latino new mothers and at 18 months for white mothers (Harrykissoon et al, 2002). The nurse must observe for physical signs of abuse, as well as for controlling or intrusive partner behavior (Giullery et al, 2012).

### Initiation of Prenatal Care

Pregnant adolescents differ remarkably from pregnant adults in initiation and compliance with prenatal care. Inadequate prenatal care has been associated with increased health risks to both the mother and the fetus. In 2003, 6.4% of pregnant 15- to 19-year-olds received late or no prenatal care (Neinstein, 2008). Teens report that the greatest barrier to care is real or perceived cost. Other barriers include denial of the pregnancy, fear of telling parents, transportation, dislike of providers' care, and offensive attitudes among clinic staff toward pregnant teens (Neinstein, 2008; Aruda et al, 2010).

Once a teen is enrolled in prenatal care, the nurse becomes an important liaison between personnel at the clinical site and the young woman. Confusion and misunderstandings occur easily when teens do not understand what a health care provider says to them. Often these misunderstandings are based on lack of knowledge about basic anatomy and physiology. For example, a teen may be told as she gets close to term that the head of the baby is down and it can be felt. This is an alarming piece of information for a young woman who imagines the entire baby could just pop out at any time!

Cooperation between the nurse and the clinical staff can also maximize the client's compliance with special health or nutritional needs. For example, a teen who has premature contractions may be restricted to bed rest and instructed to increase fluids. The nurse who makes home visits can provide additional assessment of the teen's condition and can solve problems about self-care, hygiene, meals, and schooling.

### Low-Birth-Weight Infants and Preterm Delivery

Teens are more likely than adult women to deliver infants weighing less than 5.5 lb or to deliver before 37 weeks of gestation. These low-birth-weight and premature infants are at greater risk for death in the first year of life and are at increased risk for long-term physical, emotional, and cognitive problems (Neinstein, 2008). For example, low-birth-weight and premature infants can be more difficult to feed and soothe. This challenges the limited skills of the young mother and can further strain relations with other members of the household, who may not know how to offer support or assistance.

The risk for low-birth-weight infants and premature births can be averted by the teen's early initiation into prenatal care. Although such births still occur, it is important to work closely with the teen mother as soon as she is identified as pregnant to try to promote compliance with prenatal care visits and self-care during the pregnancy. After the pregnancy, these infants and their mothers will benefit from frequent nursing supervision to ensure that their care is appropriate and that everyone in the home is coping adequately with the strain of a small infant.

### Nutrition

The nutritional needs of a pregnant teenager are especially important. First, the teen lifestyle does not lend itself to overall good nutrition. Fast foods, frequent snacking, and hectic social schedules limit nutritious food choices. Snacks, which account for approximately one third of a teen's daily caloric intake, tend to be high in fat, sugar, and sodium and limited in essential vitamins and minerals. Second, the nutritive needs of both pregnancy and the concurrent adolescent growth spurt require the adolescent to change her diet substantially. The growing teen must increase caloric nutrients to meet individual growth needs as well as to

## TABLE 35-2 Adolescent Nutritional Needs during Pregnancy

| Nutrient | Daily Requirement during Pregnancy* | Food Source |
|---|---|---|
| Calcium | 1300 mg (decrease to 1000 mg for 19-year-olds) | Macaroni and cheese; pizza; puddings, milk, yogurt; also fortified juices, water, breakfast bars and fast foods, including Taco Bell's chili cheese burrito, McDonald's Big Mac |
| Iron | 30 mg (recommendation is for 30 mg of elemental iron as daily supplement) | Meats; dried beans; peas; dark green, leafy vegetables; whole grains; fortified cereal; absorption of iron from plant foods improved by vitamin C sources taken simultaneously |
| Zinc | 15 mg | Seafood, meats, eggs, legumes, whole grains |
| Folate (folic acid) | 0.6 mg (prenatal vitamins contain 0.4-1.0 mg of folic acid) | Green, leafy vegetables; fruits |
| Vitamin A | 800 µg | Dark yellow and green vegetables, fruits |
| Vitamin B$_6$ | 2.2 mg | Chicken, fish, liver, pork, eggs |
| Vitamin D | 5 µg | Fortified milk products and cereals |

*Higher ranges are especially important for the younger pregnant teen.

allow for adequate fetal growth. Third, poor eating patterns of the teen and her current growth requirement may leave her with limited reserves of essential vitamins and minerals when the pregnancy begins. The nurse can assess the pregnant teenager's current eating pattern and provide creative guidance. Identifying good choices that a teen can consume "on the run" might include snacks of drinkable yogurt, leftover pizza, string cheese, or energy/granola bars. The teen who often eats out can boost her protein intake at fast-food establishments by ordering milkshakes instead of soft drinks and cheeseburgers or broiled chicken sandwiches instead of hamburgers (Stang and Story, 2005).

The recommended nutritional needs of the adolescent may depend on the gynecological age of the teen—that is, the number of years between her chronological age and her age at menarche, as well as her chronological age. Young women with a gynecological age of 2 years or less or under the age of 16 years may have increased nutrient requirements because of their own growth. Furthermore, the younger and still-growing teen may compete nutritionally with the fetus. Fetuses may show evidence of slower growth in young women ages 10 to 16 years (Stang and Story, 2005). The nurse, in collaboration with the WIC nutritionist, can determine the nutritional needs of the pregnant teenager to tailor education appropriately. Table 35-2 describes adolescent nutritional needs in pregnancy.

Weight gain during pregnancy is one of the strongest predictors of infant birth weight. Although precise weight gain goals in adolescence are controversial, pregnant adolescents who gain 25 to 35 lb have the lowest incidence of low-birth-weight babies. Babies born to teenagers may be at risk for being small for gestational age despite adequate weight gain if there is very slow gain in the first 24 weeks. Teenagers who begin the pregnancy at a normal weight should be counseled to begin weight gain in the first trimester and to average gains of 1 lb per week for the second and third trimesters (Stang and Story, 2005). Younger teen mothers (ages 13 to 16), because of their own growth demands, may need to gain more weight than older teen mothers (ages 17 and older) to have the same-birth-weight baby. Table 35-3 shows the recommendations established by the Institute of Medicine for adolescent gestational weight gain by pre-pregnant weight categories.

## TABLE 35-3 Gestational Weight Gain Recommendations for Adolescents*

| | RECOMMENDED TOTAL GAIN | | | |
|---|---|---|---|---|
| Prepregnant Weight Category† | kg | lb | Trimester 1 (lb) | Trimesters 2 and 3 (lb/wk) |
| Underweight (BMI 19.8) | 12.5-18 | 28-40 | 5 | 1.0 |
| Normal weight (BMI 19.9-26) | 11.5-16 | 25-35 | 3 | 1.0 |
| Overweight (BMI 26-29) | 7.0-11.5 | 15-25 | 2 | 0.66 |
| Very overweight (BMI ≥ 29) | 7.0-9.1 | 15-20 | 1.5 | 0.5 |

*Very young adolescents (14 years of age or younger, or less than 2 years postmenarche) should strive for gains at the upper end of the range.
†BMI (body mass index) is calculated as weight (in kilograms) divided by height (in meters) squared.
From Story M, Stang J, editors: *Nutrition and the Pregnant Adolescent: A Practical Reference Guide.* Minneapolis, MN, 2000, University of Minnesota, Center for Leadership, Education, and Training in Maternal and Child Nutrition. Retrieved February 2015 from http://www.epi.umn.edu/let/pubs/nmpa.shtm

It is important for the nurse to assess the attitudes of the pregnant teen about weight gain and to monitor her progress, providing feedback on adequate weight gain and counseling if weight gain is excessive. Gaining weight beyond the recommendations raises the risk for infants to be hypoglycemic, to be large-for-gestational age, and to have a low Apgar score, seizures, and polycythemia (American Dietetic Association, 2008). Family support of the pregnant teen can be a strong influence in adequate weight gain and good nutrition during the pregnancy. Nutrition education should emphasize what accounts for weight gain and how fetal growth will benefit.

Iron deficiency anemia is the most common nutritional problem among both pregnant and nonpregnant adolescent females (Stang and Story, 2005). Up to 11% of adolescents may begin a pregnancy with low or absent iron stores because of heavy menstrual periods, a previous pregnancy, growth demands, poor iron intake, or substance abuse. By the second trimester, at least 16% of pregnant adolescents will have iron deficiency anemia and even higher rates among lower income teenagers (American Dietetic Association, 2008). The increased maternal plasma volume and increased fetal demands for iron (especially in the third trimester) can further compromise the adolescent. Iron deficiency in pregnancy may contribute to increased prematurity, low birth weight, maternal cardiovascular stress, increased risk of maternal urinary tract infection, decreased maternal well-being, postpartum hemorrhage, and slower wound healing (Stang and Story, 2005). The nurse can reinforce the need for the teen to take prenatal vitamins during pregnancy and after the baby's birth. Vitamins should contain 30 to 60 mg of elemental iron daily. The nurse should educate about iron-rich foods and foods that promote iron absorption, such as those containing vitamin C.

## Infant Care

Many adolescents have cared for babies and small children and feel confident and competent. Few teens are ever prepared, however, for the reality of 24-hour care of an infant. The nurse can help prepare the teen for the transition to motherhood while she is still pregnant. The trend toward early discharge from the hospital has made prenatal preparation even more important. The nurse can enlist the support of the teen's parents in education about infant care and stimulation. Young fathers-to-be would benefit from this education as well. Family values, practices, and beliefs about child care may be deeply embedded and require the nurse to work gently and persuasively to challenge any that may be detrimental to an infant (Savio Beers and Hollo, 2009). For example, a family may believe that corporal punishment is a necessary component of child-rearing.

Adolescents often lack the self-confidence and knowledge required to positively interact with their infants. They may also have unrealistic expectations about their children's development (Ryan-Krause et al, 2009). For example, they may expect their children to feed themselves at an early age or think that their children's behavior is more difficult than an adult mother might think. Teen parents often lack knowledge about infant growth and development, as seen in their limited verbal communication with their children, limited eye contact, and the tendency to display frustration and ambivalence as mothers. Over time, adolescents can improve their ability to foster their children's emotional and social growth. Children of adolescent mothers have also been found to be at risk for academic and behavior problems as they enter school (Terry-Humen et al, 2005; Cornelius et al, 2010). These risks can be reduced when the teen mother receives professional intervention and supervision in the area of infant social and cognitive development (Ryan-Krause et al, 2009).

Abusive parenting is more likely to occur when the parents have limited knowledge about normal child development. It may also be more likely to occur among parents who cannot adequately empathize with a child's needs. Younger teens are particularly at risk for being unable to understand what their infant or child needs. This frustration may be exhibited as abusive behavior toward the child. Nurses should continually assess for child abuse risk when dealing with teens who exhibit greater psychological distress or lack social supports (Lee, 2009).

After the birth of the baby, the nurse should observe how the mother responds to infant cues for basic needs and distress. Specific techniques that the new mother can be instructed to use in early child care are listed in the How To box. Begin parenting education as early as possible. Adolescents who feel competent as parents have enhanced self-esteem, which in turn positively influences their relationship with their child. Recognizing these good parenting skills and providing positive feedback help a young mother gain confidence in her role (Ryan-Krause et al, 2009).

**HOW TO** Promote Interactions between the Teen Mother and Her Baby

*The nurse can make the following suggestions to the teen mother:*
1. Make eye contact with your baby. Position your face 8 to 10 inches from your baby's face and smile.
2. Talk to your baby often. Use simple sentences, but try to avoid baby talk. Allow time for your baby to "answer." This will help your baby to acquire language and communication skills.
3. Babies often enjoy when you sing to them, and this may help soothe them during a difficult time or help them fall asleep. Experiment with different songs and melodies to see which your baby seems to like.
4. Babies at this age cannot be spoiled. Instead, when babies are held and cuddled, they feel secure and loved.
5. Babies cry for many reasons and for no reason at all. If your baby has a clean diaper, has recently been fed, and is safe and secure, he or she may just need to cry for a few minutes. What works to calm your baby may be different from other babies you have known. You can try rocking, gentle reassuring words, soft music, or remaining quiet.
6. Make feeding times pleasant for both of you. Do not prop the bottle in your baby's mouth. Instead, sit comfortably, hold your baby in your arms, and offer the bottle or breast.
7. When babies are awake, they love to play. They enjoy taking walks and looking at brightly colored objects or pictures and toys that make noises, such as rattles and musical toys.

## Repeat Pregnancy

Teen mothers who have a closely spaced second pregnancy, or a repeat pregnancy, have poorer birth, educational, and economic outcomes than teens who do not. In 2009, 19% of teen births were a repeat birth (Ikramullah et al, 2011). Some studies have shown that the younger the teen at first birth, the more likely she will have a second teen birth within 24 months (Savio Beers and Hollo, 2009). A *Healthy People 2020* objective is to reduce the proportion of pregnancies conceived within 18 months of a previous birth. Nurses should recognize which teens are at risk for a second teen pregnancy, such as lower educational and cognitive ability, mental health issues, physical trauma, losses (such as death of a loved one), and substance use. Also, some teens who report a planned first pregnancy are more likely to have an intentional second pregnancy within 24 months to complete their family (Savio Beers and Hollo, 2009; Patchen et al, 2009).

Discussions about family planning should begin during the third trimester of the current pregnancy. Nurses should review contraceptive options and help the young woman identify the methods she is most likely to use. It is helpful to determine at this time the methods she has used in the past, her satisfaction or dissatisfaction, and reasons for use or nonuse. Many teens express unrealistic goals, such as "I am never going to have sex again" or "I need a break from guys," and they may erroneously believe that they are unable to conceive for some time after the delivery. After delivery, the nurse should follow-up on the young woman's plan. Obstacles to obtaining contraceptives may exist, and the nurse can identify these and help problem-solve with the new mother.

## Schooling and Educational Needs

Adolescents who become parents may have had limited school success before the pregnancy. However, coping with the demands of child-rearing coupled with the immaturity of the young mother may make school even less of a priority. As noted previously, the potential for a closely spaced second birth may be lessened by a return to school. Fifty-one percent of teen mothers earn a high school diploma compared with 89% of women who did not give birth during the teen years. Federal legislation passed in 1975 prohibits schools from excluding students because they are pregnant. Greater emphasis is placed on keeping the pregnant adolescent in school during the pregnancy and having her return as soon as possible after the birth. Several factors may positively influence a young woman's return to school. These include her parents' level of education and their marital stability, small family size, whether there were reading materials at home, whether her mother is employed, and whether the young woman is African American.

A practical challenge for young parents is locating and affording quality child care; difficulties with this may prevent the highly motivated teenager from returning to high school. In the past 30 years, the percentage of parenting teens who return to high school and graduate has improved significantly. Attendance in college, now becoming the career requisite, is still less attainable for women who had children as teenagers than for those who delayed childbearing, and less than 2% attain that college degree by the age of 30 (Ng and Kaye, 2012).

Young women who have pregnancy complications may seek home instruction. This decision is made according to regulations issued by the state boards of education. Some young women have difficulty attending school because of the normal discomforts of pregnancy or because of social and emotional conflicts associated with the pregnancy. Teens who leave school without parental or medical excuses may face legal problems because of truancy. This increases the potential for them to become school dropouts. The nurse can determine whether this has happened and try to coordinate with the school personnel (and school nurse, if one exists) to tailor efforts for a particular pregnant teen to keep her in school. Specific needs to be addressed include the following: (1) using the bathroom frequently, (2) carrying and consuming more fluids or snacks to relieve nausea, (3) climbing stairs and carrying heavy book bags, and (4) fitting comfortably behind stationary desks. Schools that are committed to keeping students enrolled are generally helpful and will assist in accommodating special needs.

## TEEN PREGNANCY AND THE NURSE

Nurses can influence teen pregnancy through appropriate interventions at home and in the community.

### Home-Based Interventions

Nurses can identify young women at risk for pregnancy in families currently receiving services. Younger sisters of pregnant teens are at a twofold increased risk for becoming pregnant themselves (Savio Beers and Hollo, 2009). Nurses can offer anticipatory guidance addressing sexuality issues to the parents of all preteens and teens during home visits to increase their knowledge and awareness.

Visiting the pregnant teen in her home allows the nurse to assess the facilities available at home for management of her pregnancy needs and the suitability of the environment for her child. Some specific areas to assess are adequacy of heating and cooling, a source of water, cleanliness of the home, cooking facilities, and food storage. The nurse may find it more convenient for parents and other family members to participate in education and counseling sessions in their own home. Also, the need for financial assistance and other social service support may be more easily identified. Home visiting by nurses during a young woman's pregnancy can be critical in achieving compliance with antepartum goals concerning weight gain, good nutrition, and prenatal medical concerns (Figure 35-2).

A teen pregnancy can shift the family dynamics. Families may go through stages of reactions. First, a crisis stage may occur, characterized by many emotions and conflict. By the third trimester, a honeymoon stage may occur, with greater acceptance and understanding of the teen and the impending birth. Finally, after the infant's birth, reorganization may occur, during which conflict may emerge again over issues of child care and the young woman's role. The nurse can facilitate family coping and resolution of these stages by treating the family as client and assessing each person's role and strengths. Ultimately,

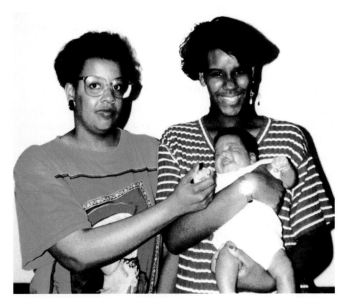

FIG 35-2 Both the teen mother and the teen's own mother can be included in health teaching.

family support for a teen parent can positively influence both mother and infant (Savio Beers and Hollo, 2009). A balance of moderate family guidance or supplementary care supports young mothers in their parenting role rather than replacing it.

## (QSEN) FOCUS ON QUALITY AND SAFETY EDUCATION FOR NURSES

### Teen Pregnancy

**Targeted Competency: Evidence-Based Practice—Integrate best current evidence with clinical expertise and client/family preferences and values for delivery of optimal health care.**

Important aspects of EBP include:

- Knowledge: Describe evidence-based practice (EBP) to include the components of research evidence, clinical expertise, and client/family values
- Skills: Locate evidence reports related to clinical practice topics and guidelines
- Attitudes: Value the need for continuous improvement in clinical practice based on new knowledge

#### Evidence-Based Practice Question

You are an RN in a community-based health clinic, conducting sports physicals for high-school aged students. You conduct a physical assessment on a female 18-year-old student, Gloria, who has been accompanied to this appointment by her mother. During the physical exam, Gloria confides in you that she is sexually active and is not currently using any form of contraception because her mother is not supportive. You ask Gloria if she would like to be using birth control and she says that she is not sure. You provide Gloria some educational materials on various contraceptive methods.

After the exam, Gloria's mother asks to speak with you privately. Gloria's mother is moderately emotional, worried that her daughter has been sexually active and might be pregnant.

- What are your legal limits around sharing information with Gloria's mother?
- Based on these limits, what information do you share with Gloria's mother?
- What might be your next step in facilitating a mother-daughter dialogue in this situation?
- Find a nursing research article about family communication with pregnant teens. Are there guidelines or outcomes from research that might be applied to this clinical scenario?
- What other patient outcome might you identify that could lead to a successful intervention in this scenario?

Prepared by Gail Armstrong, PhD©, DNP, ACNS-BC, CNE, Associate Professor, College of Nursing, University of Colorado.

## Community-Based Interventions

Many communities have broad-based coalitions and planning councils that facilitate a comprehensive approach to teen pregnancy. These groups usually include health care professionals, social workers, clergy, school personnel, businessmen, legislators, and members of other youth-serving agencies. Nurses play a significant role on this team by participating in or organizing community assessments, public awareness campaigns, group education (for professionals, parents, and youths), and interprofessional programs for high-risk youths. Community acceptance is more likely when there is a broad base of support for activities directed at the reduction of teen pregnancy or reduction of consequences.

Research has evaluated years of pregnancy prevention programs. As less funding is available, programs must stand out to

## ⟩⟩ LINKING CONTENT TO PRACTICE

Just as providing care to pregnant teens includes many of the *Healthy People 2020* objectives; this care is also consistent with the standards and competencies for public health professionals including nurses. Specifically, the nurse assesses the teen population, determines priorities for nursing actions based on the assessment, develops a plan and implements the plan by coordinating care with many appropriate agencies. In dealing with pregnant teenagers, it is essential to work with schools and many social service agencies in order to provide age-appropriate care and health education for both the teen and the baby. Skills in the core competencies such as assessment, planning, cultural competency, and communication are essential when providing care to this population.

From American Nurses Association: Scope & standards of practice: public health nursing, Silver Spring, Maryland, 2007, ANA; Public Health Foundation Council on Linkages: Core competencies for public health professionals, Washington, DC, June 11, 2009 adopted, PHF.

receive financial support. Research summaries that can be used by communities for strategic planning are available from the National Campaign to Prevent Teen and Unplanned Pregnancy (http://thenationalcampaign.org/), based in Washington, DC. Programs that have been evaluated fall into one of three categories: programs that focus on sexual factors (this includes educational programs addressing sexual behavior and STD/HIV), programs that focus on nonsexual behaviors (service learning that matches volunteerism with a didactic component), and programs that focus on both sexual and nonsexual factors (may bring other risk behaviors and/or protective factors into the curriculum). Because there is diversity available in the programs, communities can match their characteristics and needs with a program (Kirby, 2007).

The nurse can also be a valuable asset to schools. There are curriculum-based sex and STD/HIV education programs that have been evaluated and found to have positive effects on teens' sexual behavior (Kirby, 2007). Health teachers may ask nurses to provide educational materials or assistance with classroom instruction, especially in the areas of family planning, STDs, and pregnancy. Schools that do not have nurses may arrange to have a nurse from the health department available for health consultations with students during school hours. Schools may also request that nurses participate on their health advisory boards.

School-based health care clinics are operating in more than 1500 elementary, middle, and high schools in the United States. They are found primarily in urban areas (61%) but increasingly in rural (27%) and suburban (12%) regions. The services offered may include counseling, referrals, and primary care services. Some programs offer reproductive health counseling and services that can be vital in efforts to delay the onset of intercourse and increase the use of contraception. The nurse can assist school systems to design these programs as well as refer young women in need of reproductive health care services.

Nurses bring their knowledge about youth and reproductive behavior to any organization or group that has teens, their parents, or other professionals working with teens. Churches are becoming increasingly interested in addressing the needs of their youth, especially because teen sexual activity, pregnancy, and parenting are affecting more of their members.

## EVIDENCE-BASED PRACTICE

When adolescents become parents they face challenges that set them apart from adult parents. Outcomes for teen parents and their children have been generously studied and clearly stated. What has been lacking in nursing research is a better understanding of the elements of nursing intervention that can improve these outcomes.

Previous studies have identified that pregnant and parenting adolescents can benefit from visiting nursing care on many fronts. This includes decreasing hospitalizations, ER visits, repeat pregnancies, spacing between births, less domestic violence and more. These studies focused more on the improved outcomes rather than informing nursing on the process by which this happens.

This study adds to the data that helps us understand how to help teenagers become parents. It focuses on information gathered from 30 Public Health Nurses (PHN) visiting pregnant and parenting teenagers. These PHN's submitted stories about their young clients and those were analyzed to understand the basic social psychological problems experienced as well as the basic social psychological process used by the PHN to help the adolescent attain stronger parenting skills.

### Nurse Use

The data that emerged from this study confirmed that adolescents begin parenting with negative life circumstances, poor knowledge base and lack of awareness of how to attain the knowledge. The elements of the PHN interventions that improved the adolescents' role as parents were wide ranging and included case management, health education, counseling and referral. This greater understanding about the process in which PHN home visiting works is essential for targeted and effective nursing interventions

Atkinson LD, Peden-McAlpine CJ: Advancing adolescent maternal development: a grounded theory. *J Pediatr Nurs* 29:168–176, 2014.

## PRACTICE APPLICATION

A local youth-serving agency requested the assistance of a nurse, Kristen Brown, in the implementation of a new high school–based program for pregnant and parenting teen girls. The primary goal of the program is to keep these teens in school through graduation. The secondary goal is to provide knowledge and skills about healthy pregnancy, labor and delivery, and parenting. After delivery, students enrolled in this program were paid for school attendance and this money could be used to defray the costs of child care.

A nurse from the health department was the ideal choice to conduct the educational sessions. The group met weekly during the lunch hour. The curriculum that was developed included topics from early pregnancy through the toddler years. Occasionally, Ms. Brown recruited outside speakers such as a labor and delivery nurse or an early intervention specialist.

She also met individually with each enrolled student to provide case management services. Ideally, she would ensure that each student had a health care provider for prenatal care, that each was visited at home by a nurse, that each had enrolled in WIC and Medicaid if eligible, and that both the pregnant teen and her partner knew about other parenting and support groups.

One educational session that was particularly interesting was the discussion about the postpartum course—the 6 weeks after delivery. There were many lively discussions about labor experiences as well as some emotional discussions about the reality of coming home with a baby and changes in the relationship with their male partner. Accurate contraception information was provided, which helped to clarify the many myths the girls had heard from friends and older women. Many girls benefited from understanding the normalcy of postpartum blues, but one young woman recognized that she had a more serious and persistent depression and privately approached the nurse for assistance.

At the end of the first school year, the dropout rate for pregnant and parenting teens was reduced by half, and preterm labor rates had also declined. The local school board and a local youth-serving agency joined together to provide financial support to continue this program for an additional 2 years. Ms. Brown was asked to expand the educational programs and interventions she had developed.

What are some directions in which Ms. Brown might expand the program? List four.

**Answers can be found on the Evolve site.**

## KEY POINTS

- The provision of reproductive health care services to adolescents requires sensitivity to the special needs of this age group. This includes knowing about state laws regarding confidentiality and services for birth control, pregnancy, abortion, and adoption.
- Pregnant teenagers have a substantial percentage of the first births in the United States. They are more likely to deliver prematurely and have a low-birth-weight baby. This risk can be reduced by early initiation of prenatal care and good nutrition.
- Factors that can influence whether a young woman becomes pregnant include a history of sexual victimization, family

dysfunction, substance use, and failure to use birth control. Several factors may overlap.
- Nutritional needs during pregnancy can be challenged if the teenager has unhealthy eating habits and begins the pregnancy with limited reserves of vitamins and minerals. With education, the adolescent can make good food choices while still snacking or eating fast foods. Weight gain during pregnancy is a significant marker for a normal-weight baby.
- Young men need special attention and preparation as they become fathers. The interventions include information about pregnancy and delivery, declaration of paternity, care of infants and children, and psychosocial support in this role.

## KEY POINTS—cont'd

- The pregnant teen will need support during her pregnancy and in child-rearing. Families may provide most of this support. However, many communities have a variety of services available for adolescents. These services include financial assistance for medical care, nutritional programs, and school-based support groups.
- Adolescent parents often have unrealistic expectations about their children and may not know how to stimulate emotional, social, and cognitive development. The children born to adolescents are at risk for academic and behavioral problems as they become older. Teens who receive education on normal development and child care are more likely to avert these problems with their children.
- During a pregnancy, teenagers are expected to attend school. Homebound instruction is reserved for those with medical complications. Teen mothers who return to school and complete their education after the birth of their child are less likely to have a repeat pregnancy. Problems finding child care and the need to have an income can create an obstacle to school return.
- Community coalitions, which include nurses, can have a significant impact on teen pregnancy. These coalitions generally have diverse representation from the community, and therefore their activities meet with more community support.

## CLINICAL DECISION-MAKING ACTIVITIES

1. Become familiar with statistics on teen pregnancy, births, miscarriages, and abortions in your area, and collect information on use of prenatal care, low-birth-weight and premature deliveries, high school completion, and repeat pregnancies. Compare the trends in statistics to the impact and costs to the individual, her family, and the community.
2. Call or visit local schools and interview the school nurse or guidance counselors about teen pregnancy. Determine what resources are available through the schools for pregnancy prevention. Assess the family life education curriculum, and identify a teaching project for nursing students. Can pregnancy prevention and parenting education be incorporated into the learning objectives in the existing school curriculum?
3. Design and offer a childbirth preparation class for pregnant teens and their support persons. Include a plan for identifying potential participants, select a site that is accessible, and develop an evaluation method. Develop teaching tools that acknowledge adolescent development.
4. Assess reproductive health care services for young men in your community. Design an awareness campaign targeting young men on paternity issues and the prevention of pregnancy. Be specific about ways to incorporate male role models and mentors.

## REFERENCES

American Academy of Child and Adolescent Psychiatry (AACAP): *Facts for Families Pages: When Children Have Children* [Publication No. 31]. Washington, DC, 2012, AACAP. Retrieved February 2015 from: http://www.aacap.org/aacap/Families_and_Youth/Facts_for_Families/Facts_for_Families_Pages/When_Children_Have_Children_31.aspx

American College of Obstetricians and Gynecologists: Committee opinion no. 539: Adolescents and long-acting reversible contraception: implants and intrauterine devices. *Obstet Gynecol* 120:983–988, 2012.

American Dietetic Association: Position of the American Dietetic Association: nutrition and lifestyle for a healthy pregnancy outcome. *J Am Diet Assoc* 108:553–561, 2008.

Aruda M, Wadicor K, Frese L, et al: Early pregnancy in adolescents: diagnosis, assessment, options counseling, and referral. *J Pediatr Health Care* 24:4–13, 2010.

Bersamin M, Todd M, Fisher DA, et al: Parenting practices and adolescent sexual behavior: a longitudinal study. *J Marriage Fam* 70:97–112, 2008.

Brandsen CK: *A Case for Adoption.* Grand Rapids, MI, 1991, Bethany.

Centers for Disease Contol and Prevention (CDC): Youth Risk Behavior Surveillance-United States, 2013. *MMWR Morb Mortal Wkly Rep* 63:24–27, 2014.

Centers for Disease Control and Prevention (CDC): Vital Signs: Repeat Births among Teens—United States, 2007–2010. *MMWR Morb Mortal Wkly Rep* 62:249–255, 2013.

Child Trends Data Bank: *Statutory Rape: Sex between Young Teens and Older Individuals.* Washington, DC, 2013, Child Trends. Retrieved February 2015 from: http://www.childtrends.org/?indicators=statutory-rape-sex-between-young-teens-and-older-individuals.

Cornelius MD, Goldschmidt L, DeGenna NM, et al: Improvement in intelligence test scores from 6 to 10 years in children of teenage mothers. *J Dev Behav Pediatr* 31:405–413, 2010.

English A, Kenney KE: *State Minor Consent Laws: A Summary,* ed 3. Chapel Hill, NC, 2010, Center for Adolescent Health and the Law.

Finer LB, Philbin JM: Sexual initiation, contraceptive use and pregnancy among young adolescents. *Pediatrics* 131:886–891, 2013.

Guillery ME, Benzies KM, Mannion C, et al: Postpartum nurses' perceptions of barriers to screening for intimate partner violence: a cross-sectional survey. *BMC Nurs* 11(2):1–8, 2012.

Guttmacher Institute: *Fact Sheet: American Teens' Sexual and Reproductive Health.* New York, 2014, Guttmacher Institute. Retrieved February 2015 from: http://www.guttmacher.org/pubs/FB-ATSRH.html.

Guttmacher Institute: *National Reproductive Health Profile.* New York, 2015, Guttmacher Institute. Retrieved February 2015 from: http://www.guttmacher.org/datacenter/profiles/US.jsp.

Harrykissoon SD, Richert VI, Wiemann CM: Prevalence and patterns of intimate partner violence among adolescent mothers during the postpartum period. *Arch Pediatr Adolesc Med* 156:325–330, 2002.

Hatcher RA, Trussell J, Nelson AL, et al: *Contraceptive Technology,* ed 20. New York, 2011, Ardent Media.

Heavey E: Don't miss preconception care opportunities for adolescents. *MCN Am J Matern Child Nurs* 35:213–219, 2010.

Heavey EJ, Moysich KB, Hyland A, et al: Female adolescents' perceptions of male partners' pregnancy desire. *J Midwifery Womens Health* 53:338–344, 2008.

Herman JW: How teen mothers describe dating violence. *J Obstet Gynecol Neonatal Nurs* 42:462–479, 2013.

Ikramullah E, Barry M, Manlove J, et al: *Facts at a Glance: A Fact Sheet Reporting National, State, and City Trends in Teen Childbearing.* Washington, DC, 2011, Child Trends. Retrieved February 2015 from: http://www.childtrends.org/wp-content/

uploads/2011/04/2011-10FactsAtAGlance2011.pdf.

Kann L, Kinchen S, Shanklin SL, et al: Centers for Disease Control and Prevention (CDC): Youth risk behavior surveillance—United States, 2013. *MMWR Surveill Summ* 63(Suppl 4):1–168, 2014. Retrieved February 2015 from: http://www.ncbi.nlm.nih.gov/pubmed/24918634.

Kirby D: *Emerging Answers 2007: Research Findings on Programs to Reduce Teen Pregnancy and Sexually Transmitted Diseases.* Washington, DC, 2007, National Campaign to Prevent Teen and Unplanned Pregnancy.

Kost K, Henshaw S: *U.S. Teenage Pregnancies, Births and Abortions, 2010: National and State Trends by Age, Race and Ethnicity.* New York, 2014, Guttmacher Institute. Retrieved February 2015 from: http://www.guttmacher.org/pubs/USTPtrends10.pdf.

Lee Y: Early motherhood and harsh parenting: the role of human, social and cultural capital. *Child Abuse Negl* 33:625–637, 2009.

Miller E, Decker MR, McCauley HL, et al: Pregnancy coercion, intimate partner violence and unintended pregnancy. *Contraception* 81:316–322, 2010.

National Abortion and Reproductive Rights Action League Foundation (NARAL): *U.S. Supreme Court Decisions Concerning Reproductive Rights: 1927–2012.* Washington, DC, 2014a, NARAL. Retrieved February 2015 from: http://www.prochoiceamerica.org/media/fact-sheets/government-federal-courts-scotus-choice-cases.pdf.

National Abortion and Reproductive Rights Action League Foundation (NARAL): *Who Decides? The Status of Women's Reproductive Rights in the United States*, ed 23. Washington, DC, 2014b, NARAL. Retrieved February 2015 from: http://www.prochoiceamerica.org/government-and-you/who-decides/.

Neinstein LS, editor: *Adolescent Health Care*, ed 5. Philadelphia, 2008, Lippincott Williams & Wilkins.

Ng AS, Kaye K: *Why It Matters: Teen Childbearing, Education, and Economic Wellbeing.* Washington, DC, 2012, National Campaign to Prevent Teen Pregnancy. Retrieved February 2015 from: http://thenationalcampaign.org/sites/default/files/resource-primary-download/childbearing-education-economicwellbeing.pdf.

Noll JG, Shenk CE, Putnam KT: Childhood sexual abuse and pregnancy: a meta-analytic update. *J Pediatr Psychol* 34:366–378, 2009.

Office of Adolescent Health, U.S. Department of Health and Human Services [USDHHS]: *Trends in Teen Pregnancy and Childbearing.* Washington, DC, 2015, USDHHS. Retrieved February 2015 from: http://www.hhs.gov/ash/oah/adolescent-health-topics/reproductive-health/teen-pregnancy/trends.html.

Oman RF, Vesely SK, Aspy CB: Youth assets and sexual risk behavior: the importance of assets for youth residing in one-parent households. *Perspect Sex Reprod Health* 37:25, 2005.

Paschal AM, Lewis-Moss R, Hsiao T: Perceived fatherhood roles and parenting behaviors among African American teen fathers. *J Adolesc Res* 26:61–83, 2011.

Patchen L, Caruso D, Lanzi RG: Poor maternal mental health and trauma as risk factors for a short interpregnancy interval among adolescent mothers. *J Psychiatr Ment Health Nurs* 16:401–403, 2009.

Ryan-Krause P, Meadows-Oliver M, Sadler L, et al: Developmental status of children of teen mothers: contrasting objective assessments with maternal reports. *J Pediatr Health Care* 23:303–309, 2009.

Savio Beers LA, Hollo RE: Approaching the adolescent-headed family: a review of teen, parenting. *Curr Probl Pediatr Adolesc Health Care* 39:216–233, 2009.

Sipsma H, Biello KB, Cole-Lewis H, et al: Like father, like son: the intergenerational cycle of adolescent fatherhood. *Am J Public Health* 100:517–524, 2010.

Stang J, Story M, editors: *Guidelines for Adolescent Nutrition Services.* Minneapolis, MN, 2005, Center for Leadership, Education, and Training in Maternal and Child Nutrition, Division of Epidemiology and Community Health, School of Public Health, University of Minnesota. Retrieved February 2015 from: http://www.epi.umn.edu/let/pubs/img/adol_preface_materials.pdf.

Terry-Humen E, Manlove J, Moore KA: *Playing Catch-Up: How Children Born to Teen Mothers Fare.* Washington, DC, 2005, National Campaign to Prevent Teen Pregnancy.

U.S. Department of Health and Human Services (USDHHS): *Healthy People 2020.* Washington, DC, 2010, USDHHS. Retrieved February 2015 from: http://www.healthypeople.gov/.

Volpe EM, Hardie TL, Cerulli C, et al: What's age got to do with it? Partner age difference, power, intimate partner violence, and sexual risk in urban adolescents. *J Interpers Violence* 28:2068–2087, 2013.

Wisnieski D, Sieving RE, Garwick AW: Influence of peers on young adolescent females' romantic decisions. *Am J Health Educ* 44:32–40, 2013.

# 36

# Mental Health Issues

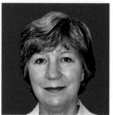

## Anita Thompson-Heisterman, MSN, PMHCNS-BC, PMHNP-BC

Anita Thompson-Heisterman earned the BSN, MSN, FNP, and PMHNP degrees and certificates from the University of Virginia. She began practicing community mental health nursing in 1983 as a psychiatric nurse in a community mental health center. Her community practice has included clinical and management activities in a psychiatric home care service, a nurse-managed primary care center in public housing, and an outreach program for rural older adults. Currently she is an assistant professor in the Division of Family, Community and Mental Health Systems at the University of Virginia School of Nursing, and her faculty practice is with the Memory and Aging Care Clinic at the University of Virginia Department of Neurology.

## ADDITIONAL RESOURCES

## OBJECTIVES

*After reading this chapter, the student should be able to do the following:*

1. Describe the history of community mental health and make predictions about the future.
2. Discuss the prevalence of mental illness in the United States and the world.
3. Describe essential mental health services and corresponding national objectives for improving mental health.
4. Evaluate standards, models, concepts, strategies, and research findings for use in community mental health nursing practice to improve community mental health.
5. Describe the role of the community mental health nurse with individuals and with groups at risk for psychiatric mental health problems.
6. Apply the nursing process in community work with clients diagnosed with psychiatric disorders, families at risk for mental health problems, and vulnerable populations.

## KEY TERMS

Americans with Disabilities Act, p. 788
assertive community treatment, p. 790
community mental health centers, p. 786
community mental health model, p. 786
Community Support Program, p. 784
consumer advocacy, p. 784
consumers, p. 788
deinstitutionalization, p. 788
institutionalization, p. 786
intensive case management models, p. 790
managed care, p. 785
mental health problems, p. 783

National Alliance for the Mentally Ill, p. 789
National Institute of Mental Health, p. 787
parity, p. 785
Patient Protection and Affordable Health Care Act, p. 785
recovery, p. 790
reinstitutionalization, p. 788
relapse management, p. 790
severe mental disorders, p. 783
systems theory, p. 789
wellness recovery action plans, p. 796
—*See Glossary for definitions*

## CHAPTER OUTLINE

Because providing community services and nursing care to people suffering from mental illness or emotional distress is complex and influenced by many individual and community factors, it requires a variety of approaches. Complicating factors include (1) the scope of emotional and mental disorders; (2) uncertainty about the specific cause, cure, and treatment for the most severe mental disorders; (3) the severe chronic disabling nature of some mental disorders; and (4) the complexity of the community mental health services sector. The scarcity of resources compounds the problems and presents challenges in community mental health work.

Cultural beliefs and economics influence the amount and types of services and treatment available in various countries. However, two universal truths exist: services for people with mental disorders are inadequate in all countries, and mental illness has a significant effect on families, communities, and nations. Therefore, specialized knowledge and skills about severe mental illness and mental health problems are necessary for effective nursing practice in the community. It is helpful to understand both the organization of mental health services from a historical perspective and the trends in current health care demands and delivery. Knowledge about populations at risk for psychiatric mental health problems and understanding illness outcomes in terms of biopsychosocial consequences are even more important. Finally, it is necessary to refine and broaden nursing process skills in treatment planning to include the impact of mental illness on families and communities.

This chapter focuses on the scope of mental disorders, the development of community mental health services, the current health objectives for mental health and mental disorders, and the role of the nurse in community settings. Conceptual frameworks useful in community mental health nursing practice are also presented. Because other chapters in this book are devoted to high-risk groups such as the homeless population and those with substance abuse problems, this chapter's focus is on the variety of mental health problems encountered in communities, with an emphasis on populations that have long-term, severe mental disorders and groups that are most vulnerable to mental health problems.

## SCOPE OF MENTAL ILLNESS IN THE UNITED STATES

Mental health is defined in *Healthy People 2020* (U.S. Department of Health and Human Services [USDHHS], 2010) as encompassing the ability to engage in productive activities and fulfilling relationships with other people, to adapt to change, and to cope with adversity. The World Health Organization (WHO) expands the definition, describing mental health as a state of well-being in which a person can realize his or her potential, and notes that mental health is essential if a person is to have health (WHO, 2008a). Mental health is an integral part of personal well-being, family and other interpersonal relationships, and contributions to community or society. Mental disorders are conditions that are characterized by alterations in thinking, mood, or behavior that are associated with distress and/or impaired functioning. Mental illness refers collectively to all diagnosable mental disorders. Severe mental disorders are determined by diagnoses and criteria that include degree of functional disability (American Psychiatric Association [APA], 2013).

Mental disorders are indiscriminate. They occur across the life span and affect persons of all races, cultures, genders, and educational and socioeconomic groups. They are the leading cause of disability in North America (WHO, 2008b). In the United States nearly 18% of adults (age 18 years and older) have a mental health condition severe enough to impair daily function, and 3.9% of these suffer from a serious mental illness such as schizophrenia (Substance Abuse and Mental Health Services Administration [SAMHSA], 2013). Nearly half of those with any mental disorder (8.1%) meet criteria for two disorders, mental health and substance abuse (National Institute of Mental Health [NIMH], 2013; SAMHSA, 2013). Fourteen percent of females and 7% of males between 12 and 17 years of age suffer from a major depressive disorder, and 11% of 13- to 18-year-old adolescents meet criteria for a lifetime substance abuse disorder (SAMHSA, 2013). By the 8th grade 24% of adolescents have ingested alcohol and by the 12th grade, 64% are drinking (SAMHSA, 2013). Adolescent mental health is a global concern as well (WHO, 2014). Nearly 17% of people over age 55 have a mood or anxiety disorder (Byers et al, 2010), and these rates will rise as the number of older Americans increases over the next two decades. Alzheimer's disease, the primary cause of dementia, is increasing. In 2014 an estimated 5.2 million Americans had Alzheimer's disease. This number includes 5 million people who were 65 years or older and approximately 200,000 individuals under age 65 who had younger-onset Alzheimer's disease (Alzheimer's Association, 2014, p. 16). The number of cases in the population doubles every 5 years of age after age 60 and is becoming a public health crisis as the "baby boomer" generation ages. Affective disorders include major depression and manic-depressive or bipolar illness. Although bipolar illness may affect only a small proportion of the population, major depression is pervasive and is the leading cause of disability among adults ages 15 to 44. Anxiety disorders, including panic disorder, obsessive-compulsive disorder, post-traumatic stress disorder (PTSD), and phobias, are prevalent, affecting 18% of American adults each year. Mental disorders can also be a secondary problem among people with other disabilities. Depression and anxiety, for example, occur more frequently among people with disabilities (NIMH, 2014).

The impact of mental illness on overall health and productivity in the United States and throughout the world is often underrecognized. In the United States, mental illness causes about the same amount of disability as heart disease and cancer. Depression is a leading cause of years of productivity loss because of disability in the United States and globally (Raviola et al, 2011; WHO, 2008b, 2012). Despite the prevalence of mental illness, only one third of persons with a mental disorder obtain help for their illness in any part of the health care system, and the majority of persons with mental disorders do not receive any specialty mental health care. Although 65% of persons with the most serious mental illnesses received treatment in 2011, 35% did not (SAMHSA, 2013). Of young people ages 4 to 17 years who have a mental disorder, 60% received help through private or community-based providers and 40% through schools (USDHHS, 2009). The World Health Organization (2008b) reports the global burden of mental health, substance abuse, and neurological diseases at 14% and noted that depression is the main cause of illness and disability in adolescents worldwide (WHO, 2014). In recognition of the lack of resources, the WHO launched a mental health global action program (mhGAP) to begin to address these needs (WHO, 2008a). Their poster "No Health Without Mental Health" effectively describes the need to integrate physical and mental health services. Given this information, it is critical that nurses recognize and provide health services for those with mental disorders in a variety of nontraditional community settings.

In addition to diagnosable mental conditions, there is growing awareness and concern about the public health burden of stress, especially after terrorist attacks at home and around the world; natural disasters such as hurricanes, tsunamis, tornados, and earthquakes; and human-made disasters. Strengthening the public health sector to respond to these events involves developing community mental health responses as well as addressing physical health concerns. Community mental health nurses (CMHNs) play an important role in identifying stressful events, assessing stress responses, educating communities, and intervening to prevent or alleviate disability and disease resulting from stress.

Although all of us are vulnerable to stressful life events and may develop mental health problems, persons with chronic and persistent mental illness have numerous problems. Mental illness is misunderstood, and those who suffer from it often experience stigma and lack of social support, which is so critical to health. Persons with mental illness are often identified by the illness as a schizophrenic instead of a person with the disease of schizophrenia. The disruptive symptoms of this illness often occur just as young persons are attempting to finish schooling and develop a career, shattering lives and driving many into a lifetime of underemployment, poverty, and lack of access to adequate health services, housing, and social supports. Many accessible and coordinated services are needed to enable that people with chronic mental illness live in the community, yet these often are not available. Despite the inadequacy of resources, advances have been made in the treatment of mental illness. Two major movements have influenced these advances: consumer advocacy and better understanding of the neurobiology of mental illness (May, 2011; Pandya and Jän Myrick, 2013; Parry, 2010). Naturally, the financing of mental health services affects access to care and influences treatment. The system known as managed care has significantly affected service delivery for the past 25 years, and passage of mental health parity and national health care reform through the Patient Protection and Affordable Health Care Act will undoubtedly influence mental health care during the next decade (Mechanic, 2012; Pearlman, 2013).

## Consumer Advocacy

Consumer advocacy movements for people with mental illness, like those for other illnesses, came about to fulfill unmet needs and to attempt to decrease the stigma associated with mental illness. Specifically, the National Alliance for the Mentally Ill (NAMI) was the first consumer group to advocate for better services. This consumer advocacy group worked to establish education and self-help services for individuals and families with mental illness. Efforts of the NAMI gained momentum in the early 1980s. Subsequently, political groups and legislative bodies responded with direct support. One example of direct support was funding for the Community Support Program (CSP) by the National Institute of Mental Health (NIMH). The CSP provided grant monies to states to develop comprehensive services for persons discharged from psychiatric institutions and invited consumers to participate. These and similar efforts have helped bring consumers, families, and professionals together to work toward improvement in the treatment and care of persons with mental illness.

## Neurobiology of Mental Illness

Mental illnesses are complex biopsychosocial disorders. Considerable emphasis in the past 20 years has focused on the biological basis of mental illness. The 1990s were declared the "decade of the brain" as advances in research in neurology, microbiology, and genetics led to understanding the structural and chemical complexity of the brain. Consequently, more is now known about the functions of the brain than at any time in history. We have learned that the brain is not a static organ. The concept of brain plasticity demonstrates that new learning actually changes brain structure. For example, traumatic experiences change brain biochemistry, as do significant positive experiences (May, 2011). This information supports the thought that both experience and psychosocial factors have effects on the etiology and on the treatment of mental illnesses. Both somatic and psychosocial interventions need to be used to treat mental illness. In addition to research, neuroradiological techniques aid diagnosis and treatment of people with psychiatric disorders. Angiography is used to screen for abnormalities of the vascular system, such as atherosclerosis and brain tumors, that can lead to behavior changes. The use of noninvasive scanning of the brain can help in making diagnoses. Computed axial tomography (CAT) scans provide a cross-sectional view of the brain, whereas nuclear magnetic resonance (NMR) imaging offers the advantage of imaging the brain from different planes. Still other techniques, such as positron emission tomography (PET) and single-photon emission computed tomography (SPECT), provide information about cerebral blood flow and brain metabolism. The information gained from these advanced technologies can lead to better understanding about mental illness and treatment and help scientists study the effects of psychotherapeutic interventions on the brain. Discoveries in psychopharmacology have also revolutionized the treatment of mental illness. New, atypical antipsychotic drugs used in the treatment of schizophrenia can improve the quality of life for many, primarily because of fewer side effects. For example, side effects of antipsychotic drugs include central and peripheral nervous system manifestations. Newer second-generation antipsychotics have reduced some of these side effects but new adverse effects, including weight gain, insulin resistance, and dangerously high blood glucose levels, collectively known as metabolic syndrome, have created fresh concerns for consumers and providers (Pramyothin and Kaodihiar, 2010). Although psychopharmacology has dramatically improved the lives of people with severe mental illness, controversies exist about the costs of monitoring treatment. Newer antidepressant medications known as selective serotonin reuptake inhibitors (SSRIs) are now considered the first choice in the treatment of depression as well as for many anxiety disorders because they lead to good responses with fewer side effects. They are now widely prescribed by primary care physicians as well as psychiatrists and are some of the most prescribed medications in the United States. Although considered safer than older agents, evidence suggests that the SSRIs may accelerate bone loss, leading to osteoporosis, and they may not be more effective than nonpharmacological interventions, such as exercise, in treating depression (Eom et al, 2012). Future directions suggest the science of pharmacogenetics will enable more individualized treatment of mental illness based on specific, genetically based responses to pharmaceuticals (Preskorn, 2010).

## SYSTEMS OF COMMUNITY MENTAL HEALTH CARE

### Managed Care

Managed care is a system of managing health care to ensure access to appropriate and cost-effective services. Managed mental health care grew rapidly during the 1990s, and by 1999 nearly 80% of Americans were enrolled in a managed health care plan. Initially a method to control costs and access to mental health care in the private insurance sector, managed care became a significant factor in public mental health, and by the turn of the century more than half of all Medicaid recipients were enrolled in a managed mental health care plan (Mechanic, 2008). Consumer outcomes such as health status, quality of life, functioning, and satisfaction are considerations in deciding whether services are effective.

Because one purpose of managed care was to control costs, often by substituting less costly services for more costly ones, the findings about consumer outcomes become critical. The provision of quality comprehensive services needed by persons with serious and persistent mental illness in the community is not inexpensive, but it is generally less costly than hospital care and frequent admissions. Services must fit the needs of the consumer, and outcomes research and consumer satisfaction can help guide care and policy decisions.

Changes continue to take place in mental health funding, and changes in one sector can have far-reaching consequences in many others. Although legislation was passed in 1996 ensuring parity for mental illness coverage in insurance plans, the implementation at the state level and the effects on insurance plans had been rather negligible for a variety of reasons, and further legislation passed in 2008 was needed to improve service access (Mental Health America, 2009).

The seemingly constant changes in mental health funding present challenges for nurses, who need to make judgments about the positive and negative outcomes of these changes on the people they care for before research findings that can be generalized to the population are readily available.

### Patient Protection and Affordable Health Care Act

The Patient Protection and Affordable Health Care Act (ACA, passed in 2010) affects both access to and funding of mental health services and will increase the need for community mental health nurses at the general and advanced practice levels (Mechanic, 2012; Pearlman, 2013). The ACA will ensure access to mental health services for 27 million more Americans who had no coverage and an additional 35.5 million who will have new or improved mental health services added to existing coverage (Pearlman, 2013). Preventive mental health services, such as depression and behavioral screening, are now required to be offered free of charge, and integration of mental health services into primary care is mandated (USDHHS, 2014). The ACA removes economic and geographic barriers and helps remove the stigma of mental illness through routine screening and treatment within a primary care visit. It is expected that earlier detection and treatment of mental health and substance abuse conditions will occur, thus improving the mental health of the population (Busch et al, 2013). Such a major change in the manner in which services are provided along with the expected increase in the number of people seeking mental health care will lead to new challenges and opportunities in the delivery of care.

### Mental Health Services

Mental health problems and mental disorders are treated by a variety of caregivers who work in diverse and loosely connected facilities. The landmark surgeon general's report on mental health, in an attempt to delineate where Americans receive mental health services, defined four major ways through which people receive assistance: (1) the specialty mental health system, both public and private, (2) the general medical or primary care sector, (3) the human service sector, and (4) the voluntary support network, including advocacy groups (USDHHS, 1999). Nurses need to understand that delivery of mental health services may occur in any of these systems. In fact, most older adults receive mental health services through the primary care sector, whereas most children and adolescents are served through human services that include schools. Those with resources, less severe mental health problems, and access to primary care are more likely to have their mental health needs addressed within the context of a visit to their primary care provider. Because of the influence of managed care, access to a specialist, if indicated for psychiatric treatment, has occurred via this route as well. The Patient Protection and Affordable Health Care Act passed in 2010 now mandates mental health screening and initiation of treatment in primary care and may have a significant effect on where mental health services are received (Mechanic, 2012; Pearlman, 2013).

The community mental health model is the primary method of care for people with serious and persistent mental illness. Components of this model include team care, case management, outreach, and a variety of rehabilitative and recovery approaches to help prevent exacerbations of illness. In most states, services are provided through comprehensive community mental health centers (CMHCs). There is great variance in how each state and locality implements mental health service delivery and each version continues to evolve in this era of health care reform, as the CMHCs react to societal, political, and fiscal pressures. As resources diminish, the focus narrows and many CMHCs are unable to provide services to populations other than those with serious and persistent mental illness. It is unclear how the growing focus on integration of mental health into primary care, parity in insurance coverage, and the passage of national health care reform might impact the community mental health system of care, but it is hoped that it will lead to more comprehensive, integrated, and less fragmented services (Garfield et al, 2011; Mechanic, 2012).

# EVOLUTION OF COMMUNITY MENTAL HEALTH CARE

## Historical Perspectives

How the community has perceived the etiology of mental and emotional illness across the ages has influenced the care and treatment of persons suffering from these disorders. These patterns were often cyclical. In ancient times, mental illness was viewed as resulting from supernatural forces, and those afflicted were sometimes shunned. During the Greco-Roman era, mental and physical illnesses were seen as interrelated and resulting from physical conditions. Treatment was aimed at curing the disease by restoring balance. A return to a belief in supernatural etiologies occurred during the Middle Ages in Europe and continued in the years in which the United States was being formed into a country. These beliefs led to poor treatment of the mentally ill, including incarceration, starvation, and torture. Near

the end of the eighteenth century, the revolution in mental health care known as Humanitarian Reform took place. This reform movement, influenced by Philippe Pinel (1759-1820) in France and Benjamin Rush (1745-1813) in North America, led to hospital expansion, medical treatment, and the community mental health movements (Boyd, 2011).

Before the Humanitarian Reform, persons with mental illness were often housed in jails because health and social services had not been developed. Even later, after the development of hospitals as a site of treatment, persons with mental disorders were neglected and mistreated. Although the first psychiatric hospital in the United States was built in Williamsburg, Virginia, in 1773, approximately 50 years passed before widespread construction of facilities in other states took place. One person in particular, Dorothea Dix, led reform efforts to correct inhumane practices (Boyd, 2011).

Dorothea Lynde Dix (1802-1887) focused attention on criminals, those with mental disorders, and victims of the Civil War. She believed that people with mental disorders needed health and social services, and her efforts influenced the improved organization of mental health services. Her work led to the development of hospitals as the primary site of care, and she influenced standards for hospital administration and nursing care. Because of her lifetime efforts, often through political action, treatment for mentally infirm persons was altered in both North America and Europe (Boyd, 2011).

## Hospital Expansion, Institutionalization, and the Mental Hygiene Movement

Psychiatric hospitals constructed during the expansion era were located in rural areas and were intended for small numbers of clients. However, they soon became overcrowded with people who had severe mental disorders, with older adults, and with immigrants who were poor and unable to speak English. Clients were essentially separated from the community and isolated from their families. Many were institutionalized for the rest of their lives, in response to both a continued fear of persons with mental disorders and a lack of community resources. Institutionalization of large numbers of people, combined with minimal information about cause, cure, and care, resulted in overcrowded conditions and exploitation of clients.

At the beginning of the twentieth century, institutional conditions were reported publicly in the United States by Clifford Beers, who had been hospitalized both in private and in public mental hospitals (Parry, 2010). Beers urged reform and influenced the founding of the National Committee for Mental Hygiene. During the mental hygiene movement, attention shifted to ideas about prevention, early intervention, and the influence of social and environmental factors on mental illness. These ideas about treatment also influenced the development of multidisciplinary approaches to treatment. The mental hygiene and community mental health movements increased understanding about mental illness.

Further understanding about the scope of mental illness was gained during the conscription process for the armed services in World War II. Many of the persons screened for military service during World War II were found to have neurological and psychiatric mental health disorders. Even more military personnel required treatment for mental health problems associated with social and environmental stress during and after the war, not only in the United States but also in Europe, Russia, and Pacific Rim countries (Boyd, 2011). At the same time, the community mental health model continued to expand slowly while populations consisting of individuals with severe mental disorders and older adult persons with dementia grew larger in the state hospitals. Demands for mental health services in communities, combined with concerns about conditions of state psychiatric hospitals, prompted federal legislation that influenced development of the community mental health concept.

## Federal Legislation for Mental Health Services

The first major piece of legislation to influence mental health services in the United States was the Social Security Act in 1935. This act, created in response to economic and social problems of the era, shifted the responsibility of care for ill people from the state to the federal government. The federal government's role expanded when the demand for mental health services increased during and after World War II. Key points of legislation that influenced the development of community mental health services are summarized in Table 36-1.

In 1946 the National Mental Health Act was passed and the National Institute of Mental Health (NIMH) administered its programs. Objectives included development of education and research programs for community mental health treatment approaches. The act also included financial incentives for training grants to increase the number of professional workers, including nurses, in mental health services. Education and research programs materialized readily, along with advances in

science and technology and the development of psychotropic medications. In 1955 the Mental Health Study Act was passed, and the Joint Commission on Mental Illness and Health was established by the NIMH. Members of the commission studied national mental health needs and submitted to Congress a report entitled *Action for Mental Health.* Recommendations of the report included continued development of research and education programs, early and intensive treatment for acute mental illness, and shifting the care of severely mentally ill persons away from the large hospitals to psychiatric wards in general hospitals and to community mental health clinics. Along with prevention and intervention, community services were to include aftercare services following hospitalization for individuals with major mental illness (Boyd, 2011). The shift in the locus of care from state hospitals to community systems was begun.

The Community Mental Health Centers Act was passed in 1963, and the CMHC concept was formalized. Federal funds were designated to match state funds to construct CMHCs and start-up programs. CMHCs were mandated to have five basic services: inpatient, outpatient, partial hospitalization, 24-hour emergency services, and consultation/education services for community agencies and professionals. In addition, regulations encouraged states to offer diagnostic and rehabilitative precare and aftercare services (Boyd, 2011). However, many CMHCs, especially those in poor and rural areas, were unable to generate adequate money for continuing their start-up programs. Funding did not follow the client to the community. The deinstitutionalization of persons with severe mental disorders was well underway before some of these shortcomings were recognized.

## TABLE 36-1   Legislation That Influenced Community Mental Health Services

| Year | Legislation | Focus |
|---|---|---|
| 1946 | National Mental Health Act | Education and research for mental health treatment approaches began (NIMH) |
| 1955 | Mental Health Study Act | Resulted in Joint Commission on Mental Illness and Health, which recommended transformation of state hospital systems and establishment of community mental health clinics |
| 1963 | Community Mental Health Centers Act | Marked beginning of community mental health centers' concept and led to deinstitutionalization of large psychiatric hospitals |
| 1975 | Developmentally Disabled Assistance and Bill of Rights Act | Addressed the rights and treatment of people with developmental disabilities and provided foundation for similar action for individuals with mental disorders |
| 1977 | President's Commission on Mental Health | Reinforced importance of community-based services, protection of human rights, and national health insurance for mentally ill persons |
| 1981 | Omnibus Budget Reconciliation Act | Rescinded much of the 1977 commission's provisions and shifted funds for all health programs from federal to state resources |
| 1986 | Protection and Advocacy for Individuals with Mental Illness Act | Legislated advocacy programs for mentally ill persons |
| 1990 | Americans with Disabilities Act | Prohibited discrimination and promoted opportunities for persons with mental disorders |
| 1996 | Mental Health Parity Act | Attempted to address discrepancy between mental health and medical-surgical benefits in employer-sponsored health plans |
| 2008 | Mental Health and Addiction Equity Act | Prohibits discrepancy in coverage between mental health and physical health benefits in employer-sponsored and private insurance plans and added substance abuse as a covered mental health condition |
| 2010 | Patient Protection and Affordable Health Care Act | Prohibits discrimination in coverage for preexisting conditions. Prohibits discontinuation of coverage because of illness |

# DEINSTITUTIONALIZATION

Deinstitutionalization involved transitioning large numbers of people from state psychiatric hospitals to communities. The cost of institutional care was perhaps the main reason for the movement; other influences included the discovery of psychotropic medications and civil rights activism (Boyd, 2011). The goal of deinstitutionalization was to improve the quality of life for people with mental disorders by providing services in the communities where they lived rather than in large institutions. To change the locus of care, large hospital wards were closed and persons with severe mental disorders were returned to the community to live. Many were discharged to the care of family members; others went to nursing homes. Still others were placed in apartments or other types of adult housing; some of these were supervised settings, and others were not.

Not surprisingly, as with any abrupt, dramatic change, problems related to unexpected service gaps between the hospitals and the CMHCs led to continuity-of-care problems. Although deinstitutionalization was a noble idea, there were not adequate resources to support the implementation. For example, families were not prepared for the treatment responsibilities they had to assume, and yet few mental health systems offered them education and support programs. Although many older adult clients were admitted to nursing homes and personal care settings, education programs were seldom available for staff members, who often lacked the skills necessary to treat persons with mental disorders. And finally, some clients found themselves in independent settings such as rooming houses and single-room occupancy hotels with little or no supervision and few skills to manage living in the community. Clients, families, communities, and the nation suffered as poor living and social conditions were associated with mental disorders. Homelessness and placement of the mentally ill in jails and prisons also occurred. These conditions may have increased the stigma associated with persons with mental illness. The placement of persons with mental illness in nursing homes, assisted living facilities, and jails was often referred to as "reinstitutionalization," because it only shifted people from one institution to another. These issues prompted additional legislation and advocacy efforts.

## Civil Rights Legislation for Persons with Mental Disorders

The development of CMHCs was based partially on the principle that persons with mental disorders had a right to treatment in the least restrictive environment (Boyd, 2011). Although CMHCs were less restrictive than institutions, they lacked necessary services. For example, people with severe mental disorders require daily monitoring or hospitalization during acute episodes of illness. Even though hospital services were available, many individuals expressed their rights to refuse treatment and resisted admission. Also, transitional care after discharge for those persons who were admitted to hospitals was not available in most communities. In addition to the right to refuse treatment, advocates for mentally ill individuals focused on such civil rights issues as segregated services, inhumane practices in psychiatric hospitals, and failure to include clients in treatment planning. Activism for minorities and handicapped persons also influenced civil rights legislation for persons with mental disorders. In particular, during the 1970s institutional conditions of persons with developmental handicaps prompted passage of the Developmentally Disabled Assistance and Bill of Rights Act. Other legislation shifted funding from the federal to the state level. The Mental Health Systems Act, was passed in 1980 to improve mental health services. However, in 1981 when Ronald Reagan took office, the Act was repeated in 1981 and replaced with a block grant program reducing the involvement of the federal government (Mechanic, 2007). This action limited the federal leadership role, shifted more costs back to the states from the federal government, and further impeded the implementation and provision of community mental health services.

State systems of mental health services developed in unique and diverse ways and were often inadequate. In general, individuals with severe mental disorders were vulnerable and neglected and either lacked or were unable to access health and social services. In an effort to offset these problems, in 1986 the federal Protection and Advocacy for Individuals with Mental Illness Act and the State Comprehensive Mental Health Services Plan Act of 1986 were passed. Advocacy programs for mentally ill persons became part of the same state advocacy systems developed earlier under the Developmental Disabled Assistance and Bill of Rights Act, and consumer involvement in CMHCs was mandated (Boyd, 2011). In spite of advocacy efforts and legislation, the CMHCs were unable to meet the increased and diverse demands for mental health services in their communities. The lack of services, combined with concerns about discrimination against all people with disabilities, led to additional legislation.

The Americans with Disabilities Act (ADA) was passed in 1990. The ADA mandated that individuals with mental and physical disabilities must not be discriminated against and must be brought into the mainstream of American life through access to employment and public services (Boyd, 2011). History reveals that past legislation promoted the rights of persons with mental disorders, but litigation was also responsible for the lack of growth, if not the decline, in community mental health services. In 1996 the Mental Health Parity Act was passed to address discrimination in insurance coverage and in 2008 the Mental Health Parity and Addiction Equity Act (MHPAEA) was passed, prohibiting differential coverage for mental health disorders (Mental Health America, 2009). The community mental health nurse can advocate for clients to ensure equality in access to health services, housing, and employment.

## Advocacy Efforts

Consumers or survivors, defined as persons who are current or former recipients of mental health services, along with their families have had a significant impact on mental health services. As in all areas of health care, the rights and wishes of consumers are important in planning and delivering services. However, consumers of mental health services have traditionally had difficulty advocating for themselves. In the past, treatment programs often fostered passivity in clients and excluded them from the treatment planning process. In addition, family members were responsible for care in the home, but they lacked resources and even information about treatment (Riesser and Schorske, 2013). Like consumers, family members suffered from the stigma of mental illness and public attitudes that contributed to self-advocacy problems. In contrast, self-advocacy and involvement in treatment planning fosters self-confidence, promotes participation in services, and may have a significant influence on policy decisions (Marchinko and Clark, 2011; Tierney and Kane, 2011). Consumer and family groups fostered these objectives.

Family members led self-advocacy efforts in the 1970s, when small groups organized to challenge and change mental health services. These early efforts resulted in the formation of the National Alliance for the Mentally Ill (NAMI), which today has both state and local affiliates. Soon, consumer groups formed to advocate for better services, changes in mental health policy, self-help programs in treatment, and empowerment. Several advocacy groups that support these consumer efforts are summarized in Box 36-1. In their assessment of resources, nurses can identify community advocacy and support groups.

## CONCEPTUAL FRAMEWORKS FOR COMMUNITY MENTAL HEALTH

The community mental health principles that are the underpinnings of practice include the right to mental health services delivered in the least restrictive environment, consumer involvement in treatment, advocacy, and rehabilitative and recovery services. Biopsychosocial theories are useful to understand the multidimensional aspects of community mental health nursing. These include theories and models that explain biological processes, systems, personality, life span development, family dynamics, and

stress and coping. Focusing on wellness or recovery, relapse prevention, or relapse management and helping the client reach a maximal level of function are useful for nursing practice.

Another helpful framework for community mental health practice is systems theory, which emphasizes the relationship between the elements of a unit and the whole. An understanding of the whole occurs through the examination of interactions and relationships that exist between the parts. A holistic view of system and subsystems can be applied in a variety of ways in community mental health practice. One example of a subsystem in a community is its cultural groups. Subsystems of the cultural groups are families; subsystems of the families are individuals. Using systems theory to explore the background, conditions, and context of situations will disclose information about the positive and negative forces that either promote or undermine the well-being of any unit in the system.

The diathesis-stress model is also useful in CMHN practice. This theory integrates the effects of biology and environment, or nature and nurture, on the development of mental illness. Certain genes or genetic combinations produce a predisposition to a disorder. When an environmental stressor challenges a predisposition to a disorder, the mental disorder may be expressed (Edmondson et al, 2014; Liu and Alloy, 2010). The integration of psychosocial and neurobiological paradigms is critical to the practice of psychiatric nursing. Nurses must recognize the effects of environment and biology on people and actively work to mitigate psychosocial as well as biological stressors through teaching strategies to promote mental health and reduce stress.

### Levels of Prevention

Health promotion and illness prevention are fundamental to community mental health practice as well as to national objectives for mental health (USDHHS, 2010). Therefore, the concepts of primary, secondary, and tertiary levels of prevention are useful in community mental health practice (see Levels of Prevention box).

Primary prevention refers to the reduction of health risks. It involves both health promotion and disease prevention. Health promotion strategies aim to enhance the well-being of healthy populations, whereas disease prevention strategies focus on the identification of populations at risk and conditions that may cause stress and illness. Providing education about stress reduction techniques to adults in the workplace is a form of mental health promotion. An example of disease prevention is to provide mental health information about depression and eating disorders to adolescents in schools.

Secondary prevention activities are aimed at reducing the prevalence or pathological nature of a condition. They involve early diagnosis, prompt treatment, and limitation of disability. Many functions of the practitioner role are aimed at secondary prevention for individuals. These include providing individual and group psychotherapy, case management, and referral. Screening members of a community for depression during National Depression Screening Day is an example of population-based secondary prevention. Counseling, referral, and treatment interventions after traumatic incidents, such as terrorist attacks or natural disasters, are other important community interventions.

Tertiary prevention efforts attempt to restore and enhance functioning. On a community level, tertiary prevention activities might include support of affordable housing, promotion of psychosocial rehabilitation and recovery programs, and involvement in advocacy and consumer groups for persons with mental illness. Many nursing role activities in community mental health are aimed at tertiary prevention with individuals. They include working with individuals to monitor illness symptoms and treatment responses, coordinating transition from the hospital to the community, and identifying respite care options for caregivers.

Relapse management with a focus on recovery is central to many of the programs and activities that enhance coping skills and competence. The nurse may participate in assertive community treatment (ACT) programs, psychosocial rehabilitation (clubhouses), and intensive case management. ACT programs differ from intensive case management approaches in that they are based more on a medical model and team approach and provide crisis and case management services 24 hours a day, 7 days a week. They are sometimes referred to as hospitals without walls (Salyers and Tsemberis, 2008). Intensive case management models vary across programs but generally include contact with clients several times a week by an individual case manager. Nurses have critical roles in both treatment programs, as they have the knowledge and skills to provide comprehensive biopsychosocial care.

For example, the nurse visits the client at home, checks medication, assesses physical and emotional functioning, and may take the client shopping for nutritional food. The nurse may accompany the consumer to the physician's office and serve as an advocate for the client in this setting.

As case managers, nurses work with consumers, family members, and other caregivers to foster coping and competency aimed at managing illness symptoms. The goal of managing illness symptoms is to offset relapse and promote recovery. Relapse management and promotion of recovery are major goals of intervention in community mental health nursing. Assessment of the frequency, intensity, and duration of symptoms for the purpose of identifying biological, environmental, and behavioral triggers that may lead to illness relapse helps the consumer manage the illness and promotes recovery. Examples of triggers are poor nutrition, poor social skills, hopelessness, and poor symptom management. Once triggers are identified, interventions aimed at fostering effective coping skills can be introduced to offset relapse of symptoms. For example, an intervention that may promote effective coping to offset social isolation is to guide the client to organized consumer group activities available in the community. Another is to promote consumer and family efforts at job training through community vocational agencies. Still another is to promote competency in family members by coordinating services that enhance their understanding of the illness, provide social support, and include respite care when needed. Finally, an alliance with the client to manage medication and side effects is an important component of relapse prevention and recovery promotion (Baker et al, 2013).

As previously discussed, scientific advances that led to the use of medications to treat mental illness revolutionized mental health care and services. Atypical antipsychotics and new antidepressants with fewer side effects have further influenced mental health care in the community. Although these new drugs have dramatically improved the lives of many people with mental disorders, they are not without problems and are not a cure. The nurse has a critical role in monitoring side effects, detecting related health problems such as diabetes, and providing education and intervention. The most effective tertiary prevention is to combine medications with other relapse management approaches including culturally sensitive social, behavioral, and psychotherapeutic interventions (Segal et al, 2010; Sterling et al, 2010).

## LEVELS OF PREVENTION
### In Community Mental Health

**Primary Prevention**
- Educate populations about mental health issues.
- Teach stress reduction techniques.
- Support and provide prenatal education.
- Provide parenting classes.
- Provide support to caregivers.
- Provide bereavement support.

**Secondary Prevention**
- Conduct screenings to detect mental health disorders.
- Provide mental health interventions after stressful events.

**Tertiary Prevention**
- Provide health promotion activities to persons with serious and persistent mental illness.
- Promote support group participation for those with mental health disabilities.
- Advocate for rehabilitation and recovery services.

## ROLE OF THE NURSE IN COMMUNITY MENTAL HEALTH

The role of the nurse in community mental health was shaped both by the evolution of services and by the work of nursing pioneers. Development of a knowledge base for the nursing discipline and the further expansion of mental health care services to nontraditional community sites called for more advanced community-based practitioners (American Academy of Nursing, 2012). Nursing practice standards reflect the values of the profession, describe the responsibilities of nurses, and provide direction for the delivery and evaluation of nursing care. These standards also describe the roles of nurses in both advanced and basic practice.

Advanced practice psychiatric nurses have graduate-level education. The psychiatric nurse practitioner title and role have been expanded to encompass primary care and specialty knowledge and skills. They provide primary, secondary, and tertiary care to individuals, groups, families, adults, children, and adolescents. Depending on state laws, some prescribe medications and have hospital admission privileges. For example, the advanced practice nurse may see clients individually to provide psychotherapy, may prescribe medications, and may conduct physical examinations or coordinate this care with other providers in primary care settings. The blended nurse practitioner role has been a response to a shift in the health care system away from specialization and toward comprehensive services that address both physical and mental health problems.

Nurses prepared at the undergraduate level provide basic primary, secondary, and tertiary services that are equally valuable. Specific roles and functions of both mental health and community nurses at the basic level (Box 36-2) are based on clinical nursing practice and standards (American Nurses Association [ANA], 2013, 2014). The functions suggest the overlapping roles of clinician, educator, and coordinator.

## Clinician

Objectives of the practitioner role are to help the client maintain or regain coping abilities that promote functioning. This involves using the nursing process to guide the diagnosis and treatment of human responses to actual or potential mental health problems (ANA, 2014). Role functions at the basic practitioner level include case management, counseling, milieu therapy, and psychobiological interventions with individuals and with groups. Clinician skills are used with individual clients in a variety of settings, including the home, and often with large groups of people in specific neighborhoods, schools, and public health districts. For example, many clients who have schizophrenia live in personal care homes. These clients require biopsychosocial interventions related to medication management, milieu management for improved social interaction, and

assistance with self-care activities for community living such as use of public transportation. Also, the practitioner increasingly coordinates these activities with both the consumer and other staff members in community settings. Therefore, coordination of care is often the means for promoting recovery plan outcomes and enhancing quality of life for clients. These activities can support positive outcomes for others in the community at large.

For example, family members are a primary support system for individuals with schizophrenia. Whether the client lives in a personal care home, a family residence, or another setting, counseling family members and the client about the illness may offset the stressors of caregiving. Moreover, educating the public may reduce the stigma and decrease social isolation for both clients and families, lead to public support for needed services, and decrease the costs of health care because of fewer hospitalizations. As suggested in these examples, clinician and educator roles overlap.

## Educator

The educator role uses teaching/learning principles to increase understanding about mental illness and mental health. The educator role is foundational to health maintenance, health promotion, and community action. Teaching clients about illness symptoms and the benefits of medications promotes health maintenance and may reduce the risk for illness relapse. Research supports similar education programs for family members to increase their ability to monitor illness symptoms and to identify events that lead to relapse (Sveinbjarnardottir et al, 2013). The nurse may facilitate a combined support and education group for parents of children with schizophrenia or for consumers with major mental illness in weekly sessions at the community mental health center. As seen in Figure 36-1 the CMHN, both at the basic and at the advanced level, may participate in developing educational groups and programs for consumers, families, and other providers either alone or in collaboration with other organizations such as the local affiliate of Mental Health America or the National Alliance for the Mentally Ill. The nurse may also teach clients primary prevention skills such as parenting as shown in Figure 36-2.

At the community level, both formal and informal teaching is important. One important objective for mental health

---

### BOX 36-2    Roles and Functions in Psychiatric/Mental Health Nursing Community Practice

**Roles**
- Clinician
- Educator
- Coordinator

**Functions**
- Advocacy
- Case finding and referral
- Case management
- Community action and involvement
- Complementary interventions
- Counseling
- Crisis intervention
- Health maintenance
- Health promotion
- Health teaching
- Home visits
- Intake screening and evaluation
- Milieu therapy
- Promotion of self-care activities
- Psychiatric rehabilitation and recovery
- Psychobiological interventions

Modified from American Nurses Association, American Psychiatric Nurses Association, and International Society of Psychiatric Mental Health Nurses: Scope and standards of psychiatric-mental health nursing, Washington, DC, 2007, American Nurses Publishing.

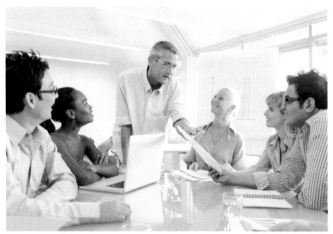

FIG 36-1 Nurse educator teaching a small group of clients. (Rawpixel Ltd, #489081731, iStock, Thinkstock)

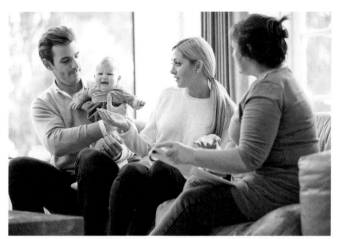

FIG 36-2 Nurse teaching a young couple parenting skills. (Monkey Business Images, #466375791, iStock, Thinkstock)

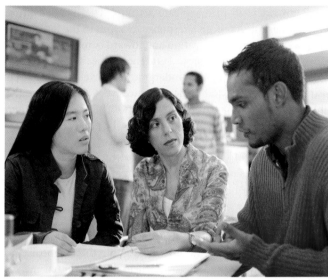

FIG 36-3 Interdisciplinary mental health planning team meeting. (Digital Vision, #200297936-001, Photodisc, Thinkstock)

promotion is to teach positive coping skills. Overmedicating is an example of an ineffective individual coping skill. Even when medications are properly used in treatment, the nurse requires specialized knowledge about drug interactions, pharmacokinetics, and pharmacodynamics. Factors that influence pharmacokinetics include anatomical and physiological changes that occur with aging or with coexisting mental and physical conditions. Use of nonprescription medications such as herbal remedies and over-the-counter drugs can influence pharmacokinetics. Because over one third of Americans use nontraditional remedies and many of these are specific for psychiatric conditions, nurses need to assess the use of these substances, be aware of interactions, and share this information with clients (Barnes et al, 2008). For example, people may use herbal remedies such as ginkgo biloba to improve memory, valerian to improve sleep, and St. John's wort to treat depression.

## Coordinator

Coordination of care is a basic principle of the multidisciplinary team approach in community mental health services. Yet there is often a lack of coordination as well as limited services in many communities. Therefore, at a minimum, the role of coordinator must include case finding, referral, and follow-up to evaluate system breakdown and deficits. Because of current system deficits, nurses in community mental health function as coordinators who carry out intake screening, crisis intervention, and home visits. The nurse coordinator also tries to improve the client's health and well-being by promoting independence and self-care in the least restrictive environment. For example, the nurse may teach the client how to fill a medication box or how to use relaxation techniques to reduce stress. Health teaching related to nutrition, smoking cessation, and sleep promotion is essential for consumers with mental illness. These functions are consistent with descriptions of clinical case management that emphasize continuity of care for individuals who need complex services and with providing information for recovery (Caldwell et al, 2010).

To achieve these objectives and improve services, nurses work with a variety of professionals, including advanced practice nurses, social workers, physicians, psychologists, occupational and vocational therapists, and rehabilitation counselors

(Figure 36-3). The nurse is often the advocate for the consumer who needs assistance making his or her needs clear and accessing both health and social services. Because nonlicensed paraprofessionals are frequently involved in direct care activities, their services must be directed, coordinated, and evaluated within the context of treatment planning. Finally, coordination also involves work with individuals who may not have formal preparation but who are essential for positive treatment outcomes. These individuals include family members, shelter volunteers, consumer support groups, and community leaders who can influence development of services. For example, the nurse can teach others about mental illness and effective interventions for times when symptoms become apparent and behaviors become difficult to manage. In the coordinator role, nurses can identify and influence health system effectiveness and ineffectiveness. To assist clients in accessing community resources and services, it is as important to develop positive relationships with other community providers as it is with clients.

## CURRENT AND FUTURE PERSPECTIVES IN MENTAL HEALTH CARE

Both nationally and internationally, too few mental health care services exist, and the available services are fragmented and often difficult to access. In the United States, large segments of the population do not have basic health care services or insurance to cover both expected and unexpected illnesses. The Patient Protection and Affordable Health Care Act passed in 2010 aims to close some of the gaps in coverage and as of March 31, 2014, an additional 8 million people had enrolled in an insurance plan. Because health insurance coverage for most Americans is linked to employment, in an economic recession when jobs are lost, insurance is often lost as well, and people are no longer able to afford health care. Also, consumers, family members, and health care providers are concerned about issues of basic treatment, continuity of care, housing, and costs for acute and long-term mental health services for persons with mental illness. As large numbers of baby boomers reach retirement age and Medicare eligibility, there is concern about whether Social Security and Medicare resources will continue to exist for older Americans. Declining state budgets and possible cuts in Medicaid funding may place community mental health services in peril. Therefore, implementation of health care reform continues to be a major political, social, and economic issue. Significant alterations in the current health care delivery system are occurring. Nurses working in communities must understand the models of care, the scope of mental illness, and the national health objectives designed to promote the health and welfare of persons with mental health problems.

Managed care and the Patient Protection and Affordable Health Care Act, as described previously, will continue to influence the delivery of mental health services. There will be a continued focus on providing services in primary care settings, attempts to reduce inpatient stays, and a more systematic evaluation of the outcomes of the care provided. The massive growth in managed care plans dramatically reduced hospital stays but also limited access to care. It is unclear how passage of national health care reform will affect the care of those with long-term care needs. Because the public mental health system is the only remaining state and federally supported treatment system for persons with serious and persistent mental disorders and Medicaid funds more than half of public mental health services, use of managed care approaches did not always provide for adequate services. The expansion of Medicaid through the ACA may improve access to mental health care for more people and improve delivery of services but could also strain systems not prepared for higher volumes of people. Differences in federal and state managed plans and services could create further barriers to care, leading to gaps in service and large holes in the safety net for vulnerable consumers suffering from mental illness.

Nurses can be important providers in community mental health because of their emphasis on wellness and health promotion, skills at teaching and case management, and lower cost for service. In communities, nurses practice primary, secondary, and tertiary prevention activities by conducting comprehensive client histories to determine health problems and interventions that improve quality of care and cost-effectiveness. In home health settings, nurses screen for ineffective coping techniques such as use of alcohol or other substances to offset the stress of traumatic life events, thereby preventing further problems and costly care. They also screen for signs of psychiatric disorders in primary care and community health care settings. Community mental health services must include access to work and school settings for families and children. These types of nursing assessments and subsequent interventions may offset costly treatment in hospital settings.

Providing the range of community services necessary to handle persistent mental illness is difficult without sufficient funds for health and social services. It is important for nurses and others working in CMHCs to recognize the impact of changes in funding, target populations, restructuring, and disagreements between professions, agencies, and levels of government. Such information enables nurses to advocate for adequate services to meet the needs of individuals with severe and persistent mental

illness. The nurse can build relationships with other providers, network with other agencies, and foster interagency collaboration to improve the quality of care for clients and their families.

## NATIONAL OBJECTIVES FOR MENTAL HEALTH SERVICES

The goals of the community mental health movement are consistent with the health promotion and disease prevention objectives outlined in *Healthy People 2020* (USDHHS, 2010). The *Healthy People 2020* box illustrates the primary objectives of the national health agenda for mental health promotion and illness prevention. The objectives of *Healthy People 2020* address both settings where people receive care (e.g., primary care, juvenile justice systems) and populations at risk (e.g., children, adults with mental illness, and older adults). Increasing cultural competency and consumer satisfaction with mental health services are further objectives of the national agenda for mental health.

The new millennium brought recognition of the importance of addressing mental health and mental illness as part of disease prevention. Recognition of the burden of mental illness and the status of mental health in the United States was clarified by a landmark report from the surgeon general's office, *Mental Health: A Report of the Surgeon General* (USDHHS, 1999), followed by a report from the Surgeon General's Conference on Children's Mental Health in 2000 (USDHHS, 2000). A national agenda for action described in *Healthy People 2010* and continued in *Healthy People 2020* (USDHHS, 2010) made mental health one of the 10 leading health indicators, which are chosen on the basis of relevance as a broad public health issue. The President's New Freedom Commission on Mental Health (2003) further highlighted the need to transform and heal system fragmentation to ensure access to quality mental health services. The goals of a transformed mental health system are found in Box 36-3.

Overall, the national goals of *Healthy People 2020* are to improve mental health and ensure access to quality and appropriate mental health services. Approaches emphasize prevention, maintenance, and restoration of mental health and independent functioning. The standards address mental health conditions of concern across the life span and with specific populations. Nurses can (1) promote the standards in the

### BOX 36-3 New Freedom Commission's Six Goals of a Transformed Mental Health System

1. Americans will understand that mental health is essential to overall health.
2. Mental health care will be consumer and family driven.
3. Disparities in mental health care will be eliminated.
4. Early mental health screening, assessment, and referral will be common practice.
5. Excellent mental health care will be delivered and research will be accelerated.
6. Technology will be used to access mental health care and information.

From President's New Freedom Commission on Mental Health: Achieving the promise: transforming mental health care in America, USDHHS Pub No SMA-03-3832, Rockville, MD, 2003, USDHHS.

agencies where they are employed, (2) use the standards in community assessment activities, and (3) introduce information about the standards to other groups and agencies, including local consumer and family organizations, to help prioritize mental health concerns. The following box lists selected objectives that pertain to mental health and mental disorders.

---

### ❤ HEALTHY PEOPLE 2020

#### *Examples of Targeted National Health Objectives for Mental Health and Mental Disorders*

Goal: Improve mental health and ensure access to appropriate, quality mental health services.
- MHMD-1: Reduce the suicide rate.
- MHMD-4: Reduce the proportion of persons who experience major depressive episode (MDE).
- MHMD-6: Increase the proportion of children with mental health problems who receive treatment.
- MHMD-9: Increase the proportion of adults with mental disorders who receive treatment.
- MHMD-10: Increase the proportion of persons with co-occurring substance abuse and mental disorders who receive treatment for both disorders.

From U.S. Department of Health and Human Services: Healthy People 2020 Objectives, Office of Disease Prevention and Health Promotion, Washington, DC, 2010, USDHHS

---

As indicated in the definitions at the beginning of this chapter, mental health is a dynamic process, influenced by both internal and external factors, that enables and promotes the individual's physical, cognitive, affective, and social functioning. In contrast, threats to mental health create stress that undermines relationships and diminishes the individual's ability to pursue and achieve life's goals. Values and beliefs influence the allocation of resources for neighborhoods and schools and can contribute to or undermine the mental health of people in communities.

Mental health problems are manifested in many ways. Untoward incidents or even anticipated life events can diminish physical, cognitive, affective, and social functioning. For example, in most situations, an anticipated or unexpected death of a family member results in grief that may temporarily interrupt the functioning of surviving family members and produce mental distress. Given adequate support and adaptation, most persons resume their lifestyles after the death of a loved one in spite of the sadness that they are likely to experience. When people do not have adequate resources, or when bereavement is complicated because of the conditions of the situation, there is an increased risk for threats to the mental health of surviving family members. Important interventions with individuals experiencing sorrow and grief are to encourage roles and activities that promote comfort and reduce isolation. Death of a family member can affect survivors of different ages in various ways. Infants and youths may be deprived of significant nurturing and care that will result in long-term emotional deficits, whereas adults are at increased risk for stress related to role changes, and older adults are vulnerable to social isolation as relatives and friends die. In any of these situations, individual or group therapy may be indicated not only for the immediate situation, but also for prevention of longer-term problems.

However, bereavement is not the only cause of diminished mental health. Other causes include, but are not limited to, physical health problems, disabilities resulting from trauma, exposure to violence in the neighborhood, job loss and unstable employment, and unanticipated environmental disasters that result in loss. Because multiple threats to mental health exist across the life span, it is useful to organize the study of problems according to life stages along life's continuum. The box that follows provides suggestions for how nurses can intervene following a community disaster.

---

**| HOW TO**  **Provide Interventions after Community Disasters**
*Community mental health nurses can intervene immediately after a mass trauma by using interventions that promote:*
- *A sense of safety*
- *Calming*
- *A sense of self and community efficacy*
- *Connectedness*
- *Hope*

*From Hobfoll SE, Watson P, Bell CC, et al: Five essential elements of immediate and mid-term mass trauma intervention: empirical evidence. Psychiatry 70:283–315, 2007.*

---

### Children and Adolescents

*Healthy People 2020* objectives aim to increase the number of children screened and treated for mental health problems. Children are at risk for disruption of normal development by biological, environmental, and psychosocial factors that impair their mental health, interfere with education and social interactions, and keep them from realizing their full potential as adults. For example, children may develop depression after a loss or behavior problems from abuse or neglect. Examples of environmental factors include crowded living conditions, violence, separation from parents, and lack of consistent caregivers. Exposure to community violence can be related to significant stress and depression in children (McClosky et al, 2008). Types of mental health problems typically diagnosed during childhood are depression, anxiety, and attention-deficit disorders. Examples of chronic disorders commonly seen are Down syndrome and autism. These problems affect growth and development and influence mental health during adolescence.

Suicide is the third leading killer of young persons between ages 15 and 24, and the second-leading cause of death in young adults, and in most cases there was a mental or substance abuse disorder (CDC, 2009, 2013). The second objective of *Healthy People 2020* is to reduce the rate of suicide attempts by adolescents. Some of the risk factors for both adolescents and adults include prior suicide attempts, stressful life events, and access to lethal methods. Increasing the number of adolescents screened for depression in primary health care settings is a new objective of *Healthy People 2020*. Early detection and treatment of depression can help prevent suicide. In addition to depression and substance abuse, adolescent problems include conduct disorders and eating disorders.

Another objective of *Healthy People 2020* is to reduce the proportion of adolescents with eating disorders. Many CMHNs do not directly work with persons with a primary eating disorder; eating disturbances often are a symptom accompanying other conditions. Because most children are not seen in the mental health system, an important role of the CMHN is to educate other community providers, teachers, parents, and children. School nurses are in an ideal position to provide primary, secondary, and tertiary interventions for children with eating disorders. Nutrition education and early recognition, intervention, referral, and follow-up can help prevent eating disorders from becoming severe and can prevent relapses. Nurses can advocate in and beyond their communities for the provision of a nurse in all schools. This can increase the chances of early recognition of and treatment for persons with eating disorders.

Effective service expansion for children, particularly for those with serious emotional disturbances, depends on promoting collaboration across critical areas of support including schools, families, social services, health, mental health, and juvenile justice. Better services and collaboration for children with serious emotional disturbance and their families will result in greater school retention, decreased contact with the juvenile justice system, increased stability of living arrangements, and improved educational, emotional, and behavioral development. One of the objectives of *Healthy People 2020* is to ensure that children in the juvenile justice system receive access to mental health assessment and treatment (USDHHS, 2010). Children and adolescents require a variety of mental health services, including crisis intervention and both short- and long-term counseling. Nurses working in community settings, well-child clinics, and home health can help to offset this problem through prevention, education, and inclusion of parents in program planning. Because many children and adolescents lack services or access to services, community mental health assessment activities are essential. Assessment activities include identifying types of programs available or lacking in places where children and adolescents spend time. Assessments should be performed in schools and in the homes of clients served, and also in day care centers, churches, and organizations that plan and guide age-specific play and entertainment programs. Assessment data are essential for planning and developing programs that address mental health problems prevalent from the prenatal period through adolescence. Preventing problems during these developmental periods can reduce mental health problems in adulthood.

## Adults

Adults suffer from varied sources of stress that contribute to their mental health status. Sources of stress include multiple role responsibilities, job insecurity, and unstable relationships. These and other conditions can undermine mental health and contribute to serious mental illness, depression, anxiety disorders, and substance abuse. *Healthy People 2020* objectives seek to help adults access treatment in order to decrease associated human and economic costs and to reduce suicide rates (USDHHS, 2010).

At some point, virtually all adults will experience a tragic or unexpected loss, a serious setback, or a time of profound sadness, grief, or distress. Major depressive disorder, however, differs both in intensity and in duration from normal sadness or grief. Depression disrupts relationships and the ability to function and can be fatal. In 2009 death by suicide surpassed that caused by motor vehicle accidents, and there has been a substantial increase in suicide rates among adults aged 35 to 64 years in the decade between 1999 and 2010 (CDC, 2013). The majority of those who kill themselves have a mental or substance abuse disorder. Other risk factors include prior suicide attempts, stressful life events, and access to lethal methods. Women are twice as likely to experience depression, and women who are poor, unemployed, or victims of domestic violence are even more at risk (USDHHS, 2008). Available medications and psychological treatment can help 80% of those with depression, yet only a few seek help. Those with depression are more likely to visit a physician for some other reason, and the mental health condition may not be noted. Therefore, it is imperative that nurses in all settings recognize and screen for depression. Community health nurses may provide treatment interventions. The Evidence-Based Practice box describes an intervention that nurses used with mothers of infants and toddlers to examine their effect on symptoms of depression.

### EVIDENCE-BASED PRACTICE

The purpose of this randomized controlled in-home interventional study was to compare interpersonal psychotherapy combined with parenting enhancement provided by advanced practice psychiatric mental health nurses with a parenting enhancement–only intervention provided by generalist nurses to determine the effect of the intervention on depressive symptoms and parenting behaviors.

Two hundred and twenty-six mothers of Early Head Start infants and toddlers from the northeastern and southeastern areas of the United States were randomized into the intervention or the control group. Depression assessments and videotaped, coded mother-child interactions were used at baseline and at 14- to 22-week and at 26-week postintervention intervals.

Mothers in both the control and intervention groups had reduction in depressive symptoms measured by the Hamilton Depression Rating Scale, but only mothers in the intervention group had significant positive interaction changes with their children. The study suggested that a combination of generalist and specialist nurses could be very effective in the treatment of maternal depression.

Nurses can provide mental health screening, support, and education for low-income mothers. Community health nurses at both the generalist and advanced practice levels can be instrumental in designing and developing programs to detect and reduce depression in mothers living in low-resourced communities. These interventions may be critical to ensuring improved mental health of both mothers and their children, as maternal depression is associated with negative emotional outcomes of their children.

Beeber LS, Schwartz TA, Holditch-Davis D, et al: Parenting enhancement, interpersonal psychotherapy to reduce depression in infants and toddlers: a randomized trial. *Nurs Res* 62:82–90, 2013.

Anxiety disorders are common both in the United States and in other countries. An alarming 18% of the adult population will experience an anxiety disorder, many with overlapping substance abuse disorders (NIMH, 2013). Anxiety disorders may have an early onset and are characterized by recurrent episodes of illness and periods of disability. Panic disorder and agoraphobia along with depression are associated with increased risks of attempted and completed suicide.

The lifetime rates of co-occurrence of mental disorders and addictive disorders are strikingly high. About one in four persons in the United States experiences a mental disorder in the course of a year, and nearly one in three adults who have a mental disorder in their lifetime also experiences a co-occurring substance (alcohol or other drugs) abuse disorder (NIMH, 2013). Individuals with co-occurring disorders are more likely to experience a chronic course and to use services than are those with either type of disorder alone; however, the services are often fragmented and treatment occurs in different segments of the system.

How can nurses intervene? The general medical sector, including primary care clinics, hospitals, and nursing homes, is typically the initial point of contact for many adults with mental disorders; for some, these providers may be the only source of mental health services. Early detection and intervention for mental health problems can be increased if persons presenting in primary care are assessed for mental health problems. Nurses who work in the general medical sector and in other community settings are in an ideal position to assess and detect mental health problems. Nurses conduct comprehensive biopsychosocial assessments and are often the professional most trusted with sensitive information by clients in these settings. The use of screening tools for depression, anxiety, substance abuse, and cognitive impairment can assist the nurse in early detection and intervention for mental health problems. Suicide can be prevented in many cases by early recognition and treatment of mental disorders, and by preventive interventions that focus on risk factors. Thus, reduction in access to lethal methods and recognition and treatment of mental and substance abuse disorders are among the most promising approaches to suicide prevention. Nurses, long respected as important population-centered providers, can work with legislators for measures to limit access to weapons such as handguns.

### LINKING CONTENT TO PRACTICE

This chapter describes the role of the nurse who works with persons with mental illness in the community. The role is diverse and complex and relies on basic nursing knowledge as well as specific knowledge about mental illness. Applying this role in the community draws on many of the recommendations of nursing and public health groups. For example, the core competencies adopted by the Council on Linkages between Academia and Public Health Practice (2010) include those related to assessment, policy development and program planning skills, communication and cultural competency skills, and involvement with the community in order to provide services effectively. The Quad Council of Public Health Nursing Organizations (2011) further develops these skills and makes clear application to nursing practice. The American Nurses Association develops and publishes scope and standards of practice documents that identify specific nursing competencies by specialty area (ANA, 2013, 2014).

## Adults with Serious Mental Illness

Objectives of *Healthy People 2020* that address tertiary prevention and are targeted to persons with serious mental illness are

to reduce the proportion of homeless adults who have serious mental illness, to increase their employment, and to decrease the number of adults with mental disorders who are incarcerated. Brief hospital stays and inadequate community resources have resulted in an increased number of persons with serious mental illness living on the streets or in jail. It is estimated that 14% of males and one third of females in jail suffer from a mental illness (Steadman et al, 2009). Some people arrested for nonviolent crimes could be better served if diverted from the jail system to a community-based mental health treatment program with linkage to mental health services. Approximately half of the homeless persons in the United States have a serious mental illness or a substance abuse problem and on any given night an astonishing 60,000 are veterans (National Coalition for Homeless Veterans, 2014). Most do not have any form of employment. At present, many people with severe mental disorders live in poverty because they lack the ability to earn or maintain a suitable standard of living. Even people who live with family caregivers or in supervised housing are at risk for inadequate services because the long-term care they need often depletes human and fiscal resources. An effective approach for helping persons with serious mental illness is to partner with consumers to facilitate recovery through intensive case management. Persistent client outreach and engagement strategies are effective in helping persons with serious mental illness (Cook et al, 2009).

CMHNs are engaged in all forms of case management activities with persons with serious and persistent mental illness. They provide important case management services, coordinate resources for consumers, and function as important members of ACT programs, which provide continuous assistance to persons with mental illness. Nurses by philosophy and training promote independent living and provide support and encouragement for persons to achieve a maximal level of wellness and function. Nurses recognize the importance of the mental health benefits of meaningful work that improves self-esteem and independence. Nurses can support development of **wellness recovery action plans** both at the individual and agency levels. Nursing health promotion interventions can be provided in shelters, soup kitchens, and other places where homeless persons receive food and protection.

## Older Adults

In the United States, the population older than 65 years has steadily increased since the year 2000. As the life expectancy of individuals continues to grow, the number experiencing mental disorders of late life will increase. This trend will present society with unprecedented challenges in organizing, financing, and delivering effective preventive and treatment services for mental health in this population. Although many older people maintain highly functional lives, others have mental health deficits associated with normal sensory losses related to aging, failing physical health, difficulty performing activities of daily living, and social deprivation or isolation. Life changes related to work roles and retirement often result in reduced social contacts and support. Other previously described losses are associated with the death of a spouse, other family members, or friends. Reduced social networks and contacts triggered by these life events can influence mood and contribute to serious states of depression. However, depression is not a normal part of aging.

The depression rate among older adults is half that of younger people, but the presence of a physical or chronic illness increases rates of depression. Depression rates for older adults in nursing homes range from 15% to 25% (Blazer, 2003). In the United States men between the ages of 65 and 74 are in the highest risk category for suicide; men account for 80% of all suicides of those older than age 65 (NIMH, 2013). Alzheimer's disease and vascular conditions can cause a severe loss of mental abilities with behavioral manifestations. Nearly half of those older than age 85 have symptoms of cognitive impairment severe enough to impair function. All these conditions affect the mental health status of individuals and their family caregivers.

Older adults, because they may be dependent on others for care, are at risk for abuse and neglect. Healthy aging activities such as physical activity and establishing social networks improve the mental health of older adults. Older adults underutilize the community mental health system and are more likely to be seen in primary care or to be recipients of care in institutions. The nurse can reach them by organizing health promotion programs through senior centers or other community-based settings. Home health care nurses can assess and intervene to protect those at risk for abuse and neglect, and mental health nurses can provide stress management education for nursing home staff. Stress management for caregivers and respite daycare programs for an older adult family member can increase coping and prevent abuse. Mental health outreach services for older adults have been very effective in reducing depressive symptoms (Tampi and Tampi, 2013). Nurses can advocate with health authorities and localities to increase awareness of the importance of meeting the mental health needs of this growing population.

Most family caregivers are women who care for a spouse, an aging parent, or a child with a long-term disabling illness. These caregivers are also at risk for health disruption. The risk is particularly great for caregivers of persons with a chronic illness. Caregivers of persons with severely disabling mental disorders often have their mental health threatened by lack of social support, the stigma of the disease, and chronic strain. During stressful life events such as these, it is important for caregivers to know how to manage the many competing demands in their lives.

Activities to improve the mental health status of adults include public education programs, prevention approaches, and provision of mental health services in primary care. Specific approaches to reduce stress include use of community support groups, education about lifestyle management, and worksite programs. Nevertheless, most programs currently available for adults, families, and caregivers with health problems primarily monitor or restore health rather than prevent problems. Therefore, the nurse can refer family caregivers and others to organizations such as the local National Alliance for the Mentally Ill for group support services. In addition, many national organizations designed for groups with specific problems (Box 36-4)

### BOX 36-4  Examples of Sources of Information and Help for People with Mental Illness and Mental Health Problems

- Alcoholics Anonymous
- Al-Anon
- Alzheimer's Association
- American Anorexia/Bulimia Association
- American Association of Suicidology
- Anxiety Disorders Association of America
- Attention Deficit Information Network
- Children and Adults with Attention Deficit Disorder
- Depressive/Manic Depressive Association
- Gamblers Anonymous
- National Center for Post-Traumatic Stress Disorder
- National Center for Learning Disabilities
- Obsessive-Compulsive Foundation Overeaters Anonymous
- Schizophrenics Anonymous

See the Evolve website at http://evolve.elsevier.com/Stanhope for more information about these organizations.

### QSEN FOCUS ON QUALITY AND SAFETY EDUCATION FOR NURSES

#### Quality and Safety Focus

**Targeted Competency: Safety—Minimizes risk of harm to clients and providers through both system effectiveness and individual performance.**

Important aspects of safety include:
- Knowledge: Examine human factors and other basic safety design principles as well as commonly used unsafe practices (such as, workarounds and dangerous abbreviations)
- Skills: Use national client safety resources for own professional development and to focus attention on safety in care settings
- Attitudes: Value the contributions of standardization/reliability to safety

#### Safety Question

Nurses engage in patient-specific interventions to keep patients safe. Nurses also regularly contribute to the development of safety approaches at the systems level. System level approaches to safety ensure standardization of processes and a consistent methodology to addressing recurring safety concerns.

You are working as an RN in home care. Your home care agency has had three patients admit to suicidal ideation and intention in the last 3 months. In all three situations, the home care nurses handled the situations very differently, with varied success. Your manager asks you to participate in a task force to develop a standard operating procedure that all home care nurses can employ to respond to a suicidal patient in the home.
- What health care team members would be helpful in addressing the development of this standardized operating procedure?
- What evidence might you look to in developing this standardized procedure?
- How might you envision most effectively training home care nurses in this standardized approach?

Prepared by Gail Armstrong, PhD©, DNP, ACNS-BC, CNE, Associate Professor, University of Colorado Denver College of Nursing.

have local chapters or information that can be accessed on the Internet. Some state activities expand mental health services to older adults, and *Healthy People 2020* has objectives designed to increase services to older adults and cultural competence within the mental health system.

## Cultural Diversity

To work effectively, health care providers need to understand the differences in how various populations in the United States perceive mental health and mental illness and treatment services. These factors affect whether people seek mental health care, how they describe their symptoms, the duration of care, and the outcomes of the care received. Various populations use mental health services in different ways. People may not seek mental health services in the formal system, they may drop out of care, or they may seek care at much later stages of illness, which typically costs more. This pattern of use may be the result of a community-based mental health service system that is not culturally relevant, responsive, or accessible to select populations. Although all socioeconomic and cultural groups have mental health problems, low-income groups are at greater risk because they often lack minimal resources for meeting basic physical and mental health needs.

In an effort to describe and remedy mental health disparities based on culture, a supplemental report was published to the landmark surgeon general's report on mental health (USDHHS, 2001). Caution is needed, however, when discussing differences among racial and ethnic groups in the rates of mental illness. Studies of the number of cases of mental health problems among racial and ethnic populations, while increasing in number, remain limited and often inconclusive. Discussion of the rates of existing cases must consider differences in how persons of different cultures and racial and ethnic groups perceive mental illness. Behavioral problems, often viewed in Western medicine as signs of mental illness, may be assessed differently by individuals in various racial and ethnic groups. The manner in which people of different cultures describe emotional distress may affect the detection and treatment of mental illness. With this caution in mind, along with the recognition that sample sizes for racial and ethnic groups may be limited, examination of existing large-scale studies for mental health trends and disparities among racial and ethnic groups remains important (Akincigil et al, 2012).

According to the surgeon general's landmark report on culture, race, and ethnicity, the predominant minority populations in the United States are African Americans, Hispanics, Asian and Pacific Islander Americans, and Native Americans including Native Alaskans (USDHHS, 2001). A notable omission from this federal report is Middle Eastern Americans, and little information could be found either in the literature or through national websites, although there is a significant and growing population, particularly in the upper Midwest. Great diversity exists among people from the Middle East, although they may share some cultural traditions with Asians, Africans, or Europeans and in some cases have been included in those classifications. However, within each of the groups identified in the federal report, there is also much diversity, as each group consists of subgroups with unique cultural differences. Therefore, it is important to avoid simplification and overgeneralization in discussions about the characteristics and problems of minorities and to examine both individual and national bias. It is critical to conduct community assessments to determine unique characteristics and factors that contribute to mental health needs within specific aggregates of the population. The information presented here is intended to stimulate thinking and awareness for developing nursing activities in individual communities. Community assessments that include data about specific populations from organized agencies such as the Indian Health Service (2014) are important because assessment data can help guide role activities during all steps of the nursing process.

Nurses provide a variety of primary, secondary, and tertiary prevention interventions with populations at risk that help meet the objectives for improving mental health. Consumers have historically influenced mental health services, and the health care industry increasingly is using consumer opinion to gain information on service needs and changes. Objectives of *Healthy People 2020* are to increase state tracking of consumer satisfaction with mental health services and to increase the number of states who incorporate plans addressing cultural competence. Nurses working within broad-based coalitions of consumers, families, other providers, and community leaders can help to achieve the goals of accessible, culturally sensitive, quality mental health services for all people.

### African Americans

African Americans are the second largest minority population in the United States. In 2012, 28.1 percent of African Americans compared to 11.0 percent of non-Hispanic whites were living at the poverty level (Office of Minority Health, USDHHS, 2012). Ethnic and racial minorities in the United States may live in an environment of social and economic discrimination and inequality, which takes a toll on mental health and places them at risk for associated mental problems. African Americans are more likely to be exposed to, or to become victims of, violence, placing them at risk for the development of post-traumatic stress disorder (PTSD). They are overrepresented both in the homeless and correctional system populations, further increasing the risk of developing mental health problems. Although they were less likely to commit suicide, the suicide rate of young African American men is now equal to that of whites (CDC, 2009). Despite these issues, African Americans are less likely to use mental health services and may have significant negative expectations about mental health services. Nurses can promote the mental health of African Americans by integrating mental health care into primary care settings, providing services in community centers, collaborating with African American faith communities, providing education to decrease the stigma, working toward the provision of safer communities, and recruiting African Americans to work as community mental health providers.

### Latino Americans

Latino Americans are the second largest minority group in America, and by 2050 they are projected to comprise 25% of the population (Office of Minority Health, USDHHS, 2012). Although they live primarily in the southwestern regions of the country, many have migrated to states in the Southeast and Midwest. Migrant farmworkers are also an important subpopulation among Latinos. As discussed in Chapter 34, migratory living patterns that are marked by low income, poor education, and lack of health services contribute to stressful living conditions. Nurses and nurse practitioners may be primary health care providers for migrant laborers and new immigrants. Their roles expand beyond traditional practice to encompass case management and interagency collaboration. Collaboration includes networking and referral to community mental health agencies and to advanced practice psychiatric nurses when either drug or alcohol abuse or mental illness is the primary health problem.

Latino Americans living in low-income urban areas are subject to many of the conditions described for low-income and disadvantaged African American families. Initially, it was reported that recent Latino immigrants had lower rates of depression than those born in the United States, but evidence from the CDC (2009) found suicide to be the eighth-leading cause of death among Latino males and even higher rates of attempts among young Latina women. There are significant relationships between suicide and having a family history of suicide, physical or sexual abuse, and environmental stress. These findings suggest serious stressful living conditions for both individuals and families. Nurses working with Latino families need knowledge and skill in both the language and cross-cultural therapies, and they also need to include consumers in planning and evaluating mental health service delivery. Focus groups can be held to involve community members in the planning and implementation of culturally relevant mental health services.

### Asian and Pacific Islander Americans

Asian and Pacific Islander Americans are a diverse and rapidly increasing population (USDHHS, 2001). This group includes both settled citizens and new refugees. The largest segment of this population lives in California. Whereas Asian and Pacific Islander Americans, like other minority groups, are represented in all socioeconomic strata, the lower-income groups include refugees and recent immigrants who are dealing with the displacement issues of loss, adjustment, and adaptation. Losses often involve forfeiture of family, traditions, and lifestyles for cultures that may seem alien. Adjustments and adaptations include those basic to daily living: learning new languages, laws,

and monetary systems and locating support systems. Finding support systems includes becoming acquainted with the health care delivery system. Our knowledge of the mental health needs of this population is limited, because they have the lowest utilization rates of mental health services of any cultural group (USDHHS, 2001). This avoidance of mental health care is associated with the stigma and shame related to having a mental disorder as well as to perceived discrimination by mental health providers (Wu et al, 2009; Spencer et al, 2010). Assessment, planning, and interventions with members of this diverse group must include information about their health beliefs, a key component in any program.

Population-focused mental health nurses need to understand existing cultural barriers and help to design culturally sensitive approaches for vulnerable populations. Nurses can work to decrease the stigma of mental illness by educating minorities about the biological basis of many mental disorders. Recruitment of a culturally diverse nursing workforce may increase use of mental health services.

### Native Americans

Native Americans represent 1.5% of the U.S. population. Although this is a small group, it is also diverse, with more than 551 tribes and more than 200 languages. Native Americans also appear to have significant rates of substance abuse, depression, and suicide (1.5 times the national rate), along with unintentional injury and homicide. They are exposed to violence at more than twice the national rate, which results in significant rates of PTSD (CDC, 2009; Indian Health Service, 2014). Use of mental health services has been difficult to determine, because only a small percentage of Native Americans use those provided by the Indian Health Service.

A promising intervention to address the needs of this diverse group is to build on the traditions of the specific tribe culture to foster identity and integration and enhance protective factors. A return to traditional values of community and group support has been shown to be effective in reducing rates of substance abuse (CDC, 2009; Indian Health Service, 2014). Nurses working with Native Americans, as with all population groups, need to learn the culture of the specific group and to mutually plan culturally sensitive mental health interventions at levels of primary, secondary, and tertiary prevention.

## ▌ P R A C T I C E   A P P L I C A T I O N

Mr. B. is an 81-year-old white widowed man living in a rural area 20 miles from a small city. The nurse practitioner who had treated Mr. B. for sinusitis referred him to the outreach nurse for an evaluation. The nurse practitioner was concerned when she noted that Mr. B. had lost weight and had started to cry when talking about his wife who had died several years before. During the initial visit, the nurse noted that Mr. B. weighed only 110 lb, was not sleeping, had stopped going to church, and was quite anxious and sad about his finances, his limitations from arthritis, his relationship with his 27-year-old stepson, Bart, and the possibility of nursing home placement.

The nurse conducted a suicide assessment, knowing that Mr. B. was at high risk because of his age, his mood, and the presence of guns in the home. Mr. B. stated that he had considered shooting himself, but he was reluctant to have the rifles removed at the nurse's suggestion because Bart used the guns for hunting. Mr. B. agreed to a family meeting with his stepson, and Bart agreed to remove the guns from the house. Both Mr. B. and Bart needed significant education about the biological basis of depression and the efficacy of using a new antidepressant, along with support to treat his condition. Mr. B., like many older adults, did not wish to see a psychiatrist or use the community mental health system. He did agree to a trial of antidepressants, however.

The nurse, through the primary care nurse practitioner, arranged for a prescription of an antidepressant (a selective serotonin reuptake inhibitor) that is safe for use with older adults, and Mr. B. started the medication within 2 weeks of the initial visit. In addition to medication and counseling, Mr. B. needed help with nutrition. Because Bart was away 10 hours a day, at work in the city, Mr. B. was alone all day. Mr. B. was not able to prepare meals because of his arthritis. The nurse arranged with the local board for aging to provide home-delivered meals. This not only helped with nutrition, but also gave Mr. B. a visit from the volunteer twice a week.

Mr. B. and Bart needed help with financial planning, as they did not want to lose the farm should Mr. B. need more assistance or nursing home placement in the future. The nurse arranged for them to talk with a social worker regarding long-term care planning.

In addition to addressing the immediate concerns, the nurse continued to provide weekly visits to Mr. B. for support and counseling, medication monitoring, and case management activities. Family meetings with Bart and Mr. B. to discuss mutual concerns were arranged every 2 months and as needed. The significant improvement of depressive symptoms (that is, sleep, appetite, weight, and mood) in Mr. B. was monitored both clinically and through use of a depression rating scale.

Psychological, physical, and social problems of older adults are closely intertwined and are best evaluated and treated by a multidisciplinary team. Psychiatric illness often presents first with physical symptoms, and physical limitations create further psychological distress. Older adults often prefer not to use formal mental health services, so careful assessment in primary care settings is critical to detect their mental health problems.

A. In addition to his stepson and the nurse, who else might notice if Mr. B.'s condition began to deteriorate?

B. What nursing measures are important in monitoring Mr. B.'s response to the antidepressant?

C. What secondary prevention measures did the nurse use?

D. What resources might be available for Bart should he need more information about depression?

**Answers can be found on the Evolve site.**

■ **K E Y   P O I N T S**

- Reform movements and subsequent federal legislation influenced the development of the current community mental health model that includes team care, case management, prevention, and rehabilitation and recovery components of service.
- During the past two decades, federal legislation in the United States focused on mainstreaming persons with mental disabilities into American life by legislating access to employment, services, and housing.
- Prevalence rates for mental health problems are very high, and people are at risk for threats to mental health at all ages across the life span. Low-income and minority groups are often at increased risk because they lack access to services and because programs may lack cultural sensitivity.
- National health objectives to promote health and services for persons who have mental health problems and severe mental disorders illustrate the scope of mental illness and provide direction for community mental health practice.
- Guidelines for attaining national health objectives were designed to help individuals at regional and local levels establish health priorities that include those for mental illness.
- The American Nurses Association standards provide a framework for the roles and functions of community mental health nurses.
- Frameworks that are useful in community mental health nursing include primary, secondary, and tertiary levels of prevention; biological theories including the effects of psychosocial factors on the brain, growth, and development; and rehabilitation and recovery models.

■ **C L I N I C A L   D E C I S I O N - M A K I N G   A C T I V I T I E S**

1. For 1 week, keep a list of incidents related to mental health problems that you learn about in the local media. Categorize the incidents according to age, sex, and socioeconomic, ethnic, or minority status. Which populations seem to have the most mental health problems?

2. Visit a local shelter or organization that offers temporary protection for persons with mental disorders. Determine services that are available or lacking for children, women, and men. Describe a nursing intervention that would improve services.

3. Visit with representatives of your local self-help organizations for consumers to determine their needs and the adequacy of resources for people with severe mental disorders and their caregivers; determine gaps in services. Develop a list of the agencies in your community that provide direct or indirect services for those with mental illness and their families.

4. Interview a school nurse, an occupational health nurse, an emergency department nurse, or a hospice nurse in your community to discuss types of mental health problems

## CLINICAL DECISION-MAKING ACTIVITIES—cont'd

they see with clients in their practice settings. Determine resources that are available or lacking for primary, secondary, and tertiary prevention. Design a primary prevention intervention.

5. Interview a nurse working in a local community mental health agency to discuss roles, functions, programs, and resources available or lacking for primary, secondary, and tertiary prevention. Compare findings about prevention programs with information obtained from the preceding interview.

6. Visit a consumer-operated program or a psychosocial rehabilitation program. Interview members to learn how they view services and resources available or lacking in this setting. Describe how your attitudes about persons in recovery from mental illness changed after your visit.

7. Accompany a community mental health nurse on home visits to clients enrolled in an assertive community outreach program, and then accompany a psychiatric nurse in a home care agency. Compare and contrast how the services, funding, populations served, and philosophies of treatment differ.

8. As a class activity, arrange for a panel of speakers representing the minority populations described in this chapter. Discuss their views about the way culture shapes thinking about mental illness, and determine types of culturally sensitive services that are available or lacking in your community.

9. Review articles in at least four research journals to determine current research findings about mental disorders and mental health problems, and compare nursing care in the United States with that of other countries. Discuss the differences in mental health care between countries.

# REFERENCES

Akincigil A, Olfson M, Siegel M, et al: Racial and ethnic disparities in depression care in community-dwelling elderly in the United States. *Am J Public Health* 102:319–328, 2012.

Alzheimer's Association: Alzheimer's disease facts and figures. *Alzheimers Dement* 10(2):18, 2014. Retrieved February 2015 from: http://www.ncbi.nlm.nih.gov/pubmed/23507120.

American Academy of Nursing Psychiatric Mental Health Substance Abuse Expert Panel: Essential psychiatric mental health and substance use competencies for the registered nurse. *Arch Psychiatr Nurs* 26:80–110, 2012.

American Nurses Association (ANA): *Public Health Nursing Standards*. Washington, DC, 2013, American Nurses Publishing. Retrieved February 2015 from: http://www.nursesbooks.org/Homepage/hot off the press/Public-Health-Nursing-2nd.aspx.

American Nurses Association, American Psychiatric Nurses Association, International Society of Psychiatric Mental Health Nurses: *Scope and Standards of Psychiatric–Mental Health Nursing*. Washington, DC, 2014, American Nurses Publishing.

American Psychiatric Association (APA): *Diagnostic and Statistical Manual of Mental Disorders*, ed 5. Washington, DC, 2013, APA.

Baker E, Fee J, Bovingdon L, et al: From taking to using medication: recovery-focused prescribing and medicines management. *Adv Psychiatr Treat* 19:2–10, 2013. Retrieved February 2015 from:

http://apt.rcpsych.org/content/19/1/2.

Barnes PM, Bloom B, Nahin RL: Complementary and Alternative Medicine Use among Adults and Children: United States, 2007. *Natl Health Stat Report* 12:1–23, 2008.

Beeber LS, Schwartz TA, Holditch-Davis D, et al: Parenting enhancement, interpersonal psychotherapy to reduce depression in infants and toddlers: a randomized trial. *Nurs Res* 62:82–90, 2013.

Blazer DG: Depression in late life: review and commentary. *J Gerontol A Biol Sci Med Sci* 58:M249–M265, 2003.

Boyd MA: Social change and mental health. In Boyd MA, editor: *Psychiatric Nursing: Contemporary Practice*, ed 5. Philadelphia, 2011, Lippincott, Williams & Wilkins.

Busch SH, Meara E, Huskamp HA, et al: Characteristics of adults with substance use disorders expected to be eligible for Medicaid under the ACA. *Psychiatr Serv* 64:520–526, 2013.

Byers AL, Yaffe K, Covinsky KE, et al: High occurrence of mood and anxiety disorders among older adults. *Arch Gen Psychiatry* 67:489–496, 2010.

Caldwell BA, Sclafani M, Swarbrick M, et al: Psychiatric nursing practice and the recovery model of care. *J Psychosoc Nurs Ment Health Serv* 48:42–48, 2010.

Centers for Disease Control and Prevention, National Center for Injury Prevention and Control: *Suicide, Facts at a Glance*, [Summer 2009]. Retrieved February 2015 from: http://www.cdc.gov.

Centers for Disease Control and Prevention (CDC): Suicide among

adults aged 35-64 years—United States, 1999–2010. *MMWR Morb Mortal Wkly Rep* 62:321–325, 2013.

Cook JA, Copeland ME, Hamilton MM, et al: Initial outcomes of a mental illness self-management program based on wellness recovery action planning. *Psychiatr Serv* 60:246–249, 2009.

Council on Linkages between Academia and Public Health Practice: *Core Competencies for Public Health Professionals*. Washington, DC, 2010, Public Health Foundation, Health Resources and Services Administration.

Edmondson D, Kronish IM, Wasson LT, et al: A test of the diathesis-stress model in the emergency department: who develops PTSD after an acute coronary syndrome? *J Psychiatr Res* 53:8–13, 2014. Retrieved February 2015 from: http://www.ncbi.nlm.nih.gov/pubmed/24612925.

Eom CS, Lee HK, Ye S, et al: Use of selective serotonin reuptake inhibitors and risk of fracture: a systematic review and meta-analysis. *J Bone Miner Res* 27:1186–1195, 2012. Retrieved February 2015 from: http://www.ncbi.nlm.nih.gov/pubmed?term=J+Bone+Miner+Res+%5BJour%5D+AND+27%5Bvolume%5D+AND+1186%5Bpage%5D&cmd=detailssearch.

Garfield RL, Zuvekas SH, Lave JR, et al: The impact of national health care reform on adults with severe mental disorders. *Am J Psychiatry* 168:486–494, 2011.

Hobfoll SE, Watson P, Bell CC, et al: Five essential elements of immediate and mid-term mass

trauma intervention: empirical evidence. *Psychiatry* 70:283–315, 2007.

Indian Health Service (IHS): *IHS Fact Sheet: Indian Health Disparities*, 2014. Retrieved February 2015 from: http://ihs.gov/newsroom/factsheets/disparities.

Liu RT, Alloy LB: Stress generation in depression: a systematic review of the empirical literature and recommendations for future study. *Clin Psychol Rev* 30:582–593, 2010.

Marchinko S, Clark D: The wellness planner: empowerment, quality of life and continuity of care in mental illness. *Arch Psychiatr Nurs* 25:284–293, 2011.

May A: Experience-dependent structural plasticity in the adult human brain. *Trends Cogn Sci* 15:475–482, 2011.

McClosky LA, Figuerdo AJ, Koss MP: The effects of systemic family violence on children's mental health. *Child Dev* 66:1239, 2008.

Mechanic D: Mental Health Services Then and Now. *Health Aff* 26(6):1548–1550, 2007.

Mechanic D: *Mental Health and Social Policy: Beyond Managed Care*, ed 5. Boston, 2008, Pearson Education.

Mechanic D: Seizing opportunities under the Affordable Care Act for transforming the mental and behavioral health system. *Health Aff* 31:376–382, 2012.

Mental Health America (MHA): *Fact Sheet: Paul Wellstone and Peter Domenici Mental Health Parity and Addiction Equity Act of 2008*. Alexandria, VA, 2009, MHA.

National Coalition for Homeless Veterans: *Background & Statistics*, 201, 2014. Retrieved February

2015 from: http://www.nchv.org/index.php/news/media/background-and-statistics.

National Institutes of Mental Health (NIMH), National Institutes of Health (NIH), U.S. Department of Health and Human Services (USDHHS): *The Numbers Count: Mental Disorders in America.* Washington, DC, 2013, NIMH. Retrieved February 2015 from: http://www.lb7.uscourts.gov/documents/12-cv-1072url2.pdf.

National Institutes of Mental Health (NIMH), National Institutes of Health (NIH), U.S. Department of Health and Human Services (USDHHS): *Statistics from the WHO.* Washington, DC, 2014, NIMH. Retrieved February 2015 from: http://www.nimh.nih.gov/healthpublications.

Pandya A, Jän Myrick K: Wellness recovery programs: a model of self-advocacy for people living with mental illness. *J Psychiatr Pract* 19:242–246, 2013.

Parry M: From a patient's perspective: Clifford Whittingham Beers' work to reform mental health services. *Am J Public Health* 100:2356–2357, 2010.

Pearlman SA: The Patient Protection and Affordable Health Care Act: impact on mental health services demand and provider availability. *J Am Psychiatr Nurses Assoc* 19:327–334, 2013.

Pramyothin P, Kaodihiar L: Metabolic syndrome with the atypical antipsychotics. *Curr Opin Endocrinol Diabetes Obes* 17:460–466, 2010.

President's New Freedom Commission on Mental Health: *Achieving the Promise: Transforming Mental Health Care in America* [USDHHS Publication No. SMA-03-3832]. Rockville, MD, 2003, USDHHS.

Preskorn SH: CNS drug development: Part II: advances from the 1960s to the 1990s. *J Psychiatr Pract* 16(6):413–415, 2010.

Quad Council of Public Health Nursing Organizations: *Competencies for Public Health Nursing Practice.* Washington, DC, 2011, ASTDN.

Raviola G, Becker AE, Farmer P: A global scope for global health, including mental health. *Lancet* 378:1613–1615, 2011.

Riesser GG, Schorske BJ: Relationships between family caregiver and mental health professionals: the American experience. In Lefley H, Wasow M, editors: *Helping Families Cope with Mental Illness,* vol 2. New York, 2013, Routledge, pp 3–26.

Salyers MP, Tsemberis S: ACT and recovery: integrating evidence based practice and recovery orientation on assertive community treatment teams. *Community Ment Health J* 44:75, 2008.

Segal SP, Siverman CJ, Temkin TL: Self-help and community mental health agency outcomes: a recovery-focused randomized controlled trial. *Psychiatr Serv* 61:905–910, 2008.

Spencer MS, Chen J, Gee GG, et al: Discrimination and mental health related service use in a national study of Asian Americans. *Am J Public Health* 100:2410–2417, 2010.

Steadman HJ, Osher FC, Robbins PC, et al: Prevalence of serious mental illness among jail inmates. *Psychiatr Serv* 60:761, 2009.

Sterling EW, von Esenwein SA, Tucker S, et al: Integrating wellness, recovery and self-management for mental health consumers. *Community Ment Health J* 46:130–138, 2010.

Substance Abuse and Mental Health Services Administration (SAMHSA): *Behavioral Health United States, 2012* [USDHHS Publication No. 13-4797]. Rockville, MD, 2013, SAMHSA.

Sveinbjarnardottir EK, Svavarsdottir EK, Wright LM: What are the benefits of a short therapeutic conversation intervention with acute psychiatric patients and their families? A controlled before and after study. *Int J Nurs Stud* 50:593–602, 2013.

Tampi RR, Tampi DJ: *Multidisciplinary teams in the continuum of care for older adults withmental illness .* Neuropsychiatry 3:555–558, 2013.

Tierney KR, Kane CF: Promoting wellness and recovery for persons with serious mental illness: a program evaluation. *Arch Psychiatr Nurs* 25:77–89, 2011.

U.S. Department of Health and Human Services (USDHHS): *Mental Health: A Report of the Surgeon General.* Rockville. MD, 1999, USDHHS.

U.S. Department of Health and Human Services; U.S. Department of Education; U.S. Department of Justice: *Report of the Surgeon General's Conference on Children's Mental Health: A National Action Agenda.* Washington, DC, 2000, U.S. Department of Health and Human Services. Retrieved February 2015 from: http://www.ncbi.nlm.nih.gov/books/NBK44233/.

U.S. Department of Health and Human Services (USDHHS): *Mental Health: Culture, Race, and Ethnicity—Supplement to Mental Health: A Report of the Surgeon General.* Rockville, MD, 2001, USDHHS.

U.S. Department of Health and Human Services (USDHHS), Health Research Services Administration, Maternal and Child Health Bureau: *Woman's Health USA, 2008.* Rockville, MD, 2008, USDHHS.

U.S. Department of Health and Human Services (USDHHS), Health Research Services Administration, Maternal and Child Health Bureau: *Child Health USA 2008–2009.* Rockville, MD, 2009, USDHHS.

U.S. Department of Health and Human Services (USDHHS): *Healthy People 2020: Mental Health and Mental Disorders.* Washington, DC, 2010, Office of Disease Prevention and Health Promotion. Retrieved February 2015 from: http://healthypeople.gov/2020.

U.S.Department of Health and Human Services (USDHHS): *Profile: Black/African American, 2012* Washington, DC, 2012. Retrieved February 2015 from: http://minorityhealth /hhs.gov/omh/browse.aspx?lvl=3&lvlid=61.

U.S. Department of Health and Human Services (USDHHS): *Patient Protection and Affordable Health Care Act, 2014.* Retrieved February 2015 from: http://www.hhs.gov./healthcare/.

World Health Organization (WHO): *mhGAP, Mental Health Action Programme: Scaling up Care for Mental, Neurological and Substance Abuse Disorders.* Geneva, Switzerland, 2008a, WHO.

World Health Organization (WHO): *The Global Burden of Disease: 2004 Update. Table A2: Burden of Disease in DALYs by Cause, Sex and Income Group in WHO Regions, Estimated for 2004.* Geneva, Switzerland, 2008b, WHO.

World Health Organization (WHO): *Depression: A Global Crisis.* Geneva, Switzerland, 2012, WHO. Retrieved February 2015 from: http://www.who.int/mental_health/management/depression/wfmh_paper_depression_wmhd_2012.pdf.

World Health Organization (WHO): *Health for the World's Adolescents: A Second Chance in the Second Decade.* Geneva, Switzerland, 2014, WHO. Retrieved February 2015 from: www.who./nt/adolescent/second-decade.

Wu MC, Kaviz FJ, Miller AM: Identifying individual and contextual barriers to seeking mental health service among Korean American immigrant women. *Issues Ment Health Nurs* 30:78, 2009.

# Alcohol, Tobacco, and Other Drug Problems

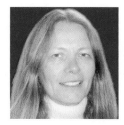

## Mary Lynn Mathre, RN, MSN, CARN

Mary Lynn Mathre earned the BSN from the College of St. Teresa in Winona, MN, and the MSN from the Frances Payne Bolton School of Nursing at Case Western Reserve University. She has 39 years of experience as an acute care nurse and has worked in the field of alcohol, tobacco, and other drugs for the past 25 years. From 1991 to 2003 she worked as the addictions consult nurse for the University of Virginia Health System and interacted with many community resources to provide appropriate referrals and aftercare for clients. From 2004 to 2007 she worked in an outpatient opioid treatment program as the executive director. Currently she works as an independent consultant on substance abuse prevention and brief interventions. She is an active member of the International Nurses Society on Addictions and serves on the editorial board for the *Journal of Addictions Nursing*.

## ADDITIONAL RESOURCES

ⓔ **Evolve website http://evolve.elsevier.com/Stanhope**
- *Healthy People 2020*
- Resource Tool 37.A: Smoking Cessation Resources
- Resource Tool 37.B: Useful Web Resources
- Resource Tool 37.C: Commonly Abused Drugs

- Quiz
- Case Studies
- Glossary
- Answers to Practice Application

## OBJECTIVES

*After reading this chapter, the student should be able to do the following:*

1. Analyze personal attitudes toward alcohol, tobacco, and other drug problems.
2. Differentiate among these terms: *substance use, abuse, dependence*, and *addiction*.
3. Discuss the differences among the major psychoactive drug categories of depressants, stimulants, marijuana, hallucinogens, and inhalants.

4. Explain the role of the nurse in primary, secondary, and tertiary prevention of alcohol, tobacco, and other drug problems as it relates to individual clients, their families, and special populations.
5. Evaluate the role of the nurse in primary, secondary, and tertiary prevention of alcohol, tobacco, and other drug problems as it relates to the community and national policies on drug control.

## KEY TERMS

addiction treatment, p. 818
Alcoholics Anonymous (AA), p. 820
alcoholism, p. 806
biopsychosocial model, p. 806
blood alcohol concentration, p. 808
brief interventions, p. 821
codependency, p. 816
cross-tolerance, p. 819
denial, p. 814
depressants, p. 806
detoxification, p. 817
drug addiction, p. 806
drug dependence, p. 806
enabling, p. 817
fetal alcohol syndrome, p. 807

hallucinogens, p. 806
harm reduction, p. 805
injection drug users, p. 816
mainstream smoke, p. 808
polysubstance use or abuse, p. 812
prohibition, p. 804
psychoactive drugs, p. 806
set, p. 811
setting, p. 811
sidestream smoke, p. 808
stimulants, p. 806
substance abuse, p. 806
tolerance, p. 808
withdrawal, p. 806
*—See Glossary for definitions*

Substance abuse is the number one national health problem, causing more deaths, illnesses, and disabilities than any other health condition. The substance abuser is not only at risk for personal health problems, but may also be a threat to the health and safety of family members, coworkers, and other members of the community.

Substance abuse and addiction affect all ages, races, sexes, and segments of society. As seen in *Healthy People 2020* (USDHHS, 2010), tobacco use and substance abuse are two major topic areas, with many objectives and subobjectives, as well as related objectives in other priority areas. The newer phrase of *alcohol, tobacco, and other drug (ATOD) problems* rather than *substance abuse* reminds us that alcohol and tobacco represent the major drugs of abuse when discussing substance abuse, drug addiction, or chemical dependency.

This chapter begins by providing a broad perspective of ATOD problems to clarify the relevant issues. A historical overview of ATOD problems and attitudes toward ATOD users and addicts is examined. Relevant terms are defined to decrease the confusion caused by frequent misuse of terms. The major drug categories are described, including information on commonly used substances and current ATOD use trends. The remainder of the chapter examines the role of the nurse in primary, secondary, and tertiary prevention and describes how the nurse can improve the outcomes for individuals, families, and various populations with ATOD problems when using a harm reduction model. It is important to apply nursing strategies to the *Healthy People 2020* objectives for ATOD problems.

## ALCOHOL, TOBACCO, AND OTHER DRUG PROBLEMS IN PERSPECTIVE

ATOD abuse and addiction can cause multiple health problems for individuals. Heavy ATOD use has been associated with many problems, including neonates with low birth weight and congenital abnormalities; accidents, homicides, and suicides; chronic diseases, such as cardiovascular diseases, cancer, lung disease, hepatitis, HIV/AIDS, and mental illness; violence; and family disruption. Factors that contribute to the substance abuse problem include lack of knowledge about the use of drugs; the war on drugs' emphasis on illicit drugs and law enforcement rather than the prevention and treatment of abuse and addiction of ATODs; lack of quality control of illegal drugs; and drug laws that label certain drug users as criminals, which encourages the negative attitudes and stigma toward these persons.

### Historical Overview

Psychoactive drug use has been part of most cultures since the beginning of humanity. Often a culture encourages use of some drugs while discouraging the use of others. Caffeine, alcohol, and tobacco are socially acceptable drugs in the United States and Canada, whereas other cultures prohibit their use. Conversely, marijuana, cocaine, and opium use are not accepted in mainstream U.S. society, although these substances are considered sacred or beneficial and their use is accepted in various other cultures.

The United States' primary solution to various "drug problems" has been **prohibition**. During alcohol prohibition from 1920 to 1933, the United States experienced a sharp increase in violent crime and corruption among law officials as a result of the illicit marketing of alcohol. Use of distilled beverages was encouraged because of the higher profit margin per bottle of liquor than for beer or wine. The high alcohol content in illicit moonshine caused severe health problems. The alcohol prohibition was eventually recognized as a failure and repealed (Rose, 1996).

Similar problems are occurring with the current war on drugs and the newer prohibition on marijuana, cocaine, and other drugs. An increase in both violent crime and reports of corruption among law officials as a result of the illicit market has become a major national problem (Common Sense for Drug Policy, 2014). Stronger drugs are pushed because of their greater profits. Some would say that drug prohibition laws have created mandatory sentences for drug offenders, violated civil liberties, and put more resources into law enforcement than into drug education and treatment (Common Sense for Drug Policy, 2014). As the drug war budget grows each year, most of that budget goes to law enforcement and punishment, leaving only a third for prevention and treatment. However, the 2014 budget is increasing its efforts in demand reduction. President Obama has requested more than $25 billion for drug control programs. Of that, 42% is designated for demand reduction: treatment, education and prevention. The remaining 58% is for supply reduction: law enforcement, interdiction, and international programs (http://www.whitehouse.gov/blog/2013/04/10/president-s-fy-2014-budget-supporting-21st-century-drug-policy).

A 3-year study by the National Center on Addiction and Substance Abuse (CASA) closely examined the 2005 federal, state, and local government budgets to measure the financial impact of ATOD problems on their health, social service, criminal justice, education, mental health, developmentally disabled, and other programs. The CASA study found that the government spent at least $467.7 billion ($238.2 billion, federal; $135.8 billion, state; and $93.8 billion, local) in 2005 on substance abuse and addiction, which amounted to 10.7% of the entire combined $4.4 trillion budgets. Of every dollar the federal and state governments spent on substance abuse and addiction, 95.6 cents was used to deal with the ATOD problems, while only 1.9 cents went to prevention and treatment, 0.4% to research, 1.4% to taxation or regulation, and 0.7% to interdiction. Almost half of this spending cannot be disaggregated by specific substance. However, of the $248 billion in ATOD-related spending, 92.3% was linked to alcohol and tobacco (National Center on Addiction and Substance Abuse, 2009). This was a landmark study to show the societal costs of drug problems, but that the funding went to dealing with the consequences rather than prevention.

## Attitudes and Myths

Attitudes are developed through cultural learning and personal experiences. Attitudes toward ATOD problems are influenced by the way society inappropriately categorizes drugs as either "good" or "bad." In the United States, good drugs are typically over-the-counter (OTC) drugs or those prescribed by a health care provider as *medicine,* but this makes them no less problematic or addictive. Bad drugs are the illegal drugs, and persons who use these drugs are considered criminals regardless of whether the drug has caused any problems.

Americans rely heavily on prescription and OTC drugs to relieve (or mask) anxiety, tension, fatigue, and physical or emotional pain. Rather than learning nonmedicinal methods of coping, many people rely on the "quick fix" and take pills to deal with their problems or negative feelings.

Addicts are often viewed as immoral, weak-willed, or irresponsible persons who should try harder to help themselves. Although alcoholism was recognized as a disease by the American Medical Association in 1954 and drug addiction was recognized as a disease some years later, much of the public and many health care professionals have failed to change their attitudes and accept alcoholics and addicts as ill persons in need of health care.

It is important for nurses to examine their attitudes toward ATOD use, abuse, and addiction before working with this health problem. To be therapeutic, the nurse must develop a trusting, nonjudgmental relationship with the client. Systematic assessment for ATOD problems is based on awareness that there may be problems with both legal and illegal drugs. If the nurse's attitude toward a client with a drug abuse problem is negative or punitive, the issue may never be directly addressed or the client may be avoided. If the client senses the negative attitude of the health care provider, either by words or from tone of voice, communication may cease and information may be withheld. To develop a therapeutic attitude, the nurse must realize that any drug can be abused, that anyone may develop drug dependence, and that drug addiction can be successfully treated.

Myths develop over years, and if myths are not questioned, many attitudes may be formed solely on the basis of fiction rather than fact. Some common myths are as follows:
- "An alcoholic is a skid row bum"—but less than 5% of persons with addictions fit this description.
- "If you teach people about drugs, they will abuse them"—although it is true that people may choose to use drugs if they have knowledge about them, it is more likely that people without knowledge about them will abuse them.
- "Addiction is a sin or moral failing"—addiction is recognized as a health problem involving biopsychosocial factors, and persons who use drugs do not do so with the intent to become addicted.

## Paradigm Shift

We can hope to see a major shift in how the United States conceptualizes ATOD problems. The old criminal justice model is based on stereotypes, misinformation, and punishment, and it uses war tactics to fight the drug users, addicts, and suppliers. Campaigns have been launched using the slogans "zero tolerance" for drug users, "just say no" to drugs, and striving for a "drug-free America"—all of which vilify the drug user or drug addict. The Obama administration's approach to the nation's drug problem is to approach it as a public health problem and not just a criminal justice problem, and the administration has put more funding into prevention and treatment ($10.7 billion) than into domestic law enforcement ($9.6 billion) (http://www.whitehouse.gov/blog/2013/04/10/president-s-fy-2014-budget-supporting-21st-century-drug-policy). Also, on the international level, experts are suggesting that national drug policies need to be more comprehensive rather than focusing on law enforcement strategies. (Box 37-1 lists Federal drug control spending by function).

The harm reduction model is a public health approach to ATOD problems initially used in Great Britain, The Netherlands, Germany, Switzerland, and Australia, and interest in it is spreading throughout Europe and in Canada. This new public health model recognizes the following:
- Addiction is a health problem.
- Any psychoactive drug can be abused.
- Accurate information can help people make responsible decisions about drug use.
- People who have ATOD problems can be helped.

---

### BOX 37-1  High-Level Principles for an Effective Drug Policy

We propose that national drug strategies should always be based on five core principles:

1. Drug policies should be developed through a structured and objective assessment of priorities and evidence.
2. All activities should be undertaken in full compliance with international human rights law.
3. Drug policies should focus on reducing the harmful consequences rather than the scale of drug use and markets.
4. Policy and activities should seek to promote the social inclusion of marginalized groups.
5. Governments should build open and constructive relationships with civil society in the discussion and delivery of their strategies.

Adapted from the Suggested principles for an effective drug policy proposed by the International Drug Policy Consortium (IDPC), published in March 2012. Available at http://idpc.net/publications/2012/03/idpc-drug-policy-guide-2nd-edition. Each chapter of the guide fully integrates the above five core principles.

---

This approach accepts the reality that psychoactive drug use is endemic, and it focuses on pragmatic interventions, especially education, to reduce the adverse consequences of drug abuse and get treatment for addicts. The United States has already taken a harm reduction approach with tobacco and alcohol. Educational campaigns are used to inform the public about the health risks of tobacco use. Warnings have appeared on tobacco product labels since 1967 as a result of the surgeon general's 1966 report on the dangers of smoking. In 1971 a ban on television and radio cigarette advertising was imposed. Cigarette smoking has declined from 42% in 1965 to 18% in 2012, which is about 43 million Americans who still smoke (USDHHS, 2014). Smoking is on the decline among eighth and twelfth graders. According to the 2012 *National Survey on Drug Use and Health: Summary of National Findings*, past month use of any tobacco product among persons aged 12 or older decreased from 30.4% on 2002 to 26.7% in 2012 and past month tobacco use among 12- to 17-year-olds fell from 15.2% to 8.6% in that same period (SAMHSA, 2013). Education is continuing to address the dangers of alcohol abuse and to establish guidelines for safe alcohol use.

Nurses need to seek the underlying roots of various health problems and plan action that is realistic, nonjudgmental, holistic, and positive. A harm reduction model for ATOD problems facilitates such an approach.

### Definitions

The terms *drug use* and *drug abuse* have virtually lost their usefulness because the public and government have narrowed the term *drug* to include only illegal drugs rather than including prescription, OTC, and legal recreational drugs. The current phrase *alcohol, tobacco, and other drugs* (ATODs) is a reminder that the leading drug problems involve alcohol and tobacco. The term *substance* broadens the scope to include alcohol, tobacco, legal drugs, and even foods. Substance abuse is the use of any substance that threatens a person's health or impairs social or economic functioning. This definition is more objective and universal than the government's definition of drug abuse, which is the use of a drug without a prescription or any use of an illegal drug. Although any drug or food can be abused, this chapter focuses on psychoactive drugs—drugs that affect mood, perception, and thought.

Drug dependence and drug addiction are often used interchangeably, but they are not synonymous. Drug dependence is a state of neuroadaptation (a physiologic change in the central nervous system [CNS]) caused by the chronic, regular administration of a drug; in drug dependence, continued use of the drug becomes necessary to prevent withdrawal symptoms. For example, when a person is given an opiate such as morphine on a regular basis for pain, management, the morphine needs to be gradually tapered rather than abruptly stopped to prevent symptoms of withdrawal.

Drug addiction is a pattern of abuse characterized by an overwhelming preoccupation with the use (compulsive use) of a drug, securing its supply, and a high tendency to relapse if the drug is removed. Frequently, addicts are physically dependent on a drug, but there also appears to be an added psychological component that causes the intense cravings and subsequent relapse. In general, anyone can develop drug dependence as a result of regular administration of drugs that alter the CNS; however, only 7% to 15% of the drug-using population will develop a drug addiction. The process of becoming addicted is complex and related to several factors, including the addictive properties of the substance, family and peer influences, personality, age of first use, cultural and social factors, existing psychiatric disorders, and genetics.

Alcoholism is addiction to the drug called alcohol. Alcoholism and drug addiction are recognized as illnesses under a biopsychosocial model. Simply stated, the disease concept of addiction and alcoholism identifies them as chronic and progressive diseases in which a person's use of a drug or drugs continues despite problems it causes in any area of life—physical, emotional, social, economic, or spiritual.

With the 2013 updated *Diagnostic and Statistical Manual of Mental Disorders* (DSM-5), the substance-related and addictive disorders classification has been replaced with a single disorder (substance use disorder) that is measured on a continuum from mild to severe and identified by the substance, such as "alcohol use disorder—moderate." The severity of the disorder is determined by the number of diagnostic criteria that are met (American Psychiatric Association, 2013).

## PSYCHOACTIVE DRUGS

Although any drug can be abused, ATOD abuse and addiction problems generally involve the psychoactive drugs. These drugs, which can alter emotions, are used for enjoyment in social and recreational settings and for personal use to self-medicate physical or emotional discomfort. Psychoactive drugs are divided into categories according to their effect on the CNS and the general feelings or experiences the drugs may induce. The Internet or a pharmacology text can provide detailed information on these drug categories (e.g., depressants, stimulants [as shown in Box 37-2], hallucinogens, inhalants [as shown in

## BOX 37-2 Cocaine and Amphetamines: Common Illicit Stimulants

The most commonly used illicit stimulants include cocaine and amphetamines (not prescribed). Cocaine comes from the coca shrub cultivated by South American Indians in the Andes Mountains for thousands of years. Purified cocaine can be snorted, smoked, or injected. Crack is a cheap form of smokable cocaine that produces an intense high, but it lasts for a short period. Street cocaine ranges in purity from 50% to 60% and may be cut with other drugs, such as procaine or amphetamine, or any white powder, such as sugar or baby powder. High doses can cause extreme agitation, paranoid delusions, hyperthermia, hallucinations, cardiac dysrhythmias, pulmonary complications, convulsions, and possibly death (Cocaine, *Merck Manual*, 2008).

Amphetamines are a class of stimulants similar to cocaine, but the effects last longer and the drugs are cheaper. Amphetamines have a chemical structure similar to adrenaline and noradrenaline and are generally used to decrease fatigue, increase mental alertness, suppress appetite, and create a sense of well-being. Historically, amphetamines have been issued to American soldiers and pilots to decrease fatigue and increase mental alertness. They are popular among people who need to stay awake for long hours to work or study. They can be taken as pills, injected, snorted, or smoked. "Ice," the smokable form of crystal methamphetamine, first appeared in Hawaii and the western states, but the market has moved across the United States. Methamphetamine is easy to manufacture on the illicit market and its effects can last up to 24 hours (Amphetamines, *Merck Manual*, 2008).

Chronic administration of these stimulants can lead to a neurotransmitter depletion (especially of dopamine), which results in an extreme dysphoria characterized by apathy, sadness, and anhedonia (lack of joy). Thus, these users can get caught up in a dangerous cycle of gaining an extreme high followed by an extreme low. To avoid that low, the person consumes more of the stimulant. Addicts who use these drugs soon are overwhelmed by their cravings and may engage in criminal activities such as theft or prostitution to get drug money.

## BOX 37-3 Inhalants

Inhalants are often among the first drugs that young children use. The primary abusers of most inhalants are adolescents who are 12 to 17 years of age. The 2012 National Survey on Drug Use and Health found that 584,000 persons aged 12 or older had used inhalants for the first time within the past 12 months and 62.5% of them were under the age of 18 (SAMHSA, 2013). Use often ends in late adolescence.

Inhalants are breathable chemicals, which include gases and solvents, and they do not fit neatly into other categories. The four categories of inhalants are volatile organic solvents, aerosols, volatile nitrites, and gases. These substances are inhaled ("huffed") from bottles, aerosol cans, or soaked cloth or put into bags or balloons to increase the concentration of the inhaled fumes and decrease the inhalation of other substances in the vapor (e.g., paint particles). (See www.inhalants.org for examples of products in these categories and specific drug information.) Inhalant users can get high several times in a short period since the inhalants are short acting and have a rapid onset. Users are predominately white. Experimental use is about equal for males and females, but males are more likely to engage in chronic use.

Depending on the dose, the user may feel a slight stimulation, less inhibition, or even lose consciousness. Other signs include paint or stains on clothes or the body; spots or sores around the mouth; red or runny eyes or nose; chemical breath odor; a drunk, dazed, or dizzy appearance; nausea and loss of appetite; and finally anxiety, excitability, and irritability. Users can die from "sudden sniffing death" syndrome, and this can occur from the first to the 100th time he or she uses the inhalant. This death appears to be related to acute cardiac dysrhythmia. Dangers with administration of gases increase when inhaling directly from pressurized tanks because the gas is very cold and can cause frostbite to the nose, lips, and vocal cords. Also, if a gas such as nitrous oxide is not mixed with oxygen, the user may die from asphyxiation (National Institute on Drug Abuse, 2012).

Box 37-3], and marijuana), and a drug chart of commonly abused drugs is provided on the Evolve site for this book. This chapter focuses on alcohol, tobacco, and marijuana since alcohol and tobacco cause the greatest harm and marijuana is the most commonly used illicit drug. (Resource Tool 37.B on the Evolve website lists useful web resources with more information on handling substance abuse and addiction.) Information on prescription drug misuse will be discussed because there has been an increase in overdose deaths from illicit use of prescription medications.

## Alcohol

Alcohol (ethyl alcohol or ethanol) is the oldest and most widely used psychoactive drug in the world. In 2012 a national survey found that young people between the ages of 12 and 20 are more likely to use alcohol than to use tobacco or illicit drugs, including marijuana. Youth tend to drink less often than adults, but they consume more alcohol per occasion. On average, youth report consuming five drinks per occasion, and they increasingly binge drink. Alcohol abuse contributes to illness in each of the top three causes of death in the United States: heart disease, cancer, and stroke. In 2012, an estimated 22.2 million persons (8.5% of the population aged 12 or older) were classified with substance dependence or abuse in the past year based on criteria specified in the *Diagnostic and Statistical Manual of Mental Disorders*, 4th edition (DSM-IV). Of these, 2.8 million were classified with dependence on or abuse of both alcohol and illicit drugs, 4.5 million were dependent on or abused illicit drugs but not alcohol, and 14.9 million were dependent on or abused alcohol but not illicit drugs (SAMHSA, 2013).

Alcohol abuse costs billions of dollars in lost productivity, property damage, medical expenses from alcohol-related illnesses and accidents, family disruptions, alcohol-related violence, and neglect and abuse of children. Chronic alcohol abuse leads to profound metabolic and physiologic effects on all organ systems. Gastrointestinal (GI) disturbances include inflammation of the GI tract, malabsorption, ulcers, liver problems, and cancers. Cardiovascular disturbances include cardiac dysrhythmias, cardiomyopathy, hypertension, atherosclerosis, and blood dyscrasias. CNS problems include depression, sleep disturbances, memory loss, organic brain syndrome, Wernicke-Korsakoff syndrome, and alcohol withdrawal syndrome. Neuromuscular problems include myopathy and peripheral neuropathy. Males may experience testicular atrophy, sterility, impotence, or gynecomastia, and females who consume alcohol during pregnancy may reproduce neonates with fetal alcohol syndrome (FAS) or fetal alcohol effects (FAE). Some of the metabolic disturbances include hypokalemia, hypomagnesemia, and ketoacidosis. Also, endocrine disturbances may result

clients identify community resources and solve problems to meet basic needs rather than avoid them.

In addition to decreasing risk factors associated with ATOD problems, it is important to increase protective or resiliency factors. Prevention guidelines to teach parents and teachers how to increase resiliency in youths include the following strategies:

- Help them develop an increased sense of responsibility for their own success.
- Help them identify their talents.
- Encourage them to dedicate their lives to helping society rather than believing that their only purpose in life is to be consumers.
- Provide realistic appraisals and feedback; stress multicultural competence; encourage and value education and skills training.
- Increase cooperative solutions to problems rather than competitive or aggressive solutions.

## Drug Education

ATOD problems include more than abuse of psychoactive drugs. Today more than 450,000 different drugs and drug combinations are available by prescription or over the counter, and in 2010 pharmaceutical drugs were involved in almost 60% of all drug-related deaths. Opiod drugs, such as oxycodone and methadone, were involved in about 3 of every 4 pharmaceutical overdose deaths. In addition, since 2007 deaths from opioids have outnumbered those for heroin and cocaine combined (http://www.pdmpexcellence.org/content/prescription-drug -abuse-epidemic-revised-1). Nurses know about medication administration, the possible dangers of indiscriminant drug use, and the inability of drugs to cure all problems. Nurses can influence the health of clients by destroying the myth of good drugs versus bad drugs. This means (1) teaching clients that no drug is completely safe and that any drug can be abused, (2) helping persons learn how to make informed decisions about their drug use to minimize potential harm, and (3) teaching them to always tell their health care provider what supplements they are taking.

Drug technology is growing, yet the public receives little information about how to safely use this technology. Harm reduction as a goal recognizes that people consume drugs and that they need to know about the use of drugs and risks involved to make decisions about their drug use. Drug education should begin on an individual basis by reviewing the client's prescription medications. Because a physician or nurse practitioner has prescribed the medication, clients often presume little risk is involved.

Is the client aware of any untoward interactions this drug may have with other drugs being used or with food? A common occurrence with drug users is taking drugs from different categories together or at different times to regulate how they feel, known as polysubstance use or abuse. For example, a person may drink alcohol when snorting cocaine to "take the edge off"; or some intravenous drug users combine cocaine with heroin (speedball) for similar reasons. Polysubstance use can cause drug interactions that can have additive, synergistic, or antagonistic effects. Indiscriminant polysubstance abuse may lead to serious physiologic consequences and can be complicated for the health care professional to assess and treat. It is important to encourage clients to ask questions about their drug use. The How To box lists key information that clients should obtain before taking a drug or medication to decrease the possible harm from unsafe medication consumption.

**HOW TO** Determine the Relative Safety of a Drug for Personal or Client Use

*Before using a drug/medication, always determine the following:*
- *The chemical being taken*
- *How and where the drug works in the body (main effects, side effects, and adverse reactions)*
- *The correct dosage and route of administration*
- *Whether there will be drug interactions, including interactions with herbal remedies or foods*
- *Awareness of the symptoms of a potential allergic reaction and know when to seek help*
- *If there will be drug tolerance*
- *If the drug will produce physical dependence*

*From Mothers Against Misuse and Abuse:* Drug consumer safety rules. *Mosier, OR. Available at http://www.mamas.org/drugSafety.htm. Accessed July 9, 2010.*

Nurses can identify references and community resources available to provide the necessary information, and they can clarify the information. User-friendly reference texts and online resources are available that describe drug interactions among medications, other drugs (including alcohol, tobacco, marijuana, and cocaine), and other substances (food and beverages); they serve as excellent guides for nurses and their clients. (See http://www.drugs.com/drug-interactions/cannabis.html for more information.) Clients should learn about and ask questions about their prescription medications, self-administered over-the-counter drugs, including supplements and herbal remedies, and recreational drugs. This does not mean that nurses should encourage other drug use but, rather, that the potential harm from self-medication can be reduced if clients have the necessary information to make more informed decisions.

Parents should seek information about their use of medications so they can act as role models for their children. It can be confusing for children and adolescents to be told to "just say no" to drugs when they see their parents trying drugs or they see drug advertisements offering to "quick fix" every health complaint, feeling of stress, anxiety, or depression with a medication. The simple "just say no" approach does not help young people for several reasons. First, children are naturally curious, and drug experimentation is often a part of normal development. Second, children from dysfunctional homes may use drugs to get attention or to escape an intolerable environment. And finally, the "just say no" approach does not address the powerful influence of peer pressure (Marijuana, *Merck Manual*, 2013).

Drug education has moved into the school curriculum with Project DARE (Drug Abuse Resistance Education), the most widely used school-based drug-use prevention program in the United States. This program uses law enforcement officers to teach the material, but recent studies find that it is less effective than other interactive prevention programs and may even result in increased drug use (Pan and Bai, 2009). Basic ATOD prevention programs for young people should combine efforts to increase resiliency factors with drug education. Nurses can serve as educators or as advisors to the school systems or community groups to ensure that all of these areas are addressed. Role-playing is useful in teaching many of these skills.

## SECONDARY PREVENTION AND THE ROLE OF THE NURSE

Screening for health problems has long been a basic tool used by public health nurses when working with various populations. There are numerous screening tools for ATOD problems that can be used independently or integrated with broader health screening tools. When drug abuse, dependence, or addiction is identified, nurses must assist clients to understand the connection between their drug use patterns and the negative consequences on their health, their families, and the community. Brief interventions include effective strategies nurses can initiate for early intervention before a person needs more extensive or specialized treatment.

One such intervention is called Screening, Brief Intervention, and Referral to Treatment (SBIRT). SBIRT is an evidence-based practice used to identify, reduce, and prevent problematic use, abuse, and dependence on alcohol, tobacco, and other drugs. The SBIRT model was incited by an Institute of Medicine recommendation that called for community-based screening for health risk behaviors, including substance use. Primary care centers, hospital emergency rooms, trauma centers, and other community settings provide opportunities for early intervention with at-risk substance users before more severe consequences occur.

- Screening quickly assesses the severity of substance use and identifies the appropriate level of treatment.
- Brief intervention focuses on increasing insight and awareness regarding substance use and motivation toward behavioral change.
- Referral to treatment provides those identified as needing more extensive treatment with access to specialty care.

A key aspect of SBIRT is the integration and coordination of screening and treatment components into a system of services. This system links a community's specialized treatment programs with a network of early intervention and referral activities that are conducted in medical and social service settings (http://www.integration.samhsa.gov/clinical-practice/SBIRT—accessed June 16, 2014).

### Assessing for Alcohol, Tobacco, and Other Drug Problems

The National Institute on Alcohol Abuse and Alcoholism (NIAAA) has published a clinician's guide for assessing problem drinking. This free booklet (NIAAA, 2005) is available in English and Spanish and provides a step-by-step guide for clinicians to use with their clients (http://www.niaaa.nih.gov/publications/clinical-guides-and-manuals/helping-patients-who-drink-too-much-clinicians-guide—accessed June 16, 2014).

Self-assessment screening tools are available online at http://www.alcoholscreening.org/Home.aspx and www.drugscreening.org. These screening tools are based on the Alcohol, Smoking, and Substance Involvement Screening Test (ASSIST) developed by the World Health Organization and allow for immediate feedback. People can participate in this screening anonymously.

During health assessment, the nurse should assess for substance abuse problems including both self-medication practices and recreational drug use when taking a medication history. Thus, all relevant drug-use history is collected and aids in the assessment of drug-use patterns. Note any changes in drug-use patterns over time. After obtaining a medication history, follow-up questions can determine if problems exist. The following are examples:

- If using a prescription drug, is the client following the directions correctly?
- Has the client increased the dosage or frequency above the prescription level?
- Is the person using any prescribed psychoactive drugs?
- If so, for how long and what is the dosage?

One useful assessment tool is to ask about the 5 As when screening for ATOD problems: (1) Ask about use; (2) Assess amount and pattern of use; (3) Advise about safe use as appropriate; (4) Assist with identifying help or resources; (5) Arrange for follow-up as needed. Also, the Levels of Prevention box shows the levels of prevention related to substance abuse that can be used by nurses.

### 📄 LEVELS OF PREVENTION

#### *Substance Use Disorders*

**Primary Prevention**
Provide community education to teach healthy lifestyles; focus on how to resist getting involved in substance abuse.

**Secondary Prevention**
Institute early detection programs in schools, the workplace, and other areas in which people gather to determine the presence of substance abuse.

**Tertiary Prevention**
Develop programs to help people reduce or end substance abuse.

When assessing self-medication and recreational or social drug-use patterns, determine the reason the person uses the drug. Some underlying health problems (e.g., pain, stress, weight, insomnia) may be relieved by nonpharmaceutical interventions. The amount, frequency, and duration of use and the route of administration of each drug should be determined. To establish the presence of a substance abuse problem, it is necessary to determine if the drug use is causing any negative health consequences or problems with relationships, employment, finances, or the legal system. The How To box lists examples of questions to ask to determine the presence of socioeconomic problems that are often a result of substance abuse. If a pattern of chronic, regular, and frequent use of a drug exists, nurses should assess for a history of withdrawal symptoms to determine if there is physical dependence on the drug. A progression in drug-use patterns and related problems warns about the possibility of addiction. Denial is a primary symptom of addiction. Methods of denial include the following:

- Lying about use
- Minimizing use patterns
- Blaming or rationalizing
- Intellectualizing
- Changing the subject
- Using anger or humor
- "Going with the flow" (agreeing that a problem exists, stating the behavior will change, but not demonstrating any behavior changes)

---

**HOW TO** Assess Socioeconomic Problems Resulting from Substance Abuse

*If the client admits to use of alcohol, tobacco, or other drugs, ask the following questions:*

1. *Do your parents, spouse, or friends worry or complain about your drinking or using drugs?*
2. *Has a family member sought help about your drinking or using drugs?*
3. *Have you neglected family obligations as a result of drinking or using drugs?*
4. *Have you missed work because of your drinking or using drugs?*
5. *Does your boss complain about your drinking or using drugs?*
6. *Do you drink or use drugs before or during work?*
7. *Have you ever been fired or quit because of drinking or using drugs?*
8. *Have you ever been charged with driving under the influence (DUI) or being drunk in public (DIP)?*
9. *Have you ever had any other legal problems related to drinking and using drugs, such as assault and battery, breaking and entering, or theft?*
10. *Have you had any accidents while intoxicated, such as falls, burns, or motor vehicle accidents?*
11. *Have you spent your money on alcohol or other drugs instead of paying your bills (e.g., telephone, electricity, rent)?*

---

A problem should be suspected if the client becomes defensive or exhibits other behavior indicating denial when asked about alcohol or other drug use.

## Drug Testing

During the 1980s, pre-employment or random drug testing in the workplace gained popularity. A person's urine, blood, saliva or hair can be examined to test for the use of drugs. The breath can be tested for alcohol. Urine testing is the most common method of drug screening. Urine testing indicates only past use of certain drugs, not intoxication. Thus, persons can be identified as having used a certain drug in the recent past, but the degree of intoxication and extent of performance impairment cannot be determined with urine testing. Also, most drug-related problems in the workplace are related to

alcohol, and alcohol is not always included in a urine drug screen. When is drug testing appropriate? Drug testing that follows documented impairment may help substantiate the cause of the impairment, and thus it serves as a backup rather than the primary screening method. It is also useful for recovering addicts. Part of their treatment is to abstain from psychoactive drug use; therefore, a urine test yielding positive results for a drug indicates a relapse.

Blood, breath, and saliva drug tests can indicate current use and amount. Any of these tests can help determine alcohol intoxication, and they are often used to substantiate suspected impairment. A serum drug screen can be useful to determine the specific drug ingested when overdose is suspected. The testing of hair is gaining attention because the results can provide a long history of drug-use patterns.

Alcohol and other drug testing should be used as a clinical and public health tool but not for harassment and punishment. For example, approximately 40% to 50% of people who are seen in trauma centers were drinking at the time of their injuries. Hence, it is recommended that breath alcohol testing should be routinely done for clients admitted to the emergency department for traumatic injuries (Physicians and Lawyers for National Drug Policy, 2008).

Employee assistance programs (EAPs) are a beneficial service in many work settings. Often a sizable number of EAP clients have substance use problems since most adults with these problems are employed. The 2012 national survey of drug use found that of the 20.7 million adults classified with dependence or abuse, 51.9% were employed full time (SAMHSA, 2013). EAP programs can identify health problems among employees and offer counseling or referral to other health care providers as necessary. Such programs provide early identification of and intervention for substance abuse problems; they also offer services to employees to reduce stress and provide health care or counseling so that they may prevent substance abuse problems from developing. Nurses frequently develop and run these programs.

## High-Risk Groups

Identifying high-risk groups helps nurses design programs to meet specific needs and to mobilize community resources.

### Adolescents

The younger a person is when beginning intensive experimentation with drugs, the more likely dependence will develop. Underage drinking is seen as the most serious drug problem for youth in the United States. Findings from the 2012 National Survey on Drug Use and Health note these drug use patterns among 12- to 17-year-olds: among 12- or 13-year-olds, 1.7% used psychotherapeutic drugs nonmedically (with 1.5% using pain relievers), 1.2% used marijuana, and 0.9% used inhalants; among 14- or 15-year-olds, 6.1% used marijuana, 2.5% used psychotherapeutic drugs nonmedically (with 2.2% using pain relievers), 0.7% used inhalants, and 0.5% used hallucinogens; among 16- or 17-year-olds, 14.0% used marijuana, 4.0% used psychotherapeutic drugs nonmedically (with 3.1% using pain relievers), 1.2% used hallucinogens, 0.7 used inhalants, and 0.2% used cocaine (SAMHSA, 2013).

People who use illicit prescription drugs are at risk of abuse and addiction as well as overdose deaths. Many teens and college youth steal them from their family members, and others buy them off the Internet. The most commonly abused opioids among teens are hydrocodone (Vicodin) and oxycodone (OxyContin), and these are sometimes crushed and snorted or injected. Friends in school share their dextroamphetamine (Adderall) or methylphenidate (Ritalin) with other students, who often use them to help them study. Benzodiazepines such as diazepam (Valium) and alprazolam (Xanax) are the depressants of choice.

A new trend called "pharming" is where young people bring prescription medications to a party to share with friends and they may take them alone, in combinations, or mixed with alcohol. Students say that prescription drugs are often cheaper and easier to obtain, and some believe that they are "cleaner" or safer than illicit drugs such as marijuana or cocaine. They generally have no idea of the toxic effects when these drugs are taken in high doses or combined.

Heavy drug use during adolescence can interfere with normal development. Note that *Healthy People 2020* objectives SA-2 and TU-3 reduce the initiation of the use of tobacco, alcohol, and other drugs (see Healthy People 2020 box) (U.S. Department of Health and Human Services, 2010). Family-related factors (genetics, family stress, parenting styles, child victimization) appear to be the greatest variable that influences substance abuse among adolescents. The co-occurrence with psychiatric disorders (especially mood disorders) and behavioral problems is also associated with substance abuse among adolescents, leaving peer pressure as a less-influential factor. Research suggests that successful social influence-based prevention programs may be driven by their ability to foster social norms that reduce an adolescent's social motivation to begin using ATODs. One particularly effective treatment approach for adolescents is the use of family-oriented therapy (SAMHSA, 2008).The Quality and Safety in Nursing Education box provides information about using information management tools to develop ATOD prevention programs in a school.

---

### ♥ HEALTHY PEOPLE 2020

**Objectives Related to Substance Abuse**
- SA-2: Increase the proportion of adolescents never using substances.
- SA-8: Increase the proportion of persons who need alcohol and/or illicit drug treatment and received specialty treatment for abuse or dependence in the past year.
- SA-17: Decrease the rate of alcohol-impaired driving (0.08+ blood alcohol content [BAC]) fatalities.

**Objectives Related to Tobacco Use**
- TU-3: Reduce initiation of tobacco use among children, adolescents, and young adults.
- TU-11: Reduce the proportion of nonsmokers exposed to second-hand smoke.
- TU-14: Increase the proportion of smoke-free homes.

From U.S. Department of Health and Human Services: *Healthy People 2020: National Health Promotion and Disease Prevention Objectives.* Washington, DC,

---

### (QSEN) FOCUS ON QUALITY AND SAFETY EDUCATION FOR NURSES

**Targeted Competency: Informatics**
Use information and technology to communicate, manage knowledge, mitigate error, and support decision making.
   Important aspects of informatics to include:
- **Knowledge:** Identify essential information that must be available in a common database to support client care.
- **Skills:** Use information management tools to monitor outcomes of care processes.
- **Attitudes:** Value technologies that support clinical decision making, error prevention, and care coordination.

**Informatics Question**
You are taking over the role of school nurse at a large regional high school. There has been a recent tragedy involving a senior from this high school drinking and driving with friends in the car, resulting in one student death, and significant injury to the driver and another passenger. You have been asked to address use of alcohol, tobacco, and other drugs (ATOD) at this high school.
1. What data should you collect to assess the scope of the ATOD problem at this school?
2. Who are some key informants you want to interview? What information will you seek from them?
3. You decide that an alcohol and drug education program is needed in the school. What data will you want to track over time to assess the effectiveness of this intervention?

From U.S. Department of Health and Human Services, 2010.

### Older Adults

Older adults (65 years of age and older) represent 13% of the U.S. population and are the fastest growing segment of U.S. society, expected to represent 21% by the year 2030. Older adults are prescribed approximately one third of all medications in the United States, and almost half of the people over 65 years of age take 3 or more prescription drugs (Basca, 2008).

Alcohol and prescription drug misuse affects as many as 17% of adults age 60 and older. Problems with alcohol consumption, including interactions with prescribed and OTC drugs, far outnumber any other substance abuse problem among older adults (SAMHSA, 2009). The free public education brochure, *As You Age … A Guide to Aging, Medicines and Alcohol* is available at http://store.samhsa.gov/product/As-You-Age-A-Guide-to-Aging-Medicines-and-Alcohol/SMA04-3940.

The increased use of prescription drugs and alcohol by older adults may be related to coping problems. Problems of relocation, possible loss of independence, retirement, illness, death of friends, and lower levels of achievement contribute to feelings of sadness, boredom, anxiety, and loneliness. Factors such as slowed metabolic turnover of drugs, age-related organ changes, enhanced drug sensitivities, a tendency to use drugs over long periods, and a more frequent use of multiple drugs all contribute to greater negative consequences from drug use among older adults. Alcohol abuse may not be identified because its effects on cognitive abilities may mimic changes associated with normal aging or degenerative brain disease. Also, depression may simply be attributed to more frequent losses rather than the depressant effects of alcohol, and the older adult may subsequently receive medical treatment for depression rather than alcoholism.

## Injection Drug Users

In addition to the problem of addiction, injection drug users (IDUs) (those who self-administer intravenously or subcutaneously) are at risk for other health complications. Intravenous (IV) administration of drugs always carries a greater risk of overdose because the drug goes directly into the bloodstream. With illicit drugs, the danger is increased because the exact dosage is unknown. In addition, the drug may be contaminated with other chemicals, such as sugar, starch, or quinine, that can cause negative consequences. Often IDUs make their own solution for IV administration, and any particles present can result in complications from emboli.

Although heroin use was at a peak in the mid-1970s, there is a new concern due to the recent surge in its use, especially in New England, the Mid-Atlantic, and Great Lakes regions in the United States. The use of heroin is up about 75% from five years ago and much of it is fueled by the low-priced drug coming in from South America and Mexico and its availability via the Internet (Pilcher and Bernard-Kuhn, 2014).

Addicts often share needles. Human immunodeficiency virus (HIV), hepatitis C, and other blood-borne diseases can be transmitted through contaminated needles. Infections and abscesses may develop as a result of dirty needles or poor administration techniques. Since the peak of the HIV epidemic among IDUs in the late 1980s, HIV incidence among IDUs has decreased by almost 80%. Despite this overall decline, IDUs continue to represent a substantial proportion of persons with new HIV diagnoses, with the highest number among African Americans (CDC, 2011). Because of this trend, emphasis is being placed on reducing the transmission of this disease through contaminated needles. Abstinence is ideal but unrealistic for many addicts. Using the harm reduction model, the nurse should provide education on cleaning needles with bleach between uses and on needle exchange programs to decrease the spread of the virus. Studies indicate that needle exchange programs have not increased injection drug abuse but have, in fact, increased the number of people entering treatment programs (Knox, 2012).

## Drug Use during Pregnancy

Most drugs can negatively affect a fetus. Thus, the use of any drug during pregnancy should be discouraged unless medically necessary. *Healthy People 2020* objectives address this issue under the Maternal, Infant and Child Health topic area with several objectives that describe recommendations to improve the health of infants, such as reducing the occurrence of fetal alcohol syndrome (FAS) (MICH-25), and increasing abstinence from alcohol, cigarettes, and illicit drugs among pregnant women (MICH-11). FAS is considered the leading preventable birth defect, causing mental and behavioral impairment. In 2011 to 2012 approximately 2.7% of pregnant women reported binge drinking and 0.3% reported heavy drinking. These low rates may be due to the extensive information available about the effects of alcohol on the fetus. Estimates of illicit drug use during pregnancy for women aged 15 to 44 were 5.9%. Tobacco remains the most-used addictive substance during pregnancy, with about 15.9% of pregnant women smoking (SAMHSA, 2013). In some states, pregnant women who are using illicit drugs are reported to child protective services because of the potential harm to the fetus.

Despite the increased focus on drug abuse interventions, many pregnant women with drug problems do not receive the help they need. This may be a result of ignorance, poverty, lack of concern for the fetus, lack of available services, and fear of the consequences of revealing drug use. The fear of criminal prosecution may push addicted women further away from the health care system, cause them to conceal their drug use from medical providers, and cause them to avoid the critical treatment and medical care that they need (Brady and Ashley, 2005).

## Persons Who Use Illicit Drugs

The strategy of "just say no" to drugs is both simplistic and misleading. Indiscriminant use of "good" drugs has caused more health problems from adverse reactions, drug interactions, dependence, addiction, and overdoses than use of "bad" drugs. However, the war on drugs focuses on illicit drugs and punishes illicit drug users. The black market associated with illicit drug use puts otherwise law-abiding citizens in close contact with criminals, prevents any quality control of the drugs, increases the risk of AIDS and hepatitis as a result of needle sharing, and hinders health care professionals' accessibility to the abuser or addict. Lack of quality control (unknown strength and purity) can cause unexpected overdoses or secondary effects of the impurities; for example, a synthetic analog of fentanyl (3-methylfentanyl) marketed as "heroin" is 6000 times as potent as morphine. Unsafe administration (contaminated needles) leads to local and systemic infections. The high cost of drugs on the black market leads to crime to support the addiction. In 2012, the highest rate of current illicit drug use was among 18- to 20-year-olds at 23.9%, with the next highest rate occurring among the 21- to 25-year-olds at 19.7%. Illicit drugs include marijuana/hashish, cocaine (including crack), heroin, hallucinogens, inhalants, or prescription-type psychotherapeutics that are used nonmedically. Marijuana was the most frequently used illicit drug (SAMHSA, 2013). See Figure 37-2 for illicit drug use by race/ethnicity.

## Codependency and Family Involvement

Drug addiction is often a family disease. One in four Americans experiences family problems related to alcohol abuse. People in a close relationship with the addict often develop unhealthy coping mechanisms to continue the relationship. This behavior is known as codependency—a stress-induced preoccupation with the addicted person's life, leading to extreme dependence and excessive concern with the addict.

Strict rules typically develop in a codependent family to maintain the relationships: don't talk, don't feel, don't trust, don't lose control, and don't seek help from outside the family. Codependents try to meet the addict's needs at the expense of their own. Codependency may underlie many of the medical

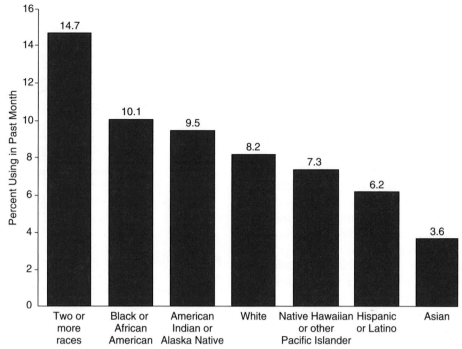

**FIG 37-2** Past month illicit drug use among persons aged 12 or older, by race/ethnicity, 2012. (From Substance Abuse and Mental Health Services Administration: *Results from the 2012 National Survey on Drug Use and Health: Summary of National Findings, Office of Applied Studies,* NSDUH Series H-46, USDHHS Pub No SMA 13-4795, Rockville, MD, 2013. See page 25 at: http://www.samhsa.gov/data/NSDUH/2012SummNatFindDetTables/NationalFindings/NSDUHresults2012.pdf)

complaints and emotional stress seen by health care providers, such as ulcers, skin disorders, migraine headaches, chronic colds, and backaches.

When the addicted person refuses to admit the problem, the family continues to adapt to emotionally survive the stress of the addict's irrational, inconsistent, and unpredictable behavior. Family members consequently develop various roles that tend to be gross exaggerations of normal family roles, and they cling irrationally to these roles, even when they are no longer functional.

One of the most significant roles a family member may assume is that of an enabler. **Enabling** is the act of shielding or preventing the addict from experiencing the consequences of the addiction. As a result, the addict does not always understand the cost of the addiction and thus is "enabled" to continue to use. Although codependency and enabling are closely related, a person does not have to be codependent to enable. Anyone can be an enabler: a police officer, a boss or coworker, and even a drug treatment counselor. Health care professionals who do not address the negative health consequences of the drug use with the addicted person are enablers.

The nurse can help families recognize the problem of addiction and help them confront the addicted member in a caring manner. Whether or not the addicted family member is agreeable to treatment, the family members should be given some guidance about the literature and services that are available to help them cope more effectively. The nurse can help identify treatment options, counseling assistance, financial assistance,

support services, and (if necessary) legal services for the family members. Children of ATOD abusers or addicts are themselves at a greater risk for developing addiction and must be targeted for primary prevention.

## TERTIARY PREVENTION AND THE ROLE OF THE NURSE

The nurse is in a key position to help the addict and the addict's family. The nurse's knowledge of community resources and how to mobilize them can significantly influence the quality of care clients receive.

### Detoxification

**Detoxification** is the clearing of one or more drugs from the person's body and managing the withdrawal symptoms. Depending on the particular drug and the degree of dependence, the time required may range from a few days to several weeks. Because withdrawal symptoms vary (depending on the drug used) and range from uncomfortable to life threatening, the setting for and management of withdrawal depend on the drug used.

Drugs such as stimulants or opiates may produce withdrawal symptoms that are uncomfortable but not life threatening. Detoxification from these drugs does not require direct medical supervision, but medical management of the withdrawal symptoms increases the comfort level. On the other hand, drugs such as alcohol, benzodiazepines, and barbiturates can produce life-threatening withdrawal symptoms. These clients should be under close medical supervision during detoxification and should receive medical management of the withdrawal symptoms to ensure a safe withdrawal. Of those who develop delirium tremens from alcohol withdrawal, 15% may not survive despite medical management; therefore, close medical management is initiated as the blood alcohol level begins to fall.

A general rule in detoxification management is to wean the person off the drug by gradually reducing the dosage and frequency of administration. Thus, a person with chronic alcoholism could be safely detoxified by a gradual reduction in alcohol consumption. In practice, however, the switch to another drug, usually a benzodiazepine, often offers a safer withdrawal from alcohol as well as an abrupt end to the intoxication from the drug of choice. For example, chlordiazepoxide (Librium) is commonly used for alcohol detoxification. Outpatient or home detoxification for persons requiring medical detoxification for alcohol withdrawal can be a cost-effective treatment. Nurses can monitor and evaluate the client's health status in the home environment to reduce the risk of medical complications related to alcohol withdrawal, and to provide encouragement and support for the client to complete the detoxification.

### Addiction Treatment

Addiction treatment differs from the management of negative health consequences of chronic drug abuse, overdose, and detoxification. Addiction treatment focuses on the addiction process. The goal is to help clients view addiction as a chronic disease and assist them to make lifestyle changes to halt the progression of the disease. According to the disease theory, addicts are not responsible for the symptoms of their disease; they are, however, responsible for treating their disease. In 2012, 22.2 million persons aged 12 or older needed treatment for an illicit drug or alcohol use problem (8.5% of the persons aged 12 or older). Of these, 4.0 million persons age 12 or older received treatment for alcohol or illicit substance use problems (SAMHSA, 2013). Figure 37-3 shows the common reasons persons do not receive treatment. Of the 2.3 million persons aged 12 or older who received substance use treatment in 2011, 898,000 were in treatment for an alcohol use disorder, 780,000 for an illicit drug use disorder, and 574,000 received treatment for both alcohol and illicit drug problems (SAMHSA, 2013).

Most treatment facilities are multidisciplinary because the intervention strategies require a wide range of approaches. Their programs involve interactions between the addict, family, culture, and community. Strategies include medical management, education, counseling, vocational rehabilitation, stress management, and support services. In addition, specific programs address the needs of various populations such as adolescents, pregnant women, specific ethnic groups, gays and lesbians, as well as health care professionals. The key to effective treatment is to match individual clients with the interventions most appropriate for them. Box 37-5 lists 13 fundamental principles for effective addiction treatment.

Total abstinence is the most recommended treatment goal for ATOD addiction. People who are addicted to a particular drug (e.g., cocaine) are advised to abstain from the use of all

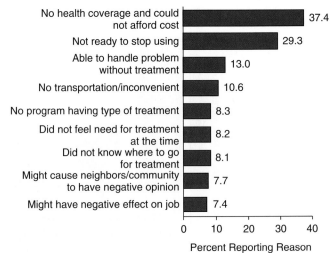

**FIG 37-3** Reasons for not receiving substance use treatment among persons aged 12 or older who needed and made an effort to get treatment but did not receive treatment and felt they needed treatment, 2009-2012 combined. *(See bottom of page 88 at: http://www.samhsa.gov/data/NSDUH/2012Summ NatFindDetTables/NationalFindings/NSDUHresults2012.pdf)* (From Substance Abuse and Mental Health Services Administration: *Results from the 2012 national survey on drug use and health: summary of national findings, Office of Applied Studies,* NSDUH Series H-46, HHS Pub No SMA 13-4795, 2013, Rockville, MD.)

psychoactive substances. The use of another drug may simply reinforce the craving for the original drug and cause relapse. More commonly, the addiction merely transfers to the replacement substance.

Treatment may be on an inpatient or outpatient basis. In general, the more advanced the disease is, the greater the need for inpatient treatment. Inpatient treatment programs usually may range from less than 1 week to as long as 90 days. Once a person has completed detoxification (considered the first phase of the treatment process), the programs use counseling and group interaction to help the client stay clean long enough for the body chemistry to rebalance. This is often a difficult time for persons recovering from addictions because they may experience mood swings and difficulty sleeping and dealing with emotions.

The goal of the educational part of the programs is to provide information about the disease and how drugs affect a person physically and psychologically. Clients are informed of the various lifestyle changes that are recommended, and they learn about tools to assist them in making these changes. Discharge planning continues throughout treatment as clients build the support systems that they will need when they leave the controlled environment of a treatment center and face pressures and temptations (triggers) that may lead to relapse.

Long-term residential programs, also called halfway houses, have been developed to ease the person recovering from an addiction back into society. These facilities provide continued support and counseling in a structured environment for persons

---

**BOX 37-5**    **Principles of Drug Addiction Treatment**

More than three decades of scientific research have yielded 13 fundamental principles that characterize effective drug abuse treatment. These principles are detailed in NIDA's *Principles of Drug Addiction Treatment: A Research-Based Guide* (April, 2009).

1. No single treatment is appropriate for all individuals. Matching treatment settings, interventions, and services to each client's problems and needs is critical.
2. Treatment needs to be readily available. Treatment applicants can be lost if treatment is not immediately available or readily accessible.
3. Effective treatment attends to multiple needs of the individual, not just his or her drug use. Treatment must address the individual's drug use and associated medical, psychological, social, vocational, and legal problems.
4. At different times during treatment, a client may develop a need for medical services, family therapy, vocational rehabilitation, and social and legal services.
5. Remaining in treatment for an adequate period of time is critical for treatment effectiveness. The time depends on an individual's needs. For most clients, the threshold of significant improvement is reached at about 3 months in treatment. Additional treatment can produce further progress. Programs should include strategies to prevent clients from leaving treatment prematurely.
6. Individual and/or group counseling and other behavioral therapies are critical components of effective treatment for addiction. In therapy, clients address motivation, build skills to resist drug use, replace drug-using activities with constructive and rewarding non–drug-using activities, and improve problem-solving abilities. Behavioral therapy also facilitates interpersonal relationships.
7. Medications are an important element of treatment for many clients, especially when combined with counseling and other behavioral therapies.

Buprenorphine, methadone, and levo-alpha-acetylmethodol (LAAM) help persons addicted to opiates stabilize their lives and reduce their drug use. Naltrexone is effective for some opiate addicts and some clients with co-occurring alcohol dependence. Nicotine patches or gum, or an oral medication, such as bupropion, can help persons addicted to nicotine.

8. Addicted or drug-abusing individuals with coexisting mental disorders should have both disorders treated in an integrated way.
9. Medical detoxification is only the first stage of addiction treatment and by itself does little to change long-term drug use. Medical detoxification manages the acute physical symptoms of withdrawal. For some individuals it is a precursor to effective drug addiction treatment.
10. Treatment does not need to be voluntary to be effective. Sanctions or enticements in the family, employment setting, or criminal justice system can significantly increase treatment entry, retention, and success.
11. Possible drug use during treatment must be monitored continuously. Monitoring a client's drug and alcohol use during treatment, such as through urinalysis, can help the client withstand urges to use drugs. Such monitoring can also provide early evidence of drug use so that treatment can be adjusted.
12. Treatment programs should provide assessment for HIV/AIDS, hepatitis B and C, tuberculosis and other infectious diseases, and counseling to help clients modify or change behaviors that place them or others at risk of infection. Counseling can help clients avoid high-risk behavior and help people who are already infected manage their illness.
13. Recovery from drug addiction can be a long-term process and frequently requires multiple episodes of treatment. As with other chronic illnesses, relapses to drug use can occur during or after successful treatment episodes. Participation in self-help support programs during and following treatment often helps maintain abstinence.

---

needing long-term assistance in adjusting to a drug-free lifestyle. The residents are expected to secure employment and take responsibility in managing their financial obligations.

Outpatient programs are similar in the education and counseling offered, but they allow the clients to live at home and continue to work while undergoing treatment. This method is effective for persons in the earlier stages of addiction who feel confident that they can abstain from drug use and have established a strong support network. The How To box provides resources to help locate treatment programs throughout the United States.

---

**HOW TO** Find an Appropriate Treatment Program

1. *Look it up in the* National Directory of Drug and Alcohol Abuse Treatment Programs *(updated annually). This directory provides information on more than 11,000 alcohol and drug treatment programs in all 50 states, the District of Columbia, Puerto Rico, and 4 U.S. territories. Free copies are available by calling SAMHSA's Clearinghouse at 1-877-726-4727.*
2. *Look it up on the Substance Abuse and Mental Health Services Administration's (SAMHSA) website. Their Substance Abuse Treatment Facility Locator Internet-based service provides an easy-to-use directory to help you locate (including road maps to each facility) and contact public and private treatment programs (http://www.findtreatment.samhsa.gov).*

---

For those addicted individuals unwilling or unable to completely abstain from psychoactive drugs, other medications can assist them in abstaining from their drug of choice. Currently there are three types of medication-assisted therapies (MAT) for treating opioid addiction: methadone, buprenorphine, and naltrexone. Methadone, when administered in moderate or high daily doses, produces a cross-tolerance to other opioids, thereby blocking their effects and decreasing the craving for the drug of choice. The advantages of methadone are that it is long acting, does not produce a "high," and is inexpensive. The oral use of methadone eliminates the danger of the spread of AIDS and other blood-borne infections that commonly occur among needle-sharing addicts. Although not recognized as a cure for heroin (or other opioid) addiction, methadone maintenance is a harm reduction intervention because it reduces deviant behavior and introduces addicted persons to the health care system (Volkow et al, 2014).

Recovery from addiction involves a lifetime commitment and may include periods of relapse. The addicted person must realize that modern medicine has not found a cure for addiction; therefore, returning to drug use may ultimately reactivate the disease process.

## Smoking Cessation Programs

Nearly 35 million Americans try to quit smoking each year. Fewer than 10% of those who try to quit on their own are able

## EVIDENCE-BASED PRACTICE

Scavone et al (2013) examined the use of cannabis prior to and during methadone maintenance treatment (MMT) for opioid dependence via a chart review of 91 patients undergoing MMT in Pennsylvania. They found that those opioid addicts with a history of cannabis use reported "significantly less daily expenditure on acquisition of opiates." In addition they found that those who used cannabis during induction had lower ratings of opiate withdrawal symptoms. The researchers concluded that these findings point to novel interventions for the treatment of opioid dependence that specifically target cannabinoid-opioid system interactions. This study supports earlier work by Reiman (2009), who found that many patients in a California cannabis dispensary reported using cannabis to help them get off and stay off of problematic drug use with alcohol, opioids, and other drugs of abuse.

### Nurse Use

With the emerging understanding of the endocannabinoid system and its overall role of maintaining homeostasis, this study supports the healing properties of cannabis as it reduces withdrawal symptoms from addictive drugs and helps addicts reach stabilization. This is not to say that a person may not have a problem with cannabis, but rather it is important to assess the reasons for drug use and the consequences of that use to determine whether or not the person has a drug use disorder.

Scavone JL, Sterling RC, Weinstein SP, et al: Impact of cannabis use during stabilization on methadone maintenance treatment. *Am J Addict* 22(4):344–351, 2013.

---

## BOX 37-6   Smoking Cessation Resources

**American Cancer Society**
"Guide to Quitting Smoking" and more
http://www.cancer.org, retrieved June 16, 2014

**American Heart Association**
"In Control: Freedom from Smoking" program
http://www.americanheart.org, retrieved June 16, 2014

**American Lung Association**
"Freedom From Smoking Online"
http://www.lung.org/stop-smoking/how-to-quit/freedom-from-smoking/joining-our-effort.html. Accessed June 16, 2014

**Centers for Disease Control and Prevention: Office on Smoking and Health**
www.cdc.gov/tobacco, retrieved June 16, 2014

**The Foundation for a Smoke-Free America**
"Quitting Tips" and more
http://www.tobaccofree.org, retrieved June 16, 2014

**National Cancer Institute (NCI)**
http://www.cancer.gov, retrieved June 16, 2014
Tobacco quit line: 1-800-784-8669 (1-800-QUIT-NOW)
Quitting information, cessation guide, and counseling is offered, as well as information on state telephone-based quit programs

**Smokefree.gov**
"Quit Smoking today! We can help"
Retrieved 6/16/2014 from http://www.smokefree.gov
Excellent source created by Tobacco Control Research Branch of NCI

**Smokefree Women**
Retrieved 6/16/2014 from http://women.smokefree.gov
NCI collaborated with:
Centers for Disease Control and Prevention—Office on Smoking and Health
Centers for Disease Control and Prevention—Division of Reproductive Health
Health Canada
American Legacy Foundation
The Robert Wood Johnson Foundation

**SmokEnders**
"The Quit Kit," an 11-week program
http://www.smokenders.com, retrieved June 16, 2014

---

to stop for a year; those who use an intervention are more likely to be successful. Interventions that involve medications and behavioral treatments appear most promising (USDHHS, 2014). For example, nicotine replacement therapy can be used to help smokers withdraw from nicotine while focusing their efforts on breaking the psychological craving or habit. Four types of nicotine replacement products are available: nicotine gum and skin patches are available over the counter, and nicotine nasal spray and inhalers are available by prescription. These products are about equally effective and can almost double the chances of successfully quitting. Other treatments include smoking cessation clinics, hypnosis, and acupuncture. The most effective way to get people to stop smoking and prevent relapse involves multiple interventions and continuous reinforcement, and most smokers require several attempts at cessation before they are successful. Many resources are available on smoking cessation programs and support groups, including those listed in Box 37-6. There is a website developed specifically for nurses to help nurses quit smoking: http://www.tobaccofreenurses.org.

## Support Groups

The founding of Alcoholics Anonymous (AA) in 1935 began a strong movement of peer support to treat a chronic illness. AA groups have developed around the world. Their success has led to the development of other support groups such as the following:

- Narcotics Anonymous (NA) for persons with narcotic addiction
- Pills Anonymous for persons with polydrug addictions
- Overeaters Anonymous
- Gamblers Anonymous

AA and NA help addicted people develop a daily program of recovery and reinforce the recovery process. The fellowship, support, and encouragement among members provide a vital social network for the person recovering from an addiction.

Al-Anon and Alateen are similar self-help programs for spouses, parents, children, or others involved in a painful relationship with an alcoholic. Nar-Anon is a support group for those in relationships with persons with narcotic addictions. Al-Anon family groups are available to anyone who has been affected by their involvement with an alcoholic person. The purposes of Alateen include providing a forum for adolescents to discuss family stressors, learn coping skills from one another, and gain support and encouragement from knowledgeable

## ≫ LINKING CONTENT TO PRACTICE

Using the tools of primary, secondary, and tertiary prevention with individuals, families, and communities in whom alcohol and other drug use is an issue incorporates both public health and public health nursing guidelines and competencies. Specifically, the core competencies of the Council on Linkages Between Academia and Public Health Practice (2010) begin by identifying the analytic and assessment skills needed by public health professionals. The 12 skills in this competency category are used in providing services to the population described in this chapter. For example, you begin by assessing the "health status of populations and their related determinants of health and stress." You next move to skill #2, which is describing the "characteristics of a population-based health problem." These competencies are described through a set of eight domains. Each domain can be used with populations dealing with alcohol and other drug problems.

Similarly, the Intervention Wheel, which is the subject of Chapter 9, has many applications with this population. The Intervention Wheel specifies that "interventions are actions that PHNs take on behalf of individuals, families, and systems, and communities to improve or protect health status (Council on Linkages, 2010, p. 1). This tool outlines 17 public health interventions. All 17 of these interventions have application with the populations described in this chapter. For example, case finding, referral and follow-up, health teaching, counseling, and policy development and enforcement are selected examples of ways in which public health nurses intervene in serving a vulnerable population with alcohol- and drug-related problems.

peers. Adult Children of Alcoholics (ACOA) groups are also available in most areas to address the recovery of adults who grew up in alcoholic homes and are still carrying the scars and retaining dysfunctional behaviors.

For some persons, the AA program places too much emphasis on a higher power or focuses too much on the negative consequences of past drinking. Women for Sobriety focuses on rebuilding self-esteem, and this is often a core issue for many women with alcoholic problems. (See www.womenforsobriety.org for additional information.) Rational Recovery has a cognitive orientation and is based on the assumption that ATOD addiction is caused by irrational beliefs that can be understood and overcome. See www.rational.org for additional information on this approach.

## Nurse's Role

Many people with alcoholism and drug addiction become lost in the health care system. If satisfactory care is not provided in one agency or the waiting list is months long, the person may give up rather than seek alternative sources of care. The nurse who knows the client's history, environment, support systems, and the local treatment programs can offer guidance to the most effective treatment modality. Brief interventions by health care professionals who are not treatment experts can be effective in helping ATOD abusers and addicts change their risky behavior. **Brief interventions** may convince the ATOD abuser or addict to reduce substance consumption or follow through with a treatment referral (SAMHSA, 2011). Box 37-7 describes six elements commonly included in brief interventions, using the acronym FRAMES. Strategies used with clients can vary depending on their readiness for change. Understanding the stages of change listed in Box 37-8 and recognizing which stage

### BOX 37-7  Brief Interventions Using the FRAMES Acronym

*Feedback.* Provide the client direct feedback about the potential or actual personal risk or impairment related to drug use.
*Responsibility.* Emphasize personal responsibility for change.
*Advice.* Provide clear advice to change risky behavior.
*Menu.* Provide a menu of options or choices for changing behavior.
*Empathy.* Provide a warm, reflective, empathetic, and understanding approach.
*Self-efficacy.* Provide encouragement and belief in the client's ability to change.

From Center for Substance Abuse Treatment: *Brief Interventions and Brief Therapies for Substance Abuse.* TIP 34, DHHS Pub No (SMA) 99-3353. Rockville, MD, 1999, USDHHS.

### BOX 37-8  Stages of Change

**Pre-Contemplation**
At this stage, the person does not intend to change in the foreseeable future. The person is often unaware of any problem. Resistance to recognizing or modifying a problem is the hallmark of pre-contemplation.

**Contemplation**
At this stage, the individual is aware that a problem exists and is seriously thinking about overcoming it but has not yet made a commitment to take action. The nurse can encourage the individual to weigh the pros and cons of both the problem and the solution to the problem.

**Preparation**
Preparation was originally referred to as *decision making.* At this stage, the individual is prepared for action and may reduce the problem behavior but has not yet taken effective action (e.g., reduces amount of smoking but does not abstain).

**Action**
At this stage, the individual modifies the behavior, experiences, or environment to overcome the problem. The action requires considerable time and energy. Modification of the target behavior to an acceptable criterion and significant overt efforts to change are the hallmarks of action.

**Maintenance**
In this stage, the individual works to prevent relapse and consolidate the gains attained during action. Stabilizing behavior change and avoiding relapse are the hallmarks of maintenance.

Modified from DiClemente CC, Schlundt D, Gemmell L: Readiness and stages of change in addiction treatment. *Am J Addict* 13(2):103-119, 2004.

a client is in are important factors for determining which interventions and programs may be most helpful to the client.

After the client has received treatment, the nurse can coordinate aftercare referrals and follow up on the client's progress. The nurse can provide additional support in the home as the client and family adjust to changing roles and the stress involved with such changes. The nurse can support addicted persons who have relapsed by reminding them that relapses may well occur, but that they and their families can continue to work toward recovery and an improved quality of life.

## OUTCOMES

Health promotion and risk reduction are basic concepts in nursing. Promoting a healthy environment in the home and local community provides individuals and families a nurturing environment in which to achieve optimal health. Individuals with high self-esteem and access to health care and information about the health risks related to drug use can be responsible for their personal health and make informed decisions about drug use. Nurses can assess the health of the community and its citizens, prioritize the needs, and identify local resources to collaborate with others to develop strategies that will improve the underlying health of the community.

Early identification and intervention for persons with ATOD problems can prevent many of the harmful physical, emotional, and social consequences that may occur if abuse continues and may also prevent abuse patterns from developing into addiction. The nurse needs to assess individual and community ATOD problems and target at-risk groups to develop strategies to increase assessment and provide appropriate interventions. Review the national health objectives (refer back to the *Healthy People 2020* box) for the tobacco and substance abuse areas and note how many can be achieved with secondary prevention strategies.

Besides saving taxpayers' money, treatment helps addicted individuals and their families recover from the devastating effects of addiction. Addicts and their families often become hopeless and helpless while actively addicted. The nurse can offer hope in affirming the addict's self-worth and can be the bridge to community resources to assist in treatment and recovery.

Many of these expected outcomes for ATOD problems have been lessened because a lack of funding has resulted from federal strategies that focus on law enforcement and punishment rather than on education and treatment. The greatest challenge for nurses is to influence policy makers to put the emphasis on health care for this major health problem.

## PRACTICE APPLICATION

Ms. Jane Doe, RN, is a home health case manager in a large, low-income housing area in her community. She designs care plans and coordinates health care services for clients who need health care at home. She makes the initial visits to determine the level and frequency of care needed and then acts as supervisor of the volunteers and nurses' aides who perform most of the day-to-day care. Single-parent families are the norm, and drug dealing is commonplace in this housing area.

Ms. Doe made a home visit to Ann Greene, a 26-year-old mother of three. She takes care of her 62-year-old maternal grandfather, Mr. Jones, who is recovering from cardiac bypass surgery. He has a smoking history of two packs per day for almost 40 years. Since his surgery, he has reduced his smoking to one pack per day, but he refuses to quit. He has a history of alcohol dependence, reportedly consuming up to a fifth of liquor a day, and a history of withdrawal seizures. Four years ago he went through alcohol detoxification, but he refused to stay at the facility for continued treatment, stating he could stay sober on his own. Since that time he has had several binge episodes, but Ann says that he has not been drinking since the surgery. A widower for 5 years, Mr. Jones now lives with his granddaughter and her three children.

Ms. Greene is a widow and has two sons, ages 3 and 9, and a daughter, age 5. The oldest son's father is an alcoholic who is currently incarcerated for manslaughter while driving under the influence of alcohol, and the father of her two youngest children was killed by a stray bullet in a cocaine bust 3 years ago. She and her husband had smoked crack cocaine for several months but both stopped when she became pregnant with their youngest child and remained cocaine free. She is angry at the system and frightened of police officers ever since the drug raid in which her husband was killed. Other residents were also hurt, and less than $500 worth of cocaine was found three apartments away from hers.

Ms. Greene does not consume alcohol, but she smokes one to two packs of cigarettes per day. She quit smoking during her pregnancies but restarted soon after each birth.

A. What type of interventions can the nurse provide for Mr. Jones regarding his smoking?
B. How can the nurse help Ms. Greene cope with the potential risk of Mr. Jones' drinking when he progresses to more independence?
C. How can the nurse help Ms. Greene with her cigarette smoking?
D. Knowing that there is a genetic link to alcoholism and being aware of the high rate of drug problems in the housing area, how can Nurse Doe help prevent this mother and her children from developing substance abuse problems?
E. What problems seem greater because of the drug laws, and what can Ms. Greene do to help make the environment safer and more nurturing?
**Answers can be found on the Evolve site.**

## KEY POINTS

- Substance abuse is the number one national health problem, linked to numerous forms of morbidity and mortality.
- Harm reduction is an approach to ATOD problems that deals with substance abuse primarily as a health problem rather than as a criminal problem.
- All persons have ideas, opinions, and attitudes about the use of drugs that influence their actions.
- Social conditions such as a fast-paced life, excessive stress, and the availability of drugs influence the incidence of substance use disorders.

## ■ KEY POINTS—cont'd

- Important terms to understand when working with individuals, groups, or communities for whom substance abuse is prevalent are *drug dependence, drug addiction, alcoholism, psychoactive drugs, depressants, stimulants, marijuana, hallucinogens,* and *inhalants.*
- Primary prevention for substance use disorders includes education about drugs and guidelines for use, as well as the promotion of healthy alternatives to drug use either for recreation or to relieve stress.
- Nurses can help develop community prevention programs.
- Secondary prevention depends heavily on careful assessment of the client's use of drugs. Such assessment should be part of all basic health assessments.

- High-risk groups include pregnant women, young people, older adults, intravenous drug users, and illicit drug users.
- Drug addiction is often a family, not merely an individual, problem.
- Codependency describes a companion illness to the addiction of one person in which the codependent member is addicted to the addicted person.
- Brief interventions by a nurse can be as effective as treatment.
- Nurses are in ideal roles to assist with tertiary prevention for both the addicted person and the family.

## ■ CLINICAL DECISION-MAKING ACTIVITIES

1. Read your local newspaper or online news for 4 days and select stories that illustrate the effects of substance abuse on individuals, families, and the community. What interventions would you use? Who would you involve in your work? Are the interventions primary, secondary, or tertiary in nature? How would you evaluate your work?

2. For each of the stories in the news related to substance abuse, describe preventive strategies that a nurse might have tried before the problem reached such a dire state.

3. Looking at your local community resources directory, the telephone book, or the Internet, identify agencies that might serve as referral sources for individuals or families for whom substance abuse is a problem.

4. Review popular magazine and television advertisements for alcohol, tobacco, and other medicines (e.g., sleep aids, analgesics, laxatives, stimulants). In small groups, discuss the messages conveyed in the advertisements, and discuss the implications of client education to reduce possible harm from misuse and abuse of these substances.

5. Attend an open AA or NA meeting and an Al-Anon meeting. Go alone if possible or with an alcoholic or a drug-addicted friend. As the members introduce themselves, give your first name and state, "I am a visitor." Plan to listen and do not attempt to take notes. Respect the anonymity of the persons present. Discuss your experiences later in a group.

6. In groups of four or five, review the national health objectives in *Healthy People 2020* (see www.healthypeople.gov) under Tobacco Use and under Substance Abuse. Pick an objective from each section, and brainstorm about possible community efforts a nurse could initiate to reach that objective.

# REFERENCES

American Psychiatric Association: *Diagnostic and Statistical Manual of Mental Disorders*, ed 5. Arlington, VA, 2013, American Psychiatric Publishing.

Amphetamines: *The Merck Manual, section 15, psychiatric disorders, chapter 198, drug use and dependence.* 2008, Merck & Co, Inc. Available at: http://www.merck.com/mmpe/sec15/ch198/ch198k.html. Accessed June 2, 2014.

Barnoya J, Glanz SA: Cardiovascular effects of secondhand smoke nearly as large as smoking. *Circulation* 111:2684–2698, 2005.

Barry M: *Health Harms from Secondhand Smoke.* 2007, National Center for Tobacco-Free Kids. Available at: http://tobaccofreekids.org/. Accessed June 17, 2014.

Basca L: *The Elderly and Prescription Drug Misuse and Abuse.* 2008, Center for Applied Research

Solutions. Available at: http://www.cars-rp.org/publications/Prevention%20Tactics/PT09.02.08.pdf.

Brady TM, Ashley OS, editors: *Women in Substance Abuse Treatment: Results from the Alcohol and Drug Services Study (ADSS), Office of Applied Studies.* DHHS Pub No SMA 04-3968, Analytic Series A-26. Rockville, MD, 2005, SAMHSA.

Centers for Disease Control and Prevention: *Prescription drug overdose in the United States: fact sheet 2014*, Available at http://www.cdc.gov/homeandrecreationalsafety/overdose/facts.html. Accessed March 5, 2015.

Centers for Disease Control and Prevention: *HIV surveillance in injection drug users (through 2011)*, 2011. Available at http://www.cdc

.gov/hiv/idu/resources/slides/index.htm. Accessed June 2, 2014.

Cocaine: *The Merck Manual, section 15, psychiatric disorders, chapter 198, drug use and dependence.* 2008, Merck & Co, Inc. Available at: http://www.merck.com/mmpe/sec15/ch198/ch198j.html. Available at Accessed June 2, 2014.

Common Sense for Drug Policy: *Drug War Facts,* updated May 30, 2014, ed 6. Available at http://www.drugwarfacts.org. Accessed June 1, 2014.

Council on Linkages Between Academia and Public Health Practice: *Core Competencies for Public Health Professionals.* Washington DC, 2010, Public Health Foundation/Health Resources and Services Administration.

Drug and Substance Use and Abuse in Adolescents: *The Merck Manual,*

*Home Health Handbook for Patients and Caregivers.* 2009, Merck & Co, Inc. Available at: http://www.merckmanuals.com/home/index.html. Accessed June2, 2014.

Kinney J, Leaton G: *Loosening the Grip,* ed 5. St Louis, 1995, Mosby.

Knox R: *Needle exchanges often overlooked in AIDS fight.* Health News from NPR: July 24, 2012. Available at http://www.npr.org/blogs/health/2012/07/24/157283038/needle-exchanges-often-overlooked-in-aids-fight. Accessed June 16, 2014.

Marijuana: *The Merck Manual, section 15, psychiatric disorders, chapter 198, drug use and dependence.* 2013, Merck & Co, Inc. Available at: http://merck.com/mmpe/sec15/ch198/ch198i.html. Accessed June 2, 2014.

Mayo Clinic Staff: *Caffeine: How Much Is too Much?* March 24, 2009. Available at http://www.mayoclinic.com/health/caffeine/NU00600/METHOD=print. Accessed June 2, 2014.

National Center on Addiction and Substance Abuse: *Shoveling Up II: The Impact of Substance Abuse on Federal, State and Local Budgets.* New York, 2009, Center on Addiction and Substance Abuse at Columbia University.

National Institute on Alcohol Abuse and Alcoholism: *Helping Patients Who Drink too Much: A Clinician's Guide (Update).* NIH Pub No 07-3769. Rockville, MD, 2005, USDHHS. Available at: http://pubs.niaaa.nih.gov/publications/Practitioner/CliniciansGuide2005/guide.pdf. Accessed June 2, 2014.

National Institute on Drug Abuse: *Research Report Series: Inhalants.* NIH Pub No 10-3818. Rockville, MD, 2012, National Clearinghouse on Alcohol and Drug Information. Available at: http://www.drugabuse.gov/publications/drugfacts/inhalants. Accessed June 2, 2014.

National Institute on Drug Abuse: *Principles of Drug Addiction Treatment: A Research Based Guide*, NIH Pub No 09-4180, Revised April 2009. ed 2. 2009.

Available at: http://www.nida.nih.gov/PODAT/. Accessed June 2, 2014.

Pacher P, Bátkai S, Kunos G: The endocannabinoid system as an emerging target of pharmacotherapy. *Pharmacol Rev* 58(3):389–462, 2006.

Pan W, Bai H: A multivariate approach to a meta-analytic review of the effectiveness of the D.A.R.E program. *Int J Environ Res Public Health* 6(1):267–277, 2009.

Physicians and Lawyers for National Drug Policy: *Policy Priorities: Summary*, 2008. Available at http://www.plndp.org/Policy_Priorities/Summary.html. Accessed June 2, 2014.

Pilcher J, Bernard-Kuhn L: Chasing the heroin resurgence. *USA Today*, 6/12/2014. Available at http://www.usatoday.com/longform/news/nation-now/2014/06/12/communities-across-usa-scramble-to-tackle-heroin-surge/9713463/. Accessed June 18, 2014.

Reiman A: Cannabis as a substitute for alcohol and other drugs. *Harm Reduct J* 6:35, 2009.

Rose KD: *American Women and the Repeal of Prohibition.* New York, 1996, New York University Press.

Scavone JL, Sterling RC, Weinstein SP, et al: Impact of cannabis use

during stabilization on methadone maintenance treatment. *Am J Addict* 22(4):344–351, 2013.

Substance Abuse and Mental Health Services Administration: *Results from the 2012 National Survey on Drug Use and Health: Summary of National Findings.* NSNUH Series H-46, HHS Publication No. (SMA) 13-4795. Rockville, MD, 2013, SAMHSA.

Substance Abuse and Mental Health Services Administration: *Screening, Brief Intervention and Referral to Treatment (SBIRT) in Behavioral Healthcare*, 4/1/2011. Available at http://bigsbirteducation.webs.com/SBIRTwhitepaper.pdf. Accessed June 25, 2014.

Substance Abuse and Mental Health Services Administration: *TIP 32: Treatment of Adolescents with Substance Use Disorders*, 2008, SAMHSA. Available at http://www.ncbi.nlm.nih.gov/bookshelf/br.fcgi?book=hssamhsatip&part=A56538. Accessed June 2, 2014.

Substance Abuse and Mental Health Services Administration, Office of Applied Studies: *Treatment Episode Data Set (TEDS). Highlights—2007, National Admissions to Substance Abuse Treatment Services.* DASIS Series:

S-45, DHHS Pub No (SMA) 09–4360. Rockville, MD, 2009.

U.S. Department of Health and Human Services: *Healthy People 2020: National Health Promotion and Disease Prevention Objectives.* Washington, DC, 2010, U.S. Government Printing Office. Available at: http://www.healthypeople.gov/HP2020/. Accessed June 2, 2014.

U.S. Department of Health and Human Services: *The Health Consequences of Smoking—50 Years of Progress: A Report of the Surgeon General.* Atlanta, 2014, USDHHS, CDC, National Center for Chronic Disease Prevention and Health Promotion, Office on Smoking and Health. Accessed June 16, 2014.

Volkow ND, Frieden TR, Hyde PS, et al: Medication-assisted therapies—tackling the opioid-overdose epidemic. *N Engl J Med* 370:2063–2066, 2014.

Werner C: *Marijuana Gateway to Health: How Cannabis Protects Us From Cancer and Alzheimer's Disease.* San Francisco, 2011, Dachstar Press.

World Health Organization: *WHO Report on the Global Tobacco Epidemic, 2008: The MPOWER Package.* Geneva, 2008, WHO.

# Violence and Human Abuse

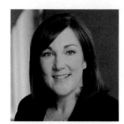

## Jeanne L. Alhusen, PhD, CRNP, RN

Jeanne L. Alhusen is an assistant professor at the Johns Hopkins University School of Nursing. Her BSN, MSN, and PhD are from Villanova University, Duke University, and Johns Hopkins University. Dr. Alhusen works as a family nurse practitioner, and her research interests are in maternal mental health and early childhood outcomes, particularly among families living in poverty. She has received funding from NIH to conduct research on the impact of domestic violence on early childhood outcomes.

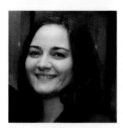

## Tina Bloom, PhD, MPH, RN

Tina Bloom is an Assistant Professor and Robert Wood Johnson Foundation Nurse Faculty Scholar at the Sinclair School of Nursing, University of Missouri-Columbia. She received a BSN from the University of Kansas in Kansas City, Kansas, and an MPH and PhD from Oregon Health and Science University in Portland, Oregon. Dr. Bloom specializes in research on intimate partner violence interventions, with a particular interest in maternal-child health and the issues of marginalized and underserved abuse survivors, and eliminating disparities in access to resources for underserved survivors.

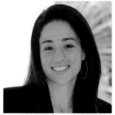

## Rosa M. Gonzalez-Guarda, PhD, MPH, RN, CPH

Rosa M. Gonzalez-Guarda is an assistant professor at the University of Miami School of Nursing and Health Studies. Dr. Gonzalez-Guard a received a bachelor of science in nursing (BSN) from Georgetown University, a master of science in nursing (MSN) and public health (MPH) from Johns Hopkins University, and an interdisciplinary PhD from the University of Miami. She has worked on community-based prevention programs and research targeting Hispanics and other health disparity populations in the areas of intimate partner violence, human immunodeficiency virus (HIV) and other sexually transmitted infections (STIs) and co-occuring health conditions. She is currently funded by the Robert Wood Johnson Foundation Nurse Faculty Scholars Program to develop and pilot test a culturally tailored teen dating violence prevention program for Hispanic youth.

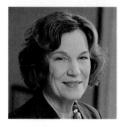

## Jacquelyn C. Campbell, PhD, RN, FAAN

Jacquelyn C. Campbell is the Anna D. Wolf Chair and Professor at the Johns Hopkins University School of Nursing with a joint appointment in the Bloomberg School of Public Health. Her BSN, MSN, and PhD are from Duke University, Wright State University, and the University of Rochester schools of nursing. Dr. Campbell has been the principle investigator on ten major National Institutes of Health, National Institute of Justice, and Centers for Disease Control and Prevention research grants and has published more than 220 articles and seven books on this subject. She is an elected member of the Institute of Medicine and the American Academy of Nursing, is Chair of the Board of Directors Family Violence Defense Fund, and was a member of the congressionally appointed U.S. Department of Defense Task Force on Domestic Violence.

## ADDITIONAL RESOURCES

Ⓔ **Evolve Website http://evolve.elsevier.com/Stanhope**
- *Healthy People 2020*
- WebLinks
- Quiz

- Case Studies
- Glossary
- Answers to Practice Application

## OBJECTIVES

*After reading this chapter, the student should be able to do the following:*

1. Discuss the scope of the problem of violence in American communities.

2. Examine at least three factors existing in most communities that influence violence and human abuse.

3. Define the four general types of child abuse: neglect, physical, emotional, and sexual.

OBJECTIVES—cont'd

## OBJECTIVES—cont'd

4. Discuss elder abuse as a crucial community health problem.
5. Discuss the principles of nursing intervention with violent families.

6. Describe specific nursing interventions with battered women.

## KEY TERMS

## CHAPTER OUTLINE

An estimated 55,000 individuals die each year in the United States as a result of violence-related injuries. While homicide rates have decreased over the last 20 years, homicide remains the second leading cause of death for individuals 15 to 24 years of age, and the third leading cause of death for individuals 1 to 4 and 25 to 34 years of age (Centers for Disease Control and Prevention [CDC], 2013). Homicides committed by intimate partners account for 14% of all U.S. homicides, and 70% of those victims were female (Smith et al, 2014). Suicide is the third leading cause of death among adolescents. In 2010, rates of suicide among male teens were highest among American Indians (24.3 per 100,000) and whites (14.2), followed by Hispanics (8.1), blacks (6.8), and Asian or Pacific Islanders at 6.3 per 100,000 (CDC, 2013). These statistics do not account for the significant morbidity associated with interpersonal violence. For every person who dies as a result of violence, many more are injured and suffer lasting physical, sexual, and mental health sequelae. As the World Health Organization has reported, when interpersonal violence results in large numbers of deaths, the issue is a significant public health concern necessitating attention from researchers, policy makers, health care providers, and the public (Krug et al, 2002).

Violence is an important public health nursing issue. Violence leads to significant mortality and morbidity. Communities across the United States are concerned about crime and violence rates. Medical, nursing, psychology, and social service professionals have been slow to develop an integrated response to violence that is part of their daily professional lives. As a result, the estimated 3.5 million victims of violence annually may not receive the best care possible. Nurses are in a unique position to develop community responses to violence, to influence public policy regarding violence, and to provide individuals, families, and communities with the necessary resources to appropriately address violence. Nurses represent a large group of health care providers who have an ethic of caring and value early intervention and health promotion. This can optimize individual, familial, community and societal health outcomes.

This chapter examines violence as a public health problem and discusses how nurses can help individuals, families, groups, and communities cope with and reduce violence and abuse. Nurses work with clients in a wide variety of settings, including the home. Because nurses are in key positions to detect and intervene in community and family violence, an understanding of how community-level influences can affect all types of violence is necessary. The *Healthy People 2020* box as follows lists five objectives for reducing violence in communities.

**HEALTHY PEOPLE 2020**

**Objectives for Reducing Violence**
- IVP-29: Reduce homicides.
- IVP-35: Reduce bullying among adolescents.
- IVP-37: Reduce child maltreatment deaths.
- IVP-39: Reduce violence by current or former intimate partners.
- IVP-40: Reduce sexual violence.

U.S. Department of Health and Human Servcies (USDHHS), 2010

## SOCIAL AND COMMUNITY FACTORS INFLUENCING VIOLENCE

Many factors in a community can support or minimize violence. Changing social conditions, multiple demands on people, economic conditions, and available social resources are predictive of the level of violence and human abuse. The following discussion of selected current social conditions helps to explain factors that influence violent behavior. The Linking Content to Practice box discusses how public health nurses can collaborate in the community to prevent violence.

**LINKING CONTENT TO PRACTICE**

According to the Quad Council Domains of Public Health Nursing Practice (Swider et al, 2013) and the American Public Health Association (2010), public health nurses must collaborate in partnership with communities to assess and identify community needs; plan, implement, and evaluate community-based programs; and assist in the setting of policy that will contribute to the needs of the community in relationship to all types of interpersonal violence. The Quad Council competencies in the analytic assessment domain direct nurses to conduct thorough health assessments of individuals, families, communities, and populations and to develop diagnoses for the population being assessed (Swider et al, 2013). Public health nurses can help the community in many ways, as is described throughout this chapter.

### Work

Productive and paid work is an expectation in mainstream American society. Work can be fulfilling and contribute to a sense of well-being; it can also be frustrating and unfulfilling, contributing to stress that may lead to aggression and violence. Unemployment and changing patterns of employment are also associated with violence both within and outside the home.

When jobs are repetitive, boring, and lacking in stimulation, frustration mounts. Some work environments discourage creativity and reward conformity and "following the rules." In many work settings, people try to get ahead regardless of the cost to others. Workers may go home feeling physically and psychologically drained. They may have worked at a back-breaking pace all day only to be yelled at by the boss for what seemed like a trivial oversight. It is hard to separate feelings generated at work from those at home. For example, a father arrives home feeling tired, angry, and generally inadequate because of a series of reprimands from his boss. Soon after he sits down, his 4-year-old son runs through the house pretending to fly a wooden airplane. After about three loud trips past his father, who keeps shouting for the child to be quiet and go outside, the airplane hits the father in the head. The father may hit the boy out of frustration and anger.

Unemployment may precipitate aggressive outbursts. The inability to secure or keep a job may lead to feelings of inadequacy, guilt, boredom, dissatisfaction, and frustration. Unemployment does not fit the image of the ideal man in American society, and these men are more likely to be violent both within and outside the family (Ellison et al, 2007; Peralta et al, 2010). Women who experience intimate partner violence (IPV) may lose their jobs because of constant harassment and stalking from the abuser and their subsequent absenteeism. Women who are stalked at work often find their jobs in jeopardy because of work interruption, continual stress, and decreased job performance. Slowly, employers are beginning to understand the implications of IPV. More women are finding support from employers when they disclose possible or actual abuse (Logan et al, 2007; Swanberg et al, 2007).

Unemployment, often linked with poverty, remains a risk factor associated with IPV (Ellison et al, 2007). Statistics from the U.S. Department of Labor (2012) showed that young, minority men have the highest rates of unemployment in the United States, ranging upward to 50% even in times of prosperity. An important theory explaining the relation between poverty and IPV is that it is mediated through stress. Living in poverty is inherently stressful, and thus it has been posited that IPV may result from stress, and poorer men have fewer available resources to reduce stress. Most analyses conclude that the differential rates of violence between African Americans and whites in the United States have more to do with socioeconomic disparities, such as poverty, unemployment, and overcrowding, than with race (Ellison et al, 2007).

### Education

In recent years, schools have assumed many responsibilities traditionally assigned to the family. Schools teach sexual development, discipline children, and often serve as a safe haven where children are fed and given the developmental support needed. Large classes often mean that teachers spend more time and energy monitoring and disciplining children than challenging and stimulating them to learn. As more and more social problems arise, it is often the expectation that the school system will teach children about these issues. One such issue is bullying. Bullying has become a major problem in U.S. schools.

According to the 2013 Youth Risk Behavior Surveillance System (CDC, 2013), 19.6% of youth were bullied on school grounds during the year, 14.8% were bullied electronically and 5.5% reported carrying a weapon on school grounds in the 30 days before the survey. Bullying can be physical and/or psychological abuse, intimidation, or verbal abuse; the exclusion of some children from group activities is another form of bullying. Bullying takes place across ethnic groups and developmental ages and is identified as an antecedent for perpetration of domestic violence (Corvo and deLara, 2010; Vervoort et al, 2010). Bullying can have devastating effects on a child's health and can lead to self-harm (Salmivalli, 2010).

Another form of aggression or bullying has emerged, labeled "cyberbullying," in which the aggression takes place via modern technological devices, and specifically mobile phones or the Internet. An issue unique to cyberbullying, which distinguishes it from most traditional forms of bullying, is the difficulty in getting away from it. Unlike traditional forms of school bullying, where the bullying can stop once the victim returns home, with cyberbullying the victim may continue to receive text messages or e-mails wherever they are located. Also, cyberbullying has the potential to reach particularly large audiences in a peer group. Cyberbullying often leads to depression, isolation, low self-esteem, and absenteeism. Many schools and parent groups are targeting bullying behavior on a larger scale by focusing on peer groups and population-based interventions (Berlan et al, 2010; Kiriakidis and Kavoura, 2010).

A substantial amount of socialization during adolescence occurs within the school setting, and thus school counselors, nurses, and other professionals play a central role in identifying and intervening in school-based violence.

## Media

The media can be instrumental in campaigns against violence. Recent television programs, both documentaries and dramatizations, and print articles have heightened public awareness about family violence. Programs that raise the social awareness of IPV may play a role in reducing violence in interpersonal relationships (Regan, 2010). Social marketing techniques and public service announcements serve as mechanisms to inform the public of community resources supporting victims of interpersonal violence and serve as mechanisms to prevent IPV (Grier and Kumanyika, 2010). Abused women and rape victims have especially benefited from media attention, which tends to lessen the stigma of such victimization. The media are also useful in publicizing services.

Conversely, research on violent television and films, video games, and music demonstrates that media violence increases the likelihood of aggressive and violent behavior, both immediately and long-term (Anderson et al, 2003). The influence of mass media is thought to be one of the many potential factors that contribute to aggressive or violent behavior. It is important to remember that violent adolescents and adults often were highly aggressive and potentially violent as children. Thus, influences that may promote aggressive behavior in children could ultimately contribute to violent behavior into adulthood. This highlights the importance of identifying factors, including media violence, that may contribute to violent behavior in childhood.

Parents and caregivers are critical in monitoring what reaches their children. Communities, including school settings, religious organizations, and parent-teacher organizations, should teach parents and children how to be more informed, healthier consumers of the media. As technology is a mainstay in most homes, parents need better tools to assist them in monitoring and modifying their children's media habits. From a policy perspective, violence prevention researchers should work with media researchers to create avenues for disseminating solutions to social and public health problems.

## Organized Religion

Historically, a seemingly contradictory relationship has existed between abuse and religion. For example, many religious groups uphold the philosophy of "spare the rod, spoil the child." Also, although divorce is socially accepted, some faiths perpetuate the victimization of people with their disapproval of divorce. Family members may stay together, although they are at emotional or physical war with one another, because of religious convictions. Although women have claimed that their spirituality has helped them in times of despair and victimization, they maintain that religious doctrine and some clergy become barriers to women seeking help in dealing with, or ending, an abusive relationship (Beaulaurier et al, 2007; Potter, 2007).

Although churches have been slow to recognize domestic violence, some positive changes are taking place. Issues of male domination over women have become a major topic of discussion in some church groups, whereas in other groups women continue to be blamed for abuse that they sustain (Levitt and Ware, 2006). Religious affiliation and religious conservatism have been identified as risk factors for family violence, particularly child abuse (Hines and Malley-Morrison, 2005). Clergy need to be taught about the nature and dynamics of violence in the family, about religious messages and the potential for support, and about the need for collaboration between the church and advocates for the prevention of domestic violence. In religious groups where there is collaboration with advocates against abuse to children, women, and elders, there is a greater recognition of the harm of abuse and the clarity of the role of the clergy in dealing with abuse (Rodriguez and Henderson, 2010).

## Population

A community's population can influence the potential for violence. Density, poverty, and diversity, particularly racial tension and overt racism, contribute to violence. In addition, one's perceptions of the safety in a community can be influenced by racism and perceptions of criminality (Lin et al, 2009; Howard et al, 2010).

High-population-density communities can positively or negatively influence violence. Those with a sense of cohesiveness may have a lower crime rate than areas of similar size that lack social and cultural groups to support unity among members. Bonds formed among church groups, clubs, and professional organizations may promote harmony among members.

Such groups provide members an opportunity to talk about stressors rather than to respond through violence. For example, residents of public housing often form neighborhood associations to deal with situations common to many or all residents. Tension can often be released in a productive way through projects carried out by the association.

Some high-population areas experience a community feeling of powerlessness and helplessness rather than one of cohesiveness. Lack of jobs and low-paying jobs may lead to feelings of inadequacy, despair, and social alienation. Social alienation and exclusion from opportunities can lead to decreased social cohesion and increased violence (Lee and Ousey, 2005; Rahn et al, 2009). Fear and apathy may cause community residents to withdraw from social contact. Withdrawal can foster crime because many residents assume someone else will report suspicious behavior, or they fear reprisals for such reports (Gracia and Herrero, 2007).

Youths often attempt to deal with feelings of powerlessness by forming gangs. Adolescents also join gangs for the safety they believe the gang provides. One of the strongest predictors of serious violence during adolescence is involvement with delinquent peers. Other significant risk factors for gang involvement include extreme poverty, disorganized neighborhoods, academic failure, high levels of family conflict, and favorable attitudes toward antisocial behavior. A number of these young adults have attempted to deal with their feelings by turning to crime against people and property to release frustration. In many cities, these gangs have been highly destructive. Through community mobilization efforts, primary prevention programs have been developed to deal with the disenfranchisement of youth and gang violence (Pitts, 2009).

Other high-population areas may be characterized by a sense of confusion, resulting in disintegration and disorganization. These areas may have transient populations with limited physical or emotional investment in the community. Lack of community concern allows crime and violence to go unchecked and may become a norm for the area. Also, as crime increases, residents who are able to move leave the area. This increases community disintegration because the residents who leave are often the most capable members of the population.

The potential for violence also tends to increase among highly diverse populations. Differences in age, socioeconomic status, ethnicity, religion, or other cultural characteristics may disrupt community stability. Highly divergent groups may not communicate effectively and neither accept nor understand one another. Many such groups become hostile and antagonistic toward one another. Each group may see the other as different and not belonging. The alienated group may become the focal point for the others' frustrations, anger, and fears. Racism, classism, and heterosexism are examples of major causes of community disintegration resulting in a vicious cycle of dishonesty, distrust, and hate.

## Community Facilities

Communities differ in the resources and facilities they provide to residents. Some are more desirable places to live, work, and raise families and have facilities that can reduce the potential for crime and violence. Recreational facilities such as playgrounds, parks, swimming pools, movie theaters, and tennis courts provide socially acceptable outlets for a variety of feelings, including aggression. Conversely, disadvantaged communities lack many of the social and economic resources for developing and maintaining secure organizations. Employers that provide employment and services are less likely to find it profitable to operate in poorer neighborhoods. Thus, basic institutions such as stores, banks, libraries, and recreational facilities, which provide both employment opportunities and social services, are less prevalent in disadvantaged communities.

Although the absence of such facilities can increase the likelihood of violence, their presence alone does not prevent violence or crime. These facilities are adjuncts and resources that residents can use for pleasure, personal enrichment, and group development. Familiarity with factors contributing to a community's violence or potential for violence enables nurses to recognize them and intervene accordingly. It is the nurse's responsibility to work with the citizens and agencies of the community to correct or improve deficits.

## VIOLENCE AGAINST INDIVIDUALS OR ONESELF

The potential for violence against individuals (e.g., murder, robbery, rape, assault) or oneself (e.g., suicide) is directly related to the level of violence in the community. Persons living in areas with high rates of crime and violence are more likely to become victims than those in more peaceful areas. The major categories of violence addressed in this chapter are described in terms of the scope of the problem in the United States and underlying dynamics.

### Homicide

Homicide is defined as a death resulting from the use of force against another person when a preponderance of evidence indicates that the use of force was intentional (Parks et al, 2014). Age-specific homicide rates are highest (11.7 deaths per 100,000 population) among those aged 20 to 24 years, followed by those aged 25 to 29 years (10.7 deaths per 100,000 population). Importantly, the homicide rate for males is nearly four times that of females (7.7 and 2.1 per 100,000, respectively). Non-Hispanic blacks account for nearly half (49.6%) of homicide deaths and have the highest rate (15.2 deaths per 100,000 population), followed by American Indians/Alaskan Natives (10.0) and Hispanics (5.1) (Parks et al, 2014). Rates of homicide for infants under the age of 1 year were highest among non-Hispanic blacks and American Indians/Alaska Natives (Parks et al, 2014). Parents perpetuate the majority of homicides of children. Strangers cause 15% of male and 9% of female homicides in the United States (Catalano, Smith, Snyder, and Rand, 2009. When strangers are involved, many of these homicides are related to the illegal substance abuse network. The majority of homicides are perpetrated by a friend, acquaintance, or family member. Therefore, prevention of homicide is at least as much an issue for the public health system as for the criminal justice system.

At least 16% of male homicides and 64% of female homicides in the United States occur in families, and half of these occur between spouses. These numbers, however, do not include unmarried couples who are living together or those who are either divorced or estranged, a group at higher risk. In total, approximately 14% of all homicides were committed by an intimate partner. Spouses or ex-spouses composed about 24% of the perpetrators in female spousal homicides. Twenty-one percent of boyfriends or girlfriends and 19% of family members were responsible for female intimate partner homicides. Female homicides are perpetrated primarily by someone whom the victim knows; only 10% of all female homicides are perpetrated by a stranger (Catalano et al, 2009).

An alarming aspect of family homicide is that small children often witness the murder or find the body of a family member (Lewandowski et al, 2004). In most communities no automatic follow-up or counseling of these children occurs through the criminal justice or mental health system. These children are at great risk for emotional turmoil and for becoming involved in violence themselves (Steeves and Parker, 2007).

The underlying dynamics of homicide within families vary greatly from those of other murders. Homicide within families is most often preceded by abuse of a family member, and homicides of intimate partners (male or female) are preceded by abuse of the female partner in 70% to 75% of cases (Campbell et al, 2000, 2003). Thus, prevention of family homicide involves working with abusive families. Homicide is the leading cause of death for pregnant and postpartum women (Nannini et al, 2008). In fact, in a study of intimate partner homicide of women, 75% of the women who were killed by their husband, boyfriend, or ex-partner had been seen in a health care setting within the year before their homicide (Woods et al, 2008). Nurses have a duty to warn family members of the possibility of homicide when severe abuse is present, just as they warn of the hazards of smoking. Other nursing care issues are further discussed in the section Family Violence and Abuse in this chapter.

## Assault

The death toll from violence is staggering, yet the physical injuries and emotional costs of assault are equally important issues in terms of the acute health care system. Twenty-two percent of females compared with 7.4% of males reported injury related to physical assault. Age is the greatest risk factor for an individual's victimization through violence, and youths are at significantly higher risk. Although more males than females are victims of homicide and assault, women are more likely to be victimized by a relative, especially a male partner (Catalano et al, 2009). In some instances the response time of emergency services and the quality of treatment facilities determine whether an assault will end as a homicide. The same community measures used to address homicide are useful to combat assault. Also, nurses often care for the long-term health problems associated with assaults such as head injuries, spinal cord injuries, and stomas from abdominal gunshot wounds in a home health care setting. In addition to providing physical care, nurses must also address the emotional trauma resulting from

a violent attack by helping victims talk through their traumatic experience to try to make some sense of the violence, and by referring them for further counseling if anxiety, sleeping problems, or depression persists after the assault.

## Rape

At present, rape is one of the most underreported forms of human abuse in the United States; only about half (47%) of rapes in the National Crime Victimization Survey (NCVS) are reported to the police (Catalano et al, 2009), although reporting rates have improved over the past 15 years. According to the NCVS (Rand, 2009), sexual assault rates fell by 52% from 1999 to 2008. The rates of completed and attempted rape are almost equivalent. The incidence of rape exceeds the prevalence of rape victims because some victims experience more than one rape in a 12-month period. In 2008, according to the NCVS, there were an estimated 182,000 rapes or sexual assaults against females 12 or older, whereas males experienced 40,000 rapes or sexual assaults. This is a rate per 1000 of approximately 1.4 and 0.3, respectively. African American females experienced higher rates of rape or sexual assault than white females and other women of color. Hispanic and non-Hispanic white females experienced comparable rates of sexual assault (Catalano et al, 2009). More than half the rapes or sexual assaults against females were committed by an offender whom they knew, and one in five was committed by an intimate partner. Strangers committed only about one third (31%) of all rapes/sexual assaults. Nearly half (47%) of the rapes and sexual assaults against females in 2009 were reported to the police. The rate of rape or sexual assault against females declined by 70% from 1993 to 2008 and by 36% during that period for males (Catalano et al, 2009).

Because the majority of violence against women is IPV and women are raped more often by someone they know than by strangers, health care providers must be alert for date and marital rape. In the National Violence Against Women Survey (Tjaden and Thoennes, 2000), 64% of rapes, physical assaults, and stalkings were committed against women by either current or former intimate partners. Official recognition of rape regardless of a victim's relationship to the perpetrator has led to an increased number of women reporting rape. Rape also happens to men, especially boys and young men, but the statistics on the incidence of male rape vary. In a survey of Air Force women, more than 50% had reported being a victim of rape at some time in their lifetime. Although the majority of rapes occurred before enlistment, 14% of women were raped for the first time in the military and 26% of women were victims of rape before and within the military (Bostock and Daley, 2007). It appears that the emotional trauma for a male rape victim is at least as serious as that for a woman.

College women are at particularly high risk for sexual victimization in the United States, with research estimating that approximately 25% of female college students will experience an attempted or completed rape at some point during their college experience (Fisher et al, 2000). Data from the Bureau of Justice Statistics demonstrate that despite arrest rates for sexual assault remaining stable, twice as many women reported a sexual assault by an intimate partner in 2010 as compared with 1994 (Catalano, 2012). The health impact of sexual assault is highly significant. Health issues include high-risk sexual behavior, substance abuse, unintended pregnancy, depression, **posttraumatic stress disorder** (PTSD), suicidal ideation, and eating disorders (Silverman et al, 2001). Nurses are well positioned to provide victims with comprehensive care including mental health services. Nurses can identify and refer clients who have experienced sexual assault. Advanced practice nurses are often providers of primary health care on college campuses, placing them in a unique position to educate and support students on the issue of dating violence.

Another form of rape is forced sexual initiations, with as many as 21% of young women in the United States whose first sexual experience is below the age of 14 reporting that this initiation was physically forced, usually by a date or boyfriend (Stockman et al, 2010). These early sexual experiences are associated with unplanned, adolescent pregnancies as well as HIV/STD risk behaviors.

Prevention of rape, like that of other forms of human abuse, requires a broad-based community focus for educating both the community as a whole and key groups such as police, health providers, educators, and social workers. Rape rates and community-level variables such as community approval and legitimization of violence (e.g., violent network television viewing and permitting corporal punishment in schools) appear related and underscore the need for community-level intervention (Casey and Lindhorst, 2009).

## Attitudes

The first priority is to change attitudes about rape and about victims or survivors. Rape is a crime of violence, not a crime of passion. The underlying issues are hostility, power, and control rather than sexual desire. The defining issue is lack of consent of the victim. When a woman or man refuses any sexual activity, that refusal means "no." People have the right to change their mind, even when they seemed initially agreeable. Pressure from physical contact, threats, or deliberate inducement of drug or alcohol intoxication is a violation of the law. The myths that women say "no" to sex when they really mean "yes" and that the victims of rape are culpable because of the way they dress or act must end.

## Pornography

Although there is evidence of a relationship between the viewing of pornographic material showing violence against women and aggressive sexual behavior, it is not clear if the relationship is causal. In other words, our current research does not yet show that viewing pornography occurs before sexual aggressiveness or that young men who are sexually violent tend to watch pornography. The current research tends to minimize the relationship between sexual assault and pornography (Ferguson and Hartley, 2009). However, there is some evidence that claims that early exposure to pornography as a child may be related to sexual offense in the future (Seto and Lalumière, 2010). Prevention programs, or more accurately labeled risk reduction or avoidance programs, also involve providing information to

women about self-protection, including using self-defense procedures, avoiding high-risk locations, and safeguarding one's home against unwanted entry. Most rape prevention programs have been oriented toward women. However, men are increasingly becoming involved in rape prevention education via anti-rape websites (Master's, 2010). Many of these websites are community-based programs that promote education about violence against women and promote a positive male role model of gender equity. They often depict examples of consensual and nonconsensual sexual behaviors.

### Victim or Survivor?

During the act of rape, **survivors** are often hit, kicked, stabbed, and severely beaten. It is this violence that is most traumatic because of the survivors' fear for their lives, helplessness, lack of control, and vulnerability.

People react to rape differently, depending on their personality, past experiences, background, and support received after the trauma. Some cry, shout, or discuss the experience. Others withdraw and fear discussing the attack. During the immediate as well as the follow-up stages, victims tend to blame themselves for what happened. When working with rape victims, help them identify the issues behind self-blame. While not placing fault on survivors, teach them to take control, learn assertiveness, and therefore believe that they can take certain actions to prevent future rapes. Survivors need to talk about what happened and to express their feelings and fears in a nonjudgmental atmosphere.

In any psychological trauma, victims should be given privacy, respect, and assurance of confidentiality. They should also be told about health care procedures conducted immediately after the rape and should be linked with proper resources for ease of reporting the crime. Nurses often provide continuous care once the victim enters the health care system. Because many victims deny the event once the initial crisis is past, a single-session debriefing should be completed during the initial examination. Specialty trainer providers should perform the physical assessment, examination, and debriefing.

As discussed in Chapter 44, in most states, nurses trained as **Sexual Assault Nurse Examiners** (SANEs), a subspecialty of **forensic** nursing, perform the physical examination in the emergency department to gather evidence (e.g., hair samples, skin fragments beneath the victim's fingernails, evidence from pelvic examinations obtained by colposcopy) for criminal prosecution of sexual assault (Sheridan, 2004). This is an important nursing intervention because physicians may not be able to take the time required for this procedure; nurses can take advantage of this opportunity to provide therapeutic communication and support. Nurses can be trained to conduct the examination either in SANE trainings or in forensic nursing programs in many schools of nursing, and their evidence is credible and effective in resultant court proceedings (Houmes et al, 2003; Campbell et al, 2006, 2007). Nurses can lobby for changes in hospital policies and state laws to make this strategy a reality in all states.

Rape is a situational crisis for which advance preparation is rarely possible. Therefore, nursing efforts are directed toward helping victims cope with the stress and disruption of their lives caused by the attack. Counseling focuses on the crisis and the concomitant fears, feelings, and issues involved. Nurses can help survivors learn how to regroup personal strengths. If PTSD occurs, professional psychological or psychiatric treatment is indicated.

Many rape victims need follow-up mental health services to help them cope with the short- and long-term effects of the crisis. The time after a rape is one of disequilibrium, psychological breakdown, and reorganization of attitudes about the safety of the world. Common, everyday tasks often tax a person's resources, and they may forget or fail to keep appointments. Nurses can make referrals and obtain the victim's permission to remain in telephone contact in order to assess support, provide encouragement, and offer resources.

## Suicide

According to the National Violent Death Reporting System (NVDRS), suicide accounted for the highest rate of violent death in 2007, taking the lives of 9245 people. Firearms accounted for 50.7%, hanging/strangulation/suffocation for 23.1%, and poisoning for 18.8% of suicides. Firearms (56%) or hanging/strangulation/suffocation (24.4%) were the most common form of suicide for men. Women used poisoning (40.8%) most frequently, followed by firearms (30.9%). Precipitating factors for suicide were mental health (45%), IPV (30%), and physical health problems (21.4%) (CDC, 2014a). The risk for death by suicide is greater than for death by homicide. Rates of completed suicide are higher for men, especially older adults, non-Hispanic whites, and Native Alaskans/American Indians (Karch et al, 2010). Affluent and educated people often have higher rates of suicide than do the economically and educationally disadvantaged except for Native Alaskan/American Indian populations, who are often poor and yet commit suicide in alarming numbers. The presence of a gun in the home is an important risk factor for both suicide and homicide (Campbell, 2007).

Suicide is the third-leading cause of death among young people ages 15 to 24. During 2005 to 2009, the highest suicide rates were among American Indian/Alaskan Native males, with 27.61 suicides per 100,000, and non-Hispanic white males, with 25.96 suicides per 100,000. Of all female race/ethnicity groups, the American Indian/Alaskan Natives and non-Hispanic whites had the highest rates with 7.87 and 6.71 suicides per 100,000, respectively. Boys and young men between the ages of 15 and 19 were five times more likely to commit suicide than females and four times more likely if between the ages of 20 and 24 (Karch et al, 2010). Attempted suicide was more prevalent for white, African American, and Hispanic females than for males of the same racial background. Leading risk factors for adolescent suicide are mental health, unintended pregnancy, and sexually transmitted disease (STD), especially HIV (Eaton et al, 2010). An important risk factor for actual and attempted suicide in adult women is IPV.

Nurses need to be involved in the reduction of suicide and the care for victims because suicide affects the community, the family, and individuals. On a community level, nurses can be involved in a coordinated response to the prevention of suicide and the care of attempted suicides. Through their roles in public health and school nursing, they can help develop policies and protocols for suicide across the life span. Nursing care may focus on family members and friends of suicide victims. Survivors may feel angry at the dead person, and turn the anger inward. They may question their own liability for the death and have difficulty dealing with their feelings toward the dead person; survivors may limit their social activities because it is difficult for them and their friends to talk about the suicide. Nurses can help survivors cope with the trauma of the loss and make referrals to a counselor or support groups.

## FAMILY VIOLENCE AND ABUSE

Family violence, including sexual, emotional, and physical abuse, causes significant injury and death. Although the rate of IPV has decreased for females and males over the last 15 years, the rate of homicides perpetrated by a known other has remained the same (Catalano et al, 2009). IPV tends to occur as part of a system of coercive control. In general, IPV is perpetrated by the most powerful against the least powerful.

The majority of IPV is directed at women, with the majority of IPV perpetrated by a male partner or ex-partner (Black et al, 2011). However, sexual minorities (LGBT; lesbian, gay, bisexuals, and transgender populations) experience violence from an intimate partner or ex-partner at similar rates as heterosexuals (Walters et al, 2013). LGBT IPV generally follows similar dynamics as heterosexual IPV (emotional, verbal, physical, and/or sexual violence, threats, isolation, and intimidation, in a context of one partner maintaining power and control over another) and results in similarly adverse health outcomes. As with heterosexual IPV, dynamics of power and control caused by race, gender expression, ability, immigration status, age, and class are methods of control in same-sex IPV (National Coalition of Anti-Violence Programs, 2012). Further, LGBT IPV survivors may face significant added barriers to help from law enforcement, health care, domestic violence agencies, and other service agencies, including a lack of appropriate services, provider stereotypes (e.g., women are not violent), discrimination, and even abuse based on their sexual minority status.

Recognizing the IPV survivor in the emergency department may be simple after the fact. It is unfortunate that, by the time medical care is sought, serious physical and emotional damage may have been done. Nurses are in a key position to predict and deal with abusive tendencies. By understanding factors contributing to the development of abusive behaviors, nurses can identify incidents of IPV.

### Development of Abusive Patterns

Perpetrators of IPV often believe that violence within an interpersonal relationship is a normal behavior pattern (Stover et al, 2010). Factors that characterize people who become involved in IPV include upbringing, living conditions, and increased stress. Understanding how these factors influence the development of abusive behavior can help the nurse manage abusive families.

## Upbringing

The most predictable factor in the background of an abuser is previous exposure to some form of violence (Whiting et al, 2009). As children, abusers were often beaten or witnessed the beating of siblings or a parent. These children learn that violence is a suitable way to manage conflict. For both men and women, witnessing abuse as a child was associated with abuse of their children. Having financial solvency and support tended to decrease the incidence of child abuse (Dixon et al, 2009; Whiting et al, 2009). Childhood physical punishment teaches children to use violent conflict resolution as an adult. A child may learn to associate love with violence because a parent is usually the first person to hit a child. Children may think that those who love them are also those who hit them. The moral rightness of hitting other family members thus may be established when physical punishment is used to train children, especially when it is used more than occasionally. These experiences predispose children ultimately to use violence with their own children.

As well as having a history of child abuse themselves, people who become abusers tend to have hostile personality styles and be verbally aggressive. They have often learned these characteristics from their own childhood experiences. Their parents may have set unrealistic goals, and when the children failed to perform accordingly, they were criticized, demeaned, punished, and denied affection. These children may have been told how to act, what to do, and how to feel, thereby discouraging the development of normal attachment, autonomy, problem-solving skills, and creativity (Dixon et al, 2005). Children raised in this way grow up feeling unloved and worthless. They may want a child of their own so that they will feel assured of someone's love.

Because of their experiences of trauma and to protect themselves from feelings of worthlessness and fear of rejection, abused children form a protective shell and grow increasingly hostile and distrustful of others. The behavior of potential abusers reflects a low tolerance for frustration, emotional instability, and the onset of aggressive feelings with minimal provocation. Because of their emotional insecurity, perpetrators of abuse often depend on a child or spouse to meet their needs of feeling valued and secure. When their needs are not met by others, they become overly critical. Critical, resentful behavior and unrealistic expectations of others lead to a vicious cycle. The more critical these people become, the more they are rejected and alienated from others. Abusive individuals tend to perceive that the target of their hostility is "out to get" them. These distorted perceptions can be detected when parents talk about an infant crying or keeping them up at night "on purpose" (Dixon et al, 2005).

## Increased Stress

A perceived or actual crisis may precede an abusive incident. Because a crisis reinforces feelings of inadequacy and low self-esteem, a number of events often occur in a short time to precipitate abusive patterns. Unemployment, strains in the marriage, or an unplanned pregnancy may precipitate violence, especially in people with other risk factors such as a history of trauma themselves.

The daily hassles of raising young children, especially in an economically strained household, intensify an already stressed atmosphere for which an unexpected and difficult event may provoke violence. Stressful life events, poverty, and cultural values and social isolation are often associated with family violence. Crowded living conditions may also precipitate abuse. The presence of several people in a small space heightens tensions and reduces privacy; tempers flare because of the constant stimulation from others.

Social isolation is associated with abuse in families (Hines and Malley-Morrison, 2005). Such isolation limits social support, decreasing a family's ability to deal with stressors. The problem may be intensified if a violent family member tries to keep the family isolated to avoid detection. Therefore, when a family chronically misses clinic or home visit appointments, nurses need to keep in mind that abuse may be present. Nurses can encourage involvement in community activities and can help neighbors reach out to neighbors to help prevent abuse.

Frequent moves disrupt social support systems, are associated with an overall increased stress level, and tend to isolate people, at least briefly. Mobility can have a serious negative effect on the abuse-prone family. These families do not readily initiate new relationships; they rely on the family for support. Resources may be unfamiliar or inaccessible to them. Because frequent moving may be both a risk factor for abuse and a sign of an abusive family trying to avoid detection, nurses should assess such families carefully for abuse.

## Types of Intimate Partner and Family Violence

Because various forms of family violence and violence outside the home often occur together, nurses who detect child abuse should also suspect other forms of family violence. When older adult parents report that their (now adult) child was abused or has a history of violence toward others, the nurse should recognize the potential for elder abuse. Physical abuse of women is frequently accompanied by sexual abuse both inside and outside the marital relationship. Severe wife abusers may have a history of other acts of violence. Families who are verbally aggressive in conflict resolution (e.g., using name calling, belittling, screaming, and yelling) are more likely to be physically abusive. Although the various forms of family violence are discussed separately, they should not be thought of as totally separate phenomena.

No member of the family is guaranteed immunity from abuse and neglect. Spouse abuse, child abuse, abuse of older adults, serious violence among siblings, and mutual abuse by members all occur. Although these examples are not inclusive, they demonstrate the scope of family violence.

### Child Abuse

A national survey estimated that in 2011, there were 742,000 unique reports of children and adolescents who were subjected to neglect, medical neglect, physical and sexual abuse, and emotional maltreatment. Of these children, 78% were victims of neglect, 18% were victims of physical abuse, 10% were sexually abused, and 8% were psychologically maltreated. The remaining 2% were medically neglected. This is probably a conservative figure, because only the most severe cases are reported. Except for sexual abuse, which is four times as high for girls as for boys, victims are equally distributed among sexually abused male and female children (U.S. Department of Health and Human Services [USDHHS], 2013).

Children also witness domestic violence (Berman et al, 2010). When children witness domestic violence, they may experience many psychological and physical problems. Long-term developmental problems, including low self-esteem, depression, anxiety, and school failure, are also more common in children who witness IPV in their home (Lichter and McCloskey, 2004). Children living in homes with parental violence are more likely to feel guilt over the abuse and suffer from post-traumatic stress syndrome than children who are not exposed to violence (Scott, 2007; Kletter et al, 2009). Victims of child abuse are also 12 times more likely to abuse their children than individuals with no history of child abuse. Bower-Russa (2005) found that attitudes about discipline and severity of abuse as a child were factors that contributed to perpetration of child abuse. Community support and intervention programs that focus on positive child-rearing practices, especially discipline and positive recognition, assist parents in a positive, developmentally appropriate approach to child rearing (Daro and Dodge, 2009).

Children who experience abuse need to understand that the abuse experience is not their fault. From a practical sense, children need to understand safety issues and what they need to do when abuse occurs (Ernst et al, 2008). Risk factors for abused children include factors such as familial financial strain, lack of social support, abuse between parents, and problems with substance abuse. Some of the risk factors are identified in Box 38-1 (USDHHS, 2013; Zimmerman and Mercy, 2010). Children who witness abuse react differently according to their age, level of development, and sex; their reactions are influenced by the severity and frequency of the abuse witnessed (Kelly et al, 2010).

Children are often abused because they are small and relatively powerless. In many families only one child may be abused.

Parents may identify with this child and be especially critical of the child's behavior. Also, this child may have certain qualities, such as looking like a relative, being handicapped, or being particularly bright and capable, that provoke the parent.

Child abuse signifies ineffective family functioning. Abusive parents who recognize their problem are often reluctant to seek assistance because of the stigma attached to being considered a child abuser and the legal ramifications of abuse. Parents with a history of abuse as a child or who have minimal education, a lack of social support, a tendency toward depression, and multiple stress factors may be at risk for abusing their children (Whiting et al, 2009). Children are often used as leverage between parents when there is a history of violence between the parents. The abusive parent is often coercive and manipulative toward the child as a mechanism to control the nonabusive parent. Abusive parents often have unrealistic expectations of a child's developmental abilities. They often use avoidance strategies to deal with behavioral issues and overreact with abusive discipline in times of stress (Rodriguez, 2010). Abusive parents use physical discipline more frequently, often in the form of physical punishment and verbal abuse. Spanking can also be considered a form of child abuse (Hines and Malley-Morrison, 2005; Straus, 2005). The nurse must not only teach appropriate parenting behavior, but also address the underlying emotional needs of the parents. These parents often experience pain and poor emotional stability and need intervention as much as their children. Following are some of the behavioral indicators of potentially abusive parents (Zimmerman and Mercy, 2010). The box that follows lists ways to recognize actual or potential signs of child abuse.

---

**HOW TO**  **Identify Potentially Abusive Parents**

*The following characteristics in couples expecting a child constitute warning signs of actual or potential abuse:*

- *Denial of the reality of the pregnancy, as seen in a refusal to talk about the impending birth or to think of a name for the child*
- *An obvious concern or fear that the baby will not meet some predetermined standard: sex, hair color, temperament, or resemblance to family members*
- *Failure to follow through on the desire for an abortion*
- *An initial decision to place the child for adoption and a change of mind*
- *Rejection of the mother by the father of the baby*
- *Family experiencing stress and numerous crises so that the birth of a child may be the last straw*
- *Initial and unresolved negative feelings about having a child*
- *Lack of support for the new parents*
- *Isolation from friends, neighbors, or family*
- *Parental evidence of poor impulse control or fear of losing control*
- *Contradictory history*
- *Appearance of detachment*
- *Appearance of misusing drugs or alcohol*
- *Shopping for hospitals or health care providers*
- *Unrealistic expectations of the child*
- *Verbal, physical, or sexual abuse of mother by father, especially during pregnancy*
- *Child is not biological offspring of male stepfather or mother's current boyfriend*
- *Excessive talk of needing to "discipline" children and plans to use harsh physical punishment to enforce discipline*

---

**BOX 38-1  Determining Risk Factors for Child Abuse**

Ask the following questions or observe the following behaviors to determine whether risk factors are present.

1. Are the parents unemployed?
2. Do the parents have the financial resources to care for a child?
3. Is there a support network that is willing to offer assistance?
4. Do one or both parents have a history of child abuse?
5. Is a parent a victim or perpetrator of intimate partner violence?
6. Do the parents have knowledge about child development?
7. Do one or both parents have problems with substance abuse?
8. Are the parents overly critical of the child?
9. Are the parents communicative with each other and the nurse?
10. Does the mother of the child seem frightened of her partner?
11. Does the child suffer from recurrent injuries or unexplained illnesses?

Data from Rodriguez CM: Personal contextual characteristics and cognitions: predicting child abuse potential and disciplinary style, *J Interpers Violence* 25(2):315-335, 2010; U.S. Department of Health and Human Services, Administration for Children and Families, Administration on Children, Youth and Families, Children's Bureau: *Child maltreatment, 2008*, 2010a. Available at http://www.acf.hhs.gov/programs/cb/stats_research/index.htm#can. Accessed August 20, 2010; Zimmerman F, Mercy JA: A better start: child maltreatment prevention as a public health priority, *Zero to Three* 30(5):4-10, 2010.

*Foster Care.* When child abuse is discovered, the child is often placed in a foster home. It is the legal responsibility of the nurse to report all cases of child abuse. Ideally, the initial report begins a process in which both the child and the family can receive the care needed. Although the focus of care should be on the best interests of the child and the parents, the primary attention should be on the health and safety of the child. While in foster care the abused child should receive continuous nursing care. The nurse is often the one consistent person abused children can relate to as they are transferred from their home to foster care and hopefully back to their home. Abused children generally want to return to their parents, and the goal of most agencies is to help natural families stay together as long as it is safe for the child. However, a family preservation approach may not always keep children safe (O'Reilly et al, 2010). Often the nurse's role is to help monitor a family in which a formerly abused child is returned from foster care. Keen judgment and close collaboration with social services are necessary in these situations. The nurse must ensure the safety of the child while working with the parents in an empathetic way. The nurse's goal is to enhance parenting skills through education on child care and development, communication, and principles of social learning theory. Parents must also be given positive support and reassurance about their ability to provide proper care to their child.

One of the most distressing outcomes of child abuse is depression and other mental health problems, especially suicide. Adolescents who have been placed in the social service system many times or who move from one foster home to another are at risk for delinquency, severe depression, alcohol and substance abuse, and suicide. Nurses need to understand the dynamics of adolescent suicide and substance abuse (Fletcher, 2010; Ford et al, 2010).

*Indicators of Child Abuse.* It is essential that nurses recognize the physical and behavioral indicators of abuse and neglect. Child abuse ranges from violent physical attacks to passive neglect. Violence such as beating, burning, kicking, or shaking may lead to severe physical injury. Passive neglect may result in insidious malnutrition or other problems. Abuse is not limited to physical maltreatment but includes emotional abuse such as yelling at or continually demeaning and criticizing the child. Children who come from a family where IPV occurs are at greater risk for physical and psychological abuse and child neglect (Hines and Malley-Morrison, 2005; Whiting et al, 2009; Fletcher, 2010).

Emotional abuse involves extreme debasement of feelings and may lead the child to feel inadequate, inept, uncared for, and worthless. These children learn to hide their feelings to avoid more scorn. They may act out by performing poorly in school, becoming truant, and being hostile and aggressive. Children who are abused or who witness domestic violence can suffer developmentally (Kletter et al, 2009; Rodriguez, 2010). Major responses of adolescents to physical and sexual abuse are substance abuse, severe depression, and running away from home (Fletcher, 2010; Ford et al, 2010).

Physical symptoms of physical, sexual, or emotional stress may include hyperactivity, withdrawal, overeating, dermatological

---

**HOW TO** Recognize Actual or Potential Child Abuse

*Be alert to the following:*
- *An unexplained injury*
- *Skin: burns, old or recent scars, ecchymosis, soft tissue swelling, human bites*
- *Fractures: recent, or older ones that have healed*
- *Subdural hematomas*
- *Trauma to genitalia*
- *Whiplash (caused by shaking small children)*
- *Dehydration or malnourishment without obvious cause*
- *Provision of inappropriate food or drugs (alcohol, tobacco, medication prescribed for someone else, foods not appropriate for the child's age)*
- *Evidence of general poor care: poor hygiene, dirty clothes, unkempt hair, dirty nails*
- *Unusual fear of nurse and others*
- *Considered to be a "bad" child*
- *Inappropriate dress for the season or weather conditions*
- *Reports or shows evidence of sexual abuse*
- *Injuries not mentioned in history*
- *Seems to need to take care of the parent and speak for the parent*
- *Maternal depression*
- *Maladjustment of older siblings*
- *Current or history of intimate partner violence in the home*

---

problems, vague physical complaints, stuttering, enuresis (bladder incontinence), and encopresis (bowel incontinence). Ironically, bedwetting is often a trigger for further abuse, thereby creating a vicious cycle. When a child displays physical symptoms without clear physiological origin, the nursing assessment should rule out the possibility of abuse.

*Child Neglect.* The four categories of child neglect include physical, emotional, medical, and educational neglect. Physical neglect is failure to provide adequate food, proper clothing, shelter, hygiene, or necessary medical care and is most often associated with extreme poverty. In contrast, emotional neglect is the lack of the basic nurturing, acceptance, and caring essential for healthy personal development. These children are largely ignored or treated as nonpersons, which affects the development of self-esteem. A neglected child has difficulty feeling self-worth because the parents have not shown that they value the child. Medical and educational neglect consist of the failure to provide for a child's basic medical and educational needs. Children with disabilities may be neglected because of inadequate resources. Medical neglect may be due to an inability to buy basic drugs needed for common diseases. All forms of neglect may be involved when a parent fails to teach children about risky behaviors such as smoking and substance abuse (Hines and Malley-Morrison, 2005). Astute observations of children, their homes, and the family can assist in a proper assessment of neglect and possible recommendations for care.

*Sexual Abuse.* Child abuse also includes sexual abuse. Approximately 1 in 4 female children and 1 in 10 males in the United States experiences some form of sexual abuse by the time he or she reaches 18 years of age. It is difficult to determine the exact prevalence because not all children have the cognitive ability to describe these experiences. Rates based on reports to child protective services estimate that 50 in every 1000 children suffer from child abuse and/or neglect (USDHHS, 2013). This abuse ranges from unwanted sexual touching to intercourse. The child generally knows and trusts the person who perpetrates the sexual abuse. One third to one half of all sexual abuse involves a family member (Hines and Malley-Morrison, 2005; USDHHS, 2013). A child's risk for abuse is highest with parents, immediate family members, and nonrelated caregivers, although coaches, scout leaders, and even priests and other church workers have been reported as sexual abusers. The long-term effects of sexual abuse include depression, sexual disturbances, suicide, and substance abuse. Individuals with a history of both physical and sexual abuse tend to experience more severe symptoms than children who experience one form of abuse (Fletcher, 2010; Stevenson, 2009). Physically and sexually abusive parents share many of the same characteristics, including unhappiness, loneliness, and rigidity. However, sexually abused children have more gastrointestinal symptoms and post-traumatic stress disorders than physically abused children (Drossman, 2011).

Father–daughter incest is the type of incest most often reported; however, mothers do engage in child sexual abuse. In recent years more males have discussed their experiences of child sexual abuse. It is estimated that one in five children is a victim of child sexual abuse. Cases of father–daughter, father–son, mother–daughter, and mother–son incest have been reported (Hines and Malley-Morrison, 2005). Many cases of parental sexual abuse go unreported because victims fear punishment, abandonment, rejection, or family disruption if the problem is acknowledged. Although stepfathers are considered the most common perpetrator of father–daughter incest, we know little about female perpetrators. Incest occurs in all races, religious groups, and socioeconomic classes. Incest is receiving greater attention because of mandatory reporting laws, yet all too often its incidence remains a family secret.

Nurses must be aware of the incidence, signs and symptoms, and psychological and physical trauma of incest. Symptoms include low self-esteem, depression, anxiety, and somatic symptoms of headaches, eating and sleeping disorders, menstrual problems, and gastrointestinal distress (Drossman, 2011). Sexually abused children often exhibit premature sexual behavior, such as masturbation. Children often try to avoid or escape the abusive behavior. Avoidance can be through either behavioral or mental reactions, such as dressing to cover one's body or pretending that the abuse is not taking place. The child can escape either physically by running away or emotionally by withdrawing into other activities and thereby placing the sexual abuse in the background (Stevenson, 2009).

Adolescents may display inappropriate sexual activity or truancy or may run away from home. Running away is usually considered a sign of delinquency; however, an adolescent who runs away may be exhibiting a healthy response to a violent family situation. Therefore, the assessment should include questions about sexual and physical abuse at home and a plan for appropriate intervention.

The effects of childhood sexual abuse can be mitigated by continual professional support. At different developmental stages, children may need assistance to overcome negative feelings about their own sexuality (Stevenson, 2009). Adult survivors of sexual abuse often are socially isolated and have significant health problems that need to be addressed in terms of the ongoing effects of their childhood and adult experiences (Mapp, 2006).

## Abuse of Female Partners

Neither the term wife abuse nor the term spouse abuse takes into account violence in dating or cohabiting relationships or violence in same-sex relationships. IPV, a more inclusive term, refers to all kinds of violence between partners. IPV is not a rare event, with one in three women and one in four men reporting physical violence, rape, and/or stalking by a current or former intimate partner at some point in their life (Black et al, 2011). However, these figures do not include psychological forms of IPV, which also could have severe consequences. Recently, more attention has been given to female-perpetrated IPV and bidirectional violence (i.e., male-to-female violence concurrent with female-to-male violence), especially in the context of teen dating violence. Nevertheless, female victims of IPV are more likely to report severe IPV and experience more negative individual, family, and community consequences than their male counterparts, and a greater potential for intimate partner homicide (Black et al, 2011; Campbell, 2007).

IPV appears early in life. In fact, approximately 22% of victims of rape, physical abuse, and/or stalking by an intimate partner report their first experience when they were between the ages of 11 and 17. Nearly half (47%) report their first incident between the ages of 18 and 24 (Black et al, 2011). As in adulthood, IPV experienced by adolescents and young adults is associated with poor mental health outcomes such as depression and suicidality, are linked to risky behaviors such as substance abuse and risky sexual behaviors, and can set the stage for unhealthy relationships in adulthood (Coker et al, 2000; Fredland and Burton, 2011).

*Signs of Abuse.* Battered women often have bruises and lacerations of the face, head, and trunk of the body. Attacks are often carefully inflicted on parts of the body that are disguised by clothing. This pattern of proximal location of injuries (e.g., breasts, abdomen, upper thighs, and back) rather than distal and patterned injuries (in various stages of healing, in particular configurations matching the body part or object used as a weapon) is characteristic of abuse (Campbell and Sheridan, 2004; Sheridan and Nash, 2009). When a woman has a black eye or bruises about the mouth, the nurse should ask, "Who hit you?" rather than, "What happened to you?" The latter implies that the nurse is neither knowledgeable nor comfortable with violence, and this may prompt the woman to fabricate a more acceptable cause of her injury.

Once abused, women tend to exhibit low self-esteem and depression, and even PTSD (Humphreys and Campbell, 2010). They have more physical health problems than other women, such as chronic pain (back, head, abdominal), neurological problems, problems sleeping, gynecological symptoms, urinary tract infections, and chronic gastrointestinal problems (Campbell, 2002). Victims of IPV are also at greater risk for HIV and other STIs, which appear to be both a risk factor and consequence of the abuse (Coker et al, 2009). In addition, female victims of IPV are more at risk for chronic diseases such as cardiovascular disease, atherosclerosis, and autonomic nervous system disorders (Symes et al, 2010). Although the focus tends to be on the victim of the abuse, it is important to note that there are health consequences to the perpetrator and children witnessing the abuse as well. These physical and mental health consequences incur health care costs that are preventable (Rivara et al, 2007).

*Abuse as a Process.* Nursing research by Ford-Gilboe and colleagues (2010) suggests that there is a process of response to battering over time wherein the woman's emotional and behavioral reactions change. At first there is a great need to minimize the seriousness of the situation. The violence usually starts with a slight shove in the middle of a heated argument. If there is any physical aggression, both the man and the woman tend to blame the incident on something external such as a stressful day at work or drinking too much. The male partner usually apologizes for the incident, and as with any problem in a relationship, the couple tries to improve the situation. Although marital counseling may be useful at this early stage, it is generally contraindicated at all other stages because of the risk to the woman's safety. Unfortunately, abuse tends to escalate in frequency and severity over time, often leading to severe physical injuries and even death (Piquero et al, 2006), and the man's remorse tends to lessen. Similar power and control dynamics and risks have been documented in same-sex relationships, yet these dynamics may be more difficult to assess because screening and services for IPV are often designed for heterosexual relationships (Alhusen et al, 2010).

Because women have often been taught to take responsibility for the success of a relationship, they usually go through a period in which they try to change their behavior to end the violence. They may even blame themselves for infuriating their partner. Women who blame themselves for provoking the abuse are more likely to have low self-esteem and be depressed than those who do not blame themselves. Some women experience a moral conflict between their need to leave an abusive relationship and their sense that it is their responsibility to maintain a relationship (Flinck et al, 2005). She is also typically concerned about her children, which may create barriers to a woman's ability to leave or to remain out of the relationship. The frequency of abuse, severity of power and control tactics used by the perpetrator, feelings of guilt, and social and financial responsibility are additional influences on a woman's decision about how she responds to the abuse and whether she stays or leave the relationship (Sonis and Langer, 2008; Rhodes et al, 2010).

Although leaving the abusive partner may ultimately contribute to a decrease in the woman's risk for further victimization, the moment in which she leaves the relationship is the time in which there is the greatest risk for intimate partner homicide (Campbell, 2007). This creates a Catch-22 situation, in which the woman feels she will die whether she stays or leaves. Consequently, battered women often try several times to leave a relationship. The safety of the woman and her children is a nursing priority during these attempts.

## EVIDENCE-BASED PRACTICE

Sharps and colleagues (2013) conducted a multistate longitudinal study testing the effectiveness of a structured intimate partner violence (IPV) intervention integrated into health department perinatal home visitation programs in rural and urban locations. All women (n = 239) enrolled in the randomized clinical trial were pregnant at the time of enrollment and reported a positive history of IPV in the perinatal period. The research partners included individuals from two schools of nursing, an urban East Coast health department, and 13 rural Midwestern health departments. The Domestic Violence Enhanced Home Visitation (DOVE) intervention, based on an empowerment model, combined two evidence-based interventions: a 10-minute brochure-based IPV intervention and perinatal nurse home visitation. Quantitative and qualitative data revealed that women in both the intervention group and control group demonstrated a significant decrease in IPV over time. However, women receiving the DOVE intervention had significantly lower levels of IPV than did control subjects at 24 months. Home visitors in both groups (e.g., intervention and control) were taught how to screen for IPV and how to coordinate appropriate referrals, ensuring that each woman received basic safety information.

**Nurse Use**

Nurses need to be able to work with survivors of IPV as well as providers within communities who work with abused women. Community-based partnerships are essential to most effectively develop and implement evidence-based IPV interventions such as DOVE. To best address IPV in a community, nurses must understand cultural differences among women who experience IPV as well as among community advocates who may also be assisting abused women. Public health nurses are well positioned to forge such partnerships and take an active role in planning, implementing, and evaluating programmatic change.

*Partnering with the Community.* Nurses need to be able to work to address IPV on various levels of intervention. Community-based partnerships are essential collaborative actions that will assist in the reduction of IPV. To do so, nurses must understand cultural differences related to IPV, as well as the needs and strengths of the communities with which they partner. Public health nurses can take an active role in leading groups and planning, implementing, and evaluating programmatic change. There are various examples of nurse-led community partnerships to prevent and address IPV. For example, both Belknap and VandeVusse (2010) and Gonzalez-Guarda and colleagues (2013) partnered with community agencies, schools, and community members to identify needs and preferences for IPV prevention and services for the Hispanic/Latino community. This work has led to the development, implementation, and evaluation of dating violence prevention programs for Hispanic/Latino youth.

The Centers for Disease Control and Prevention (CDC) has launched an initiative called Dating Matters. The purpose of this program is to teach parents and adolescents about healthy relationships and to give them tools to deal with unhealthy relationships such as teen dating violence (CDC, 2014b). Dating Matters focuses on 11- to 14-year-olds in high-risk, urban communities, and includes prevention strategies for individuals, peers, families, schools, and neighborhoods. The Migrant Clinicians Network, an organization to help migrant and other poor transient workers, has developed a natural helper model for migrant workers, to work within their own community to identify and teach about IPV (Kugel et al, 2009). On the basis of models developed in the 1980s, communities are developing a coordinated response in which multiple agencies work together to assist with preventing IPV.

*Screening.* Given the high prevalence of IPV and the negative physical, psychological, social, and economic consequences associated with this public health problem, adolescents and adults should be screened for violence in their primary intimate relationship. The U.S. Preventive Services Task Force recommends screening women of childbearing age for IPV and referring or providing women who disclose abuse to intervention services (U.S. Preventive Services Task Force, 2013). The use of effective screening protocols, institutional support for implementing screening, initial and ongoing staff training, and access to services onsite or through a strong referral system are recommended as part of a comprehensive screening program (O'Campo et al, 2011).

*Safety Planning.* Victims of IPV are at high risk for severe injuries and homicide, especially at the moment they decide to leave an abusive relationship (Campbell, 2007). As such, nurses should work with women victims in creating a safety plan. This plan may include the following: (1) an order of protection (a legal document to keep the abuser away from her); (2) help in getting to a safe place, such as a domestic violence shelter in an anonymous location; (3) access to individual advocacy and support groups/or the criminal justice system (Harding and Helweg-Larsen, 2009); and (4) a carefully calculated plan for escape that includes keeping a bag with a copy of important documents and other resources (e.g., keys, phone, contact information) for emergencies. Although leaving an abusive relationship has been shown to be protective in the long term (Campbell, 2007), it is important to avoid pushing women into actions they are not ready to take. Cultural factors that influence responses to IPV are also important to consider in the development of interventions addressing the safety of victims (Ward and Wood, 2009; Belknap and VandeVusse, 2010).

*Batterer's Interventions.* The male partner may attend a program for batterers as an alternative to ending the relationship. These programs appear to be effective for some individuals. These programs are most effective if they are part of a coordinated community response, involve appropriate risk assessment and management practices, are of adequate structure (e.g., duration), are court-mandated and closely monitored, and involve training and close supervision of the staff implementing the program (Salcido Carter, 2009).

## Intimate Partner Sexual Abuse

Battered women are often forced into sexual encounters. This sexual abuse is usually but not always accompanied by physical abuse. Women who are sexually abused are at risk for STDs (Coker et al, 2009). Sexual abuse increases the risk for mental health problems for all women who are involved in physically abusive relationships. Women who experience child abuse are at even greater risk for depression than those not exposed to abuse as a child (Fogarty et al, 2009).

The belief that men have a right to force their wives to have sex comes from traditional English law that said a woman gave irrevocable and perpetual consent to her husband on marriage to have sex whenever and however he wanted. Marital rape was not considered a crime in the United States until 1993 (Yllo, 1999). Marital rape leads to serious physical and emotional damage. Women who suffer from IPV may not consider forced sex a form of abuse. It is essential when women come to the emergency room with injuries that they are assessed for the presence of both physical and sexual abuse (Catallo, 2006).

To assess for sexual assault, the following question should be used in all nursing assessments to determine whether marital rape, date rape, or rape of a male has occurred: "Have you ever been forced into sex you did not wish to participate in?"

## Abuse during Pregnancy

Battering during pregnancy has serious implications for the health of women and their children. As a conservative estimate, 3% to 8% of pregnant women in the United States are physically battered during pregnancy, with a larger proportion of women abused during the year before pregnancy. Even more (up to 20%) adolescents are abused during pregnancy than adult women (Bloom et al, 2010). Although abuse during pregnancy occurs across ethnic groups, Puerto Rican, white, and African American women experience a significantly higher severity of physical abuse than Hispanic women from Mexico and Central America (Bloom et al, 2010). Women abused during pregnancy are at risk for spontaneous abortion, premature delivery, low-birth-weight and small-for-gestational age infants, substance abuse during pregnancy, and depression (Alhusen et al, 2013; McFarlane and Parker, 2005). A man's control of contraception, a form of abusive controlling, may lead to unintended pregnancy and subsequent abuse. In addition, a man's refusal to use a condom places a woman at increased risk of STDs, including infection with HIV (Campbell et al, 2008).

Women who are abused during pregnancy are more likely to experience health problems and are at risk for alcohol and drug abuse (Blake et al, 2007). This group of infants could be anticipated to be at particularly high risk of child abuse after they are born. Clearly, all pregnant women should be assessed for abuse at each prenatal care visit, and postpartum home visits should include assessment for child abuse and partner abuse. There is a significant overlap in wife abuse and child abuse, and in more than half of families where there is severe wife abuse, there is also child abuse (Humphreys and Campbell, 2010).

## Elder Abuse

The World Health Organization defines **elder abuse** broadly, as "a single or repeated act or lack of appropriate action, occurring within any relationship where there is an expectation of trust which causes harm or distress to an older person" (World Health Organization, 2002, p. 29). Research findings regarding the prevalence of elder abuse vary widely, depending on the population that is studied (e.g., community-dwelling elders versus those who are institutionalized), the study methods (e.g., review of service provider and protective service records versus population-based surveys of elders themselves), and the specific definition of elder abuse that was used in the research (Acierno et al, 2010; Mysyuk et al, 2013). Even the definition of who may be considered an "elder" is not consistent across research studies (Acierno et al, 2010) or across cultures (Mysyuk et al, 2013). Large, longitudinal national studies that describe the prevalence of elder abuse, its risk and protective factors, and its consequences to health over time are needed (Dong and Simon, 2011).

Regardless, it is clear that elder abuse is common. In a recent random-digit dial survey of 5777 community-dwelling U.S. elders at least 60 years of age, 1 in 10 reported past-year emotional, physical, or sexual mistreatment or potential neglect (i.e., an identified need for assistance that no one was addressing) (Acierno et al, 2010). Elder abuse has significant implications for public health, as it is associated with significant consequences to mental and physical health; increasing risk of physical injury; gastrointestinal, gynecological, and musculoskeletal issues; delusions, dementia, anxiety, and depression; and mortality (Daly, 2011). Elder abuse is underreported across virtually all cultures, and constitutes a violation of elders' basic human rights (World Health Organization, 2002).

*Types of Elder Abuse.* Specific types of elder abuse include the following (Daly, 2011):
- *Physical abuse:* The use of physical force, potentially resulting in injury, pain, or impairment
- *Sexual abuse:* Nonconsensual sexual contact of any kind
- *Emotional abuse:* Verbal or nonverbal acts that inflict psychological anguish, pain, or distress
- *Financial or material abuse:* Illegal or improper use of the elder's money, property, or assets
- *Neglect:* Refusing or failing to fulfill one's obligations or duties to an elder
- *Abandonment:* Desertion by a caregiver or custodian

Perpetrators of elder abuse may include family members, caregivers in home or institutional settings, and intimate partners. In addition, "resident-to-resident" verbal, sexual, and/or physical aggression within long-term care settings has been described (Daly, 2011). Although resident-to-resident aggression may not clearly fall under the World Health Organization definition of elder abuse (which implies a trusting or caregiver relationship), this type of violence also has obvious potential for harm to vulnerable elders.

*Prevention of Elder Abuse.* Effectively addressing elder abuse requires the involvement of multiple sectors and disciplines. Increasing awareness and recognition of elder abuse among professionals and the public, and training of service providers, are key areas for intervention (Daly, 2011; World Health Organization, 2002), as is improving education for health professionals on management and reporting guidelines for elder abuse (Dong and Simon, 2011).

*Screening for Elder Abuse.* The U.S. Preventive Services Task Force (USPSTF) has recommended that clinicians routinely screen all women of childbearing age for IPV. In the same report, the USPSTF concluded that there is insufficient evidence to support universal screening of elders for abuse. However, the Task Force also noted that elder abuse is both common and underreported, suggesting potential benefits for universal

screening, and that the existing evidence regarding the lack of harm resulting from IPV screening suggests that screening for elder abuse may also represent a small risk of harm (U.S. Preventive Services Task Force, 2013). More research is needed in this area. In the absence of support for universal screening, evidence-based guidelines for nurses published in 2010 indicate that certain groups of elders are particularly likely to benefit from assessment for abuse or risk for abuse (Daly, 2011). More recently, a systematic review of studies of community-dwelling elders by Johannesen and LoGiudice (2013) suggested that living with others (versus living alone) was correlated with overall abuse but not financial abuse; this may be another factor that warrants added attention to risk assessment.

For nurses, in-depth evidence-based guidelines for the prevention of elder abuse and numerous risk assessment tools for elder abuse are available from the University of Iowa College of Nursing's Hartford/Csomay Center for Geriatric Nursing Excellence. See, *www.nursing.uiowa.edu/hartford*. If a nurse is working with an elder and abuse or risk of abuse is identified, the nurse should create an individualized plan of care and service, using such evidence-based practice guidelines. To be effective, these plans should focus on both the elder and their caregiver (Daly, 2011).

Nurses also can play a key role in facilitating primary and secondary prevention interventions. More research is needed regarding the effectiveness of such interventions, including evaluation of outcomes related to mandatory reporting laws. However, evidence to date suggests that there are a number of promising interventions, including educational programs (for elders, the general public, care providers including nursing assistants, or for mandatory reporters), home visitation, caregiver skill-building, counseling or social support interventions, respite care, and batterer intervention (for intimate partners who are violent) (U.S. Preventive Services Task Force, 2013; Daly, 2011). Nurses can also play a role in advocating for vulnerable elders with policy makers, working to ensure adequate funding of state and federal legislation that addresses elder abuse; in the United States these include the Older American Act, the Violence Against Women Act, and the Elder Justice Act (Dong and Simon, 2011).

## NURSING INTERVENTIONS

### Primary Prevention

A community approach is essential to prevent violence and human abuse. Public health nurses can help the community in the following areas.

First, the community can take a stand against violence and make sure their elected officials and the local media consider nonviolence a priority. Public education programs can educate communities about various forms of violence and ways to get help and intervene (Campbell and Manganello, 2006; Post et al, 2010). Nurses, as community advocates, should be integral in this process. In the legislative arena, laws are needed to outlaw physical punishment in schools and marital rape. Nurses can become involved with faith-based communities and schools to implement and evaluate prevention programs aimed at decreasing violence. Policies for the various kinds of abuse should become standardized (Miller, 2005).

Strong community sanctions against violence in the home can reduce abuse levels (Sullivan et al, 2005). Neighbors can watch what is happening and work together to address problems in other families; this is not an invasion of privacy but a sign of community cohesiveness. Nurses can work with advocacy groups to make sure law enforcement personnel deal with assault within marriage as swiftly, surely, and severely as assault between strangers (Stover et al, 2010). Nurses can encourage others to intervene when they witness children beaten in a grocery store, notice that an older adult is not being properly cared for, see a neighborhood bully beat up his or her classmates, or hear a neighbor hitting his wife.

## (QSEN) FOCUS ON QUALITY AND SAFETY EDUCATION FOR NURSES

### *Quality and Safety Focus*

**Targeted Competency: Teamwork and Collaboration**—Function effectively within nursing and interprofessional teams, fostering open communication, mutual respect, and shared decision making to achieve quality client care.

Important aspects of teamwork and collaboration include:

- **Knowledge:** Recognize contributions of other individuals and groups in helping client/family achieve health goals
- **Skills:** Assume role of team member or leader, based on the situation
- **Attitudes:** Respect the unique attributes that members bring to a team, including variations in professional orientations and accountabilities

**Teamwork and Collaboration Question**

If you learned, after careful assessment of your community, that family violence is a significant community health problem, what plan of action could you take to intervene? Remember that the goal is to promote health. Are there other individuals in the community whose collaboration you could enlist? Might there be insights and assistance that could be offered by leaders in church organizations, educators in schools, primary care providers, or social workers? Outline a plan of action with objectives, timetables, implementation strategies, and evaluation plans for intervening in family violence in your community. Include the unique contributions of other team members.

Prepared by: Gail Armstrong, PHD©, DNP, ACNS-BC, CNE, Associate Professor, University of Colorado Denver College of Nursing.

Second, people can take measures to reduce their vulnerability to violence by improving the physical security of their homes and learning personal defense measures. Nurses can encourage people to keep windows and doors locked, trim shrubs around their homes, and keep lights on during high-crime periods. Many neighborhoods organize crime watch programs and post signs to that effect. One sign, often posted in a window, shows a hand and indicates that people in this home will assist children who need help. Also, many neighbors informally agree to monitor one another's property and safety, and many law enforcement agencies evaluate homes for security and teach individual or neighborhood safety programs.

Unfortunately, handguns are far more likely to kill family members than intruders (Hahn et al, 2005). Firearm accidents are a leading cause of death for young children, and handguns

kept in the home are easy to use when people are either depressed or very angry. A handgun is used in the majority of homicides between family members and in most suicides. Nursing assessments should include a question about guns kept in the home. The family should be made aware of the risk that a handgun holds for family members. If the family thinks that keeping a gun is necessary, safety measures should be taught, such as keeping the gun unloaded and in a locked compartment, keeping the ammunition separate from the gun and also locked away, and teaching children about the dangers of firearms. Lobbying for handgun control laws is a primary prevention effort that can significantly decrease the rate of death and serious injury caused by handguns in the United States.

### Assessment for Risk Factors

Identification of risk factors is an important component of primary prevention. Although abuse cannot be predicted with certainty, several factors influence the onset and support the continuation of abusive patterns. Nurses can identify potential victims of abuse because they care for clients in a variety of settings. Factors to include in an assessment for individual or family violence, or the potential for family violence, are identified in Figure 38-1. Both individual and familial factors must be assessed within the context of the larger community (Straus et al, 2009). Factors that must be included are found in Box 38-2.

---

**BOX 38-2   Assessing for Violence in a Community Context**

**Individual Factors**
- Signs of physical abuse (e.g., abrasions, contusions, burns)
- Physical symptoms related to emotional distress
- Developmental and behavioral difficulties
- Presence of physical disability
- Social isolation
- Decreased role performance within the family, and in job- or school-related activities
- Mental health problems such as depression, low self-esteem, and anxiety
- Fear of intimate others
- Substance abuse

**Familial Factors**
- Economic stressors
- Presence of some form of family violence
- Poor communication
- Problems with child rearing
- Lack of family cohesion
- Recurrent familial conflict
- Lack of social support networks
- Poor social integration into the community
- Multiple changes of residence
- Access to guns
- Homelessness

**Community Characteristics**
- High crime rate
- High levels of unemployment
- Lack of neighborhood resources and support systems
- Lack of community cohesiveness

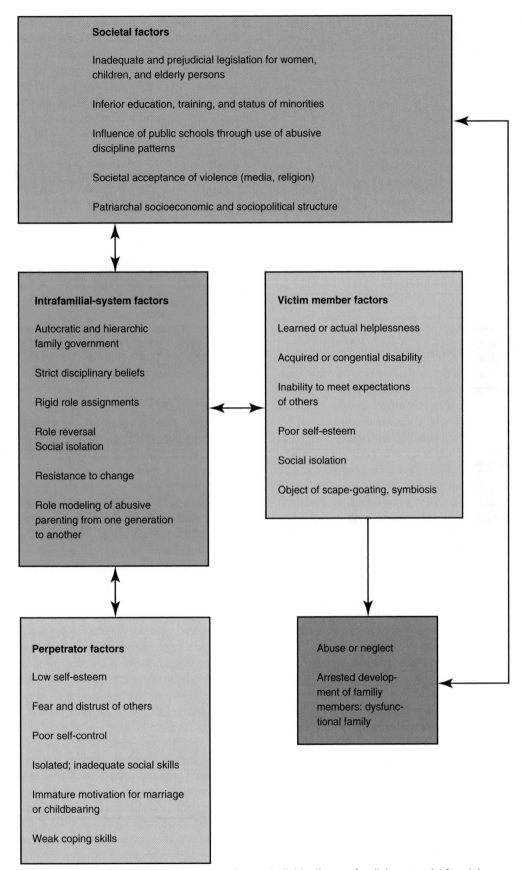

FIG 38-1 Factors to include when assessing an individual's or a family's potential for violence.

---

### BOX 38-3    Prevention Strategies for Violence

**Individual and Family Levels**
- Provide education on developmental stages and needs of children (primary).
- Teach parenting techniques (primary).
- Teach stress-reduction techniques (primary).
- Provide assessment during routine examination (secondary).
- Assess for marital discord (secondary).
- Provide counseling for at-risk parents (secondary).
- Encourage assistance with controlling anger (secondary).
- Provide treatment for substance abuse (tertiary).

**Community Level**
- Develop policy.
- Conduct community resource mapping.
- Collaborate with community to develop systemic response to violence.
- Develop media campaign.
- Develop resources such as transition housing and shelters.

---

### Individual and Family Strategies for Primary Prevention

Primary prevention of violence can take place through community, family, and individual interventions (Box 38-3). Nurses, in their work with schools, community groups, employee groups, daycare centers, and other community institutions, can foster healthy developmental patterns and identify signs of potential abuse. For example, nurses may take part in media campaigns that identify risk factors for abuse. Nurses can lead in developing after-school programs and late-night programs that support young people to work toward positive goals and to develop a constructive support network. These primary prevention efforts should be broad-based, to include vulnerable youth populations such as sexual minorities, that is, a group whose sexual orientation and practices are different from the majority in a given society (Walters et al, 2013). Nurses can identify community needs and resources by capacity mapping. The identification of strengths and weaknesses can assist in determining future goals and needed interventions for the good of the community.

Primary prevention of abuse includes strengthening individuals and families so they can cope more effectively with multiple life stressors and demands, and mitigating the risk factors in the community that increase the risk of violence. Providing support and psychological enrichment to at-risk individuals and families often prevents the onset of health disruption. For example, nurses can strengthen and teach parenting abilities. A class, clinic, or home visiting services can include basic skills such as diapering, feeding, quieting, and even holding and rocking. Parents also need to learn acceptable and effective ways to discipline children so that limits are maintained without causing the child emotional or physical harm. The Nurse–Family Partnership model of professional nurse home visitation for at-risk pregnant women has been shown to significantly reduce the risk of child abuse and is being adapted to work toward primary and secondary prevention of IPV (Niolon et al, 2009).

Mutual support groups are valuable for new parents, families of children with special needs, or abused people themselves. Such groups have variable formats and can provide information, support, and encouragement to facilitate positive outcomes. Nurses can help establish such groups, refer clients, or serve as group leaders. Chapter 16 describes the role of the nurse in working with community groups.

---

### 📄 LEVELS OF PREVENTION

#### *Violence*

**Primary Prevention**
Strengthen individual and family by teaching parenting skills.

**Secondary Prevention**
Reduce or end abuse by early screening; teach families how to deal with stress and how to have fun and enjoy recreation.

**Tertiary Prevention**
When signs of abuse are evident, refer client to appropriate community organizations.

---

## Secondary Prevention

When abuse occurs, nurses can initiate measures to reduce or end further abuse. Both developmental and situational crises present opportunities for abusive situations to develop. On a community level, nurses must form collaborative relationships to provide health services for battered women (McFarlane et al, 2005). There is a critical lack of appropriate services and resources available for many violence survivors, such as LGBT persons (Walters et al, 2013); nurses are key change agents in reaching vulnerable subpopulations. Researchers must work effectively with community agencies to use current research to screen for domestic violence and to use model treatments that have a positive effect on decreasing domestic violence (Humphreys and Campbell, 2010).

Nurses can be primary leaders in the development of screening practices in the health care arena (Higgins and Hawkins, 2005). The development of training programs for health care providers can be an effective step in identifying and treating victims of violence. Nurses can work closely with domestic violence shelters in identifying the needs of individuals who seek sanctuary from abusive situations.

On a family level, nursing intervention can help family members discuss problems and seek ways to deal with the tension that led to the abusive situations. Injured persons must be temporarily or permanently placed in a safe location. Secondary preventive measures are most useful when potential abusers recognize their tendency to be abusive and seek help. For children, there is often a need for 24-hour child protection services or caregivers who can take care of the child until the acute family or individual crisis is resolved. Respite care is extremely important in families with frail older adult family members. Telephone crisis lines can be used to provide immediate emergency assistance to families.

Effective communication with abusive families is important. Typically, these families do not want to discuss their problems and many are embarrassed to be involved in an abusive situation. Often a lot of guilt is involved. Effective communication must be preceded by an attitude of acceptance. It is often difficult for nurses to value the worth of an individual who willfully abuses another. The behavior, not the person, must be condemned.

In addition, families do not always know how to have fun. Nurses can assess how much recreation is integrated into the family's lifestyle. Through community assessment, nurses know what resources and facilities are available and how much they cost. Families may need counseling about the value of recreation and play in reducing tension and appropriately channeling aggressive impulses.

## Tertiary Prevention: Therapeutic Intervention with Abusive Families

Although it may be difficult for abusive families to form trusting relationships with health care providers, nurses can act as a case manager, coordinating the other agencies and activities involved. Principles of giving care to families who are experiencing violence include the following:

- Intolerance for violence
- Respect and caring for all family members
- Safety as the first priority
- Absolute honesty
- Empowerment

Nurses must clearly indicate that any further violence, degradation, and exploitation of family members will not be tolerated, and that all family members are respected, valued human beings. However, everyone must understand that the safety of every family member is the first priority.

Abusers often fear they will be condemned for their actions, making it difficult to maintain contact with abusive families. Although nurses convey an attitude of caring and concern for them, families may doubt the sincerity of this concern. They may avoid being home at the scheduled visit time out of fear of the consequences of the visit or an inability to believe that anyone really wants to help them. If the victim is a child, parents may fear that the nurse will try to remove the child.

Nurses are mandatory reporters of child abuse, even when only suspected, in all states. They are also mandatory reporters of elder abuse and abuse of other physically and cognitively dependent adults as well as of felony assaults on anyone in most states. The mandatory reporting laws also protect reporters from legal action on cases that are never substantiated. Even so, physicians and nurses are sometimes reluctant to report abuse. They may be more willing to report abuse in a poor family than in a middle-class one, or they may think that an older adult or child is better off at home than in a nursing home or foster home. Referral to protective service agencies should be viewed as enlisting another source of help, rather than as an automatic step toward removal of the victim or criminal justice action. This same attitude can be communicated to families, so that reporting is done with families rather than without their knowledge and prior input. Absolute honesty about what will be

reported to officials, what the family can expect, what the nurse is entering into records, and what the nurse is feeling is essential.

To further empower the family, the nurse needs to recognize and capitalize on the violent family's strengths, as well as to assess and deal with its difficulties. The nurse must use a nurse–family partnership rather than a paternalistic or authoritarian approach. Families can often generate many of their own solutions, which tend to be more culturally appropriate and individualized than those the nurse generates. Victims of direct attack need information about their options and resources, and they need reassurance that abuse is unfortunately rather common and that they are not alone in their dilemma. They also need reassurance that their responses are normal and that they do not deserve to be abused. Continued support for their decisions must be coupled with nursing actions to ensure their safety.

### Nursing Actions

The nurse can meet the family's therapeutic needs in a variety of ways. Besides referral to appropriate community agencies, nurses can act as role models for the family. During clinic and home visits, nurses can demonstrate constructive adult–child interactions. Nurses often teach mothers childcare skills such as proper feeding, calming a fretful child, effective discipline, and constructive communication.

Nurses can demonstrate good communication skills and discipline by teaching both parents and children in a calm, respectful, and informative manner. Caregivers, especially those caring for children, people with special needs, or older adults, may need to learn age-appropriate expectations. It is unreasonable to expect a 14-month-old infant to differentiate between right and wrong. Children at this age do not deliberately annoy caregivers by breaking delicate pieces of china. Likewise, a person with poor sphincter control does not willingly soil clothes or bedding.

Role modeling can be used with abuse victims of all ages. When providing nursing care to abused spouses or to older adults, nurses can demonstrate communication skills, conflict resolution, and skill training. For example, adult children often become abusive toward their older parents when they become frustrated in trying to care for them. During home visits, nurses can show how to physically and psychologically care for the relative. The nurse can work with caregivers to help them develop approaches that are acceptable to the individual older adult. Assessment, creativity, and critical thinking help the nurse, family, and client learn how to meet client and family needs without causing undue stress and frustration.

Working with abusers and victims of abuse can be emotionally intensive and physically draining. Abusers present difficult clinical challenges because they are often reluctant to seek help or to remain actively involved in the helping process.

Referral is an important part of tertiary prevention. Nurses should know about available community resources for abuse victims and perpetrators. Some of these resources are listed in Box 38-4. If community attitudes and resources are inadequate, it is often helpful to work with local radio and television stations

---

**BOX 38-4  Common Community Services**

- Child protective services
- Child abuse prevention programs
- Adult protective services
- Parents Anonymous
- Domestic violence shelters
- Programs for children of battered women
- Community support groups
- 24-hour hotline
- Legal advocacy or information
- State/county coalition against domestic violence
- Batterer treatment
- Victim assistance programs
- Sexual assault programs
- Transition housing

---

and newspapers to provide information about the nature and extent of human abuse as a community health problem. This also helps to acquaint people with available services and resources. Frequently, people do not seek services early in an abusive situation because they simply do not know what is available to them. Ideally, a program or plan for abused people begins with a needs assessment to identify potential clients and to determine how to effectively serve this group. Nurses can help to get programs started and provide public education.

### Nursing Interventions Specific to Female Partner Abuse

Women in abusive relationships may seek care for injuries in an emergency setting, a physician's office, or a prenatal clinic. These women may be seeking assistance for injuries sustained during physically abusive episodes (McFarlane et al, 2005), but more often they are in the health care system for other health problems. Despite the overall prevalence of battering and its resultant physical and emotional health problems for women, health professionals, even those working in emergency departments, often fail to identify abused women. Some health care professionals are perceived as paternalistic, judgmental, insensitive, and less effective and helpful than they could be (Alhusen et al, 2010).

Because of the stigma and unease involved, women and health care providers may hesitate to initiate discussion about abuse. However, the majority of battered women claim they would have liked to talk about the issue with a health care professional if they were asked (Higgins and Hawkins, 2005). Because abuse develops slowly, starting with minor psychological abuse and building to more severe physical incidents, victims and health care providers alike may not recognize the abuse until a severe episode occurs.

The quality of health care that a battered woman receives often determines whether she follows through with referrals to legal, social service, and health care agencies. The emergency department is the point of entry for many women in abusive relationships. Care in the emergency department is often fragmented and necessarily oriented toward addressing the most acute illness or injury. Therefore, women may not be adequately

assessed and often receive little or no support or referral to services to assist in dealing with the abuse. A cycle persists in which women seek care and receive either no interventions or ineffective interventions. This cycle perpetuates feelings of anger and inadequacy in health care providers, resulting in blame placed on women for their lack of compliance with remedies offered.

Managed care and clinic settings may be the best places to routinely screen for domestic violence. Ideally a clinical nurse specialist who is an expert in screening for IPV should be available to coordinate efforts in the different health care settings. If battered women can be identified, perhaps effective interventions can be provided that will prevent the kind of serious injury that later results in emergency department visits or even a homicide.

However, some battered women hesitate to identify themselves as victims of domestic violence for several reasons. They may fear that revelation will further jeopardize their safety by increasing the violence, and they may also think that it will increase their sense of shame and humiliation. In addition, the nature of the systems in which victims of violence introduce themselves can be barriers. Emergency departments, clinics, managed care settings, and health departments are busy places. Staff members work hard to maintain the functioning of these facilities. Sometimes it is difficult in such chaotic settings for staff members to realize their importance as the first or only health provider to recognize violence in their clients' lives, and that women need them to take the time to deal with this issue (Straus et al, 2009).

Studies have found that only a small percentage of battered women in emergency departments and other health care settings were identified as such and treated for the abuse, despite the significant prevalence (Furniss et al, 2007). Battered women present for treatment in a number of ways, including physical complaints (such as inability to sleep or chronic pain) related to the chronic stress of living in an abusive situation or to old injuries. They may be unaware of the relationship of their symptoms to the violence in their lives. Therefore, professional nursing organizations (American Nurses Association, Emergency Nurses Association, Association of Women's Health, Obstetric and Neonatal Nurses, American College of Nurse-Midwives) recommend that all women be routinely screened for domestic violence each time they come to a health care setting. For the battered woman and the staff to begin to make the connection between her life situation and the presenting complaints, the nurse needs to ask direct questions in a supportive, open, and concerned manner (Straus et al, 2009). Computerized inquiry is also effective in identifying abused women in health care settings (Trautman et al, 2007).

*Assessment.* Assessment for all forms of violence against women should therefore take place for all women entering the health care system. The assessment should be ongoing and confidential. A thorough assessment gathers information on physical, emotional, and sexual trauma from violence, risk for future abuse, cultural background and beliefs, perceptions of the woman's relationships with others, and stated needs. Conduct the assessment in private and direct other adults who are present to the waiting area and tell them that it is policy that initially women are seen alone. Women should be asked directly if they were in an abusive relationship as a child or are currently in an abusive relationship as an adult. They should also be asked whether they have ever been forced into sex. Shame and fear often make disclosure difficult. Verbal acknowledgment of the situation and emotional and physical support assist women in talking about past or current circumstances (Humphreys and Campbell, 2010).

Women can be categorized into three groups: no, low, or moderate to high risk. Women with no signs of current or past abuse are considered at no risk. However, every future visit should include questioning a woman about whether there have been any changes in her life or whether she has additional information or questions about topics discussed at previous visits. If there is a new intimate partner in her life, she should again be screened for abuse. The Abuse Assessment Screen (AAS) is a four-question screen that has been successfully used in almost every kind of health care setting and can be downloaded from the Nursing Network on Violence Against Women International (NNVAWI) website (http://www.nnvawi.org).

Women at low risk show no evidence of recent or current abuse. Education that helps a woman gain perspective on her situation and her needs should be discussed. Resource materials including group and individual formats can be suggested. The risk level should be recorded and preventive measures and teaching should be documented.

Assessment of moderate to high risk includes evaluation of a woman's fear of both psychological and physical abuse. Lethality potential should be assessed (Campbell et al, 2009) and can be done with the Danger Assessment, also available at the NNVAWI website. Risk factors for lethality include behaviors such as stalking or frequent harassment, threats or an escalation of threats, use of weapons or threats with weapons, excessive control and jealousy, and forced sex. Statements from an abuser such as "If I can't have you, no one can" should be taken seriously. In all cases, a history of abuse and alcohol and drug use should be collected and carefully documented. The determined risk level should also be documented along with any past or present physical evidence of abuse from prior or current assault; this evidence should be photographed, shown on a body map, or described narratively. It is important that the assailant be identified in the record; this can take the form of either quotes from the woman or subjective information. These records can be very important for women in future assault or child custody cases, even if the woman is not ready to make a police report at the present time.

Immediate care for a woman in a potentially harmful or present abusive situation involves the development of a safety plan. A woman can be assisted to look at the options available to her (Dienemann et al, 2009). Discuss shelter information, access to counseling, and legal resources. If a woman wants to return to her partner, she can be helped in the development of plans that can be carried out if the abuse continues or becomes more serious. The Domestic Violence Abuse Survivor Assessment is an assessment tool that can help providers assist women in decision making and the identification of services to meet needs. The assessment covers discussion about the relationship and assessment of psychosocial needs, safety and danger issues, speaking with children, and issues of substance abuse. The assessment can be found at the NNVAWI website.

Whenever there is evidence of sexual assault within the prior 24 to 48 hours, a rape kit examination should be performed. Lists of resources such as rape crisis clinics and support groups for survivors of physical and emotional abuse should be made available.

*Prevention.* Prevention, public policy, and social attitudes are intertwined. Our society has taken a major step toward the secondary prevention of abuse through the establishment of programs that encourage women and children to speak about their experiences. Nurses need to support these programs further by supporting individuals and families confronted with violence. In the development of laws that punish perpetrators of child and women abuse, society has given some support to the victims of abuse. Often, however, the victims are again victimized by disbelief of their experiences, a devaluing of the effects of these assaults, and a focus on assisting the perpetrators of the crimes. Primary prevention includes a social attitudinal change. Both girls and boys need to be taught human values of interdependence, respect for human life, and a commitment to empathy and strength in the development of the human species regardless of sex, race, or socioeconomic status. We must urge continued progress toward eliminating the feminization of poverty and ensuring gender parity in economic resources. In addition, local communities must make it clear that violence against women is not tolerated by eliminating pornography, mandating arrests of abusers, and creating a general climate of nonviolence.

Abused women need assistance in making decisions and taking control of their lives. Public health nurses, prenatal nurses, Planned Parenthood, primary care, and emergency department nurses are involved with women when they can be screened for the presence or absence of abuse. There are mechanisms for routinely asking women who are either abused or at risk for abuse (Higgins and Hawkins, 2005; Dienemann et al, 2009). To intervene effectively, nurses must understand abuse as a cumulative process that must be examined as a continuum within the context of a relationship. During this process, the abuse, the relationship, and a woman's view of changes within herself require time-specific interventions. Women are often blamed and held responsible for the abuse inflicted on them by their male partners (Weaver et al, 2007; Copel, 2008; Saito et al, 2009; Ting and Panchanadeswaran, 2009). When this happens, either they are assisted in a way that discounts their feelings and further devalues them, or the abuse is ignored.

*Strategies for Addressing Education for Health Professionals.* Various strategies have been reported that address the knowledge deficit of health practitioners on abuse issues. The National March of Dimes Birth Defects Foundation has sponsored a variety of training sessions for health professionals and produced an excellent training manual that addresses violence against women and battering during pregnancy (McFarlane and Parker, 2005). The program covers the assessment and planning of interventions to assist pregnant women in abusive relationships.

More and more nursing programs are implementing courses on how to intervene with IPV. Wallace (2009) developed and implemented a two-credit elective course focusing on attitudes, knowledge, and interventions in a structured learning environment to help nursing students acquire the expertise needed to work with women in abusive relationships. An educational program for nurses was developed in order to initiate system-wide routine inquiry in an urban health care system (Schoening et al, 2004). The program consisted of a mandatory 1-hour program for all nurses with an optional 3-hour program for nurses working in obstetrics. The program focused on the dynamics of abuse, screening procedures, and nursing interventions. The program showed an increase in positive responses to battered women for nurses involved in the 3-hour program and for nurses in the 1-hour program only if they had previous education on abuse. Short programs with skills education as well as discussion can be a benefit to both nurses and the clients they serve.

Nurses are also joining in community-based efforts to prevent and intervene with IPV and child abuse. Nurses work in public health collaborating with shelters for women, community mental health centers, criminal justice and advocacy institutions, and community-based health care. Bloom and colleagues (2009) developed a program to assist Latinas experiencing IPV. The program was developed specifically for the cultural and linguistic needs of the population. Emphasis was placed on assisting the Hispanic community in developing the knowledge and background to deal with the issue. At the same time, community efforts focused on expanding the knowledge base of the community at large about IPV.

## PRACTICE APPLICATION

Mrs. Smith, a 75-year-old bedridden woman, became consistently rude and combative when her daughter Mary attempted to bathe her and change her clothes each morning. During a home visit, Mary told the nurse, Mrs. Jones, that she had become so frustrated with her mother on the previous morning that she had hit her. Mary felt terrible about her behavior. She stressed that her mother's incontinence made it essential that she be kept clean; her clothes had to be changed every day for her own safety and physical well-being.

A. How should Mrs. Jones respond to this disclosure?
B. What specific nursing actions should be taken?
C. What ongoing services does the nurse need to provide?
**Answers can be found on the Evolve site.**

## KEY POINTS

- Violence and human abuse are not new phenomena, but they have increasingly become community health concerns.
- Communities throughout the United States are angry and frustrated about increasing levels of violence.
- Nurses can evaluate and intervene in incidents of community and family violence; to intervene effectively, the nurse must understand the dynamics of violence and human abuse.
- Factors influencing social and community violence include changing social conditions, economic conditions, population density, community facilities, and institutions within a community, such as organized religion, education, the mass communication media, and work.
- The potential for violence against individuals or against oneself is directly related to the level of violence in the community. Identification and correction of factors affecting the level of violence in the community constitute one way of reducing violence against family members and other individuals.

- Violence and abuse of family members can happen to any family member: spouse, older adult, child, or developmentally disabled person.
- People who abuse family members were often themselves abused and react poorly to real or perceived crises. Other factors that characterize the abuser are the way the person was raised and the unique character of that person.
- Child abuse can be physical, emotional, or sexual. Incest is a common and particularly destructive form of child abuse.
- Spouse abuse is usually wife abuse. It involves physical, emotional, and, frequently, sexual abuse within a context of coercive control. It usually increases in severity and frequency and can escalate to homicide of either partner.
- Nurses are in an excellent position to identify potential victims of family abuse because they see clients in a variety of settings, such as schools, businesses, homes, and clinics. Treatment of family abuse includes primary, secondary, and tertiary prevention and therapeutic intervention.

## CLINICAL DECISION-MAKING ACTIVITIES

1. For 1 week, keep a log or diary related to violence.
   A. Make a note of each time you feel as though you are losing your temper. Consider what it might take to cause you to react in a violent way.
   B. Think back. When was the last time you had a violent outburst? What precipitated it? What were your thoughts? What were your feelings? How might you have handled the situation or those feelings without reacting in a violent way?
   C. During this same week, make note of the episodes of violent behaviors you observe. For example, do parents hit children in the supermarket? What seems to precipitate such outbursts? What alternatives might exist for reacting in a less violent way?

## CLINICAL DECISION-MAKING ACTIVITIES—cont'd

2. If you learned, after a careful assessment of your community, that family violence is a significant community health problem, what plan of action might you take to intervene? Remember that the goal is to promote health. Outline a plan of action with objectives, timetables, implementation strategies, and evaluation plans for intervening in family violence in your community.

3. Complete a partial community assessment to determine the actual incidence and types of violence in your community.

4. What resources are available in your community for victims of violence? Interview a person who works in an agency that

seeks to aid victims of violence. What is the role of the agency? Do its services seem adequate? Who is eligible? Is there a waiting list? What is the fee scale?

5. Cut out all stories about violence that you find in your local newspaper every day for 2 weeks. Note the patterns. Is the majority of the violence perpetrated by strangers or family members? How are the victims portrayed? What kinds of families are involved? What kinds of stories and families get front-page treatment rather than a few lines in the back of the paper?

## REFERENCES

Acierno R, Hernandez MA, Amstadter AB, et al: Prevalence and correlates of emotional, physical, sexual, and financial abuse and potential neglect in the National Elder Mistreatment Study. *Am J Public Health* 100:292–297, 2010.

Alhusen JL, Baty M, Glass N: Perceptions of and experiences with system responses to female same-sex intimate partner violence. *Partner Abuse* 1:443–462, 2010.

Alhusen JL, Lucea M, Bullock L, et al: Intimate partner violence and adverse neonatal outcomes among urban women. *J Pediatr* 163:471–476, 2013.

American Public Health Association: *10 Essential Public Health Services*, 2010. Retrieved March 2015 from: http://www.apha.org/about-apha/centers-and-programs/quality-improvement-initiatives/national-public-health-performance-standards-program/10-essential-public-health-services.

Anderson CA, Berkowitz L, Donnerstein E, et al: The influence of media violence on youth. *Psychol Sci Public Interest* 4:81–110, 2003.

Beaulaurier RL, Seff LR, Newman FL, et al: External barriers to help seeking for older women who experience intimate partner violence. *J Fam Violence* 22:747–755, 2007.

Belknap RA, VandeVusse L: Listening sessions with Latinas: documenting life contexts and creating connections. *Public Health Nurs* 27:337–346, 2010.

Berlan ED, Corliss HL, Field AE, et al: Sexual orientation and bullying among adolescents in the Growing Up Today Study. *J Adolesc Health* 46:366–371, 2010.

Berman H, Hardesty H, O'Connor A, et al: Children of abused women. In Humphreys J, Campbell JC,

editors: *Family Violence and Nursing Practice*, ed 2. New York, 2010, Springer, pp 154–185.

Black MC, Basile KC, Breiding MJ, et al: *The National Intimate Partner and Sexual Violence Survey (NISVS): 2010 Summary Report*. Atlanta, GA, 2011, National Center for Injury Prevention and Control, Centers for Disease Control and Prevention.

Blake SM, Kiely M, Gard CC, et al: Pregnancy intentions and happiness among pregnant black women at high risk for adverse infant health outcomes. *Perspect Sex Reprod Health* 39:194–205, 2007.

Bloom T, Bullock L, Sharps PW, et al: Intimate partner violence during pregnancy. In Humphreys J, Campbell JC, editors: *Family Violence and Nursing Practice*, ed 2. New York, 2010, Springer, pp 279–398.

Bloom T, Wagman J, Hernandez R, et al: Partnering with community-based organizations to reduce intimate partner violence. *Hisp J Behav Sci* 31:244–257, 2009.

Bostock DJ, Daley JG: Lifetime and current sexual assault and harassment victimization rates of active-duty United States Air Force women. *Violence Against Women* 13:927–944, 2007.

Bower-Russa M: Attitudes mediate the association between childhood disciplinary history and disciplinary responses. *Child Maltreat* 10:272–282, 2005.

Campbell JC: Health consequences of intimate partner violence. *Lancet* 359:1331–1336, 2002.

Campbell JC: *Assessing Dangerousness: Violence by Batterers and Child Abusers*, ed 2. New York, 2007, Springer.

Campbell R, Long SM, Townsend SM, et al: Sexual assault nurse examiners' experiences providing

expert witness court testimony. *J Forensic Nurs* 3:7–14, 2007.

Campbell JC, Manganello J: Changing public attitudes as a prevention strategy to reduce intimate partner violence. *J Aggress Maltreat Trauma* 13:13–39, 2006.

Campbell R, Patterson D, Adams AE, et al: A participatory evaluation project to measure SANE nursing practice and adult sexual assault patients' psychological well-being. *J Forensic Nurs* 4:19–28, 2008.

Campbell JC, Sharps PW, Glass NE: Risk assessment for intimate partner homicide. In Pinard GF, Pagani L, editors: *Clinical Assessment of Dangerousness: Empirical Contributions*. New York, 2000, Cambridge University Press, pp 136–157.

Campbell JC, Sheridan DJ: Assessment of intimate partner violence and elder abuse. In Jarvis C, editor: *Physical Assessment for Clinical Practice*. Philadelphia, 2004, Elsevier Science, pp 74–82.

Campbell R, Townsend SM, Long SM, et al: Responding to sexual assault victims' medical and emotional needs: a national study of the services provided by SANE programs. *Res Nurs Health* 29:384–398, 2006.

Campbell JC, Webster DW, Glass NE: The Danger Assessment: validation of a lethality risk assessment instrument for intimate partner femicide. *J Interpers Violence* 24:653–674, 2009.

Campbell JC, Webster D, Koziol-McLain J, et al: Risk factors for femicide in abusive relationships: results from a multi-site case control study. *Am J Public Health* 93:1089–1097, 2003.

Casey EA, Lindhorst TP: Toward a multi-level, ecological approach to the primary prevention of sexual assault: prevention in peer and

community contexts. *Trauma Violence Abuse* 10:91–114, 2009.

Catalano S: *Intimate Partner Violence: Attributes of Victimization, 1993-2011*. Washington, DC, 2012, Bureau of Justice Statistics. Retrieved March 2015 from: http://www.bjs.gov/content/pub/pdf/ipvav9311.pdf.

Catalano S, Smith E, Snyder H, et al: *Female Victims of Violence*. Washington, DC, 2009, Bureau of Justice Statistics Selected Findings. Retrieved March 2015 from: http://bjs.ojp.usdoj.gov/content/pub/pdf/fvv.pdf.

Catallo C: Review: meta-analysis of qualitative studies generated recommendations for healthcare professionals meeting with women who had experienced intimate partner violence. *Evid Based Nurs* 9:125–134, 2006.

Centers for Disease Control and Prevention (CDC): *Youth Risk Behavior Surveillance System (YRBSS)*, 2013. Retrieved March 2015 from: www.cdc.gov.mmwr/pds/ss/ss6304.pdf.

Centers for Disease Control and Prevention (CDC): *Web-Based Injury Statistics Query and Reporting System (WISQARS)*, 2013. Retrieved March 2015 from: http://www.cdc.gov/injury/wisqars/index.html.

Centers for Disease Control and Prevention (CDC): *National Suicide Statistics at a Glance*, 2014a. Retrieved March 2015 from: http://www.cdc.gov/violenceprevention/suicide/statistics/index.html.

Centers for Disease Control and Prevention (CDC): *Dating Matters Initiative*, 2014b. Retrieved March 2015 from: http://www.cdc.gov/violenceprevention/datingmatters/index.html.

Coker AL, Hopenhayn C, DeSimone CP, et al: Violence against women raises risk of cervical cancer.

*J Womens Health* 18:1179–1185, 2009.

Coker AL, McKeown RE, Sanderson M, et al: Severe dating violence and quality of life among South Carolina high school students. *Am J Prev Med* 19:220–227, 2000.

Copel LC: The lived experience of women in abusive relationships who sought spiritual guidance. *Issues Ment Health Nurs* 29:115–130, 2008.

Corvo K, deLara E: Towards an integrated theory of relational violence: is bullying a risk factor for domestic violence? *Aggress Violent Behav* 15:181–190, 2010.

Daly JM: Elder abuse prevention: evidence-based practice guidelines. *J Gerontol Nurs* 37:11–17, 2011.

Daro D, Dodge KA: Creating community responsibility for child protection: possibilities and challenges. *Future Child* 19:67–93, 2009.

Dienemann J, Neese J, Lowry S: Psychometric properties of the Domestic Violence Survivor Assessment. *Arch Psychiatr Nurs* 23:111–118, 2009.

Dixon L, Browne K, Hamilton-Giachritsis C: Patterns of risk and protective factors in the intergenerational cycle of maltreatment. *J Fam Viol* 24:111–122, 2009.

Dixon L, Hamilton-Giachritsis C, Browne K: Risk factors of parents abused as children: a mediational analysis of the intergenerational continuity of child maltreatment. *J Child Psychol Psychiatry* 46:59–68, 2005.

Dong X, Simon MA: Enhancing national policy and programs to address elder abuse. *JAMA* 305:2460–2461, 2011.

Drossman AD: Abuse, trauma, and GI illness: is there a link? *Am J Gastroenterol* 106:14–25, 2011.

Eaton DK, Kann L, Kinchen S, et al: Youth risk behavior surveillance—United States, 2009. *MMWR Surveill Summ* 59:1–42, 2010.

Ellison CG, Trinitapoli JA, Anderson KL, et al: Race/ethnicity, religious involvement, and domestic violence. *Violence Against Women* 13:1094–1112, 2007.

Ernst AA, Weiss SJ, Enright-Smith S, et al: Positive outcomes from an immediate and ongoing intervention for child witnesses of intimate partner violence. *Am J Emerg Med* 26:389–394, 2008.

Ferguson CJ, Hartley RD: The pleasure is momentary...the expense damnable? The influence of pornography on rape and sexual assault. *Aggress Violent Behav* 14:323–329, 2009.

Fisher BS, Cullen FT, Turner MG: *The Sexual Victimization of College*

*Women.* Washington, DC, 2000, U.S. Department of Justice. Retrieved March 2015 from: https://www.ncjrs.gov/pdffiles1/nij/182369.pdf.

Fletcher J: The effects of intimate partner violence on health in young adulthood in the United States. *Soc Sci Med* 70:130–135, 2010.

Flinck A, Paavilainen E, Åstedt-Kurki P: Survival of intimate partner violence as experienced by women. *J Clin Nurs* 14:383–393, 2005.

Fogarty CT, Fredman L, Heeren TC, et al: Synergistic effects of child abuse and intimate partner violence on depressive symptoms in women. *Prev Med* 46:463–469, 2009.

Ford JD, Elhai JD, Connor DF, et al: Poly-victimization and risk of posttraumatic, depressive, and substance use disorders and involvement in delinquency in a national sample of adolescents. *J Adolesc Health* 46:545–552, 2010.

Ford-Gilboe M, Varcoe C, Wuest J, et al: Intimate partner violence and nursing practice. In Humphreys J, Campbell JC, editors: *Intimate Partner Violence and Nursing Practice*. New York, 2010, Springer, pp 115–153.

Fredland NM, Burton C: Nursing care and teen dating violence: promoting healthy relationship development. In Humphreys J, Campbell J, editors: *Intimate Partner Violence and Nursing Practice*, ed 2. New York, 2011, Springer, pp 225–252.

Furniss K, McCaffrey M, Parnell V, et al: Nurses and barriers to screening for intimate partner violence. *Am J Matern Child Nurs* 32:238–243, 2007.

Gonzalez-Guarda RM, Cummings AM, Becerra M, et al: Needs and preferences for the prevention of intimate partner violence among Hispanics: a community's perspective. *J Prim Prev* 34:221–235, 2013.

Gracia E, Herrero J: Perceived neighborhood social disorder and attitudes toward reporting domestic violence against women. *J Interpers Violence* 22:737–752, 2007.

Grier SA, Kumanyika S: Targeted marketing and public health. *Annu Rev Public Health* 31:349–369, 2010.

Hahn RA, Bilukha O, Crosby A, et al: Firearms laws and the reduction of violence: a systematic review. *Am J Prev Med* 28(Suppl 1):40–71, 2005.

Harding H, Helweg-Larsen M: Perceived risk for future intimate partner violence among women in a domestic violence shelter. *J Fam Violence* 24:75–85, 2009.

Higgins LP, Hawkins JW: Screening for abuse during pregnancy:

implementing a multisite program, MCN. *Am J Matern Child Nurs* 30:109–114, 2005.

Hines DA, Malley-Morrison K: *Family Violence in the United States.* Thousand Oaks, CA, 2005, Sage.

Houmes BV, Fagan MM, Quintana NM: Violence: recognition, management and prevention: establishing a Sexual Assault Nurse Examiner (SANE) program in the emergency department. *J Emerg Med* 25:111–121, 2003.

Howard KAS, Budge SL, McKay KM: Youth exposed to violence: the role of protective factors. *J Community Psychol* 38:63–79, 2010.

Humphreys JC, Campbell JC: *Family Violence and Nursing Practice.* New York, 2010, Springer.

Johannesen M, LoGiudice D: Elder abuse: a systematic review of risk factors among community-dwelling elders. *Age Ageing* 42:292–298, 2013.

Karch DL, Dahlberg LL, Patel N: Surveillance for violent deaths—National Violent Death Reporting System, 16 states, 2007. *MMWR Surveill Summ* 59:1–50, 2010.

Kelly UA, Gonzalez-Guarda RM, Taylor J: Theories of intimate partner violence. In Humphreys J, Campbell JC, editors: *Intimate Partner Violence and Nursing Practice*, ed 2. New York, 2010, Springer, pp 253–278.

Kiriakidis SP, Kavoura A: Cyberbullying: a review of the literature on harassment through the Internet and other electronic means. *Fam Community Health* 33:82–93, 2010.

Kletter H, Weems CF, Carrion VG: Guilt and posttraumatic stress symptoms in child victims of interpersonal violence. *Clin Child Psychol Psychiatry* 14:71–83, 2009.

Kugel C, Retzlaff C, Hopfer S, et al: Familias con Voz: community survey results from an Intimate Partner Violence (IPV) Prevention Project with migrant workers. *J Fam Viol* 24:649–660, 2009.

Krug EG, Dahlberg LL, Mercy JA, et al: *World Report on Violence and Health.* Geneva, Switzerland, 2002, World Health Organization.

Lee MR, Ousey GC: Institutional access, residential segregation, and urban Black homicide. *Sociol Inq* 75:31–54, 2005.

Levitt HM, Ware K: "Anything with two heads is a monster": religious leaders' perspectives on marital equality and domestic violence. *Violence Against Women* 12:1169–1190, 2006.

Lewandowski L, McFarlane J, Campbell JC, et al: "He killed my mommy!" Murder or attempted murder of a child's mother. *J Fam Violence* 19:211–220, 2004.

Lichter EL, McCloskey LA: The effects of childhood exposure to marital violence on adolescent

gender-role beliefs and dating violence. *Psychol Women Q* 28:344–357, 2004.

Lin J, Thompson MP, Kaslow NJ: The mediating role of social support in the community environment—psychological distress link among low-income African American women. *J Community Psychol* 37:459–470, 2009.

Logan TK, Cole J, Capillo A: Sexual Assault Nurse Examiner program: characteristics, barriers, and lessons learned. *J Forensic Nurs* 3:24–33, 2007.

Mapp SC: The effects of sexual abuse as a child on the risk of mothers physically abusing their children: a path analysis using systems theory. *Child Abuse Negl* 30:1293–1310, 2006.

Masters NT: "My strength is not for hurting": men's anti-rape websites and their construction of masculinity and male sexuality. *Sexualities* 13:33–46, 2010.

McFarlane JM, Groff JY, O'Brien JA, et al: Prevalence of partner violence against 7,443 African American, white, and Hispanic women receiving care at urban public primary care clinics. *Public Health Nurs* 22:98–107, 2005.

McFarlane J, Parker B: *Abuse during Pregnancy: A Protocol for Prevention and Intervention.* White Plains, NY, 2005, March of Dimes Birth Defects Foundation.

Miller C: Elder abuse: the nurse's perspective. *Clin Gerontol* 28:105–133, 2005.

Mysyuk Y, Westendorp RG, Lindenberg J: Added value of elder abuse definitions: a review. *Ageing Res Rev* 12:50–57, 2013.

Nannini A, Lazar J, Berg C, et al: Physical injuries reported on hospital visits for assault during the pregnancy-associated period. *Nurs Res* 57:144–149, 2008.

National Coalition of Anti-Violence Programs: *Lesbian, Gay, Bisexual and Transgender Domestic Violence in the United States in 2012.* Retrieved March 2015 from: avp.org/storage/documents/ncavp_2012_ipvreport.final.pdf.

Niolon PH, Whitaker DJ, Feder L, et al: A multicomponent intervention to prevent partner violence within an existing service intervention. *Prof Psychol Res Pr* 40:264–271, 2009.

O'Campo P, Kirst M, Tsamis C, et al: Implementing successful intimate partner violence screening programs in health care settings: evidence generated from a realist-informed systematic review. *Soc Sci Med* 72:855–866, 2011.

O'Reilly R, Wilkes L, Luck L, et al: The efficacy of family support and family preservation services on reducing child abuse and neglect: what the literature reveals. *J Child Health Care* 14:82–94, 2010.

Parks SE, Johnson LL, McDaniel DD, et al: Surveillance for violent deaths—National Violent Death Reporting System, 16 States, 2010. *MMWR Surveill Summ* 63:1–33, 2014.

Peralta RA, Tuttle LA, Steele JL: At the intersection of interpersonal violence, masculinity, and alcohol use: the experiences of heterosexual male perpetrators of intimate partner violence. *Violence Against Women* 16:387–409, 2010.

Piquero AR, Brame R, Fagan J, et al: Assessing the offending activity of criminal domestic violence suspects: offense specialization, escalation and de-escalation evidence from the Spouse Assault Replication Program. *Public Health Rep* 121:409–418, 2006.

Pitts J: Youth gangs, ethnicity and the politics of estrangement. *Youth Policy* 102:101–113, 2009.

Post LA, Klevens J, Maxwell CD, et al: An examination of whether coordinated community responses affect intimate partner violence. *J Interpers Violence* 25:75–93, 2010.

Potter H: Battered black women's use of religious services and spirituality for assistance in leaving abusive relationships. *Violence Against Women* 13:262–284, 2007.

Rahn WM, Yoon KS, Garet M, et al: Geographies of trust. *Am Behav Sci* 52:1646–1663, 2009.

Rand MR: *National Crime Victimization Survey: Criminal Victimization, 2008* [Bureau of Justice Statistics Bulletin], 2009. Retrieved March 2015 from: http://bjs.ojp.usdoj.gov/content/pub/pdf/cv08.pdf.

Regan ME: Implementation and evaluation of a youth violence prevention program for adolescents. *J Sch Nurs* 25:27–33, 2010.

Rhodes K, Cerulli C, Dichter M, et al: "I didn't want to put them through that": the influence of children on victim decision-making in intimate partner violence cases. *J Fam Violence* 25:485–493, 2010.

Rivara FP, Anderson ML, Fishman P, et al: Intimate partner violence and health care costs and utilization for children living in the home. *Pediatrics* 120:1270–1277, 2007.

Rodriguez CM: Personal contextual characteristics and cognitions: predicting child abuse potential and disciplinary style. *J Interpers Violence* 25:315–335, 2010.

Rodriguez CM, Henderson RC: Who spares the rod? Religious orientation, social conformity, and child abuse potential. *Child Abuse Negl* 34:84–94, 2010.

Saito AS, Cooke M, Creedy DK, et al: Thai women's experience of intimate partner violence during the perinatal period: a case study analysis. *Nurs Health Sci* 11:382–387, 2009.

Salcido Carter L: Batterer intervention: doing the work and measuring the progress: a report on the December 2009 expert round table. Retrieved March 2015 from: https://www.futureswithout violence.org/userfiles/file/Children_and_Families/Batterer%20Intervention%20Meeting%20Report.pdf.

Salmivalli C: Bullying and the peer group: a review. *Aggress Violent Behav* 15:112–120, 2010.

Schoening AM, Greenwood JL, McNichols JA, et al: Effect of an intimate partner violence educational program on the attitudes of nurses. *J Obstet Gynecol Neonatal Nurs* 33:572–579, 2004.

Scott ST: Multiple traumatic experiences and the development of posttraumatic stress disorder. *J Interpers Violence* 22:932–938, 2007.

Seto MC, Lalumière ML: What is so special about male adolescent sexual offending? A review and test of explanations through meta-analysis. *Psychol Bull* 136:526–575, 2010.

Sharps P, Alhusen JL, Bullock L, et al: Engaging and retaining abused women in perinatal home visitation programs. *Pediatrics* 132:S134–S139, 2013.

Sheridan D: Legal and forensic nursing responses to family violence. In Humphreys J, Campbell JC, editors: *Family Violence and Nursing Practice*. Philadelphia, 2004, Lippincott, Williams & Wilkins, pp 385–406.

Sheridan DJ, Nash KR: Acute injury patterns of intimate partner violence victims. *Trauma Violence Abuse* 8:281–289, 2009.

Silverman JG, Raj A, Mucci LA, et al: Dating violence against adolescent girls and associated substance use, unhealthy weight control, sexual risk behavior, and suicidality. *JAMA* 286:572–579, 2001.

Smith SG, Fowler KA, Niolon PH: Intimate partner homicide and corollary victims in 16 states: National Violent Death Reporting System, 2003-2009. *Am J Public Health* 104:461–466, 2014.

Sonis J, Langer M: Risk and protective factors for recurrent intimate partner violence in a cohort of low-income inner-city women. *J Fam Violence* 23:529–538, 2008.

Steeves RH, Parker B: Adult perspectives on growing up following uxoricide. *J Interpers Violence* 21:1270–1284, 2007.

Stevenson M: Perceptions of juvenile offenders who were abused as children. *J Aggress Maltreat Trauma* 18:331–349, 2009.

Stockman J, Campbell J, Celentano D: Sexual violence and HIV risk behaviors among a nationally representative sample of heterosexual American women: the importance of sexual coercion. *J Acquir Immune Defic Syndr* 53:136–143, 2010.

Stover CM, Berkman M, Desai R, et al: The efficacy of a police-advocacy intervention for victims of domestic violence: 12 month follow-up data. *Violence Against Women* 16:410–425, 2010.

Straus M: Children should never, ever, be spanked no matter what the circumstances. In Loseke DR, Gelles R, Cavanaugh M, editors: *Current Controversies on Family Violence*. Thousand Oaks, CA, 2005, Sage, pp 137–157.

Straus H, Cerulli C, McNutt LA, et al: Intimate partner violence and functional health status: associations with severity, danger, and self-advocacy behaviors. *J Womens Health* 18:625–631, 2009.

Sullivan M, Bhuyan R, Senturia K, et al: Participatory action research in practice: a case study in addressing domestic violence in nine cultural communities. *J Interpers Violence* 20:977–995, 2005.

Swanberg J, Macke C, Logan TK: Working women making it work: intimate partner violence, employment, and workplace support. *J Interpers Violence* 22:292–311, 2007.

Swider SM, Krothe J, Reyes D, et al: The Quad Council practice competencies for public health nursing. *Public Health Nurs* 30:519–536, 2013.

Symes L, McFarlane J, Frazier L, et al: Exploring violence against women and adverse health outcomes in middle age to promote women's health. *Crit Care Nurs Q* 33:233–243, 2010.

Ting L, Panchanadeswaran S: Barriers to help-seeking among immigrant African women survivors of partner abuse: listening to women's own voices. *J Aggress Maltreat Trauma* 18:817–838, 2009.

Tjaden P, Thoennes N: *Full Report of the Prevalence, Incidence, and Consequences of Violence against Women: Findings from the National Violence Against Women Survey* [National Institutes of Justice, CDC]. Washington, DC, 2000, U.S. Department of Justice.

Trautman D, McCarthy ML, Miller N, et al: Intimate partner violence and emergency department screening: computerized screening versus usual care. *Ann Emerg Med* 49:526–534, 2007.

U.S. Department of Health and Human Services (USDHHS): *Healthy People 2020: Objectives*. Washington, DC, 2010, Office of Disease Prevention and Health Promotion, USDHHS.

U.S. Department of Health and Human Services, Administration for Children and Families, Administration on Children, Youth and Families, Children's Bureau: *Child Maltreatment 2012*, 2013. Retrieved March 2015 from: http://www.acf.hhs.gov/sites/default/files/cb/cm2012.pdf.

U.S. Department of Labor, Bureau of Labor Statistics: *Demographics*, 2012. Retrieved March 2015 from: http://www.bls.gov/cps/demographics.htm#race.

U.S. Preventive Services Task Force: *Screening for Intimate Partner Violence and Abuse of Elderly and Vulnerable Adults* [U.S. Preventive Services Task Force Recommendation Statement]. 2013. Retrieved March 2015 from: http://www.uspreventiveservicestaskforce.org/uspstf12/ipvelder/ipvelderfinalrs.htm.

Vervoort MH, Scholte RH, Overbeek G: Bullying and victimization among adolescents: the role of ethnicity and ethnic composition of school class. *J Youth Adolesc* 39:1–11, 2010.

Wallace CM: Measuring changes in attitude, skill and knowledge of undergraduate nursing students after receiving an educational intervention in intimate partner violence [doctoral dissertation]. College of Saint Mary, 2009.

Walters ML, Chen J, Breiding MJ: *The National Intimate Partner and Sexual Violence Survey (NISVS): 2010 Findings on Victimization by Sexual Orientation*. Atlanta, GA, 2013, National Center for Injury Prevention and Control, Centers for Disease Control and Prevention.

Ward C, Wood A: Intimate partner violence: NP role in assessment. *Am J Nurs Pract* 13:9–15, 2009.

Weaver TL, Turner PK, Schwarze N, et al: An exploratory examination of the meanings of residential injuries from intimate partner violence. *Women Health* 45:85–102, 200, 2007.

Whiting JB, Simmons LA, Havens JR, et al: Intergenerational transmission of violence: the influence of self-appraisals, mental disorders and substance abuse. *J Fam Viol* 24:639–648, 2009.

Woods SJ, Hall RJ, Campbell JC, et al: *J Midwifery Womens Health* 53:538–546, 2008.

World Health Organization: *Active Ageing: A Policy Framework*. Geneva, 2002, World Health Organization.

Yllo K: Wife rape. *Violence Against Women* 5:1059–1063, 1999.

Zimmerman F, Mercy JA: A better start: child maltreatment prevention as a public health priority. *Zero Three* 30:4–10, 2010.

# PART 7

# Nurses' Roles and Functions in the Community

At one time, the role of the public health nurse was primarily visiting clients at home and identifying cases of communicable disease. Over the decades, the role has become complex and now involves population-centered practice. The role of the community-based nurse focuses on improving the health of individuals and families through the delivery of personal health services, with an emphasis on primary prevention, health promotion, and health protection. Community-oriented, or population-focused, nursing practice emphasizes the delivery of services and interventions aimed at improving health and protecting entire populations from illness, disease, and injury. As the health care system has changed, the need for a comprehensive, population-focused public health system has become more evident. Nurses are able to provide care to individuals, families, and populations including aggregates and communities in a variety of settings and roles.

With increasing emphasis being placed on the community as the client, nurses recognize that to address community health issues, they must be able to meet the needs of the individuals, families, and groups that are the nucleus of the community. In recent decades, the primary practice setting for the nurse was the hospital, but now nurses are caring for clients in many settings. Regardless of the type of client, practice setting, specialty area of practice, or the functional role of the nurse, nurses act as advocates for clients in meeting their needs through the health care system.

This section discusses the roles of manager, consultant, clinical nurse specialist, and nurse practitioner, with particular emphasis on the development of the advocacy role in population-centered practice. Throughout the text, content is applicable to a variety of practice settings, including the more traditional public health practice areas such as the health department. A few other practice settings with close association to population-centered nursing have been highlighted, such as school health, occupational health, home health/hospice, and congregational settings. In the community setting, the field of forensics is receiving increasing attention as an area of practice for public health nurses. This area of practice is a highlight of this text.

# 39

# The Advanced Practice Nurse in the Community

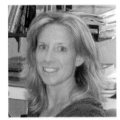

*Kellie A. Smith, RN, EdD*
Kellie A. Smith is an Assistant Professor at Thomas Jefferson University in Philadelphia, Pennsylvania, and is the coordinator of the graduate community health/public health nursing program entitled Community Systems Administration. She is a clinical nurse specialist in community health nursing. She has been involved in NIH/NIDDK (National Institute of Health/National Institute of Diabetes and Digestive and Kidney Diseases) research for type 2 diabetes prevention, the Diabetes Prevention Program. Dr. Smith was also involved with the trial's translational campaign, "Small Steps. Big Rewards," directed by The National Diabetes Education Program (NDEP). Dr. Smith has participated in health care professions' interprofessional education initiatives, including a chronic disease health mentor program. She has assisted students in community activism and philanthropy as the nursing student government faculty advisor.

## ADDITIONAL RESOURCES

Ⓔ **Evolve Website http://evolve.elsevier.com/Stanhope**
- *Healthy People 2020*
- WebLinks
- Quiz

- Case Studies
- Glossary
- Answers to Practice Application

## OBJECTIVES

*After reading this chapter, the student should be able to do the following:*

1. Briefly discuss the historical development of the roles of the advanced public health nurse and the nurse practitioner.
2. Describe the educational requirements for population-focused advanced practice nurses.
3. Discuss certification/credentialing mechanisms in nursing as they relate to the role of the advanced practice nurse.
4. Compare and contrast the various role functions and practice arenas of population-focused advanced practice nurses.
5. Explore current issues and concerns related to practice.
6. Identify five stressors that may affect nurses in expanded roles.

## KEY TERMS

A special thanks to Molly Rose for the many contributions to this chapter in edition 8 of the text.

This chapter explores the roles of the advanced practice nurse in the community. Why, one might ask, is this chapter in the text? For a few good reasons, because it is the intent to provide the bachelor of science in nursing (BSN) student with an understanding of the career opportunities that may be chosen for continuing one's education to the graduate level. For the nurse in a graduate program, this chapter provides an in-depth understanding of the role in the specialty area that has been chosen. The advanced practice nurse roles described in this chapter offer excellent choices for exciting careers, which will ensure satisfaction that a major contribution can be made to making a difference in health outcomes and improved health status of clients at all levels.

The advanced practice nurse is a licensed professional nurse prepared at the master's level or doctoral level to take leadership roles in applying the nursing process and public health sciences to achieve specific health outcomes for the community; this nurse is often referred to as an advanced public health nurse (APHN). Because both the American Nurses Association (ANA, 2013) and the Association of Community Health Nursing Educators (ACHNE, 2007) refer to this specialized role as APHN, this is the title that is used in this chapter. On the other hand, the advanced practice nurse in the community may be a nurse practitioner (NP). A nurse practitioner is generally a nurse with a master's or doctoral degree, who autonomously and in collaboration with health care professionals and other individuals provides a range of primary, acute, and specialty health care services (American Association of Nurse Practitioners [AANP], 2014b). The APHN and NP often work in similar settings. However, their client focuses differ. The NP's client is an individual or family, usually in a fixed setting, who has the opportunity to identify individual trends in their practices. The APHN's clients may be individuals, families, groups at risk, or communities, but the ultimate goal is the health of the community as a whole (ANA, 2013; Swider et al, 2014). The APHN always has a population focus and obtains knowledge from nursing, social, and public health sciences to achieve goals of

| TABLE 39-1   How to Distinguish Similarities and Differences in Functions of Advanced Public Health Nurses and Nurse Practitioners | | |
|---|---|---|
| Function | NP Program | APHN Program |
| Comprehensive assessment | Always | Often |
| Physiology and pharmacology | Almost always | Often |
| Diagnosis and management | Always | Often |
| Systems | Individual/family focus | More systems focused |
| Leadership | Usually | Almost always |
| Program planning and evaluation | Less often | Always in community and public health |
| Research | Generally | Generally |

Association of Community Health Nursing Educators (ACHNE): *Graduate Education for Advanced Practice in Community/Public Health Nursing: at the Crossroads.* Latham, NY, 2007, ACHNE. American Nurses Association (ANA): *Public Health Nursing: Scope and Standards of Practice*, ed 2. Washington, DC, 2013, ANA.

promoting and protecting the health of populations by creating conditions in which people can optimize their health (ACHNE, 2007; ANA, 2013). Table 39-1 compares the functions taught to the APHN and the NP in their educational programs.

This chapter provides a history of the educational preparation of the advanced practice nurse. Functions in advanced practice and arenas for practice are discussed. Issues and concerns, role negotiation, and areas of role stress relative to the APHN and the NP in the community are also discussed.

## HISTORICAL PERSPECTIVE

Changes in the health care system and nursing have occurred in the past few decades because of a shift in societal demands and needs. Trends that have influenced the roles of the APHN and NP include a shift from institution-based health care to population-focused health care, improvements in technology, self-care, cost-containment measures, accountability to the client, third-party reimbursement, and demands for making technology-related care more responsive to the client. It is anticipated that the 2010 Patient Protection and Affordable Care Act will significantly impact health care delivery to the previously uninsured and cause a need for more health care professionals and their roles (Japsen, 2013).

The clinical nurse specialist (CNS) role began in the early 1960s and grew out of a need to improve client care. In addition to providing direct patient care, CNSs influence care outcomes by providing expert consultation for nursing staffs and by implementing improvements in health care delivery systems (National Association of Clinical Nurse Specialists, 2014). Concurrently in the 1960s, a shortage of physicians occurred, and there was an increasing tendency among physicians to specialize. The number of physicians who might have provided medical care to communities and families across the nation was reduced. As this trend continued, a serious gap in primary health care services developed. Primary health care includes both public health and primary care services.

The NP movement began in 1965 at the University of Colorado, led by Dr. Loretta Ford, a nurse, and Dr. Henry Silver, a pediatrician. They determined that the morbidity among medically deprived children could be decreased by educating nurses to provide well-child care to children of all ages. Nursing practice for these pediatric nurse practitioners included the identification, assessment, and management of common acute and chronic health problems, with appropriate referral of more complex problems to physicians (Silver et al, 1967). The priorities of the nursing profession have traditionally been to care for and support the well, the worried well, and the ill, offering physical care services previously provided only by physicians. Preparing nurses as primary health care providers was responsive to society's critical need for primary health care services, including health promotion and illness prevention (Institute of Medicine, 2011).

In 1965, the physician assistant (PA) role was initiated at Duke University. This program was intended to attract former military corpsmen for training as medical extenders. Nurse practitioners are often combined into a single category with other nonphysician providers and are mistakenly portrayed as physician extenders. This misinterpretation of the intended role is addressed by one of the founders, Dr. Loretta Ford:

> As conceptualized, the nurse practitioner was always intended to be a nursing model focused on the promotion of health in daily living, on growth and development of children in families, and on the prevention of disease and disability. Nursing as a discipline and a profession evolved not because there was a shortage of physicians but because of societal needs. The early plans did not include preparing nurses to assume medical functions. The interests were in health promotion and disease prevention for aggregate populations in community settings, including underserved

> groups. These were the hallmarks of community-oriented nursing (Ford, 1986).

A report issued by the U.S. Department of Health, Education, and Welfare (now the U.S. Department of Health and Human Services [USDHHS]), Extending the Scope of Nursing Practice (1971), helped convince Congress of the value of NPs as primary health care providers. The Nurse Training Act of 1971 (PL 92-158) and the comprehensive Health Manpower Act of 1971 (PL 92-157) provided education monies for many NP and PA programs through the 1970s and into the 1980s. Similarly, in the 1970s the concept of an expanded practice role for nurses was garnering interest in Canada. The United Kingdom has increased their advanced practice nurse programs to educate and monitor the role, which has been in place for about 20 years. Graduate education for nursing is changing. In 2007 the American Association of Colleges of Nursing (AACN) called for the creation of a new nursing role, clinical nurse leader (CNL) (AACN, 2014a). The clinical nurse leader is defined as a nurse who is a master's degree–prepared generalist who functions at the microsystem level and assumes accountability for health care outcomes for a specific group of clients within a unit or area (Commission on Nurse Certification, 2012; Foster et al, 2011). The AACN has determined that the preferred preparation for specialty advanced practice nurses should be the doctor of nursing practice (DNP) (AACN, 2014a). In 2013, there were 241 DNP programs in the United States. A task force is in progress to uncover barriers and facilitators for schools transitioning their master's level advanced practice programs to the DNP (Kirschling, 2014).

## COMPETENCIES

The Quad Council of Public Health Nursing Organizations, in 2003, developed a set of national public health competencies specific for public health nursing practice that are based on the Core Competencies for Public Health Professionals authored by the Council on Linkages between Academia and Public Health Practice. The core competencies were designed to serve as a starting point for academic and practice organizations to understand, assess, and meet training and workforce needs for health professionals practicing in public health; they were updated in 2011 (Quad Council, 2011). The Quad Council competencies are more specific to public health nursing and were developed to assist agencies that employ public health nurses, as well as academic settings that prepare public health nurses, to facilitate education, orientation, training, and lifelong learning (Quad Council, 2011) (see the Linking Content to Practice box). The ANA (2013) published Public Health Nursing: Scope and Standards of Practice, which includes population-focused standards of care in the following areas: assessment, population diagnosis and priorities, outcome identification, planning, implementation, evaluation, and standards for professional performance in ethics, education, evidence-based practice and research, quality of practice, communication, leadership, collaboration, professional practice evaluation, and resource utilization, environmental health, and advocacy. This document is based on a collaboration between the ANA and the American Public Health Association (APHA)-Public Health Nursing Section (2013) definition and role of public health nursing practice. The second edition includes competencies that appear at the end of each of the standards of practice for the advanced public health nurse. For example, under Standard 1: Assessment, additional competencies for the advanced practice nurse include the following: gathers data from multiple interdisciplinary sources as well as synthesizes qualitative and quantitative data during data analysis for a comprehensive population assessment (ANA, 2013).

### ⏩ LINKING CONTENT TO PRACTICE

In this chapter, emphasis is placed on the role of the advanced public health nurse (APHN) in the community. The Quad Council Public Health Nursing Competencies (Quad Council, 2011) were developed by four organizations (Association of Community Health Nursing Educators, Association of State and Territorial Directors of Nursing, American Public Health Association Public Health Nursing Section, and American Nurses Association Congress on Nursing Practice and Economics). The competencies are categorized into eight domains and are applied to three tiers of public health nursing practice:

- Tier 1: Generalist public health nurses who carry out day-to-day functions in state and local public health organizations, including clinical, home visiting, and population-based services and who are not in management positions
- Tier 2: Public health nurses with an array of program implementation, management, and/or supervisory responsibilities, including responsibility for clinical services, home visiting, and community-based and population-focused programs
- Tier 3: Public health nurses at an executive/senior management level and leadership levels in public health organizations.

The domains are core areas of analytic and assessment skills, policy development/program planning, communication, cultural competency, community dimensions of practice, public health science, financial planning and management, and leadership and systems thinking skills (Quad Council, 2011). The latter tiers include a higher level mastery of skills and competencies. As an example, their fifth domain, Community Dimensions of Practice Skills, lists a tier 1 competency as: identifies community partners for PHN practice with individuals, families, and groups; a tier 2 competency as: identifies need for community involvement and partners to create community groups/coalitions; and a tier 3 competency as: establishes organizational relationships, processes, and system improvements to enhance collaboration and cooperation among stakeholders in population-focused health policies (Quad Council, 2011). The tier 2 and tier 3 competencies/skills are clearly consistent with the APHN role and are at an advanced mastery level. This is in contrast to the generalist/staff public health nurse, where the expected level of performance mastery for this domain is more at the knowledge/identification level. Thus, if an agency planned to conduct health education programs within a community, the APHN would take leadership roles in developing, implementing, and evaluating a needs assessment and interacting with community stakeholders to assist with conducting the health education programs that would be most relevant and accessible to the community.

## EDUCATIONAL PREPARATION

Educational preparation for the APHN includes a minimum of a master's degree and is based on a synthesis of current knowledge and research in nursing, public health, and other scientific disciplines. In addition to performing the functions of the generalist in population-focused nursing, the specialist possesses clinical experience in interprofessional planning, organizing, community empowerment, delivering and evaluating service, political and legislative activities, and assuming a leadership role in interventions that have a positive effect on the health of the community. ACHNE recommendations for graduate nursing education for the public health nurse specialty are guided by the report *Who Will Keep the Public Healthy?* (Institute of Medicine, 2003), the ANA's *Public Health Nursing: Scope and Standards of Practice* (2013), and the AACN's *Essentials of Doctoral Education for Advanced Practice Nursing* (2006).

The ACHNE identified five role characteristics of APHNs: (1) population-level health care focus; (2) ecological view; (3) responsibility for health outcomes for populations; (4) partnership/collaboration, using an interprofessional approach; and (5) leadership in practice. The curriculum areas for the APHN that were identified are population-centered nursing theory and practice, interprofessional practice, leadership, systems thinking, biostatistics, epidemiology, environmental health sciences, health policy and management, social and behavioral sciences, public health informatics, genomics, health communication, cultural competence, community-based participatory research, global health, policy, and law, and public health ethics. In addition to didactic content, graduate education for the APHN must include practicum experience that takes place at the population level, be grounded in the ecological perspective, and include the measurement of outcomes (ACHNE, 2007).

In contrast to the APHN, educational preparation of the NP has not always been at the graduate level. Early NP programs were continuing education certificate programs, and the baccalaureate degree was not always a requirement. At present, however, NPs are required to hold master's degrees and encouraged to obtain a practice doctorate (AACN, 2014a). The curriculum prepares NPs to perform a wide range of professional nursing functions including assessing and diagnosing, conducting physical examinations, ordering laboratory and other diagnostic tests, developing and implementing treatment plans for some acute and chronic illnesses, prescribing medications, monitoring client status, educating and counseling clients, and consulting and collaborating with and referring to other providers (American Nurses Credentialing Center [ANCC], 2014).

A 2006 AACN position statement calls for DNP education for advanced practice nurses and nurses seeking top systems/organizational roles. The eight foundational essentials for DNP programs are knowledge with a scientific underpinning, organizational and systems leadership, clinical scholarship, information systems, policy, collaboration, prevention and population health, and advanced nursing practice (AACN, 2006). Future recommendations of doctoral programs in nursing continue to be reviewed and discussed (Kirschling, 2014). The Academic Partnerships to Improve Health (APIH) is a collaborative between the AACN and the Centers for Disease Control and Prevention to help build capacity in the public health nursing workforce. This program supports faculty development in the area of population health and connects nursing students with hands-on experiences at the community level to enhance their preparation for professional practice (AACN, 2014b).

## CREDENTIALING

Certification examinations for advanced practice nurses are offered by the American Nurses Credentialing Center (ANCC). The purpose of professional certification is to confirm knowledge and expertise and provide recognition of professional achievement in a defined area of nursing. Certification is a means of assuring the public that nurses who claim to be competent at an advanced level have had their credentials verified through examination (ANCC, 2014). Although certification itself is not mandatory, many state boards of nursing require that nurses in advanced practice, particularly those in an NP role, be nationally certified to practice.

The American Nurses Association (ANA) began its certification program in 1973 and has offered NP certification examinations since 1976. The ANCC was opened in 1991 and offers certification in NP, advanced practice, and CNS specialty areas. Until 2009 a nurse could also be certified as a generalist or as a BSN-prepared specialist in community health. Since 1985, the basic qualifications for certification as an NP have been a baccalaureate degree in nursing and successful completion of a formal NP program. As of 1992, a master's or higher degree in nursing is required for NP certification through the ANCC. NPs are required to maintain certification by renewing every 5 years.

A number of nurse practitioner certifications are available at the ANCC. The examination topics vary, based on the specialty area (ANCC, 2014). The American Association of Nurse Practitioners (AANP) also has national competency-based certification examinations in three areas: family, adult, and adult-gerontology primary care nurse practitioners (AANP, 2014a).

The certification examination for CNS in public/community health nursing was first offered in October 1990 and required a master's or higher degree in nursing with a specialization in community/public health nursing practice. Effective in 1998, eligibility requirements included holding a master's or higher degree in nursing with a specialization in community/public health nursing or holding a baccalaureate or higher degree in nursing and a master's degree in public health with a specialization in community/public health nursing. In 2009, the ANCC Commission changed the certification examination from clinical nurse specialist in public/community health to either advanced public health nursing or public health clinical nurse specialist. However, as of December 31, 2013, these examinations are no longer available. If one already holds these certifications through examination, they may be renewed with professional development and practice hours. Effective January 1, 2014, an advanced public health nurse–board certified (APHN-BC) credential can be obtained by the "certification through portfolio assessment" method (ANCC, 2014).

To complete the portfolio assessment, one must hold a current, active RN license in a state or territory of the United States, have the equivalent of at least 2 years of full-time practice as a registered nurse, possess a graduate degree (master's, postgraduate, or doctorate) in nursing or hold a graduate degree in public health and a bachelor's in nursing, have a minimum of 2000 practice hours in the specialty area of advanced public health nursing in the past 3 years, have completed 30 hours of continuing education in advanced public health nursing in the past 3 years, and fulfill two additional professional development categories (e.g., academic credits, presentations, publication or research, preceptor, or professional service) (ANCC, 2014).

## ADVANCED PRACTICE ROLES

APNs holding a master's degree in nursing or DNP and specializing in public health nursing, in community health nursing, or as a nurse practitioner have many roles, some of which are described here. It should be noted that the "nursing role in APPHN [advanced practice public health nursing] is not distinguished by the sites at which nurses practice, but rather by the perspective, knowledge base, and principles that focus on care of populations" (ACHNE, 2007, p. 16). The APHN's role characteristics include a focus on population health such as population and community assessment; advocacy and policy setting at the organizational, community, and state levels; ecological view for large-scale program planning and project management; and leadership and partnership building. APHNs deliver population-focused services, programs, and research (ACHNE, 2007; APHA, 2013).

### Clinician

Most of the differences between the roles of the APHN and the NP are seen in clinical practice. Although the APHN's practice includes nursing directed at individuals, families, and groups, the primary responsibility is to take a leadership role in the overall assessment, planning, development, coordination, and evaluation of innovative programs to meet identified community health needs. The APHN provides the direction for population-focused health care by identifying and documenting health needs and resources in a particular community and in collaborating with population-focused nurse generalists, other health professionals, and consumers (ACHNE, 2007; APHA, 2013). Practicing within the role of clinician, the APHN is involved in conducting community assessments; identifying needs of populations at risk; and planning, implementing, and evaluating population-focused programs to achieve health goals, including health promotion and disease prevention activities. The APHN ultimately works toward the goals of promoting and protecting the health of populations by creating conditions in which people can optimize their health (ANA, 2013; APHA, 2013).

The NP applies advanced practice nursing knowledge and physical, psychosocial, and environmental assessment skills to manage common health and illness problems of clients of all ages and both sexes. The NP's primary client is the individual and family. In the direct role of clinician, the NP assesses health risks and health and illness status, as well as the response to illness of individuals and families. The NP also diagnoses actual or potential health problems; decides on treatment plans jointly with clients; intervenes to promote health, to protect against disease, to treat illness, to manage chronic disease, and to limit disability; and evaluates with the client and other primary care team members about how effective and comprehensive the nursing intervention may be in providing continuity of care (AACN, 2011). Despite the setting of the practice nurse practitioner, the practice can be population focused. These interventions often include community assessment and analysis, case finding, an emphasis on prevention, and participation in public policy. An advanced practice nurse in the community may work in an agency or setting where the caseload consists of individuals who present themselves for services. The APHN goal would be to identify others in the community who may be at risk and in need of the services. Outreach activities can accomplish this while also trying to accomplish the goals and objectives of *Healthy People 2020* (Box 39-1).

The ability of NPs to diagnose and treat has increased the provision of health care, teaching, and client compliance with treatment plans. The amount of physician involvement in the NP's practice is generally directed through state legislation (AANP, 2014b). Frequently, the NP will use protocols or algorithms that have been previously agreed on by the physician and the NP. These documents, required by some states, serve as standing orders for the management of certain illnesses. As of 2010, all states have passed legislation, either partial or full, granting NPs supervisory, collaborative, or independent authority to practice. Each state has differing regulatory and legislative mandates regarding NP areas of practice authority, reimbursement, and prescriptive authority (Phillips, 2014). The most up-to-date information on state nurse practitioner practices and laws is through the American Association of Nurse Practitioners (AANP) website (http://www.aanp.org/).

An important area for both APHNs and NPs to include in their advanced practice is health promotion/disease prevention. Within the past several decades, there has been a growing belief that the most effective way of dealing with major health problems is through prevention. This requires refocusing the health care system, identifying aggregates (populations) at risk, introducing risk reduction interventions, teaching people that they

control their own health, and encouraging health promotion and disease prevention behaviors. The goals of the Patient Protection and Affordable Care Act (PPACA, 2010), such as improvement of the individual health care experience, reduction of the cost of health, and improvement of the health of populations, create the potential for new public health nursing roles and responsibilities. Public health nurses in the community (through their assessment skills, primary care focus, and system-level perspectives) are vital to the interprofessional teams needed to ensure that all people have equitable access to high-quality care and healthy environments through health system reform (APHA, 2013). The USDHHS (2014a) develops national objectives for promoting health and preventing disease. Since 1997, this initiative, called *Healthy People,* has set and monitored national health objectives to meet a broad range of health needs, encourage collaboration across sectors, guide individuals toward making informed health decisions, as well as measure the impact of prevention activities. This campaign is essential for APHNs and NPs working toward the goal of a healthier nation. Nurses and advanced practice nurses may also use *The Guide to Clinical Preventive Services* to address health promotion and disease prevention (USDHHS/AHRQ/USPSTF, 2014). NPs and APHNs are especially involved in helping to meet the proposed objectives in the access to health services, educational and community-based programs, and public health infrastructure domains.

### Population-Focused Intervention

The following example illustrates a population-focused intervention. An APHN was recently hired at a community hospital in the hospital's community health department. Traditionally, this department provided excellent health education and screening programs to individuals in the surrounding communities. However, outreach activities did not occur. After reviewing the data on attendance at community health events, the APHN developed and implemented a needs assessment in three neighboring communities not attending the events. In one neighborhood, consisting of 1800 apartments, 85% of the population was middle-income African Americans of all ages. The needs assessment revealed a strong interest in health promotion and disease prevention but nevertheless a lack of participation. The APHN developed a collaborative relationship with churches and community groups in the neighborhood. Health fairs and events were initiated (see the Levels of Prevention box).

### Educator

Nurses in advanced practice function in several indirect nursing care roles, including that of educator. The role of the APHN and NP includes health education within a nursing framework (as opposed to health educators, who may not have a nursing background) and professional nurse educator (faculty) roles.

The APHN identifies groups at risk within a community and implements, for example, health education interventions. The APHN and NP increase wellness and contribute to maintaining and promoting health by teaching the importance of good nutrition, physical exercise, stress management, and a healthy lifestyle. They provide education about disease processes and

---

**BOX 39-1** **Example of a *Healthy People 2020* Objective and Selected Advanced Practice Nursing Activities**

**Objective**
- Under Mental Health (objective MHMD-1): Reduce suicide rate to no more than 10.2 suicide deaths per 100,000 people.

**Activities**
- Review recent literature and epidemiology of suicide.
- Provide in-service education programs to groups of health professionals related to groups at risk for suicide and related assessment and screening tools for early detection and treatment of depression.
- Become active in legislation activities related to firearm access.
- Assess individual clients for depression and suicide risk.

U.S. Department of Health and Human Services (USDHHS): *Healthy People 2020.* Washington, DC, 2014a, U.S. Government Printing Office. Retrieved March 2015 from http://www.healthypeople.gov/

## LEVELS OF PREVENTION
### Population-Focused APHN Activities

**Primary Prevention**
- Flu immunizations at churches
- Classes on breast self-examination
- Education on the need for early detection of breast cancer

**Secondary Prevention**
- "Men's Night Out" event with screenings for blood pressure and cholesterol (at neighborhood sites)
- Health fair at neighborhood sites with screenings

**Tertiary Prevention**
- Identified need and follow-up at clinics for groups with chronic diseases (diabetes, cancer, hypertension)

the importance of following treatment regimens. In addition, they provide anticipatory guidance and educate clients on the use of medications, diet, birth control methods, and other therapeutic procedures (ACHNE, 2007; ANA, 2013; APHA, 2013). They also counsel clients, families, groups, and the community on the importance of assuming responsibility for their own health. This education may occur on an individual, family, or group level, in an institutional, ambulatory, or home setting, or it may occur in the community with vulnerable at-risk populations.

As professional nurse educators, the APHN and NP provide formal and informal teaching of staff nurses and undergraduate and graduate students in nursing and other disciplines (Figure 39-1). They also serve as role models by instructing (or being a preceptor to) students in advanced practice in the clinical setting.

## Administrator

The APHN and NP may function in administrative roles. As a health **administrator**, they may be responsible for all

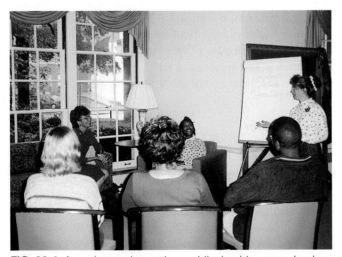

**FIG 39-1** An advanced practice public health nurse leads a training session for a group of congregational nurses.

administrative matters within an agency setting. They may be responsible for and have direct or indirect authority and supervision over the organization's staff and client care. In this capacity, nurses in advanced practice serve as decision-makers and problem solvers. They may also be involved in other business and management aspects such as supporting and managing personnel; budgeting; establishing quality control mechanisms; and program planning and influencing policies, public relations, and marketing (ACHNE, 2007; Drennan, 2012; Quad Council, 2011).

## Consultant

Consultation is an important part of practice for APHNs and NPs. The consultant problem-solves with an individual, family, or community to improve health care delivery. Steps of the consultation process include assessing the problem, determining the availability and feasibility of resources, proposing solutions, and assisting with implementing a solution, if appropriate (AACN, 2011; APHA, 2013). The APHN and NP may serve as a formal or informal **consultant** to other nurses, providing them with information on improving client care. They may also consult with physicians and other health care providers or with organizations or schools to improve the health care of clients. For example, nurse consultants are often used at the district or state level of public health departments. APHNs and NPs work closely with nurse supervisors, other nurse practitioners, and staff public health nurses to develop programs and improve the services provided to clients at clinics and in the home. Nurse consultants in the public health arena may work with all other public health nurses or may work in departments as members of an interprofessional team such as maternal–child health, chronic diseases, or family planning (University of Michigan Center of Excellence, 2013).

## Researcher

Improvement in nursing practice depends on the commitment of nurses to developing and refining knowledge through research. Practicing APHNs and NPs are in ideal positions to identify researchable nursing problems related to the communities they serve. They can apply their research findings to the community health practice setting.

All APHNs and most NPs are trained in the research process and, as **researchers**, can conduct their own investigations and collaborate with doctorate-prepared nurses, answering questions related to nursing practice and primary health care. The acts of identifying, defining, and investigating clinical nursing problems and reporting findings encourages peer relationships with other professions and contributes to health care policy and decision making (Harne-Britner and Schafer, 2009). For example, APHNs in administrative, consultant, or practitioner roles encounter situations daily that need further investigating (e.g., noncompliance with certain public health regimens or immunization schedules). They may, anecdotally or through needs assessments, identify a trend that, if examined, could be dealt with through population-based strategies (see the Evidence-Based Practice box). APHNs and NPs may collaborate with population-focused nurses at all levels to develop the research design, collect and analyze the data, and determine the implications for further use of nursing interventions identified. APHNs play a critical role in ensuring that evidence-based research is shared and integrated into health care practice (APHA, 2013; Harne-Britner and Schafer, 2009; Issel et al, 2011; Kulbok and Ervin, 2012).

---

## EVIDENCE-BASED PRACTICE

A retrospective cohort analysis of Latina clients (n = 680) served by public health nurses in an urban Midwest public health agency was conducted. The purpose was to evaluate outcomes of a public health nursing family home visiting program for Latina mothers with and without mental health problems. The program served at-risk Latina mothers by providing resources and support. The early intervention program provided foundational knowledge and skills development that encouraged healthy parenting practices and care for new babies. Researchers used the Problem Rating Scale for Outcomes to evaluate client progress, using a five-point, Likert-type scale that measured the dimensions of knowledge, behavior, and status based on problems identified and addressed by public health nurses. Comparisons were made between Latina mothers with documented mental health programs and mothers without. Of the 680 mothers, 158 had mental health problems and 522 did not. Mothers with mental health problem had more problems and received more visits than mothers without. However, across the length of service, mothers improved for all three outcome dimensions (knowledge, behavior, status) ($p < 0.001$). Findings demonstrated significant improvements over the course of the public health nurse home visiting intervention. Public health nurses provided valuable interventions and services that contributed to improving the health and outcomes of mothers and their children.

### Nurse Use

This study supports the need for targeting home visiting interventions to underserved groups such as Latina mothers. It also highlights the role of the advanced public health nurse in evaluating and assessing similar programs for effectiveness.

Garcia G, McNaughton D, Radosevich D, et al: Family home visiting outcomes for Latina mothers with and without mental health problems. *Public Health Nurs* 30:429–438, 2013.

---

## ARENAS FOR PRACTICE

Regardless of where public health nurses work (e.g., schools, homes, clinics, jails, shelters, or mobile vans), the core interventions to accomplish the goals of promoting and protecting the health of populations are similar across all practice arenas. Positions for NPs and APHNs vary greatly in terms of scope of practice, degree of responsibility, power and authority, working conditions, and innovation. These factors and the effects on practice are influenced by nurse practice acts and other legislation (e.g., reimbursement and prescriptive privileges) that govern the legal practice in each state (Phillips, 2014). The following areas include traditional as well as alternative practice settings for APHNs and NPs.

### Primary Care

Research indicates that the opportunities for APNs in primary care settings has increased, and this trend is expected to continue (APHA, 2013; Fairman et al, 2011). Primary care settings such as private practices, large health systems, community health centers, patient-centered medical homes, and others, provide various roles for the advanced practice nurse. For example, many practices employ NPs, physicians assistants, RNs, licensed practical nurses, pharmacists, behavioral health providers, community health workers, and physicians to provide care in a formal or informal team structure (Ladden et al, 2013). Evidence indicates that appropriately trained nurses in primary care can produce the same high-quality care and achieve equally positive health outcomes for clients as physicians. In general, preliminary research found no appreciable differences between physicians and nurses in health outcomes for clients, process of care, resource utilization, or cost (Laurant et al, 2005; Newhouse et al, 2011).

### Independent Practice

Nurses form an **independent practice** for several reasons, including a personal or professional desire to break new ground for nursing and to meet health care needs within a community. It is important to investigate the state's nurse practice act to determine the limitations and laws related to this arrangement. For example, NPs may provide a more comprehensive array of health services in states where they have legislative authority to prescribe drugs. Nurses in many states have successfully lobbied for third-party reimbursement for all RNs who provide direct care services to individual clients (Phillips, 2014). The independent practice option is more likely to be chosen by NPs and APHNs in states that have established legislation to provide for this nursing practice.

Another option for NPs and APHNs interested in independent practice is to contract with physicians or organizations to provide certain services for their clients or staff. Nurses need to define a service package and market it attractively. An example is providing a home visit to new parents after 2 weeks to assess the newborn, respond to parental concerns, and provide counseling and anticipatory guidance about nutrition, development, and immunization needs. This service may be marketed to pediatricians and family practice physicians who would offer or recommend the service to their clients as an option. An NP may negotiate with a local school board to provide preschool children with health examinations or physical assessments before the children participate in sports. Under a contract, APHNs may develop and implement health and safety programs on accident prevention and health promotion activities for small companies.

### Nursing Centers

**Nursing centers** or nurse-managed health clinics, a type of joint practice developed by advanced practice nurses to address vulnerable populations, provide opportunities for collaborative relationships for APHNs, NPs, baccalaureate-prepared nurses, other health care professionals, and community members (National Nursing Centers Consortium, 2014; Paterson et al, 2009). Primary health services may be provided by NPs, depending on state legislation. Community APHNs, along with nurses and nursing students, focus on the neighborhood level and understand community needs. A central mission of nurse-managed clinics is community development such as health care accessibility and resources; public involvement; interprofessional practice; and health promotion and disease prevention supported by the principles of primary health care (National Nursing Centers Consortium, 2014; Paterson et al, 2009). Nursing center models are discussed in more detail in Chapter 21.

## Retail Clinics

Retail clinics are staffed primarily by nurse practitioners with convenient hours. The first retail clinic opened in Minneapolis in 2000, but their growth between 2006 and the present has been substantial. They offer routine preventive and acute care services. Although still generally operated by large retail pharmacies, involvement of hospital systems in retail clinic ownership is a more recent phenomenon (Aiken, 2011; Kaissi and Charland, 2013).

## Faith Community Nursing/Parish Nursing

Faith community nursing, also known as parish nursing, is a concept that began in the late 1960s in the United States when increasing numbers of churches employed registered nurses to provide holistic, preventive health care to congregation members. Faith community nursing is a model of care that uses nurses based within faith communities such as churches and synagogues to provide health services to the members of those communities. Faith community nursing is a practice specialty that focuses on the intentional care of the spirit, promotion of an integrative model of health, and prevention and minimization of illness within the context of a faith community. Although primarily for faith community nurses and the nursing profession, it is also aimed at other health care providers, spiritual leaders, families, and members of faith communities (ANA, 2012).

Because these activities are complementary to the population-focused practice of APHNs, faith community nurses either have a strong public health background or work directly with both baccalaureate-prepared nurses and APHNs. Faith community nurses positively affect client outcomes by providing health services in health promotion and disease prevention, chronic disease management, and culturally sensitive services (Roberts, 2014). See Chapter 45 for further discussion about faith community/parish nursing.

## Institutional Settings
### Ambulatory/Outpatient Clinics

NPs and APHNs may be employed in the primary care unit of an institution (e.g., the ambulatory center or outpatient clinic). These centers/clinics generally provide hospital referral, hospital follow-up care, and health maintenance and management for nonemergency problems. The population served is usually more culturally and economically diverse and represents a larger geographic area than that served by private practices. In these outpatient settings, NPs typically practice jointly with physicians to provide acute and chronic primary care. Hospital acute care outpatient services may include clinics for general medicine or family practice, or specialty-oriented clinics, such as pediatric, obstetric-gynecologic, and ear, nose, and throat clinics. Outpatient clinics organized for chronic care may be problem oriented (e.g., hypertension, diabetes, or acquired immunodeficiency syndrome [AIDS] clinics).

## Emergency Departments

Persons without access to health care, such as the medically uninsured and the homeless, often do not seek health care services until they become ill. Hospital emergency departments (EDs) are increasingly used for nonemergency primary care. Although this is an inappropriate use of expensive health services, it is a result of the current system, which limits access to routine and preventive health care. Emergency department care is one of the most expensive services offered in health care today (Wood et al, 2010).

Emergency services often require long waits for persons who have nonemergency problems. Fast-track/nonemergency sections (sometimes called urgent care) of EDs have become commonplace to accommodate these situations. NPs in these settings see clients with nonemergency problems and provide the necessary treatment and appropriate counseling. APHNs may also help educate clients on the importance of health care and how to gain access to the preventive health care system. APHNs, with their knowledge of community health resources, can help ensure that psychosocial needs are assessed and met. APHNs can act as liaisons or go-betweens for community programs that serve the needs of special populations.

## Long-Term Care Facilities

The elderly age group represents the fastest growing population (especially those over 85 years of age) in the United States (Administration on Aging, 2012). The data reveal a long anticipated trend that we are living longer, resulting in higher percentages of elderly Americans. By 2030, it is projected that one in five people will be aged 65 or older. Statistics reveal a shortage of advanced practice nurses specializing in gerontological nursing to care for the growing older adult population (Donald et al, 2013).

Gerontology is an increasingly important field of study, and many courses are available on the health needs of older adults. NPs and APHNs with an interest in geriatrics need to continue their education in this area to increase their knowledge and skills specific to this at-risk aggregate (Donald et al, 2013). Many NPs and APHNs view long-term care facilities as exciting areas for practice and a way of increasing quality of care while containing costs for older adults and the disabled. U.S. federal legislation provides reimbursement for NPs and APHNs to provide care to clients in Medicare-certified nursing homes and to recertify eligible clients for continued Medicare coverage. In long-term care facilities where clients are not ambulatory, NPs and APHNs may make regular nursing home rounds, assess the health status of clients, and provide care and counseling as appropriate. In long-term care facilities in which the residents are more ambulatory, NPs and APHNs may also provide health maintenance and other primary health care services to the nursing home clients.

form, to the local Medicare insurance carrier agency for each visit or procedure.

## Institutional Privileges

Because of their direct care role, NPs in the community are more concerned than APHNs about institutional privileges. Traditionally it has been difficult for NPs to obtain hospital privileges within institutions where their clients are admitted. However, with the broadening scope of practice and professional responsibilities, more nurse practitioners are obtaining hospital privileges (often referred to as credentialing). An application process is generally required and reviewed by a group of physicians in the department of medicine. The criteria for nurse practitioners wishing to obtain hospital privileges vary by hospital and state; however, most hospitals require that nurse practitioners have national certification.

## Employment and Role Negotiation

For NPs and APHNs to collaboratively provide comprehensive primary health care, they must understand and develop negotiating skills. Positive working relationships with health professionals, organizations, and clients require role negotiation, particularly when few guidelines exist for a role or a role is new and undeveloped. NPs and APHNs need to assess the internal politics of the organization as part of their role negotiation. Networking is another necessary skill. Forums, joint conferences, collaborative practice, and research provide opportunities to expand their functions.

Because NPs and APHNs in some locations often seek employment, as opposed to being sought by employers, assertiveness is needed. Increased financial constraints have reduced the number of job opportunities. NPs and APHNs should feel comfortable about marketing their skills. Marketing strategies should be designed to project an image that shows a nurse's individual achievement. In assessing and analyzing the needs of target markets, nurses must consider professional and institutional goals, and the target client group's goals.

Methods of obtaining positions and negotiating future roles include providing portfolios of credentialed documents and samples of professional accomplishments such as audiovisual materials, program plans and evaluations conducted, client education packets, and history and physical assessment tools developed. Portfolios are folders that contain all of these documents to showcase the nurse's abilities. NPs and APHNs should keep current portfolios containing examples of their professional activities. Names, addresses, and telephone numbers of professional and personal references should be furnished in the portfolios (but only after the referring persons have granted permission). A new application that can assist in keeping portfolios current is an electronic portfolio, or e-portfolio, where information is housed on the Internet and can be easily updated and shared/transmitted to employers and others. Many websites provide e-portfolio management and services, such as Decision Critical website (www.healthstream.com).

## ROLE STRESS

Factors causing stress for advanced practice nurses include legal issues (as discussed previously), professional isolation, liability, collaborative practice, conflicting expectations, and professional responsibilities. NPs and APHNs will want to identify self-care strategies to cope with predictable stressors, some of which are discussed here.

## Professional Isolation

Professional isolation is a source of conflict for NPs and APHNs. Because they practice across all age groups, NPs and APHNs are likely to be hired in remote practice employment sites. Rural communities unable to support a physician, for example, may find the NP an affordable and logical alternative for primary care services. The autonomy of practice in these sites attracts many NPs and APHNs, who may fail to consider the disadvantages of isolated practice. Long drives, long hours, lack of social and cultural activities, and lack of opportunity for professional development are often experienced by these rural practitioners. These sources of stress, which could lead to job dissatisfaction, can be reduced or eliminated by negotiating the employment contract to include educational and personal leaves.

## Liability

All nurses are liable for their actions. Because more legal action is appearing in the judicial system, specifically concerning NPs, the importance of liability and/or malpractice insurance cannot be overemphasized (AANP, 2014b). Although malpractice insurance may not be required to function as an NP or an APHN, most nurses carry their own liability insurance. It is in the best interest of NPs and APHNs to thoroughly investigate the coverage offered by various companies rather than to assume that the coverage is adequate. Practitioners who function without a physician on site are particularly vulnerable. The scope of the NP's and APHN's authority determines the liability standards applied. The limits of each practitioner's authority are legislated by individual states (Phillips, 2014).

## Interprofessional Collaborative Practice

The future of NPs and APHNs depends on whether they make a recognized difference in the health of families and communities, and on their ability to practice collaboratively with physicians. Interprofessional collaborative practice defines a peer relationship with mutual trust and respect. Working out a collaborative practice takes a considerable amount of time and energy. Until such practice relationships evolve within joint practice situations, the quality health care that nursing and medicine can collaboratively provide will not be achieved. The arrangement demands the professional maturity to work together without territorial disputes, and the structure and philosophy of the organization must support joint practice as a mechanism for health care delivery. The growing pains of establishing such a practice produce stress for all involved; however, the results and benefits to clients and professionals are worth the effort (Interprofessional Education Collaborative Expert Panel, 2011).

Interprofessional collaborative practice for APHNs and NPs involves more disciplines than just medicine. Advanced practice nurses work with baccalaureate-prepared nurses and other nurses, social workers, public health professionals, nutritionists, occupational and physical therapists, and community leaders and members to meet their goals for the health of individuals, families, groups, and communities. To work toward the *Healthy People 2020* objectives, collaboration of multidisciplinary groups is essential. APHNs, NPs, and baccalaureate-prepared nurses can provide leadership in attaining this collaborative effort.

## Conflicting Expectations

Services provided by NPs and APHNs in health promotion and maintenance are often more time consuming and complex than just the management of clients' health problems. NPs and APHNs frequently experience conflict between their practice goals in health promotion and the need to see the number of clients required to maintain the clinic's financial goals. The problem becomes worse when the clinic administrator or physician views NPs and APHNs only as medical extenders and limits reimbursement to the nurse. A practice model that can assist nurses in including health promotion and maintenance activities as well as medical case management into each client visit uses (1) flexible scheduling, (2) health maintenance flow sheets, and (3) problem-oriented recording with nursing goals and plans prominently displayed in the health record. For APHNs, program planning and evaluation based on systematic needs assessments conducted with communities are methods to show the needs and benefits of health promotion/disease prevention. Being an educator and role model in carrying out *Healthy People 2020* objectives emphasizes the importance of health promotion and disease prevention in the health care system.

## Professional Responsibilities

Professional responsibilities contribute to role stress. Most states require NPs and APHNs in expanded roles to be nationally certified and to maintain certification. Recertification requires documentation of continuing education hours. Because there may not be many nurse practitioners in an area, continuing education may not be locally available and may require travel and lodging expenses in addition to time away from the practice site. Anticipating professional responsibilities and travel expenses in financial planning decreases these concerns. Negotiating with the employer for educational leave and expenses should be part of any contract.

Quality of client care, however, cannot be measured or ensured by continuing education or the nurse's credentials. Professional responsibility includes monitoring one's own practice according to standards established by the profession and protocols, if used, and a personal feeling of responsibility to the community. Continuous quality improvement is another professional responsibility for NPs and APHNs. This process should evaluate need, cost, and effectiveness of care in relation to client outcomes (Kelly et al, 2014).

## TRENDS IN ADVANCED PRACTICE NURSING

Advanced practice nurses are prominent in multiple health care arenas today, and this is unlikely to change in the future (Naylor and Kurtzman, 2010). With the goals of the Patient Protection and Affordable Care Act (PPACA, 2010) and *Healthy People 2020* objectives, a substantial need for health care providers exists. The prominence of interprofessional education and practice, along with team-based and patient-centered care, is congruent with the PPACA and *Healthy People 2020*. APHNs and NPs have the knowledge and skills base to lead the health care team in both individual- and population-based outcomes in prevention and population health.

APHNs and NPs, in collaboration with nurses, community agencies and members, and other disciplines, have the potential to make an impact on health promotion and disease prevention at the individual, family, group, and community levels. Population-focused APHNs and NPs are in excellent positions to use the *Healthy People 2020* National Health Promotion and Disease Prevention objectives and the Healthy People in Healthy Communities model in planning their advanced practice nursing interventions (Zanzano et al, 2011).

### (QSEN) FOCUS ON QUALITY AND SAFETY EDUCATION FOR NURSES

#### The Advanced Practice Nurse in the Community

**Targeted Competency: Informatics**—Use information and technology to communicate, manage knowledge, mitigate error, and support decision making.

Important aspects of informatics include:

- **Knowledge:** Describe examples of how technology and information management are related to the quality and safety of patient care
- **Skills:** Use information management tools to monitor outcomes of care processes
- **Attitudes:** Value nurses' involvement in design, selection, implementation, and evaluation of information technologies to support patient care

**Informatics Question**

You are an adult/geriatric NP who has just been hired at a nursing center, where that targeted patient population is patients over the age of 65, covered by Medicare insurance. Because your nursing center provides primary care for a substantial portion of your community's Medicare population, you have been approached by the local hospital and home care agency to help them track ER visits (not resulting in admission) and hospital readmission rates, within 30 days of a hospitalization.

- What data points will you want to track to establish a preintervention baseline for these data?
- Assuming you are involved in developing an educational module for at-risk patients, families, and home care nurses, what data points will you want to track after implementing this educational module?
- Which EHR (hospital, home care, nursing center) might contain these data points?
- How might you envision shared documentation/communication among the hospital, home care agency, and nursing center to effectively manage the targeted patients?

Prepared by Gail Armstrong, PhD(c), DNP, ACNS-BC, CNE, Associate Professor, University of Colorado Denver College of Nursing

Home health, palliative, and hospice nursing are rapidly expanding practice specialties. Assessment, planning, intervention, and evaluation are the focus of the services. For the purposes of this chapter, home health, palliative, and hospice nursing refer to a wide variety of holistic services typically provided to clients of all ages in their residences and other noninstitutional settings. Note that some agencies have agreements with work and school settings as well as residential and acute care facilities so that nurses provide services in locations in addition to homes. Mergers and collaborative agreements that cause practice boundaries to blur are increasing rapidly.

Numerous references in this chapter describe home health research, finances, and client personal preference, suggesting that the home is the optimal location for diverse health and nursing services (Buhler-Wilkerson, 2007; Beales and Edes, 2009; Hospice Association of America [HHA], 2010; Ferrante et al, 2010; National Association for Home Care and Hospice [NAHC], 2010; Sternberg et al, 2011; Moorman and Macdonald, 2013; Oguh et al, 2013; Nurse Family Partnership [NFP], 2014; Rockoff, 2014). Client residences include houses, apartments, trailers, boarding and care homes, hospice houses, assisted living facilities, shelters, and cars. Home health, palliative, and hospice services are provided by formal caregivers who include nurses, social workers, physical and occupational therapists, home health aides, chaplains, physicians, and others. Because of the nature of home health, palliative, and hospice

practice, a team approach and interprofessional collaboration are required. The specific disciplines involved vary with the program, the intensity of the client and family's needs, and the location of the program and home.

The Triple Aim model for health care was published in 2008 (Berwick, Nolan, & Whittingham, 2008). However, the primary concepts of the model have been the foundation and core values of home health and related community-based services from their inception: services that are client centered, that involve or engage the client and family, and are of high quality, efficient, and cost effective. The Triple Aim is a good strategy to encourage health promotion, prevention, and healthier lifestyles. However, all illness, including chronic illness, cannot be prevented or cured. As the population ages in this country and internationally, the need for home health, palliative, and hospice services is expected to continue and increase.

Access to other health care professionals, resources, and equipment is very different when home and institutional care settings are compared. Many nurses find home health, palliative, and hospice practice very rewarding because they observe the impact of their services and practice with a high degree of autonomy. Nurses who make home visits need to have good organizational, communication, critical thinking, and documentation skills. They need to understand ever-changing reimbursement regulations. Competence, integrity, adaptability, and creativity are essential characteristics. Home health nurses need the effort (Interprofessional Education Collaborative Expert Panel, 2011).

Interprofessional collaborative practice for APHNs and NPs involves more disciplines than just medicine. Advanced practice nurses work with baccalaureate-prepared nurses and other nurses, social workers, public health professionals, nutritionists, occupational and physical therapists, and community leaders and members to meet their goals for the health of individuals, families, groups, and communities. To work toward the *Healthy People 2020* objectives, collaboration of multidisciplinary groups is essential. APHNs, NPs, and baccalaureate-prepared nurses can provide leadership in attaining this collaborative effort.

## Conflicting Expectations

Services provided by NPs and APHNs in health promotion and maintenance are often more time consuming and complex than just the management of clients' health problems. NPs and APHNs frequently experience conflict between their practice goals in health promotion and the need to see the number of clients required to maintain the clinic's financial goals. The problem becomes worse when the clinic administrator or physician views NPs and APHNs only as medical extenders and limits reimbursement to the nurse. A practice model that can assist nurses in including health promotion and maintenance activities as well as medical case management into each client visit uses (1) flexible scheduling, (2) health maintenance flow sheets, and (3) problem-oriented recording with nursing goals and plans prominently displayed in the health record. For APHNs, program planning and evaluation based on systematic needs assessments conducted with communities are methods to show the needs and benefits of health promotion/disease prevention. Being an educator and role model in carrying out *Healthy People 2020* objectives emphasizes the importance of health promotion and disease prevention in the health care system.

## Professional Responsibilities

Professional responsibilities contribute to role stress. Most states require NPs and APHNs in expanded roles to be nationally certified and to maintain certification. Recertification requires documentation of continuing education hours. Because there may not be many nurse practitioners in an area, continuing education may not be locally available and may require travel and lodging expenses in addition to time away from the practice site. Anticipating professional responsibilities and travel expenses in financial planning decreases these concerns. Negotiating with the employer for educational leave and expenses should be part of any contract.

Quality of client care, however, cannot be measured or ensured by continuing education or the nurse's credentials. Professional responsibility includes monitoring one's own practice according to standards established by the profession and protocols, if used, and a personal feeling of responsibility to the community. Continuous quality improvement is another professional responsibility for NPs and APHNs. This process should evaluate need, cost, and effectiveness of care in relation to client outcomes (Kelly et al, 2014).

## TRENDS IN ADVANCED PRACTICE NURSING

Advanced practice nurses are prominent in multiple health care arenas today, and this is unlikely to change in the future (Naylor and Kurtzman, 2010). With the goals of the Patient Protection and Affordable Care Act (PPACA, 2010) and *Healthy People 2020* objectives, a substantial need for health care providers exists. The prominence of interprofessional education and practice, along with team-based and patient-centered care, is congruent with the PPACA and *Healthy People 2020*. APHNs and NPs have the knowledge and skills base to lead the health care team in both individual- and population-based outcomes in prevention and population health.

APHNs and NPs, in collaboration with nurses, community agencies and members, and other disciplines, have the potential to make an impact on health promotion and disease prevention at the individual, family, group, and community levels. Population-focused APHNs and NPs are in excellent positions to use the *Healthy People 2020* National Health Promotion and Disease Prevention objectives and the Healthy People in Healthy Communities model in planning their advanced practice nursing interventions (Zanzano et al, 2011).

---

**QSEN FOCUS ON QUALITY AND SAFETY EDUCATION FOR NURSES**

### The Advanced Practice Nurse in the Community

**Targeted Competency: Informatics**—Use information and technology to communicate, manage knowledge, mitigate error, and support decision making.

Important aspects of informatics include:

- **Knowledge:** Describe examples of how technology and information management are related to the quality and safety of patient care
- **Skills:** Use information management tools to monitor outcomes of care processes
- **Attitudes:** Value nurses' involvement in design, selection, implementation, and evaluation of information technologies to support patient care

**Informatics Question**

You are an adult/geriatric NP who has just been hired at a nursing center, where that targeted patient population is patients over the age of 65, covered by Medicare insurance. Because your nursing center provides primary care for a substantial portion of your community's Medicare population, you have been approached by the local hospital and home care agency to help them track ER visits (not resulting in admission) and hospital readmission rates, within 30 days of a hospitalization.

- What data points will you want to track to establish a preintervention baseline for these data?
- Assuming you are involved in developing an educational module for at-risk patients, families, and home care nurses, what data points will you want to track after implementing this educational module?
- Which EHR (hospital, home care, nursing center) might contain these data points?
- How might you envision shared documentation/communication among the hospital, home care agency, and nursing center to effectively manage the targeted patients?

Prepared by Gail Armstrong, PhD(c), DNP, ACNS-BC, CNE, Associate Professor, University of Colorado Denver College of Nursing

## PRACTICE APPLICATION

### Case 1: APHN

Martha Corley is an APHN who coordinates the after-care services for a community hospital's early discharge clients. Martha has worked with the nursing staff to develop a nursing history form to identify family and social supports available to clients who are likely to need nursing or supportive care for a limited time after discharge. With this and additional information from head nurses, Martha visits selected clients to begin discharge planning. She consults with each client and family to validate assessed needs. The physician is also consulted about medical therapies to be continued at home. Martha has access to nurses and other resources throughout the community that accept cases on contract. She outlines the initial care plan with nurse case managers assigned to the client and receives regular progress reports. An essential aspect of her practice is to evaluate outcomes of her interventions.

Which of the following is the best example of evaluation of Martha's nursing care?

A. Assessment of client and family satisfaction with her services
B. Reported medical complications of her caseload
C. Review of related literature about home care programs
D. Collected data on hospital readmissions of her clients

### Case 2: Family Nurse Practitioner

Julie Andrews is an NP who practices with two board-certified family practice physicians in an urban office. Julie has her own appointment schedule and sees 12 to 20 adults and children on an average day. Although she sees some acutely ill clients, most of her appointments are for routine health maintenance visits. The two physicians also refer clients to Julie for management of stable chronic health problems such as hypertension and diabetes. She has received a number of referrals from Martha Corley (see case 1) of clients with hypertension and diabetes. Assignment of these clients to Julie by the physicians did not begin until Julie had been with the practice for about a year. During the first months of practice, Julie assessed the numbers and types of client problems seen in a typical week. She found that hypertension was the most frequent chronic problem. Julie reviewed a sample of records of clients with hypertension and found that many had recorded blood pressures indicating uncontrolled hypertension.

On the basis of this information, what advanced practice nursing intervention could Julie provide?

A. Continue to see the clients referred to her through the physicians and Martha.
B. Conduct an in-service education program on hypertension for the staff in the office.
C. Provide nurse practitioner visits for hypertensive clients and compare the outcomes with those of hypertension clients seen by the physicians in the office.
D. Provide care for all hypertensive clients in the office.

**Answers can be found on the Evolve site.**

## KEY POINTS

- Changes in the health care system and nursing have occurred in the past few decades because of a shift in society's demands and needs.
- Trends such as a shift of health care from institution-based sites to the community, an increase in technology, self-care, cost-containment measures, accountability, third-party reimbursement, and demands for humanizing technical care have influenced the new roles of the APHN and NP.
- Educational preparation of the APHN has always been at the graduate level, whereas this has not been true of the NP; however, there are implications that both the NP and APHN educational preparation may be at the doctorate of nursing practice level.
- Specialty certification began through the ANA in 1976 for NPs, and through the ANCC in 1990 for APHNs.
- The major role functions of the NP and APHN in community health are clinician, consultant, administrator, researcher, and educator; typically, the NP spends a greater amount of time in direct care clinical activities and less time in indirect activities than the APHN.
- Major arenas for practice for NPs and APHNs in community health include primary care practice, institutional settings, industry, government, public health agencies, schools, home health, correctional health, nursing centers, retail clinics, and health ministry settings.
- Legal status, reimbursement, institutional privileges, and role negotiation are important issues and concerns to nurses who practice in an advanced role in public health nursing.
- Major stressors for NPs and APHNs include professional isolation, liability, collaborative practice, conflicting expectations, and professional responsibilities.
- The use of *Healthy People 2020* objectives is important in emphasizing health promotion and disease prevention in advanced practice nursing and in improving the health of the nation.

## CLINICAL DECISION-MAKING ACTIVITIES

1. Explore the development of the NP and APHN in the community. Give details about the differences in the roles.
2. Investigate graduate programs in public health in a state or region to determine the requirements for admission, the type of degree awarded, and whether or not NP and/or APHN preparation is available. Do the similarities and differences make sense to you? Why?

## CLINICAL DECISION-MAKING ACTIVITIES—cont'd

3. Review your state's nurse practice act and any rules and regulations governing advanced practice roles. Are rules different for NPs and APHNs? Give examples.

4. Negotiate a clinical observation experience with an NP and an APHN in community and public health, and compare and contrast their roles. Discuss the roles as you see them with the NP and APHN. When you consider your thoughts about the roles, have you considered what the APHN and NP have told you about their roles? How has their input changed your views?

## REFERENCES

Administration on Aging: *A Profile of Older Americans*: 2012. Retrieved March 2015 from: http://www.aoa.gov/Aging_Statistics/Profile/2012/docs/2012profile.pdf.

Aiken LH: Nurses for the future. *N Engl J Med* 364:196–198, 2011.

Almost J, Doran D, Ogilvie L, et al: Exploring worklife issues in correctional settings. *J Forensic Nurs* 9:3–13, 2013.

American Association of Colleges of Nursing (AACN): *The Essentials of Doctoral Education for Advanced Practice Nursing*. Washington, DC, 2006, AACN.

American Association of Colleges of Nursing (AACN): *The Essentials of Master's Education in Nursing*. Washington, DC, 2011, AACN.

American Association of Colleges of Nursing (AACN): *CNL and DNP Program Updates*, 2014a. Retrieved March 2015 from: http://www.aacn.nche.edu/.

American Association of Colleges of Nursing (AACN): *AACN and CDC Partner to Advance the Public Health Nursing Workforce*, 2014b. Retrieved March 2015 from: www.aacn.nche.edu/public-health-nursing.

American Association of Nurse Practitioners (AANP): *Certification*, 2014a. Retrieved March 2015 from: http://www.aanpcert.org/ptistore/control/certs/index.

American Association of Nurse Practitioners (AANP): *State Practice Environment*, 2014b. Retrieved March 2015 from: http://www.aanp.org/legislation-regulation/state-legislation-regulation/state-practice-environment.

American Nurses Association (ANA): *Faith Community Nursing: Scope and Standards of Practice*. Washington, DC, 2012, ANA.

American Nurses Association (ANA): *Public Health Nursing: Scope and Standards of Practice*, ed 2. Washington, DC, 2013, ANA.

American Nurses Credentialing Center (ANCC): *Advanced Practice Certification Information*. Washington, DC, 2014, ANA. Retrieved March 2015 from: www.nursecredentialing.org/publichealthadvportofolio.

American Public Health Association (APHA), Public Health Nursing Section: *The Definition and Practice of Public Health Nursing*. Washington, DC, 2013, APHA, Public Health Nursing Section.

Association of Community Health Nursing Educators (ACHNE): *Graduate Education for Advanced Practice in Community/Public Health Nursing: at the Crossroads*. Latham, NY, 2007, ACHNE.

Commission on Nurse Certification: *Clinical Nurse Leader Career Resource Guide*. Washington, DC, 2012, AACN. Retrieved March 2015 from: www.aacn.nche.edu/CNL.

Donald F, Martin-Misener R, Carter N, et al: A systematic review of the effectiveness of advanced practice nurses in long-term care. *J Adv Nurs* 69:2148–2161, 2013.

Drennan J: Master's in nursing degrees: an evaluation of management and leadership outcomes using a retrospective pre-test design. *J Nurs Manage* 20:102–112, 2012.

Fairman JA, Rowe JW, Hassmiller S, et al: Broadening the scope of nursing practice. *N Engl J Med* 364:193–196, 2011.

Ford LC: *Nurses, Nurse Practitioners: The Evolution of Primary Care* [book review]. *Image J Nurs Scholar* 18:177, 1986.

Foster J, Clark AP, Heye ML, et al: Differentiating the CNS and CNL roles. *Nurs Manage* 42:51–54, 2011.

Garcia G, McNaughton D, Radosevich D, et al: Family home visiting outcomes for Latina mothers with and without mental health problems. *Public Health Nurs* 30:429–438, 2013.

Harne-Britner S, Schafer D: Clinical nurse specialists driving research and practice through research roundtables. *Clin Nurse Spec* 23:305–308, 2009.

Institute of Medicine: *Who Will Keep the Public Health?* Washington, DC, 2003, National Academies Press.

Institute of Medicine: *The Future of Nursing: Leading Change, Advancing Health*. Washington, DC, 2011, National Academies Press.

Interprofessional Education Collaborative Expert Panel: *Core Competencies for Interprofessional Collaborative Practice: Report of an Expert Panel*. Washington, DC, 2011, Interprofessional Education Collaborative.

Issel LM, Bekemeier B, Baldwin KA: Three population-patient care outcome indicators for public health nursing: results of a consensus project. *Public Health Nurs* 28:24–34, 2011.

Japsen B: Doctor, nurse vacancies soar amid Obamacare rollout. *Forbes Magazine*, December 8, 2013. Retrieved March 2015 from: www.forbes.com/sites/brucejapsen.

Kaissi A, Charland T: The evolution of retail clinics in the United States, 2006-2012. *Health Care Manag (Frederick)* 32:336–342, 2013.

Kelly P, Vottero BA, Christie-McAuliffe C: *Introduction to Quality and Safety Education for Nurses: Core Competencies*. New York, 2014, Springer.

Kirschling JM: *Reflections on the future of doctoral programs in nursing*. Presented at the AACN Doctoral Education Conference, Naples, FL, January 30, 2014. Retrieved March 2015 from at: http://www.aacn.nche.edu/dnp/JK-2014-DNP.pdf.

Kulbok PA, Ervin NE: Nursing science and public health: contributions to the discipline of nursing. *Nurs Sci Q* 25:37–43, 2012.

Kvedar J, Coye MJ, Everett W: Connected health: a review of technologies and strategies to improve patient care with telemedicine and telehealth. *Health Aff (Millwood)* 33:194–199, 2014.

Ladden MD, Bodenheimer T, Fishman NW, et al: The emerging primary care workforce: preliminary observations from the primary care team: learning from Effective Ambulatory Practices Project. *Acad Med* 88:1830–1834, 2013.

Laurant M, Reeves D, Hermens R, et al: Substitution of doctors by nurses in primary care. *Cochrane Database Syst Rev* (18):CD001271, 2005.

Levin PF, Swider SM, Breakwell S, et al: Embracing a competency-based specialty curriculum for community-based nursing roles. *Public Health Nurs* 30:557–565, 2013.

National Association of Clinical Nurse Specialists: *History of Clinical Nurse Specialist*, 2014. Retrieved March 2015 from: www.nacns.org/html/cns-faqs.php.

National Nursing Centers Consortium: *NNCC: Keeping our nation healthy (home page)*, 2014. Retrieved March 2015 from: http://www.nncc.us/.

Naylor MD, Kurtzman ET: The role of nurse practitioners in reinventing primary care. *Health Aff (Millwood)* 29:893–899, 2010.

Nelson R: School nurses are needed more than ever. *Am J Nurs* 109:25–27, 2009.

Newhouse R, Stanik-Hutt J, White K, et al: Advanced practice nurse outcomes 1990-2008: a systematic review. *Nurs Econ* 29:230–250, 2011.

Paterson B, Duffett-Leger L, Cruttenden K: Contextual factors influencing the evolution of nurses' roles in a primary health care clinic. *Public Health Nurs* 26:421–429, 2009.

Patient Protection and Affordable Care Act, Public Law No. 111-148, Section 2702, 124 Stat 119, 318-319, 2010.

Pearson LJ: Annual update of how each state stands on legislative issues affecting advanced nursing practice. *Nurse Pract* 23:14–16, 19–20, 25–26, 1998.

Phillips S: 26th legislative update: progress for AORN authority to practice. *Nurs Pract* 39:29–52, 2014.

Public Health Accreditation Board: *Standards and Measures*, 2014. Retrieved March 2015 from: http://www.phaboard.org/wp-content/uploads/SM-Version-1.5-Board-adopted-FINAL-01-24-2014.docx.pdf.

Quad Council of Public Health Nursing Organizations: *Quad Council Public Health Nursing Competencies*, 2011. Retrieved March 2015 from: www.phf.org/resourcestools/Pages/Public_Health_Nursing_Competencies.aspx.

Riggs JS, Madigan EA, Fortinsky RH: Home health nursing visit intensity and heart failure patient outcomes. *Home Health Care Manag Pract* 23:412–420, 2011.

Roberts ST: Parish nursing: providing spiritual, physical, and emotional care in a small community parish. *Clin Nurs Studies* 2:118–122, 2014.

Silver HK, Ford LC, Stearly SA: A program to increase health care for children: the pediatric nurse practitioner program. *Pediatrics* 39:756, 1967.

Swider SM, Levin PF, Kulbok P: *Quad Council of Public Health Nursing Organizations Invitational Forum on the Role and Future of Nurses in Public Health: Final Report*, 2014. Retrieved March 2015 from: http://www.achne.org/files/Quad%20Council/PHNInvitational ConferenceReportFINAL03102014 .pdf.

University of Michigan Center of Excellence in Public Health Workforce Studies: *Enumeration and Characterization of the Public Health Nurse Workforce: Findings of the 2012 Public Health Workforce Surveys*. Ann Arbor, MI, 2013, University of Michigan.

U.S. Department of Defense/Today's Military: *Health Care Practitioners*, 2014. Retrieved March 2015 from: http://todaysmilitary.com/careers/career-fields/officer/health-care -practitioners.

U.S. Department of Health, Education, and Welfare: *Extending the Scope of Nursing Practice*. Washington, DC, 1971, U.S. Government Printing Office.

U.S. Department of Health and Human Services, Agency for Healthcare Research and Quality, U.S. Preventive Services Task Force (USDHHS/AHRQ/USPSTF): *The Guide to Clinical Preventive Services*, 2014. Retrieved May 2015 from: http://www.ahrq.gov/professionals/clinicians-providers/guidelines-recommendations/guide/cpsguide.pdf.

U.S. Department of Health and Human Services (USDHHS): *Healthy People 2020*. Washington, DC, 2014a, U.S. Government Printing Office. Retrieved March 2015 from: http://www.healthy people.gov/.

U.S. Department of Health and Human Services (USDHHS): *National Health Service Corps*, 2014b. Retrieved March 2015 from: http://nhsc.hrsa.gov/index .html.

Wasem C: The Rural Health Clinic Services Act: a sleeping giant of reimbursement. *J Am Acad Nurse Pract* 2:85–87, 1990.

Wood C, Wettlaufer J, Shaha SH, et al: Nurse practitioner roles in pediatric emergency departments: a national survey. *Pediatr Emerg Care* 26:406–407, 2010.

Zanzano T, Allan JD, Bigley MB, et al: The roles of health care professionals in implementing clinical prevention and population health. *Am J Prev Med* 40:261–267, 2011.

# 40

# The Nurse Leader in the Community

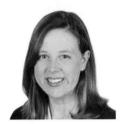

*Lisa Pedersen Turner, PhD, RN, PHCNS-BC**

Lisa Pedersen Turner felt called to the field of public and community health nursing while obtaining her BSN degree, inspired by the focus on preventing disease and helping underserved populations. Since then, she has provided care for a wide variety of vulnerable populations, including children in the schools, adults who are homeless, low-income families, and elders in long-term care facilities. She served as a nurse and clinic coordinator of the Good Samaritan Nursing Center at the University of Kentucky for twelve years. Her work at the Good Samaritan Nursing Center focused on providing school health services to underserved populations as well as developing a K-12 school health curriculum for a county in rural Kentucky. She has lectured and supervised students studying public health nursing in a myriad of community settings, including school clinics, homeless shelters, and free clinics for adults and children. She has contributed to several projects to evaluate school health services and has presented at national and international symposia on nursing clinics in the community. Her research interests are in the areas of vulnerable populations, access to health care, and obesity prevention. Dr. Turner currently serves as an assistant professor at Berea College, Berea, Kentucky.

## ADDITIONAL RESOURCES

**Evolve Website http://evolve.elsevier.com/Stanhope**
- *Healthy People 2020*
- WebLinks
- Quiz
- Case Studies

- Glossary
- Answers to Practice Application
- Resource Tools
  - Resource Tool 3.A: Declaration of Alma Ata

## OBJECTIVES

*After reading this chapter, the student should be able to do the following:*

1. Explain why nurses need effective leadership, management, and consultation skills in today's public health care environment.
2. Explore what is meant by partnership and interprofessional practice and describe how these concepts are related to nursing leadership, management, and consultation.
3. Analyze what is meant by systems thinking in community-based and public health settings.
4. Describe the major competencies required to be effective as a nurse leader, manager, and consultant in community-based and public health settings.
5. Examine nursing leadership strategies to enhance client safety and reduce health care errors in community settings.
6. Explain how nurses provide leadership in care coordination in the community.

## KEY TERMS

alliances, p. 875
budget, p. 880
business plan, p. 880
coaching, p. 878
coalitions, p. 875
collaborative, p. 869
complex adaptive systems, p. 872
conflict resolution, p. 879
consultation, p. 870
consultation contract, p. 873
contracting, p. 873
cost–effectiveness analysis, p. 881
delegation, p. 876

distribution effects, p. 871
empowerment, p. 875
external consultant, p. 872
internal consultant, p. 874
leadership, p. 870
learning organizations, p. 871
managed care organizations, p. 868
management, p. 870
microsystems, p. 872
negotiation, p. 873
partnerships, p. 868
political skills, p. 869
power dynamics, p. 879

*Dr. Turner would like to acknowledge the author of this chapter in edition 8 of the text, Dr. Juliann G. Sebastian, PhD, RN, FAAN, for her many contributions that will continue to appear in this chapter.

The profession of nursing has consistently ranked highly in public surveys as the most trusted profession (Jones, 2011). As such, the general public looks to nurses to act as leaders, providing guidance on health care choices. With more than 3 million nurses employed in the United States (American Nurses Association [ANA], 2011a), the nursing profession has the potential to greatly influence the health of the nation. It is therefore imperative that nurses understand how to be leaders, not only with their professional colleagues, but also within their communities. Leadership as a role for nurses began to emerge as the profession became more structured in the mid-1800s, moving from a loosely defined trade to an organized, educated profession (Smith, 2012). Florence Nightingale (1912), the founder of modern nursing, devoted a chapter in her book, *Notes on Nursing*, to what she called "petty management," defining the importance of a nurse being able to think critically, act proactively, and take charge of a situation in an efficient manner, all essential leadership skills. Since then, the concept of nursing leadership has evolved to include such qualities as developing relationships, facilitating communication between individuals and groups, providing guidance and direction, inspiring groups and organizations, and demonstrating vision (Huber, 2014). Agencies, localities, and professional organizations increasingly recognize the need for effective leadership in public health and community life.

Population-focused nurses have a responsibility to provide leadership in creating a new future for healthier communities. Members of the public ask whether better approaches to health care delivery might be developed that will ensure that all people around the world live in health-promoting communities and have access to quality health care as well as to health promotion and illness prevention services. Population-focused nurses practice in a variety of settings, including public health departments, community-based clinics, occupational health settings, schools, and managed care organizations. Leadership, management, and consulting skills are important to the success of client outcomes that depend heavily on cost-effective, efficient delivery of care. Care coordination and managing care transitions throughout the community, including acute and long-term care settings, are important to promoting a healthy community. Nurses need effective skills in communication, negotiation, and interprofessional practice and good leadership, management, and consultation skills, even if they do not have formal positions as managers or consultants.

Nurses must focus attention not only on the populations that are served by their organizations, but also on those that are not. Because they concern themselves with the total public, their focus is always on the future and on the interacting factors that influence the health of the public. Nurses work with partnerships of community members and community organizations. Partnerships can be complex and require time and thoughtful attention. This chapter examines the roles and functions of nurse leaders, managers, and consultants in the twenty-first century. It emphasizes nursing leadership in public health and community-based nursing practice, personnel management, and consultation with groups and individuals.

## MAJOR TRENDS AND ISSUES

Ensuring client safety and quality of care, performing evidence-based practice, eliminating disparities in health care access and outcomes, and focusing on consumer participation in and satisfaction with care are key trends in health care.

The Institute of Medicine report titled *To Err Is Human* (Kohn et al, 2000) focused attention on the incidence of health care errors. The issue of reducing health care errors continues to be a topic of interest for health leaders. In 2011, the Secretary of the U.S. Department of Health and Human Services

(USDHHS), Kathleen G. Sebelius, followed up on this report in a presentation describing new measures the USDHHS is implementing to improve patient safety, including monetary incentives for hospitals providing quality care and resources for providers to form accountable care organizations (National Research Council, 2011a). This is a concern in the community just as in hospitals and long-term care agencies. For example, studies in the United States (Lancaster, 2010), Europe (Gusdal et al, 2011; McCann et al, 2012), and Australia (Kalisch et al, 2012) show that older adults living in the community are at high risk for medication errors. Sometimes this is because they are taking high-risk medications (Gusdal et al, 2011; Kalisch et al, 2012), or because they cannot read instructions for medications (McCann et al, 2012), or because of medication complexity (polypharmacy) and not understanding how to take medications that have been prescribed for them (Kalisch et al, 2012; Lancaster, 2010).

Evidence-based practice is another trend important for public health nurses. Basing clinical practice patterns and community programs on research and other forms of evidence such as best practice data is a key strategy for ensuring high-quality care. One example of evidence-based practice in a community setting is a social media intervention developed by a group of community nurses aimed at educating 15- to 24-year-olds to reduce the incidence of risky sexual behaviors (Jones et al, 2012). In this program, the researchers evaluated the effectiveness of delivering education about the signs, symptoms, screening, treatment, and prevention of *Chlamydia* through a Facebook site. The researchers concluded that the use of social media sites may be an effective mechanism for delivering health information and promoting behavioral changes for adolescents and young adults.

The health system in some local areas has been reorganized to provide a full continuum of services in a seamless system of care. Large, vertically integrated systems are able to do this. Vertical integration means that the system owns all of the services that clients might need (e.g., clinics, hospitals, and home health agencies). In other cases, free-standing agencies collaborate and contract with one another to achieve seamlessness. The goal is to reduce fragmentation, which should be helpful for vulnerable populations. Nurses coordinate clients' care across agencies, but this new trend in the health care system places added emphasis on relationships, such as alliances, agency partnerships, joint programs, and participation in service delivery networks (Berry et al, 2013). Nurses actively participate in these groups and need good negotiating and political skills to be effective.

Another important trend is related to the movement toward more community partnerships (Plumb et al, 2012). Partnerships with community members and community agencies are essential to effective public and community health practice. The public has an increasing interest in becoming involved in planning for health services and in being active partners in their own care. Partnerships succeed when strong communication mechanisms are in place to ensure definition of needs and problems, timely problem resolution, and ongoing development of shared visions. In public and community health, the development of shared visions and goals and the operational mechanisms to make those goals a reality is the key to success. Nurses need to be able to listen well and collaborate with lay community members, whose goals and ideas may differ from those of health care professionals. For example, a successful community partnership was created between the public grade schools and two schools of nursing to explore the implementation of a school-based obesity prevention program (Tucker et al, 2011). The program sought input from school personnel, parents, students, and other relevant partners in order to tailor the intervention to the community. A win-win situation resulted where the school community benefited from having an obesity program implemented without extra demands on their faculty, and the nursing schools benefited by having a clinical learning opportunity for their students. Above all, the students enrolled in the intervention benefited by successfully learning healthy habits for life.

The public is increasingly using the Internet, a wide variety of publications, and lay support groups to obtain health information. People need help deciding which information is good and how best to work with their health care providers to adapt information to their own health profiles. Those with low health literacy (see Chapter 16) need special help in obtaining the health information necessary to be effective partners in health care (National Research Council, 2011b).

To know whether an agency is performing as expected, nurses must be familiar with their professional standards of care, the standards held by accrediting bodies, such as The Joint Commission, and guidelines for practice, such as those published by the federal Agency for Healthcare Research and Quality, the U.S. Clinical Preventive Services Task Force (2014), and the Task Force on Community Preventive Services (Centers for Disease Control and Prevention [CDC], 2013a). Nurse leaders also need to know how to use electronic health records and management information systems to link client outcomes with clinical and administrative processes. Registries are examples of clinical databases dedicated to certain population groups, such as people with cancer, diabetes, injuries, or population groups such as women. Nurses should know how to work with the taxonomies for nursing diagnoses, interventions, and outcomes of nursing actions (Bulechek et al, 2013) because these are being included in electronic health records and will help nurses identify changing health needs (Englebright et al, 2014).

One trend that combines the idea of partnerships with a structured method for rapid performance improvement is the use of collaboratives. A collaborative is a group of similar organizations that agree to use common processes for providing clinical care and share certain types of data so all may learn. A well-known example is the Health Care Disparities Collaboratives (HDCs) used by the Federal Bureau of Primary Health Care. The HDCs are a nationwide initiative to improve care for people with chronic conditions (Bureau of Primary Health Care, 2014). Community health centers may apply to participate in HDCs that target certain chronic health problems, such as diabetes or cardiovascular disease.

A major trend in public health is a stronger focus on implementing the core functions of public health and providing the essential services of public health (Council on Linkages between Academia and Public Health Practice, 2010). Competencies have been identified for generalist public/community health nurses that build on the core function and essential services (Education Committee of the Association of Community Health Nurse Educators, 2010).

---

### EVIDENCE-BASED PRACTICE

A systematic review of studies (Wong et al, 2013) examined the relationship between nursing leadership practices and patient outcomes. Twenty English-only research articles examining leadership practices of nurses in formal leadership roles and patient outcomes were included in the review. Leadership was defined as "the process through which an individual attempts to intentionally influence another individual or a group in order to accomplish a goal" (p. 710). The researchers further classified leadership into two styles, either relationally oriented (focusing on people and relationships) or task-oriented (focusing on structures and tasks). The findings suggest relationships between positive relational leadership styles and higher patient satisfaction and lower patient mortality, medication errors, restraint use, and hospital-acquired infections. Relational leadership styles were also positively and indirectly related to nurse's motivation to perform and improve work environments.

#### Nurse Use

The development of leadership skills among nurses may successfully improve a variety of patient and work outcomes. Relationally oriented leadership styles appear to be especially effective in the current health care environment, thereby reinforcing the importance of emotional intelligence competencies among nurse leaders. Studies should continue to be done to show evidence of the relationship between leadership and patient outcomes. Further research is also needed to evaluate the effectiveness of other leadership styles.

Wong CA, Cummings GG, Ducharme L: The relationship between nursing leadership and patient outcomes—a systematic review update. *J Nurs Manag* 21:709-724, 2013.

---

## DEFINITIONS

**Leadership** can be defined as the process of influence that occurs between a leader and an individual, group, organization, community, or society, often by inspiring, enlivening, and engaging others to participate in the achievement of goals (Kelly and Tazbir, 2013). Therefore, nursing leadership refers to the influence that nurses exert on improving client health, whether clients are individuals, families, groups, or entire communities. **Management**, on the other hand, refers to "the process of planning, organizing, coordinating, and controlling resources and staff to achieve organizational goals" (Kelly and Tazbir, 2013, p. 510). For nurses, these resources might be people, as when a nurse coordinates an interprofessional team, or financial resources. An example of managing financial resources is when a nurse monitors the budget for an immunization program to make sure that personnel time, supplies, and equipment are being used efficiently. Nurses also manage time. For example, home health nurses must manage their time in order to provide clients with direct and indirect nursing services, such as health education and making referrals, respectively.

It is important to point out that leadership and management are two different skills. Leadership sets the direction, and management ensures that goals will be achieved. Nurses must possess strong clinical leadership and management skills to be effective, whether or not they hold management positions.

**Consultation** in nursing refers to the process that occurs when a nurse works with an individual, group, organization, or community with the specific purpose of assisting them to solve actual or potential problems related to the health status of patients or to the health care organization (Wilson, 2008). Clinical consultation increasingly focuses on ways to better coordinate the care delivery process across sites of care. Population-focused nurses have a breadth of knowledge that makes them desirable consultants for colleagues both inside and outside the organizations in which they work. For example, a nurse working in a home health agency might be called on by a school nurse to give suggestions about the most effective way to intervene for a child using a respirator. Another example that occurs frequently is the informal consultation provided by nurses in the community, who help nurses working in hospitals make effective community referrals. At the population level, nurses who consult with a local health department about developing a program for obesity prevention in school-age children are focusing their efforts on a particular target population. An example would be the nurse leader of a community-based diabetes program who works with clinical colleagues in a hospital to improve the self-management education for people with diabetes.

Consultation is closely linked with the ideas of empowerment and self-management. When consultants help clients identify and work through problems and learn new skills that clients see as most important, they are enabling clients to solve more of their own problems. This is very similar to the traditional nursing philosophy of helping people to solve their own problems, whether they are individuals, families, groups, or communities. Empowerment is consistent with Jean Watson's theory of human caring (Watson, 2008), in which the nurse may advocate for the client but also may assist the client to advocate for themselves (Smith et al, 2013).

## LEADERSHIP AND MANAGEMENT APPLIED TO POPULATION-FOCUSED NURSING

### Goals

Nursing leaders work with others to ensure a healthy community. They serve as an advocate for vulnerable and high-risk populations and work toward achieving health equity, eliminating disparities, and improving the health of all groups. Nurse leaders also participate in establishing public and organizational policies and programs that promote a healthy living and working environment; and work with interprofessional teams to design ways to coordinate care across sites and over time, in order to evaluate and continually improve health care outcomes.

One way nurses lead is by participating in a *Healthy Communities Program* (CDC, 2013b) at the local level. Working with others to develop policies for smoke-free public spaces is an example of promoting healthy living and working environments. Another example is collaborating with consumers and professionals from other disciplines to evaluate root causes of medication errors in home-bound elders and design a process improvement strategy to reduce errors.

Nursing managers use a systems perspective to achieve agency and professional goals for client services and clinical outcomes. Managers help personnel perform their responsibilities effectively and efficiently; and they mentor other staff members, and foster lifelong learning. Furthermore, nurse managers develop new services that will enable the agency to respond to emerging community health needs, monitor health outcomes for particular population groups, and identify changes or variances suggesting new problems.

An example of how nurses show management abilities occurs when they develop plans for broad-based immunization clinics, such as smallpox vaccination clinics. Doing this in advance of confirmed bioterrorism is a way of preparing to meet an emerging community health need that achieves goals of protecting the public's health and helping personnel work effectively and efficiently. Table 40-1 shows examples of ways population-focused nurse leaders and managers facilitate primary, secondary, and tertiary preventive services.

## Theories of Leadership and Management

Leadership and management theories help explain individual and group behavior as well as organizational and system dynamics. Theories that help explain and predict individual behavior often focus on employee motivation and job satisfaction. Some theories address interpersonal issues such as leadership, communication, conflict resolution, and group dynamics. Working with consumers, staff members, and other health professionals in an adult daycare facility to design a memory improvement program for participants highlights the use of these theories. This type of project requires knowledge of motivation and

leadership, team work, change theory, and project planning, management, and evaluation. Organizational and systems theories explain issues at a broader agency or community level. These theories focus on the best ways to organize work, on how to obtain the resources necessary to accomplish agency goals, on organizational level change, on power dynamics, and understanding systems. Systems theories help explain the dynamics of rapid, interconnected change and the emergence of patterns of activity (Weberg, 2012).

Good leadership skills are essential for nurse leaders and are among the key competencies for generalist public/community health nurses recommended by the Quad Council of Public Health Nursing Organizations (2011) and for "entry level public health professionals" by the Council on Linkages between Academia and Public Health Nursing Practice (2010, p. 4).

The transformational leader is able to transform, or change, the situation to one that differs from the status quo (Luzinski, 2011). Transformational leaders are sometimes found in learning organizations, or agencies that create cultures that support ongoing learning, experimentation, and creation of new knowledge (Roussel, 2011). Transformational leadership is essential to promoting a culture of safety and positive work environments for others (Institute of Medicine [IOM], 2011).

Systems theories and systems thinking emphasize the interdependence of multiple parties. Nurses often recognize interdependence of units within an agency but may be less aware of agency interdependence. Economists analyze how distribution of resources affects policies, which players in a system will be influenced by policies, and how they will be influenced. These are called distribution effects. For example, if the federal government reduces money for health and social services, the clients of those services may be negatively affected. Employees of service agencies are also affected because agencies are likely to downsize to manage the reduced funding. Consequently, employees may either lose their jobs or experience wage cuts.

## TABLE 40-1  Examples of Levels of Prevention and Population-Focused Nursing Leadership and Management

| Levels of Prevention | Nursing Leadership (Sets Goals) | Nursing Management (Directs Use of Resources) |
|---|---|---|
| Primary (prevention of illnesses or problems before they begin) | Works with a community coalition to design a broad-based strategy for ensuring health and social needs of uninsured and underinsured populations are met. Works with nurses and interprofessional colleagues to develop goals related to preventing health care errors and ensuring client safety | Develops policies and procedures for a referral program for low-income mothers and children to obtain nutrition services. Ensures that individuals and families understand care routines to promote adherence and reduce chances of health care error |
| Secondary (screening for illness and treatment of health problems before they worsen) | Works with local government and health department to design lead screening and abatement programs in high-risk census tracts. Monitors data about a caseload of clients to determine whether patterns are developing that might indicate a health problem or issue needs to be resolved | Designs protocols for lead screening program and hires staff to implement program. Works with other members of care team to design protocols to improve specific health outcomes |
| Tertiary (treatment of health problems to foster stabilization or delay exacerbation) | Participates on a planning commission with local health department, hospitals, police, and political leaders to update a community-wide disaster response plan that accounts for bioterrorism. Collaborates with interprofessional teams to set goals for performance improvement and rapid changes in quality of care problems | Serves as chair of a committee that organizes, staffs, and monitors budget for a smallpox vaccination program. Monitors implementation of performance improvement activities to ensure timely and appropriate completion or revision as necessary |

Table developed by J. Sebastian (2010) for the 8th edition of *Public Health Nursing.*

Others likely to be affected include voluntary agencies and religious groups, which might be expected to provide more services.

Roy's adaptation model of nursing has been extended to include nursing management (Alligood, 2014). Roy argues that agencies are composed of interdependent systems. The role of nurse managers is to help the agency adapt to changing circumstances in the most effective way possible. Roy's model is particularly helpful for explaining and predicting how nurse managers and consultants can help agencies adapt to change. Nurse leaders should analyze how well interdependent units function to achieve agency goals. Furthermore, nurse leaders function as change agents because they foster agency adaptation. Complexity leadership theory accounts for the unpredictability of the behavior of people and organizations (Weberg, 2012). The combination of unpredictability and interdependence leads to disequilibrium and potentially to adaptation and growth. Communities exemplify complex adaptive systems. Nurse leaders must understand the analytical, political, and communication skills needed to work effectively in these systems.

Clinical microsystems are the systems, people, information, and behaviors that take place at the point of client care (Pardini-Kiely et al, 2010). Evidence-based clinical improvements can be implemented quickly in a clinical microsystem that has sufficient data about the practice, information systems that support clinical decision making, and a well-functioning team. For example, nurses working in a mobile health unit are part of a clinical microsystem. The team can make rapid changes in responses to quality problems if team members work well together and the mobile health clinic has an information system that makes it possible to track population health outcomes and clinical practice patterns.

Population-focused nurse leaders should assess the systems within which they work to evaluate risks to client safety. In the community these risks might be related to communication problems, inadequate follow-up, or lack of continuity of care. Nurses should maintain accountability for the outcomes of individuals, families, and groups and should do their best to ensure that complete care is provided across the continuum and that clients feel empowered to manage their own care.

### Nurse Leader and Manager Roles

First-line nurse managers may be team leaders or program directors (e.g., director of a satellite occupational health clinic or director of a small migrant health clinic), whereas mid- or executive-level nurse managers may be division directors (including multiple programs or departments), local or state commissioners of health, or directors of large home health agencies with multiple offices. They function as coaches, facilitators, role models, evaluators, advocates, visionaries, community health program planners, teachers, and supervisors. Population-focused nurse leaders have ongoing responsibilities for the health of clients, groups, and communities, as well as for personnel and fiscal resources under their supervision. Nurse

leaders may have positions as managers or they may be excellent clinicians and change agents who are seen as opinion leaders.

## CONSULTATION

### Goal

The goal of consultation is to help others empower themselves to take more responsibility, feel more secure, deal with their feelings and with others in interactions, and use flexible and creative problem-solving skills (Hamric et al, 2014). The functions of a consultant differ from those of a manager because consultation is typically a temporary and voluntary relationship between a professional helper and a client. The similarities between consultants and leaders are in the emphasis on empowerment and helping others develop. Consulting relationships are based on cooperation and respect between consultants and clients, who share equally in problem solving (Hamric et al, 2014).

The nurse's job responsibilities may include internal and external consultation. Internal consultants are members of the organization who work in a temporary capacity to help the client create or sustain change. For example, a nurse may be employed to consult with other nurses in the agency about client care problems or, as an employee of the health department, may serve as a consultant to a local community retirement center about the public health care needs of its residents. If the nurse is an internal consultant, the nurse is employed on a full-time salaried basis by a community agency in which the consultation takes place. If the nurse is an external consultant, the nurse is employed temporarily on a contractual basis by the client. The client of the external nurse consultant may be a colleague, another health provider, or a community group or agency. Consulting may occur informally when a staff nurse asks a colleague for advice or help in solving a problem. The nature of the consultation relationship, whether it is internal or external, should not change the goal of consultation.

### Theories of Consultation

Several models of consultation have been developed. Although nurses often consult with individuals about their own health care, or with another nurse or health professional about the needs of an individual client, this section emphasizes population-based consultation. At this level, the nurse focuses on the needs of a group, organization, or community. The client in this case is an organization or group. Content models emphasize the role of consultant as the expert who provides specific answers to problems or issues identified by the client. This approach has the advantage of being relatively quick and often responsive to client requests, but it does not help engage the client in problem solving and learning how to address similar issues in the future (Schein, 2011). This chapter focuses on Edgar Schein's model of process consultation because it is consistent with the nursing process and with nursing values of empowering clients and collaboratively working as partners with clients. The process model consultation focuses on the process of problem solving and collaboration between consultant and the client. The major goal of the process model is to help the client assess both the problem and the kind of help needed to solve it (Schein, 2011). Process consultation includes assessing the underlying agency culture that influences the problem and its solution (Schein, 2010). Both consultant and client participate in the problem-solving steps that lead to changes or to actions for problem solution.

Although consultants should emphasize process consultation, they should be willing to share their expert knowledge when appropriate. Because process consultation is collaborative, Schein (2011) recommends that consultants be willing to offer opinions and advice at all stages of the consultation process. Thus, although the major emphasis should be on process consultation, consultants may find it effective to integrate both context and process.

In the process model, the consultant is a resource person whose primary goal is to provide the client with choices for decision making. Process consultation includes the same steps as the nursing process: establishing a nurse–client relationship based on trust to assess the problem, planning and implementing actions, and evaluating the outcomes of nursing interventions. Nursing interventions may be described as direct client care or as consultation activities, depending on the goal of the intervention.

Consultation may occur before a problem occurs or after a problem exists. For example, a parent–teacher council developing a school-based family center contacts the nurse to assist with options for future nursing and health care for the students and their families. The board wishes to be proactive and plan for the needs of high-risk students and families. The administrator of a minimum-security prison has found that inmates are missing work for minor health problems and that health costs are skyrocketing. The nurse is asked to help explore solutions to the problem. Prison administration is reacting to an existing problem requiring immediate intervention.

The client is identified by determining who in the situation has the problem and needs to change. The following vignette illustrates this point:

Barry Henderson, RN, has been asked by the pastor of his congregation to consult with the parish council regarding the potential establishment of a health ministry. Barry decides that the consultation contract needs to include representatives of the parish council and parishioners themselves to find effective answers to the question. He realizes that time would be wasted and resistance to change would still be present if the focus were on only one group at a time. If he met separately with the parish council, they may decide such a program should include only one set of services. The parishioners either may want a different set of services or may desire to have services and programming organized in a very different manner. For example, the parish council may be especially interested in blood pressure screening, whereas the parishioners may be interested in wellness classes to keep the congregation healthy and in-home visiting for those who are ill. After spending much energy meeting with both groups separately, Barry believes that by being a messenger between the two groups rather than a facilitator for problem solving, the consultant role has been diluted. On the other hand, by meeting with both groups together, Barry could serve as a

resource, helping them explore all viewpoints and alternatives for developing the new program. In this case, both the parish council and the parishioners are Barry's clients.

## Consultation Contract

The consultation relationship is based on expectations. The consultant has expectations concerning time, money, resources, and the participation of the client in the process. Clients have expectations about what they will gain from the consultation relationship. Discussing the terms of a consultation contract makes expectations explicit, lessens the likelihood of violations of contract terms, and reduces the risk of additional demands being made on either party. Contracting involves identifying expectations and responsibilities by both parties. Some contracts are informal, verbal agreements between individuals, whereas others (such as the consulting contract) are formal, written agreements. Areas to include in the written consultation contract are as follows:

- Client and consultant goals
- The identified problem
- The time commitment
- Limitations of the contract
- Cost
- Conditions under which the contract may be broken or renegotiated
- Intervention strategies suggested
- Expected benefits for the client
- Methods of data collection to be used
- Potential interventions
- Evaluation methods to be used
- Confidentiality

Writing a contract for consultation relationships has a number of advantages. The contract terms assist the consultant in determining the number of hours that must be devoted to the interaction and in identifying needed resources and out-of-pocket expenses required to complete the interaction. Negotiation of the contract assists the client in identifying realistic expectations of the consultant and firmly establishes what the consultant will and will not do. The client has the opportunity during the negotiation to place limits on what the consultant can do, and the contract allows for future renegotiation of terms. Pricing methods for consultation services vary with the nature of the services. Consultants may price their services on the basis of the actual number of billable hours required to perform the service, or they may set a flat fee during the contract negotiation phase. Flat fees are more attractive to clients because they reduce uncertainty over the total cost of the consultation. They create an incentive for consultants to be efficient and to use an accurate method of estimating their services before the contract negotiation meeting.

The initial contact is made when the client or someone in a family, group, agency, or community communicates with the nurse about a potential problem that requires intervention. The communication may be a person-to-person contact during a home visit, may be written, or may occur by telephone. On initial contact, the client and the nurse have an exploratory meeting to define the problem, assess the nurse's interest and ability to help, and formulate future actions. If the nurse has little experience with the type of problem presented, the client may wish to seek assistance elsewhere. The nurse may also conclude that the situation is not within the nurse's expertise and will want to recommend someone else to work with the client.

Next, the terms of the relationship are discussed. The nurse consultant finds out what the client expects to gain from the relationship and develops terms for the interaction. Finally, in the initial exploratory meeting, the setting for the consultation is decided, the time schedule is set, the goals of the interaction are established, and the mode of intervention is chosen.

When the terms of the contract are agreed on, the data-gathering methods will be part of the agreement. Data-gathering methods used by consultants include direct observation, individual and group interviews, use of questionnaires or surveys, and tape recordings. While data are being gathered and after the diagnosis has been finalized, the nurse implements the intervention. After fulfilling the terms of the contract, the nurse must disengage or reduce the amount of involvement with the client. Decreased contacts allow each side to evaluate the effectiveness of the intervention. During disengagement, the nurse reassures the client that future interactions are possible at the client's discretion. When the agreed-on period of disengagement has passed, the relationship is terminated. The nurse typically provides the client with a written summary of the findings and recommendations resulting from the interactions during the disengagement and termination phases (Zuzelo, 2010).

An example of an internal consultative intervention follows:

*The director of nursing in a local health department telephoned the state public health nursing consultant for alcohol and other substance abuse prevention and requested a meeting at the local health department. The purpose of the meeting was to help staff analyze the evidence base and develop the protocols for a community-wide substance abuse prevention program they wished to provide. Several departments within the health department had been providing different aspects of substance abuse prevention but a coordinated effort was not in place. The nurse consultant, Paula, met with the client, Maggie, and reviewed her findings, sharing her analysis of the current situation and contributing factors. The central issue was defined as an organizational culture that did not promote interprofessional teamwork. This resulted in difficulties providing comprehensive and coordinated substance abuse prevention initiatives. Maggie then spoke with the other department directors to identify barriers and facilitators to interprofessional teamwork. Each director agreed to speak with staff in their departments to obtain their input on barriers and facilitators. One suggestion made by staff members was to hold an off-site retreat for team-based planning related to transitional care programs such as this one. Paula worked with Maggie to help develop suggestions for the agenda and logistics that Maggie shared with the other directors. The directors asked Paula to facilitate the retreat. After revision of the program plan during the retreat, Paula met with Maggie and the other directors to help them develop*

*additional strategies to foster an organizational culture that promoted interprofessional teamwork. She maintained contact with Maggie until the updated evidence base and program plan had been approved by the health department board and termination of the consultation occurred.*

---

**QSEN  FOCUS ON QUALITY AND SAFETY EDUCATION FOR NURSES**

**Targeted Competency: Teamwork and Collaboration**—Function effectively within nursing and interprofessional teams, fostering open communication, mutual respect, and shared decision-making to achieve quality patient care. Important aspects of teamwork and collaboration include the following:

- **Knowledge:** Describe own strengths, limitations, and values in functioning as a member of a team.
- **Skills:** Initiate plan for self-development as a team member.
- **Attitudes:** Acknowledge own potential to contribute to effective team functioning.

**Teamwork and Collaboration Question**

You have been selected to lead a task force aimed at reducing obesity rates in your community. Although you feel you are knowledgeable about obesity prevention and have several ideas for nursing interventions to reduce the obesity rate, you feel somewhat overwhelmed to be the person in charge of the task force. What can you do to feel more confident in your new leadership role?

**Answer**

First, reflect on what knowledge, values, and skills you bring to the task force that are strengths and identify areas that you feel less confident in. For example, you may feel you have a good understanding of obesity prevention but lack experience in team building and conflict resolution. Next, make a plan for how you can improve your weaknesses. For example, you could attend a continuing education workshop about team building or read the current literature on strategies for conflict resolution. Consider inviting people and organizations to join your taskforce who are proficient in the areas you feel weakest in. By reminding yourself of your strengths and actively working to improve your weaknesses, you are taking the steps to seeing your potential to being an effective leader on the task force.

---

## Nurse Consultant Role

An agency whose delivery of care is similar to that of an official public health service will most likely employ a nurse who provides traditional or nursing consultation for a broad range of community health activities (e.g., a community or public health nurse clinical specialist). A community health agency that provides a program approach to the delivery of community health services, such as family planning, maternity, child health, handicapped children's services, school health, or home health, will tend to employ specialist consultants. These consultants may have skills and training in specific clinical areas (e.g., a nurse with expertise in maternal and child health). Agencies providing primary health care require a consultant with both general knowledge of public health practice and specialized knowledge in a primary care clinical area. This is also a requirement in agencies involved in long-term and home health care.

The nurse consultant employed in an official public health agency functions as an internal consultant to the employing agency. As a representative of the agency, the nurse provides nursing and consultation to colleagues, other disciplines, agency administration, and other health and human service agencies and/or community groups. Two primary roles of the internal consultant are resource person and facilitator.

With knowledge of available resources, the nurse consultant can identify gaps in service, identify the critical services provided by the health care delivery system, and promote services for meeting health or social needs of the population. The consultant facilitates staff nurse problem solving about individual client and family needs, health needs of a group of clients, or professional concerns and attitudes. The consultant may assist managers and administrators in solving problems about personnel, program needs, organizational goals, community relationships, and client population needs. The consultant may also facilitate communication across agencies by working with interagency coalitions or alliances.

Consultants from federal agencies are often used as external nurse consultants. The nurse consultant from the federal agency may come to the local or state agency to serve on request as facilitator or resource person helping with program planning, development, and implementation. The primary role function of this consultant is to serve as a resource person, although the consultant may facilitate movement toward identifying actual program objectives.

An example of a vital role nurse consultants can play is in helping a community agency or a coalition conduct community needs assessments and develop strategic plans and associated action plans for achieving *Healthy People 2020* goals (see the *Healthy People 2020* box) (USDHHS, 2010).

 **HEALTHY PEOPLE 2020**

### *Objectives Related to the Four Overarching Goals*

The following are examples of some of the proposed objectives related to leadership, management, and consultation by public health nurses:

- AHS-2: (Developmental) Increase the proportion of persons with coverage of appropriate evidence-based clinical preventive services.
- HC/HIT-11: (Developmental) Increase the proportion of meaningful users of health information technology.
- PHI-1: Increase the proportion of federal, tribal, state, and local public health agencies that incorporate core competencies for public health professionals into job descriptions and performance evaluations.
- PHI-14: Increase the proportion of national and local public health jurisdictions that conduct a public health system assessment based on national performance standards.

*AHS,* Access to health services; *HC/HIT,* health communication/health information technology; *PHI,* public health infrastructure.
From U.S. Department of Health and Human Services: *Healthy People 2020,* Washington, DC, 2010. Available at http://www.healthypeople.gov/HP2020/Objectives/TopicAreas.aspx. Accessed September 2, 2010.

## COMPETENCIES FOR NURSE LEADERS

Nurses should watch for opportunities to participate in leadership development institutes or consider ongoing formal education through advanced public health nursing degree programs. Leadership development programs are available at various levels and are provided by civic and professional organizations. Civic programs introduce participants to the full range of leadership and quality-of-life issues in a community, including

health, education, politics, the arts, and business. This breadth of concerns is consistent with nurses' understanding that health results from the interaction of many facets of social and economic influences. Other leadership development opportunities are provided by professional organizations (e.g., the International Honor Society for Nursing, the American Public Health Association), continuing education, and local groups. Graduate degree programs in public health nursing provide systematic academic development of public and leadership competencies and prepare nurses to sit for advanced nursing certification through the American Nurses Credentialing Center, such as the Nurse Executive Certification. Nurses should take advantage of opportunities such as these for lifelong learning and the strengthening of leadership skills.

The following section describes essential competencies that nurses must master in order to become effective leaders in the community.

### Leadership Competencies

Nurses need effective leadership, interpersonal, political, organizational, fiscal, analytical, and information competencies. Some competencies are similar to those required for leadership in other clinical areas, such as good communication skills and the ability to delegate effectively. Working in the community means being able to work with populations and groups, to build coalitions and work with partnerships. Leadership essential to these roles involves identifying a shared vision and influencing others to achieve the vision, emphasizing that client needs are the basis for health services, empowering others, delegating tasks and managing time appropriately, and making decisions effectively. Public health nurse managers should be involved in developing agency-level vision, mission, and goal statements.

#### Empowerment

Leaders help others empower themselves to make organizations more responsive to client needs. This means removing barriers to decision making and allowing staff nurses the authority to make client decisions in "real time," as needs demand, rather than requiring nurses to obtain numerous approvals. Empowerment is more than simply increasing nurses' authority—it includes ensuring that they have the necessary knowledge, skills, and resources to effectively make the decisions for which they are held accountable. For example, nurse managers who are responsible for preparing their own department or program budgets and for approving program spending must be given the opportunity to learn budgetary concepts. Nurses are likely to feel more empowered to do their work in a less bureaucratic environment that supports clinical autonomy and collaborative professional relationships (Spence Laschinger et al, 2010).

The concept of empowerment underpins the consulting process. Consultants assist others in identifying solutions to problems and, more importantly, in developing the ability to manage problems independently in the future.

#### Delegation

Effective delegation is a key competency of public health nurses. The Education Committee of the Association of Community

Health Nurse Educators (2010) listed delegation among the competencies for community/public health nurses. This group noted that delegation is part of ensuring that care is appropriately coordinated within an interprofessional health care team. It has become increasingly necessary because of the complexity of care in public health and community settings (Resha, 2010).

Agency efficiency increases when tasks are assigned to the first level in the hierarchy where employees possess the necessary skills and knowledge to complete the task and where the task is related to the goals of those positions. Delegation develops others' talents and can contribute to job satisfaction. Asking a nurse in a nursing clinic for homeless families to develop a booklet describing community resources for this population

helps the staff nurse learn more about community resources, the gaps that exist in local resources, and where opportunities exist for interagency collaboration. The nurse is also likely to learn about visual presentation, layout and brochure design issues, and how to present material at the appropriate reading level. Finally, delegation is an important tool in time management. A school nurse may delegate locating resources for a screening clinic to the parent–teacher association, and the time saved can be spent on developing a teaching plan for volunteers who will help with the actual screening. Strategies for delegating responsibilities are listed in Box 40-1. Figure 40-1 provides a sample timetable for conducting a health fair, showing how the nurse might decide which activities need to be completed and suggesting those that might be delegated.

Delegation has become an increasingly important skill for nurses, whether they have official roles as managers or not. As more agencies increase their use of unlicensed assistive personnel and lay community workers, nurses are increasingly delegating selected aspects of practice to others and supervising the completion of those tasks. Two types of delegation occur in clinical practice. Direct delegation involves speaking to an individual personally and transferring responsibility for a task to that person (ANA and National Council of State Boards of Nursing [NCSBN], 2006). Indirect delegation results when an

### BOX 40-1 Delegating Responsibility

Nurse managers share responsibility for any tasks they delegate to others. The nurse manager delegates responsibility for a task but retains final accountability for the safe, effective outcome of the task (ANA, 2010). It is critical, then, that nurse managers know that the individuals to whom they are delegating responsibility are both prepared and capable of effectively performing the tasks. Nurse managers should provide clear guidelines and plan specific times to obtain progress reports on task completion. This will allow the opportunity to manage problems as they arise and to provide staff with helpful feedback or instruction if needed.

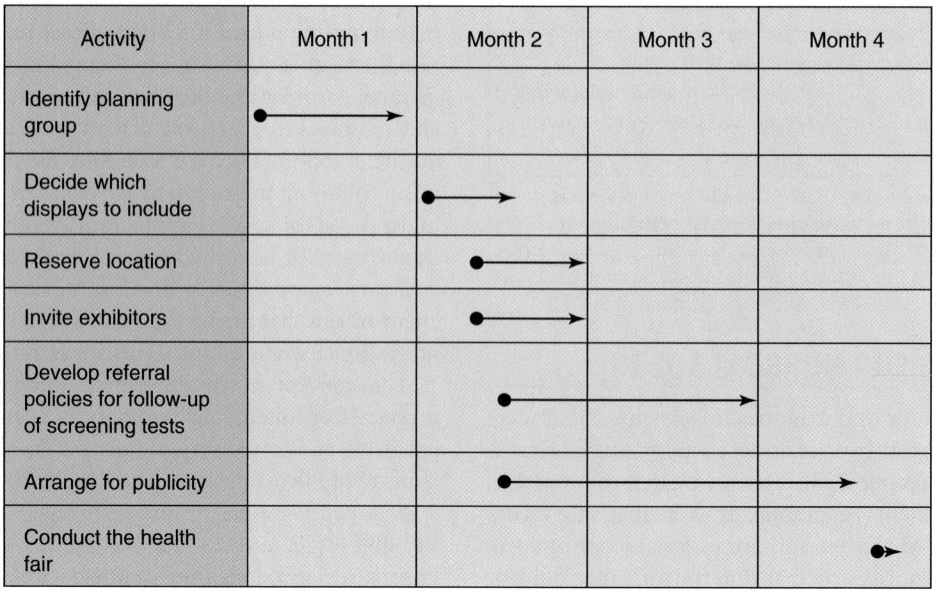

| Activity | Month 1 | Month 2 | Month 3 | Month 4 |
|---|---|---|---|---|
| Identify planning group | ●——→ | | | |
| Decide which displays to include | | ●——→ | | |
| Reserve location | | ●——→ | | |
| Invite exhibitors | | ●——→ | | |
| Develop referral policies for follow-up of screening tests | | ●————————→ | | |
| Arrange for publicity | | ●——————————→ | | |
| Conduct the health fair | | | | ●—→ |

FIG 40-1 Sample timetable for conducting a health fair.

agency has policies and procedures in place that allow tasks to be performed by someone other than the person who is accountable (ANA and NCSBN, 2006). Sometimes nurses mistakenly think that they are not accountable for tasks that are indirectly delegated through agency policies (e.g., policies for cross-training). However, if nursing care has been delegated, then nurses and their organizations are accountable for the safe and effective completion of that care (ANA and NCSBN, 2006). Organizations are responsible for ensuring that staffing is sufficient to allow for safe and appropriate delegation of care (ANA and NCSBN, 2006; Cipriano, 2010).

The first source of guidance for delegating tasks to unlicensed individuals is the state nurse practice act (ANA and NCSBN, 2006). The next source of assistance comes from specialty professional organizations. For example, the National Association of School Nurses and the ANA included care coordination, and working with parents, teachers, community members, and "adjunct personnel" (ANA, 2011b, p. 39) in the standards of professional performance for school nurses. Related responsibilities include ensuring optimal outcomes and quality of care.

To delegate effectively, public health nurses must understand the differences between responsibility, accountability, and authority (Weydt, 2010). The nurse may have the authority to delegate certain tasks to another individual or group. That individual or group accepts the responsibility to complete the task, but the nurse retains accountability to ensure the safety and quality of the outcome.

For example, a school nurse has the responsibility to assess a child with physical disabilities and develop a plan of care for that child. Selected aspects of that plan of care, such as assisting with feeding or emptying a catheter bag and recording output, could be delegated to an assistant, provided that person had received appropriate training and was competent to perform the task. This means that it is not adequate that the nurse know the individual has been certified as a nursing assistant; the nurse also needs to know that the individual is competent to safely perform the delegated task. It is important to ensure that those to whom certain tasks have been delegated have been trained to accept the responsibility and carry it out effectively. Public health nurses must also provide adequate time to plan the delegation process and to communicate with the person or group to whom a task is being delegated (ANA and NCSBN, 2006). Communication should occur throughout the process to allow for feedback and clarifications when needed. The nurse retains the legal accountability for safe client care. This responsibility may be shared with the person to whom one is delegating, but accountability is never transferred (ANA and NCSBN, 2006; ANA, 2010).

## Critical Thinking

Public health nursing leaders and consultants must be adept at critical thinking. Critical thinking includes analyzing and synthesizing data, using knowledge and values in making judgments, and using creative approaches in decision making and problem solving (Michelangelo, 2013). It includes reflection about the connections between sociocultural and biophysiological aspects of health status and services. Critical thinking may be fostered through the use of guided group discussions, in which group members are assisted to think about the connections just described and about the distribution effects that decisions may have on others. It is also fostered through activities to stimulate creativity, such as brainstorming. In the example of the occupational wellness program, the nurse manager would need to critically think about ways to increase program quality.

## Decision Making

Finally, a core leadership skill is the ability to make decisions effectively. Decision making and problem solving are critical aspects of nursing practice in complex clinical environments (Michelangelo, 2013). This is a two-stage process in which the nurse first must decide how much input to seek from others and second must generate alternatives for the decision and choose among the alternatives. Including others in the decision-making process is beneficial in part because others may have information and ideas that would lead to a better decision, and also because others may support the decision more if they are involved in making it. This also fosters team building and collaboration, which are two competencies for public health nurses (Quad Council of Public Health Nursing Organizations, 2011; Council on Linkages between Academia and Public Health Practice, 2010).

A decision tree can be used for selecting a leadership style that varies from a unilateral, independent decision process, to progressively more participative styles, with the most participative style involving delegating authority to a group that will be responsible for making the decision. Although many assume that autocratic decision making is not effective, in fact it may be both effective and efficient under certain circumstances, such as emergencies. In other situations, it is better to seek input from others, individually or as a group, to seek suggestions for solutions from the group, or to simply turn a problem over to a group to solve on their own.

The next stage of the decision-making process is to generate alternative solutions and to choose among those solutions. Both risk and cost are important dimensions in most situations. The goal involves low cost and low risk to clients and staff. Other dimensions might be unique to the situation. For example, if the nurse is trying to decide whether to develop an in-house wellness program for an occupational setting or to contract with a consulting group for that service, the nurse could compare the risks and benefits of both alternatives. The occupational health nurse might decide that the advantages of an in-house wellness program are that (1) it allows for staff participation in identifying key dimensions and goals and brainstorming creative solutions, (2) participants' values are built into the dimensions and goals, and (3) it allows for both creative and logical thinking processes.

## Interpersonal Competencies

Nurse leaders, managers, and consultants need effective interpersonal skills in communicating, motivating, appraising and coaching, contracting, supervising, team building, and promoting diversity.

## Communication

Good communication skills, including skills in the use of assertiveness techniques and conflict resolution (P. Kritek, quoted in IOM, 2010, p. 44) as well as communicating through the media and professional and scientific literature, are essential to being effective in leadership roles. Nurses have a particular challenge in communicating because many of those with whom they work may be in a different health profession or in a different field altogether. Nurses often communicate with lay workers or with the public through media outlets such as newspaper columns, television and radio interviews, blogs, and public service announcements. It is especially critical to listen carefully, to make underlying assumptions clear, and to speak in the other's language. This may mean avoiding the use of professional jargon and speaking in more commonly shared language or speaking in the listener's primary language. It is increasingly important for nurses to be bilingual or multilingual, depending on the ethnic composition of the community.

Communication must be culturally competent to be effective. Because communication involves words, tone of voice, posture, eye contact, and spatial relationships, cultural norms often influence the meanings given to different aspects of body language. For example, whereas most advise direct eye contact when communicating, in some cultures this may be viewed as aggressive, especially when the eye contact is prolonged. Some cultures prefer the closer-space relationships that may make others feel they are being crowded. Other aspects of communication are important as well, such as the appropriate place for reprimands. It is never appropriate to reprimand or criticize in public, although public praise is usually an excellent idea. Nurse managers and consultants should be sensitive to the power of written communication and be aware that, although putting a message in writing is a good way to avoid confusion, it also may be seen as aggressive, distrustful, or a bid for power. The key is to make certain that the message that is communicated is the message that was intended. Effective communication skills are listed in Box 40-2.

## Creating a Motivating Workplace

One of the more difficult skills to master is motivating other people; in fact, one cannot ever really motivate others, because motivation is internal. However, the skillful leader can create a motivating environment, working to make certain that both individual and agency goals are met to the extent possible.

---

**BOX 40-2    Effective Communication Skills**

- Listen actively.
- Restate the main points.
- Speak in the listener's language.
- Maintain culturally appropriate eye contact and body language.
- Provide an appropriate environment.
- Be aware of the power of written communication.
- Use simple, direct words.
- Use "I" statements and say how you feel.
- Provide frequent feedback.
- Reflect on the meaning of the message.

---

Sometimes individual motivation may be low because employees do not believe they have the skills necessary to achieve their goals, or they believe that the system will not allow them to do so. The effective nurse leader identifies which perceptions are inaccurate and helps individuals develop plans for improving their personal capacities for achieving goals. Although adequate salaries are important, compensation is not the only way to create a motivating environment for professionals. One home health aide supervisor is known for the high level of morale among her staff and the unusually low level of turnover. She makes a point of being available for discussion before the aides leave the agency in the morning and on their return in the afternoon. She always gives each person a birthday card, and thanks them for a job well done. For the long-term good, leaders should work with others in the community to increase salaries if they are not competitive.

## Appraisal and Coaching

Employee appraisal and coaching are closely related to motivation and individual development (Mackenzie, 2013). The purpose of performance evaluation is to assist employees to more effectively meet the objectives of their roles and to help them develop their potential in ways that facilitate achieving agency goals. Performance evaluation should not take place just before an annual appraisal interview is scheduled. It should be a regular part of the job, with the manager providing regular feedback on employee progress toward goals. Performance appraisal is particularly challenging for nurse managers because so many community health workers practice independently in the field. For example, nurse managers in home health must plan either to make visits with the nursing staff on a regular basis or to obtain other forms of input on employee performance, such as planning telephone or office conferences with staff.

Coaching involves working one-on-one with others to improve clinical care delivery (Kalkbrenner, 2012). With coaching, managers retain responsibility for decisions but request input and explain decisions. They support progress by helping the employee break the tasks into manageable parts, providing resources for accomplishing tasks and for acquiring the necessary skills, and praising task accomplishment. Coaching is most useful with people who may not yet be skillful in a particular area and who are not confident about their skills.

## Supervision

Nurse managers who delegate tasks to others must supervise the completion of those tasks and build in mechanisms to make certain that the tasks are completed safely and effectively (ANA, 2010; ANA and NCSBN, 2006). Supervision means decision making and implementation of activities in an ongoing relationship. It may occur either on site when the nurse manager is present and while the activity is being performed, or off site when the nurse is providing care in a community setting. It is important for nurse managers to build effective means of providing off-site supervision because so many community health activities do not take place within a single agency (e.g., home health care occurs in individual homes, and school health services are provided in individual schools).

Handling criticism is a difficult skill that involves both the giving and the taking of criticism related to job performance. Nurse managers should provide constructive critique as close as possible to the time they observe a problem with an employee's job performance. Constructive criticism focuses on the behaviors necessary to meet the job expectations and helps identify sources of problems, resources for managing problem behavior, and feedback. For example, if an employee is chronically tardy, the nurse manager should speak privately with the employee about the job expectation for promptness, identify why the employee is frequently tardy, establish a behavioral goal with time frames and consequences of achieving or not achieving the goal, and assist the employee to develop a plan for achieving the goal. The employee may be unaware of the importance of being punctual and can easily change the behavior. On the other hand, a behavior modification plan may be useful to help change the behavior. Behavioral consequences may include both positive reinforcers, such as praise, and disciplinary measures, such as oral and written warnings, limited raises, suspension, and termination. Suspension and termination are normally used only with problems related to safety, inability to perform job duties, breach of confidentiality, and illegal acts; they are detailed in agency policies and procedures.

### Team Building

Finally, team building and managing diversity are group-level skills needed by nurse leaders, managers, and consultants (Armitage and Hingham, 2011). Interprofessional teams increasingly are used to assess clients, plan client care or services, and manage quality improvement activities. Teams may include members of multiple health disciplines as, for example, with community health coalitions. They also may include people from other backgrounds, including lay community health workers. Nurse managers and consultants can facilitate team building by assisting the team to develop goals and ground rules, identifying who will fill various roles and determining how to share leadership, developing strategies for ongoing cooperation and recognition of contributions of each member, and resolving conflict.

### Promoting Diversity

A key challenge to nurse managers is promoting and managing diversity in positive ways that value different perspectives and provide insights into culturally competent strategies to eliminate disparities. By 2060, minorities are projected to comprise 57% of the U.S. population (U.S. Census Bureau, 2012). Nurse leaders must work with others to create workplaces that build on the strengths of a diverse workforce to provide excellent health care and eliminate disparities in outcomes. Nurses should partner with schools, faith communities, health care agencies, and universities to encourage minority group members who are interested in nursing careers. This will help build a community nursing workforce that better reflects the population as a whole (Loftus, 2010; Sullivan Commission, 2004). Nurse managers must understand cultural values and norms to communicate effectively and interpret behavior accurately. They must know how to prevent any form of racial, sexual, or ethnic harassment and ensure a positive and welcoming environment in the workplace.

### Power Dynamics and Conflict Resolution

Power imbalances can occur within groups, community organizations, and policy-making bodies, and affect health care professionals and community members. Managing power dynamics effectively requires that public health nurses understand community systems, collaboration, and strategies for providing information to empower others to work on their own behalf. Public health nurses work closely with community groups to build capacity for assessing strengths and needs, developing solutions to community health problems and promoting health and wellness, and managing long-term approaches for healthier communities. This is particularly important when working with vulnerable populations (Zandee et al, 2013).

Effective conflict resolution requires negotiation skills as well as skills in recognizing and managing power dynamics. Principled negotiation (Mafalo, 2012) emphasizes collaborative problem solving and development of mutually agreeable ways of achieving goals. Conflict resolution strategies can result in win–win, win–lose, or lose–lose outcomes. Strategies most likely to create win–win situations include collaborating, confronting problems directly, building consensus, and ensuring that all parties have an adequate opportunity for input (Mafalo, 2012).

Population-focused nurse leaders must understand power dynamics. Because nurses possess altruistic values, they may believe that being powerful is not necessary. However, it is impossible to create health-promoting public health services without some legitimacy in decision-making arenas. Membership on community agency boards and advisory committees puts nurse managers in the position to influence service delivery.

Consultants' advice may be followed because the client feels that the consultant possesses superior knowledge or skills and is trustworthy and credible. Internal nurse consultants may have power resulting from their roles in the organization. The client may not feel obligated to implement the recommendations of external consultants. On the other hand, external consultants may be viewed as influential because of an affiliation with other well-known consultants or a national organization. The consultant's ability to persuade clients by offering reasons, new techniques, or methods of problem solving may motivate clients to follow the consultant's advice.

### Organizational Competencies

Nurses use organizational skills, such as planning, organizing, implementing, and coordinating as well as monitoring, evaluating, and improving quality. Nurses use these skills when managing programs and projects and when coordinating care for individuals, families, and groups.

### Planning

Planning includes prioritizing daily activities to achieve goals. It also includes long-range planning, such as working with nurses in a department to plan a new program. Planning is a collaborative activity that can involve interprofessional teams, community groups, and policy makers. Developing a shared vision, goals, and measurable objectives provides the foundation for a plan. Nurses must be able to anticipate the cost of providing nursing services to a certain population over a period of time and to develop a proposal (or a **business plan**) for a contract to provide the services. Because planning is primarily a cognitive activity, nurse managers and consultants may tend to lessen its importance and allow little time for adequate planning. However, planning is the basis for direct nursing services and it is an essential competency for population-focused nurse care (ANA, 2013; Quad Council of Public Health Nursing Organizations, 2011), so it is important to make adequate time for planning.

Several documents are available to help nurse managers and consultants plan nursing services. *Healthy People 2020* (USDHHS, 2010) defines the national health goals for the United States by the year 2020 and should be the basis for program planning. The *Healthy Communities Program* (CDC, 2013b) describes strategies for working with community groups to achieve *Healthy People* goals at a local level. The Task Force on Community Preventive Services wrote *The Guide to Community Preventive Services* (CDC, 2013a) to provide evidence-based strategies for community health planning.

### Organizing

Organizing involves determining appropriate sequencing and timelines for the activities necessary to achieve goals and arranging for the appropriate people to carry out the plan. Flow sheets and timetables are helpful tools that allow nurse managers and consultants to visualize how tasks are organized and to identify gaps in the planning. Figure 40-1, as shown earlier, illustrates a timetable for conducting a health fair.

### Implementing and Coordinating

Implementing and coordinating a plan includes not only following the timelines, but also making certain that the relevant regulations and policies are adhered to, that activities are appropriately documented, and that the work of all team members is coordinated. One strategy that helps ensure coordination is use of an action plan (Mauksch and Safford, 2013). This is a table that includes the program goals and objectives, activities to meet the objectives, identification of those responsible for each activity, the timeframe for completing the activities, and the plan for evaluating achievement of the objectives. Team members should review the action plan at regular meetings and make changes as necessary. Action plans are also used to coordinate care for people with chronic illnesses such as obesity (see, e.g., Mullersdörf et al, 2010). Nurse managers and consultants should give sufficient attention to the change process by helping those involved identify the need for change, keeping them informed, soliciting their input, and making modifications in the plan as necessary.

### Monitoring, Evaluating, and Improving

Monitoring, evaluating, and making improvements are critical to nursing services. Nurses should monitor nursing services on a regular basis and make improvements as soon as the need for improvements becomes apparent. Professional standards and the standards of various accrediting bodies guide the focus of monitoring and evaluating. The Joint Commission standards for home health and ambulatory care clinics (http://www .jointcommission.org/) provide detailed and explicit minimal standards that all such agencies should be expected to meet.

In addition to professional standards of practice available from the ANA and specialty nursing organizations, the Agency for Healthcare Research and Quality has published clinical guidelines for prevention and treatment of selected health problems, such as wound care, pain, and tobacco cessation. Using evidence-based clinical guidelines is a key way to improve the quality of care. Finally, nurses should evaluate and monitor changes in client health outcomes. Effective outcomes management programs using information systems can be applied for ongoing planning and program improvements for target populations such as women and children (Monsen et al, 2010).

## Fiscal Competencies
### Forecasting Costs

Nurse leaders must be skilled in the area of fiscal management. Nurse managers and consultants must be able to project the cost of public health nursing services. This is especially important in today's tight economic environment because the forecast should include an assessment of the risk rating of the likely health and illness experiences of a target population. Combining community health assessment skills, epidemiologic projections, and consultation are key steps in this process and make it possible to design health programs to reduce health risks among various populations. After developing a profile of the anticipated health and illness experiences of a target population, the next step is anticipating the amount and kind of nursing resources needed by the population. These skills are basic to the development of proposals for new nursing services and contracts with external groups.

### Develop and Monitor Budgets

Nurse managers have taken on more responsibility for developing and monitoring their own department budgets as agencies have decentralized. They must be able to develop a justifiable **budget** and monitor how actual spending compares with planned spending. Expenses commonly included in an operating budget are salaries and benefits, equipment, supplies, travel, and overhead. It is helpful to obtain staff input when developing a budget in order to make financial projections as realistic as possible. Nurse managers should review program action plans with staff to determine the resources necessary to implement the program. Combining anticipated volume, revenues, and expenses allows the nurse manager to anticipate a breakeven point for new services (i.e., determining when a new program can be expected to be financially self-sufficient).

**Variance analysis** means identifying the difference between actual and planned results, determining the cause of the variation, and correcting problems when they exist. Spending more than anticipated is not always negative; it may simply indicate that client or service volume was higher than anticipated. This could, however, be of concern in an agency that is fully capitated and receives a set amount of money to see a client for usually a year, regardless of the cost of the services the client needs. Additional services do not bring in additional revenues.

Nurses in fully capitated environments have more opportunity than ever before to focus on health promotion and illness prevention services.

Higher expenses than planned are not always under the control of the nurse manager. For example, if the prevailing wage increases because of changes in the labor market, an agency may spend more than expected on salaries. On the other hand, spending less than predicted does not always indicate that a program is running efficiently; client volume may be down, or staff may not be providing adequate services. The most important thing for a public health nurse to do initially is to monitor expenses carefully and analyze why expenses might differ from the original plan.

For example, if a nurse manager observes that more has been spent on salaries and supplies than originally budgeted, and less on travel, should he or she think this is desirable or undesirable? To analyze the variance, the nurse should ask if the prices for labor and supplies were higher than expected or if the agency has used more nursing time or supplies than planned (Finkler et al, 2012; Talley et al, 2013). The answers to these questions will help determine whether the variance resulted from factors under the manager's control, such as inefficiency, or from factors outside of the manager's control, such as higher wages or higher prices than expected. The answers will also help determine whether the variance resulted from an increase in client volume or an alteration in case mix, with the agency serving sicker clients.

### Conduct Cost–Effectiveness Analysis

Regardless of the type of reimbursement system in place, nurses should be able to conduct a simple cost–effectiveness analysis of their interventions. Such analyses are not measurements of the efficiency of a program (see Chapter 25 for a discussion of this distinction) but are comparisons of the money spent for the outcomes across two or more interventions. Cost–effectiveness analyses compare alternative approaches for achieving the same goals. The nurse should measure the full costs and benefits (or savings) of each alternative intervention and construct ratios to compare the alternatives. The final result might be stated as the number of people who were able to achieve a desired health outcome (e.g., losing weight or adhering to an exercise program) for each additional dollar spent. The results of cost–effectiveness analyses sometimes raise new questions that must be analyzed. For example, in a study of the cost-effectiveness of varying levels of worksite wellness programs in rural employment sites (Saleh et al, 2010), investigators found that the lower intensity interventions of screening and general awareness were more cost-effective than higher intensity interventions. However, the higher intensity interventions yielded better health outcomes in many areas. What would you recommend to management in an occupational setting, based on these results?

### Analytical and Information Competencies

It is increasingly important for nurses to have excellent analytical competencies and competencies in the use of information. For example, access to useful and needed data helps nurses and other health professionals monitor clinical outcomes, identify systems issues that can result in health care errors, and plan to better meet the health needs of their populations. Population-focused nurses need a good understanding of descriptive and clinical epidemiology as well as the ability to analyze graphical data displays such as histograms, flowcharts, and line graphs. Use of aids such as checklists, reminders, and clinical decision support are all good ways to improve the quality of care and prevent errors (Pardini-Kiely et al, 2010). Because nurses are interested in identifying patterns of health problems, care delivery, and outcomes in community settings, more nurses are including nursing taxonomies (or languages) in electronic client records. Nursing leaders who participate in incorporating electronic records and information systems should have a conceptual framework to guide the project (Englebright et al, 2014).

## FUTURE OF NURSING LEADERSHIP

As noted at the beginning of this chapter, as the most trusted profession, nursing is in a position of influence. Using that power in a responsible and effective way is the task of the nurse leader.

With the passage and implementation of the Affordable Care Act of 2010 (ACA), nurses have the opportunity to take a pivotal leadership role in leading the nation in transforming the health care system (Wakefield, 2013). In 2013, Kathleen G. Sebelius, Secretary of the U.S. Department of Health and Human Services, expressed the vital role nurses can play in whether or not the ACA is successful, stating nurses are "at the heart of our healthcare system" (Nurse.com News, 2013). Nurse leaders are needed to provide education to individuals and communities about the ACA and assist them in navigating the health insurance marketplace. The ACA could impact nursing in a variety of ways, including the following: (1) increased nursing workforce needs, (2) an expansion of nursing roles outside of acute care, (3) a need for more nurse practitioners, (4) increased accountability for health care quality and value, and (5) opportunities for the development of innovative nursing care delivery models (Sherman, 2012). Nurse leaders are needed to address these potential influences and to develop innovative solutions to the challenges that arise.

In 2010, the IOM released its landmark report, *The Future of Nursing: Leading Change, Advancing Health*. In this report sponsored by the Robert Wood Johnson Foundation (RWJF), the committee described a vision of a transformed health care system in which quality care is accessible to the diverse populations of the United States, wellness and disease prevention are promoted, health outcomes improve, and compassionate care is provided across the life span (IOM, 2010). To achieve this health care system, the IOM (2010) recommends that the nursing workforce become prepared to "assume leadership positions across all levels" and suggests that nursing have representatives on boards, executive management teams, and in other key leadership positions. By working with policy makers, government leaders at all levels, and advocacy organizations, nurse leaders have the power to change the health care system to provide accessible, quality, evidence-based care to individuals and populations.

## PRACTICE APPLICATION

The nurse manager of a nursing clinic in a residential facility for frail older adults approached the local college of nursing for assistance with health promotion and health monitoring activities for the residents. The facility was undergoing renovation and was expected to more than triple its capacity by the time the renovation was completed. The nurse manager thought the health promotion activities that were already in place would be inadequate to serve the growing needs. Most of the residents were more than 70 years of age and had several chronic illnesses. The residential complex was 10 to 15 miles away from health care facilities.

Shirley, the nurse manager, supervised a staff of three nurses and one homemaker aide. She contracted with a local physical therapy firm for services as needed for the residents. Shirley had asked the staff if they thought they could realistically expand their services, and they suggested consultation. The staff commented that residents needed nurses who could provide health monitoring and skilled nursing services in their apartments, because so many were increasingly homebound. Staff members were hesitant about expanding into home care themselves because they feared it would mean a cutback in the health promotion activities they currently offered. They thought the needs, and the resources that would be required to meet the needs, should be evaluated before making any final decision.

What should the staff do to complete the evaluation of the problem?

A. Call a meeting of persons affected by the problem and decide on using an internal or external consultant to help evaluate the problem.

B. Write a contract and indicate how they want the evaluation to be done.

C. Develop a plan to implement home health services because the plan would include an analysis of needs and resources.

D. Continue with their health promotion activities and decide about home health services when more resources could be identified.

**Answers can be found on the Evolve site.**

## KEY POINTS

- Nurse leaders may function in formal roles as managers or consultants, or they may use managerial and consulting skills in their everyday clinical practice.
- Nurse leaders, managers, and consultants should work with organizations, coalitions, and community groups to design local strategies that will help achieve the *Healthy People 2020* goals.
- The goals of nursing leadership and management are (1) to achieve organization and professional goals for client services and clinical outcomes, (2) to empower personnel to perform their responsibilities effectively and efficiently, (3) to develop new services that will enable the organization to respond to emerging community health needs, and (4) to work with others for a healthy community.
- Systems thinking promotes sensitivity to the interdependence of parts of a system and the potential causes and consequences of organizational actions.
- Nurse managers may be team leaders or program directors, directors of home health agencies or community-based clinics, or commissioners of health. They function as visionaries, coaches, facilitators, role models, evaluators, advocates, community health and program planners, and teachers. They have ongoing responsibilities for clients, groups, and community health and for personnel and fiscal resources under their direction.
- The goal of consultation is to stimulate clients to take responsibility, feel more secure, deal constructively with their feelings and with others in interaction, and internalize skills of a flexible and creative nature.
- Consultation models can be categorized as content or process models. Process model consultation helps the client assess both the problem and the kind of help needed to solve the problem.
- Consultation involves seven basic phases: initial contact, definition of the relationship, selection of setting and approach, data collection and problem diagnosis, intervention, reduction of involvement and evaluation, and termination.
- Nurse consultants may function as internal consultants within an organization or external consultants outside the client organization.
- Nurse managers and consultants need a wide variety of competencies, including leadership, interpersonal, organizational, and political skills. Leadership skills include abilities to influence others to work toward achieving a vision, empower others, delegate tasks, manage time, and make decisions effectively.
- Interpersonal skills include communication, motivation, appraisal and coaching, contracting, team building, and diversity management skills.
- Organizational skills include planning, organizing, and implementing community nursing services; monitoring and evaluating services; quality improvement; and managing fiscal resources.
- Political skills are those used in negotiation and conflict management and managing power dynamics among health care teams and within the community.
- Population-focused nurses need analytical and informatics skills to be able to identify and monitor trends, improve health care safety, and evaluate outcomes.
- In general, both nurse managers and consultants must hold a minimum of a baccalaureate degree in nursing.

## KEY POINTS—cont'd

Organizations employing nurses without this credential should help them obtain additional education in the areas of community or nursing, management theories and principles, and theories and principles of consultation.

- By working with policy makers, government leaders at all levels, and advocacy organizations, nurse leaders have the power to change the health care system to provide accessible, quality, evidence-based care to individuals and populations.

## CLINICAL DECISION-MAKING ACTIVITIES

1. Discuss with your class members the implications that managed care and discounted fee-for-service preferred provider organizations have for nurse managers and consultants in community-based organizations and in the public health departments. What other implications can you think of in addition to those described in the text?
2. Draft a vision and mission statement for a nursing clinic with your classmates. Develop goals and objectives that follow the vision and mission you selected. What type of employees would you need to hire? List some of the policies and procedures you would need to have in such a clinic on the basis of your vision, mission goals, and objectives.
3. Have several class members obtain the vision, mission, and philosophy statements from agencies in which students have community health clinical experiences. Compare these statements in terms of the agencies' target populations, basic values, and essential functions.
4. Interview one or more practicing staff nurses working with populations. Ask them to describe the activities of their jobs that could be categorized as consultation. During the interview, attempt to determine the following:
   A. How they define consultation
   B. The goals they are attempting to achieve with their consulting activities

C. The model they seem to be applying in their consulting activities
D. The intervention strategies they use
E. Whether their activities are of a generalist or a specialist nature and of an internal or external consultative nature
F. The strengths and limitations they perceive in themselves regarding their consultative functions (e.g., education, experiential, organizational, relational, economic)

5. Interview one or more nurse consultants. During the interview, attempt to determine the answers to the preceding questions. Compare the responses of the two groups (public health nurse consultants and population-focused staff nurses). Analyze the factors you think account for the similarities and differences.
6. Visit a nurse-managed clinic for underserved populations. Talk with nurses and other staff members about how they work together as a team and what they do to promote client involvement in determining needed clinic services. Develop a case analysis of the microsystem within the clinic and how clinical care delivery is continuously monitored, evaluated, and improved within the system. What recommendations might you have for strengthening the clinical information system in the clinic?

# REFERENCES

Alligood MR: Nursing Theorists and Their Work, ed 8. St. Louis, 2014, Elsevier.

American Nurses Association (ANA): Scope and Standards for Nurse Administrators, ed 2. Silver Spring, MD, 2010, ANA.

American Nurses Association (ANA): Fact Sheet. Silver Spring, MD, 2011a, ANA. Retrieved March 2015 from: http://nursingworld.org/FunctionalMenuCategories/MediaResources/MediaBackgrounders/NursingbytheNumbers.pdf.

American Nurses Association (ANA): Scope and Standards of Professional School Nursing Practice, ed 2. Washington, DC, 2011b, American Nurses Association and the National Association of School Nurses.

American Nurses Association (ANA): Public Health Nursing: Scope and

Standards of Practice, ed 2. Silver Spring, MD, 2013. Nursesbooks.org.

American Nurses Association (ANA); National Council of State Boards of Nursing (NCSBN): Joint Statement on Delegation, 2006. Retrieved March 2015 from https://www.ncsbn.org/Delegation_joint_statement_NCSBN-ANA.pdf.

Armitage C, Hingham P: The productive ward: encouraging teambuilding and innovation. Nurs Manage (Lond) 18:28–31, 2011.

Berry LL, Rock BL, Smith Houskamp B, et al: Care coordination for patients with complex health profiles in inpatient and outpatient settings. Mayo Clin Proc 88:184–194, 2013.

Bulechek GM, Butcher HK, Dochterman JM, et al: Nursing Interventions Classification, ed 6. St. Louis, 2013, Mosby.

Bureau of Primary Health Care: Report to Congress: Efforts to Expand and Accelerate Health Center Program Quality Improvement. Washington, DC, 2014, U.S. Department of Health and Human Services. Retrieved March 2015 from: http://bphc.hrsa.gov/ftca/riskmanagement/healthcenterqualityimprovement.pdf.

Centers for Disease Control and Prevention (CDC): The Guide to Community Preventive Services: What Works to Promote Health? Atlanta, GA. 2013a, CDC.

Centers for Disease Control and Prevention (CDC): Healthy Communities Program. Atlanta, GA. 2013b, CDC. Retrieved March 2015 from: http://www.cdc.gov/nccdphp/dch/programs/healthycommunities program/.

Cipriano PF: Overview and summary: delegation dilemmas: standards

and skills for practice. Online J Issues Nurs 15(9):2010.

Council on Linkages between Academia and Public Health Practice: Core Competencies for Public Health Professionals. Atlanta, GA, 2010, Centers for Disease Control and Prevention, Health Resources and Services Administration, and the Public Health Foundation. Retrieved March 2015 from: http://www.phf.org/resourcestools/Pages/Core_Public_Health_Competencies.aspx.

Education Committee of the Association of Community Health Nurse Educators: Essentials of baccalaureate nursing education for entry-level community/public health nursing. Public Health Nurs 27:371–382, 2010.

Englebright J, Aldrich K, Taylor CR: Defining and incorporating basic nursing care actions into the electronic health record. *J Nurs Scholarsh* 46:50–57, 2014.

Finkler SA, Kovner CT, Jones C: *Financial Management for Nurse Managers and Executives*, ed 4. St. Louis, 2012, Saunders.

Gusdal AK, Beckman C, Wahlström R, et al: District nurses' use for an assessment tool in their daily work with elderly patients' medication management. *Scand J Public Health* 39:354–360, 2011.

Hamric AB, Hanson CM, Tracy MF, et al: *Advanced Practice Nursing: An Integrative Approach*, ed 5. St. Louis, 2014, Elsevier.

Huber D: *Leadership and Nursing Care Management*, ed 5. St. Louis, 2014, Elsevier.

Institute of Medicine (IOM): *A Summary of the February 2010 Forum on the Future of Nursing: Education*. Washington, DC, 2010, National Academies Press. Retrieved April 2015 from: http://www.iom.edu/Reports/2010/A-Summary-of-the-February-2010-Forum-on-the-Future-of-Nursing-Education.aspx.

Institute of Medicine (IOM): *The Future of Nursing: Leading Change, Advancing Health*. Washington, DC, 2011, National Academies Press. Retrieved March 2015 from: http://www.thefutureofnursing.org/IOM-Report.

Jones JM: *Record 65% Rate Honest, Ethics of Members of Congress Low: Rating of Nurses, Pharmacists, and Medical Doctors Most Positive*. 2011, Gallup Politics. Retrieved March 2015 from: http://www.gallup.com/poll/151460/Record-Rate-Honesty-Ethics-Members-Congress-Low.aspx.

Jones K, Baldwin KA, Lewis PR: The potential influence of a social media intervention on risky sexual behavior and *Chlamydia* incidence. *J Community Health Nurs* 29:106–120, 2012.

Kalisch LM, Caughey GE, Barratt JD, et al: Prevalence of preventable medication-related hospitalizations in Australia: an opportunity to reduce harm. *Int J Qual Health Care* 24:239–249, 2012.

Kalkbrenner AC: Coaching strategies for clinical learning: a strengths-based approach to student development. *Nurse Educ* 37:185–186, 2012.

Kelly P, Tazbir J: *Essentials of Nursing Leadership and Management*, ed 3. Clifton Park, NY, 2013, Cengage Learning.

Kohn L, Corrigan J, Donaldson M, editors: *To Err Is Human: Building a Safer Health System*. Washington, DC, 2000, National Academies Press.

Lancaster RJ: Factors that contribute to medication discrepancy errors and nurse time in community dwelling older adults [doctoral dissertation], 2010. Abstract available at http://search.proquest.com/docview/741708731; full text retrieved from CINAHL website.

Loftus J: Educating ethnic minority students for the nursing workforce: facilitators and barriers to success. *J Natl Black Nurses Assoc* 21:7–16, 2010.

Luzinski C: Transformational leadership. *J Nurs Adm* 41:501–502, 2011.

Mackenzie R: Supervision and appraisal: how to support staff performance. *Nurs Residential Care* 15:452–454, 2013.

Mafalo E: Conflict resolution. *Nurs Update* 37:44–45, 2012.

Mauksch L, Safford ML: Engaging patients in collaborative care plans. *Fam Pract Manag* 20:35–39, 2013.

McCann RM, Jackson AJ, Stevenson M, et al: Help needed in medication self-management for people with visual impairment: case-control study. *Br J Gen Pract* 62:e530–e537, 2012.

Michelangelo L: Emotional intelligence, emotional competency, and critical thinking skills in nursing and nursing education [doctoral dissertation], 2013. Full text retrieved from CINAHL website.

Monsen KA, Fulkerson JA, Lytton AB, et al: Comparing maternal child health problems and outcomes across public health nursing agencies. *Matern Child Health J* 14:412–421, 2010.

Mullersdörf M, Zuccato LM, Nimborg J, et al: Maintaining professional confidence—monitoring work with obese schoolchildren with support of an action plan. *Scand J Caring Sci* 24:131–138, 2010.

National Research Council: *The Richard and Hinda Rosenthal Lecture 2011: New Frontiers in Patient Safety*. Washington, DC, 2011a, National Academies Press. Retrieved March 2015 from: http://www.nap.edu/catalog/13217/the-richard-and-hinda-rosenthal-lecture-2011-new-frontiers-in.

National Research Council: *Promoting Health Literacy to Encourage Prevention and Wellness: Workshop Summary*. Washington, DC, 2011b, National Academies Press. Retrieved March 2015 from: http://www.nap.edu/catalog.php?record_id=13186.

Nightingale F: *Notes on Nursing*. 1859. Reprint, New York, 1912, D. Appleton and Company.

Nurse.com News: *Sebelius Lauds Nurses, Pledges Continued Support*. 2013. Retrieved March 2015 from: http://news.nurse.com/article/20130506/NATIONAL02/105130026/-1/frontpage#.U0uTwVVdXy8.

Olson LG: Public health leadership development: factors contributing to growth. *J Public Health Manag Pract* 19:341–347, 2013.

Pardini-Kiely K, Greenlee E, Hopkins J, et al: Improving and sustaining core measure performance through effective accountability of clinical microsystems in an academic medical center. *Jt Comm J Qual Patient Saf* 36:387–398, 2010.

Plumb J, Weinstein LC, Brawer R, et al: Community-based partnerships for improving chronic disease management. *Prim Care* 39:433–447, 2012.

Quad Council of Public Health Nursing Organizations: *Core Competencies for Public Health Nurses*. Clifton Park, NY, 2011, ASTDN.

Resha C: Delegation in the school setting: is it a safe practice? *Online J Issues Nurs* 15(2):2010.

Roussel LA: *Management and Leadership for Nurse Administrators*, ed 6. Sudbury, MA, 2011, Jones & Bartlett.

Saleh SS, Alameddine MS, Hill D, et al: The effectiveness and cost-effectiveness of a rural employer-based wellness program. *J Rural Health* 26:259–265, 2010.

Schein E: *Organizational Culture and Leadership*. San Francisco, 2010, John Wiley.

Schein E: *Helping: How to Offer, Give, and Receive Help*. San Francisco, 2011, Berrett-Koehler.

Sherman RO: *5 Ways the Affordable Care Act Could Change Nursing, 2012*. Retrieved March 2015 from http://www.emergingrnleader.com/5-ways-the-affordable-care-act-could-change-nursing/.

Smith MC, Turkel MC, Wolf ZR: *Caring in Nursing Classics—an Essential Resource*. New York, 2013, Springer.

Smith N: Nurses as leaders—the past, present and future of nursing leadership. *ArticleMyriad*, 2012. Retrieved March 2015 from http://www.articlemyriad.com/nurses-leaders-present-future-nursing-leadership/.

Spence Laschinger HK, Gilbert S, Smith LM, et al: Toward a comprehensive theory of nurse/patient empowerment: applying Kanter's empowerment theory to patient care. *J Nurs Manag* 18:4–13, 2010.

Sullivan Commission: *Missing Persons: Minorities in the Health Professions: a Report of The Sullivan Commission on Diversity in the Healthcare Workforce*.

Washington, DC, 2004, The Sullivan Commission.

Talley LB, Thorgrimson DH, Robinson NC: Financial literacy as an essential element in nursing management practice. *Nurs Econ* 31:77–82, 2013.

Tucker S, Lanningham-Foster L, Murphy J, et al: A school based community partnership for promoting health habits for life. *J Community Health* 36:414–422, 2011.

U.S. Census Bureau: *U.S. Census Bureau projections show a slower growing, older, more diverse nation a half century from now* [CB12-243], 2012. Retrieved March 2015 from http://www.census.gov/newsroom/releases/archives/population/cb12-243.html.

U.S. Clinical Preventive Services Task Force: *Guide to Clinical Preventive Services, 2014: Recommendations of the U.S. Preventive Services Task Force*. AHRQ Publication No. 14-05158. Rockville, MD, 2014, Agency for Healthcare Research and Quality. Retrieved May 2015 from: http://www.ahrq.gov/professionals/clinicians-providers/guidelines-recommendations/guide/cpsguide.pdf.

U.S. Department of Health and Human Services (USDHHS): *Healthy People 2020*. Washington, DC, 2010, Office of Disease Prevention and Health Promotion. Retrieved March 2015 from: http://www.healthypeople.gov/2020/default.aspx.

Wakefield M: Nurses and the Affordable Care Act: a call to lead. *Reflect Nurs Leadersh* 39(3):2013. Retrieved March 2015 from: http://www.reflectionsonnursingleadership.org/Pages/Vol39_3_Wakefield_Obamacare.aspx.

Watson J: *Nursing—the Philosophy and Science of Caring*. Boulder, CO, 2008, University Press of Colorado.

Weberg D: Complexity leadership: a healthcare imperative. *Nurs Forum* 47:268–277, 2012.

Weydt A: Developing delegation skills. *Online J Issues Nurs* 15(1):2010.

Wilson DW: Multiple relationships in nursing consultation. *Nurs Forum* 43:63–71, 2008.

Zandee GL, Bossenbroek D, Slager D, et al: Teams of community health workers and nursing students effect health promotion of underserved urban neighborhoods. *Public Health Nurs* 30:439–447, 2013.

Zuzelo PR: *The Clinical Nurse Specialist Handbook*. Sudbury, MA, 2010, Jones & Bartlett.

# The Nurse in Home Health, Palliative Care, and Hospice

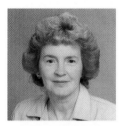

## Karen S. Martin, RN, MSN, FAAN

Karen S. Martin is a health care consultant who has been in private practice since 1993. She works with clinicians, managers, administrators, educators, researchers, and software developers nationally and internationally. Her focus is evaluation and improvement of practice, documentation, and information management systems to meet quality, data exchange, and interoperability standards for electronic health records. Karen has been employed as a staff nurse, director of a combined home care/public health agency, and, from 1978 to 1993, the Director of Research of the Visiting Nurse Association of Omaha, Nebraska, where she was the principal investigator of Omaha System research.

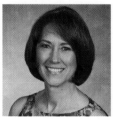

## Kathryn H. Bowles, RN, PhD, FAAN

Kathryn H. Bowles is the van Ameringen Professor of Nursing Excellence at the University of Pennsylvania School of Nursing and the Director of the Center for Integrative Science in Aging. For several years, Dr. Bowles was the Director of Nursing Research at the Visiting Nurse Association of Greater Philadelphia and is currently the Beatrice Renfield Visiting Scholar at the Visiting Nurse Service of New York, with a focus on bringing evidence-based practice to home care. Her program of research focuses on improving the care of adults using information technology such as decision support for hospital discharge planning and referral decision making, as well as testing telehealth technologies in community-based settings.

## ADDITIONAL RESOURCES

Ⓔ **Evolve website http://evolve.elsevier.com/Stanhope**
- *Healthy People 2020*
- WebLinks
- Quiz
- Case Studies

- Glossary
- Answers to Practice Application
- Resource Tools
  - Resource Tool 41.A: The Living Will Directive
  - Resource Tool 41.B OASIS-C: Start of Care Assessment

## OBJECTIVES

*After reading this chapter, the student should be able to do the following:*

1. Compare different practice models for home and community-based services.
2. Summarize the basic roles and responsibilities of home health, palliative, and hospice nurses.
3. Explain the professional standards and educational requirements for nurses in home health, palliative care, and hospice.
4. Describe the three components of the Omaha System.
5. Analyze how nurses in home health, palliative care, and hospice use best practices, evidence-based practice, and quality improvement strategies to improve the care they provide.
6. Cite examples of trends and opportunities in home health, palliative care, and hospice involving technology, informatics, and telehealth.

## KEY TERMS

accreditation, p. 901
benchmarking, p. 901
client engagement, p. 895
client outcomes, p. 896
documentation, p. 894
electronic health record (EHR), p. 894
evidence-based practice, p. 889
family caregiver, p. 887
home health care, p. 887

home health nursing, p. 887
hospice and palliative care, p. 887
hospice care, p. 888
information management, p. 894
interoperability, p. 905
interprofessional collaboration, p. 889
meaningful use, p. 905
medical home, p. 890
Medicare-certified, p. 890

Home health, palliative, and hospice nursing are rapidly expanding practice specialties. Assessment, planning, intervention, and evaluation are the focus of the services. For the purposes of this chapter, home health, palliative, and hospice nursing refer to a wide variety of holistic services typically provided to clients of all ages in their residences and other noninstitutional settings. Note that some agencies have agreements with work and school settings as well as residential and acute care facilities so that nurses provide services in locations in addition to homes. Mergers and collaborative agreements that cause practice boundaries to blur are increasing rapidly.

Numerous references in this chapter describe home health research, finances, and client personal preference, suggesting that the home is the optimal location for diverse health and nursing services (Buhler-Wilkerson, 2007; Beales and Edes, 2009; Hospice Association of America [HHA], 2010; Ferrante et al, 2010; National Association for Home Care and Hospice [NAHC], 2010; Sternberg et al, 2011; Moorman and Macdonald, 2013; Oguh et al, 2013; Nurse Family Partnership [NFP], 2014; Rockoff, 2014). Client residences include houses, apartments, trailers, boarding and care homes, hospice houses, assisted living facilities, shelters, and cars. Home health, palliative, and hospice services are provided by formal caregivers who include nurses, social workers, physical and occupational therapists, home health aides, chaplains, physicians, and others. Because of the nature of home health, palliative, and hospice

practice, a team approach and interprofessional collaboration are required. The specific disciplines involved vary with the program, the intensity of the client and family's needs, and the location of the program and home.

The Triple Aim model for health care was published in 2008 (Berwick, Nolan, & Whittingham, 2008). However, the primary concepts of the model have been the foundation and core values of home health and related community-based services from their inception: services that are client centered, that involve or engage the client and family, and are of high quality, efficient, and cost effective. The Triple Aim is a good strategy to encourage health promotion, prevention, and healthier lifestyles. However, all illness, including chronic illness, cannot be prevented or cured. As the population ages in this country and internationally, the need for home health, palliative, and hospice services is expected to continue and increase.

Access to other health care professionals, resources, and equipment is very different when home and institutional care settings are compared. Many nurses find home health, palliative, and hospice practice very rewarding because they observe the impact of their services and practice with a high degree of autonomy. Nurses who make home visits need to have good organizational, communication, critical thinking, and documentation skills. They need to understand ever-changing reimbursement regulations. Competence, integrity, adaptability, and creativity are essential characteristics. Home health nurses need to anticipate danger from people and circumstances in the physical environment to be savvy about their own safety as well as the safety of their clients (Humphrey and Milone-Nuzzo, 2010; Marrelli, 2012).

Home health care is a broad concept and approach to services. It includes a focus on primary, secondary, and tertiary prevention; the primary focus can involve aggregates, similar to other population-focused nurses. (See the Levels of Prevention box.) Initiatives involving primary and secondary prevention have always been important to home health care.

## LEVELS OF PREVENTION

### Home Health

**Primary Prevention**
The nurse (a) administers seasonal and H1N1 flu vaccine or (b) provides case management interventions so clients obtain the vaccines at convenient locations.

**Secondary Prevention**
The nurse monitors clients in their homes for early signs of new health problems in order to initiate prompt treatment. When the nurse works collaboratively with the physician and/or nurse practitioner, effective interventions can be provided. An example is monitoring clients for medication side effects.

**Tertiary Prevention**
The nurse provides instruction about dietary modifications and insulin injections to newly diagnosed diabetic clients. The purpose of these interventions is to prevent development of complications from diabetes. Diabetic clients and their families implement the therapeutic plan with the goal of maintaining the highest possible level of health.

Home health nursing is "a specialty area of nursing practice that promotes optimal health and well-being for patients, their families, and caregivers within their homes and communities. Home health nurses use a holistic approach aimed at empowering patients/families/caregivers to achieve their highest levels of physical, functional, spiritual, and psychosocial health. Home health nurses provide nursing services to patients of all ages and cultures and at all stages of health and illness, including end of life" (American Nurses Association [ANA], 2014, p. 7). Home health nurses include generalist nurses, public health nurses, clinical nurse specialists, and nurse practitioners. They and their interprofessional team members provide diverse services to target populations such as new parents, frail elders, and clients who have injuries, surgery, disabilities, and acute or chronic health problems. Some home health agencies include wellness programs, health fairs, school nurses, communicable disease, and other programs that are similar to public health department.

Hospice and palliative care are equally broad concepts and approaches to care. Hospice and palliative nursing are specialized areas of practice designed to "provide evidence-based physical, emotional, psychosocial, and spiritual or existential care to individuals and families experiencing life-limiting, progressive illness" (HPNA/ANA, 2007, p. 1). The Hospice

and Palliative Nurses Association (HPNA) did not define their specialty in their new 2014 publication, but, instead, endorsed the National Consensus Project of Palliative Care's (NCP) definition. "Palliative care means patient and family-centered care that optimizes quality of life by anticipating, preventing, and treating suffering. Palliative care throughout the continuum of illness involves addressing the physical, intellectual, emotional, social, and spiritual needs and [facilitating] patient autonomy, access to information, and choice" (NCP, 2013, p. 9). The HPNA and others refer to palliative care as a broad term occurring over a longer period of time, and hospice as a subset with a short time period (ANA/HPNA, 2014; Gomes et al, 2013).

In the United States, funding sources determine many aspects of hospice and palliative care. As of 2012, 67% of hospitals were able to support inpatient palliative care programs, an increase from 24.5% in 2000 (Center to Advance Palliative Care (CAPC), 2013; ANA/HPNA, 2014). Lack of funding may decrease the continuity and comprehensive nature of palliative and hospice programs and services and often separate them. Palliative services can be initiated whether or not cure is possible and can be considered a continuum of care. Services are more flexible and reimbursed based on the client's individual coverage, making funding more challenging. In contrast, hospice involves supportive services when a life-limiting illness does not respond to curative treatment, is the end-of-life portion of the continuum, and is regulated as a 6-month time period by Medicare. The time period is divided into two 90-day certification periods that must be authorized by physicians (Perry and Parente, 2010; Centers for Medicare and Medicaid Services [CMS], 2014a). Advanced practice hospice and palliative nursing are emerging roles. Nurses work closely with members of other disciplines to provide comprehensive interprofessional care; volunteers are important team members.

When entering a home, the home health, palliative, or hospice nurse is a guest and needs to earn the trust of the family and establish a partnership with the client and family (Figure 41-1). It is essential that clients and families are involved in making decisions for home-based services to be efficient and effective. Family is defined by the individual client and includes any caregiver or significant other who assists the client with care at home. Family caregiving involves transportation, helping clients meet their basic needs, and providing care such as personal hygiene, meal preparation, medication administration, and simple as well as complex treatments. Today's clients and family caregivers provide many aspects of care in the home that were previously provided in hospitals or in home by professional caregivers. Care can be confusing, challenging, stressful, and frightening for family caregivers (Buhler-Wilkerson, 2007; Gorski, 2010; Carcone et al, 2012; Moorman and Macdonald, 2013; Oguh et al, 2013; Utens et al, 2014). Clients need to be monitored regularly, and some require 24-hour care. It is likely that family members are grieving when clients receive end-of-life care. Nurses need to identify support services that enable family caregivers to provide care while maintaining their own physical and emotional health status.

Focus of care

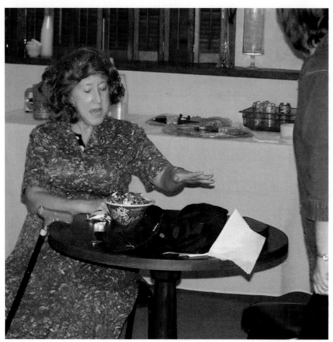

FIG 41-1 Nurses are guests in clients' homes. (From www
.omahasystem.org/photogallery.html. Used with permission
from Karen S. Martin, RN, MSN, FAAN.)

## EVOLUTION OF HOME HEALTH, PALLIATIVE CARE, AND HOSPICE

Home health care provided by formal caregivers in the United
States originated in the nineteenth century. In many communities, the initial programs evolved into visiting nurse associations. The movement expanded rapidly in the United States,
resulting in the formation of 71 agencies prior to 1900, and 600
organizations by 1909. Additional historical details are described
in Chapter 2 and other publications (Buhler-Wilkerson, 2002;
Donahue, 2011).

Home health services were included as a major benefit when
Medicare and Medicaid legislation was passed in 1965 and
implemented in 1966. (See Chapter 5, Economics of Health
Care Delivery.) Both resulted in significant changes nationally.
The Medicare benefit was designed to provide intermittent,
shorter visits with temporary lengths of stay to people age 65
and older. Medicaid covered a wider range of services than
Medicare, and included children, pregnant women, parents of
certain Medicaid-eligible children, and persons with certain disabilities. For clients who qualified for Medicare or Medicaid
services, the home health agency was required to develop a plan
of care for clients and obtain the signature of a physician.

During the next 30 years, the number of Medicare-certified
agencies grew rapidly as a result of the aging population and
prospective payment legislation that decreased the length of
hospital stays. This trend changed when the Balanced Budget
Act of 1997 was enacted, changing the home health payment
system from a fee-of-service model to prospective payment
based on a standardized assessment completed at admission.
The Act prompted the closure of more than 30% of

the country's Medicare-certified home health agencies and a
dramatic decline in the number of clients served (NAHC, 2010;
Zerwekh and Warner, 2014).

Hospice care was introduced in the United States in the
1970s by Florence Wald, often referred to as the mother of the
hospice movement. Before establishing Connecticut Hospice in
1974, Dr. Wald collaborated with Dame Cicely Saunders, a
British nurse, physician, and social worker who founded
St. Christopher's Hospice in England in 1967 (Zerwekh, 2006;
ANA/HPNA, 2014; Zerwekh and Warner, 2014). During the
same era, Dr. Elisabeth Kübler-Ross, a physician, published *On
Death and Dying* (1969), a book that was widely read by the
public and health care professionals. Dr. Ross described the
inhumanity of a death-denying society such as the United
States, the need to provide sensitive end-of-life care and involve
clients in choices, and an emphasis on the quality of life
(Zerwekh, 2006; Malloy et al, 2008; Perry and Parente, 2010;
Sanders et al, 2010; ANA/HPNA, 2014).

In 1987, the first comprehensive, integrated palliative care
program was established at the Cleveland Clinic. In 1999, the
Robert Wood Johnson Foundation funded the Center to
Advance Palliative Care (CAPC) to stimulate the development
of high-quality palliative care programs in hospitals and other
health care settings. In 2010, the CAPC convened a consensus
panel to establish criteria for palliative care assessment components at hospital admission and during the hospital stay (Weissman and Meier, 2011; CAPC, 2013). Assessment items include
recent history of the illness, pain and symptom assessment,
patient-centered goals of care, and transition of care plans. The
Center's goal is to help clinicians identify those individuals and
their families who need palliative care consultation and then
palliative care.

Both home-based and inpatient hospice as well as palliative
models share a focus on comfort, pain relief, and mitigation of
other distressing symptoms. The purpose of the hospice movement is to humanize the end-of-life experience and provide
palliative care. However, because of reimbursement requirements in this country, palliative services are not restricted based
on the disease or progress, and may be appropriate for those
with a serious, complex illness regardless if they are expected to
recover fully, live with a chronic illness for an extended time, or
experience serious disease progression (Perry and Parente,
2010; Sanders et al, 2010; Levine et al, 2013; Wiener et al, 2013;
Hill et al, 2014). Medicaid reimbursement for hospice care
began in 1980 and Medicare in 1983; reimbursement determines many aspects of the programs, including the types and
length of services. For hospice services, physicians need to indicate that clients have six months or less to live, and clients
acknowledge that they have a terminal prognosis and select care
that is comfortable, not life-extending. Because the time of
death is difficult to predict and many people in this country are
reluctant to acknowledge a terminal prognosis, hospice care
often begins late in the disease process. Barriers and stigmas
continue to be associated with hospice for some clients, families,
and physicians; because they equate hospice with hopelessness
and giving up, they will not consider hospice. A number of the
same people are receptive to the concept of palliative care, and

will accept those services (Zerwekh, 2006; HAA, 2010; Perry and Parente, 2010; Levine et al, 2013; Sacco et al, 2013; Hill et al, 2014; Rockoff, 2014).

## DESCRIPTION OF PRACTICE MODELS

Population-focused home care, transitional care, home-based primary care, home health, and hospice/palliative care are models in current use. All involve interprofessional collaboration as well as a focus on care coordination, critical thinking, best practices, and evidence-based practice. Best practices suggest using credible, established evidence from a variety of sources including research, experience, and expert clinicians; evidence-based practice suggests increased emphasis on programs of research that demonstrate consistently good outcomes. The models vary regarding the size and extent of participation, focus of the services, target population, research, political involvement, and funding. With each model, nurses have essential roles in the provision of care, documentation of services, program development and management, outcome and effectiveness analysis, and public education.

### Population-Focused Home Care

Using an evidence-based and data-driven approach to population-focused home care, certain models of care delivery have produced superior outcomes. These models usually include structured approaches to regular visits with assessment protocols, focused health education, counseling, and health-related support and coaching.

The Nurse-Family Partnership (NFP) was initiated in 1977 by a researcher, David Olds, and a nurse, Harriet Kitzman; it is probably the best known and well-funded nurse home visit program in the United States (Olds et al, 1997; Kitzman et al, 2000; NFP, 2014). The Partnership involves nurses who provide structured education and case management during regularly scheduled home visits to pregnant women; visits continue until the children's second birthday. Recipients of care have been ethnically diverse, low-income, first-time mothers and their families who lived in New York, Tennessee, and Colorado. The goals of the program are to improve pregnancy outcomes, improve child health and development, and improve economic self-sufficiency of the families. Longitudinal, randomized controlled trials documented numerous life-long improvements in health outcomes that were statistically significant and economically sound. Mothers had fewer children, were more likely to become employed, and were less likely to enter the criminal justice system; children were less likely to be abused; and both mothers and children demonstrated improved health and development. The researchers estimate that nurses visited more than 28,000 families in 43 states in 2013. Testing is beginning internationally. Federal and private funding continues to increase as the program maintains successful outcomes and grows (Olds et al, 1997; Kitzman et al, 2000; Donelan-McCall et al, 2009; Eckenrode et al, 2010; NFP, 2014; Olds et al, 2014).

The Program of All-Inclusive Care for the Elderly (PACE) began in 1972, and is a managed care model of integrated health and personal care services for noninstitutionalized individuals aged 55 and older who meet frailty criteria (Dobell and Newcomer, 2008; National PACE Association, 2014). Interprofessional care is provided in adult daycare centers with home-based assessments and supportive services also provided as needed. Nurses are essential team members (Madden et al, 2014). Home health care and hospice can be services offered through this model. Because of the model's success and ongoing research, it is now included in Medicare and Medicaid capitation plans. Outcomes include lower rates of hospitalization, readmission, and potentially avoidable hospitalization (Segelman et al, 2014). As of 2014, 104 PACE programs operated in 31 states (National PACE Association, 2014).

### Transitional Care

As a result of a fragmented health care system, increasing complexity of client care, and rising costs, transitional care has gained much needed attention in this country and internationally (Meadows et al, 2014). Transitional care is defined as "a set of actions designed to ensure the coordination and continuity of health care as clients transfer between different locations and different levels of care in the same location" (Coleman and Berenson, 2004, p. 1). Challenges to quality care originate from a lack of depth, accuracy, and timeliness of information received from the referring site; the need for complex medication reconciliation; and difficulties with communication and coordination among community-based providers.

Transitional care programs that involve home health have emerged as low- and high-intensity interventions that include, but vary from, traditional home care interventions. Low-intensity interventions include coaching, telephone follow-up, and specific disease management programs (Boling, 2009). High-intensity transitional care programs are designed for populations who have complex or high-risk health problems. An example is the Transitional Care Model, where advanced practice nurses perform transitional care from hospital to home providing in-hospital visits and discharge planning followed with home visits, primary care office visits, and telephone follow-up for 1 to 3 months after discharge (Brooten et al, 2001; Naylor, 2004). Numerous studies have been conducted to test the Model with additional high-risk groups (Naylor et al, 1999; Naylor et al, 2007). The research model is currently implemented in practice settings in collaboration with major insurance companies and home care agencies (Naylor et al, 2013).

Outcomes achieved with the Transitional Care Model consistently show cost savings and improvements in clinical and quality outcomes for clients receiving the intervention compared with usual care (Naylor et al, 2011). The most common outcome across all populations is a consistent reduction in readmissions to a hospital. The Transitional Care Model strategies emphasize screening in acute care for high-risk clients; engaging the elder/caregiver in designing personalized goals and the plan of care; managing symptoms; educating and promoting self-management; and collaborating with the multidisciplinary team members to assure continuity and a team approach. Both the low and high intensity transitional care programs have spread rapidly into practice as hospitals seek ways to avoid the financial penalties instituted through the

Readmission Reduction Program enacted through the 2010 Patient Protection and Affordable Care Act (CMS, 2013a; Kaiser Family Foundation, 2013).

There are additional transitional care interventions that home health nurses can adopt to improve the safe transition of clients they are admitting to service. For example, home health agencies should work closely with the acute care interprofessional team to educate them about the benefits of home health, and how to identify clients for referral (Bowles et al, 2009; Meadows et al, 2014). Evidence-based discharge decision support software is now available to help those in acute care. The software helps identify patients who need home health care and is having an impact on readmissions (Bowles et al, 2014). Once the referral is made, the home health nurse should request specific information about the hospitalization and what the client was taught to help establish a baseline and develop a care plan (Bowles et al, 2010). Finally, because clients and family caregivers often find it difficult to learn during hospitalization, home health nurses should ask hospital staff what clients were taught about their conditions, medications, self-care, and symptoms. The home health nurse can reinforce information, evaluate the client's ability to adhere to the treatment plan, prioritize the first home visit, and prevent unnecessary rehospitalization.

## Home-Based Primary Care

The goal of home-based primary care is to offer clients an alternative to receiving services in a primary care clinic, community center, or physician's office. These clients have functional or other health problems that make the trip from their homes to other care sites very difficult.

The Veterans Health Administration Hospital-Based Home Care Program targets individuals who have complex chronic disabling diseases with the goal of maximizing the independence of the client and reducing preventable emergency room visits and hospitalizations (Beales and Edes, 2009; Marsteller et al, 2009; Sperber et al, 2014; Schectman and Stark, 2014; True et al, 2014). An interprofessional team provides comprehensive longitudinal primary care that incorporates telehealth and electronic health records (EHRs). Nurses serve as case managers, continually evaluate clients' needs, and deliver care. Approximately three fourths of Veterans Health Administration facilities offer the Home Care Program. The program has produced positive outcomes, but many authors describe mixed evidence. They cite veterans' hesitation to use the services; describe the investment of time and effort to create and maintain the provider teams, and challenges with communication; and question if telehealth and telephone contacts are adequate substitutes for in-person care or are supplements to in-person interaction (Beales and Edes, 2009; Marsteller et al, 2009; Chang et al, 2009; Sperber et al, 2014; Bidassie et al, 2014).

In 1967, the American Academy of Pediatrics originated the concept of a medical home in an attempt to establish centralized, accessible health care records for medically complex, chronically ill children (Friedberg et al, 2009; Sternberg et al, 2011). Although there are distinct variations of medical homes, the models typically include superb access to care; patient engagement in care; EHRs that may be client controlled; care coordination; integrated, comprehensive care; ongoing, routine client feedback; and publicly available information about practices (Davis and Stremikis, 2010; Ferrante et al, 2010; Sternberg et al, 2011; Swartwout et al, 2014). More recently, the Centers for Medicare and Medicaid Services (CMS) and politicians supported the medical home as a model to decrease costs and incorporated the concept into health care reform. Nurse practitioners are especially interested in the policy implications and in participating as leaders in this movement (Swartwout et al, 2014). As noted with the Veterans Health Administrations' experiences, the model continues to have supporters, but the effectiveness of the evidence is limited; some medical home interventions may lead to modest improvements in outcomes and moderate cost savings (Leff et al, 2009; Arend et al, 2012; Evans et al, 2013).

## Home Health

Staff members of home health agencies provide care at home and help clients and their families achieve improved health and independence in a safe environment. According to CMS (2012a) and NAHC (2010), approximately 12 million clients received Medicare-certified home health services in 2010. An unknown number of additional clients receive services from non-Medicare-certified agencies. Persons who were 65 years and older accounted for more than 70% of all home health clients; agencies provide care to twice as many women as men. Recipients of home health services had diverse needs, but circulatory disease was the most common diagnosis, followed by neoplasms and endocrine diseases, especially diabetes. It was estimated that 10,581 Medicare-certified home health agencies employed over one million employees; approximately half of those were clinical staff. In 2012, the estimated number of agencies increased to 12,253 (CMS, 2013b). The size of individual agencies varied from those that employ a few nurses to the Visiting Nurse Service of New York with its 2,600 nurses, more than 20,000 employees, 35,000 census, and 2,425,000 annual visits (VNSNY, 2014).

Annual national expenditures for home health care in 2009 were over 72 billion. Home health accounted for approximately 3% of the country's total health expenditures in contrast to 37% for hospitals and 26% for physicians and clinical services. As the largest payer, Medicare accounted for 41% of total home health reimbursement. In addition to Medicare, state and local governments accounted for 15% of home health reimbursement, Medicaid for 24%, private insurance for 8%, out-of-pocket or private pay 10%, and other sources 2% (CMS, 2012a; NAHC, 2010).

Home health agencies can be divided into six general categories although the distinctions continue to blur as more agency mergers and purchases occur. A description of each follows:
- Official/public: approximately 13% of total home health agencies
- Visiting Nurse Association: approximately 5% of total home health agencies
- Private and voluntary: approximately 6% of total home health agencies

*Medicare Criteria*

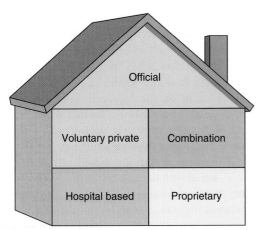

**FIG 41-2** Types of home health agencies.

- Combination: approximately 0.3% of total home health agencies
- Hospital based: approximately 12% of total home health agencies
- Proprietary: approximately 62% of total home health agencies (Figure 41-2)

Official or public agencies receive tax revenue and are operated by state, county, city, or other local government units, such as health departments. Typically, official agencies also offer well-child clinics, immunizations, health education programs, and home visits for preventive health care.

Visiting Nurse Associations are usually freestanding, voluntary, nonprofit organizations governed by a board of directors, and usually financed by earnings and tax-deductible contributions. Sometimes they are categorized with combination agencies because of their similar characteristics.

Voluntary and private agencies are nonprofit home health agencies and usually receive some funds from United Way, donations, and endowments. Currently, there are about the same number of voluntary and private agencies.

Combination agencies have characteristics of both governmental and voluntary agencies. The number of combination agencies continues to decrease although some are large agencies.

Hospital-based agencies grew rapidly during the 1970s and 1980s when the advent of diagnostic-related groups led to earlier hospital discharges. Some hospitals and their home health agencies are separating because of recent changes in Medicare reimbursement.

Proprietary agencies are free-standing, for-profit agencies that are required to pay taxes. Many are part of large chains. Proprietary agencies now dominate the industry.

In addition to Medicare-certified home health agencies, there are other agencies that are not certified. These are often private agencies, governed by individual owners or corporations that offer private duty, home health aide, and homemaker services.

Although the programs, size, administration, organization, and board structures of Medicare-certified agencies differ, they must meet ever-changing licensure, certification, and accreditation regulations established by national and state groups (Buhler-Wilkerson, 2007; NAHC, 2010; Fazzi et al, 2010a; Fazzi Associates, 2010b). The primary source of those regulations is CMS (2012b; NAHC, 2010). To be Medicare-certified, key criteria identified in the Conditions of Participation are (a) the client must be home-bound; (b) services must be intermittent and include a skilled service provided by a nurse, physical therapist, or speech and language pathologist; (c) a plan of care must be initiated and followed; and (d) Medicare forms, physician orders, and client records must be completed on a timely basis. Skilled nursing services is the Medicare term that describes the duties of the registered nurse, and refers to the requirement of nursing judgment. Those services involve assessment, teaching, and selected procedures. Using Omaha System terms, the focus of assessment is Environmental, Psychosocial, Physiological, and Health-related Behaviors while interventions are categorized as Teaching, Guidance, and Counseling; Treatments and Procedures; Case Management; and Surveillance (Martin, 2005; Monsen et al, 2011; Omaha System, 2014).

The Conditions of Participation are lengthy, complex, and subject to change. OASIS was mandated as one portion of the conditions in 1999 and is described later in this chapter. Beginning in 2011, the physician or the allowed nonphysician practitioner need to have a face-to-face encounter prior to signing orders and initiating care. Agencies provide orientation and review sessions for all clinicians, but often employ one or more nurses as experts to ensure that their agencies are compliant. These nurses need to be detail oriented, and develop skills by reading and rereading the Conditions, attending workshops or classes, and communicating with peers. In addition to their daily responsibilities, these nurses usually serve as leaders when surveyors, accreditors, and auditors visit.

## Hospice and Palliative Care

*Similar*

Hospice and palliative care are similar and, yet, very different. Similarities that are described throughout this chapter include a client-focused approach, holistic and evidence-based practice, emphasis on ethics, communication skills, interprofessional collaboration, care coordination, focus on transitions of care, and caregiving skills including symptom management and pain control. The Hospice and Palliative Nurses Association (HPNA) is an umbrella organization that represents hospice and palliative nurses and other members of the team employed in home-based organizations as well as acute and long-term care, outpatient, and other settings (ANA/HPNA, 2014). The organization's mission is to advance expert care during serious illness; it is based on four pillars of education, advocacy, leadership, and research. Differences between hospice and palliative care include the length of care, frequency and intensity of services; the maturity of the practice within agencies; and funding sources and regulations that directly impact care. Hospice is a formalized program in hospice and home health agencies. For that reason, it is the focus of this section of the chapter. Palliative care has no specific federal designation as a specialty; rather it exists as a consultative discipline delivering a philosophy of care. Palliative care clinicians must meet the regulatory requirements for home health or other setting where they practice (ANA/HPNA, 2014).

The Trajectories of Palliative Care includes similarities and differences between hospice and palliative care. Palliative care is an extended continuum of chronic serious illness to acute serious illness during which stabilization and exacerbations may occur. Services and treatment will vary during this time. The continuum encompasses diagnosis and limited signs and symptoms, increasing severity of signs and symptoms, onset of a relatively short period of hospice care, death, and bereavement care for family members.

Hospice programs are usually operated and staffed as independent entities or corporations even when they are part of a larger organization because of the specialized nature of the practice and the complex regulations and financial requirements. An increasing number of home health agencies are establishing palliative programs as a subspecialty of their home health program or a subspecialty in their hospice program. In neither case is there a Medicare, Medicaid, or other funding source specific to palliative care as there is to hospice. Similarly to home health, hospice and palliative providers introduce clinicians to the regulations, but employ nurse experts who are responsible for current knowledge of the ever-changing clinical and financial rules. Responsibilities of the experts include orientation, performance improvement, documentation, and compliance.

More than 1 million clients received Medicare-certified hospice services in 2010 with an average stay of 71 days. The average length of stay will rise if home health nurses and others provide information about end-of-life hospice care to clients and families, and hospice becomes more widely accepted by the public. Health care professionals and the media are making slow progress to introduce palliative care and hospice services (Candy et al, 2011; Weissman and Meier, 2011; CAPC, 2013; Sacco et al, 2013; Rockoff, 2014). However, because of the hospice stigma, more home health agencies are developing palliative care programs that do not include the 6-month admission requirement. Even when nurses, physicians, and others discuss quality of life and encourage the transition from palliative services to hospice, clients and/or families may continue in denial and not accept hospice until the last several days of life. Brief stays make it difficult for the hospice team to provide comprehensive, more cost-effective services to clients and families. For many in this country, death is not viewed as a normal or natural part of the life cycle (Rockoff, 2014).

Initially, cancer was the primary diagnosis of most clients in hospice programs. Currently, cancer is the diagnosis of about one third of hospice clients, and various neurologic, cardiac, and other end-stage diseases comprise two thirds of the diagnoses. Palliative care expanded from the hospice model. Clients who receive palliative care have diverse chronic illness diagnoses (Zerwekh, 2006; NAHC, 2010; HAA, 2010; Perry and Parente, 2010; Candy et al, 2011; ANA/HPNA, 2014).

Medicare, Medicaid, managed care, private insurance, and private donations fund most hospice services. Medicare reimbursement accounts for almost 85% of the total while private insurance is approximately 8%, Medicaid is 5%, and other

sources are 3%. The number of Medicare-certified hospices grew from 31 in 1984 to 3,407 in 2010. Hospice services account for approximately 2.8% of the total Medicare budget, just less than home health services (CMS, 2013b). Typically, services are provided nationally based on Medicare criteria although there are differences based on the Medicare intermediaries. More diversity occurs with non-Medicare sources of reimbursement. For example, each state administers and funds its own Medicaid programs, and criteria for hospice admission, types and locations of services, types of clinician providers, number of visits, and length of stay vary.

Medicare-certified hospice programs are not required to complete OASIS. Instead, the industry has been developing quality measures that will be reported by providers. CMS has mandated that hospices begin their data set reporting process with two measures: one that is client related and one that is structural. It is expected that the number of measures will increase as the industry identifies, proposes, and refines a data set. It is likely that new CMS regulations will include a Hospice Information Set (HIS) and that hospice reimbursement will be reduced just as home health reimbursement is scheduled for reduction (CMS, 2014a; Fazzi Associates, 2014; Martin and Utterback, 2014).

After the client acknowledges a terminal prognosis and selects comforting care rather than life-extending or curative care, hospice organizations coordinate services in partnership with the client and family and provide financial case management. The four types of care and the percentage used were (1) routine home care with intermittent visits, 96.5%; (2) continuous home care when condition is acute and death is near, 1.1%; (3) general inpatient/hospital care for symptom relief, 2.2%; and (4) respite care in a nursing home of no more than 5 days at a time to relieve family members, 0.2% (NAHC, 2010; HAA, 2010).

Medicare-certified hospice providers can be divided into the following four general categories:
- Home health agencies: approximately 17% of total hospice providers
- Hospital-based facilities: approximately 16% of total hospice providers
- Skilled nursing facilities: approximately 0.6% of total hospice providers
- Free-standing facilities: approximately 67% of total hospice providers (NAHC, 2013a)

The focus of hospice care is comfort, peace, and a sense of dignity at a very difficult time, a focus that is similar to palliative care. Comprehensive services emphasize continuity of care. According to Zerwekh (2006), hospice addresses four foci: (1) attention to the body, mind, and spirit; (2) death is not a taboo topic; (3) health care technology should be used with discretion; and (4) clients have a right to truthful discussion and participation in treatment decisions. Hospice is the only Medicare benefit that includes medications, medical equipment, 24-hour/seven-day-a-week access to care, and support for family members after death. Those who receive Medicare-certified hospice services are evaluated during the 6-month period to determine if they are eligible to continue.

The client's family and friends are essential hospice team members who are involved in symptom and medication management, personal care, and the use of supplies. Death produces intense emotions even when family members have prepared for it. Bereavement services that are part of hospice involve attending the funeral or other services for the deceased client, and contact at anniversaries of death, holidays, and the client's birthday for 13 months after the client's death. Hospice organizations usually offer support group opportunities for families or refer them to support groups in the area (Malloy et al, 2008; Levine et al, 2013; Wiener et al, 2013).

The interprofessional hospice team includes nurses, physicians, social workers, therapists, chaplains, counselors, aides, pharmacists, and volunteers. Volunteers are an important part of the team. In 2009, there were approximately 102,000 employees and 50,000 volunteers; nurses, aides, and social workers were the largest groups of employees (NAHC, 2010). Most agencies and team members consider conferences and continuing education essential to develop and renew their skills involving topics such as end-of-life comfort measures, new medications and treatments, compassion fatigue, spirituality, complex family dynamics, and cultural awareness. Working with clients who are dying involves unique emotional stress; hospice programs address the team's well-being as well as that of the clients and families (Hinds et al, 2005; Zerwekh, 2006; ANA/HPNA, 2014; HAA, 2010; Mack and Joffe, 2014).

### Home Care of Dying Children

"The death of a child alters the life and health of others immediately and for the rest of their lives" (Hinds et al, 2005, p. S70). The needs of dying children and their families are unique because of the degree of emotional impact, and because the young are not expected to die or precede the death of their parents. It is essential that nurses understand the child's physical, cognitive, psychosocial, and spiritual development and family dynamics, cultural heritage, and spiritual beliefs in order to provide appropriate pain management, assist the child and family to communicate with each other, advocate for their needs in the community, and provide case management and continuity of care (Hinds et al, 2005; Hinds et al, 2012; Levine et al, 2013; Wiener et al, 2013; Hill et al, 2014; Mack and Joffe, 2014).

Bereavement programs as described for hospice programs are especially important for families who have lost a child. Parents, grandparents, and siblings can participate in a variety of support groups offered by the hospice program or other bereavement organizations (Levine et al, 2013; Wiener et al, 2013).

## SCOPE AND STANDARDS OF PRACTICE

Nursing is a theory and practice-based profession that incorporates art and science. Examples of nursing, family, and systems theories are mentioned and summarized in other chapters of this book. Chapter 7 focuses on cultural diversity. Many publications are available, including an article about students and cultural awareness (Mager and Grossman, 2013). Chapter 15

---

> **HOW TO** Use a Hospice Approach to Care in Any Setting
>
> *The hospice philosophy of care means providing comfort measures to individuals before death and support for their families before and after death. Individuals may be any age. Death may occur in the individual's home, a hospital setting, or an uncontrolled setting such as the community. How does one adapt nursing care in any situation? What basic skills can professional caregivers use that can be applied in any situation or setting? How do professional caregivers adapt to the death of a hospice client, inpatient death, or a sudden, unexpected death where, for example, many people have died as a result of a natural disaster or a terrorist act?*
>
> - *Be prepared. Consider your own philosophy of death so that you can assist others without distraction when that time comes.*
> - *Cultures vary in their beliefs about and responses to death. Know the differences in cultural responses so that you can effectively help people in their time of need.*
> - *Death events cannot be totally controlled even in a hospice environment where the eventual death has been illustrated to family and friends and the dying individual before the death. Expect the unexpected and take cues from the client and the loved ones regarding their needs.*
> - *Shock, disbelief, and crisis reactions occur even with prepared, hospice deaths. Ask family and caregivers what they need; provide them with the basics such as food or blankets; provide comfort; if it is not contraindicated, provide the family/friends with personal effects or mementos of the individual; give sensitive, caring support. Sit with them and listen.*
> - *In a disaster, the philosophy of care is to provide the greatest good to the greatest number of people. Using triage, the needs of those with less severe injuries have priority over the needs of those who are closer to death. Responsibilities of caregivers and health professionals will be stretched to the maximum. A leader for a group of clients needs to be identified and must delegate responsibility to a caregiver who can assist the dying and their loved ones.*
>
> *From Mistovich JJ, Karren KJ: Prehospital Emergency Care, ed 10, Upper Saddle River, NJ, 2014, Pearson Education.*

addresses evidence-based practice; the concept is addressed frequently in this chapter, and two examples are included. Melnyk is one of the most prolific authors on this topic (Melnyk and Fineout-Overholt, 2011; Malloch and Melnyk, 2013; Melnyk et al, 2014). Several chapters of this book describe the Quad Council's (2011) eight domains of practice; those domains are linked to information in this chapter in the Linking Content to Practice box.

The nursing process is the theoretical framework used by the ANA, which notes that the nursing process is the essential methodology by which client goals are identified and achieved. Their scope and standards publications, including those for home health nursing and palliative nursing, are organized according to the nursing process and contain two sections: the Standards of Care and the Standards of Professional Performance (ANA, 2014; ANA/HPNA, 2014). Both include the six steps of the nursing process: assessment, diagnosis, outcomes identification, planning, implementation, and evaluation; the steps are linked to standards and more specific measurement criteria that are stated in behavioral objectives. The standards address quality of care, performance appraisal, critical thinking

▶▶  **LINKING CONTENT TO PRACTICE**

### The Nurse in Home Health, Palliative Care, and Hospice

The individuals, families, and communities served by home health, palliative, and hospice nurses are described throughout this chapter as are the knowledge, skills, and attitudes of nurses who function well in those settings. The descriptions are evident in the text, clinical examples, boxes/figures/tables, references, and other parts of the chapter. The competencies in this chapter are congruent with the following core competencies of the Quad Council's Domains of Public Health Nursing (2011): (1) Analytic/assessment skills, (2) Policy development/program planning skills, (3) Communication skills, (4) Cultural competency skills, (5) Community dimensions of practice skills, (6) Basic public health sciences skills, (7) Financial planning and management skills, and (8) Leadership and systems thinking skills. Students and new graduates cannot be expected to have developed all of these skills when they begin home health or hospice practice (Mager and Grossman, 2013). However, as nurses proceed in their career development and gain valuable work experience, they will progress along the novice to expert continuum.

skills, education, collegiality, ethics, collaboration, research, and resource use.

## OMAHA SYSTEM

According to Clark and Lang (1992), "If we cannot name it, we cannot control it, finance it, teach it, research it or put it into public policy" (p. 27). The Omaha System was initially developed to operationalize the nursing process and provide a practical, easily understood, computer-compatible guide for daily use in diverse community settings. It is the only ANA-recognized terminology developed inductively by and for nurses who practice in the community. Approximately 21,000 multiprofessional clinicians, educators, and researchers use Omaha System point-of-care electronic health records (EHRs) across the continuum in the United States and other countries, and 2000 more use paper-and-pen records. EHRs are longitudinal collections of clinical and demographic client-specific data that are stored in a computer-readable format. By 2005, 85% of all counties in Minnesota had one or more public health or home care agencies or schools/colleges of nursing using Omaha System software. That number continues to increase. During 2014, Minnesota became the first state to recommend that the Omaha System be used as a standardized terminology in the EHRs of all community health care settings in the state. Details about Omaha System application, users, case studies, inclusion in reference terminologies, research, best practices/evidence-based practice, and listserv are described in publications and on the website (Martin, 2005; Martin et al, 2011; Omaha System, 2014; Topaz et al, 2014).

## Description of the Omaha System

As early as 1970, the nurses, other staff, and administrators of the Visiting Nurse Association (VNA) of Omaha, Nebraska, began addressing nursing practice, documentation, and information management concerns. Information management is the integration of clinical, demographic, financial,

administrative, and staffing data; manipulation or processing of these data; and production of various reports that transform data into meaningful information for decision making (Martin, 2005). At that time, clinicians were not using computers, and there was no systematic nomenclature or classification of client problems and concerns, interventions, or client outcomes to quantify clinical data and integrate with a problem-oriented record system. Between 1975 and 1993, the VNA of Omaha staff conducted four extensive, federally funded development and refinement research studies that established reliability, validity, and usability of the Omaha System. The result of the research was the Problem Classification Scheme, the Intervention Scheme, and the Problem Rating Scale for Outcomes. These three components of the Omaha System were designed to be used together, be comprehensive, relatively simple, hierarchical, multidimensional, and computer compatible. The Omaha System has existed in the public domain since the initial research in 1975. Because it is not held under copyright, software companies can use it as the foundation of their software without obtaining licenses or paying fees. They are expected to replicate the structure, terms, and codes as presented, and cite their source (Martin, 2005; Martin et al, 2011; Omaha System, 2014).

As depicted in Figure 41-3, the Omaha System conceptual model is based on the dynamic, interactive nature of the nursing or problem solving process, the practitioner–client relationship, and concepts of diagnostic reasoning, critical thinking, and quality improvement. The client as an individual, a family, or a community appears at the center of the model. This location suggests the range of Omaha System application, client-centered care, and the essential partnership between clients and practitioners. More recently, the term

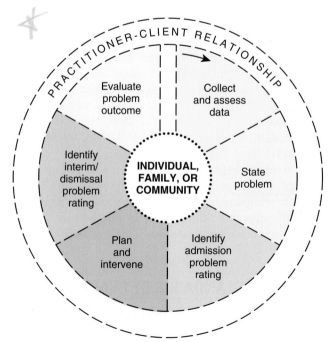

**FIG 41-3** Omaha System model of the problem-solving process. (From Martin KS: *The Omaha System: a key to practice, documentation, and information management,* reprinted ed 2, Omaha, NE, 2005, Health Connections Press.)

*Client engagement* has been used to describe this partnership, especially in acute care practice. Most nurses and other clinicians employed in community settings recognized that partnership was essential from the beginning of their employment. The outer circle is the practitioner–client relationship. Additional details about the conceptual model are described in the following paragraphs.

The Omaha System was intended for use by nurses and all members of the health care delivery team. The goals of the research were to (1) develop a structured and comprehensive system that could be both understood and used by members of various disciplines, and (2) foster collaborative practice. Therefore, the Omaha System was designed to guide practice decisions, sort and document pertinent client data uniformly, and provide a framework for an agency-wide, multidisciplinary clinical information management system capable of meeting the daily needs of clinicians, managers, and administrators (Martin, 2005; Garvin et al, 2008; Correll and Martin, 2009; Westra et al, 2010; Martin et al, 2011; Monsen et al, 2011; Omaha System, 2014).

## Problem Classification Scheme

The Omaha System Problem Classification Scheme is a comprehensive, orderly, nonexhaustive, mutually exclusive taxonomy designed to identify diverse clients' health-related concerns. Its simple and concrete terms are used to organize a comprehensive assessment, an important standard of nursing practice. The Problem Classification Scheme consists of four levels. Four domains appear at the first level and represent priority areas. Forty-two terms, referred to as client problems or areas of client needs and strengths, appear at the second level. The third level consists of two sets of problem modifiers: health promotion, potential and actual, as well as individual, family, and community. Clusters of signs and symptoms describe actual problems at the fourth level. The content and relationship of the domain and problem levels depicted in Box 41-1 are further illustrated by the case example at the end of this chapter. Understanding the meaning of and relationships among the terms is a prerequisite to using the scheme accurately and consistently to collect, sort, document, analyze, quantify, and communicate client needs and strengths.

## Intervention Scheme

The Omaha System Intervention Scheme is an important standard of nursing practice in providing interventions. Four broad categories of interventions appear at the first level of the Intervention Scheme. An alphabetical list of 75 targets or objects of action and 1 "other" appear at the second level. Client-specific information generated by clinicians is at the third level. The contents of the category and target levels are depicted in Boxes 41-2 and 41-3, respectively. The Intervention Scheme provides the terms for care plans and services. It enables

---

**BOX 41-1  Domains and Problems of the Omaha System Problem Classification Scheme**

**Environmental Domain**
Material resources and physical surroundings both inside and outside the living area, neighborhood, and broader community:
- Income
- Sanitation
- Residence
- Neighborhood/workplace safety

**Psychosocial Domain**
Patterns of behavior, emotion, communication, relationships, and development:
- Communication with community resources
- Social contact
- Role change
- Interpersonal relationship
- Spirituality
- Grief
- Mental health
- Sexuality
- Caretaking/parenting
- Neglect
- Abuse
- Growth and development

**Physiological Domain**
Functions and processes that maintain life:
- Hearing
- Vision
- Speech and language
- Oral health
- Cognition
- Pain
- Consciousness
- Skin
- Neuro-musculo-skeletal function
- Respiration
- Circulation
- Digestion-hydration
- Bowel function
- Urinary function
- Reproductive function
- Pregnancy
- Postpartum
- Communicable/infectious condition

**Health-Related Behaviors Domain**
Patterns of activity that maintain or promote wellness, promote recovery, and decrease the risk of disease:
- Nutrition
- Sleep and rest patterns
- Physical activity
- Personal care
- Substance use
- Family planning
- Health care supervision
- Medication regimen

---

From Martin KS: The Omaha System: *A Key to Practice, Documentation, and Information Management*, reprinted ed 2, Omaha, NE, 2005, Health Connections Press.

---

**BOX 41-2**   **Categories of the Omaha System Intervention Scheme**

**Teaching, Guidance, and Counseling**

Activities designed to provide information and materials, encourage action and responsibility for self-care and coping, and assist the individual, family, or community to make decisions and solve problems.

**Treatments and Procedures**

Technical activities such as wound care, specimen collection, resistive exercises, and medication prescriptions that are designed to prevent, decrease, or alleviate signs and symptoms for the individual, family, or community.

**Case Management**

Activities such as coordination, advocacy, and referral that facilitate service delivery; promote assertiveness; guide the individual, family, or community toward use of appropriate community resources; and improve communication among health and human service providers.

**Surveillance**

Activities such as detection, measurement, critical analysis, and monitoring intended to identify the individual, family, or community's status in relation to a given condition or phenomenon.

From Martin KS: The Omaha System: *A Key to Practice, Documentation, and Information Management,* reprinted ed 2, Omaha, NE, 2005, Health Connections Press.

---

**BOX 41-3**   **Targets of the Omaha System Intervention Scheme**

| | |
|---|---|
| anatomy/physiology | medication administration |
| anger management | medication coordination/ordering |
| behavior modification | medication prescription |
| bladder care | medication set-up |
| bonding/attachment | mobility/transfers |
| bowel care | nursing care |
| cardiac care | nutritionist care |
| caretaking/parenting skills | occupational therapy care |
| cast care | ostomy care |
| communication | other community resources |
| community outreach worker services | paraprofessional/aide care |
| continuity of care | personal hygiene |
| coping skills | physical therapy care |
| daycare/respite | positioning |
| dietary management | recreational therapy care |
| discipline | relaxation/breathing techniques |
| dressing change/wound care | respiratory care |
| durable medical equipment | respiratory therapy care |
| education | rest/sleep |
| employment | safety |
| end-of-life care | screening procedures |
| environment | sickness/injury care |
| exercises | signs/symptoms-mental/emotional |
| family planning care | signs/symptoms-physical |
| feeding procedures | skin care |
| finances | social work/counseling care |
| gait training | specimen collection |
| genetics | speech and language pathology care |
| growth/development care | spiritual care |
| home | stimulation/nurturance |
| homemaking/housekeeping | stress management |
| infection precautions | substance use cessation |
| interaction | supplies |
| interpreter/translator services | support group |
| laboratory findings | support system |
| legal system | transportation |
| medical/dental care | wellness |
| medication action/side effects | other |

From Martin KS: The Omaha System: *A Key to Practice, Documentation, and Information Management,* reprinted ed 2, Omaha, NE, 2005, Health Connections Press.

---

clinicians to describe, quantify, and communicate their practice, including improving or restoring health, describing deterioration, or preventing illness.

### Problem Rating Scale for Outcomes

The Omaha System Problem Rating Scale for Outcomes consists of three five-point, Likert-type scales for measuring the entire range of severity for the concepts of Knowledge, Behavior, and Status. Each of the subscales is a continuum providing a framework for measuring and comparing problem-specific client outcomes at regular or predictable times, because evaluation is an important standard of nursing practice. Suggested times include admission, specific interim points, and discharge. The content and relationships of the scale are depicted in Table 41-1. Using the Problem Rating Scale for Outcomes with the Problem Classification Scheme and the Intervention Scheme creates a comprehensive problem solving model for practice, education, and research.

## PRACTICE GUIDELINES

Nursing practice is based on education, experience, and evidence. Because home health, palliative, and hospice nurses usually work with clients and their families in their homes, they must develop skills to conduct home visits efficiently, effectively, and safely (Box 41-4). A positive attitude about client-centered care, the nurse–client partnership, and patient engagement is essential. Critical thinking skills are also essential. Effective care coordination requires familiarity with community resources. Knowledge and skills involving medications, treatments, documentation, and equipment nures necessary. Excellent strategies include accompanying skilled home health, palliative, and hospice nurses when they make home visits as well as having

expert mentors. However, novice nurses also need a commitment to life-long learning, practice, and self-evaluation (Zerwekh, 2006; Humphrey and Milone-Nuzzo, 2010; Abele and Nies, 2011; Marrelli, 2012). The following is a brief summary of steps included in a home visit; these steps can be modified slightly for other noninstitutional settings:

- Review client data, including the referral from the intake department, hospital discharge summary, orders, and plan of care to become familiar with the client's history, purpose of the visit, and expectations.
- Contact the client or family by calling the telephone number listed on the referral information to obtain agreement for the visit, schedule the day and time, and discuss the address.
- Gather agency and Medicare forms, a nursing bag, cellular phone or pager, portable computing device, teaching

## TABLE 41-1   Omaha System Problem Rating Scale for Outcomes

| Concept | 1 | 2 | 3 | 4 | 5 |
|---|---|---|---|---|---|
| Knowledge: Ability of client to remember and interpret information | No knowledge | Minimal knowledge | Basic knowledge | Adequate knowledge | Superior knowledge |
| Behavior: Observable responses, actions, or activities of client fitting occasion or purpose | Not appropriate behavior | Rarely appropriate behavior | Inconsistently appropriate behavior | Usually appropriate behavior | Consistently appropriate behavior |
| Status: Condition of client in relation to objective and subjective defining characteristics | Extreme signs/symptoms | Severe signs/symptoms | Moderate signs/symptoms | Minimal signs/symptoms | No signs/symptoms |

From Martin KS: *The Omaha System: A Key to Practice, Documentation, and Information Management*, reprinted ed 2, Omaha, NE, 2005, Health Connections Press.

### BOX 41-4   Guidelines for Home Health and Hospice

- You are a guest in your client's home and neighborhood. Your behavior and your manners must convey that you recognize this role.
- Respect the client's cultural, religious, and ethnic heritage. Hesitate before contradicting that heritage. Clients are more likely to follow their heritage than your advice.
- The client may not respect your cultural, religious, and ethnic heritage. If you are a male nurse, the client may expect, and even request, a female nurse. Develop interpersonal skills—and a tough skin.
- Almost every home health client has family members, significant others, or friends who offer advice and can serve as either your advocate or your foe. Try to enlist them as your advocate.
- The client "owns" the health-related problem that initiated your services. That problem is just one portion of the client's past, present, and future. Thus it is the client who experiences, learns to understand, and ultimately solves the problem. It is your goal to help clients and their families become independent as quickly as possible. Talk to your peers and supervisors if you sense that you may be losing that perspective.
- Enjoy the unique autonomy and challenges of providing highly complex care in the home and community setting. Home health practice requires integration of high-technology skills, teaching, case management, and monitoring. Remember the need and benefits of collaboration with other members of the health care team. The nurse is usually responsible for judging whether or not the client can safely remain at home. However, data and information to support this and other decisions need to be communicated with team members orally and through the electronic health record.
- Maintain your sense of humor. You will need it!

Adapted from Black JM, Hawks JH: *Medical Surgical Nursing*, ed 8, St Louis, 2009, Saunders, p. 94.

materials, and supplies; understand the client's location; follow the agency policy when checking-out for the visit.

- Observe the neighborhood for resources and safety when approaching the client's home.
- Greet the client/family to begin developing a positive, appropriate professional relationship; involve them as much as possible during the visit and post-visit activities.
- Obtain signatures and complete needed forms.
- Provide care by completing a comprehensive assessment, identifying client problems, providing interventions, and evaluating client outcomes. Interventions may include teaching, guidance, and counseling; treatments and procedures; case management; and surveillance (Martin, 2005).
- Discuss the plan of care with the client and family during informal or formal conferences; modify as needed.
- Document some or all of the visit details in the home, preferably while using a portable computing device and an EHR.
- Discuss the next visit as well as follow-up activities and referrals.
- Proceed to the next scheduled visit after checking in, according to the agency policy.
- Complete remaining visit documentation, submit forms, coordinate referrals to other community resources, and communicate with agency colleagues, the referral source, physicians, and others as appropriate. Obtain revised orders if needed.
- Revisit to reassess the client and provide care.

### Clinical Example from Community-Focused Practice

The example describes an innovative and collaborative community-focused program developed in Tucson, Arizona, by the Pima County Health Department and the Pima County Public Library (Innes, 2012; Robert Wood Johnson Foundation (RWJF), 2013). The Library requested that the Health Department hire a social worker to increase safety and a welcoming environment in five high-risk libraries. Concerns included loitering, behavioral health concerns, encampment, and abandonment. Many patrons were homeless and/or had chronic diseases that were not being managed. Children and elders were left at the library by family members while they completed errands or went to work.

After a root-cause analysis was conducted and a logic model developed, the decision was made by Kathleen Malkin, Public Health Nursing Division Manager, and the Health Department and Library management staff to hire one full-time public health nurse in January 2012, a first in this country. It was decided that a nurse could better meet the identified needs of the patrons and library staff. In addition to increasing safety and a welcoming environment, a goal was to coordinate with community resource agencies to provide nutritious snacks for children and reduce hunger concerns.

During the first year, the program expanded to include five public health nurses working in six high-risk libraries. They made 180 visits to the libraries and had 2,181 patron encounters. Client problems and clinician interventions were documented. The most frequently identified problems were health care supervision, nutrition, circulation, hearing, personal care, and cognition. The nurses instructed the library staff on communicable disease prevention topics. During the first year, calls made to the police and 911 were reduced by 6% and calls to 911 for medical emergencies were reduced by 20%.

In the second year, the program expanded to 13 library sites, including two bookmobile sites serving rural communities. Student nurses assisted the public health nurses as they completed community assessments and tailored services to the needs of each library. Working with library patrons, nurses completed 3,746 encounters and 1,160 assessments; 1,420 health education sessions; and 192 referrals for services. They also provided health education to 76 library staff members. During the third year, nurses provided diverse health education and services to patrons. Services include assistance applying for public or private insurance, diabetes education, flu vaccine, and health education for library staff.

Using the Omaha System and an automated documentation system to capture community-level data had numerous benefits. Included were communication between the nurses and between the nurses and their health department; an evidence-based approach to practice; a standardized method of assessment, care planning, services, and evaluation; and a process that generated accurate and consistent data capable of conversion to information and useful reports.

## PRACTICE LINKAGES

There are no limits to the diversity of clients who live in the community, their problems, and their strengths; the interventions that nurses provide; and the client outcome data that are generated. Although many examples are diverse, as can be seen in the practice application on page 907, they represent a small fraction of the actual roles and responsibilities of home health, palliative, and hospice nurses. The examples illustrate fundamental principles of professional practice: (1) a holistic approach to the steps of the nursing or problem solving process; (2) client engagement or a partnership with clients as unique individuals, families, and communities; and (3) a focus on outcomes.

The following sections of the chapter are designed to increase the reader's understanding about the links between systematic best practices, evidence-based practice, and other aspects of the home health, palliative, and hospice milieu. The typical nurse will not be involved with the theme of each section daily, but will over a period of months.

Setting short- and long-term goals provides criteria for evaluation and increases continuity of care and the potential for improved outcomes. Research has shown that goals set with the client rather than for the client are more successful regarding self-motivation, adherence, and attainment (Evans et al, 2013; Sacco et al, 2013; Naylor et al, 2013; Bowles et al, 2014b).

### Outcome and Assessment Information

The Centers for Medicare and Medicaid Services (CMS) mandated the Outcome and Assessment Information Set (OASIS) as part of the Conditions of Participation for Medicare-certified home health agencies in 1999 (Fazzi Associates, 2010b; CMS,

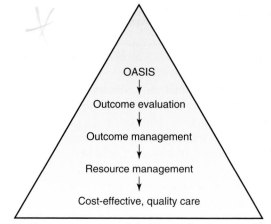

**FIG 41-4** The outcome model. (From Centers for Medicare and Medicaid Services: *Outcome-based quality improvement [OBQI] implementation manual,* August 2010, p. 2.9.)

2012b; O'Connor and Davitt, 2012). Completion of OASIS provides a systematic comparative measurement of client outcomes at two points in time. The goal of OASIS is to demonstrate improved, cost-effective client outcomes as a result of home health services for agency reports and for public reporting. It was designed to represent selected core items that are a part of a comprehensive assessment for an adult, nonmaternity home health client, and form the basis for measuring client outcomes for outcome-based quality improvement. OASIS also provides data for calculating the agency's reimbursement, and promotes a standardized approach to surveys (Figure 41-4) (CMS, 2012b; Fazzi Associates, 2010b; NAHC, 2013a; Fazzi Associates, 2014).

OASIS-C has had major revisions to improve its comprehensiveness, ease of use, reliability, and validity. The current version has 114 data elements or structure/process/outcome items, each followed by a list of choices or fill-in-the-blanks. The next revision, OASIS-C1, consists of approximately 110 data elements and is compatible with ICD-10. OASIS-C1 was scheduled to replace OASIS-C late in 2014. However, due to delays in the implementation of ICD-10, a modified OASIS-C1 (referred to as OASIS-C1/ICD-9 version) was created and implemented January 2015 (CMS, 2015). OASIS-C1/ICD-10 version will go into effect when the ICD-10 is implemented (CMS, 2015). (See Resource Tool 41.A on the Evolve website for one part of this assessment.)

OASIS is a complex and important component of home health practice. A nurse or other clinician provides care in the client's residence. While providing care, the clinician collects and completes the functional, demographic, and clinical data assessment items, the primary sections of OASIS. The goal of data collection is to use an evidence-based approach to care; generate outcomes data across time; improve communication among the agency's clinicians, other agency staff, and external groups; and improve reimbursement.

Registered nurses or physical, occupational, or speech and language pathology therapists complete OASIS items at the start of care, after hospitalization, at the 60-day recertification date following admission, at discharge, and at other points in time.

Clinicians need to complete the initial OASIS accurately and consistently to reflect a client's actual status, and integrate OASIS with the other portions of the agency's comprehensive assessment. They or their colleagues compare initial data to future versions as do Medicare surveyors and reimbursement reviewers. Many home health agencies use a computerized clinical information system so that the clinician completes OASIS electronically; regardless, final data from OASIS must be submitted to CMS electronically.

OASIS offers a challenging assignment for those who provide direct care, and one that requires extensive orientation and review. In many agencies, nurse experts serve as compliance officers to help ensure accurate and consistent completion. Not only is evidence of the quality of care related to OASIS, but so is agency reimbursement and a publically available comparison to other agencies. Agencies may receive sanctions or be denied payment by CMS for services already provided based on claims data, audits, or surveys that reflect responses on OASIS. More recently, agencies have received Additional Development Requests (ADRs) generated by CMS. ADRs require agencies to submit extensive verification that the services they provided were essential; if verification is not adequate, agencies must initiate a legal appeal or return funds to CMS.

Target areas for emphasis on OASIS mirror challenges identified by nurses and home health agencies. Included are diabetic foot care, fall prevention, depression intervention, pain, pressure ulcers, safety, medication management, and infection control. Box 41-5 illustrates M2000 from OASIS, one of the items related to medication management. Although all target areas are important, the latter two are of special concern to many nurses employed in hospice and palliative programs as well as diverse public health and other health care settings; they are summarized below.

## Medication Management

Medication management is an important component of home health practice. The goal is to assist clients and family caregivers to become independent and reliable in managing medication administration at home, and prevent rehospitalizations. However, home health clients experience many challenges including the complexity of their chronic conditions, cognitive status, coordination of their medical care, drug–drug interactions and side effects of medications, and cost. Many home health clients are expected to take ten to thirty prescription and over-the-counter medications throughout the day. Too often, the number of medications is more than is clinically indicated, and results in increased confusion, urinary incontinence, increased weakness, and changes in sleeping patterns. Riker and Setter (2012) describe this as *polypharmacy*, and discuss its assessment, causes, and management.

Corbett et al (2010) found that medication discrepancies were astoundingly widespread during the transition from hospital to home. In their study of 101 subjects, 94% had at least one discrepancy, most had 3.3, and some had more; discrepancies were identified in almost all classes of medications. Home health nurses expect to spend considerable time with medication reconciliation, and address medications during initial and subsequent home visits. Unlike clients in residential settings, home health clients may or may not have all of their medications, may not take them as ordered, and may store them inappropriately. When nurses ask to see medications, they are often given a box or bag that includes current medications and ones that are extremely outdated or were prescribed for other family members.

Home health nurses use numerous interventions including those that are evidence-based. Teaching clients to use a medication organizer for oral medications is frequently an initial intervention. However, that does not ensure that medications will be taken appropriately; subsequent teaching, return demonstrations, and surveillance are essential. In addition, clients and caregivers need diverse materials about medication benefits, interactions, and side-effects as well as the steps they should take to communicate that information to others. Materials need to be simple, understandable, and in the appropriate language. Clients who cannot read need graphic materials.

Many tools are available in addition to those specific for home health nurses. Morisky and his colleagues (1986) were early researchers who established concurrent and predictive validity for a four-item self-reported medication scale; they continued to expand their research. Corbett et al (2010) emphasized the need for sufficient medication teaching at hospital discharge, accurate assessment at home care admission, and the use of more sophisticated Agency for Healthcare Research and Quality (AHRQ) toolkits. The 17 toolkits are designed for professionals, clients, and consumers for use in acute care settings and at home (AHRQ, 2011). Reidt et al (2014) conducted a study to explore the benefit of a pharmacist serving as a home health agency team member; findings included a positive clinical impact on clients. An excellent, comprehensive resource is the Medication Adherence Educators Toolkit, the product of a competition by schools of pharmacy (AACP/NCPA, 2013). It consists of four sections: assessing medication adherence, improving medication adherence through the use of aids, empowering patients to improve medication adherence, and resolving barriers to medication adherence. The toolkit includes evidence-based detailed information that addresses literacy, e-reminders, interprofessional practice, and cultural awareness.

> ### BOX 41-5    Example of an Item from OASIS-C
>
> M2000 Drug Regimen Review: Does a complete drug regimen review indicate potential clinically significant medication issues (for example: adverse drug reactions, ineffective drug therapy, significant side effects, drug interactions, duplicate therapy, omissions, dosage errors, or noncompliance [non-adherence])?
>
> 0—Not assessed/reviewed [Go to M2010]
> 1—No problems found during review [Go to M2010]
> 2—Problems during drug review
> NA—Patient is not taking any medications [Go to M2040]
>
> Centers for Medicare and Medicaid Services (CMS): *OASIS C1.* 2015. Available at http://www.cms.gov/Medicare/Quality-Initiatives-Patient-Assessment-Instruments/HomeHealthQualityInits/OASIS-C1.html. Accessed April 24, 2015.

As experienced in an evidence-based practice improvement project at a large home care agency in the northeastern United States, other factors such as dementia and medication nonadherence present challenges. Home care nurses searched and critically evaluated the literature to find and use evidence-based screening tools to identify clients with cognitive impairment and medication adherence issues and created plans of care based on the latest published evidence to address these issues (Ferrar et al, 2012).

## Infection Prevention

Infection prevention is an important priority in home health and hospice practice. Infection prevention usually focuses on wound care, and invasive devices such as urinary and intravenous catheters as well as chest, tracheostomy, gastrostomy, and other tubes. Preventing infection by promoting appropriate vaccinations such as flu and pneumonia is also a priority. Most importantly, nurses need to assume that every client is potentially infected or colonized with an organism that can be transmitted, and recognize that all blood and body secretions may contain transmissible agents. They need to be familiar with the infectious process, research evidence and best practices, bag technique, personal protective equipment, cleaning equipment, medical waste management, and infection control programs. Nurses need to practice sound technique during each and every client encounter (see How To box).

---

**HOW TO**   **Promote Infection Prevention Standards**

*The practice of standard precautions means that all blood and body fluids must be treated as potentially infectious. Standard precautions are implemented to prevent exposure and infection of family caregivers and health care providers.*

- *Use extreme care to prevent injuries when handling needles, scalpels, and razors. Do not recap, bend, break, or remove needles from syringes before disposal. Discard needles and syringes in puncture-resistant containers made of plastic or metal and dispose of them as directed by agency policy or community guidelines.*
- *Wear barrier precautions such as gloves, masks, eye covering, and gowns when contact with blood and body fluids is expected. Use masks in combination with eye protection to eliminate contact with respiratory secretions or sprays of blood or body fluids during invasive respiratory procedures or wound irrigations.*
- *Use aseptic technique with all sterile injection equipment.*
- *Double bag and discard soiled dressings or other materials contaminated with body fluids in polyethylene garbage bags.*
- *Clean kitchen counters, dishes, and laundry with warm water and detergent after use. Clean bathrooms with a household disinfectant.*
- *Hand hygiene is the single most important practice in preventing infections. Hand hygiene should be performed before and after providing client care and before and after preparing food, eating, feeding, or using the bathroom.*
- *For clients with multidrug resistant organisms, limit the amount of nondisposable equipment brought into the home; use disposable stethoscopes, etc. when possible.*

---

Nurses need to become familiar with evidence-based practice literature specific to infection prevention. The Centers for Disease Control and Prevention (CDC) offers a variety of materials including guidelines to prevent the most frequent infections (CDC, 2014). Publications by other authors describe home health and hospice infection prevention and control programs and lessons learned as well as nosocomial and health care acquired infections (Swanson and Jeanes, 2011; McGoldrick, 2013; Poff et al, 2014). Evidence-based publications are also available that target specific therapies and illustrate the translation of research into practice. Gorski (2004, 2010) is a home infusion therapy expert and has published extensively about central venous access devices (CVADs). Gorski states that infections are preventable when four topics are implemented consistently: attention to hand hygiene, site assessment and care, use of aseptic technique with all infusion-related procedures, and thorough education for the client and family. In 2013, the American Society for Parenteral and Enteral Nutrition (ASPEN) published a comprehensive set of recommendations about parenteral nutrition safety (Ayers et al, 2014). Specific details about parenteral nutrition infusion and blood samples are described in the Evidence-Based Practice box.

---

### EVIDENCE-BASED PRACTICE BOX

The question "What practices maintain patient safety during the infusion of parenteral nutrition?" is included in ASPEN's parenteral nutrition safety publication. One of the 18 recommendations for this question is vascular access devices used for parenteral nutrition administration should not be used to obtain blood samples for laboratory tests unless no peripheral access is available. Evidence indicates that vascular access devices are a leading cause of serious adverse complications, in particular, central-line associated bloodstream infection. In addition, blood specimens drawn from vascular access devices have resulted in incorrect values and inappropriate treatment. When the recommendation was followed in recent years, infection rates were reduced substantially. Many home care organizations have added this recommendation to their protocols; all should do so.

**Nurse Use:** Nurses who provide parenteral nutrition care in the home should become familiar with this comprehensive publication.

From Ayers et al: A.S.P.E.N. parenteral nutrition safety consensus recommendations. *JPEN J Parenter Enteral Nutr* 38:296–333, 2014.

---

## ACCOUNTABILITY AND QUALITY MANAGEMENT

### Evidence-Based Quality/Performance Improvement

All providers, whether they are within community-based settings, hospitals, long-term care, or private practices, are accountable to their clients, reimbursement sources, and professional standards. Accountability is directly linked to quality or the degree to which health services for individuals, families, and communities increase the likelihood of desired health outcomes, and are consistent with current professional knowledge. Florence Nightingale is often credited with establishing standards of care, demonstrating the value of evidence-based practice, and analyzing health-related outcome data successfully.

Most home health, palliative, and hospice providers have a long history of evaluating the quality of care they provided to their clients. Often, agencies use a systematic, triangulated approach in their pursuit of excellence that includes hiring qualified personnel, new employee orientation, mentoring programs, case conferences, supervisory shared visits, record audits, utilization reviews, quality studies, client satisfaction surveys, in-service education, recognition for outstanding performance, and annual evaluations. Some agencies became accredited as a way to distinguish themselves from other providers.

The sophistication of quality and performance improvement strategies used in home health, palliative care, and hospice has dramatically improved in recent years. Changes were prompted by the interest in research-based practice that has evolved into programs of research and evidence-based practice, use of computers and the Internet, guidelines developed by the National Quality Forum (2014), and the mandate from Medicare to use OASIS and Outcome-Based Quality Improvement. Nurses should have access to current research literature, critique that research, and apply it to their practice (Melnyk and Fineout-Overholt, 2011; O'Connor and Davitt, 2012; CMS, 2014b; Melnyk et al, 2014). Several frameworks have been described to guide evidence-based practice projects (Levin et al, 2010; Melnyk and Fineout-Overholt, 2011; Malloch and Melnyk, 2013).

Evaluating the quality of care professionally and legally should be done in many ways, but documentation is of special significance. The steps of the nursing process must be documented and include communication with team members, physicians, and community resources. It is through the clinical record that nurses demonstrate that they are delivering quality care and identifying strategies to improve the quality of care.

## Outcome-Based Quality Improvement

Outcome measurement and cost control are the focus of the CMS Outcome-Based Quality Improvement (OBQI) program. Their definition of outcomes is (1) health status changes between two or more time points, where the term "health status" encompasses physiologic, functional, cognitive, emotional, and behavioral health; (2) changes that are intrinsic to the client; (3) positive, negative, or neutral changes in health status; and (4) changes that result from care provided or natural progression of disease and disability, or both (CMS, 2014b).

Data from OASIS-C are part of the two-stage CMS OBQI framework to produce various reports (see Figure 41-5). The first stage, outcome analysis, enables an agency to compare its performance to a national sample, note factors that may affect outcomes, and identify final outcomes that show improvement in or stabilization of a client's condition. Comparing agency data and trends to a national sample is also known as benchmarking, an analysis process that has been used by many businesses but is relatively new to health care. CMS collects and publishes Health Compare Scores publically. The second stage, known as outcome enhancement, enables the agency to select specific client outcomes and determine strategies to improve care. Reports include agency-client–related characteristics (case mix), potentially avoidable events (adverse event outcomes), and end-result and utilization outcomes. The reports are for a

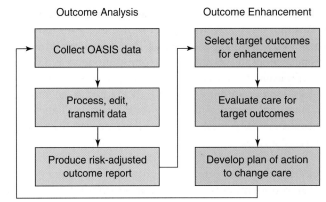

Outcome Analysis        Outcome Enhancement

**FIG 41-5** Two-stage Outcome-Based Quality Improvement framework. (From Centers for Medicare and Medicaid Services: *OASIS-C guidance manual*, December 2012b, p. F.3.)

12-month period, the agency's previous 12-month period, and national reference or comparative data. Comparisons are risk adjusted for client differences, both over time for the agency and between the agency and the reference group. Similarly to OASIS, a detailed manual describes the OBQI program; the most recent manual was published in 2010 (CMS, 2014b).

## Accreditation

Home health and hospice providers participate in several different continuous quality improvement options. They may elect to meet the accreditation standards of one of the following groups and complete the Medicare survey according to their guidelines: the Joint Commission, the Community Health Accreditation Program of the National League for Nursing, or the Accreditation Commission for Health Care. If providers do not seek accreditation, Medicare surveyors will conduct regular reviews. In 2007, the Public Health Accreditation Board was established to offer national public health accreditation. Because some home health and hospice programs are integrated with health departments, they will participate in public health accreditation (PHAB, 2014).

After an agency applies for accreditation, a lengthy self-study must be completed that addresses all aspects of the agency's operation, and an accreditation team schedules a site visit. Both accrediting organizations review agencies' organizational structure, compliance with Medicare Conditions of Participation, care provided during home visits and documentation of those visits, and the outcomes of client care with a focus on improved health status. Site visitors accompany nurses and other clinicians on home visits to observe the steps of the problem-solving process in action. To maintain accreditation, agencies must follow guidelines and undergo periodic reviews. In the future, accreditation may become a requirement for licensure of all home health agencies.

## PROFESSIONAL DEVELOPMENT AND COLLABORATION

### Education, Certification, and Roles

Nurses are employed in home health, palliative care, and hospice from a variety of educational and practice backgrounds. They should be educated to function at a high level of competency so that they can be relied on not only by their professional colleagues, but also by the community. They have diverse roles and responsibilities in their practice settings; autonomy is a fundamental characteristic that was mentioned earlier in this chapter. Nurses are responsible for basing their practice on research evidence. A growing number of home health, palliative, and hospice nurses are conducting research; some are members of interprofessional research teams. Their studies add to the body of knowledge for evidence-based practice, especially when the focus is outcomes of care. The application of existing evidence and generation of new research must be priorities to increase the quality and cost-effectiveness of care (Smith, 2012; Mager and Grossman, 2013; ANA, 2014; ANA/HPNA, 2014).

The educational preparation of the 132,400 nurses employed in home health agencies varies greatly (NAHC, 2010). According to the ANA (2014), a baccalaureate degree in nursing should be the minimum requirement for entry into professional practice. According to the 2014 Home Health Nursing Scope and Standards, completion of a baccalaureate degree is the appropriate and preferred educational preparation. Roles for nurses include care management and coordination of care, education, advocacy, administration, supervision, and quality improvement. The nurse with a baccalaureate degree functions in the role of a generalist, providing skilled nursing and coordinating care for a variety of clients. Nurses with a master's degree are prepared for roles as clinical specialists, nurse practitioners, researchers, administrators, or educators. Educational programs are increasing to prepare nurses for advanced practice roles in home health. As home health continues to expand, the need for specialized nurse clinicians will also increase to meet the highly technological and complex care needs of individuals, families, and communities. In managed care, more clinical specialists will be needed to provide case management and to develop programs to meet the needs of the population served by the managed care network. Nurse practitioners can provide primary care to frail older adults and other homebound clients.

The Hospice and Palliative Nurses Association (HPNA) offers many conferences, certification examinations, and credentialing (ANA/HPNA, 2014). There are approximately 14,000 credentialed registered hospice and palliative nurses. Licensed registered nurses may qualify for two levels of specialty practice certification that are differentiated by education, complexity of practice, and performance of certain nursing functions. Generalists provide direct care, function as educators, case managers, nurse clinicians, administrators, and other roles. The advanced practice certification is for a nurse prepared at the master's level or higher as a clinical nurse specialist or nurse practitioner. Roles of the advanced practice nurse include expert clinician, leader and facilitator of interprofessional teams, educator, researcher, consultant, collaborator, advocate, case manager, or administrator.

## Interprofessional Collaboration

Typically, home health, palliative, and hospice nurses are members of interprofessional teams. The primary goal of the team is to help clients achieve their maximum level of health,

> **BOX 41-6 Factors for Successful Interprofessional Collaboration**
>
> **Knowledge**
> 1. Understand how the group process can be used to achieve group goals.
> 2. Understand problem solving.
> 3. Understand role theory.
> 4. Understand what other professionals do and how they view their roles.
> 5. Understand the differences between client levels of acuity across levels of care, including acute care, home care, ambulatory care, and long-term care.
>
> **Skills**
> 1. Use principles of group process effectively.
> 2. Communicate clearly and accurately.
> 3. Communicate without using the profession's jargon.
> 4. Express self clearly and concisely in writing.
>
> **Attitudes**
> 1. Feel confident in role as a professional.
> 2. Trust and respect other professionals.
> 3. Share tasks with other professionals.
> 4. Work effectively toward conflict resolution.
> 5. Be flexible.
> 6. Adopt an attitude of inquiry.
> 7. Be timely.

self-care, and independent functioning in a safe environment. Medicare regulations, professional organizations, and state licensing boards influence team composition and functions. Box 41-6 shows successful interprofessional collaboration depending on the knowledge, skills, and attitudes of each team member. When team members work collaboratively in partnership with clients, families, and volunteers, the plan of care can be implemented effectively and reinforced by all. Although each team member has a specific responsibility, any overlap in responsibilities can be beneficial for reinforcement. Team members communicate through e-mail, phone calls, and face-to-face case conferences to review the plan of care, client progress, and team effectiveness (Martin, 2005; Zerwekh, 2006; Humphrey and Milone-Nuzzo, 2010; Marrelli, 2012).

Details about the role of nurses have been described in other sections of this chapter. Nurses often serve as the team leader or care manager in part because nursing service may be the client's primary need. Larger agencies may expand their nursing services to include wound and ostomy, intravenous, psychiatric/mental health, nurse practitioner, and other nursing specialists.

Physicians are an integral part of interprofessional teams; they submit initial and interim orders and review and sign the initial and updated plan of care. Many agencies hire a physician on a part-time basis or have an agreement with a physician who serves as a voluntary consultant. Because state laws are changing rapidly, nurse practitioners are increasingly involved and may have responsibilities similar to physicians. In addition, agencies may have specialized services such as podiatrists, pharmacists, registered dietitians, respiratory therapists, music therapists, psychologists, and chaplains.

Physical therap. other occupations LEGAC
LEGAL...

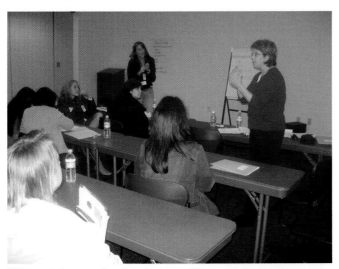

FIG 41-6 Interprofessional team. (From www.omahasystem .org/photogallery.html. Used with permission from Karen S. Martin, RN, MSN, FAAN.)

The services of physical therapists, occupational therapists, speech and language pathologists, social workers, and home health aides are available in most agencies. They may be employed by the agency or hired through contractual agreements. Their roles are summarized below.

- Physical therapists: Provide maintenance, and preventive and restorative treatment that includes strengthening muscles, restoring mobility, controlling spasticity, gait training, and teaching active and passive resistive exercises.
- Occupational therapists: Focus on upper extremities to restore muscle strength and mobility for functional skills and performance of activities of daily living.
- Speech and language pathologists: Evaluate speech and language abilities, develop a plan of care, and teach clients to improve their communication involving speech, language, or hearing.
- Social workers: Help clients and families manage social, emotional, and environmental factors that affect their well-being through identification and referral to appropriate community resources.
- Home health aides: Provide personal care and assist with activities of daily living under the supervision of nurses or physical therapists. Home health aides or homemakers may also help with light housekeeping, laundry, meal preparation, and shopping.

## LEGAL, ETHICAL, AND FINANCIAL ISSUES

The potential for human error as well as illegal and unethical activity exists in every health care organization. Examples of Medicare fraud and abuse in home health and hospice include inappropriate use of services, excessive payments to administrative staff or owners, "kickbacks" for referrals, and billing for visits and/or medical supplies that are not authorized or not provided. In addition, the complex regulations of CMS are difficult to understand and have not been interpreted consistently by Medicare surveyors.

Nurses are confronted with legal and ethical issues regularly. They need to be familiar with the living will, power of attorney for health care and do-not-resuscitate documents. In addition, they need to be informed about local, state, and federal regulations that govern their profession and nursing license; and those that govern their employers. They need to be alert for potential problems or violations and identify solutions in a proactive manner. The privacy guidelines of the Health Insurance Portability and Accountability Act of 1996 (USDHHS, 2014a) ensures protection of clients' personal health information and includes provisions about informed consent. The legislation also allows clients full access to their health care records (Marquis and Huston, 2011; Smith, 2012).

Nurses are expected to follow professional, legal, and ethical standards to deliver care to clients, develop trusting relationships, act as client advocates, and help clients and families increase their self-advocacy skills. Because these responsibilities can produce tension, nurses need to recognize their personal values and biases to make certain they do not interfere with those of clients and families. Nurses should continually reassess client and family needs to avoid inappropriate use and overuse of services. The safety of clients who live alone as well as family caregiver neglect and/or abuse are ethical concerns. If the clients' needs are greater than what reimbursement allows, nurses need to talk to the clients, their families, and agency personnel to consider alternatives. In addition, many agencies have established ethics committees to assist with ethical dilemmas.

Home health, palliative, and hospice nurses are at risk for malpractice claims related to the complexity of care, failure to adhere to standards of practice, and other errors (Marquis and Huston, 2011; Smith, 2012). Nurses and their employers need to be proactive by taking responsibility for personal and agency actions. A focus on communication with clients, families, and the health care team; commitment to providing quality care; documentation refresher sessions; performance improvement programs; use of evidence-based practice guidelines; and appropriate use of information technology and telehealth are strategies that can help reduce risks.

Reimbursement for home health, palliative care, and hospice is complex and tenuous; historical milestones are described earlier in this chapter, and more details about economics and reimbursement are included in Chapter 5. Medicare, state and local governments, Medicaid, and managed care are the principal funding sources for home health and hospice (Buhler-Wilkerson, 2007; HAA, 2010; NAHC, 2010; Fazzi et al, 2010b; NAHC, 2013a; Zerwekh and Warner, 2014; Fazzi Associates, 2014). If clients meet the eligibility criteria for the Conditions of Participation, Medicare is used as their primary payment source. When clients no longer meet those criteria and still require care, their services may be reimbursed by Medicaid, private insurance, donations, or the agency's United Way and other special needs funds. Home health and hospice providers are watching closely to see what impact the 2010 Patient Protection and Affordable Care Act (ACA) will have on their clients and programs (Kaiser Family Foundation, 2013; Zerwekh and Warner, 2014; Fazzi Associates, 2014). Several provisions may be beneficial to rural agencies, improve transitions of care, provide more preventive services, and offer more options to those who are disabled to live at home rather than in long-term care facilities. Other provisions may be negative: hospice providers have new regulations involving medications, reimbursement for visits is being questioned more aggressively, and Medicare funding to home health is scheduled to decrease. In addition, the increasing speed of consolidation and merger of health care systems is resulting in closures of facilities or reduction of services that include home health agencies.

Nurses who work in home health, palliative care, and hospice are involved with financial aspects of care to a greater extent than most other nurses. Nurses and their social work colleagues must be well informed about services that are covered by Medicare and other funding sources, and recognize how tenuous those funding sources are. Clients and families often ask for help to understand decisions about care and the numerous notices and bills that they receive. Nurses participate directly in decisions about the frequency, length, and type of client services, and their documentation needs to accurately support those decisions. Nurses must be knowledgeable about the reimbursement of medical supplies and should discuss problematic situations with clients, families, and agency personnel. Clients and families may be unhappy when their specific requests cannot be granted.

## TRENDS AND OPPORTUNITIES

### National Health Objectives

The overarching goals of the *Healthy People 2020* objectives (USDHHS, 2014b) are as follows:

- Attain high-quality, longer lives free of preventable disease, disability, injury, and premature death.
- Achieve health equity, eliminate disparities, and improve the health of all groups.
- Create social and physical environments that promote good health for all.
- Promote quality of life, healthy development, and healthy behaviors across all life stages.

Nurses who work with clients and families in the home and community have opportunities to promote achievement of key objectives. They can assess client status, identify available resources and gaps to meet client needs, encourage clients and families to use resources, and coordinate care with other providers and community agencies. They can participate in numerous population-level projects and campaigns.

The Healthy People 2020 box highlights objectives relevant to home health and hospice nurses. Note that many objectives relate to lifestyle issues. With appropriate health education, referral to community resources, and follow-up, there is a potential to reduce morbidity and mortality and decrease chronic disabilities. Nurses can make important contributions on one-to-one and population-focused levels.

### Organizational and Professional Resources

It is increasingly important for nurses to be involved in political, economic, and regulatory issues at the local, state, and national

**HEALTHY PEOPLE 2020**

**Examples of National Health Objectives for the Year 2020**
- AOCBC-11: Reduce hip fractures among older adults.
- C-1: Reduce the overall cancer death rate.
- C-13: Increase proportion of cancer survivors beyond 5 years.
- CKD-9: Reduce kidney failure due to diabetes.
- HD-3: Reduce stroke deaths.
- HDS-1: (Developmental) Increase overall cardiovascular health in the U.S. population.
- HDS-5: Reduce the proportion of persons in the population with hypertension.
- IID-4: Reduce invasive pneumococcal infections.

U.S. Department of Health and Human Services: *Healthy People 2020: 2020 Topics and Objectives-Objectives A-Z.* 2014b. Available at http://www.healthypeople.gov/2020/topicsobjectives2020/default.aspx. Accessed May 6, 2014.

levels before they affect practice and services to clients. Joining organizations, reviewing the Internet, networking with colleagues, and reading professional literature provide opportunities to become informed and influence decisions.

Nationally, several prominent home health organizations have extensive resources and websites. The National Association for Home Care & Hospice (NAHC) is a trade organization formed in 1982. A few years later, the Hospice Association of America (HAA) and NAHC developed an organizational partnership. Many agencies join as members, but nurses can also participate in the nursing section after joining as individual members. Lobbying is NAHC's primary focus; it also schedules an annual meeting, publishes a journal (*Caring*), and offers educational opportunities. The Visiting Nurse Association of America, formed in 1983, has a similar focus, but membership is limited to community-based, nonprofit home health and hospice providers. *Home Healthcare Nurse, Home Health Care Management and Practice, Family and Community Health, Journal of Community Health Nursing,* and *Home Health Care Services Quarterly* are additional journals for home health clinicians and managers.

Hospice and palliative care organizations also have extensive resources and websites. The National Hospice and Palliative Care Organization was formed in 1978 to stimulate public and professional interest. The Hospice Foundation of America was founded in 1982; its initial mission was fundraising. The Hospice Nurses Association was formed in 1986. About 12 years later, the organization expanded and became the Hospice and Palliative Nurses Association (HPNA), and also changed the name of its national certification board. HPNA now has more than 11,000 members. The organization schedules conferences, publishes the *Journal of Hospice and Palliative Nursing,* and offers certification and credentialing. The *American Journal of Hospice and Palliative Care, Journal of Pediatric Oncology Nursing, International Journal of Palliative Nursing,* and other related journals address nursing practice, pain control, oncology, and medical practice. It is interesting to note that the title of the organization's publication changed from *Hospice and Palliative Nursing Scope and Standards of Practice* in 2007 to *Palliative Nursing: Scope and Standards of Practice—An Essential*

*Resource for Hospice and Palliative Nurses* in 2014 (HPNA/ANA, 2007; ANA/HPNA, 2014).

Home health, palliative, and hospice nurses belong to a variety of specialty organizations such as Infusion Nurses Society; Wound, Ostomy, and Continence Nurses Society; American Public Health Association; and Healthcare Information and Management Systems Society along with nurses employed in diverse settings. It is important that they share their knowledge about community-focused practice by being active members, speaking, and writing for publication.

## Technology, Informatics, and Telehealth
### Technology

Advances in technology, informatics, and telehealth are pervasive in health care and nursing practice; they are a window to the present and future. Many home health and hospice nurses have developed specialized skills with the following: extensive dressing changes, parenteral nutrition, chemotherapy, intravenous therapy for hydration and antibiotics, intrathecal pain management, ventilators, and apnea monitors. As mentioned earlier in the chapter, clients and family caregivers must learn to complete procedures and manage equipment frequently. It is the responsibility of the nurse and fellow team members to determine if such procedures and equipment can be used safely; when the answer is yes, team members must provide sufficient education, demonstrations, and monitoring so that care continues safely. Advances in technology, informatics, and telehealth should not be viewed as replacements for nurses and team members, but as tools to improve the quality of their practice. The tools are evolving rapidly, influencing the practice of home health nurses, and transforming home health operations.

### Informatics

Informatics is one of the most important new tools for nurses, including those employed in community settings (Sensmeier, 2011; Cipriano et al, 2013; Friedman et al, 2013; Nelson and Staggers, 2014; Sockolow et al, 2014; HealthIT.gov, 2014). Nurses face urgent information management challenges that include the need for timely, reliable, and valid quantified data and information about clients, the services they receive, and their outcomes of care. They also need verbal and automated methods to communicate with other nurses and health care providers wherever they are in the community. Increasingly, agencies require clinicians to document care during the visit rather than in their office or other location (Martin, 2005; Correll and Martin, 2009; Westra et al, 2010; Martin et al, 2011; Monsen et al, 2011; Martin and Utterback, 2014; Sockolow et al, 2014; Topaz et al, 2014; Fazzi Associates, 2014).

The American Nurses Association anticipated the impact of information technology on the profession, and took the first step early in the 1990s. They began to recognize standardized terminologies that could be used by nurses and other health care disciplines to describe, document, and quantify their daily practice accurately and consistently (ANA, 2012; ANA, 2014; Omaha System, 2014). The Omaha System and 11 more interface or point-of-care and reference terminologies have been recognized. The Omaha System is an interface or point-of-care terminology; clinicians see it imbedded in their clinical documentation systems and need to learn to use it accurately and consistently.

The second step involves interoperability—the exchange of coded data and ability to use those data (ANA, 2012; Sensmeier, 2011; Bowles et al, 2013). SNOMED CT and Logical Observation Identifiers, Names, and Codes (LOINC) are examples of reference terminologies that facilitate interoperability by sharing data generated by the interface terminologies. Minnesota is the first state to recommend that health care providers use both ANA-recognized standardized point-of-care and reference terminologies. In 2014, Minnesota released their decision that the Omaha System should be the point-of-care terminology for the software used by all home health, public health, and other community-based providers (Omaha System, 2014).

The third step is meaningful use. This suggests that better health care does not come solely from the adoption of technology itself, but through the exchange and use of electronic health information to best inform clinical decisions at the point-of-care (Martin et al, 2011; HealthIT.gov, 2014; Omaha System, 2014). Meaningful use incorporates complex processes and workflow involving nurses and all health care clinicians, and it requires data integration and accessibility. Minnesota's requirement is part of their eHealth and Integrating the Healthcare Enterprise (IHE) strategy to actualize meaningful use through the use of the Consolidated Continuity of Care Document (C-CDA). Their mandate indicates that all providers will have interoperable EHRs by 2015. When more states proceed, there will be a nation-wide health information network.

Health care providers throughout the United States are converting to EHRs rapidly. EHRs are becoming ubiquitous, and the Office of the National Coordinator was established for that reason (HealthIT.gov, 2014). As part of the 2009 American Recovery and Reinvestment Act (ARRA), and the Health Information Technology for Economic and Clinical Health (HITECH) Act, CMS provides reimbursement incentives for eligible professionals and hospitals to become "meaningful users" (Sensmeier, 2011; Friedman et al, 2013; Kaiser Family Foundation, 2013). In physician practices, EHR use increased from approximately 48% in 2009 to 72% in 2012 (CDC, 2012). The percentage of use in hospitals more than doubled in two years, increasing from 16% in 2009 to 35% in 2013 (Paddock, 2012). Although home health agencies cannot obtain funding through AARA, their reported use of EHRs was 43% in 2007, and exceeded 58% in 2013 (NAHC, 2013b). The privacy guidelines of HIPAA (USDHHS, 2014a) ensure protection of clients' personal health information and include provisions about informed consent.

Personal health records (PHRs) are another important development (Anderson et al, 2012; HealthIT.gov, 2014). A PHR is also an electronic collection of health-related information, but individuals manage and control their own health information rather than clinicians and agencies. Typically, a PHR includes a health history, medications, allergies, and results from laboratory and other tests.

The Blue Button is a PHR initiative that began in 2010 by the Department of Veterans Affairs. Soon an online patient portal was launched. While their initiative is limited to veterans, many other groups use the Blue Button symbol. Usage of the Blue Button logo and brand is free, but must conform to user guidelines (The Blue Button, 2014). The goal is to encourage as many people as possible to use a Blue Button site to download their own health information.

Increasingly, individuals and families served by home health, palliative, and hospice nurses have informatics skills. They may use the Internet frequently and be well informed about diagnoses, treatments, and medications. They may also use smart phones, other mobile devices, and social media. Nurses need to inquire about their clients' skills rather than make assumptions based on their age or other factors.

### Telehealth

Telehealth supports long-distance health care, client and professional health-related education, and public health and health administration using electronic information and telecommunications technologies (Institute of Medicine (IOM), 2012; Schlachta-Fairchild et al, 2014). The technology used varies to include videoconferencing, the Internet, store-and-forward imaging, streaming media, satellite, wireless communications, and plain old telephone systems. Telehealth equipment and program components include telephone triage and advice, and biometric telemonitoring equipment to measure vital signs, weight, cardiac function, and point-of-care diagnostics. The system may or may not include video technology for live interaction (IOM, 2012; Schlachta-Fairchild et al, 2014).

The increased availability of telehealth coincides with trends described in this and other chapters in this book: an aging population, increased chronic illness and costs, and changes in health care reimbursement. New trends promote new opportunities: home health, palliative, and hospice nurses can use innovations such as telehealth in combination with in-person visits. They can monitor health status and symptom recognition, provide education, increase communication, and enable clients to become active partners in their own care (Fazzi et al, 2010; IOM, 2012; Madigan et al, 2013; Schlachta-Fairchild et al, 2014; Fazzi Associates, 2014). Telehealth has emerged as a viable and acceptable way to supplement the delivery of health care economically.

Numerous studies have confirmed that telehealth is used successfully to improve physical, emotional, and financial health outcomes for diverse home health clients. Chen et al (2011) studied those who had multiple chronic conditions. Many researchers explored the relationship between telehealth and circulatory problems. The study by Wakefield et al (2011) focused on diabetes and hypertension, Gellis et al (2012) on heart or chronic respiratory failure, Madigan et al (2013) on heart failure, Woods and Snow (2013) on circulatory and/or respiratory diagnoses, Hoban et al (2013) on heart failure, and Heeke et al (2014) on heart failure. Gellis and colleagues (2014) also studied elders with depression. Woods and Snow (2013) found that those who participated in a telemonitoring intervention had significantly lower rates of rehospitalization and emergency room use. When Heeke and colleagues (2014) completed their pilot study, no clients had been readmitted to the hospital.

Telemonitoring is increasingly being used with infants, women with high-risk pregnancies, and adults with various health problems. Smart homes are emerging to help the older adult to "age in place" (Rantz et al, 2013). Sensors can monitor activities and detect adverse events such as a fall or lack of movement and trigger a call for help. Medication management devices remind clients to take their medications, dispense medications, and send alerts to providers if devices are not accessed as expected (Marek et al, 2013). The next generation of devices is expected to focus on handheld devices such as smartphone technology, making telemonitoring even more ubiquitous.

## SUMMARY

These are changing times for home health, palliative care, and hospice. The need for nurses prepared to practice in these specialties is expected to grow as the population ages, chronic illness rises, and more care is delivered in the community. Practice will become ever more complex and diverse as individuals and their families request more choices and personalized care. Practice will require a strong educational background and a commitment to life-long learning. It will require the use of enhanced critical thinking and sound judgment as well as interpersonal, communication, and technological skills. It is a good time to celebrate the past, embrace the present, and look forward to the future.

---

**(QSEN) FOCUS ON QUALITY AND SAFETY EDUCATION FOR NURSES**

**Targeted Competency**

Client-Centered Care: Recognize the client or designee as the source of control and full partner in providing compassionate and coordinated care based on respect for client's preferences, values, and needs.

Important aspects of client-centered care include:

- **Knowledge:** Demonstrate comprehensive understanding of the concepts of pain and suffering, including physiologic models of pain and comfort.
- **Skills:** Elicit expectations of client and family for relief of pain, discomfort, or suffering.
- **Attitudes:** Recognize that client expectations influence outcomes in management of pain or suffering.

**Client-Centered Care Question**

Visit a community-based hospice or palliative care unit. Spend time observing the care provided in this setting.

1. How is care provided in this setting different from care you have seen in the acute care setting? In the home care setting?
2. Notice how nurses and nursing assistants assess pain in this environment.
3. Discuss with the nurses how they address concerns around pain and suffering with clients and families in this environment. How do nurses evaluate clients' and families' expectations around pain?
4. Discuss with the nurses differences in care approaches between a community-based hospice or palliative care versus care approaches for home hospice and palliative care. Is there additional education that is required for the client and family, because the family often provides some aspects of care for home hospice and palliative care?

Prepared by Gail Armstrong, PhD(c), DNP, ACNS-BC, CNE, Associate Professor, University of Colorado Denver College of Nursing.

## PRACTICE APPLICATION

The first example is an individual who lives alone, the second is an individual whose family includes an involved spouse, and the third and fourth clients are the community. Ideally, the student who visits Martha P. and the home health nurse who visits Mr. and Mrs. Jones use portable computing devices and document in the EHRs in the home. The childcare health consultants use a single electronic documentation system, can communicate easily about practice, and are creating a state-wide database. The public health nurses who are part of the Library Nurse Project use laptops for documentation.

Martha P. is an older woman who lives in a deteriorating home. She is a relatively typical client for a student or home health nurse to visit. Box 41-7 consists of a story and answers designed to promote independent learning and group discussion. Note that the story and answers should be congruent: all pertinent data in the story should be reflected in the answers and all answers should match pertinent details in the story.

Mr. Jones, the second clinical example, is also a relatively typical client. After reading the example, identify the Omaha System problems, interventions, and ratings that are illustrated in the story. Discuss key characteristics of practice during this visit and an appropriate care plan for the next visit.

Mr. Jones, 70 years old, was discharged from the hospital yesterday after heart surgery for coronary artery disease and was referred to the local home health agency. Today, the home health nurse admitted him for skilled nursing care services. The nurse assessed Mr. Jones' cardiovascular status, the healing of his incisions, adjustment to his postsurgical status, and level of self-care. The nurse talked to Mr. and Mrs. Jones about exercise, nutrition, the signs and symptoms of possible postoperative cardiac problems, and their coping. Together, they looked at his medications. Mrs. Jones indicated that they were getting along well, but were concerned about the high cost of his new medications. They reviewed Mr. Jones' discharge packet. The nurse emphasized the need to maintain close communication with his physician and nurse practitioner, and the need to participate in the local exercise and nutrition rehabilitation program that they had prescribed. Mr. and Mrs. Jones indicated that they would do so. Before the visit ended, the nurse completed the necessary forms, documented the visit, and offered to call a local social service agency about financial assistance for medications. They made an appointment for the nurse's return visit.

The third clinical example describes the Arizona childcare health consultant program. In 1987, two public health departments in Arizona began to offer childcare health consultation services to childcare programs. They recognized that if the health and safety of young children in childcare environments was not addressed, related efforts to advance quality standards for children could not succeed (Ford and Linker, 2002). The nurses from Pima and Maricopa counties scheduled regular visits to childcare centers, family childcare homes, and Head Start centers. They worked collaboratively with providers to impact issues such as communicable disease, playground safety, safe infant sleep, medication management, and the inclusion of children with special health needs in the group setting. The nurses kept anecdotal notes and frequency counts for the number of consultation visits they made and how many staff members attended their educational programs. In time, they and their health departments realized that they had an information overload: their data were inconsistent and difficult to access, and were not organized in a way to produce meaningful reports.

In 2005, Kathi Ford and the Pima County Health Department participated in a pilot childcare quality improvement project that involved childcare health consultants. Such a consultant is a "licensed health professional with education and experience in child and community health and childcare and preferably specialized training in child care health consultation" (AAP/APHA, 2011, p. 33). The Omaha System and an automated clinical information system were used to capture their data. Although their nursing practice did not change, the data collection, analysis, and reporting changed dramatically. Using community as the modifier, it was possible to describe and quantify common problems, interventions, and changes in Knowledge, Behavior, and Status.

Arizona has voluntary quality improvement and rating system for child care, First Things First's "Quality First" program. Early in 2010, all First Things First–supported child care health consultants began to document their services in a single web-accessed charting system based on the Omaha System. Soon, data from the Omaha System's Problem Rating Scale for Outcomes suggested needed modifications in the service delivery model (Ramler et al, 2006; Banghart and Kreader, 2012).

The home visit is the hallmark of nursing in home health and hospice. Nurses are guests when they enter a client's home, and must recognize that their services can be accepted or rejected. The interpersonal relationship established during the first visit is critical, as is the initial assessment of the client, support system, and environment.

A. What strategies should the nurse use to develop a positive relationship during the first visit?

B. What are the most important elements to assess in the home environment?

C. What should the nurse do to establish a partnership with the client?

D. What is necessary for the nurse to include in the client contract?

E. How can the nurse determine the client's preferred learning style?

**Answers can be found on the Evolve site.**

## BOX 41-7   Martha P.: Older Woman Living in a Deteriorating Home

Joan B. Castleman, RN, MS, Clinical Associate Professor
College of Nursing, University of Florida
Gainesville, Florida

### Information Obtained During the First Visit/Encounter

Martha P. was a 93-year-old woman who lived by herself in a deteriorating house. She had kyphosis and arthritis that contributed to her unsteady gait. Martha rarely used her cane in her house, but steadied herself by holding on to furniture.

When a student nurse arrived, Martha was shivering under a thin blanket. Boxes filled with old papers were stacked along the walls. The student nurse asked Martha if she had wood for the stove that heated the house. She replied that she ran out of wood yesterday and said, "I don't know what I'm going to do, but I'm not leaving this house." She reported that people from a church had brought the last load of wood. The student asked permission to contact Concerned Neighbors, a volunteer organization that could provide firewood. Martha was pleased. The student expressed concern that the boxes of paper, especially those near the stove, were a fire hazard. "Those boxes have been there for years, and I use them to light the stove," Martha said. When the student asked if she could help Martha move the four boxes near the stove to the other wall, she grudgingly agreed.

The student nurse noted that Martha was wearing a "Lifeline necklace," a fall alert system, and asked about her history of falls. Martha described how she moved around her home and fell in the bathroom last week when she was trying to take a sponge bath. She pushed the button, and "two nice gentlemen from the fire department came to pick me up." The student and Martha walked around her house. They talked about where she fell in the past, how fortunate she was not to have injuries, and ways to decrease her risk of falling in the future. Martha was willing to have a personal care assistant visit weekly to help her with a bath and shampoo as long as there was no charge. Before leaving, the student took Martha's vital signs and blood pressure and noted that they were within normal limits. The student called Concerned Neighbors and arranged for firewood to be delivered that day; the student also telephoned a local health assistance organization to schedule a home health aide to provide personal care for the next week. Although Martha sounded grumpy, she asked the student to return.

### Application of the Omaha System

Problem: Residence (High Priority)

### Problem Classification Scheme

Modifiers: Individual and Actual
Signs/symptoms of Actual:
   Inadequate heating/cooling
   Cluttered living space
   Unsafe storage of dangerous objects/substances

### Intervention Scheme

Category: Teaching, Guidance, and Counseling
Targets and Client-specific Information: Safety (moved boxes away from stove; Martha unwilling to dispose of papers)
Category: Case Management
Targets and Client-specific Information: Other community resources (referred to Concerned Neighbors; arranged delivery of firewood)
Category: Surveillance
Targets and Client-specific Information: Home (needed wood)

### Problem Rating Scale for Outcomes

Knowledge: 2—minimal knowledge (not aware/unwilling to recognize fire hazards)
Behavior: 2—rarely appropriate behavior (unable/unwilling to make changes)
Status: 2—severe signs/symptoms (residence was livable but needed changes)
Domain: Physiological

### Problem: Neuro-Musculo-Skeletal Function (High Priority)

### Problem Classification Scheme

Modifiers: Individual and Actual
Signs/symptoms of Actual:
   Limited range of motion
   Decreased balance
   Gait/ambulation disturbance

### Intervention Scheme

Category: Teaching, Guidance, and Counseling
Targets and Client-specific Information: Mobility/transfers (ways to decrease risk of falling, absence of injuries, continue wearing "Lifeline necklace")
Category: Surveillance
Targets and Client-specific Information:
   mobility/transfers (how, when falls occurred)
   signs/symptoms—physical (falls/injuries; vital signs, blood pressure)

### Problem Rating Scale for Outcomes

Knowledge: 2—minimal knowledge (knew few options to decrease falls)
Behavior: 2—rarely appropriate behavior (had not used cane in house; did wear and use "Lifeline necklace")
Status: 3—moderate signs/symptoms (activities restricted, fell last week)
Domain: Health-Related Behaviors

### Problem: Personal Care (High Priority)

### Problem Classification Scheme

Modifiers: Individual and Actual
Signs/symptoms of Actual:
   Difficulty with bathing
   Difficulty shampooing/combing hair

### Intervention Scheme

Category: Teaching, Guidance, and Counseling
Targets and Client-specific Information: Personal hygiene (needed help with bathing, shampoo)
Category: Case Management
Targets and Client-specific Information: Paraprofessional/aide care (referred to health assistance organization for home health aide)

### Problem Rating Scale for Outcomes

Knowledge: 3—basic knowledge (knew she needed to bathe, but not aware of assistance)
Behavior: 3—inconsistently appropriate behavior (tried to take a sponge bath)
Status: 3—moderate signs/symptoms (cannot bathe safely without help)

This case illustrates use of the Omaha System with a client in the home. Talk with your classmates and other colleagues about how use of the Omaha System can guide your practice and documentation and can generate aggregate data to promote high-quality home health service. Identify Martha P.'s strengths and how to maximize those when providing care.

From Martin KS: The Omaha System: *A Key to Practice, Documentation, and Information Management*, Omaha, NE, 2005, Health Connections Press.

## KEY POINTS

- Home health, hospice, and palliative nursing practice provided in the client's home differ from care in institutional settings. The home setting affects practice in unique ways including establishing trust, developing care partnerships (patient engagement), selecting interventions, collecting outcomes and data, ensuring client safety, and promoting quality.
- Family members, including caregivers and significant persons who provide assistance and/or care, are essential members of the health care team.
- Home health has its roots in public health nursing, with an emphasis on health promotion, illness prevention, and caring for people in their communities.
- Home health and hospice practice and reimbursement changed when they became major Medicare benefits.
- Five models of care are described in this chapter: population-focused home care, transitional care, home-based primary care, home health, and palliative care/hospice. Home health, palliative, hospice, and all other nurses should become familiar with the models to inform clients and their families about options and educate providers who are potential referral sources.
- Medicare-certified home health and hospice agencies are divided into various types of administrative and organizational structures. However, many aspects of nursing practice are the same in the various types.
- Standards of home nursing practice originate from the ANA and specialty organizations, and encourage adoption of evidence-based practice.
- Consistently demonstrating professional competency is essential for home health, hospice, and palliative nurses.
- Home health nurses practice in accordance with the ANA (2014) *Home Health Nursing Scope and Standards of Practice*.

- Hospice and palliative nurses use the *Palliative Nursing: Scope and Standards of Practice—An Essential Resource for Hospice and Palliative Nurses* published by the ANA and Hospice and Palliative Nurses Association (2014).
- Interprofessional collaboration is inherent in home health, palliative care, and hospice.
- The Omaha System was developed and refined through a process of research. Reliability and validity were established for the entire system.
- The Omaha System is unique in that it is the only comprehensive vocabulary developed initially by and for nurses practicing in the community.
- The Omaha System consists of the Problem Classification Scheme (assessment), Intervention Scheme (care plans and services), and Problem Rating Scale for Outcomes (client change/evaluation).
- The Omaha System is designed to enhance practice, documentation, and information management. These areas are of concern to community health educators and students as well as clinicians and administrators.
- Interprofessional clinicians employed in Medicare-certified home health agencies use OASIS-C at designated intervals; it is the outcome measurement tool mandated by the Centers for Medicare and Medicaid Services' conditions of participation.
- Evidence-based quality/performance improvement is important in all home health and hospice agencies. Currently, Medicare's Outcome-Based Quality Improvement program is used for outcome measurement and cost control.
- Exciting trends and opportunities are pervasive in home health, palliative, and hospice care. Many nurses are developing skills using technology, informatics, and telehealth; a commitment to life-long learning is necessary.

## CLINICAL DECISION-MAKING ACTIVITIES

1. Make a home visit with an experienced home health or hospice nurse and do the following:
   A. Evaluate the process and content of the nurse–client interaction to determine what aspects of the visit were based on evidence-based practice; describe the process of the visit.
   B. Compare actual roles and functions with the *Home Health Nursing: Scope and Standards of Practice* (ANA, 2014), the *Palliative Nursing: Scope and Standards of Practice—An Essential Resource for Hospice and Palliative Nurses* (ANA/ HPNA, 2014), or other specialty standards as appropriate for the client population.
   C. Observe and discuss whether that nurse uses a client problem/nursing diagnosis, intervention, or outcome measurement system or framework. Is it important to use a system or framework approach? Explain.

2. Work with a partner or in a small group. Select a client you have visited or invent a fictitious client, and list data for a typical referral and initial visit. Independently apply the three parts of the Omaha System to the client data. Compare each portion of your selections with that of your partner or group members.
3. Make a joint home visit with another health care professional and assess as in the preceding activity. Attend a client/ family–provider conference and write a summary of the group process. Has your attitude changed after you listened to the opinions expressed by family members?
4. Review a client record. What client outcomes were met through home health care? What specific outcomes showed an improvement or a stabilizing condition?
5. Interview a home health or hospice nurse who uses electronic health records (EHRs). Ask about the advantages of

## CLINICAL DECISION-MAKING ACTIVITIES—cont'd

EHRs and challenges associated with them. How can aggregate clinical data generated by EHRs help nurses better understand the needs of their clients? How might knowing the needs of their clinical population assist in reviewing the research literature and planning new interventions?

6. Review your state's laws governing advance directives. Consider the legal and ethical advantages and disadvantages of

having such directives. How would you write an advance directive for yourself?

7. Participate in a telehomecare visit using video technology or observe the analysis of data from remote monitoring. Trace the nurse's decision making and changes in the plan of care based on the telemonitoring data. Determine what outcomes might be expected from this type of care.

## REFERENCES

Abele CL, Nies MA: Home health and hospice. In Nies MA, McEwen M, editors: *Community/Public Health Nursing: Promoting the Health of Populations*, ed 5. St Louis, 2011, Elsevier, pp 649–666.

Agency for Healthcare Research and Quality (AHRQ): *Patient Safety Tools: Improving Safety at the Point of Care*. 2011. Available at: http://www.ahrq.gov/professionals/quality-patient-safety/patient-safety-resources/pips/index.html. Accessed May 5, 2014.

American Academy of Pediatrics, American Public Health Association (AAP/APHA), National Resource Center for Health and Safety in Child Care and Early Education: *Caring for Our Children: National Health and Safety Performance Standards: Guidelines for Early Care and Education Programs*, ed 3. Elk Grove Village, IL, 2011, American Academy of Pediatrics. Available at: cfoc.nrckids.org/WebFiles/CFOC3-color-small.pdf. Accessed April 24, 2014.

American Association of Colleges of Pharmacy and National Community Pharmacists Association (AACP/NCPA): *Medication Adherence Educators toolkit*. 2013. Available at: http://www.aacp.org/resources/education/Documents/AACP%20NCPA%20Medication%20Adherence%20Educators%20Toolkit.pdf. Accessed May 4, 2014.

American Nurses Association (ANA): *ANA Recognized Terminologies That Support Nursing Practice*. 2012. Available at: http://www.nursingworld.org/MainMenuCategories/ThePracticeofProfessionalNursing/NursingStandards/Recognized-NursingPractice-Terminologies.pdf. Accessed April 26, 2014.

American Nurses Association (ANA): *Home Health Nursing: Scope and Standards of Practice,*, ed 2. Silver Spring, MD, 2014. Nursesbooks.org.

American Nurses Association and Hospice and Palliative Nurses Association (ANA/HPNA): *Palliative*

*Nursing: Scope and Standards of Practice—An Essential Resource for Hospice and Palliative Nurses*. Silver Spring, MD, 2014. Nursesbooks.org.

Anderson C, Hull S, Murphy J, et al: Ask for your health records week campaign. *Comput Inform Nurs* 30:577–578, 2012.

Arend J, Tsang-Quinn J, Levine C, et al: The patient-centered medical home: history, components, and review of the evidence. *Mt Sinai J Med* 79:433–450, 2012.

Ayers P, Adams S, Boullata J, et al: A.S.P.E.N. parenteral nutrition safety consensus recommendations. *JPEN J Parenter Enteral Nutr* 38:296–333, 2014.

Banghart P, Kreader JL: *What Can CCDF Learn from the Research on Children's Health and Safety in Child Care?* Washington, DC, 2012, Office of Planning, Research, and Evaluation/Urban Institute. Available at: http://www.acf.hhs.gov/sites/default/files/opre/synthesis_brief_1.pdf. Accessed April 21, 2014.

Beales JL, Edes T: Veteran's Affairs home based primary care. *Clin Geriatr Med* 25:149–154, 2009.

Berwick DM, Nolan TW, Whittington J: The Triple Aim: care, health, and cost. *Health Aff* 27:759–769, 2008.

Bidassie B, Davies ML, Start R, et al: VA experience in implementing patient-centered medical home using a breakthrough series collaborative. *J Gen Intern Med* 29(Suppl 2):S563–S571, 2014.

Black JM, Hawks JH: *Medical Surgical Nursing*, ed 8. St Louis, 2009, Saunders, p 94.

Boling PA: Care transitions in home health. *Clin Geriatr Med* 25:135–148, 2009.

Bowles KH: Developing evidence-based tools from EHR data. *Nurs Manage* 45:18–20, 2014.

Bowles KH, Holmes JH, Ratcliffe SJ, et al: Factors identified by experts to support discharge referral

decision making. *Nurs Res* 58:115–122, 2009.

Bowles KH, Pham J, O'Connor M, et al: Information deficits in home care: a barrier to evidence-based disease management. *Home Health Care Manag Pract* 22:278–285, 2010.

Bowles KH, Potashnik S, Ratcliff SJ, et al: Conducting research using the electronic health record across multi-hospital systems. *J Nurs Adm* 43:355–360, 2013.

Bowles KH, Hanlon AL, Holland DE, et al: Impact of discharge planning decision support on time to readmission among older adult medical patients. *Prof Case Manag* 19:29–38, 2014.

Brooten D, Youngblut JM, Brown L, et al: A randomized trial of nurse specialist home care for women with high risk pregnancies: outcomes and costs. *Am J Manag Care* 7:793–803, 2001.

Buhler-Wilkerson K: No place like home: a history of nursing and home care in the U.S. *Home Healthc Nurse* 20:641–647, 2002.

Buhler-Wilkerson K: Care of the chronically ill at home: an unresolved dilemma in health policy for the United States. *Milbank Memorial Fund Q* 85:611–639, 2007.

Candy B, Holman A, Leurent B, et al: Hospice care delivered at home, in nursing home and in dedicated hospice facilities: a systematic review of quantitative and qualitative evidence. *Int J Nurs Stud* 48:121–133, 2011.

Carcone AL, Ellis DA, Naar-King S: Linking caregiver strain to diabetes illness management and health outcomes in a sample of adolescents in chronically poor metabolic control. *J Dev Behav Pediatr* 33:343–351, 2012.

Center to Advance Palliative Care (CAPC): *Growth of Palliative Care in U.S. Hospitals: 2013 Snapshot*. 2013. Available at: http://www.capc.org/capc-growth-analysis-snapshot-2013.pdf. Accessed May 6, 2014.

Centers for Disease Control and Prevention (CDC): *Use and Characteristics of Electronic Health Records Systems among Office-based Physician Practices: United States, 2001-2012*. 2012. Available at: http://www.cdc.gov/nchs/data/databriefs/db111.htm. Accessed May 5, 2014.

Centers for Disease Control and Prevention (CDC): *Healthcare-associated Infections (HAIs)-Guide to infection prevention for outpatient settings: Minimum expectations for safe care*. 2014. Available at: http://www.cdc.gov/HAI/settings/outpatient/outpatient-care-guidelines.html. Accessed April 24, 2015.

Centers for Medicare and Medicaid Services (CMS): *National Health Expenditure Accounts: Methodology Paper*. 2012a. Available at: http://www.cms.gov/Research-Statistics-Data-and-Systems/Statistics-Trends-and-Reports/NationalHealthExpendData/downloads/dsm-12.pdf. Accessed April 23, 2014.

Centers for Medicare and Medicaid Services (CMS): *2012 OASIS-C Guidance Manual*. 2012b. Available at: http://www.cms.gov/Medicare/Quality-Initiatives-Patient-Assessment-Instruments/HomeHealthQualityInits/HHQIOASISUserManual.html. Accessed May 4, 2014.

Centers for Medicare and Medicaid Services (CMS): *Readmissions Reduction Program: Readmissions Reduction Program*. 2013a. Available at: http://www.cms.gov/Medicare/Medicaid-Fee-for-Service-Payment/AcuteInpatientPPS/Readmissions-Reduction-Program.htm. Accessed April 27, 2014.

Centers for Medicare and Medicaid Services (CMS): *2013 CMS Statistics*. 2013b. Available at: http://www.cms.gov/Research-Statistics-Data-and-Systems/Statistics-Trends-and-Reports/CMS-Statistics-Reference-Booklet/Downloads/CMS_Stats_2013_final.pdf. Accessed April 24, 2015.

Centers for Medicare and Medicaid Services (CMS): *FY 2015 Hospice Payment Rate Update.* 2014a. Available at: http://www.cms.gov/Medicare/Medicare-Fee-for-Service-Payment/Hospice/Hospice-Regulations-and-Notices-Items/cms-1609-P.html?DLPage=1&DLSort=38DLSortDir=descending. Accessed May 6, 2014.

Centers for Medicare and Medicaid Services (CMS): *OASIS OBQI.* 2014b. Available at: http://www.cms.gov/Medicare/Quality-Initiatives-Patient-Assessment-Instruments/HomeHealthQualityInits/HHQIOASISOBQI.html. Accessed May 6, 2014.

Centers for Medicare and Medicaid Services (CMS): *OASIS C1.* 2015. Available at: http://www.cms.gov/Medicare/Quality-Initiatives-Patient-Assessment-Instruments/HomeHealthQualityInits/OASIS-C1.html. Accessed April 24, 2015.

Chang C, Jackson SS, Bullman TA, et al: Impact of a home-based primary care program in an urban Veterans Affairs medical center. *J Am Med Directors Assoc* 10:133–137, 2009.

Chen HF, Kalish MC, Pagan JA: Telehealth and hospitalizations for Medicare home healthcare patients. *Am J Manag Care* 17(6 Spec No.):e224–e230, 2011.

Cipriano PF, Bowles K, Dailey M, et al: The importance of health information technology in care coordination and transitional care. *Nurs Outlook* 61:475–489, 2013.

Clark J, Lang N: An international classification for nursing practice. *Int Nurs Rev 39* 27:109, 1992.

Coleman EA, Berenson RA: Lost in transition: challenges and opportunities for improving the quality of transitional care. *Ann Intern Med* 140:533–536, 2004.

Corbett CF, Setter SM, Daratha KB, et al: Nurse identified hospital to home medication discrepancies: implications for improving transitional care. *Geriatr Nurs* 31:188–196, 2010.

Correll PJ, Martin KS: The Omaha System helps a public health organization find its voice. *CIN Comp Inform Nurs* 27:12–15, 2009.

Davis K, Stremikis K: Family medicine: preparing for a high performance health care system. *J Am Board Fam Med* 23(Suppl 1):S11–S16, 2010.

Dobell LG, Newcomer RJ: Integrated care: incentives, approaches, and future considerations. *Social Work Public Health* 23:25–47, 2008.

Donahue MP: *Nursing, the Finest Art,* ed 3. St Louis, 2011, Elsevier.

Donelan-McCall N, Eckenrode J, Olds DL: Home visiting for the prevention of child maltreatment: lessons learned during the past 20 years. *Pediatr Clin North Am* 56:389–403, 2009.

Eckenrode J, Campa M, Luckey DW, et al: Long-term effects of prenatal and infancy nurse home visitation on the life course of youths 19-year follow-up of a randomized trial. *Arch Pediatr Adolesc Med* 164:9–15, 2010.

Evans JM, Baker GR, Berta W, et al: The evolution of integrated health care strategies. *Adv Health Care Manag* 15:125–161, 2013.

Fazzi R, Ashe T, Reissig M: The same but different: three insider's views of hospital-based, hospital affiliated, and freestanding agencies. *Caring* 29:32–36, 2010a.

Fazzi Associates: *OASIS-C Best Practice Manual: Developed at the National OASIS-C Best Practice Forum.* 2010b. Available at: http://www.fazzi.com/+1_files/documents/research-and-resources/OASIS-C_Best_Practice_Manual.pdf. Accessed May 4, 2014.

Fazzi Associates: *2013-2014 National State of the Home Care Industry Study for Home Health and Hospice.* 2014. Available at: http://www.fazzi.com/tl_files/documents/Fazzi%20State%20of%20the%20Industry%20Study%20Report.pdf. Accessed September 7, 2014.

Ferrante JM, Balasubramanian BA, Hudson SV, et al: Principles of the patient-centered medical home and preventive services directory. *Ann Fam Med* 8:108–116, 2010.

Ferrar L, Lauder B, Levin R, et al: Implementing an evidence-based practice improvement program in a community health agency: the Visiting Nurse Service of New York experience, Part II. In Levin R, Feldman H, editors: *Teaching Evidence-based Practice,* ed 2. New York, 2012, Springer.

First Things First: *Who we are.* 2010. Available at: http://www.azftf.gov/whoweare/pages/default.aspx. Accessed April 24, 2015.

Ford KM, Linker LA: Compliance of licensed child care centers with the American Academy of Pediatrics' recommendations for infant sleep positions. *J Community Health Nurs* 19:83–91, 2002.

Friedberg MW, Lai DJ, Hussey PS, et al: A guide to the medical home as a practice-level intervention. *Am J Manag Care* 15:S291–S299, 2009.

Friedman DJ, Parrish RG, Ross DA: Electronic health records and US public health: current realities and future promise. *Am J Public Health* 103:1560–1567, 2013.

Garvin JH, Martin KS, Stassen DL, et al: The Omaha System: coded data that describe patient care. *J AHIMA* 79:44–49, 2008.

Gellis ZD, Kenaley B, McGinty J: Outcomes of a telehealth intervention for homebound older adults with heart or chronic respiratory failure: a randomized controlled trial. *Gerontologist* 52:541–552, 2012.

Gellis ZD, Kenaley BL, Ten Have T: Integrated telehealth care for chronic illness and depression in geriatric home care patients: the Integrated Telehealth Education and Activation of Mood (I-TEAM) Study. *J Am Geriatr Soc* 62:889–895, 2014.

Gomes B, Calanzani N, Curiale V, et al: Effectiveness and cost-effectiveness of home palliative care services for adults with advanced illness and their caregivers. *Cochrane Database Syst Rev* Issue 6, Arto. No. CD007760, 2013.

Gorski LA: Making a commitment to clinical data. *Home Health Care Manag Pract* 16:206–211, 2004.

Gorski LA: Central venous access device associated infections. *Home Healthc Nurse* 28:221–229, 2010.

HealthIT.gov: *About ONC.* 2014. Available at: http://www.healthit.gov/newsroom/about-onc. Accessed May 6, 2014.

Heeke S, Wood F, Schuck J: Improving care transitions from hospital to home: standardized orders for home health nursing with remote telemonitoring. *J Nurs Care Qual* 29:E21–E28, 2014.

Hill DL, Miller V, Walter JK, et al: Regoaling: a conceptual model of how parents of children serious illness change medical care goals. *BMC Palliat Care* 13:9, 2014.

Hinds PS, Oakes LL, Hicks J, et al: Parent-clinician communication intervention during end-of-life decision making for children with incurable cancer. *J Palliat Med* 15:916–922, 2012.

Hinds PS, Schum L, Baker JN, et al: Key factors affecting dying children and their families. *J Palliat Med* 8(Suppl 1):S70–S78, 2005.

Hoban MB, Fedor M, Reeder S, et al: The effect of telemonitoring at home on quality of life and self-care behaviors of patients with heart failure. *Home Healthc Nurse* 31:368–377, 2013.

Hospice Association of America (HAA): *Hospice Facts and Statistics.* Washington, DC, 2010, HAA. Available at: http://www.nahc.org/assets/1/7/HospiceStats10.pdf. Accessed April 22, 2014.

Hospice and Palliative Nurses Association and American Nurses Association (HPNA/ANA): *Hospice and Palliative Nursing: Scope and Standards of Practice.* Silver Spring, MD, 2007, Nursesbooks.org.

Humphrey CJ, Milone-Nuzzo P: Transitioning nurses to home care. In Harris MD, editor: *Handbook of Home Health Care Administration,* ed 5. Sudbury, MA, 2010, Jones and Bartlett, pp 515–527.

Innes S: *Library nurses look after those in need, Arizona Daily Star.* Tucson, AZ, 2012. Available at: http://azstarnet.com/news/science/health-med-fit/library-nurses-look-after-those-in-need/article_6ee73756-17a6-50ff-afb1-d3921b85e8b2.html. Accessed April 21, 2014.

Institute of Medicine (IOM): *The Role of Telehealth in an Evolving Health Care Environment: Workshop Summary.* Washington, DC, 2012, National Academies Press. Available at: http://books.nap.edu/openbook.php?record_id=13466.

Kaiser Family Foundation: *Focus on Health Reform: Summary of the Affordable Care Act.* 2013, Kaiser Family Foundation. Available at: http://kaiserfamilyfoundation.files.wordpress.com/2011/04/8061-021.pdf. Accessed May 5, 2014.

Kitzman H, Olds DL, Sidora K, et al: Enduring effects of nurse home visitation on maternal life course: a 3-year follow-up of a randomized trial. *JAMA* 283:1983–1989, 2000.

Kübler-Ross E: *On Death and Dying.* New York, 1969, McMillan.

Leff B, Burton L, Mader SL, et al: Comparison of functional outcomes associated with hospital at home care and traditional acute hospital care. *J Am Geriatr Soc* 57:273–278, 2009.

Levin R, Keefer JM, Marren J, et al: Evidence-based practice: merging two paradigms. *J Nurs Care Qual* 25:117–126, 2010.

Levine D, Lam CG, Cunningham MJ, et al: Best practices for pediatric palliative cancer care: a primer for clinical providers. *J Support Oncol* 11:114–125, 2013.

Mack JW, Joffe S: Communicating about prognosis: ethical responsibilities of pediatricians and parents. *Pediatrics Suppl* 1:S24–S30, 2014.

Madden KA, Waldo M, Cleeter D: The specialized role of the RN in the Program of All-inclusive Care for the Elderly (PACE) interdisciplinary care team. *Geriatr Nurs* 35:199–204, 2014.

Madigan E, Schmotzer BJ, Struk CJ, et al: Home health care with telemonitoring improves health status for older adults with heart failure. *Home Health Care Serv Q* 32:57–74, 2013.

Mager DR, Grossman S: Promoting nursing students' understanding and reflection on cultural awareness with older adults in home care. *Home Healthc Nurse* 31:582–590, 2013.

Malloch K, Melnyk BM: Developing high-level change and innovation agents: competencies and challenges for executive leadership. *Nurs Adm Q* 37:60–66, 2013.

Malloy P, Paice J, Virani R, et al: End-of-life nursing education consortium: 5 years of educating graduate nursing faculty in excellent palliative care. *J Prof Nurs* 24:352–357, 2008.

Marek KD, Stetzer F, Ryan PA, et al: Nurse care coordination and technology effects on health status of frail older adults via enhanced self-management of medication: randomized clinical trial to test efficacy. *Nurs Res* 62:269–278, 2013.

Marquis BL, Huston CJ: *Leadership Roles and Management Functions in Nursing: Theory and Application,* ed 7. Philadelphia, 2011, Lippincott, Williams & Wilkins.

Marrelli TM: *The Handbook of Home Health Standards: Quality, Documentation, and Reimbursement,* ed 5. St. Louis, 2012, Elsevier.

Marsteller JA, Burton L, Mader SL, et al: Health care provider evaluation of a substitutive model of hospital at home. *Med Care* 47:979–985, 2009.

Martin KS: *The Omaha System: A Key to Practice, Documentation, and Information Management,* reprinted, ed 2. Omaha, NE, 2005, Health Connections Press.

Martin KS, Monsen KA, Bowles KH: The Omaha System and meaningful use: applications for practice, education, and research. *Comput Inform Nurs* 29:52–58, 2011.

Martin KS, Utterback KB: Home health and related community-based systems. In Nelson R, Staggers N, editors: *Health Informatics: An Interprofessional Approach.* St. Louis, 2014, Elsevier, pp pp147–pp163.

McGoldrick M: Surveillance, identification and reporting of infections. In *Home Care Infection Prevention and Control Program. Home Health Systems.* St. Simons Island, GA, 2013, Author.

Meadows CA, Fraser J, Camus S, et al: A system-wide innovation in transition services: transforming the home care liaison role. *Home Healthc Nurse* 32:78–86, 2014.

Melnyk BM, Fineout-Overholt E: *Evidence-based Practice in Nursing and Healthcare: A Guide to Best Practice.* Philadelphia, 2011, Lippincott, Williams & Wilkins.

Melnyk BM, Gallagher-Ford L, Long LE, et al: The establishment of evidence-based practice competencies for practicing registered nurses and advanced practice nurses in real-world clinical settings: proficiencies to improve healthcare quality, reliability, patient outcomes, and costs. *Worldviews Evid Based Nurs* 11:5–15, 2014.

Mistovich JJ, Karren KJ, Hafen B: *Prehospital Emergency Care,* ed 10. Upper Saddle River, NJ, 2014, Pearson Education.

Monsen KA, Westra BL, Oancea SC, et al: Linking home care interventions and hospitalization outcomes for frail and non-frail elderly patients. *Res Nurs Health* 34:160–168, 2011.

Moorman SM, Macdonald C: Medically complex home care and caregiver strain. *Gerontologist* 53:407–417, 2013.

Morisky DE, Green LW, Levine DM: Concurrent and predictive validity of a self-reported measure of medication adherence. *Med Care* 24:67–74, 1986.

National Association for Home Care & Hospice (NAHC): *Basic Statistics About Home Care.* Washington, DC, 2010. Available at: http://www.nahc.org/assets/1/7/10HC_Stats.pdf. Accessed April 22, 2014.

National Association for Home Care & Hospice (NAHC): *Home Health Survey and Certification.* Washington, DC, 2013a. Available at: http://www.nahc.org/assets/1/7/104.pdf. Accessed May 4, 2014.

National Association for Home Care & Hospice (NAHC): *Voluntary Long-term Post-acute Care (LTPAC) Clectronic Health Record (EHR) Certification Program.* Washington, DC, 2013b, Home Care Technology Association of America. Available at: http://www.nahc.org/search/keywords=Adoption%20of%20EHRs. Accessed May 3, 2014.

National Consensus Project for Quality Palliative Care (NCP): *Clinical Practice Guidelines for Quality Palliative Care,* ed 3. Pittsburgh, PA, 2013, Author.

National PACE Association: *Who, What and Where Is PACE?* Available at: http://www.npaonline.org/website/article.asp?id=12&title=Who,_What_and_Where_Is_PACE? Accessed April 26, 2014.

National Quality Forum: *About Us.* 2014. Available at: http://www.qualityforum.org/Home.aspx. Accessed May 4, 2014.

Naylor MD: Transitional care for older adults: a cost-effective model. *LDI Issue Brief* 9:1–4, 2004.

Naylor MD, Aiken LH, Kurtzman ET, et al: The care span: the importance of transitional care in achieving health reform. *Health Aff* 30:746–754, 2011.

Naylor MD, Bowles KH, McCauley KM, et al: High-value transitional care: translation of research into practice. *J Eval Clin Pract* 19:727–733, 2013.

Naylor MD, Brooten D, Campbell R, et al: Comprehensive discharge planning and home follow-up of hospitalized elders: a randomized trial. *JAMA* 282:613–620, 1999.

Naylor MD, Hirschmann KB, Bowles KH, et al: Care coordination for cognitively impaired older adults and their caregivers. *Home Health Care Serv Q* 26:57–78, 2007.

Nelson R, Staggers N: *Health Informatics: An Interprofessional Approach.* St. Louis, 2014, Elsevier.

Nurse Family Partnership (NFP): *Proven effective through extensive research.* 2014. Available at: http://www.nursefamilypartnership.org/proven-results. Accessed April 25, 2014.

O'Connor M, Davitt JK: The Outcome and Assessment Information Set (OASIS): a review of validity and reliability. *Home Health Care Serv Q* 31:267–301, 2012.

Olds DL, Eckenrode J, Henderson CR Jr, et al: Long-term effects of home visitation on maternal life course and child abuse and neglect: fifteen year follow-up of randomized trial. *JAMA* 278:637–643, 1997.

Olds DL, Holmberg JR, Donelan-McCall N, et al: Effects of home visits by paraprofessionals and by nurses on children: follow-up of a randomized trial at ages 6 and 9 years. *JAMA Pediatr* 168:114–121, 2014.

Omaha System: 2014. Available at http://www.omahasystem.org. Accessed May 3, 2014.

Oguh O, Kwasny M, Carter J, et al: Caregiver strain in Parkinson's disease: National Parkinson Foundation Quality Initiative Study. *Parkinson Relat Disord* 19:975–979, 2013.

Paddock C: *Electronic Health Record Use in US Hospitals has Doubled in Last Two Years.* 2012, Medical News Today. Available at: http://www.medicalnewstoday.com/articles/241871.php. Accessed May 6, 2014.

Perry KM, Parente CA: Integrating palliative care into home care practice. In Harris MD, editor: *Handbook of Home Health Care Administration,* ed 5. Sudbury, MA, 2010, Jones and Bartlett, pp 863–875.

Poff RM, Browning SV: Creating a meaningful infection control program. *Home Healthc Nurse* 32:167–171, 2014.

Public Health Accreditation Board: *Advancing Public Health Performance.* 2014. Available at: info@phaboard.org. Accessed July 24, 2014.

Quad Council: *Quad Council Public Health Nursing Competencies.* 2011. Available at: http://www.phf.org/resourcestools/Pages/Public_Health_Nursing_Competencies.aspx. Accessed May 4, 2014.

Ramler M, Nakatsukasa-Ono W, Loe C, et al: *The Influence of Child Care Health Consultants in Promoting Children's Health and Well-Being: A Report on Selected Resources.* Newton, MA, 2006, Healthy Child Care Consultant Network Support Center. Available at: http://www.ecetp.pdp.albany.edu/hcc/wp-content/uploads/2010/10/Influence%20of%20Child%20Care%20Health%20Consultants%20Aug%202006%20Study.pdf. Accessed May 3, 2014.

Rantz MJ, Skubic M, Miller SJ, et al: Sensor technology to support aging in place. *J Am Med Dir Assoc* 14:386–391, 2013.

Reidt SL, Larson TA, Hadsall RS, et al: Integrating a pharmacist into a home healthcare agency care model. *Home Healthc Nurse* 32:146–152, 2014.

Riker GI, Setter SM: Polypharmacy in older adults in home: what it is and what to do about it. *Home Healthc Nurse* 30:474–487, 2012.

Robert Wood Johnson Foundation (RWJF): *Public Health Nurses Bringing Care to Libraries.* 2013. Available at: http://www.rwjf.org/en/blogs/human-capital-blog/2013/04/public_health_nurses.html. Accessed May 3, 2014.

Rockoff JD: A new ending for terminally ill patients: palliative-care programs aim to both improve care and cut costs. *Wall St J* R5, 2/24/14.

Sacco J, Deravin Carr DR, Viola D: The effects of the Palliative Medicine Consultation on the DNR status of African Americans in a safety-net hospital. *Am J Hosp Palliat Care* 30:363–369, 2013.

Sanders S, Mackin ML, Reyes J, et al: Implementing evidence-based practices: considerations for the hospice setting. *Am J Hosp Palliat Care* 27:369–376, 2010.

Schectman G, Stark R: Orchestrating large organizational change in primary care: the Veterans' Health Administration experience implementing a patient-centered medical home. *J Gen Intern Med* 29(Suppl 2):S550–S551, 2014.

Schlachta-Fairchild L, Rocca M, Cordi V, et al: Telehealth and applications for delivering care at a distance. In Nelson R, Staggers N, editors: *Health Informatics: An Interprofessional Approach.* St. Louis, 2014, Elsevier, pp 125–146.

Segelman M, Szydlowski J, Kinosian B, et al: Hospitalizations in the program of all-inclusive care for the elderly. *J Am Geriatr Soc* 62:320–324, 2014.

Sensmeier J: Transforming nursing practice through technology and informatics. *Nurs Manage* 42:20–23, 2011.

Smith MH: *The Legal, Professional, and Ethical Dimensions of Education in Nursing*, ed 2. New York, 2012, Springer.

Sockolow PS, Bowles KH, Adelsberger MC, et al: Impact of homecare electronic health record on timeliness of clinical documentation, reimbursement, and patient outcomes. *ACI* 5:445–462, 2014.

Sperber NR, King HA, Steinhauser K, et al: Scheduled telephone visits in the Veterans Health Administration patient-centered medical home. *BMC Health Serv Res* 14:145, 2014.

Sternberg SB, Co JP, Homer CJ: Review of quality measures of the most integrated health care settings for children and the need for improved measures: recommendations for initial care measurement set for CHIPRA. *Acad Pediatr* 11(3 Suppl):S49–S58, 2011.

Swanson J, Jeanes A: Infection control in the community: a pragmatic approach. *Br J Community Nurs* 16:282–288, 2011.

Swartwout K, Murphy MP, Dreher MC, et al: Advanced practice nursing students in the patient-centered medical home: preparing for a new reality. *J Prof Nurs* 30:139–148, 2014.

The Blue Button: 2014. Available at http://www.healthit.gov/patients-families/blue-button/about-blue-button. Accessed May 3, 2014.

Topaz M, Golfenshtein N, Bowles KH: The Omaha System: A systematic review of the recent literature. *J Am Med Inform Assoc* 21:163–170, 2014.

True G, Stewart GL, Lampman M, et al: Teamwork and delegation in medical homes: primary care staff perspectives in the Veterans Health Administration. *J Gen Intern Med* 20(Suppl 2):S632–S639, 2014.

U.S. Department of Health and Human Services (USDHHS): *Understanding Health Information Privacy: HIPAA*. 2014a. Available at: http://www.hhs.gov/ocr/privacy/hipaa/understanding/index.html. Accessed May 6, 2014.

U.S. Department of Health and Human Services: *Healthy People 2020: 2020 Topics and Objectives-Objectives A-Z*. 2014b. Available at: http://www.healthypeople.gov/2020/topicsobjectives2020/default.aspx. Accessed May 6, 2014.

Utens CM, van Schayck OC, Goossens LM, et al: Informal caregiver strain, preference and satisfaction in hospital-at-home and usual hospital care for COPD exacerbations: results of a randomised controlled trial. *Int J Nurs Stud* 51:1093–1102, 2014.

Visiting Nurse Service of New York (VNSNY): *Our services*. 2014. Available at: http://www.vnsny.org. Accessed May 3, 2014.

Wakefield BJ, Holman JE, Ray A, et al: Effectiveness of home telehealth in comorbid diabetes and hypertension: a randomized, controlled trial. *Telemed J* 17:254–261, 2011.

Westra BL, Oancea C, Savik K, et al: The feasibility of integrating the Omaha System data across home care agencies and vendors. *Comput Inform Nurs* 28:162–171, 2010.

Weissman DE, Meier DE: Identifying patients in need of a palliative care assessment in the hospital setting. *J Palliat Med* 14:1–7, 2011.

Wiener L, McConnell DG, Latella L, et al: Cultural and religious considerations in pediatric palliative care. *Palliat Support Care* 11:47–67, 2013.

Woods LW, Snow SW: The impact of telehealth monitoring. *Home Healthc Nurse* 31:39–45, 2013.

Zerwekh JV: *Nursing Care at the End of Life: Palliative Care for Patients and Families*. Philadelphia, 2006, FA Davis.

Zerwekh J, Warner KD: Clients receiving home health and hospice care. In Allender JA, Rector C, Warner KD, editors: *Community and Public Health Nursing*, ed 8. Philadelphia, 2014, Wolters Kluwer, pp 1041–1061.

# The Nurse in the Schools

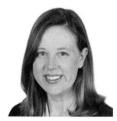

## Lisa Pedersen Turner, PhD, RN, PHCNS-BC

Lisa Pedersen Turner felt called to the field of public and community health nursing while obtaining her BSN degree, inspired by the focus on preventing disease and helping underserved populations. Since then, she has provided care for a wide variety of vulnerable populations, including children in the schools, adults who are homeless, low-income families, and elders in long-term care facilities. She served as a nurse and clinic coordinator of the Good Samaritan Nursing Center at the University of Kentucky for twelve years. Her work at the Good Samaritan Nursing Center focused on providing school health services to underserved populations as well as developing a K-12 school health curriculum for a county in rural Kentucky. She has lectured and supervised students studying public health nursing in a myriad of community settings, including school clinics, homeless shelters, and free clinics for adults and children. She has contributed to several projects to evaluate school health services and has presented at national and international symposia on nursing clinics in the community. Her research interests are in the areas of vulnerable populations, access to health care, and obesity prevention. Dr. Turner currently serves as an assistant professor at Berea College, Berea, Kentucky.

## ADDITIONAL RESOURCES

(e) **Evolve website http://evolve.elsevier.com/Stanhope**
- *Healthy People 2020*
- WebLinks
- Quiz

- Case Studies
- Glossary
- Answers to Practice Application

## OBJECTIVES

*After reading this chapter, the student should be able to do the following:*

1. Discuss professional standards expected of school nurses.
2. Differentiate between the many roles and functions of school nurses.
3. Describe the different variations of school health services and coordinated school health programs.
4. Discuss common health problems of children and adolescents seen in the school setting.
5. Analyze the nursing care given in schools in terms of the primary, secondary, and tertiary levels of prevention.
6. Anticipate future trends in school nursing.

## KEY TERMS

advanced practice nurses, p. 917
Americans with Disabilities Act, p. 916
case manager, p. 920
Child Nutrition and WIC Reauthorization Act, p. 916
community outreach, p. 920
consultant, p. 920
counselor, p. 920
crisis teams, p. 925
direct caregiver, p. 919
do-not-attempt-resuscitate orders, p. 932
Education for All Handicapped Children Act, p. 916
emergency plan, p. 925
health educator, p. 919
Healthy, Hunger-Free Kids Act, p. 916
Health Insurance Portability and Accountability Act (HIPAA), p. 924

Individuals with Disabilities Education Act (IDEA), p. 916
individualized education plans (IEPs), p. 916
individualized health plans (IHPs), p. 916
National Association of School Nurses, p. 917
No Child Left Behind Act, p. 916
primary prevention, p. 923
researcher, p. 920
Safe Kids Campaign, p. 923
school-based health centers, p. 922
School Health Policies and Practices Study, p. 922
school-linked program, p. 922
school nursing, p. 915
secondary prevention, p. 923
Section 504 of the Rehabilitation Act, p. 916
tertiary prevention, p. 923
*—See Glossary for definitions*

With thanks to Erin G. Cruise, PhD, RN, NCSN, Assistant Professor, Radford University School of Nursing, Radford, VA 24142

In the fall of 2013, approximately 50.1 million children attended a public school in the United States (35.3 million in elementary and middle schools, 14.8 million in high schools), and an additional 5.2 million students attended a private school (U.S. Department of Education, 2013). These children and adolescents need health care during their school day, and this is the job of the school nurse. There were, in 2010, approximately 73,600 registered nurses currently working as school nurses (Health Resources and Services Administration [HRSA], 2010). The school nurse serves an important role in providing health services and health promotion in the school setting (Board et al, 2011; National Association of School Nurses, 2011).

A common misperception is that school nurses only put bandages on cuts and soothe children with stomachaches. However, that is not their major role. The National Association of School Nurses (NASN) defines school nursing as "a specialized practice of professional nursing that advances the well-being, academic success and lifelong achievement and health of students" (Board et al, 2011). School nurses give comprehensive nursing care to the children and the staff at the school (NASN, 2011). At the same time, they coordinate the health education program of the school, consult with school officials to help identify and care for other persons in the school community, and provide leadership in promoting health and safety (NASN, 2011). The school nurse provides care to the children not only in the school building itself, but also in other settings where children are found—for example, in juvenile detention centers, in preschools and daycare centers, during field trips, at sporting events, and in the children's homes (Nic Philibin et al, 2010). The school nurse, therefore, must be flexible in giving nursing care, education, and help to those who need it.

This chapter discusses the history of nursing in the schools and the functions of school nurses today. In addition, the standards of practice for school nurses are discussed, as the nurse takes on a variety of roles. Different types of school health services are reviewed, including government-financed programs. The primary, secondary, and tertiary levels of nursing care that nurses give to children in the schools are presented. The most common health problems that the school nurse finds in children are also discussed under their appropriate prevention levels. The chapter ends with a discussion of the ethical dilemmas that may arise for school nurses, and the future of nursing in the schools is predicted for ever-changing communities.

## HISTORY OF SCHOOL NURSING

### The 1800s and Beyond

The history of school nursing began with the earliest efforts of nurses to care for people in the community. In the late 1800s in England, the Metropolitan Association of Nursing provided medical examinations for children in the schools of London (Wright, 2011). By 1892 nurses in London were responsible for checking the nutrition of the children in the schools (Wright, 2011). These ideas spread to the United States where, in 1897, nurses in New York City schools began to identify ill children. They then excluded these children from classes so that other children would not be infected (Earles and Jones, 2011). Health education was also important during this time. Many states had laws in the late 1800s mandating that nurses teach within the schools about the abuse of alcohol and narcotics (Earles and Jones, 2011).

In the early 1900s in the United States, the main health problem in the community was the spread of infectious diseases. On October 2, 1902, in New York City, Lillian Wald's Henry Street Settlement nurses began going into homes and schools to assess children. These public health nurses were at first in only four schools caring for about 10,000 children. They made plans to identify children with lice and other infestations and those with infected wounds, tuberculosis (TB), and other infectious diseases (Earles and Jones, 2011; Judd et al, 2010).

The need for school nurses was immediately recognized by the health care community. By 1910, Teachers College in New York City added a course on school nursing to their curriculum for nurses. In 1916 a school superintendent requested that a public health nurse be sent to the schools to care for children of immigrants (Judd et al, 2010). By the 1920s school nurse teachers were employed by most municipal health departments. As the years went by and communities struggled with serious economic issues and hardships during the Depression, school nurses continued to provide health care to children in the schools through the federal Works Progress Administration program (WPA) (Judd et al, 2010).

In the 1940s the nurses were mostly employed by the school districts directly. The nurses also provided home nursing and health education for the children and their parents (Earles and Jones, 2011). In addition, school nurses became concerned with the condition of school buildings (Judd et al, 2010).

After World War II and into the 1950s, as a result of the increased use of immunizations and antibiotics, the number of children with communicable disease in the schools fell. School nurses then turned their attention to screening children for common health problems and for vision and hearing. School nurses were less likely to teach health concepts in the children's classrooms and more likely to consult with teachers about health education (Earles and Jones, 2011). However, there was an increased emphasis on employee health, and school nurses began screening teachers and other school staff for health problems (Earles and Jones, 2011).

The 1960s saw an upsurge in the call for higher levels of education for school nurses. A position paper delivered at the 1960 American Nurses Association (ANA) convention called for the Bachelor of Science in nursing degree as the minimum educational preparation for school nurses. By 1970 the first school nurse practitioner program was started at the University of Colorado. There, school nurses learned advanced concepts of school nursing practice to provide primary health care to children (Earles and Jones, 2011).

Table 42-1 gives the highlights of school nursing history over the last century.

## Federal Legislation in the 1970s, 1980s, 1990s, and 2000s

Community involvement in health in schools was a major thrust in the 1970s and 1980s. Counseling and mental health services were added to the responsibilities of school nurses, who began to directly teach children concepts of health. Children were no longer just being screened for illnesses (Earles and Jones, 2011). Because of federal laws that required schools to make accommodations for handicapped children, medically fragile children were attending schools, often for the first time. One of these laws, PL 93-112, Section 504 of the Rehabilitation Act of 1973, was an important step in helping all children enjoy a normal educational experience (Robert Wood Johnson Foundation, 2010). This law was followed by PL 94-142, Education for All Handicapped Children Act, which required that children with disabilities have services provided for them in the schools.

Following the passage of the Americans with Disabilities Act in 1992, PL 105-17 Individuals with Disabilities Education Act (IDEA) passed in 1997. Both of these laws required that more children be allowed to attend schools. Schools had to make allowances for their special needs, which included ensuring that their school experience was in balance with their health care needs by developing individualized education plans (IEPs) and individualized health plans (IHPs). That meant that more children with human immunodeficiency virus (HIV), acquired immunodeficiency syndrome (AIDS), chronic illnesses, or mental health problems were in the classrooms and needed more attention from the school nurse (Robert Wood Johnson Foundation, 2010).

### TABLE 42-1   High Points In School Nursing History

| Decade | Major Events in School Nursing |
|---|---|
| 1890s | English and American nurses are used in schools to examine children for infectious diseases and to teach about alcohol abuse. |
| 1900s | Henry Street Settlement in New York City sends nurses into schools and homes to investigate children's overall health. |
| 1910s | School nursing course added to Teachers College nursing program. |
| 1920s and 1930s | School nurses are employed by community health departments. |
| 1940s | School districts employ school nurses. |
| 1950s | Children are screened in schools for common health problems. |
| 1960s | Educational preparation for school nurses is debated. |
| 1970s | School nurse practitioner programs began. Increased emphasis put on mental health counseling in schools. |
| 1980s | Children with long-term illness or disabilities attend schools. |
| 1990s | School-based and school-linked clinics are started. Total family and community health care is offered. |
| 2000s | School nurses give comprehensive primary, secondary, and tertiary levels of nursing care. |

From Schlachta-Fairchild L, Varghese SB, Deickman A, et al: Telehealth and telenursing are live: APN policy and practice implications. *J Nurse Pract* 6:98-106, 2010.

The No Child Left Behind Act of 2001 requires a healthy environment in the schools, which also affects children who have health problems (Ringwalt et al, 2011).

Also during the 1990s, the responsibilities of the school nurse were extended to include the development of complete clinics and health care agency centers within or attached to the schools (Earles and Jones, 2011). These school-based clinics will be discussed later in this chapter. By 2002, some school nurses were responsible for several schools, and they provided care under a variety of nursing roles. To address obesity and to promote healthy eating and physical activity through changes in school environments, Congress passed the Child Nutrition and WIC Reauthorization Act of 2004 (PL 108.265, Section 204). This act designated that each local education agency (LEA) participating in federal school meal programs, such as the National School Lunch or Breakfast Program, must establish a local school wellness policy.

The Healthy, Hunger-Free Kids Act of 2010 authorizes funding and sets policy for the National School Lunch Program, the School Breakfast Program, the Summer Food Service Program, and other child and adult food programs (Office of the Press Secretary, 2010). This law seeks to reform the foods available at school so that healthier, more nutritious foods are

## TABLE 42-2   Federal Legislation Affecting School Nursing

| Law | Effect on School Nurses and Children |
|---|---|
| 1973: PL 39-112, Section 504 of Rehabilitation Act | Children cannot be excluded from schools because of a handicap. The school must provide health services that each child needs. |
| 1975: PL 94-142, Education for All Handicapped Children Act | All children should attend school in least restrictive environment. Requires school district's committee on handicapped to develop individualized education plans (IEPs) for children. |
| 1992: Americans with Disabilities Act | Persons with disabilities cannot be excluded from activities. |
| 1997: PL 105-17, Individuals with Disabilities Education Act (IDEA) with updates in 2004 | Educational services must be offered by schools for all disabled children from birth through age 22 years. |
| 2001: No Child Left Behind Act of 2001 | All children must receive standardized education in a healthy environment. |
| 2004: Child Nutrition and WIC Reauthorization Act of 2004 | Every local education agency (LEA) participating in federal school meal programs must establish a local school wellness policy. |
| 2010: Healthy, Hunger-Free Kids Act of 2010 | Reform of the National School Lunch Program and National School Breakfast Program through increased funding and setting policy on nutritional quality of foods served on school grounds. Also opens eligibility requirements to improve access to the free and reduced-price lunch program. |

Compiled from Betz CL: Use of 504 plans for children and youth with disabilities: nursing application. *Pediatr Nurs* 27:347–352, 2001; Whalen LG, Grunbaum JA, Kann L, et al: *Profiles 2002. School Health Profiles. Surveillance for Characteristics of Health Programs among Secondary Schools.* Washington, DC, 2004, Centers for Disease Control and Prevention, USDHHS.

served. In recent times this law has become controversial because schools are having difficulty complying with the terms of the Act.

Table 42-2 summarizes the effects of these laws on school nurses and schoolchildren.

## STANDARDS OF PRACTICE FOR SCHOOL NURSES

The professional body for school nurses is the National Association of School Nurses (NASN), headquartered in Washington, DC. This association provides the general guidelines and support for all school nurses. It revised the standards of professional practice for school nurses in 2011. These standards require that all school nurses use the nursing process throughout their practice: assessment, analysis, planning,

implementation, and evaluation. The major concepts addressed in the standards include the following:
- Give and evaluate appropriate up-to-date nursing care.
- Collaborate well with other health providers and school staff.
- Maintain school health office policies, including privacy and safety of health records.
- Teach health promotion and maintenance to children, families, and communities.(NASN, 2011)

In addition, the professional standards rely on nurses to give care based on 11 criteria (NASN, 2011). These criteria include the ability to do the following:
- Develop school health policies and procedures.
- Evaluate their own nursing practice.
- Keep up with nursing knowledge.
- Interact with the interprofessional health care team.
- Ensure confidentiality in providing health care.
- Consult with others to give complete care.
- Use research findings in practice.
- Ensure the safety of children, including when delegating care to other school personnel.
- Have good communication skills.
- Manage a school health program effectively.
- Teach others about wellness.

## EDUCATIONAL CREDENTIALS OF SCHOOL NURSES

School nursing requires the nurse to be able to practice independently, supervise others, and delegate care in a community (Board et al, 2011; Sheets et al, 2012). The NASN recommends that school nurses be registered nurses who also have bachelor's degrees in nursing and a special certification in school nursing (Board et al, 2011; NASN, 2011; Sheets et al, 2012). However, not all school nurses have been educated this way. There are no general laws regarding the educational background of school nurses. School nurses in some states are required to be registered nurses, and others require specialty certification for school nurses. Yet, licensed practical nurses are also seen in some schools. Table 42-3 lists the education requirements for school nurses for each state.

School nurses in some schools may be advanced practice nurses who specialize in caring for children. They may be nurse practitioners who have specialized in child health nursing (pediatrics), in family nursing, or in the school nurse practitioner role. Clinical nurse specialists who are school nurses may also be found in child health nursing or community or public health nursing. The higher the educational level of the school nurse, the better that nurse is able to give complete care to children and their families. These advanced practice nurses may be certified by professional organizations, such as the ANA, or their own professional organization. Most hold master's degrees in nursing.

Most school nurses do not start their nursing careers in the schools. Rather, the majority have prior experience in nursing, most from working either in hospitals or with communities. It is helpful if their previous experience entailed working with

## TABLE 42-3    States' Requirements for School Nurses

| State | Minimum Education Standard Mandated by Law | | | Requires Previous Nursing Experience in a Clinical Nursing Setting | Requires School Nurse Certificate or Professional Development Training for School Health | Nurse-to-Student Ratio |
|---|---|---|---|---|---|---|
| | Minimum not mandated | Licensed Practical Nurse | Registered Nurse | | | |
| Alabama | | X[a] | X | | | Goal: 1:500 |
| Arkansas | | X | | | | Goal: 1:750 |
| Arizona | | | X[b] | | Yes | |
| California | | | X[b] | | | |
| Colorado | | | X[b] | | Yes, if baccalaureate degree is not in nursing | |
| Connecticut | | | X | | Yes | At least one school nurse or nurse practitioner per local or regional board of education |
| District of Columbia | X | | | | | |
| Delaware | | | X[b] | Min. 3 years | Yes | At least one full-time nurse per school |
| Florida | | X[c] | | | Encouraged | |
| Georgia | | X | | | | Goal: 1:750 |
| Hawaii | X | | | | | |
| Iowa | | | X[b] | | | Goal: 1:750 |
| Idaho | | | X[b] | Min. 2 years | Yes | |
| Illinois | | | X[b] | | Yes | |
| Indiana | | | X[d] | | | Goal: 1:750 |
| Kansas | | | X | | | |
| Kentucky | | | X[e] | | Provisional certificate for non-BSN prepared RN | |
| Louisiana | | | X | Min. 2 years | | 1:1500 |
| Massachusetts | | | X[b] | Min. 2 years | | At least one nurse per school |
| Maryland | | | X | | Yes | |
| Maine | | | X[b] | Min. 3 years | | 1:800 |
| Michigan | | | X | | | |
| Minnesota | | | X[b] | | Yes | 1:1000 |
| Missouri | X | | | | | Goal: 1:750 |
| Mississippi | | X | | | Yes | |
| Montana | X | | | | | |
| North Carolina | | | X | | | 1:3000 |
| North Dakota | X | | | | | |
| Nebraska | | | X | | Yes | Goal: 1:750 |
| New Hampshire | | | X[b] | | | |
| New Jersey | | | X[b] | | Yes | At least one nurse per district |
| New Mexico | | | X[f] | If LPN: Min. 1 year | | |
| Nevada | | | X[b] | | | |
| New York | | | X[b] | | | |
| Ohio | | | X[b] | | Yes | |
| Oklahoma | | | X[b] | | | |
| Oregon | | | X[b] | Min: Practicum in a school setting | Yes | 1:225 "medically complex" students 1:125 "medically fragile students" Goal: 1:750 students in district |
| Pennsylvania | | | X[b] | | Yes | 1:1500 |
| Rhode Island | | | X | | Yes | |

## TABLE 42-3   States' Requirements for School Nurses—cont'd

| State | Minimum Education Standard Mandated by Law | | | Requires Previous Nursing Experience in a Clinical Nursing Setting | Requires School Nurse Certificate or Professional Development Training for School Health | Nurse-to-Student Ratio |
|---|---|---|---|---|---|---|
| | Minimum not mandated | Licensed Practical Nurse | Registered Nurse | | | |
| South Carolina | | | X | | | |
| South Dakota | | | X | | | |
| Tennessee | | | X | | | 1:3000 or 1:school system |
| Texas | X | | | | Yes | |
| Utah | X | | | | | 1:5000 |
| Virginia | | X | | | | 1:1000 |
| Vermont | | | X[b] | Min. 4 years | | |
| Washington | | | X[b] | | | |
| Wisconsin | | | X | | | |
| West Virginia | | | X[b] | | Yes | 1:1500 for grades K-7 |
| Wyoming | | | X[b] | | Yes | |

[a]Requires there may not be more than five LPNs for each RN within each school system.
[b]Requires bachelor's degree.
[c]Preferred entry is a BSN or higher.
[d]Requires at least one BSN prepared RN to coordinate health services.
[e]Requires nurse must at least be working toward completion of a bachelor's degree.
 Requires school nurses in supervisory positions to have a master's degree in nursing.
Data from: National Association of State Boards of Education: *State School Health Policy Database: Requirements For School Nurses*, 2013. Available at http://www.nasbe.org/healthy_schools/hs/bytopics.php?topicid=2130. Accessed April 15, 2014.

children, so that they are aware of children's special health needs. While it is common that school nurses come to the field with prior nursing experience, it is possible for newly graduated nurses to work in the schools, depending on the entry criteria of their state and local health departments and schools. Ideally, the less-experienced nurses should complete an extended orientation period until they feel comfortable practicing alone.

## ROLES AND FUNCTIONS OF SCHOOL NURSES

School nurses give care to children as direct caregivers, educators, counselors, consultants, and case managers. They must coordinate the health care of many students in their schools with the health care that the children receive from their own health care providers.

In *Healthy People 2020 Objectives*, goal ECBP-5 states that there should be one full-time registered nurse for every 750 children in each school (USDHHS, 2010). The NASN supports the 1:750 nurse-to-student ratio, but also notes that a 1:1 ratio may be necessary for individual students who require daily and continuous nursing services (DuRant et al, 2010). Table 42-3 lists the nurse-to-student ratio for each state, if specified by the state. However, only approximately 45% of the nation's schools have met that standard (USDHHS, 2010). Having fewer nurses in the schools means that the nurses are expected to perform many different functions. It is therefore possible that they are unable to give the amount of comprehensive care that the students need (Maughan and Adams, 2011).

## School Nurse Roles
### Direct Caregiver

The school nurse is expected to give immediate nursing care to the ill or injured child or school staff member. Direct caregiver is the traditional role of the school nurse.

Although most school nurses are in public or private schools and give care only during school hours, the nurse in a boarding school provides nursing care to children 24 hours a day and 7 days a week. In boarding schools, the children live at school and go home only for vacations. The nurse also lives at the school and may be on call all the time. The nurse in the boarding school is very important to the children because this nurse is the gatekeeper to their complete health care (Earles and Jones, 2011). The nurse makes all of the health care decisions for the child and has a referral system to contact other health care providers, such as physicians and psychological counselors, if needed.

### Health Educator

The school nurse in the health educator role may be asked to teach children both individually and in the classroom. The nurse uses different approaches to teach about health, such as teaching proper nutrition or safety information. Many school nurses teach the older elementary girls and boys about the coming changes in their bodies as puberty arrives. Other school nurses may teach the health education classes that are required by the states to be included in the programs.

## Case Manager

The school nurse is expected to function as a case manager, helping to coordinate the health care for children with complex health problems. This may include the child who is disabled or chronically ill and who may be seen by a physical therapist, an occupational therapist, a speech therapist, or another health care provider during the school day. The nurse sets up the schedule for the child's visits so that those appointments do not unnecessarily impact negatively on the child's academic day.

## Consultant

The school nurse is the person best able to provide health information to school administrators, teachers, and parent–teacher groups. As a consultant, the school nurse can provide professional information about proposed changes in the school environment and their impact on the health of the children. The nurse can also recommend changes in the school's policies or engage community organizations to help make the children's schools healthier places (Nic Philibin et al, 2010). This is a population-level role for the school nurse; the population consists of all children, families, staff, and the surrounding community.

## Counselor

The school nurse may be the person whom children trust to tell important secrets about their health. It is important that, as a counselor, the school nurse have a reputation as being a trustworthy person to whom the children can go if they are in trouble or if they need to confide about a personal matter (Nic Philibin et al, 2010). Nurses in this situation should tell children that if anything they reveal points out that they are in danger, the parents and school officials must be told. However, privacy and confidentiality, as in all health care, are important.

In addition, the school nurse may be the person to help with grief counseling in the schools. (See later discussion on the school crisis team.)

## Community Outreach

When participating in community outreach, nurses can be involved in community health fairs or festivals in the schools, using that opportunity to teach others. They can be part of an influenza immunization program for the school staff and can promote a health education fair and do blood pressure screenings. They can initiate a liaison, coordinating with local health charities to provide education to the schools (Avery et al, 2013).

## Researcher

Little research has been done on nurses caring for children in the schools. The school nurse is responsible for making sure that the nursing care given is based on solid, evidence-based practice. Outcomes regarding school nurse services need to be studied (Nic Philibin et al, 2010). Therefore, the school nurse, as an educator, is in the right position to do studies as a researcher that advance school nursing practice.

---

### EVIDENCE-BASED PRACTICE

Because of the obesity epidemic in the United States, interventions to increase physical activity and reduce sedentary behaviors have become a priority for public health practitioners. This research study evaluated the feasibility and efficacy of a school nurse–delivered intervention aimed at improving diet and activity and reducing body mass index (BMI) among overweight and obese adolescents. This study used a pair-matched cluster-randomized controlled school-based trial. Six high schools were randomized into either the six-session counseling intervention or the control group. The intervention, "Lookin' Good Feelin' Good" consisted of six one-on-one school nurse–led counseling sessions conducted over two months during school hours. Those in the control group had six one-on-one visits with the school nurse over two months to be weighed and review informational pamphlets on weight management. Although there was no significant difference in BMI, activity, or caloric intake between the groups at two months, those in the intervention group ate breakfast on more days of the week and had a lower intake of sugar than the control group.

#### Nurse Use

This study indicates that a school-nurse–delivered obesity intervention is feasible and may improve select behaviors that may result in obesity.

Pbert L, Druker S, Gapinski MA, et al: A school nurse-delivered intervention for overweight and obese adolescents. *J Sch Health* 83(3):182-193, 2013.

## SCHOOL HEALTH SERVICES

School health services vary in their scope. However, there are common parts to the programs.

### Federal School Health Programs

The federal government, through the coordination of the Centers for Disease Control and Prevention, has developed a plan that school health programs are encouraged to follow (CDC, 2013a) (Figure 42-1).

This plan was originally developed in 1987 after the CDC began funding schools for HIV-prevention education programs. By 1992 this educational system was so successful that it was expanded to include school health programs to teach children prevention of other chronic illnesses. These include diseases caused in part by risk factors such as poor diet, lack of exercise, and smoking.

Then, in 1998, the government expanded the program again to include a more complete school health education program that included the parents and the community in the children's care. By 2009, 22 states had been funded for their school health programs by the CDC. The funding has paid for the development of health education plans of study, or curricula, which include policies, guidelines, and training for these health programs. The states then use these courses to teach the children. The schools are actively involved in helping the children practice problem solving, communication, and other life skills so they can reduce their risk factors (CDC, 2009).

According to the CDC (2009), two states in particular have been very successful with these programs. West Virginia has developed a program called the Instructional Goals and Objectives for Health Education and Physical Education, which increased the ability of the children to pass the President's

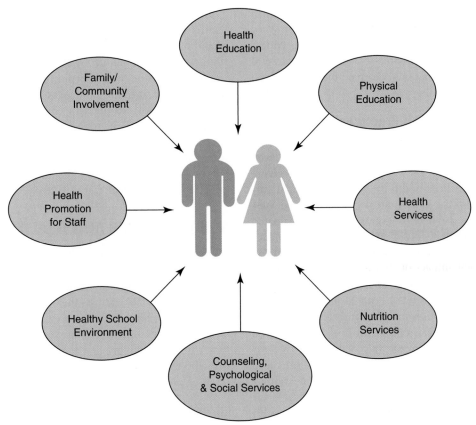

**FIG 42-1** The eight components of a coordinated school health program. (From Centers for Disease Control and Prevention: *Adolescent and School Health: Components of Coordinated School Health*, 2013b, CDC. Available at http://www.cdc.gov/healthyyouth/cshp/components. htm. Accessed April 15, 2014.)

## ⟫ LINKING CONTENT TO PRACTICE

School nurses play a primary role in the implementation of the CDC School Health Program components. These components are described below and addressed throughout this chapter. The emphasis in this program design is working with the school as a population or community. This plan has eight parts:

- *Health education*—This section includes teaching children about how to stay healthy and how to prevent becoming ill or being injured. The health education is offered in a planned, sequential, K-12 curriculum that addresses all dimensions of health.
- *Physical education*—Taking part in physical activity during the school day is recommended for all children. This is to provide regular exercise as well as to provide sports programs outside the normal school day. This, it is hoped, may help reduce obesity, high blood pressure, and other diseases later in life (CDC, 2013b).
- *Health services*—The purpose of this segment is to reduce illness in children. Specifically, the schools can provide services to ensure access or referral to primary care, prevent and control communicable disease, provide emergency care for illness or injury, and provide educational and counseling opportunities for promoting and maintaining health across all settings (CDC, 2013a). This is also the section of comprehensive school health that promotes the school nurse to student ratio of 1:750 as discussed earlier in this chapter (USDHHS, 2010).
- *Nutrition services*—Information on nutrition and diet should be taught to all children. In addition, the schools should provide healthy food choices for

students in their meal programs (both breakfast and lunch). The U.S. Department of Agriculture's Team Nutrition Program called *Making It Happen* is a federal program that encourages schools to have nutritious foods available for all students (CDC, 2013b).

- *Counseling, psychological, and social services*—This section promotes the health of children who receive special education services (IDEA), as well as children who have mental health needs. Working with families at risk because of socioeconomic needs is also part of this area (Kanter and Abramson, 2014).
- *Healthy school environment*—The emphasis in this area is to reduce tobacco use in teenagers as well as reducing violence overall in the schools. Education regarding the prevention of HIV/AIDS is also a part of this section (Jackson, 2011).
- *Health promotion for staff*—Nurses can help provide health care for teachers and other staff members in the schools. Staff can ask nurses about their health and obtain health education at school during their workday (Baisch et al, 2011).
- *Family/community involvement*—The school health program should contact families and community leaders to find out what health services are needed the most and how they can work together to emphasize health education for all. This includes being involved as health educators when adolescents take part-time jobs.

Physical Fitness Test. In Michigan, the Governor's Council on Physical Fitness, Health, and Sports developed an Exemplary Physical Education Curriculum project that made up educational materials and plans for children to achieve high physical fitness scores. All of these programs were paid for by the federal school health program funding.

## School Health Policies and Practices Study 2012

After the CDC began funding educational programs about prevention of HIV in the schools in 1987, there was clearly a need to expand these programs. By 1992 the CDC began giving money to fund other school health programs that taught students about heart disease, cancer, stroke, diabetes, and substance abuse prevention. These programs have been evaluated by the School Health Policies and Practices Study 2012 (CDC, 2013c), which looked at all eight parts of the school health program in all 50 states and the District of Columbia. The study found that 12.5% of districts had at least one school-based health center (SBHC) that offered both health services and mental health or social services to students. It also found that 67.5% of districts prohibited all tobacco use in all locations. The study noted that 14.8% of districts required and 26.5% recommended that schools offer a self-serve salad bar. Results also showed that 93.6% of districts required physical education in elementary schools, 91.9% for middle schools, and 92.4% for high schools. Nearly three fourths of states had adopted health education standards based on the 2007 National Health Education Standards (NHES) (CDC, 2013c).

## School-Based Health Programs

Because many schoolchildren may not receive health care services other than screening and first aid care from the school nurse, the U.S. government began funding school-based health centers (SBHCs) during the 1990s. These are family-centered, community-based clinics run within the schools. These clinics give expanded health services, including mental health and dental care, as well as the more traditional health care services (Bannister and Kelts, 2011). The SBHCs can range in size from small to large; some school clinics are open to the community only during the school year and others are open 24 hours a day all year round. An example of the more limited clinic is the SBHC in Worchester, MA, where six clinics are run in the schools (elementary through high school) by the Family Health Center of Worchester, Inc. during the school year months of August through May (Family Health Center, 2010).

Another example of a clinic is the school-linked program, which is coordinated by the school but has community ties (Bannister and Kelts, 2011). An example of this is the Collaborative Model for School Health in Pitts County, North Carolina. The nurses employed by the local hospital in that area provide health care for children in kindergarten through fifth grade. There is collaboration between the county health department, the local university's nursing school, and other private health care providers to give primary, secondary, and tertiary nursing care. An evaluation of the program has shown that the children's school attendance and learning has increased as a result of the presence of more complete school health services (Trapp, 2010).

At a center in Texas, an urban SBHC is located in a school district where many of the children lack health insurance. The school nurses there are assisted by three part-time nurse practitioners and one public health nurse. The school nurse is responsible for the record keeping on the children's immunizations, does the screening, and gives first aid to injured children. Then the school nurse refers children who need additional health care to the SBHC in the school. Parents like the program because they trust the school nurse. They also like its location inside the school because everyone can receive health care without having to travel far to get to a clinic (Texas Association of School-Based Health Centers, 2010).

## SCHOOL NURSES AND *HEALTHY PEOPLE 2020*

Many *Healthy People 2020* proposed objectives are directed toward the health of children. In addition, several point directly at the care that nurses give to children in the schools. The *Healthy People 2020* box lists the objectives that involve school-age children. These objectives are concerned with the children with disabilities in the schools, the number of children with major health problems, and the ratio of nurses to children in the schools. Nurses can accomplish the goals using the three levels of prevention, as discussed next.

### ♥ HEALTHY PEOPLE 2020

#### *Objectives Related to School Health and School Nursing*

- AH-5: Increase educational achievement of adolescents and young adults.
- AH-9: (Developmental) Increase the percentage of middle and high schools that prohibit harassment based on a student's sexual orientation or gender identity.
- ECBP-2: Increase the proportion of elementary, middle, and senior high schools that provide comprehensive school health education to prevent health problems in the following areas: unintentional injury; violence; suicide; tobacco use and addiction; alcohol or other drug use; unintended pregnancy, HIV/AIDS and STD infection; unhealthy dietary patterns; and inadequate physical activity.
- ECBP-5: Increase the proportion of the nation's elementary, middle, and senior high schools that have a nurse-to-student ratio of at least 1:750.
- IID-10: Maintain vaccination coverage levels for children in kindergarten.
- IID-11: Increase routine vaccination coverage levels for adolescents.
- IVP-27: Increase the proportion of public and private schools that require students to wear appropriate protective gear when engaged in school-sponsored physical activities.
- NW-2: Increase the percentage of schools that offer nutritious foods and beverages outside of school meals.
- RD-5: Reduce the number of school days or work days missed among persons with current asthma.
- TU-15: Increase tobacco-free environments in schools, including all school facilities, property, vehicles, and school events.

From U.S. Department of Health and Human Services: *Healthy People 2020 Objectives*, 2010. Available at http://www.healthypeople.gov/hp2020/Objectives/TopicAreas.aspx. Accessed April 15, 2014.

## THE LEVELS OF PREVENTION IN SCHOOLS

The three levels of prevention—primary, secondary, and tertiary—have always been a part of health care in the schools

Levels of Prev.

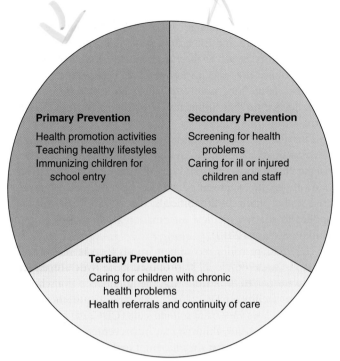

**Primary Prevention**
Health promotion activities
Teaching healthy lifestyles
Immunizing children for
school entry

**Secondary Prevention**
Screening for health
problems
Caring for ill or injured
children and staff

**Tertiary Prevention**
Caring for children with chronic
health problems
Health referrals and continuity of care

FIG 42-2 Levels of prevention in schools.

(Selekman, 2012). **Primary prevention** provides health promotion and education to prevent health problems in children. **Secondary prevention** includes the screening of children for various illnesses, monitoring their growth and development, and caring for them when they are ill or injured. **Tertiary prevention** in the schools is the continued care of children who need long-term health care services, along with education within the community (Figure 42-2).

## Primary Prevention in Schools

Children need continued health services in the schools. The school nurse sees them on an almost daily basis and is the person who is usually given the role of teaching them about and promoting their health.

The school nurse may have the opportunity to go into the classroom to teach health promotion concepts, such as handwashing or tooth-brushing skills. He or she may spend time with the teachers, giving them the latest information on healthy lifestyles for children or ways to spot a child who may be ill or in need of counseling.

> **HOW TO  Teach Young Children in School**
> *When teaching children in preschools and elementary schools, keep the lesson to no more than 10 minutes. Use a lot of examples, pictures, and stuffed animals in the talk. Always remember the developmental stage of the children when teaching them.*

In addition, nurses can teach healthy food choices and encourage school districts that allow vending machines to have nutritious foods instead of "junk food" available in the machines (CDC, 2013b). The Food-Safe Schools (FSS) project sponsored by the American Nurses Foundation and the CDC Division of

Adolescent School Health has educated many school nurses on how to promote proper food storage and preparation in the schools. The hope is to reduce the incidence of foodborne diseases in the schools (CDC, 2010a). These are examples of population-level health care for schools.

School nurses use the nursing process while they care for children in the schools. In their primary prevention efforts, they assess children and families to determine their level of knowledge about health issues. Finding out whether children are at risk for preventable problems is also completed. The nurse then analyzes the assessment findings. Plans are made to develop teaching plans or health promotion activities. Once these activities are implemented, the nurse can evaluate and revise the plan.

The areas of primary prevention that the school nurse focuses on include preventing childhood injuries, preventing substance abuse behaviors, reducing the risk of the development of chronic diseases, and monitoring the immunization status of children. These primary prevention activities are completed for the population of children in the school. The activities for the population are determined by the analysis of the assessments completed on all of the children in the school to determine the most pressing priorities for the population.

### Prevention of Childhood Injuries

Accidents (unintentional injuries) are the leading cause of death among children and teenagers (Heron, 2013). The school nurse educates children, teachers, and parents about preventing injuries. Working with the national Safe Kids Campaign, the school nurse can provide educational programs reminding children to use their seat belts or bicycle helmets to prevent injuries. Other classes can be on crossing the street, water safety, and fire safety. The school nurse, as the trusted person at school, is able to quickly give information to help prevent injuries from occurring, since most injuries are preventable (Diaz and Wyckoff, 2012; Rains and Robinson, 2012).

School nurses also provide health promotion to prevent playground injuries, which number over 100,000 injuries to children per year. School nurses assess school playgrounds for equipment safety on the basis of the U.S. Consumer Product Safety Commission (2010) guidelines. School sports also have the potential to cause injuries to children, and the school nurse is usually involved in deciding with parents and coaches on how to best prevent injuries on the sports field (Rains and Robinson, 2012).

Scooter and skateboard injuries have been increasing (AAP, 2009). School nurses also promote skateboard and scooter safety by providing health educational workshops to children and their families.

The nurse can implement these programs on a community-wide scale. Research has shown that once behaviors of children related to safety are taught, their effects spread quickly throughout the community. This makes the entire community safer (Selekman, 2012).

### Substance Abuse Prevention Education

Primary prevention interventions by the school nurse include educating children and adolescents about the effects of drugs and alcohol on their bodies. Preventing use of and "saying no" to drugs have been part of the school health program for many years. Teenagers are taught by the school nurse to stay away from street drugs (such as marijuana, cocaine, crack, and heroin) and alcohol.

There has been an increase in the use of "club drugs" such as lysergic acid (LSD), ketamine, gamma hydroxybutyrate (GHB), Rohypnol, and Ecstasy (MDMA). The school nurse can provide instruction about the serious side effects of Ecstasy, especially that it causes a very high body temperature that can lead to death. Teaching the teenagers about the dangers of all drugs is the responsibility of the school nurse. In addition, the school nurse can teach parents and other members of the community about the latest drug fads, increasing everyone's awareness of these dangerous trends (Embrey, 2012).

### Disease Prevention Education

The nurse has the opportunity to teach children healthy lifestyles to reduce their risk of disease later in life. For example, children can be taught ways to reduce their risk of becoming obese by teaching and reinforcing healthy nutrition and exercise (Morrison-Sandberg et al, 2010). The school nurse can then reinforce the teachers' educational plans or develop the program further for other age groups to teach them how to take care of their heart.

Dissemination of health promotion information to the parents of the children is often a challenge for the school nurse. In Newark, Delaware, the school nurse at one of the elementary schools has a "School Nurse's Corner" webpage (Laudorn, 2010). On this page, the nurse shares important health information related to school-age children, such as immunization requirements and childhood obesity. In this way, the school nurse is able to promote the health of not only the schoolchildren, but also the community.

### Vaccinations for Schoolchildren

All states have laws that require that children receive immunizations, or vaccinations, against communicable diseases before they attend school (CDC, 2010b). School nurses must be up to date on the latest laws on immunizations for children in their own state. For children entering kindergarten, these vaccinations include diphtheria, pertussis, and tetanus (the DTaP series); measles, mumps, and rubella (the MMR series); polio; and others. Chapters 13 and 14 have a more complete discussion of communicable diseases and immunizations in children.

The school nurse must keep a complete file of all of the children's vaccination records in order to meet the state's laws. These files will contain the student's name, date of birth, address and telephone number, parents'/guardians' names, and contact information. They will also include the student's primary health care provider's name, telephone number, and address. Most important, the information should include all the vaccinations with the dates the child received booster shots. This makes it easy for the school nurse to find out which children still need immunizations or boosters.

The Health Insurance Portability and Accountability Act (HIPAA) of 1996 requires that all health information be private.

This Act presents a challenge for the school nurse and personnel within the school and the school system. Teachers and school administrators as well as interprofessional health care partners feel they have the right to know about health issues of their students. Thus, they often challenge the school nurse if the nurse declines to share information to protect the child's privacy. (Cruise, 2015).

There is conflicting information on whether the immunization status of children is covered by the law. Whereas some believe that school clinics and school nurses are allowed to have that information without permission because they are considered to be public health officials, others state that this only applies to sharing medical information (Office of Health and Human Services, 2010).

The CDC provides recommendations for vaccinations, but it is up to each individual state to determine which immunizations are required for enrollment and attendance at a school or childcare facility (CDC, 2012). Vaccine requirements and exemptions laws vary from state to state (CDC, 2012). Depending on the state's law, children may be prevented from enrolling in or attending school if they have not had the required immunizations or have not provided the required paperwork for exemptions (either for medical, religious, or philosophical/conscientious belief reasons) (CDC, 2012).

Each school nurse must be aware of the vaccine requirements for their state and make every effort to find missing data in the student's immunization record. The nurse will need to contact the parents to get the immunization history for the child. Written notes will need to be sent to each child's home at least one year before each new immunization is needed so that the parents have time to get the child to his or her health care provider for the shots. If the parents or guardians do not speak English, these notes will need to be translated into the family's language. If the parents have lost the information that gives the child's immunization history, they should be encouraged to contact their physician or nurse practitioner to get it.

Many problems with children not being immunized or having incomplete vaccination records may arise in families who have moved a great deal or who may not have a regular physician. The parents may have no idea whether the child has even received the shots. Families may also be without health care insurance to pay for the immunizations, or they may have insurance that does not pay for preventive care. In these cases, the parents have to pay for the immunizations, which can be expensive. Certain low-income families without health care insurance may qualify for federal programs that provide free immunizations to children. Each state has its own program, so school nurses will want to become familiar with what their state provides.

Some parents may request that their child be exempted from the required immunizations because of their belief that not all immunizations are good for their children, for medical reasons, or for religious or philosophical reasons. The school nurse will want to be aware of the laws in the state regarding acceptable reasons for immunization exemption. At the same time, the nurse has the opportunity to teach parents and the rest of the community about the overall benefits to society from the use of immunizations. It is important, in light of the measles outbreak at Disneyland in 2014-15, that school nurses be alert to the development of vaccine preventable diseases in their communities or schools so that unvaccinated children may be sent home from school for their protection against the disease outbreak (Cruise, 2015).

School nurses can also play an important role in immunizing children against seasonal flu. The American Academy of Pediatrics (AAP, 2013) recommends that all people who are six months of age and older receive an annual seasonal influenza vaccination, especially children younger than five years of age and all children with chronic medical conditions. Vaccination against influenza should begin as soon as that season's vaccine becomes available (Li and Freedman, 2009). During the 2009 H1N1 influenza outbreak, school nurses were at the front line of the epidemic. In fact, it was a school nurse in Queens, New York, who first notified the CDC that the influenza epidemic had reached U.S. soil (Robert Wood Johnson Foundation, 2010). School nurses were challenged to reduce the spread of the epidemic among school-age children. School nurses may administer the influenza vaccine to children at the school with the parents' permission and can educate students, families, and school staff about the vaccine itself (Bobo et al, 2013).

## Secondary Prevention in Schools

Because secondary prevention involves caring for children when they need health care, this is the largest responsibility for the school nurse. This includes caring for ill or injured students and school employees. It also involves screening and assessing children, and referral to appropriate health agencies or providers. The school nurse uses the nursing process during secondary prevention activities. When an ill or injured child comes to the school's health office, the nurse must immediately assess the child for the degree of illness or injury.

Children seek out the school nurse for a variety of different needs:
- Headaches
- Stomachaches
- Diarrhea
- Anxiety over being separated from the parents
- Cuts, bruises, or other injuries

In addition, children may seek reassurance from the school nurse or even appear to hide in the nurse's office. This may be a result of harassment or bullying from other children in the school (Frisen and Bjarnelind, 2010).

Once the assessment data are gathered, the nurse determines the course of action and follows it through the implementation and evaluation phases. This occurs for direct child health care as well as for screening children for other health problems. If assessment data identify a child as having a health problem, the school nurse continues to follow the nursing process to further care for that child.

## Nursing Care for Emergencies in the School

Events that occur in or near schools may cause a crisis for children, teachers, and staff. The school nurse must have an **emergency plan** in place so that a routine can be followed when

emergencies occur. Disaster planning in the schools includes becoming prepared for natural disasters (such as fire or severe weather), man-made disasters (such as school shooting or structure collapse), as well as health condition emergencies (such as asthma attack or seizure) (Doyle, 2011). The NASN recommends that school nurses provide leadership to schools in all phases of emergency preparedness and management (Cagginello et al, 2011).

The following summarizes the NASN's recommendations of the role of the school nurse during each phase of disaster planning (Cagginello et al, 2011):
- Prevention/Mitigation: perform an ongoing assessment to identify hazards
- Preparedness: serve on planning groups, establish emergency response plans, provide training to school personnel
- Response: perform triage, coordinate the first-aid response team, provide direct hands-on care to victims, act as a counselor to help everyone cope with the emotional aspects of this serious event (Box 42-1)
- Recovery: provide direct support, act as liaison between community resources and those in need; school may become an emergency shelter for community-at-large

The U.S. Department of Education (2010) recommends that all schools have crisis plans in place to help the children, teachers, parents, and community cope with the sudden event. Crisis teams are prepared to help everyone respond quickly to the crisis, to ensure the safety of the school, and to follow up on the effects of the crisis on the members of the school (Lerner et al, 2013. The crisis plan includes an administrative policy made either for the entire school district or, if the schools are large, for each individual school. The plan includes the names of the persons on the crisis team: the superintendent of the school district, the school nurse, the guidance counselor, the school psychologist or social worker, teachers, police or school security, clergy from the community, and parents. Plans to obtain and share information can be made quickly (Lerner et al, 2013).

The nurse can help the crisis team make a checklist for everyone to follow that explains what to do in every possible crisis situation. Then, at the end of the crisis, the crisis team will want to take time to counsel all of the people who helped in the crisis, including the teachers, emergency personnel, and parents,

---

### BOX 42-1    Dealing with a Disaster: Responsibilities of the School Nurse

- Provide triage.
- Communicate with emergency medical personnel.
- Assess the school community for the presence of shock and stress.
- Recommend reduced television viewing of the disaster.
- Provide grief counseling.
- Communicate with the children, parents, and school personnel.
- Follow up with assessment of children for anxiety, depression, regression, and post-traumatic stress disorder.

Modified from Lerner MD, Lindell B, Volpe J: *A Practical Guide for Crisis Response in Our Schools*. 2010, American Academy of Experts in Traumatic Stress. Available at http://store.nc-cm.org/servlet/Detail?no=1. Accessed March 19, 2011.

as well as the children. That way everyone can talk about the crisis. The crisis plan should be reviewed every year to see what parts of the plan need updating. Drills take place to act out the plan to see how it works and how it can be revised to make it more workable (Lerner et al, 2013).

Individualized emergency plans are made for all students who may have a health problem that could result in an emergency situation in the school (Doyle, 2011). This plan could be for the child with food allergies (e.g., to peanuts), one who has sensitivity to insect bites that could result in anaphylactic shock, or those with chronic illnesses such as asthma, diabetes, or hemophilia. The individualized emergency plan should include the student's medical history, list of medications, location of emergency medication, and list of personnel trained to administer emergency medication. It is important that the school nurse communicate with school personnel about students requiring emergency medication to ensure quick access to emergency medications at all times.

The nurse may not always be at the school and the emergency may have to be handled by a teacher, administrator, secretary, custodian, or coach (Doyle, 2011). This issue is especially applicable to school nurses in rural settings, who may have several schools for which they are responsible when such schools may be far apart. Therefore, all emergency procedures are written and easily accessible to anyone in the school. Along with

the procedures and an emergency manual written or obtained by the school nurse, an injury or illness log is available for personnel to fill out so that there is an accurate record of what happened. Along with this form, procedures for notifying the parents or legal guardians about the emergency are spelled out and include what was done for the child and where the child was sent if transfer to a hospital or other medical agency was required.

Because the school nurse may have to give nursing care to a child or adult in respiratory or cardiac arrest, the nurse must have current certification in cardiopulmonary resuscitation (CPR) and the use of the automated external defibrillator (AED), which should be available to all school nurses. All fifty states have passed laws requiring that public gathering places have AEDs available, some requiring them in the schools (AED Brands, 2010). Other education in the area of emergency nursing would also be helpful to the school nurse, including pediatric advanced life support (PALS) or emergency nursing for pediatrics (ENPC) certification (USDE, 2010).

### Emergency Equipment in the School Nurse's Office

The school nurse needs a great deal of equipment to deal with emergencies in the school. These needs are based on the guidelines of the NASN (Pontius and Doyle, 2012). The school office will need to have basic emergency items on hand (Box 42-2).

---

### BOX 42-2   Emergency Items for Schools With and Without a School Nurse Present

**Supplies for Schools WITHOUT a School Nurse Present**

- Accessible keys to locked supplies
- Accessible list of phone resources
- Automated external defibrillator (AED) if school meets the AHA guidelines
- AED supplies stored with AED (razor, alcohol pads, dry towel, scissors, electrode pads)
- Biohazard waste bags
- Blunt scissors
- Clock with a second hand
- CPR trained staff on-site when students are on the premises
- Disposable blankets
- Emergency cards on all staff
- Emergency cards on all students
- Established relationship with local EMS personnel
- Eye protection (full peripheral glasses or goggles, face shield)
- Ice (not cold packs)
- Individual care plans/emergency plans for students with specialized needs
- First aid tapes
- Nonlatex gloves
- One-way resuscitation mask
- Cell phone or other two-way communication device
- Posters with CPR/abdominal or chest thrusts instructions
- Refrigerator or cooler
- Resealable plastic bags
- School-wide emergency operations/response plan

- Sharps container
- Soap and source of water/hand sanitizer for hand and wound cleansing
- Source of oral glucose (i.e., frosting gel, glucose tablets, juice box)
- Splints
- Staff names who have received basic first aid training
- Variety of bandages and dressings
- Water source/normal saline for wound/eye irrigation

**Additional Supplies for Schools WITH a School Nurse Present**

- C-spine immobilizers of different sizes
- Glucose monitoring device*
- Medications**
  - Albuterol
  - Epinephrine (auto injector preferred)
- Oxygen
- Nebulizer
- Penlight
- Self-inflating resuscitation device in two sizes (500 ml and 1 liter) with appropriate sized masks to meet needs of population being served
- Stethoscope
- Sphygmomanometer and cuffs in pediatric, adult regular, and adult large sizes
- Suction equipment (minimal source, does not have to be electric, i.e. bulb suction or v-vac type device)

*Committee acknowledges challenges with maintenance and expense of test strips. Monitoring of machine must also be in compliance with CLIA (Clinical Laboratory Improvement Amendments).
**All medications including oxygen should be in accordance with state laws, pharmacy, and nurse practice acts.
From: Pontius D, Doyle J: Emergency Preparedness and Response in the School Setting—The Role of the School Nurse: National Association of School Nurses. Available at https://www.nasn.org/PolicyAdvocacy/PositionPapersandReports/NASNPositionStatementsFullView/tabid/462/ArticleId/117/Emergency-Preparedness-The-Role-of-the-School-Nurse-Adopted-2011. Accessed April 15, 2014.

Additional equipment may be obtained if a nurse is present in the school (Box 42-3). Various sizes of these items are needed since children may be of different ages in the school. Another recommended item for the nurse's office includes an epinephrine auto injector kit (EpiPen auto injector) in case a child goes into anaphylactic shock after exposure to an allergen (Pontius and Doyle, 2012). This should be locked in a medication cabinet because of the needle in the kit. The school nurse will need to teach other school personnel how to use the EpiPen auto injector in an emergency (Kruger et al, 2009).

Gloves to meet standard precautions guidelines and a telephone available for calling emergency personnel and parents are essential. Next to the telephone, paper and pen should be available so that instructions from the emergency personnel can be written down. The AED should be located in a central location at the school for easy access in an emergency. It should not be locked in the nurse's office but available for school staff to obtain in case the nurse is off site that day.

## Giving Medication in School

The school nurse, as part of secondary prevention, may be responsible for giving medications to children during the school day (Zacharski et al, 2012). These may include prescribed medications, medications that the parents have asked the school's nurse to give (such as cold remedies), or vitamins. In all instances, the nurse will want to develop a series of guidelines to help with the legal administration of medications in the school. The school nurse will inquire of parents if the child is taking any medications (Zacharski et al, 2012). HIPAA requires that all of this information be confidential (Nic Philibin et al, 2010). A current, signed parental consent form for giving the medication is essential for the student's file (Zacharski et al, 2012).

The prescribed drug must have the original prescription label on it and be in the original container so that there are no errors. A current drug reference in the nurse's office is necessary so that it can be consulted for information. The nurse is responsible for giving the medication and is expected by state law to know its action, side effects, and implications. The school nurse must have a means of contacting a pharmacist to ask questions regarding the medication if needed.

*Delegation.* Some states allow school nurses to delegate medication administration to unlicensed assistive personnel (UAP) or to a licensed practical nurse (Zacharski et al, 2012). There are several benefits and challenges associated with delegation in the school setting. On the positive side, delegation allows services to be provided in the absence of a school nurse, which is especially helpful if a nurse is covering multiple schools (Resha, 2010). Also, delegation gives the ability to provide one-on-one care for children with complex medical needs (Resha, 2010). The challenge with delegation is ensuring the UAPs receive adequate training, and regular supervision and monitoring of the UAP (Resha, 2010). Delegation can be done safely in the school environment provided the nurse has clear policies and procedures to follow, understands the "Five Rights of Delegation," understands the scope of practice under the state's Nurse Practice Act, and has a trusting relationship with the UAP and school administrators (Board et al, 2010; Resha, 2010).

### QSEN FOCUS ON QUALITY AND SAFETY EDUCATION FOR NURSES

**Targeted Competency: Safety**

Safety minimizes risk of harm to patients and providers through both system effectiveness and individual performance.

Important aspects of safety include:

- **Knowledge:** Describe factors that create a culture of safety (such as open communication strategies and organizational error reporting systems).
- **Skills:** Communicate observations or concerns related to hazards and errors to patients, families, and the health care team.
- **Attitudes:** Value own role in preventing errors.

**Safety Question**

Imagine you are working as a nurse in an elementary school. Due to budget cuts, you are only at the school two days a week. Juan, a student in the third grade, is newly diagnosed with asthma and will have an inhaler at school for emergencies. Your state allows nurses to delegate the administration of inhaler medications to unlicensed personnel. You decide to delegate the administration of Juan's emergency inhaler to his classroom teacher, Mr. Smith. What steps would you take to ensure you safely delegated this medication?

*Answer*

First, you would need to establish open communication between Mr. Smith and yourself. After the initial medication training, you can maintain open communication by checking in with Mr. Smith on a regular basis to assess his knowledge and comfort level in administering Juan's inhaler. Second, in the event that Mr. Smith gives Juan a dose from the inhaler, have a system in place to document when and why the medication was given. Periodically review the records to ensure that everything was documented correctly and that the medication was given for appropriate reasons. Last, in the event of a medication error, reflect on what you can do differently to prevent future errors.

## Assessing and Screening Children at School

Children should receive screening for vision, hearing, height and weight, oral health, tuberculosis, and scoliosis in the schools. For each of these areas, the school nurse will keep a confidential record of all of the screening results for the children in the school according to the HIPAA rules. In addition, each state has different laws regarding the screenings and the nurse will need to be aware of these laws.

Screening for tuberculosis (TB) in schoolchildren is also done in several states. This can be problematic because the nurse cannot read the Mantoux test, or the TST test, until three days after it is administered. Often nurses are part time and may not be at the school on the day the child's test needs to be read. In some states, school nurses are required to participate in a training program to read the tests (Cruise, 2015). It may be more efficient to have the children screened for TB at a health clinic and then have the school nurse read the test and send that information to the health clinic for follow-up. If the site is positive, the child has been exposed to TB and needs further health screening.

The school nurse can also screen children and adolescents for hypertension, or high blood pressure. One study found that of the adolescent students whom the school nurse referred to a family physician for follow-up for elevated cholesterol or blood pressure, 60% actually went to the doctor, 58% had further tests, 10% were referred to specialists, and 3% were prescribed medication (Kilty and Prentice, 2010). These findings indicate the importance of the school nurse in providing effective prevention strategies related to screening, follow-up, and treatment.

Physical examinations to participate in a school sport also may be given in the school. The school nurse arranges for the sports physicals and helps to monitor the examinations being done by the school's physician or nurse practitioner. In addition, some children may not have a regular physician or other primary health care provider such as a nurse practitioner to give them health care. For these children, the AAP recommends that children have a physical and developmental examination in the school setting. This would include obtaining information on their language skills and their motor abilities. Their social abilities and their height and weight are also tested. As the children grow up, their level of physical growth can be noted as well as their sexual maturation. Dental assessments are also to be made. Some states are passing laws requiring these assessments and giving nurses the right to complete the assessment and refer to a dentist.

## Screening Children for Pediculosis (Lice)

School nurses must screen children for lice infestation. Prevalence of head lice in U.S. schools ranges from 10% to 40%, being found most commonly in school-aged children, typically in late summer and autumn (Wolfram, 2010). Lice are found most often in white middle-class children because of their oval hair shafts. Lice also are more often seen in clean hair. Therefore, the suggestion that lice are associated with unclean homes in poverty areas is incorrect (Wolfram, 2010). The school nurse needs to check children for lice because in many areas, children with lice are excluded from school. During the "lice check," the nurse must check the children's hair for both lice and nits (Pontius and Teskey, 2011).

It is the responsibility of the school nurse to teach children, parents, and teachers how to prevent lice and treat cases of infestation. The nurse can do this by teaching children not to share combs and hats, and teaching parents to completely treat the child with anti-lice medications. Parents also need to be told to remove all nits from the head with a fine-toothed comb and to wash all bed linens and clothing (Pontius and Teskey, 2011).

## Identification of Child Abuse or Neglect

The school nurse is mandated by state laws to report suspected cases of child abuse or neglect. These laws differ from state to state and the nurse must be aware of the particular requirements for reporting in his or her state.

When the nurse identifies a child who may be abused, or receives information from a teacher or other staff member that leads to the belief that a child has been abused, the nurse must contact the appropriate legal authorities as well as the school's principal. A confidential file should be made about the incident. However, the nurse contacts the government authorities, usually the state or county child protection department, who look into the suspected case. In all cases, the child must be protected from

harm, and those who have no right to know that child abuse or neglect is suspected should not be given any information.

## Communicating with Health Care Providers

The school nurse often makes an assessment of a child that requires referral to the child's family physician or other health care provider. The findings from these assessments must be communicated accurately to the child's parent and the provider. The nurse must be able to disseminate the information quickly and accurately to the child's parents. Again, HIPAA privacy rules must be followed (Nic Philibin et al, 2010).

One way to do this is to write a detailed report about the findings. This information can be given to the child to give to his or her parents. However, the child may lose the report on the way home. The information can be mailed to the parents, but this takes more time. There is also an issue, in some instances, that are related to parental literacy issues.(Cruise, 2015). Perhaps the best way is to telephone the parents, telling them that the child needs to see the physician or nurse practitioner and that the child will be bringing the information home that day. In this way, the parents can ask the child for the report, the parent can read the report, or if unable to do so can provide it to the child's physician or nurse practitioner. With the phone call the child is aware that the parents expect the report.

---

**HOW TO** **Develop Good Relationships with Families**

*School nurses need to have good relationships with families. The school nurse can make this possible by doing the following:*
1. *Being visible at school events.*
2. *Sending home invitations for parents and guardians to call the nurse at any time.*
3. *Inviting parents to visit the school health office.*
4. *Calling parents or guardians to ask about ill children.*
5. *Offering to help families cope with children who have long-term illnesses.*
6. *Acting as a referral source for families with health care needs.*
7. *Including parents and members of the community in health education activities.*

---

## Efforts to Prevent Suicide and Other Mental Health Problems

Suicide is the third leading cause of death in teenagers. Recommendations have been made about reducing the incidence of suicide in teenagers. A suicide prevention program developed in one school district (see later discussion) contains ideas for the school nurse to use. Suicide prevention must be addressed by school nurses. Nurses can lead educational programs within the schools to emphasize coping strategies and stress management techniques for children and adolescents who have problems, and to teach about the risk factors. The school nurse can teach faculty members to look for the risk factors. The school nurse can also help organize a peer assistance program to help teenagers cope with school stresses (Ramos et al, 2013).

If a student threatens suicide at school, the school nurse can intervene by ensuring the safety of the student and by removing him or her from the school situation immediately. While parents are being notified, the nurse is able to assess the child's suicide risk and refer the child or teenager to crisis intervention or mental health services.

In the unfortunate instance in which a teenager who attended the school has committed suicide, the school nurse is called upon to help the school population, both students and teachers, cope with the death. Grief counseling is set up and coordinated by the school nurse, usually in collaboration with guidance counselors and school administrators. In addition, further assessments can be made regarding the suicide potential among the deceased teenager's friends, since suicide clusters have been noted.

Other mental health problems may affect students. Adolescents may have early signs of mental or emotional problems such as behavior problems in class or severe class or test anxiety. Families may be in crisis, and this translates into problems for the children. Sometimes, children with mental health issues come to the school nurse with somatic complaints and nothing can be found on assessment. The nurse should be alert to the possibility that the child is experiencing emotional, hunger, or family problems in such cases and look further for the source of the complaints (Cruise, 2015).

Children who are homeless have special problems. Because these children do not have a stable address, this also means that they probably have frequently moved from school to school. Children whose parents are addicted to drugs or alcohol can also benefit from support from the school nurse. This lack of a stable environment may increase chances that they may develop a mental or emotional problem. The school nurse can be an advocate for these children and their families.

## Violence at School

In 2009, in the previous 30 days prior to the survey, approximately 5.6% of high school students carried a weapon on school property and 5% of high school students missed at least one day of school because they felt unsafe (CDC, 2010c). Approximately 38% of public schools reported to police at least one incident of violence during the 2005-2006 school year (CDC, 2010c). In 2007, 23% of students reported gangs at their schools (CDC, 2010c). In 2006, there were 29 violent crimes (including rape, sexual and aggravated assault, and robbery) at school per 1000 students (CDC, 2010c). In the past several years, there have been school shootings by students or other attackers against other students and teachers.

Bullying is at the center of attention among child and adolescent advocates. Approximately 20% of high-school students experience bullying in the U.S. (CDC, 2011). Since 2007, the incidence of cyber bullying has risen (Patchin and Hinduja, 2013). Physical injury, social and emotional distress, and even death can result from bullying (CDC, 2011). Students may come to the school nurse complaining of psychosomatic illnesses, such as headaches and stomachaches, due to bullying (CDC, 2011). Students who are being bullied may feel sad or lose hope and begin considering harming themselves (CDC, 2011). The school nurse needs to be knowledgeable about bullying and provide leadership to implement bullying prevention strategies, such as increased supervision and anti-bullying policies (DeSisto and Smith, 2014). In an effort to reduce the prevalence of bullying, 49 states now have anti-bullying laws (Clark, 2013).

The school nurse's primary goal is to prevent violence from occurring and prioritize the safety of everyone on the school's campus (Tuck et al, 2013). Interventions that the nurse can implement to prevent violence include (Tuck et al, 2013):

- Facilitate student connectedness to the school community.
- Engage parents in school activities that promote connections with their children, and foster communication, problem solving, limit setting, and monitoring of children.
- Support activities and strategies to help establish a climate that promotes and practices respect for others and for the property of others.
- Support policies of zero tolerance for weapons on school property, including school buses.
- Advocate for adult monitoring in the hallways between classes and at the beginning and end of the school day, and the assignment of staff to monitor the playground, cafeteria, and school entrances before and after school.
- Serve as positive role models, developing mentoring programs for at-risk youth and families.
- Educate students and their parents about gun safety.

If violence occurs, the school nurse should do the following (Tuck et al, 2013):

- Coordinate emergency response until rescue teams arrive;
- Provide nursing care for injured students;
- Apply crisis intervention strategies that help de-escalate a crisis situation and help resolve the conflict;
- Identify and refer those students who require more in-depth counseling services; and
- Participate in crisis intervention teams.

By helping to identify the student who might be considering school violence or by teaching students and teachers about these warning signs in students, the school nurse may be able to help prevent violent actions through education and follow-up of children who need help. The U.S. federal government has many agencies that can be used as resources to help school nurses develop programs in their schools (CDC, 2010d).

## Tertiary Prevention in Schools

Using the nursing process, the school nurse gives nursing care related to tertiary prevention when working with children who have long-term or chronic illnesses or special needs. As prevalence of chronic conditions such as asthma and diabetes increases among children, today's school nurse faces a school population that is more medically diverse than ever seen in the past (Robert Wood Johnson Foundation, 2010). The nurse participates in developing an individual education plan (IEP) for students with long-term health needs (Box 42-3).

For example, nurses must have information about children's medications to be administered during school hours. They also need to know if the children need any therapy during the school day, such as physical or occupational therapy. If the child has a hearing or vision problem, the nurse may need to ask the teacher to seat the child in the best place in the classroom so the child can see or hear better. If a child is in a wheelchair or uses crutches, the school building itself may need to be altered so that the child can get around the school and use the restrooms. It is the responsibility of the nurse to tell the school's administrators about any needs such as these.

### Children with Allergies

Food and insect sting allergies that result in anaphylaxis are being diagnosed more frequently (Zacharski et al, 2012). Anaphylaxis is a severe allergic reaction that occurs quickly and can be life-threatening. Food allergies affect approximately 4% to 6% of children in the United States (CDC, 2013d). Milk, eggs, fish, shellfish, wheat, soy, peanuts, and tree nuts account for 90% of serious allergic reactions in the United States (CDC, 2013d).

The school nurse must take a leadership role in coordinated care for these students. The school nurse must develop a plan for preventing exposure to a known allergen and responding to an allergy emergency, collaborating with the student, the student's parents, and school personnel to determine the best plan of action (Zacharski et al, 2012). The school nurse must provide annual training to school personnel who are involved with the student (Zacharski et al, 2012). Most states have laws that allow students to carry emergency medication and, if developmentally appropriate, self-administer as needed (Zacharski et al, 2012). Some states allow trained unlicensed assistive personnel to administer the emergency medication if the student is unable to do so and a nurse is not available.

### Children with Asthma

Asthma is the leading cause of children being absent from school because of a chronic illness (CDC, 2013e). Children may be hospitalized with an asthma attack or they may have just returned home from the hospital. Asthma can also be caused by allergic triggers that affect children in the school. Possible culprits are chalk dust from the blackboards, molds or mildew in the school, or dander from pets that live in some classrooms (CDC, 2013e).

There may also be concerns about the quality of the air in the school building because many doors are shut. Industrial arts classes and other sources of air pollution can occur in the school (U.S. EPA, 2010). The school nurse can keep track of the indoor air quality of the school so that school administrators have data about what can affect the children. Figure 42-3 contains the questions developed by the U.S. Environmental Protection Agency that the school nurse should answer regarding the air quality of the school.

The nurse uses tertiary prevention when helping children who have asthma. This includes administering, or helping them use, their inhalers or other asthma rescue medications (NASN, 2013). It also includes instructing the teachers, children, and parents about asthma and ways to reduce allergens in the classroom (NASN, 2013). The nurse will also want to be seek information about the types of cleaning solutions used in schools. Many school systems are going with non-toxic cleaners, but many still use chemicals, such as bleach-based solutions, that can be dangerous to children if not properly stored and used (Cruise, 2015). Schools have management programs in place to help children with asthma (NASN, 2013).

### Children with Diabetes Mellitus

Diabetes is one of the most common chronic diseases in children and adolescents; about 151,000 people below the age of 20 years have diabetes (CDC, 2013f). Every year, more than 13,000 children and adolescents are diagnosed with type 1 diabetes (CDC, 2013f). In the last couple of decades, type 2 diabetes (formerly known as adult-onset diabetes) has been reported among U.S. children and adolescents with increasing frequency (CDC, 2013f). Case management and coordination of care are critical roles for the school nurse in caring for diabetic students (Butler et al, 2012). The school nurse must establish a plan of care for children with diabetes. This includes methods of monitoring blood glucose levels and administering insulin or other medications during the school day (Butler et al, 2012). Special nutritional needs also need to be discussed with parents, teachers, and cafeteria staff. There may be significant challenges getting the child's nutritional restrictions met due to the institutional nature of most school food services and lack of education of staff about nutrition-related health concerns (Butler et al, 2012; Cruise, 2015).

### Children Who Are Autistic or Who Have Attention-Deficit/ Hyperactivity Disorder

Because all children are expected to attend some school regardless of their illness, children with autism go to regular schools in most cases. Because a child with autism has severe communication problems, the school nurse provides help for the child, the teachers, and the parents so that the child's school day is pleasant and productive. The nurse can give the child prescribed medications for mood or prevention of seizures. The nurse is also responsible for preparing the teachers about the communication problems that the child may have. The nurse may recommend the use of sign language, picture boards, or other types of communication devices that are used by the child. In addition, the nurse can teach the parents about autism. The

# Health Officer/School Nurse

*This checklist discusses three major topic areas:*
Student Health Records Maintenance
Public Health and Personal Hygiene Education
Health Officer's Office

**Instructions:**
1. Read the IAQ *Backgrounder*.
2. Read each item on this Checklist.
3. Check the diamond(s) as appropriate or check the circle if you need additional help with an activity.
4. Return this checklist to the IAQ Coordinator and keep a copy for future reference.

Name: _____

Room or Area: _____

School: _____

Date Completed: _____

Signature: _____

### MAINTAIN STUDENT HEALTH RECORDS

There is evidence to suggest that children, pregnant women, and senior citizens are more likely to develop health problems from poor air quality than most adults. Indoor Air Quality (IAQ) problems are most likely to affect those with preexisting health conditions and those who are exposed to tobacco smoke. Student health records should include information about known allergies and other medically documented conditions, such as asthma, as well as any reported sensitivity to chemicals. Privacy considerations may limit the student health information that can be disclosed, but to the extent possible, information about students' potential sensitivity to IAQ problems should be provided to teachers. This is especially true for classes involving potential irritants (e.g., gaseous or particle emissions from art, science, industrial/vocational education sources). Health records and records of health-related complaints by students and staff are useful for evaluating potential IAQ-related complaints.

**Include information about sensitivities to IAQ problems in student health records**
- Allergies, including reports of chemical sensitivities.
- Asthma.
◇ Completed health records exist for each student.
◇ Health records are being updated.
○ Need help obtaining information about student allergies and other health factors.

**Track health-related complaints by students and staff**
- Keep a log of health complaints that notes the symptoms, location and time of symptom onset, and exposure to pollutant sources.
- Watch for trends in health complaints, especially in timing or location of complaints.
◇ Have a comprehensive health complaint logging system.
◇ Developing a comprehensive health complaint logging system.
○ Need help developing a comprehensive health complaint logging system.

**Recognize indicators that health problems may be IAQ**
- Complaints are associated with particular times of the day or week.
- Other occupants in the same area experience similar problems.
- The problem abates or ceases, either immediately or gradually, when an occupant leaves the building and recurs when the occupant returns.
- The school has recently been renovated or refurnished.
- The occupant has recently started working with new or different materials or equipment.
- New cleaning or pesticide products or practices have been introduced into the school.
- Smoking is allowed in the school.
- A new warm-blooded animal has been introduced into the classroom.
◇ Understand indicators of IAQ-related problems.
○ Need help understanding indicators of IAQ-related problems.

### HEALTH AND HYGIENE EDUCATION

Schools are unique buildings from a public health perspective because they accommodate more people within a smaller area than most buildings. This proximity increases the potential for airborne contaminants (germs, odors, and constituents of personal products) to pass between students. Raising awareness about the effects of personal habits on the well-being of others can help reduce IAQ-related problems.

**Obtain *Indoor Air Quality: An Introduction for Health Professionals***
- Contact IAQ INFO, 800-438-4318.
◇ Already have this EPA guidance document.
◇ Guide is on order.
○ Cannot obtain this guide.

**Inform students and staff about the importance of good hygiene in preventing the spread of airborne contagious diseases**
- Provide written materials to students (local public health agencies may have information suitable for older students).
- Provide individual instruction/counseling where necessary.
◇ Written materials and counseling available.
◇ Compiling information for counseling and distribution.
○ Need help compiling information or implementing counseling program.

**Provide information about IAQ and health**
- Help teachers develop activities that reduce exposure to indoor air pollutants for students with IAQ sensitivities, such as those with asthma or allergies (contact the American Lung Association [ALA], the National Association of School Nurses [NASN], or the Asthma and Allergy Foundation of America [AAFA]). Contact information is also available in the IAQ Coordinator's Guide.
- Collaborate with parent-teacher groups to offer family IAQ education programs.
- Conduct a workshop for teachers on health issues that covers IAQ.
◇ Have provided information to parents and staff.
◇ Developing information and education programs for parents and staff.
○ Need help developing information and education program for parents and staff.

**Establish an information and counseling program regarding smoking**
- Provide free literature on smoking and secondhand smoke.
- Sponsor a quit-smoking program and similar counseling programs in collaboration with the ALA.
◇ "No Smoking" information and programs in place.
◇ "No Smoking" information and programs in planning.
○ Need help with a "No Smoking" program.

### HEALTH OFFICER'S OFFICE

Since the health office may be frequented by sick students and staff, it is important to take steps that can help prevent transmission of airborne diseases to uninfected students and staff (see your IAQ Coordinator for help with the following activities).

**Ensure that the ventilation system is properly operating**
- Ventilation system is operated when the area(s) is occupied.
- Provide an adequate amount of outdoor air to the area(s). There should be at least 15 cubic feet of outdoor air supplied per occupant.
- Air filters are clean and properly installed.
- Air removed from the area(s) does not circulate through the ventilation system into other occupied areas.
◇ Ventilation system operating adequately.
○ Need help with ventilation-related activities.

☐ **No Problems to Report.** I have completed all the activities on this checklist, and I do not need help in any areas.

**FIG 42-3** Indoor air quality checklist. (From U.S. Environmental Protection Agency: *School and Child Care-Based Asthma Education Programs,* 2010. Available from http://www.epa.gov/asthma/school-based.html. Accessed April 15, 2014.)

nurse can also help parents work with others in the health care system, such as speech-language therapists and developmental specialists, so that the child can have a positive learning experience at school (Bellando and Lopez, 2009; Blackborow et al, 2013).

Children with attention-deficit/hyperactivity disorder (ADHD) also attend school. As of 2011, 6.4 million children between 5 and 17 years of age have been diagnosed with ADHD (CDC, 2013g). The school nurse can help these children learn appropriate behaviors to reduce classroom disruptions. An example of a common disruption is medication management at school (Blackborow et al, 2013).

## Children with Special Needs in the Schools

Children who need urinary catheterization, dressing changes, peripheral or central line intravenous catheter maintenance, tracheotomy suctioning, gastrostomy or other tube feedings, or intravenous medication also attend schools. The nurse may supervise a health aide who is assigned to the child to care for complex nursing needs. In all these cases, the school nurse provides tertiary care to maintain the child's health. The nurse has the skills needed to assess the child's well-being. In addition, the nurse may have to teach another person in the school how to care for the child in case the nurse is not in the building when the child needs help. It is the responsibility of the school nurse to keep up with the latest health care information through in-service programs.

An example of how a school nurse can help an injured child return to school after long absences follows. Enrique, a sixth-grade boy who had received serious facial burns, is preparing to return to school. Enrique is afraid of how the children will respond to the pressure mask he wears to minimize future scarring. The nurse has a meeting with Enrique's mother and the school's principal and also contacts nurses from the hospital's burn unit to determine a plan to Enrique's reentry to school. According to their plan, the school nurse first teaches a lesson to the boy's classmates about burns and their treatment. After the lesson, Enrique joined the class with the nurse and showed his classmates his face with and without his pressure mask. Both Enrique and the nurse answered the children's questions. In addition to the education provided, changes were made in Enrique's schedule so he could be out of the sun during the school day and during gym time. The nurse found that Enrique's burns were soon forgotten and he was accepted by his friends.

Children with HIV or AIDS may also attend school. Because of privacy and confidentiality laws, the school nurse may not even know that the child attends the school. In these cases, the nurse may be aware of the child's HIV status either by direct notification from the parents or physician or just by knowing that certain drugs the child is prescribed during the school day are anti-HIV medications. In all cases, the nurse must maintain confidentiality. This means that information cannot be released to anyone, including teachers, other health professionals, other students, or staff.

As part of regular health education in the school, the school nurse can provide education about HIV/AIDS prevention and risks to the children, school employees, and community. The school nurse should also be part of the school health advisory committee to develop an HIV/AIDS health curriculum that teaches not only about HIV/AIDS prevention, but also about the disease itself, so that children and families are not afraid to go to school with children who have the disease.

## Children with DNAR Orders

As part of tertiary prevention, the school nurse also maintains the health of children with terminal diseases who go to school. These children have been largely mainstreamed into the regular school population. The PL 94-142 Education for All Handicapped Children Act stated that all children should go to school in the "least restrictive environment" (AAP, 2010). Therefore, there may be children who have do-not-attempt-resuscitate orders (DNAR orders) at school, and some may die at school. DNAR orders are signed by the parents and the physician according to the state's law. Under law, the school nurse is bound to obey the DNAR order; however, it is not clear how the schools view them.

The AAP's committees on school health and bioethics reaffirmed a set of guidelines to help school health providers and the schools decide what to do when a child with a DNAR order attends the school (AAP, 2010). A formal request to the school and the school board from the physician is a must regarding the written DNAR order. The school nurses should be involved in discussions regarding when to use the DNAR order. The decision not to do anything for a dying child, and how to function if the child were to suddenly face death, is made in advance of discussions between the school nurse, the parents, the physician, and the school officials (Tuck et al, 2014).

When a child dies in school, the nurse is responsible for helping the children who witnessed the death. The nurse becomes a grief counselor and helps the children and teachers cope with the death. Further education about death and dying given by the school nurse would also help the school community cope with death in the schools. (Tuck et al, 2014).

## Homebound Children

Even though the laws regarding disabled persons state that all children should go to school, some children cannot. Instead, they may be taught in the home or in another institutional setting such as the hospital. In these situations, the school nurse can be a liaison between the child's teacher, physician, school administrators, and parents regarding the child's needs. The nurse helps these individuals develop the child's IEP so that it is appropriate for the child and does not remove necessary learning from the plan. The child should be allowed to go to school when he or she is able, at which point the school nurse coordinates the child's health care needs and classes.

## Pregnant Teenagers and Teenage Mothers at School

Many teenage girls who are pregnant attend school. Therefore, the school nurse may provide ongoing care to the mother as well as coordination of care the teen may need outside the school system, ie, visits to the physician or nurse practitioner (Brewin et al, 2013; Norris et al, 2009). Although this may appear to be primary prevention, it is tertiary prevention because adolescent pregnancies are considered to be high risk. This is discussed in more detail in Chapters 29 and 35.

## CONTROVERSIES IN SCHOOL NURSING

School nursing has evolved into a complex health care role, and some areas of the field still cause controversy, such as birth control education and giving out birth control to students in the schools. Although differences in opinion exist relating to sex education, reproductive services, and screening for sexually transmitted diseases in the schools, the literature supports a comprehensive approach to sexual health education (Bradley et al, 2012). The school nurse should make an effort to communicate with the community, school board, teachers, parents, and students about what they think about different types of services in the schools.

## ETHICS IN SCHOOL NURSING

The school nurse may be faced with ethical issues in the schools. For example, a child may have a DNAR order that the parents wish to be used if the child dies at school (see earlier text), but following the DNAR order may be against the nurse's personal beliefs. Perhaps a girl asks the nurse where she can get an abortion and wishes to talk to the school nurse about how she feels, but the nurse is against abortions. Alternatively, a teenager asks for emergency contraception, which the nurse cannot condone. In these cases, the nurse must give nursing care to the student client and keep personal beliefs out of the discussion. However, if the nurse feels so strongly that he or she cannot work with the situation, another school nurse should be called for help, or the student should be referred to other health providers who can give the care the student needs. Care should never be denied or ignored; referral is a good option.

### TABLE 42-4　Online Resources for School Nurses

| Organization | Internet Address |
|---|---|
| The American Academy of Child and Adolescent Psychiatry | http://www.aacap.org |
| American Academy of Pediatrics | http://www.aap.org |
| National Association of School Nurses | http://www.nasn.org |
| Center for Health and Health Care in the Schools | http://www.healthinschools.org |
| National Youth Violence Prevention Resource Center | http://www.safeyouth.org |
| U.S. Department of Education Emergency Preparedness | http://www2.ed.gov/admins/lead/safety/emergencyplan/index.html |
| Healthy Schools Network | http://www.healthyschools.org |

## FUTURE TRENDS IN SCHOOL NURSING

The future of school nursing is strong. The amount of health care being given in the schools is increasing. In the future, school nursing will entail telehealth and telecounseling to teach health education (Hoffmann et al, 2012; Schlachta-Fairchild et al, 2010). The Internet will be used by school nurses to work with children and parents. Teleclinics operated out of the schools will be seen more frequently (Hoffman et al, 2012; Schlachta-Fairchild et al, 2010). Online resources are listed in Table 42-4. The school nurse is responsible for keeping up with the latest changes in health care and health practice so that the health of children in the schools can be enhanced by new trends in health care.

## PRACTICE APPLICATION

The elementary school principal has notified the school nurse that Melissa and John, 8-year-old twins who receive daily physical therapy for mild cerebral palsy, have transferred to the school. The nurse must comply with federal laws related to providing education and services to all children with disabilities.

A. What nursing responsibilities should the school nurse carry out?

B. What factors must be considered when the nurse coordinates the IEP and IHP plans?

C. How will this situation impact other children at school?

D. What is the central focus of Melissa's and John's education?
**Answers can be found on the Evolve site.**

## KEY POINTS

- School nurses provide health care for children and families.
- In the early 1900s school nurses screened children for infectious diseases.
- By 2005 school nurses provided direct care, health education, counseling, case management, and community outreach.
- The National Association of School Nurses (NASN) is the professional organization for school nurses.
- School nurses have varying educational levels depending on state laws.

- The U.S. government supports school-based health centers, school-linked programs, and full-service school-based health centers.
- *Healthy People 2020* has objectives to enhance the health of children in schools.
- Primary prevention provides health promotion and education to prevent childhood injuries and substance abuse.
- The school nurse monitors the children for all of their state-mandated immunizations for school entry.

## KEY POINTS—cont'd

- HIPAA privacy rules regarding the health information of children apply in schools.
- Secondary prevention involves screening children for illnesses and providing direct nursing care.
- School nurses develop plans for emergency care in the schools.
- Giving medications to children in the school must be monitored carefully to prevent errors.
- School health nurses are mandated reporters to tell the authorities about suspected cases of child abuse and/or neglect.

- Disaster-preparedness plans should be set up for all schools with the school nurse as a member of the crisis response team.
- Tertiary prevention includes caring for children with long-term health needs, including asthma and disabling conditions.
- School nurses carry out catheterizations, suctioning, gastrostomy feedings, and other skills in the schools.
- Some ethical dilemmas in the schools are related to women's health care.
- Some school nurses use the Internet to help communicate with children and their families.

## CLINICAL DECISION-MAKING ACTIVITIES

1. For the state where you live, make a list of the immunizations required for children attending schools. Then contrast this to the immunizations you received when in school. How has this changed over the years?
2. Contact the nurse in your former high school. Interview the nurse, focusing on the major focus of the role. Describe what the nurse likes best and least about the role. What changes can be made to make the responsibilities easier?
3. Arrange to visit an elementary school health office during screening activities. Observe the interaction between the nurse and the children. Describe how the nurse is using the nursing process during the screening process.
4. Organize a group of nursing students to volunteer at a school health fair. Develop a health education booth for the fair.

Describe how the health information can be used by the children, families, and the community.
5. Attend the annual school board meeting that discusses the budget for the next year. Analyze the budget for health services. How will this be adequate to care for the children? What issues influence the budgetary process?
6. On the Internet, focus on your state's health department. What trends do you see relating to health in the schools?
7. Volunteer as a participant in your school district's emergency response drill. How did the school nurse's responsibilities work to help reduce confusion and increase the provision of emergency care?

## REFERENCES

AED Brands: *AED State Laws & Legislation.* 2010. Available at: http://www.aedbrands.com/resource-center/implementation/aed-state-laws/. Accessed April 15, 2014.

American Academy of Pediatrics, Committee on Injury and Poison Prevention: Skateboard and scooter injuries. *Pediatrics* 109:542–543, 2002. Reaffirmed 2009.

American Academy of Pediatrics, Council on School Health and Committee on Bioethics: Honoring do-not-attempt-resuscitation requests in schools. *Pediatrics* 125(5):1073–1077, 2010.

American Academy of Pediatrics, Committee on Infectious Diseases: Recommendations for prevention and control of influenza in children, 2013-2014. *Pediatrics* 132(4):e1–e16, 2013. Available at: http://pediatrics.aappublications.org/content/early/2013/08/28/peds.2013-2377. Accessed April 15, 2014.

Avery G, Johnson T, Cousins M, et al: The school wellness nurse: a model for bridging gaps in school wellness programs. *Pediat Nurs* 39(1):13–17, 2013.

Baisch MJ, Lundeen SP, Murphy MK: Evidence-based research on the value of school nurses in an urban school system. *J Sch Health* 81(2):74–80, 2011.

Bannister A, Kelts S: NASN position statement: the role of the school nurse and school-based health centers. *NASN Sch Nurse* 26(3):196–197, 2011.

Bellando J, Lopez ML: The school nurse's role in treatment of the student with autism spectrum disorders. *J Spec Pediatr Nurs* 14(3):173–182, 2009.

Blackborow M, Tuck C, Lambert P, et al: *Mental Health of Students—Position Statement.* 2013, National Association of School Nurses. Available at: http://www.nasn.org/PolicyAdvocacy/PositionPapersandReports/NASNPositionStatementsFullView/

tabid/462/smid/824/ArticleID/36/Default.aspx. Accessed April 15, 2014.

Board C, Bushmiaer M, Davis-Alldritt L, et al: *Delegation—Position Statement.* 2010, National Association of School Nurses. Available at: https://www.nasn.org/PolicyAdvocacy/PositionPapersandReports/NASNPositionStatementsFullView/tabid/462/smid/824/ArticleID/21/Default.aspx. Accessed April 15, 2014.

Board C, Bushmiaer M, Davis-Alldritt L, et al: *Role of the School Nurse: Position Statement.* 2011, National Association of School Nurses. Available at: http://www.nasn.org/portals/0/positions/2011psrole.pdf. Accessed April 14, 2014.

Bobo N, Rose KC, Tuck C, et al: *School-Located Vaccination—Position Statement.* 2013, National Association of School Nurses. Available at: https://www.nasn.org/PolicyAdvocacy/PositionPapersandReports/

NASNPositionStatementsFullView/tabid/462/smid/824/ArticleID/487/Default.aspx. Accessed April 15, 2014.

Bradley BJ, Mancuso P, Cagginello JB, et al: *School Health Education about Human Sexuality—Position Statement.* 2012, National Association of School Nurses. Available at: http://www.nasn.org/PolicyAdvocacy/PositionPapersandReports/NASNPositionStatementsFullView/tabid/462/smid/824/ArticleID/43/Default.aspx. Accessed April 15, 2014.

Brewin D, Koren A, Morgan B, et al: Behind closed doors—school nurses and sexual education. *J Sch Nurs* 30(1):31–41, 2013.

Butler S, Fekaris N, Pontius D, et al: *Diabetes Management in the School Setting—Position Statement.* 2012, National Association of School Nurses. Available at: http://www.nasn.org/PolicyAdvocacy/PositionPapersandReports/NASNPositionStatementsFullView/

tabid/462/smid/824/ArticleID/22/Default.aspx. Accessed April 15, 2014.

Cagginello JB, Clark S, Compton L, et al: *Emergency Preparedness— The Role of the School Nurse— Position Statement.* 2011, National Association of School Nurses. Available at: https://www.nasn.org/PolicyAdvocacy/PositionPapersandReports/NASNPositionStatementsFullView/tabid/462/ArticleId/117/Emergency-Preparedness-The-Role-of-the-School-Nurse-Adopted-2011. Accessed April 15, 2014.

Centers for Disease Control and Prevention: *Healthy Youth! Funded Partners: State, Territorial, and Local Agencies and Tribal Governments Coordinated School Health Programs (CSHPs).* 2009. Available at: http://www.cdc.gov. Accessed March 19, 2011.

Centers for Disease Control and Prevention: *Healthy Youth! Food Safety.* 2010a. Available at: http://www.cdc.gov/HealthyYouth/foodsafety/index.htm. Accessed April 14, 2014.

Centers for Disease Control and Prevention: *State Vaccination Requirements.* 2010b. Available at: http://www.cdc.gov/vaccines/imz-managers/laws/state-reqs.html. Accessed April 14, 2014.

Centers for Disease Control and Prevention, Youth Risk Behavior Survey: *Behaviors that Contribute to Violence on School Property.* 2010c. Available at: http://www.cdc.gov/HealthyYouth/yrbs/trends.htm. Accessed April 14, 2014.

Centers for Disease Control and Prevention: *Understanding School Violence: Fact Sheet.* 2010d. Available at: www.cdc.gov/violenceprevention. Accessed April 14, 2014.

Center for Disease Control and Prevention: *Understanding Bullying: Fact Sheet.* 2011. Available at: http://www.cdc.gov/violenceprevention/pdf/bullying_factsheet-a.pdf. Accessed April 15, 2014.

Centers for Disease Control and Prevention: *Vaccines and Immunizations: State Vaccination Requirements.* 2012. Available at: http://www.cdc.gov/vaccines/imz-managers/laws/state-reqs.html#other. Accessed July 29, 2014.

Centers for Disease Control and Prevention: *Adolescent and School Health: Components of Coordinated School Health.* 2013a. Available at: http://www.cdc.gov/healthyyouth/cshp/components.htm. Accessed April 15, 2014.

Centers for Disease Control and Prevention: *Make a Difference at Your School.* 2013b. *Chronic Disease,* Paper 31. Available at: http://digitalcommons.hsc.unt.edu/disease/31. Accessed April 15, 2014.

Centers for Disease Control and Prevention: *Results from the School Health Policies and Practices Study 2012.* Atlanta, 2013c, CDC, USDHHS. Available at: http://www.cdc.gov/HealthyYouth/shpps/index.htm. Accessed April 14, 2014.

Centers for Disease Control and Prevention: *Food Allergies in Schools.* 2013d. Available at: http://www.cdc.gov/HealthyYouth/foodallergies/. Accessed April 15, 2014.

Centers for Disease Control and Prevention: *Asthma and Schools.* 2013e. Available at: http://www.cdc.gov/HealthyYouth/asthma/. Accessed April 15, 2014.

Centers for Disease Control and Prevention: *Children and Diabetes—More Information.* 2013f, Division of Diabetes Translation, National Center for Chronic Disease Prevention and Health Promotion. Available at: http://www.cdc.gov/diabetes/projects/cda2.htm. Accessed April 15, 2014.

Centers for Disease Control and Prevention: *Attention-Deficit/Hyperactivity Disorder (ADHD).* 2013g, Division of Human Development, National Center on Birth Defects and Developmental Disabilities. Available at: http://www.cdc.gov/ncbddd/adhd/data.html. Accessed April 15, 2014.

Clark M: *49 States Now Have Anti-bullying Laws. How's That Working Out?* November 4, 2013, Governing.com. Available at: http://www.governing.com/news/headlines/49-States-Now-Have-Anti-Bullying-Laws-Hows-that-Working-Out.html. Accessed April 15, 2014.

Cruise EG: *Contributions to the Chapter.* 2015, Radford University School of Nursing Radford. VA 24142.

DeSisto MC, Smith S: *Bullying Prevention in Schools—Position Statement.* 2014, National Association of School Nurses. Available at: http://www.nasn.org/PolicyAdvocacy/PositionPapersandReports/NASNPositionStatementsFullView/tabid/462/ArticleId/638/Bullying-Prevention-in-Schools-Adopted-January-2014. Accessed April 15, 2014.

Diaz AL, Wyckoff LJ: *Concussions— The Role of the School Nurse: Position Statement.* Silver Spring, 2012, National Association of School Nurses. Available at: https://www.nasn.org/PolicyAdvocacy/PositionPapersandReports/NASNPositionStatementsFullView/tabid/462/ArticleId/218/Concussions-The-Role-of-the-School-Nurse-Adopted-January-2012. Accessed April 15, 2014.

Doyle J: *Disaster Preparedness— Guidelines for School Nurses.* Silver Springs, 2011, National Association of School Nurses.

DuRant BM, Gibbons LJ, Poole C, et al: *Caseload Assignments.* 2010, National Association of School Nurses. Available at: http://www.nasn.org/PolicyAdvocacy/PositionPapersandReports/NASNPositionStatementsFullView/tabid/462/smid/824/ArticleID/7/Default.aspx. Accessed April 14, 2014.

Earles C, Jones S: School nursing. In Davies R, Davies A, editors: *Children and Young People's Nursing: Principles for Practice.* Boca Raton, 2011, CRC Press, pp 212–236.

Embrey ML: Gaining insights from students in recovery from prescription drug abuse: did school nurses report an influence on their practice? Outcomes results from a live symposium. *NASN Sch Nurse* 27:166, 2012.

Family Health Center: *Our programs and services.* 2010. Available at: http://www.fhcw.org. Accessed April 15, 2015.

Frisen A, Bjarnelind S: Health-related quality of life and bullying in adolescence. *Acta Paediatr* 99(4):597–603, 2010.

Health Resources and Services Administration: *The Registered Nurse Population: Initial Findings from the 2008 National Sample Survey of Registered Nurses.* 2010, U.S. Department of Health and Human Services. Available at: http://bhpr.hrsa.gov/healthworkforce/rnsurveys/rnsurveyinitial2008.pdf. Accessed April 14, 2014.

Heron M: Deaths: Leading causes for 2010. *Nat Vital Stat Rep* 62(6):1–97, 2013. Available at: http://www.cdc.gov/nchs/data/nvsr/nvsr62/nvsr62_06.pdf. Accessed April 15, 2014.

Hoffmann S, Dolatowski R, McDowell B, et al: *The Use of Telehealth in Schools—Position Statement.* 2012, National Association of School Nurses. Available at: http://www.nasn.org/PolicyAdvocacy/PositionPapersandReports/NASNPositionStatementsFullView/tabid/462/smid/824/ArticleID/52/Default.aspx. Accessed April 15, 2014.

Jackson V: What is the role of the school nurse in sexual health education? *NASN Sch Nurse* 26(3):146–147, 2011.

Judd D, Sitzman S, Davis M: *A History of American Nursing: Trends and Eras.* Sudbury, MA, 2010, Jones & Bartlett.

Kanter RK, Abramson D: School interventions after the Joplin tornado. *Prehospital Disaster Med* 21:1–4, 2014.

Kilty HL, Prentice D: Adolescent cardiovascular risk factors: a follow-up study. *Clin Nurs Res* 19(1):6–20, 2010.

Kruger BJ, Toker KH, Radjenovic D, et al: School nursing for children with special needs: does number of schools make a difference? *J Sch Health* 79(8):337–346, 2009.

Laudorn C: *School nurse's corner.* 2010. Available at: http://www.christina.k12.de.us/downes/resources/nurse.html. Accessed March 19, 2011.

Lerner MD, Lindell B, Volpe J: *A practical guide for crisis response in our schools,* ed 4. American Academy of Experts in Traumatic Stress, 2013.

Li C, Freedman M: Seasonal influenza: an overview. *J Sch Nurs* 25(Suppl 1):4s–10s, 2009.

Maughan E, Adams R: Educators' and parents' perceptions of what school nurses do: the influence of school nurse/student ratios. *J Sch Nurs* 27(5):355–363, 2011.

Morrison-Sandburg LF, Kubik MY, Johnson KE: Obesity prevention practices of elementary school nurses in Minnesota: findings from interviews with licensed school nurses. *J Sch Nurs* 27(1):13–21, 2011.

National Association of School Nurses and the American Nurses Association: *Scope and Standards of Professional School Nursing Practice,* ed 2. Washington, DC, 2011, Nursebooks.

National Association of School Nurses: *Asthma Online Tool Kit.* 2013, NASN. Available at: http://www.nasn.org/ToolsResources/Asthma. Accessed April 15, 2014.

National Association of State Boards of Education: *State School Health Policy Database: Requirements for School Nurses.* 2013. Available at: http://www.nasbe.org/healthy_schools/hs/bytopics.php?topicid=2130. Accessed April 15, 2014.

Nic Philibin CA, Griffiths C, Byrne G, et al: The role of the public health nurse in a changing society. *J Adv Nurs* 66(4):743–752, 2010.

Norris J, Howell E, Wydeven M, et al: Working with teen moms and babies at risk: the power of partnering. *Am J Matern Child Nurs* 34(5):308–315, 2009.

Office of Health and Human Services: *Frequently Asked Questions on HIPAA and School Health.* 2010. Available at: http://www.mass.gov. Accessed March 19, 2011.

Office of the Press Secretary: *President Obama signs Healthy, Hunger-free Kids Act of 2010 into Law.* 2010. Available at: http://www.whitehouse.gov/the-press-office/2010/12/13/president-obama-signs-healthy-hunger-free-kids-act-2010-law. Accessed April 14, 2014.

Patchin J, Hinduja S: *Words Wound: Delete Cyberbullying and Make*

experiencing rapid growth, due in large part to the aging of the baby-boom generation, who will require more medical care. In addition, some health care occupations will be in greater demand for other reasons. As health care costs continue to rise, work is increasingly being delegated to lower-paid workers in order to cut costs. For example, tasks that were previously performed by doctors, nurses, dentists, or other health care professionals increasingly are being performed by physician assistants, nursing and medical assistants, dental hygienists, and physical therapist aides. In addition, clients increasingly are seeking home care as an alternative to costly stays in hospitals or residential care facilities, causing a significant increase in demand for home health aides. Although not classified as health care workers, personal and home care aides are being affected by this demand for home care as well (Bartsch, 2009).

## Characteristics of Work

There has been a dramatic shift in the types of jobs held by workers. Following the evolution from an agrarian economy to a manufacturing society and then to a highly technological workplace, the greatest proportion of paid employment was in the occupations of trade, transportation, and utilities with 25 million workers (BLS, 2008b). During the 1996 to 2000 period, service-providing industries accounted for virtually all of the job growth. Only construction added jobs in the goods-producing business sector, offsetting declines in manufacturing and mining.

The nature of work has been accompanied by many new occupational hazards, such as complex chemicals, nanotechnology, nonergonomic workstation design (requiring the adaptation of the workplace or work equipment to meet the employee's health and safety needs), and many issues related to work organization such as job stress, burnout, and exhaustion. In addition, the emergence of a global economy with free trade and multinational corporations presents new challenges for health and safety programs that are culturally relevant.

## Work–Health Interactions

The influence of work on health, or work–health interactions, is shown by statistics on illnesses, injuries, and deaths associated with employment. Employers reported 3.4 work injuries and occupational illnesses per 100 workers in 2011 (BLS, 2012). Occupational injuries alone are reported to cost over $100 billion in lost wages and lost productivity, administrative expenses, health care, and other costs (BLS, 2006). This figure does not include the cost of occupational diseases. These figures are often described as the "tip of the iceberg," because many work-related health problems go unreported. However, even the recorded statistics are significant in describing the amount of human suffering, financial loss, and decreased productivity associated with workplace hazards. Laborers, truck drivers, construction, health care, manufacturing, transportation, and service providing industries (Figure 43-2) were among the top occupations representing days away from work due to injury or illness in 2007 (BLS, 2014).

The high number of work injuries and illnesses can be drastically reduced. In fact, significant progress has been made in

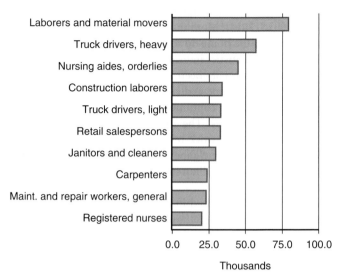

**Occupational injuries and illnesses involving days away from work for selected occupations, 2007 (thousands)**

**FIG 43-2** Occupational injuries and illnesses involving days away from work for selected occupations, 2007 (thousands). (From Bureau of Labor Statistics, 2014)

improving worker protection since Congress passed the 1970 Occupational Safety and Health Act. For example, vinyl chloride–induced liver cancers and brown lung disease (byssinosis) from cotton dust exposure have been almost eliminated. Reproductive disorders associated with certain glycol ethers have been recognized and controlled. Fatal work injuries have declined substantially through the years. Notably, from 1970 to 1995, fatal injury rates in coal miners were reduced by more than 75%, and the disease prevalence was reduced by 90%. However, since 1995 there has been a doubling of the disease incidence (NIOSH, 2008).

The U.S. workplace is rapidly changing and becoming more diverse. Major changes are also occurring in the way work is organized, with increased shift work, reduced job security, and part-time and temporary work as realities of the modern workplace. In addition, new chemicals, materials, processes, and equipment (such as nanotechnology and fermentation processes in biotechnology) continue to be developed and marketed at an accelerating pace creating new work-related hazards.

## APPLICATION OF THE EPIDEMIOLOGIC MODEL

The Epidemiologic Triangle can be used to understand the relationship between work and health (Figure 43-3). The reader is referred to Chapter 12, Epidemiology for a fuller description. With a focus on the health and safety of the employed population, the **host** is described as any susceptible human being. Because of the nature of work-related hazards, nurses must assume that all employed individuals and groups are at risk of being exposed to occupational hazards. The **agents**, factors associated with illness and injury, are occupational exposures that are classified as biological, chemical, enviromechanical, physical, or psychosocial (Box 43-1). The third element, the

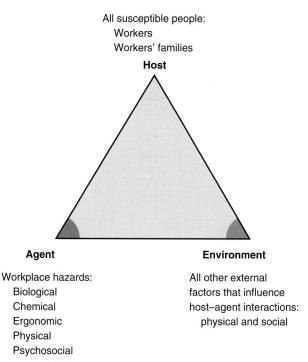

All susceptible people:
Workers
Workers' families
**Host**

**Agent**

Workplace hazards:
Biological
Chemical
Ergonomic
Physical
Psychosocial

**Environment**

All other external
factors that influence
host–agent interactions:
physical and social

**FIG 43-3** The epidemiologic triangle.

---

**BOX 43-1    Categories of Work-Related Hazards**

Biological and infectious hazards—Infectious/biological agents, such as bacteria, viruses, fungi, or parasites, that may be transmitted via contact with infected clients or contaminated body secretions/fluids to other individuals

Chemical hazards—Various forms of chemicals, including medications, solutions, gases, vapors, aerosols, and particulate matter, that are potentially toxic or irritating to the body system

Enviromechanical hazards—Factors encountered in the work environment that cause or potentiate accidents, injuries, strain, or discomfort (e.g., unsafe/inadequate equipment or lifting devices, slippery floors, workstation deficiencies)

Physical hazards—Agents within the work environment, such as radiation, electricity, extreme temperatures, and noise, that can cause tissue trauma

Psychosocial hazards—Factors and situations encountered or associated with one's job or work environment that create or potentiate stress, emotional strain, or interpersonal problems

Rogers B: *Occupational Health Nursing: Concepts and Practice.* In Press, 2015.

---

environment, includes all external conditions that influence the interaction of the host and agents. These may be workplace conditions such as temperature extremes, crowding, shift work, and inflexible management styles. The basic principle of epidemiology is that health status interventions for restoring and promoting health are the result of complex interactions among these three elements. To understand these interactions and to design effective nursing strategies for dealing with them in a proactive manner, nurses must look at how each element influences the others.

## Host

Each worker represents a host within the worker population group. Certain host factors are associated with increased risk of adverse response to the hazards of the workplace. These include age, sex, health status, work practices, ethnicity, and lifestyle factors (Rogers, 2015. For example, the population group at greatest risk for experiencing work-related accidents with subsequent injuries is new workers with less than one year of experience on the current job. Most nonfatal injuries and illnesses involving days away from work occur among new workers (the highest percentages were in mining [44%]; agriculture, forestry, and fishing [43%]; construction [41%]; and wholesale and retail trade [34%]). Thirty-five percent of injury and illness cases with days away from work occurred among workers with 5 or fewer years of service with their employer (BLS, 2012). The host factors of age, sex, and work experience combine to increase this group's risk of injury because of characteristics such as risk taking, lack of knowledge, and lack of familiarity with the new job.

Older workers may be at increased risk in the workplace because of diminished sensory abilities, the effects of chronic illnesses, and delayed reaction times. Another population group that may be very susceptible to workplace exposure is women in their child-bearing years. The hormonal changes during these years (along with the increased stress of new roles and additional responsibilities) and transplacental exposures are host factors that may influence this group's response to potential toxins.

In addition to these host factors, there may be other, less well-understood individual differences in response to occupational hazard exposures. Even if employers maintain exposure levels below the level recommended by occupational health and safety standards, 15% to 20% of the population may have health reactions to the "safe" low-level exposures (Levy and Wegman, 2011). This group has been termed *hypersusceptible*. A number of host factors appear to be associated with this hypersusceptibility: light skin, malnutrition, compromised immune system, glucose-6-phosphate dehydrogenase deficiency, serum alpha1-antitrypsin deficiency, chronic obstructive pulmonary disease, sickle cell trait, and hypertension. Individuals who have known hypersusceptibility to chemicals that are respiratory irritants, hemolytic chemicals, organic isocyanates, and carbon disulfide may also be hypersusceptible to other agents in the work environment (Levy and Wegman, 2011). Although this has prompted some industries to consider preplacement screening for such risk factors, the associations between these individual health markers and hypersusceptible response are speculative and require further research.

## Agent

Work-related hazards, or agents (see Box 43-1), present potential and actual risks to the health and safety of workers in the millions of business establishments in the United States. Any worksite commonly presents multiple and interacting exposures from all five categories of agents. The following paragraphs discuss each of these five agents in more detail.

**TABLE 43-1** Selected Job Categories, Exposures, and Associated Work-Related Diseases and Conditions

| Job Categories | Exposures | Work-Related Diseases and Conditions |
|---|---|---|
| All workers | Workplace stress | Hypertension, mood disorders, cardiovascular disease |
| Agricultural workers | Pesticides, infectious agents, gases, sunlight | Pesticide poisoning, "farmer's lung," skin cancer |
| Anesthetists | Anesthetic gases | Reproductive effects, cancer |
| Automobile workers | Asbestos, plastics, lead, solvents | Asbestosis, dermatitis |
| Butchers | Vinyl plastic fumes | "Meat wrappers' asthma" |
| Caisson workers | Pressurized work environments | Caisson disease ("the bends") |
| Carpenters | Wood dust, wood preservatives, adhesives | Nasopharyngeal cancer, dermatitis |
| Cement workers | Cement dust, metals | Dermatitis, bronchitis |
| Ceramic workers | Talc, clays | Pneumoconiosis |
| Demolition workers | Asbestos, wood dust | Asbestosis |
| Drug manufacturers | Hormones, nitroglycerin, etc. | Reproductive effects |
| Dry cleaners | Solvents | Liver disease, dermatitis |
| Dye workers | Dyestuffs, metals, solvents | Bladder cancer, dermatitis |
| Embalmers | Formaldehyde, infectious agents | Dermatitis |
| Felt makers | Mercury, polycyclic hydrocarbons | Mercurialism |
| Foundry workers | Silica, molten metals | Silicosis |
| Glass workers | Heat, solvents, metal powders | Cataracts |
| Hospital workers | Infectious agents, cleansers, radiation | Infections, latex allergies, unintentional injuries |
| Insulators | Asbestos, fibrous glass | Asbestosis, lung cancer, mesothelioma |
| Jack-hammer operators | Vibration | Raynaud's phenomenon |
| Lathe operators | Metal dusts, cutting oils | Lung disease, cancer |
| Office computer workers | Repetitive wrist motion on computers | Tendonitis, carpal tunnel syndrome, tenosynovitis, eye strain |

Table 43-1 lists some of the more common workplace exposures, their known health effects, and the types of jobs associated with these hazards.

## Biological Agents

Biological agents are living organisms whose excretions or parts are capable of causing human disease, usually by an infectious process. Biological hazards are common in workplaces such as health care facilities and clinical laboratories where employees are potentially exposed to a variety of infectious agents, including viruses, fungi, and bacteria. Of particular concern in occupational health is infectious diseases transmitted by humans (e.g., from client to worker or from worker to worker) in a variety of work settings. Bloodborne and airborne pathogens represent a significant class of exposures for U.S. health care workers at risk. Occupational transmission of bloodborne pathogens (including the hepatitis B and C viruses and the human immunodeficiency virus [HIV]) occurs primarily by means of needlestick injuries as well as through exposures to the eyes or mucous membranes (Dupler et al, 2013). The risk of hepatitis B virus infection following a single needlestick injury with a contaminated needle varies from 2% to greater than 40%, depending on the antigen status of the source person and the nature of the exposure. The risk of hepatitis C virus transmission depends on the same factors and ranges from 3.3% to 10% (Dupler et al, 2013).

Transmission of tuberculosis (TB) within health care settings (especially multidrug-resistant TB) has reemerged as a major public health problem (USDHHS, CDC, NIOSH, 2009). Since 1989 outbreaks of this type of TB have been reported in hospitals, and some workers have developed active drug-resistant TB. In addition, among workers in health care, social service, and corrections facilities who work with populations at increased risk of TB, hundreds have experienced tuberculin skin test conversions. Reliable data are lacking on the extent of possible work-related TB transmission among other groups of workers at risk for exposure. Many workers in these settings were employed as maintenance workers, security guards, aides, or cleaning people, who were not well protected from inadvertent exposure. Education should be provided to all health care workers, including those not having direct client care, in the proper handling and disposal of potentially contaminated linens, soiled equipment, and trash containing contaminated dressings or specimens (Gonzalez and Conlon, 2013) (See Evidence-Based Practice box).

## Chemical Agents

More than 300 billion pounds of chemical agents are produced annually in the United States. Of the approximately 2 million known chemicals in existence, less than 0.1% have been adequately studied for their effects on humans. Of those chemicals that have been linked to carcinogens, approximately half test positive as animal carcinogens. Most chemicals have not been studied epidemiologically to determine the effects of exposure on humans (Levy and Wegman, 2011). As a consequence of general environmental contamination with chemicals from work, home, and community activities, a variety of chemicals have been found in the body tissues of the general population. These tissue loads may result in part from the accidental release of chemicals into the environment, such as that which occurred

## EVIDENCE-BASED PRACTICE

The aim of this study was to investigate occupational exposures of health care workers to blood and body fluids in eastern Ethiopia (Reda et al, 2010). Health care workers still fail to adhere to standard precaution guidelines despite evidence that such a failure increases the risk of mucocutaneous blood and body fluid exposure resulting in bloodborne infection. The major infectious occupational hazards in the health care sector are hepatitis B and C viruses (HBV, HCV) and human immunodeficiency virus (HIV).

A total of 475 health care workers were surveyed working in 10 hospitals in eastern Ethiopia with an 84.4% response rate. Lifetime needlestick risk was 30.5% and lifetime blood/body fluid exposure risk was 28.8%. Only 80.8% followed standard precautions regularly while 46.9% recapped and 5.9% reused syringes. 44.8% of health care workers reported they were dissatisfied by the supply of personal protective equipment and 70.9% perceived they were at risk in the workplace.

### Nurse Use

Training programs and better provision of PPE are critically needed. Compliance with PPE must be emphasized along with effective teaching in infection control and safe work practice behavior.

Reda AA, Fisseha S, Mengistie B, et al: Standard precautions: occupational exposure and behavior of health care workers in Ethiopia, *PLoS One*, 5(12): e14420, 2010. doi:10.1371/journal.pone.0014420.

in Love Canal when chemicals leached out from buried industrial wastes.

In many workplaces, significant exposure to a daily, low-level dose of workplace chemicals may be below the exposure standards but may still create a potentially chronic and perhaps cumulative assault on workers' health. Predicting human responses to such exposures are further complicated because multiple chemicals often combine and interact to create a new chemical agent. Human effects may be associated with the interaction of these agents rather than with a single chemical. Another concern about occupational exposure to chemicals is reproductive health effects. Workplace reproductive hazards have become important legal and scientific issues. Toxicity to male and female reproductive systems has been demonstrated from exposure to common agents such as lead, mercury, cadmium, nickel, and zinc, as well as in antineoplastic drugs. Because data for predicting human responses to many chemical agents are inadequate, workers should be assessed for all potential exposures and cautioned to work preventively with these agents. High-risk or vulnerable workers, such as those with a latex allergy—a widely recognized health hazard—should be carefully screened and monitored for optimal health protection (USDHHS, CDC, NIOSH, 2009). To accurately assess and evaluate the exposure and recommend changes for abatement, it is essential that the nurse have a good understanding of the basic principles of toxicology, including routes of exposure (i.e., inhalation, skin absorption, and ingestion), dose–response relationships, and differences in effects (i.e., acute versus chronic toxicity).

## Enviromechanical Agents

**Enviromechanical agents** are those that can potentially cause injury or illness in the workplace. They are related to the work process or to working conditions, and they can cause postural or other strains that can produce adverse health effects when certain tasks are performed repeatedly. Examples are repetitive motions, poor or unsafe workstation–worker fit, slippery floors, cluttered work areas, and lifting heavy loads. Severity of illness or injury can be estimated from the number of days away from work. Sprains and strains, bruises/contusions, cuts/lacerations, fractures, and multiple injuries accounted for more days away from work than for all types of injury and illness. In 2011 (BLS, 2012), sprains, strains, and tears accounted for 38% of total injury and illness cases (n = 447,200) resulting in of days away from work. Twenty-two percent of these occurred as a result of overexertion in lifting or lowering (Figure 43-4). The back was the body part most often affected by disabling work incidents.

Back pain/injury is one of the most common and significant musculoskeletal problems in the world (USDHHS, CDC, NIOSH, 2009). In 2011, back injuries and disorders accounted for 36% of all nonfatal occupational injuries and illnesses involving days away from work in the United States. Although the exact cost of back disorders is unknown, the estimates are

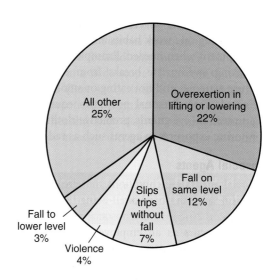

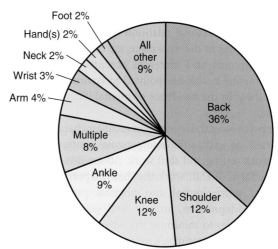

**FIG 43-4** Types of occupational injuries. (From Bureau of Labor Statistics, 2014.)

In industries that have exposures regulated by law, certain programs are required, such as respiratory protection or hearing conservation. The ability of a company to offer additional programs depends on employee needs, management's attitudes and understanding about health and safety, acceptance by the workers, and the economic status of the company. A significant increase in the number of health promotion and employee assistance programs offered in industry has occurred over the past few years. Health promotion programs focus on lifestyle choices that cause risks to health (e.g., job stress, obesity, smoking, stress responses, or lack of exercise) (O'Donnell, 2009). Employee assistance programs are designed to address personal problems (e.g., marital/family issues, substance abuse, or financial difficulties) that affect the employee's productivity. Since such efforts are cost-effective for businesses, they should continue to increase.

Similar types of occupational health and safety programs are available on a contractual basis from community-based providers. These may be offered by free-standing occupational health clinics, health maintenance organizations, hospitals, emergency clinics, and other health care organizations. In addition, consultants in each discipline work in the private sector (self-employed, in group practice, or in insurance companies) and in the public sector (in local and state health departments or departments of labor and industry). These services may be provided on-site, delivered at a specific location in the community, or offered through a mobile van that visits companies. These multiple resources have increased the options for companies that need occupational health and safety services, and they have also broadened the employment opportunities for health and safety professionals.

## NURSING CARE OF WORKING POPULATIONS

The nurse is often the first health care provider seen by an individual with a work-related health problem. Consequently, nurses are in key positions to intervene with working populations at all levels of prevention (see the Levels of Prevention box). Prevention may be accomplished in the prepathogenesis period by measures designed to promote general optimal health, by protection against specific disease agents, or by the establishment of barriers against agents in the environment. These procedures have been termed *primary prevention*.

### LEVELS OF PREVENTION

#### Occupational Health

**Primary Prevention**
Nurse provides education on use of personal protective equipment in the workplace to prevent injury/exposure.

**Secondary Prevention**
Nurse screens for hearing loss resulting from noise levels in the plant.

**Tertiary Prevention**
Nurse works with chronic diabetic workers to ensure appropriate medication use and blood glucose screening to avoid lost work days.

As soon as the disease is detectable, early in pathogenesis, secondary prevention may be accomplished by early diagnosis and prompt and adequate treatment. When the process of pathogenesis has progressed and the disease had advanced beyond its early stages, secondary prevention may be accomplished by means of adequate treatment to prevent sequelae and limit disability. Later, when defect and disability have been resolved, tertiary prevention may be accomplished by rehabilitation.

The occupational health nurse practices all levels of prevention (Rogers, 2015). Delivery of primary prevention services to employees is directed toward promoting health and averting a problem. In the occupational health setting, the purpose of health promotion is to maintain or enhance the well-being of individuals or groups of employees, and the company in general. This may include programs designed to enhance coping skills or good nutrition and knowledge about potential health hazards both inside and outside of the workplace.

Health protection (i.e., taking primary prevention measures) is designed to eliminate or reduce the risk of disease in order to prevent the development of an illness or injury. Walk-throughs by the occupational health nurse and/or other team members to identify workplace hazards are aimed at health protection.

Specific protection programs or interventions often require active participation on the part of the employee. Participation in an immunization program, employment of personal protective equipment such as respirators or gloves, and cessation of smoking are examples of specific health protection measures.

Secondary prevention occurs after a disease process has already begun. It is aimed at early detection, prompt treatment, and prevention of further limitations. For employees, early detection involves health surveillance and periodic screening to identify an illness at the earliest possible moment in its course, and elimination or modification of the hazard-producing situation. Interventions aimed at disability limitation are intended to prevent further harm or deterioration, and they include referral for counseling and treatment of an employee with an emotional or mental health problem whose work performance has deteriorated, as well as removal of workers from heavy-metal exposure who manifest neurologic symptoms.

Tertiary prevention is intended to restore health as fully as possible and assist individuals to achieve their maximum level of functioning. Rehabilitation strategies such as return-to-work programs after a heart attack or limited duty programs after a cumulative trauma injury are examples of tertiary prevention.

### Worker Assessment

The initial step of assessment involves the traditional history and physical assessment, emphasizing exposure to occupational hazards and individual characteristics that may predispose the client to the increased health risk of certain jobs. The occupational health history is an indispensable component of the health assessment of individuals (Rogers, 2015). Because work is a part of life for most people, including an occupational health history in all routine nursing assessments is essential. Many workers in the United States do not have access to health care services in their workplaces, yet it is not unusual to find health care providers in the community who have little or no knowledge about workplaces or expertise in occupation-related illnesses and injuries. Because of the large number of small businesses that do not have the resources for maintaining on-site health care, injured and ill workers are first seen in the public and private health care sector (e.g., in clinics, emergency departments, physicians' offices, hospitals, health maintenance organizations, and ambulatory care centers). Nurses are often the first-line assessors of these individuals and perhaps the only contact for education about self-protection from workplace hazards.

Identifying workplace exposures as sources of health problems may influence the client's course of illness and rehabilitation and may also prevent similar illnesses among others with potential for exposure (Levy and Wegman, 2011). Including occupational health data into client assessments begins with recognizing the possible relationship between health and occupational factors. The next step is to integrate into the history-taking procedure some routine assessment questions that will provide the data necessary to confirm or rule out occupationally induced symptoms.

Symptoms of hazardous workplace exposures may be indicated by vague complaints involving any body system. These complaints are often similar to common medical problems. Three points that occupational health histories should include are a list of current and past jobs the client has held; questions about exposures to specific agents and relationships between the symptoms and activities at work, job titles, or history of exposures; and other factors that may influence the client's susceptibility to occupational agents (e.g., lifestyle history such as smoking, underlying illness, previous injury, or disabling condition).

Questions about the employee's occupational history can be included in existing assessment tools. The more complete the data collected, the more likely the nurse is to notice the influence of work–health interactions. All employees should be questioned about their employment history. To describe only a current status of "retired" or "housewife" may lead to the omission of needed data. The nurse should be aware that not all workers are well informed about the materials with which they work or about potential hazards. For this reason, the nurse must develop basic knowledge about all of the types of jobs held by clients and the possible hazards associated with them. Because there is an increased likelihood of multiple exposures from other environments such as the home and the community that may interact with workplace exposures, the nurse should extend the questioning to include this information.

Identifying work-related health problems should be an integrated focus of any assessment effort. A systematic approach for evaluating the potential for workplace exposures is the most effective intervention for detecting and preventing occupational health risks. Figure 43-5 shows one short assessment tool that can be incorporated into routine history taking. Similar questions can be included in the assessment of workers' spouses and dependents, who may receive second-hand or indirect exposure to occupational hazards.

## (QSEN) FOCUS ON QUALITY AND SAFETY EDUCATION FOR NURSES

**Targeted Competency: Evidence-based Practice**
Integrates the best current clinical evidence with client and family preferences and values to provide optimal client care
- **Knowledge:** Explain the role of evidence in determining best clinical practice
- **Skill:** Read original research and evidence reports related to area of practice
- **Attitude:** Appreciate the importance of reading relevant professional journals

**Evidence-based Practice Question**
The PHN Quad Council competency of leadership and systems thinking skills recommends the beginning PHN provide data to measure, report, and improve organizational performance. You are working as an occupational health nurse. You have noticed there are a lot of work days lost because of work-related injuries or exposure to some type of hazard in the workplace. In this chapter you will see which of the injuries and exposures are more likely to occur in industry. Choose one of the hazard categories and read the evidence available about this hazard category. What does the evidence suggest in terms of organizational changes that could help reduce the risk for this hazard? How can the occupational health nurse promote changes in practice using the evidence available?

Prepared by Gail Armstrong, PhD(c), DNP, ACNS-BC, CNE, Associate Professor, University of Colorado Denver College of Nursing.

During these health assessments, the nurse has the opportunity to teach about workplace hazards and prevention measures the worker can use. At the same time, the nurse is obtaining information that will be valuable in optimizing the fit between the job and the worker. Such assessments can be done during preplacement examinations before the client begins a job, on a periodic basis during employment, or when a work-related health problem or exposure becomes apparent. One important group to consider are the nearly 15 million truck drivers who face health hazards from long work hours and fatigue, shift work, sleep deprivation, chemical exposure, and sedentary work and lifestyle (Apostolopoulos et al, 2010). Life expectancy for these workers is only 63 years (Heron et al, 2009). The occupational health nurse can help identify physical and psychosocial health and life-threatening issues for this workforce and develop interventions to mitigate the risk. Work-related health assessments should also be conducted when an employee is being transferred to another job with different requirements and exposures. The goal of these assessments is to identify agent and host factors that could place the employee at risk and to determine prevention steps that can be taken to eliminate or minimize the exposure and potential health problem.

When the health data from such assessments are considered collectively, the nurse may determine some patterns in risk factors associated with the occurrence of work-related injuries and illnesses in a total population of workers. For example, a nurse practitioner in a clinic noted a dramatic increase in the number of dermatitis cases among her clients. When she looked at factors in common among these individuals, she determined that they all worked at a company with solvent exposure commonly associated with dermal irritations. She worked with the union and the company to assess the environment/agent exposure to the employees. This nursing intervention led to a safer

I.   **Present Job**

    A.   What is your job title? _____

    B.   What do you do for a living? _____

    C.   How long have you had this job? _____

    D.   Describe the specific tasks of this job: _____
          _____

    E.   What product or service is produced by the company where you work? _____
          _____

    F.   Are you exposed to any of the following on your present job?

| Metals | Radiation | Stress |
|---|---|---|
| Vapors, gases | Vibration | Others: _____ |
| Dusts | Loud noise | |
| Solvents | Extreme heat or cold | |

    G.   Do you feel you have any health problems that may be associated with your work?
          If yes, describe: _____
          _____

    H.   How would you describe your satisfaction with your job? _____
          _____

    I.   Have any of your co-workers complained of illness or injuries that they associate with their jobs?
          If yes, describe: _____
          _____

II.  **All Past Work**

    Starting with your first job, please provide the following information:

| Job title | Years held | Description of work | Exposures | Injuries/Illnesses | Personal protection equipment used |
|---|---|---|---|---|---|
| | | | | | |
| | | | | | |
| | | | | | |
| | | | | | |
| | | | | | |

III. **Other Exposures**

    A.   Do you have any hobbies that involve exposure to chemicals, metals, or any of the other agents mentioned
          before? If yes, describe: _____

    B.   Are any other members of your household exposed to any of the substances listed above? If yes, describe:
          _____

    C.   Do you live near any factories, dump sites, or other sources of pollution? If yes, describe: _____
          _____

**FIG 43-5** Occupational health history form.

work environment and a decrease in dermatitis in this population group. Such an approach can be used at the company, industry, and community levels. The initial collection of data and the questioning about workplace exposures are vital steps for any intervention.

## Workplace Assessment

The nurse may conduct a similar assessment of the workplace itself. The purpose of this assessment, known as a **worksite walk-through** or survey, is to become knowledgeable about the work processes and the materials, the requirements of various jobs, the presence of actual or potential hazards, and the work practices of employees (Rogers, 2015). Figure 43-6 shows a brief outline that can be used to guide a worksite assessment. More complex surveys are performed by industrial hygienists and safety professionals when the purpose of the walk-through is environmental monitoring using sampling techniques or a safety audit. However, most occupational health nurses have developed expertise in these areas and include such tasks as part of their functions. For all health care providers who assess workers, this information makes an important database. In addition, for the on-site health care provider, worksite walk-throughs assist the professional in developing rapport with and being seen as a credible worker among the employees.

A worksite survey begins with an understanding of the type of work that occurs in the workplace. All business organizations are classified within the North American Industry Classification System (NAICS) with a numerical code. This code, usually a two- to four-digit number, indicates a company's product and, therefore, the possible types of **occupational health hazards** that may be associated with the processes and materials used by its employees. NAICS codes are used to collect and report data on businesses. For example, illness and injury rates of one company are compared with the rates of other companies of similar size with the same code to determine whether the company is having an excess of illness or injury. In addition, by knowing the NAICS code of a company, a health care professional can access reference books that describe the usual processes, materials, and by-products of that kind of company.

The nurse will want to review the work processes and work areas by jobs or locations in the workplace. These preliminary data provide clues about what hazards may be present and an understanding of the types of jobs and health requirements that may be involved in a particular industry. A description of the work environment is next and provides an overall picture of general appearances, physical layout, and safety of the environment. Are safety signs posted and readable where needed? Is there clutter or dampness on the floor that could cause slips or falls?

A description of the employee group is necessary information to understand the demographics and the work distribution in the company. Knowing about shift work and productivity can be helpful in pinpointing potential stressors. Human resources' management and corporate commitment to health and safety are needed to develop a supportive culture for effective and efficient programming. Reviewing the status of policies and procedures and assessing opportunities for input into

improving service are important to establish the organization's strength in occupational health and safety management. Gathering data about the incidence and prevalence of work-related illnesses and injuries and the cost patterns for these conditions provides useful epidemiologic trend data and helps to target high-cost areas. The types of occupational safety and health services and programs are important to know. This will show whether required programs are being offered and includes health promotion and disease prevention strategies.

---

> **HOW TO**    **Assess a Worker and the Workplace**
>
> *Assessing the worker for a work-related problem is a critical practice element. You need to do the following:*
> - *Complete general and occupational health history-taking with emphasis on workplace exposure assessment, job hazard analysis, and list of previous jobs.*
> - *Conduct a health assessment to identify agent and host factors that interact to place workers at risk.*
> - *Identify patterns of risk associated with illness/injury.*
>
> *Assessing the work environment is necessary to determine workplace exposures that create worker health risk. You need to do the following:*
> - *Understand the work being done.*
> - *Understand the work process.*
> - *Evaluate the work-related hazards.*
> - *Gather data about incidence/prevalence of work-related illness/ injuries and related hazards.*
> - *Conduct a walk-though of the work environment.*
> - *Examine prevention and control strategies in place for eliminating exposures.*

---

Finally, examining control strategies that are effective in eliminating or reducing exposure is important in determining risk reduction. Control strategies follow a hierarchical approach. Engineering controls can reduce worker exposure by modifying the exposure source, such as putting needles in a puncture-proof container. Work practice controls include good hygiene and proper waste disposal and housekeeping. Administrative controls reduce exposure through job rotation, workplace monitoring, and employee training and education. Finally, personal protective control is the last resort and requires the worker to actively engage in strategies for protection such as use of gloves, masks, and gowns to prevent exposures (Rogers, 2015).

The more information that can be collected before the walk-through, the more efficient the process of the survey will be. After the survey is conducted, the nurse can use the information with the aggregate health data to evaluate the effectiveness of the occupational health and safety program and to plan future programs.

## HEALTHY PEOPLE 2020 DOCUMENT RELATED TO OCCUPATIONAL HEALTH

In an attempt to meet the goal of attaining high-quality, longer lives free of preventable disability, injury, and premature death for Americans, health promotion and protection strategies are

Name of company: _____   Date: _____

Address: _____

Telephone: _____

Parent company (if any): _____

Location of corporate offices: _____

SIC code: _____

**The Work**

Major products: _____

Major processes and operations, raw materials, by-products: _____

_____

Type of jobs: _____

_____

Potential exposures: _____

_____

**Work Environment**

General conditions: _____

Safety signs: _____

Physical environment: _____

**Worker Population**

Employees

Total number: _____ Number in production: _____ Others: _____

% Full-time: _____ % Men: _____ % Women: _____

% First shift: _____ % Second shift: _____ % Third shift: _____

Age distribution: _____

% Unionized: _____ Names of unions: _____

**Human Resources Management**

Corporate commitment to health

Personnel

Policies/procedures

Input/surveys/committees

Record keeping

**Health Data**

Work-related illnesses, injuries, deaths per annum: _____

OSHA recordable: _____ Workers' compensation: _____

Other: _____ Most frequent complaints: _____

Average number of monthly calls to the health unit: _____

Absenteeism rate: _____

**Occupation Health and Safety Services**

Examinations

Employee assistance

Treatment of illness/injury

Health education

Physical fitness, health promotion activities

Mandatory programs

Safety audits

Environmental monitoring

Health risk appraisal

Screenings

Health promotion

**Control Strategies**

Engineering

Work practice

Administrative

Personal protective equipment

**FIG 43-6** Worksite assessment guide.

proposed to address the needs of large population groups such as the American workforce. As part of the *Healthy People 2020* document (USDHHS, 2010), occupational safety and health objectives were identified to promote good health and well-being among workers, including the elimination and reduction of elements in occupational environments that cause death, injury, disease, or disability. In addition, this document promotes the minimizing of personal damage from existing occupationally related illness.

 **HEALTHY PEOPLE 2020**

*Objectives Related to Occupational Health*

- OSH-1: Reduce deaths from work-related injuries.
- OSH-2: Reduce nonfatal work-related injuries.
- OSH-3: Reduce the rate of injuries and illness cases.
- OSH-4: Reduce pneumoconiosis deaths.
- OSH-5: Reduce deaths from work-related homicides.
- OSH-6: Reduce work-related assault.
- OSH-7: Reduce the proportion of persons who have elevated blood lead concentrations from work exposures.
- OSH-8: Reduce occupational skin diseases or disorders among full-time workers.
- OSH-9: (Developmental) Increase the proportion of employees who have access to worksites that provide programs to prevent or reduce employee stress.
- OSH-10: Reduce new cases of work-related noise-induced hearing loss.

U.S. Department of Health and Human Services: *Healthy People 2020*. Washington, DC, 2010, U.S. Government Printing Office.

# LEGISLATION RELATED TO OCCUPATIONAL HEALTH

The occupational health and safety services provided by an employer are influenced by specific legislation at federal and state levels. Although the relationship between work and health has been known since the second century (Ramazzini, 1713), public policy that effectively controlled occupational hazards was not enacted until the 1960s. The Mine Safety and Health Act of 1968 was the first legislation that specifically required certain prevention programs for workers. This was followed by the Occupational Safety and Health Act of 1970, which established two agencies, OSHA and NIOSH, each with discrete functions (Box 43-3) to carry out the act's purpose of ensuring "safe and healthful working conditions for working men and women" (PL 91-596, 1970). The reader is also referred to Chapters 3 and 5, the Affordable Care Act, for additional information on employer mandates.

In the context of the Occupational Safety and Health Act, OSHA, a federal agency within the U.S. Department of Labor, was created to develop and enforce workplace safety and health standards and regulations on workers' exposure to potentially toxic substances, enforcing these at the federal and state levels.

Specific standards and information about compliance can be obtained from federal, regional, and state OSHA offices, which

---

**BOX 43-3  Functions of Federal Agencies Involved in Occupational Safety and Health**

**Occupational Safety and Health Administration (OSHA)**

Determines and sets standards and permissible exposure limits (PELs) for hazardous exposures in the workplace.

Enforces the occupational health standards (including the right of entry for inspection).

Educates employees and employers about occupational health and safety.

Develops and maintains a database of work-related injuries, illnesses, and deaths.

Monitors compliance with occupational health and safety standards.

**National Institute for Occupational Safety and Health (NIOSH)**

Conducts research and reviews findings to recommend exposure limits for occupational hazards to OSHA.

Identifies and researches occupational health and safety hazards.

Educates occupational health and safety professionals.

Distributes research findings relevant to occupational health and safety.

U.S. Department of Health and Human Services, National Institute for Occupational Safety and Health: *National Occupational Research Agenda*. Cincinnati, OH, 2010, USDHHS.

---

**BOX 43-4  National Occupational Research Agenda (NORA) Sectors**

Agriculture, Forestry, and Fishing
Construction
Healthcare and Social Assistance
Manufacturing
Mining
Oil and Gas Extraction
Public Safety
Services
Transportation, Warehousing, and Utilities
Wholesale and Retail Trade

U.S. Department of Health and Human Services, National Institute for Occupational Safety and Health: *National Occupational Research Agenda*. Cincinnati, OH, 2010, USDHHS.

---

can be found on the OSHA website. The **National Institute for Occupational Safety and Health (NIOSH)** was established by the Occupational Safety and Health Act of 1970 and is part of the Centers for Disease Control and Prevention (CDC). In 1996 NIOSH and its partners unveiled a ten-year **National Occupational Research Agenda (NORA)**, a framework to guide occupational safety and health research into the following decade. The NIOSH agency identifies, monitors, and educates about the incidence, prevalence, and prevention of work-related illnesses and injuries and examines potential hazards of new work technologies and practices (USDHHS, NIOSH, 2010). The second decade of NORA (Box 43-4) is focused on targeted sectors to reduce the still significant toll of workplace illness and injury.

Many standards have been established by OSHA and promulgated to protect worker health. One example is the **Hazard Communication Standard**. This standard is based on the premise that while working to reduce and eliminate potentially toxic agents in the work environment, an important line of defense is to provide the work community with information about hazardous chemicals in order to minimize exposures. The Hazard Communication Standard, which was first established in 1983, requires that all worksites with hazardous substances inventory their toxic agents, label them, and provide information sheets, called material safety data sheets (MSDSs), for each agent. In addition, the employer must have in place a hazard communication program that provides workers with education about these agents. This education must include agent identification, toxic effects, and protective measures. Numerous standards have been established by OSHA for specific chemicals and programs. A standard familiar to all health care professionals is the *Bloodborne Pathogens Standard.*

**Workers' compensation acts** are important state laws that govern financial compensation to employees who suffer work-related health problems. These acts vary by state, and each state sets rules for the reimbursement of employees with occupational health problems for medical expenses and lost work time associated with the illness or injury. Workers' compensation claims and the experience-based insurance premiums paid by industry have been important motivators for increasing the health and safety of the workplace.

## ▶▶ LINKING CONTENT TO PRACTICE

### *Disaster Planning and Management*

Although disaster planning and management have been functions of occupational health and safety programs, this is an area of legislation that affects businesses and health professionals. The legislation of the Superfund Amendment and Reauthorization Act (SARA) requires that written disaster plans be shared with key resources in the community, such as fire departments and emergency departments. Concern about disasters—such as the terrorist attacks on the World Trade Center and Pentagon on September 11, 2001; the methyl isocyanate leak in Bhopal, India; effects of hurricanes such as Katrina and Sandy; or the community exposure to chemicals at Times Beach, Missouri, and exposure to radiation from crippled nuclear plants in Japan—has mandated more attention to disaster planning.

In occupational health, the goals of a disaster plan are to prevent or minimize injuries and deaths of workers and residents, minimize property damage, provide effective triage, and facilitate necessary business activities. A disaster plan requires the cooperation of different personnel within the company and community. The nurse is often a key person on the disaster planning team, along with safety professionals, physicians, industrial hygienists, the fire chief, and company management. The potential for disaster (e.g., explosions, floods, fires, leaks) must be identified, and this is best achieved by completing an exhaustive chemical and hazard inventory of the workplace. The material safety data sheet and plant blueprints are critical for correctly identifying substances and work areas that may be hazardous. Worksite surveys are the first step to completing this inventory. The reader is also referred to Chapter 23 on the PHN and disasters management.

Effective disaster plans are designed by those with knowledge of the work processes and materials, the workers and workplace, and the resources in the community. Specific steps must be detailed for actions to be put in place by specific individuals in the event of a disaster. The written plan must be shared with all who will be involved. Employees should be prepared in first aid, cardiopulmonary resuscitation, and fire brigade procedures. Plans must be clear, specific, and comprehensive (i.e., covering all shifts and all work areas) and must include activities to be conducted within the worksite and those that require community resources. Transportation plans, fire response, and emergency response services should be coordinated with the agencies that would be involved in an actual disaster. The disaster plan, emergency and safety equipment, and the first response team's abilities should be tested at least annually with a drill. Practice results should be carefully evaluated, with changes made as needed.

Hospitals and other emergency services, such as fire departments, should be involved in developing the disaster plan and should receive a copy of the plan and a current hazard inventory. It is imperative that the plan and hazard inventory be periodically updated. The occupational health nurse or another company representative should provide emergency health care providers with updated clinical information on exposures and appropriate treatment. It should never be presumed that local services will have current information on substances used in industry. Representatives of these agencies should visit the worksite and accompany the nurse on a worksite walk-through so that they are familiar with the operations.

In disaster planning, the nurse is often assigned or assumes the responsibility for coordinating the planning and implementing efforts, working with appropriate key people within the company and in the community to develop a workable, comprehensive plan. Other tasks include providing ongoing communication to keep the plan current; planning the drills; educating the employees, management, and community providers; and assessing the equipment and services that may be used in a disaster.

In the event of a disaster, the nurse should play a key role in coordinating the response. Principles of triage may be used as the response team determines the extent of the disaster and the ability of the company and community to respond. Postdisaster nursing interventions are also critical. Examples include identifying the ongoing disaster-related health needs of workers and community residents, collecting epidemiologic data, and assessing the cause and the necessary steps to prevent a recurrence.

Occupational health nursing is a broad, dynamic specialty practice. The Public Health Foundation provides the basis for practice, supporting a health promotion and protection and prevention model. The occupational health nurse must have interprofessional skills and linkages to provide the most effective care and service. Occupational health nurses are involved in all levels of prevention in their practice.

## ▎PRACTICE APPLICATION

An insurance company recently renovated its claims processing office area and fitted the workstation with new computers. The company's occupational health nurse noticed an increase in visits to the health unit for complaints of headaches, stiff neck muscles, and visual disturbances consistent with computer usage.

To conduct a complete investigation of this problem, the nurse assessed the workers, the agent (computer), previously existing potential agents, and the work environment. Interventions focused on designing the health hazard out of the work process, if possible. In the present example, the first level of

## PRACTICE APPLICATION—cont'd

intervention was to refit the workstation for better worker use of the computer.

Minimizing the possible hazards of the agent involved recommendations for desks, chairs, and lighting designs that would accommodate the individual worker and allow shielding of the monitor. The nursing interventions included strengthening the resistance of the host by prescribing appropriate rest breaks, eye exercises, and relaxation strategies. Recognizing that previous cervical neck injury or impaired vision may increase the risk of adverse effects from computer work, the nurse would include assessment for these factors in employees' preplacement and periodic health examinations.

For the environmental concerns, the nurse educated the manager about the health risks of paced, externally controlled work expectations and recommended alternatives.

This case is an example of which of the following?
A. The application of the occupational health history
B. A worksite assessment or walk-through
C. A work–health interaction
D. The use of the epidemiologic triangle in exploring occupational health problems
**Answers can be found on the Evolve site.**

## KEY POINTS

- Occupational health nursing is an autonomous practice specialty.
- The scope of occupational health nursing practice is broad, including worker and workplace assessment and surveillance, case management, health promotion, primary care, management/administration, business and finance skills, and research.
- The workforce and workplace are changing dramatically, requiring new knowledge and new occupational health services.
- The type of work has shifted from primarily manufacturing to service and technological jobs.
- Workplace hazards include exposure to biological, chemical, enviromechanical, physical, and psychosocial agents.
- The Occupational Safety and Health Act of 1970 states that workers must have a safe and healthful work environment.
- The interprofessional occupational health team consists of the occupational health nurse, occupational medicine physician, industrial hygienist, and safety specialist.

- Work-related health problems must be investigated and control strategies implemented to reduce exposure.
- Control strategies include engineering, work practice, administration, and personal protective equipment.
- The Occupational Safety and Health Administration enforces workplace safety and health standards.
- The National Institute for Occupational Safety and Health is the education and research agency that provides grants to investigate the causes of workplace illness and injuries.
- Workers' compensation acts are important laws that govern financial compensation of employees who suffer work-related health problems.
- The occupational health nurse should play a key role in disaster planning and coordination.
- Academic education in occupational health nursing is generally at the graduate level.

## CLINICAL DECISION-MAKING ACTIVITIES

1. Arrange to visit a local industry to observe work processes and discuss working conditions. See if you can identify the work-related hazards and make recommendations for eliminating them.
2. Interview the occupational health nurse in an industry setting and ask questions about scope of practice, job functions, and contributions to the business. Compare and contrast what you have learned about this nurse role to that of the school health nurse.
3. Contact the American Association of Occupational Health Nurses and ask what the most pressing trends are in the

specialty. What are some of the complex issues related to these trends?
4. Obtain a proposed standard from the Occupational Safety and Health Administration, critique it, and submit your comments.
5. Attend a workers' compensation hearing, analyze the problem, and critique the outcome. How is your critique affected by what you thought the outcome should be?

# REFERENCES

American Association of Occupational Health Nurses: *The Nurse in Industry*. New York, 1976, AAOHN.

American Association of Occupational Health Nurses: *Foundation Blocks XII: Developing Occupational Health Job Description*. Pensacola, 2007, Florida.

American Association of Occupational Health Nurses: *Code of Ethics*. Atlanta, 2009, AAOHN.

American Association of Occupational Health Nurses: *Standards of Occupational Health Nursing Practice*. Atlanta, 2012, AAOHN.

Apostolopoulos Y, Sonmez S, Shattell M, et al: Worksite-induced morbidities among truck drivers in the United States. *AAOHN J* 58(7):285–296, 2010.

Bartsch KJ: The Employment Projections for 2008–18. 2009. Available at www.bls.gov/opub/mlr/2009/11/art1exc.htm. Accessed March 19, 2011.

Brown M: *Occupational Health Nursing*. New York, 1981, MacMillan.

Bureau of Labor Statistics: *Lost Work Time Injuries and Illnesses: Characteristics and Resulting Time Away From Work*. Washington, DC, 2006, U.S. Department of Labor.

Bureau of Labor Statistics: *Older Workers*. 2008a. Available at www.bls.gov/spotlight/2008/older workers. Accessed August 5, 2010.

Bureau of Labor Statistics: *Overview of 2008-2018 Population Projection, Occupational Outlook Handbook*. 2008b. Available at www.bls.gov. Accessed August 5, 2010.

Bureau of Labor Statistics: *Non-fatal Occupational Injuries and Illnesses Requiring Days Away From Work, 2011*. Washington, DC, 2012, U.S. Department of Labor.

Bureau of Labor Statistics: *Handbook of Labor Statistics*. Washington, DC, 2014, U.S. Department of Labor.

Dupler AE, Postma J, Sanders A: Minimizing nurses' risks for needlestick injuries in the hospital setting. *Workplace Health Saf* 61(5):197–2023, 2013.

Felton J: The genesis of American occupational health nursing, part 1. *Occup Health Nurs* 33:615, 1985.

Gonzalez M, Conlon H: Updating a tuberculosis surveillance program: Considering all of the variables. *Workplace Health Saf* 61(6):271–278, 2013.

Gordis L: *Epidemiology*, ed 4. St Louis, 2008, Elsevier.

Health Resources and Services Administration: *The Registered Nurse Population: Findings from the 2008 National Sample Survey of Registered Nurses*. 2010. Available at http://bhpr.hrsa.gov/healthworkforce/rnsurveys/rnsurveyfinal.pdf. Accessed April 16, 2015.

Heron MP, Hoyert DL, Murphy SL, et al: *Deaths: Final Data for 2006*. 2009. Available at www.cdc.gov/nchs/datalnvsr57/nvsr57_14.pdf. August 5, 2010.

Hollmann FW, Mulder TJ, Kallan JE: *Methodology and Assumptions for Population Projections of the United States: 1999-2100,*

*Population Division Working Paper No 38*. Washington, DC, 2000, Bureau of Census, U.S. Department of Commerce.

Levy BS, Wegman DH: *Occupational Health: Recognizing and Preventing Occupational Disease*. Philadelphia, 2011, Lippincott Williams & Wilkins.

McGrath B: Fifty years of industrial nursing. *Public Health Nurs* 37:119, 1945.

Mosisa A, Hipple S: Trends in labor force participation in the U.S. *Mon Labor Rev* 129:35–57, 2006. Available at: www.bls.gov. Accessed August 5, 2010.

National Institute for Occupational Safety and Health: *Occupational Respiratory Disease Surveillance*. 2008. Available at www.cdc/niosh.gov. Accessed March 19, 2011.

O'Donnell M: Definition of health promotion: Embracing passion, enhancing motivation, recognizing dynamic balance, and creating opportunities. *Am J Health Promot* 24(1):IV, 2009.

Public Law 91-596: *The Occupational Safety and Health Act*. Washington, DC, 1970, U.S. Department of Labor.

Ramazzini B: *De Morbis Artificum* [Diseases of Workers], 1713, Translated by Wright WC. Chicago, 1940, University of Chicago Press.

Reda AA, Fisseha S, Mengistie B, et al: Standard precautions: occupational exposure and behavior of health care workers in Ethiopia. *PLoS One* 5(12):e14420, 2010. doi: 10.1371/journal.pone.0014420.

Rogers B: Perspectives on occupational health nursing. *AAOHN J* 36:100–105, 1988.

Rogers B, Randolph S, Mastroianni K: *Occupational Health Nursing Guidelines for Primary Clinical Conditions*. Beverly, MA, 2009, OEM Press.

Rogers B: Occupational Health Nursing: Concepts and Practice. In Press, 2015.

U.S. Census Bureau: *World and Population Clocks*. 2009. Available at http://www.census.gov/popclock/. Accessed April 16, 2015.

U.S. Department of Health and Human Services: National Institute for Occupational Safety and Health: *The Changing Organization of Work and the Safety and Health of Working People, Pub No 2002-116*. Cincinnati, OH, 2002, USDHHS.

U.S. Department of Health and Human Services: *Healthy People 2020*. Washington, DC, 2010, U.S. Government Printing Office.

U.S. Department of Health and Human Services: National Institute for Occupational Safety and Health: *National Occupational Research Agenda*. Cincinnati, OH, 2010, USDHHS.

USDHHS, CDC, NIOSH: *State of the Sector/Healthcare and Social Assistance, Pub No 2009-139*. Washington, DC, 2009, Author.

# Forensic Nursing in the Community*

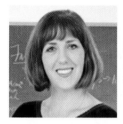

## Natalie McClain, PhD, RN, CPNP

Dr. McClain earned her bachelor and master's degrees from the University of Texas Health Sciences Center-Houston and the PhD from the University of Virginia. She has worked at the Children's Assessment Center, an advocacy center providing services for child victims of sexual abuse in Houston, Texas. At the Assessment Center and later in Charlottesville, Virginia, Dr. McClain performed medical forensic exams in cases of sexual assault, testified in both civil and criminal trials, and served as an expert witness for the FBI. Dr. McClain served on the 2012-2013 Committee on Commercial Sexual Exploitation and Sex Trafficking of Minors in the U.S. Dr. McClain is currently a Clinical Associate Professor at Boston College William F. Connell School of Nursing in Boston, MA.

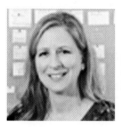

## Melissa Sutherland, PhD, FNP-BC

Dr. Sutherland earned the bachelor and master's degrees from Binghamton University in New York, and the PhD from the University of Virginia. She is a Board Certified Family Nurse Practitioner and an Associate Professor at the William F. Connell School of Nursing. Her major areas of research and practice are interpersonal violence and women's health. She serves as treasurer of the Nursing Network Violence Against Women, International and is a member of the International Association of Forensic Nurses. Most recently she was appointed a member of the Board Committee for Community Service at Boston Children's Hospital, Boston, MA.

## ADDITIONAL RESOURCES

ⓔ **Evolve Website http://evolve.elsevier.com/Stanhope**
- Healthy People 2020
- Quiz
- Case Studies
- Glossary
- Answers to Practice Application

## OBJECTIVES

*After reading this chapter, the student will be able to do the following:*

1. Describe the specialized competencies and skills of the forensic nurse within the nursing process.
2. Discuss the relationship of the forensic nurse with public health professionals in addressing injury as a public health concern.
3. List the health risks that result from incidents of injury.
4. Identify how forensic nurses deal with injuries in the three levels of prevention.
5. Discuss the health disparities that contribute to the occurrence and poor outcomes in marginalized groups who experience injury.
6. Explain the contribution of theoretical underpinnings to current models of forensic nursing practice.
7. Identify client populations and clinical arenas in the community where forensic nurses practice.
8. Define the key terms and concepts within forensic nursing theory.
9. Identify professionals who commonly work in collaboration with the forensic nurse in addressing injury care and prevention.

## KEY TERMS

adjudication, p. 960
forensic, p. 958
forensic nurse examiner, p. 958
forensic nursing, p. 958
injury, p. 958
justice, p. 963

legal nurse consultants, p. 960
perceptivity, p. 963
sexual assault nurse examiner (SANE), p. 958
victimization, p. 963
—*See Glossary for definitions*

---

*Special thanks goes to Dr. Susan Patton, who authored this chapter in the 8th edition of the textbook. Appreciation is given to Drs. Karen Landenburger and Jacquelyn Campbell for providing some content related to forensic nursing that was moved from Chapter 38, which discusses violence in the community.

## PERSPECTIVES ON FORENSICS AND FORENSIC NURSING

Injuries resulting from crime and victimization cause pain and suffering and may cause disability, economic failure, and "distress of the human spirit" (Lynch, 2011, p. 15). However, such injuries have often taken a back seat to treatment of disease and infection. Today forensic nurses expertly care for victims of injuries, largely as a community-based specialty, from a medical as well as a legal perspective. Whether the injury is caused by intentional violence or unintentional accident, forensic nurses are involved with not only the treatment but also the prevention of what is the leading cause of death in the first four decades of life (CDC, 2011; CDC, 2013). The burden of injuries to individuals ranges from minimal and brief to debilitating or fatal. The economic burden worldwide is tremendous. Each year in the United States more than 2.8 million people are hospitalized and 31.7 million people receive treatment in emergency departments as a result of violence and injuries (CDC, 2011). The total costs, for both fatal and nonfatal injuries and violence, are estimated to be more than $405 billion in medical care and lost productivity each year (Finkelstein et al, 2006). Because injuries result from a wide variety of physical, environmental, and behavioral causes, risk reduction comes from a variety of approaches. Forensic nurses have a unique set of skills for dealing with injury, and these skills will be discussed in this chapter.

Forensic means pertaining to the law. Forensic nursing synthesizes the biopsychosocial and spiritual aspects of nursing care with an expert understanding of forensic science and the criminal justice process (International Association of Forensic Nurses, 2014). Forensic nursing has a unique body of knowledge and set of skills. It also has unique practice arenas and the client population served. The skill set is defined by the scope and standards of practice, which includes skills such as collection, documentation, and preservation of evidence and other findings that may later be used in the prosecution of a crime. Practice standards also reflect care given to both the living and the dead, victims of trauma and perpetrators of crime, as well as individuals and groups within a community. Forensic nurses often have experience in emergency and trauma services and can provide an expert analysis of wounding patterns and physiological response to injury. They are able to compassionately care for individuals and families who experience emotional

reactions to trauma from a variety of causes. While the majority of forensic nurses in the United States are sexual assault nurse examiners (SANEs), other roles exist to care for survivors of other crimes, liability-related injury, and deaths. These include the clinical forensic nurse, forensic nurse examiner or investigator, forensic psychiatric nurse, forensic correctional nurse, legal nurse consultant, nurse attorney, and nurse coroner or death investigator. Arenas of care include but are not limited to emergency departments and community-based urgent care clinics, offices of the medical examiner and coroner, investigative units of law enforcement and criminal justice agencies, and governmental programs of safety prevention.

Forensic nursing care largely occurs in collaboration with professionals, both within and outside of nursing, including but not limited to public health professionals including epidemiologists, law enforcement and corrections officers, emergency department providers, and psychiatric practitioners. Forensic nurses also work collaboratively with public health nurses who bring a population focus to injury prevention programs. As part of a public health approach to crime, forensic nurses serve as content experts, clinician advisors, and/or the clinical managers of care facilities that may contribute to a community response to injury prevention.

## INJURY PREVENTION

Not surprisingly, the health determinants of injury, identified in *Healthy People 2020*, mirror disease occurrence in a community. The rate of injury and crime is lower in communities that promote good health. Where inequities of resources and education exist, health disparity, violence, and other crimes rise and accidental injuries occur more often. Trauma victims are overrepresented in minority, disenfranchised, and disadvantaged groups. Disparity can also be seen in the prosecution, conviction, and incarceration of individuals of minority groups in many countries. In the United States, one in three African American males and one in six Latinos will be incarcerated sometime in their lives (Mauer, 2009). Populations that experience more disease also experience more violent as well as accidental injury, and more events that lead to prosecution. The measures that improve overall health, lower risk, and reduce disparity also reduce physical and emotional injury. Injury now joins certain categories of disease, disability, and premature death as a major preventable health state. Reducing injury reflects the goals of *Healthy People 2020* as well as goals of other organizations such as the U.S. Public Health Service, the Centers for Disease Control and Prevention (CDC), the World Health Organization (WHO), and the International Association of Forensic Nurses (IAFN).

The National Center for Injury Prevention and Control, within the CDC, was established in 1997 to coordinate prevention of injuries, violence, and their consequences. The work of this center includes providing grants that fund prevention programs, dissemination of research findings, and maintenance of a website, blogs, podcasts, and electronic newsletters. This funding helps to inform the public of the epidemiology of injury and to provide other resources for professionals. The Center's website includes a wide variety of information on injury prevention and violence prevention, home and recreational safety, traumatic brain injury, injury data and statistics, injury response, motor vehicle safety, and violence prevention (CDC, 2013). The database of the International Association of Forensic Nurses (http://www.iafn.org) lists over 700 sexual assault centers in the United States, Canada, and Australia. Forensic Nurse Death Investigators serve as trainers for the CDC's National Sudden Unexpected Infant Death Investigation program.

## HEALTHY PEOPLE 2020 GOALS, PREVENTION, AND FORENSIC NURSING

The *Healthy People 2020* goals that deal with reducing injury and violence in the United States reflect the breadth of concerns and problems that result in injury, both intentional and unintentional, in communities. Objectives related to safety, violence, injury, and sexual assault are incorporated throughout the *Healthy People 2020* document. These objectives relate to injuries that are both intentional and unintentional. The box that follows lists selected objectives related to violence.

### HEALTHY PEOPLE 2020
#### Objectives Pertaining to Injury

The following proposed objectives are examples that pertain to injury and are relevant in forensic nursing:
- IVP-29: Reduce homicides.
- IVP-30: Reduce firearm-related deaths.
- IVP-33: Reduce physical assaults.
- IVP-34: Reduce physical fighting among adolescents.
- IVP-36: Reduce weapon carrying by adolescents on school property.
- IVP-40: Reduce sexual violence (U.S. Department Health and Human Services, 2010).

U.S Department of Health and Human Services: Healthy People 2020. Available at http://www.healthypeople.gov/2020/default.aspx. Accessed June 8, 2011.

Nurses who work in the area of forensics use all three levels of prevention. For example, forensic nurses (FNs) promote safety in their involvement with projects that aim to prevent domestic violence, sexual assault, child abuse, and accidental injuries before they occur (primary prevention) and in program development and management of care centers. Community awareness of violent crimes is achieved in concert with certain programs and the community-based professionals who work there. Secondary prevention is practiced following the occurrence of injuries and crime. Forensic nurses provide direct care to both victims and perpetrators. Their expertise serves the individual as well as the community in the collection of evidence for the legal justice system. Goals of compassionate holistic care are to minimize the spiritual, psychological, physical, and social trauma, as well as the financial burden. Although the World Health Organization (WHO) guidelines recommend against routine intimate partner screening (WHO, 2013), the 2013 U.S. Preventive Services Task Force recommends "that clinicians screen women of childbearing age for intimate partner violence…." (Feder et al, 2013; Moyer, 2013). Worth noting is that the WHO does recommend that health care providers ask about IPV exposure in situations involving injuries or that may have been caused or complicated by IPV. FNs are often the first providers to assess a patient's medical situation and to have contact with victims.

If disability, incarceration, or death occurs, FNs provide tertiary care in settings appropriate to address rehabilitation or identify factors that have put individuals at risk. Evidence should be collected in such a way that the collection itself protects rather than destroys or alters the evidence.

### LEVELS OF PREVENTION
#### Intentional Injury

**Primary Prevention**
Develop programs that promote safety and avoidance of violence, including both intentional violence and unintentional accidents.

**Secondary Prevention**
Provide timely, sensitive, direct care to both victims of injury and perpetrators of crime and violent behavior.

**Tertiary Prevention**
When injury has occurred, refer clients to appropriate community services for appropriate follow-up care and rehabilitation of the effects of trauma.

## FORENSIC NURSING AS A SPECIALTY AREA THAT PROVIDES CARE IN THE COMMUNITY

Within communities, the growing prevalence of "criminal and negligence-based trauma" indicates a need for health professionals who can intercede with skills that address social justice as well as care for social offenders (Lynch, 2011, p. 17). Thus, forensic nurses respond to sexual assault, drug- and alcohol-related crimes, incidents of human trafficking, elder mistreatment, child abuse, gang violence, as well as mass disaster, automobile accidents, and work-related injuries. In each situation, forensic nurses look for historical, behavioral, and physical indicators that a crime has been committed and intentional injury has occurred. For example, children who are abused may have cigarette burns, bite marks, pressure sores, and other physical signs that parents may claim to be the result of accidents. Munchausen syndrome by proxy is a form of child abuse in

---

**BOX 44-1** **Emergency Response to Assault Victims**

1. Use standardized medical treatment and forensic protocols.
2. Assess for sexual assault using "forced sex" terminology rather than "rape" or "sexual assault," and call a sexual assault nurse examiner if appropriate.
3. Support privacy of assault victim.
4. Explain procedures clearly to the assault victim.
5. Document location, date, and time of assault.
6. Collect evidence in a systematic format; take pictures if necessary.
7. Take care not to destroy evidence while giving care.
8. Maintain chain of evidence.
9. Maintain evidence integrity.
10. Document the following:
    a. Injuries
    b. Emotional state
    c. Medical history
    d. Victim's account of assault
11. Identify and refer to resources that can be used after the assault.

From U.S. Department of Justice, Office on Violence Against Women: A national protocol for sexual assault medical forensic examinations adults/adolescents, 2004. Available at http://www.ncjrs.gov/pdffiles1/ovw/206554.pdf. Accessed August 20, 2010.

---

which the primary caregiver uses the child as a mechanism to gain attention. The caregiver often causes illnesses and subsequent symptoms in the child (Finn, 2011).

A client who is admitted to a hospital with traumatic injuries should be evaluated as to the potentially forensic nature of the injuries (Sheridan and Nash, 2009). The response to victims of assault includes a number of steps, as outlined in Box 44-1. The nurse most often comes in contact with police, victims, and perpetrators of violence or crime in the emergency department. The nurse provides a vital link between the investigative process, health care, and the court (Sachs et al, 2008). Nurses should take specific actions when they come in contact with victims. It is important that evidence be carefully collected and that the person who is doing the collection be systematic in this process.

One example of appropriate forensic care is to avoid cutting through the bullet hole in the shirt when cutting a shirt off a victim who has been shot in the chest. Rather, it should be cut to the side of the hole to protect the point of origin of the bullet for later criminal investigation. The collection of DNA provides a significant role in criminal investigations. It is essential that DNA be collected correctly and that elimination samples of DNA be collected from authorized people at the crime scene and from the victim (USDOJ/Office on Violence Against Women, 2013).

The most common types of trace evidence of victims of violence, including those who are raped, are clothing, bullets, bloodstains, hairs, fibers, and small pieces of material such as fragments of metal, glass, paint, and wood. In the investigation of sexual assault, an evidence kit should be used within 72 hours of the assault with specimens collected and preserved according to state crime lab procedures. Only the victim or a nurse wearing protective gloves should handle the clothing. Throughout the collection process, the nurse takes every opportunity to show compassion to the victim of the assault while maintaining objectivity in recording observations (Houmes et al, 2003).

Laughon et al (2004) provide a useful guide to assessment of all forms of violence, including child abuse and neglect, elderly abuse, and intimate partner violence. The authors state that documentation should include written documentation as well as forensic photography. Written forms of documentation should be as verbatim as possible, with the use of declarative statements and body maps. When possible, use a 35-mm or digital camera to take the necessary photographs. The photographs should be taken in context, with two or more photos focusing clearly on the injury. Injuries should also be depicted on diagrams and recorded in the nurses' notes. The How To box describes how to label photographs taken after the injury.

---

**HOW TO** **Label Photos**

*All photos should be clearly labeled with the following information:*
- *Client's name*
- *Client's medical identification number*
- *Client's date of birth*
- *The date and time of the photograph*
- *The name of the photographer*
- *The body location of the injury*
- *The forensic case number*

*From Sheridan DJ: Legal and forensic nursing responses to family violence. In Humphrey J, Campbell JC, editors: Family violence and nursing practice, Philadelphia, 2004, Lippincott Williams & Wilkins.*

---

Forensic nurses may have alternative specialties that are combined for a special population. Advanced practice nurses (APNs) such as psychiatric, pediatric, geriatric, and acute care nurse practitioners bring to forensic nursing skills that allow them to provide advanced assessment and prescription of medications and treatments needed by forensic clients. Notably, forensic psychiatric nurses treat both victims of post-traumatic stress disorder and seriously emotionally disturbed clients incarcerated for violent crimes. APNs in correctional facilities may identify themselves as forensic nurses when they manage acute and chronic illness, promote wellness, and work in these systems to develop policies around legal and ethical issues.

The specialty also incorporates three subspecialties of nursing practice that are located within the criminal justice system: forensic nurse, nurse attorney, and legal nurse consultant. Forensic nurses employed in the criminal justice arena generally provide care to individuals who are either victims of injury or perpetrators of a crime that is under investigation. Legal nurse consultants provide expert consultation regarding health care to attorneys in either civil or criminal court but do not render direct client care in that setting. Some of these situations might include medical malpractice, personal injury, workers' compensation, and probate. Nurse attorneys hold a license from a state bar association in addition to a nursing license and generally use their nursing knowledge for adjudication. Adjudication refers to a judicial decision or a sentence.

Finally, forensic nurses are advocates for programs that prevent injuries, which occur as a result of both intentional injury and health hazards related to environments that create injury. Relying on an understanding of epidemiology, these nurses have knowledge of occurrence as well as the mechanisms of injury in a community. Forensic nurses partner with public health professionals including nurses to design, implement, and evaluate projects and programs that have a forensic focus.

## History of Forensic Nursing

Early writings about the evolution of modern nursing, particularly with regard to care given to victims of war, mental illness, and abuse, lay a foundation for the advent of forensic nurses in the twentieth century (Nutting and Dock, 1907). Chapter 2 discusses the history of public health nursing; this section emphasizes nursing history's linkages to forensic nursing. With public health nurses, forensic nurses celebrate the early pioneers working in communities that brought medical care to the most vulnerable and marginalized. They worked to develop national and international organizations such the National Organization for Public Health Nursing (1912), National Society of Nurses (later the American Nurses Association [ANA], 1912), the International Congress of Nursing (1912), and the WHO (1948). These organizations were designed to give structure and standards for care and education regarding issues of violence and neglect. These issues pertain to public health, mental health, and forensic nurses who are experts in dealing with the effects of trauma, and who advocate for care of the wounded, both physically and emotionally.

Contemporary practice of forensic nursing in the United States was largely propelled by early efforts to identify and prevent child abuse and neglect and sexual assault of women. In the 1940s through the 1960s, radiologists identified fractures that they linked to assault and pediatricians began describing indicators of "battered child syndrome" (Gurevich, 2010). Subsequently, nurses became aware of their role in identifying indicators of assault. In emergency departments, forensic nurses assisted in "rape" kit collection. The nurses showed compassion and competence in preserving crucial evidence and had a strong understanding of the "rape trauma syndrome" first described by Burgess in 1973. Burgess and other advanced practice nurses initiated previously undescribed care with forensic clients. The first nurse-run sexual assault clinics opened in Memphis and Minneapolis in 1974 (Speck, n.d.) with subsequent development of the first protocols for sexual assault care (Ledray, 1998). In 1985 the U.S. Surgeon General identified violence as a health care issue, and health care providers such as nurses working with victims and perpetrators of crimes, as key agents in ameliorating the effects of violence in our communities (International Association of Forensic Nurses (IAFN), 2010.). In 1990 Virginia Lynch published her dissertation on the role description and Integrated Model of Forensic Nursing care of both living and deceased victims of trauma and perpetrators of crime (Lynch, 1990). By 1992, The Joint Commission began to require hospitals to develop protocols for the treatment of victims of sexual assault. At the present time most victims of sexual assault go to emergency departments. The lack of availability of trained providers spurred the development of SANE programs.

Today, the Integrated Model of Forensic Nursing is recognized internationally as the basis for practice as well as education of forensic nurses. Following efforts to describe the unique contribution of forensic nursing (Lynch, 1986), the specialty was recognized by the American Academy of Forensic Science in 1991. The following year SANEs from the United States and Canada established the International Association of Forensic Nurses (IAFN). In 1995 the ANA designated forensic nursing as a specialty, and it is now recognized as one of the fastest growing specialties in nursing. IAFN boasts a membership of over 3000 nurses worldwide and has members in over 22 countries (IAFN, 2012).

## Educational Preparation

Historically, forensic nurses refined and developed their forensic skills through clinical practice and continuing education. Today, there are three primary routes for training in forensic nursing. First, nurses can gain additional skills and knowledge through continuing education courses or basic concepts introduced in generalist education. Second, certificate programs include specific content, entrance requirements, and many have clinical opportunities. Third, graduate nursing academic programs are offering minors or concentrations in forensic nursing.

Formal graduate course work on forensic nursing began at the University of Texas, Arlington in 1986. To begin a specialty by starting with graduate preparation is both uncommon and courageous; more often content is introduced in the undergraduate studies, and graduate study assists in refining and developing the content until it is formalized in courses and majors. By 2000 there were 12 graduate programs preparing clinical nurse specialists and nurse practitioners with a focus on forensic nursing. The development of the scope and standards of practice and a core curriculum for graduate study in 2004 facilitated the development of new programs of study and formed the basis for advanced practice credentialing of students and practicing clinicians. A forensic focus in research became more prevalent in both master's and doctoral studies, which facilitated the opening of the first doctor of nursing practice (DNP) program focused on forensic nursing in 2002 at the University of Tennessee Health Science Center in Memphis. Now, new DNP programs are opening based on this model of advanced nursing practice.

The inclusion of forensic nursing content into undergraduate generalist education remains controversial. The American Association of Nurse Attorneys (TAANA) and the IAFN have recommended coursework regarding public and private legal proceedings. Students need to develop a working understanding of laws and procedures applicable to nursing practice and certain client situations, such as mandated reporting of child abuse (Feng et al, 2012). In addition, nurses are prepared to care for families experiencing trauma. Many educators in the United States believe the complexity of forensic content has evolved so that the skills and competencies required to differentiate the specialty are not appropriate in a generalist educational curriculum.

## Theoretical Foundations of Forensic Nursing

Humans seek stability; they seek safety from physical trauma and emotional wounding from violent relationships; and they seek protection of their finances and freedom from fears that threaten their very understanding of human existence. Theories that contribute to our understanding of what constitutes safety and well-being have been extrapolated from a variety of sources outside of nursing. Maslow, an American psychologist,

for entry-level licensure, certification examination, peer review, and personal reflection. Reflection should be on practice as well as during practice. As part of professional expectations and standards, forensic nurses are encouraged to participate in continuous quality improvement using the best evidence for practice or promising practice methods under evaluation (Nayduch and Fitzpatrick, 1999; Harkins, 2006). Scientific research in forensic nursing is in its infancy. Although a large majority of the published research consists of descriptive studies of the forensic nursing role and the client populations (Evans, 2000; Lewis-O'Connor, 2009; Shelton, 2009), there is a growing number of studies examining forensic practice and outcomes. For example, research on sexual assault response teams supports the use of these approaches to practice and recommends outcome measurement of both short-term outcomes such as client satisfaction and long-term outcomes such as prosecution rates (Campbell et al, 2006; Johnston, 2005; Speck, 2005; Campbell et al, 2005; Bechtel et al, 2008; Campbell et al, 2008). Studies in collaboration with other disciplines are currently underway to test the basis for distinctions among injuries such as bruising (Wiglesworth et al, 2009; Pierce et al, 2010). Forensic nurses are producing valuable information regarding DNA sampling (Maguire et al, 2008; Ledray, 2010). Scholarly contributions to forensic nursing practice have increased since professional journals such as the *Journal of Forensic Nursing* have increased publication of forensic specific content. The following Evidence-Based Practice example describes the ways in which DNA evidence can be accurately obtained.

## EVIDENCE-BASED PRACTICE

An essential step in a forensic evaluation following an alleged sexual assault is the collection of trace evidence including DNA. In addition to the history of the assault, alternative light sources (ALS) have been used to assist examiners in identifying areas of potential DNA evidence. A common ALS used is the Wood's lamp. The goal of this project was to determine the best practice using an alternative light source (ALS) to aid in the identification of trace DNA evidence in sexual assault forensic exams.

The authors reviewed the limited data available on this topic (7 studies) and concluded that the Wood's lamp should no longer be used as the ALS. However, ALS with wavelengths able to detect DNA should be used. Most importantly, examiners must be educated about the advantages and disadvantages and proper use of the use of ALS. Further research is necessary on the use of ALS in forensic evaluations along with development of new techniques to assist in identification of semen in forensic exams.

**Nurse Use**
SANEs play a key role in providing care for victims of sexual assault. The training to become a SANE is specialized and growing in importance and the recognition of its value to victims, their families, and the criminal justice system (International Association of Forensic Nurses (IAFN) 2014.). Evidence-based practice ensures patients receive the highest quality of care supported by research.

Eldredge K, Huggins E, Pugh LC: Alternate light sources in sexual assault examinations: An evidence-based practice project. *J Forensic Nurs* 8:39–44, 2012.

## Certification

The scope and standards of forensic nursing practice have been used for the development of the certification examination and other credentials that are intended to demonstrate competence of the practitioner. Credentialing within forensic nursing, as with all new professional specialties, has become an increasingly important issue. Different types of credentials pertain to nursing, both within and outside the discipline. While all nurses should have an understanding of credentialing and the implications and responsibilities that accompany such a designation, it is uniquely important for FNs who maintain close relationships to both the medical and the legal communities. FNs provide care when health and the law intersect and must therefore have credentials that speak to their unique qualifications to give that specialized care (Patton, 2011).

Certification examination for pediatric, adolescent, and adult sexual assault nurse examiners (SANE A and SANE P) is available through the International Association of Forensic Nurses. This certification along with the Legal Nurse Consultant, Corrections Nurse, Death Investigators, and Forensic Examiner are offered by other organizations to registered nurses meeting entry criteria but generally do not require a graduate degree. Recognition of the Advanced Forensic Nurse (AFN) by the American Nurses Credentialing Center through a portfolio method of credentialing was used to establish a way to provide board certification for APNs specializing in forensic nursing (http://www.nursecredentialing.org/ForensicNursing-Advanced). Seen in light of the APRN Consensus Model for Regulation, forensic nursing is a specialty focus, beyond the role and population focus of the four categories of advanced practice (APRN Joint Dialogue Group et al, 2008). Although the AFN credential represents a specialty focus for APNs, it is currently not an avenue for advanced practice certification or advanced practice licensure. Forensic Nurse Examiners are most often referred to as Forensic Examiners, Medicolegal Death Investigators and Coroners, Sexual Assault Nurse Examiners, or Advanced Forensic Nurses.

## ETHICAL ISSUES

Ethical considerations in the practice of forensic nursing are unique because of the implications to not only a client's health, but in some cases, his or her freedom. Practice outcomes affect individuals and families, as well as society as a whole. Ethics and law are closely tied but are not equivalent. Ethical nursing practice involves adherence to law in most cases, but also to the ethics of nursing and the dictates of one's conscience (Walsh, 2005). Nurses maintain a different code of conduct than do certain colleagues. For example, law enforcement personnel answer singly to the law for their standard. Knowledge and understanding of these considerations is core to the specialty of forensic nursing (International Association of Forensic Nurses Ethics Committee, 2008).

Olsen (2013) organized ethical principles into five categories: respect for person, beneficence, distributive justice, respect for community, and contextual caring. Each of these categories reflects examples of the tension that may arise when the forensic nurse faces a dilemma imposed by conflicting interests. An overriding consideration is the need to respect each person and to develop contextual caring within the art of nursing. Respect for person means respect for autonomy while protecting vulnerable persons. The right of each human to self-determination is recognized within nursing but may not be respected by all societies. Therefore, respect for human rights may involve advocacy to some degree. Laws, cultural norms, and considerations of safety, which limit the liberty of an individual, may constrain the nurse's ability to fully exercise a therapeutic relationship. Questions raised pose dilemmas in a variety of medical and psychiatric settings.

Forensic environments include courtrooms, jails, prisons, and psychiatric facilities for the criminally insane. When criminal action or trauma to an individual requires care, the need for coercion is likely. Certain situations may make medical coercion necessary. These situations include incapacity (or inability) to make decisions and making decisions that could result in harm to self or harm to others in the absence of interventions. Paternalism has been defined as "the principle that allows one person to make decisions for another" (Williams, 2007, p. 93). This may be necessary in the case of minors or older adults. Paternalistic intervention was viewed by the U.S. Supreme Court as lawful in the case of *Washington v Harper* (1990), when it ruled that mentally ill inmates could be compelled to take psychotropic medications against their will if the mental disorder is serious, the inmate is dangerous to himself, and the medication prescribed is in the inmate's best medical interest. Therefore, the ability of a psychiatric forensic nurse practicing in an advanced role to make a determination of rational autonomy is crucial in questions of coercion: to make judgments without being judgmental (Rose, 2005).

This same principle may be applied to clients who refuse treatment of infectious disease, whether or not they are incarcerated, in much the same way that public health law is used to guide treatment in community settings. Instructive guidelines on involuntary treatment are available from the American Correctional Association, the CDC, and the American Public Health Association (Finkelstein et al, 2006).

Beneficence (care) and the complementary principle of nonmaleficence (without harm) go beyond autonomy in the responsibility of the nurse to not only support an individual's choices but to perform actions that enhance the health of others. Nurses provide care without prejudice of the circumstance or individual characteristics. They provide care to the injured, marginalized, and poor whether the individuals are victims or offenders. Nurses who care for pregnant teens in a youth facility or collect evidence from drug addicts each hold the same ethical responsibility as described previously (Muster, 1992; Hufft and Peternelj-Taylor, 2008). Questions may arise when the resources to achieve adequate health are not plentiful enough for all to receive adequate care. When economic restraints limit funds to process sexual assault evidentiary kits, treat victims of assault, and provide dental care to methamphetamine addicts in prison, where should the funds be applied? Principles of distributive justice address such questions in deciding what goods will be distributed to which persons in what proportions. Forensic nurses may find themselves in a policy-making position to answer such questions to ensure that their clients given similar circumstances are treated no better or worse than others in the application of protection and medical care. Also, when there are questions of retribution, whether withholding provisions or threatening harm, forensic nurses never participate in the punishment, however subtle, of another being.

Ethical decisions can be exceedingly difficult when the safety of a society is at risk. One approach to making decisions with respect for the community is utilitarianism, which appeals exclusively to outcomes or consequences in determining which choice to make. Williams (2009) explains:

> Utilitarianism, with its mandate for the general good, rather than a specific interest, would place the safety of the community above the rights of any one individual. The forensic nurse expert, hired by the court to evaluate a client, as an example, testifies on behalf of society, not the individual. To that end, it may be argued that the nurse expert uses a utilitarian perspective that may not serve the interests of the client but instead, serves the interests of society. Traditional nursing mandates that the correct focus (and therefore the right moral choice) be placed on the individual. However, the burden of responsibility often shifts in forensic nursing from the individual to the community, a correct moral choice under utilitarianism (p. 50).

During a forensic examination, the potential exists for withholding vital information in the investigation of wrongdoing. The temptation to "assist" the perceived victim's case may be justified by a desired outcome for that individual as well as the ultimate safety of a community. This dilemma of information can be carried to situations of privacy protection. The entitlement to privacy may be changed when someone's safety is at stake. If a specimen for DNA is collected during the investigation of a crime, should that information remain in the Combined DNA Index System (CODIS) for use in future crimes, regardless of the outcome of prosecution of that case and when there is the potential for repeat offense (Hackenschmidt, 2004)? Do hospitals have the right to videotape parents who are suspected of Munchausen syndrome, or is this a violation of Fourth Amendment rights (Morrison, 1999)? When victims give information to sexual assault examiners, are they informed that records may be released to law enforcement and attorneys? Should they consent to the release of photographs that depict intimate areas of their body for anyone in law enforcement, attorneys, and juries to see, even in the name of full disclosure (Ledray, 2008)?

Finally, there are always questions regarding the relationship between forensic clients and nurses. Caring is the essence and core value of nursing (Watson, 2008). Olsen (2013) recognized that caring as well as ethics is influenced in the context of relationships and that nurses' "emotion is inextricably bound to moral good" (p. 51). Contextual caring is not synonymous with beneficence but "entreats the forensic nurse to interact with each client, whether criminal or victim, as a person within an ethical relationship of caring concern grounded in the nurse's personal values" (Olsen, 2013, p. 51). The care goes beyond the "obligatory dictates" of client rights. Unique problems are posed when the client is in denial about the role he or she plays in the problem or poses a safety risk to the nurse. In addition, forensic nurses must overcome the societal bias of establishing relationships with individuals believed to have injured another, perhaps intentionally. Finally, when personal bias or issues of conscience impair the ability to prescribe or participate in particular medical interventions, objections may be raised. Examples of situations at risk for bias in forensics include collection of trace evidence from individuals who have impaired consciousness or are coerced into consent, prescription of birth control following sexual assault, participation in capital punishment, and the use of unnecessary physical or medical restraint. Nurses and other health care professionals have well-established codes of ethics and other examined statements to guide practice and inform care (Walsh, 2005; Ferguson, 2006; Committee on Bioethics, 2009; Lynch and Duval, 2011). It is imperative to view these statements that guide practice as a basis for conduct as well as for reflective dialogue in real client situations. The following two case studies demonstrate some of the aspects of forensic nursing care.

*Case #1:* Tamara Lynch is a 6-year-old child who lives in a busy household of four children, her grandmother, mother, and stepfather. She is a client of the local pediatric clinic and has an appointment today for a school-related examination. She has been very interested in school in the past but recently her grades have declined and her mother describes her behavior as withdrawn. Shirley Meres is the pediatric nurse practitioner who has seen Tamara for her most recent health care. She too has noted the change in Tamara's affect. Based on the health history, Ms. Meres uses developmentally appropriate questions to ask Tamara about situations in which she may not feel safe or situations with adults that have made her feel uncomfortable about her body. Tamara describes repeated episodes with her stepfather during which she was inappropriately touched and fondled. The nurse meets with Tamara's mother and explains her role as a forensic nurse. She explains that Tamara will need a specialized physical examination with collection of evidence, including laboratory specimens and photographs. After obtaining permission from the mother, the evaluation is performed using enhanced lighting and visualization equipment to collect photographic evidence, and body fluids for diagnostic and forensic testing. The nurse tells Tamara and her mother that the examination is normal for her age; no indications of trauma are noted. All evidence is packed for preservation according to crime lab protocols. Following the interview and examination, Ms. Meres counsels the child and mother about predictable psychological reactions to child sexual assault and disclosure even though no evidence of abuse was found in the nurse's examination. The mother is given information on advocacy, the legal process that follows a report to law enforcement agencies, and mental health counseling that is available locally. Tamara is given an appointment at the clinic in 2 weeks. The nurse makes contact with law enforcement to report the child's disclosure and make arrangements for transfer of all evidence. Ms. Meres continues to follow the health care of the family in the months to follow for evaluation and prevention of common problems that present to families who experience child abuse.

*Case #2:* Mike Post is an 18-year-old male who is taken to the emergency department by ambulance for what appeared to be a motor vehicle collision. His condition is considered serious. Following resuscitative measures, he is pronounced dead. Staff members at the emergency department contact the medical examiner's office to report the death. Sean Miller is the forensic nurse investigator on duty who receives the call. When Mr. Miller arrives at the emergency department, he interviews paramedics and emergency department clinicians about the accident site and the appearance of the decedent on arrival. He photographs the body, clothing, and other sources of trace evidence, including items in the decedent's pockets. Mr. Miller performs a thorough examination of Mike Post and discovers a small bullet hole in the left postauricular tissue. All items are individually bagged, sealed, and labeled for further analysis by the crime laboratory. The nurse then meets with the family to explain the need for investigation of all sudden, unexpected deaths. He describes the process involved in the investigation and preparation of the body prior to transfer to a funeral home. Copies of the medical record and x-rays obtained at the facility are transported with the body for autopsy. Mr. Miller reports his findings to the forensic pathology team and law enforcement officers. The autopsy is performed and the ballistics analysis of the recovered bullet leads to the arrest of the alleged assailant. When the case goes to court, the nurse is subpoenaed to testify about the investigation and collection of evidence. The nurse maintains contact with the family to keep them informed of the progress of the case and the resources for legal and family grief counseling available in their community. See the Quality and Safety in Nursing Education box that follows to learn ways in which nurses partner with families to coordinate care.

## FUTURE PERSPECTIVES

Forensic nursing is predominantly a community-oriented specialty. Practice arenas are associated with health care facilities such as private clinics and emergency departments, criminal justice centers for victims of crime, medical examiner offices, police departments, correctional facilities, and mental health centers. What is consistent in each of these practice sites is the care of individuals who have experienced the effects of injury, either intentional or unintentional. Increasingly it is being recognized that hospitals need forensic nursing services. Clients routinely enter hospitals with conditions that have overlying legal implications (Markowitz et al, 2005). In addition, injuries occur as a result of medical incidents and errors. Forensic nurses use their expert understanding of cause and effects of trauma and are in a position to investigate the circumstances in order to design a plan of care for individual as well as special groups of clients. They serve as a liaison between the hospital and the medical-legal community to reduce the effects of trauma.

## QSEN FOCUS ON QUALITY AND SAFETY EDUCATION FOR NURSES

### Quality and Safety Focus

**Targeted Competency: Client-Centered Care**

Recognize the client or designee as the source of control and full partner in providing compassionate and coordinated care based on respect for client's preferences, values, and needs.

Important aspects of client-centered care include:

- **Knowledge:** Describe strategies to empower clients or families in all aspects of the health care process.
- **Skills:** Assess level of client's decisional conflict and provide access to resources.
- **Attitudes:** Value active partnership with clients or designated surrogates in planning, implementation, and evaluation of care.

**Client-Centered Care Question**

You are an RN at a correctional facility, where system-focused updates have recently been implemented to ensure provider safety. A metal detector has been

implemented that all inmates must pass through before entering the clinic. A standardized frisk procedure has also been implemented. The presence of a security guard has been standardized for all clinic visits. The clinic environment has been modified so that all sharp objects or potentially dangerous objects have been locked up. Extra surveillance cameras have been added to each clinical examination room, and panic buttons have been added as extra security for providers in each exam room.

- Which system updates might impact patients' experience of care?
- Amidst all of the identified heightened security approaches, how do you communicate client-centered care to your clients?
- How do you address client safety in this new environment?
- How do you protect client confidentiality and privacy in this new environment?

Prepared by Gail Armstrong, PhD(c), DNP, ACNS-BC, CNE, Associate Professor, University of Colorado Denver College of Nursing.

## PRACTICE APPLICATION

A 26-year-old woman arrived unaccompanied to the emergency department of an academic medical center with cuts on her face, hands, legs, and pelvic area. She was crying and said that she had been attacked and was afraid to have an examination or to provide the name of her attacker. What is the first action that the nurse should take?

1. Explain to her the importance of reporting this crime immediately.

2. Listen closely to her and reflect back to her the fear, anger, and other feelings you hear in her voice.

3. Immediately call law enforcement officials yourself.

   Once you select the first action that you would take, explain your rationale and outline your exact actions.

   **Answers can be found on the Evolve site.**

## KEY POINTS

- Forensic nursing is a community-oriented specialty that addresses the prevention and treatment of accidental injury and violent crimes.
- The specialty reflects an integration of nursing, forensic science, and the law.
- Forensic nursing is needed whenever injury has legal implications.
- Forensic nurses need to maintain objectivity in rendering care to both victims of injury and perpetrators of crime.
- The scope and standards of forensic nursing practice guides forensic nurses with unique skills of the specialties such as

expert courtroom testimony and documentation and security of evidence.

- Forensic nurses work in cooperation with public health professionals, including nurses, in developing programs of prevention such as automobile safety and intimate partner violence prevention.
- Educational programs for forensic nurses are offered through continuing education offerings and formal graduate degree programs.
- Credentialing for forensic nurses include Sexual Assault Nurse Examiners and Advanced Practice Forensic Nurses.

## CLINICAL DECISION-MAKING ACTIVITIES

1. Think about injuries you have experienced and answer the following questions:
   A. How did the injury affect my ability to perform normal activities of my daily routine?
   B. What injury patterns did I have that would lead me to conclude it was violent or accidental?

   C. What could I have done to prevent the injury from occurring?
2. Discuss the effects of violence in your community with a fellow student. What situations exist that increase the risk that someone will be assaulted?

## CLINICAL DECISION-MAKING ACTIVITIES—cont'd

3. Write a list of the types of evidence that can be collected at a crime scene or in an emergency room based on a scenario of crime involving a young woman who is the victim of sexual assault.

4. In a short paragraph, explore how you might feel toward someone who commits a crime and needs nursing care. What ethical standards of nursing will influence your treatment of this individual?

## REFERENCES

American Nurses Association: *Recognition of a Specialty, Approval of Scope Statements and Acknowledgement of Nursing Practice Standards.* Washington, DC, 2004, American Nurses Association.

APRN Joint Dialogue Group, The APRN Consensus Work Group, & Committee, NAA: *Consensus Model for APRN Regulation: Licensure, Accreditation, Certification and Education.* Washington, DC, 2008, APRN.

Bechtel K, Ryan E, Gallagher D: Impact of sexual assault nurse examiners on the evaluation of sexual assault in a pediatric emergency department. *Pediatr Emerg Care* 24(7):442–447, 2008.

Brown D, Butchart A, Harvey A, et al: *Third Milestones of a Global Campaign for Violence Prevention Report 2007: Scaling Up.* Geneva, 2007, WHO.

Burgess AW, Holmstrom LL: Rape trauma syndrome. *Am J Psychiatry* 131(9):981–986, 1974.

Campbell JC, Humphreys JC: *Family Violence and Nursing Practice.* Baltimore, 2003, Lippincott, Williams & Wilkins.

Campbell R, Patterson D, Adams AE, et al: A participatory evaluation project to measure SANE nursing practice and adult sexual assault patients' psychological well-being. *J Forensic Nurs* 4(1):19–28, 2008.

Campbell R, Townsend SM, Long SM, et al: Organizational characteristics of sexual assault nurse examiner programs: results from the National Survey Project. *J Forensic Nurs* 1(2):57–64, 88, 2005.

Campbell R, Townsend SM, Long SM, et al: Responding to sexual assault victim's medical and emotional needs: a national study of the services provided by SANE programs. *Res Nurs Health* 29:384–398, 2006.

Centers for Disease Control and Prevention: *National Center for Injury Prevention and Control.* 2013. Available at http://www.cdc.gov/injury/. Accessed April 13, 2014.

Centers for Disease Control and Prevention: National Center for Injury Prevention and Control: *Web-based Injury Statistics Query and Reporting System (WISQARS).* 2011: Available at http://www.cdc.gov/injury/wisqars. Accessed April 14, 2014.

Committee on Bioethics: Physician refusal to provide information or treatment on the basis of claims of conscience. *Pediatrics* 124(6):1689–1693, 2009.

Council on Linkages Between Academia and Public Health Practice: *Core Competences for Public Health Professionals: Tier 2012.* 2012. Available at www.phf.org/programs/core competencies. Accessed April 23, 2014.

Eldredge K, Huggins E, Pugh LC: Alternate light sources in sexual assault examinations: An evidenced-based practice project. *J Forensic Nurs* 8:39–44, 2012.

Evans N: Special focus: mental health nursing: developing forensic nursing. *Nurs Manage* 6(10):14–17, 2000.

Feder G, Wathen CN, MacMillian HL: An evidence-based response to intimate partner violence, WHO guidelines. *JAMA* 310(5):479–480, 2013.

Feng J, Chen Y, Fetzer S, et al: Ethical and legal challenges of mandated child abuse reporters. *Child Youth Services Rev* 34(1):276–280, 2012.

Ferguson C: Providing quality care to the sexual assault survivor: education and training for medical professionals. *J Midwifery Womens Health* 51(6):486–492, 2006.

Finkelstein EA, Corso PS, Miller TR: *The Incidence and Economic Burden of Injury in the United States.* 2006. Available at http://www.ncbi.nlm.nih.gov/pmc/articles/PMC2652974/. Accessed May 19, 2014.

Finn C: Child maltreatment: forensic biomarkers. In Lynch VA, Duvall JB, editors: *Forensic Nursing Science,* ed 2. St Louis, 2011, Elsevier.

Gurevich L: Parental child murder and child abuse in Anglo-American legal system. *Trauma Violence Abuse* 11(1):18–26, 2010.

Hackenschmidt A: Advancing justice for sexual assault survivors and innocent inmates, or threat to privacy? A controversial DNA technology. *J Emerg Nurs* 30(6):575–577, 2004.

Haddon W: A logical framework for categorizing highway safety phenomena and activity. *J Trauma* 12:193–207, 1972.

Hammer RM, Moynihan B, Pagliaro E: *Forensic Nursing: A Handbook for Practice.* Sudbury, MA, 2006, Jones and Bartlett.

Harkins T: Forensic nursing and quality assurance: a perfect match. *On the Edge* 12(3):5, 2006.

Houmes BV, Fagan MM, Quintana NM: Violence: recognition, management, and prevention: establishing a sexual assault nurse examiner (SANE) program in the emergency department. *J Emerg Med* 25:111–121, 2003.

Hufft AG: Theoretical foundations for advanced practice nursing. In Hammer RH, Moynihan B, Pagliano EM, editors: *Forensic Nursing: a Handbook for Practice.* Sudbury, MA, 2006, Jones and Bartlett.

Hufft AG, Peternelj-Taylor C: Ethical care of pregnant adolescents in correctional settings. *J Forensic Nurs* 4(2):94–96, 2008.

International Association of Forensic Nurses (IAFN): *History of IAFN.* IAFN website. Available at http://www.iafn.org/displaycommon.cfm?an=1&subarticlenbr=149. Accessed May 18, 2014.

International Association of Forensic Nurses (IAFN): *2012 IAFN Annual Report.* 2012. IAFN website. Available at http://www.iafn.org/displaycommon.cfm?an=1&subarticlenbr=802. Accessed April, 2014.

International Association of Forensic Nurses Ethics Committee: *The vision of ethical practice.* 2008. Available at http://www.iafn.org/displaycommon.cfm?an=1&subarticlenbr=56. Accessed May 15, 2014.

James SH, Nordby JJ, editors: *Forensic Science: An Introduction to Scientific and Investigative Techniques,* ed 3. Boca Raton, 2009, CRC Press.

Johnston BJ: Outcome indicators for sexual assault victims. *J Forensic Nurs* 1(3):118, 2005.

Krug EG, Dahlberg LL, Mercy JA, et al: *World Report on Violence and Health.* Geneva, 2002, WHO.

Laughon K, Amar AF, Sheridan DJ, et al: Legal and forensic nursing responses to family violence. In Humphrey J, Campbell JC, editors: *Family Violence and Nursing Practice.* Philadelphia, 2004, Lippincott Williams & Wilkins.

Ledray L: *SANE Development and Operation Guide.* Washington, DC, 1998, Sexual Assault Resource Service, U.S. Department of Justice, Office of Justice Programs, and Office of Victims of Crime.

Ledray LE: Consent to photograph: how far should disclosure go? *J Forensic Nurs* 4(4):188–189, 2008.

Ledray L: Expanding evidence, collection time: Is it time to move beyond the 72 hour rule? How do we decide? *J Forensic Nurs* 6(1):47–50, 2010.

Lewis-O'Connor A: The evolution of SANE/SART—are there differences? Sexual Assault Nurse Examiner/Sexual Assault Response Team. *J Forensic Nurs* 5(4):220–227, 2009.

Lynch VA: *Forensic Nursing: A New Field for the Profession.* Paper presented at the 38th Annual Meeting of the American Academy of Forensic Science, 1986.

Lynch VA: *Clinical Forensic Nursing: A Descriptive Study in Role Development.* Arlington, TX, 1990, University of Texas.

Lynch VA: Concepts and theory of forensic nursing science. In Lynch VA, Duvall JB, editors: *Forensic Nursing Science,* ed 2. St Louis, 2011, Elsevier.

Lynch VA, Duval JB, editors: *Forensic Nursing Science,* ed 2. St Louis, 2011, Elsevier.

Maguire S, Ellaway B, Bowyer VL, et al: Retrieval of DNA from the faces of children aged 0–5 years: a technical note. *J Forensic Nurs* 4(1):40–44, 2008.

Markowitz JR, Steer S, Garland M: Hospital-based intervention for intimate partner violence victims: a forensic nursing model. *J Emerg Nurs* 31(2):166–170, 2005.

Maslow AH: A theory of human motivation. *Psychol Rev* 50:370–396, 1943. Available at: http://psychclassics.yorku.ca/Maslow/motivation.htm. Accessed May 15, 2014.

Mason T, Mercer D, editors: *Critical Perspectives in Forensic Care: Inside Out.* Hampshire, London, 1998, Macmillan.

Mauer M: *Racial Disparities in the Criminal Justice System.* Washington, DC, 2009, The Sentencing Project.

Morrison CA: Cameras in hospital rooms: the fourth amendment to the constitution and Munchausen syndrome by proxy. *Crit Care Nurs Q* 22(1):65–68, 1999.

Moyer VA: U.S. Preventive Services Task Force, Screening for intimate partner violence and abuse of elderly and vulnerable adults: U.S. preventive services task force recommendation statement. *Ann Intern Med* 158(6):478–486, 2013.

Muster NJ: Treating the adolescent victim-turned-offender. *Adolescence* 27(106):441, 1992.

Nayduch DA, Fitzpatrick MK: The application of forensic findings to the trauma quality management process. *J Trauma Nurs* 6(4):98–102, 1999.

Nutting MA, Dock LL: *A History of Nursing: The Evolution of Nursing Systems from the Earliest Times to the Foundation of the First English and American Training Schools for Nurses,* vol 1. New York, 1907, G.P. Putnam's Sons.

O'Neill B: Accidents or crashes: highway safety and William Haddon Jr. *Contingencies* 24(1):30–32, 2002.

Olsen D: Ethical considerations in forensic nursing. In Hammer RH, Moynihan B, Pagliaro EM, editors: *Forensic Nursing: A Handbook for Practice,* ed 2. Sudbury, MA, 2013, Jones and Bartlett, pp 45–71.

Patton SB: Credential development for forensic nurses. In Lynch VA, Duval JB, editors: *Forensic Nursing Science,* ed 2. St Louis, 2011, Elsevier Mosby.

Peden M, Oyegbite K, Ozanne-Smith J, et al: *World Report on Child Injury Prevention.* Geneva, 2009, WHO.

Pierce MC, Kaczor K, Aldridge S, et al: Bruising characteristics discriminating physical child abuse from accidental trauma. *Pediatrics* 125(1):67–74, 2010.

Rose DN: Respect for patient autonomy in forensic psychiatric nursing. *J Forensic Nurs* 1(1):23–27, 2005.

Sachs CJ, Weinberg E, Wheeler MW: Sexual assault nurse examiners' application of statutory rape reporting laws. *J Emerg Nurs* 34(5):410–413, 2008.

Shelton D: Forensic nursing in secure environments. *J Forensic Nurs* 5(3):131–142, 2009.

Sheridan DJ, Nash KR: Acute injury patterns of intimate partner violence victims. *Trauma Violence Abuse* 8:281–289, 2009.

Speck PM: *Program Evaluation of Current SANE Services to Victim Populations in Three Cities.* Memphis, 2005, University of Tennessee Heath Science Center.

Speck PM: *The Lived History of Forensic Nursing.* Memphis, n.d., PowerPoint presentation.

U.S. Department of Justice, Office on Violence Against Women: *A national protocol for sexual assault medical forensic examinations adults/adolescents,* 2004. Available at: http://www.ncjrs.gov/pdffiles1/ovw/206554.pdf. Accessed August 20, 2010.

U.S. Department of Health and Human Services, Office of Disease Prevention and Health Promotion: *Healthy People 2020,* 2010. Available at http://www.health.gov/healthypeople/url/. Accessed May 30, 2013.

Walsh SJ: Legal perceptions of forensic DNA profiling: Part I: a review of the legal literature. *Forensic Sci Int* 155(1):51–60, 2005.

*Washington v Harper,* 494 U.S., 1990.

Watson J: Social justice and human caring: a model of caring science as a hopeful paradigm for moral justice for humanity. *Creat Nurs* 14(2):54–61, 2008.

Wiglesworth A, Austin R, Corona M, et al: Bruising as a marker of physical elder abuse. *J Am Geriatr Soc* 57(1):1191–1196, 2009.

Williams D: Forensic nursing and utilitarianism: the quest for being right. *J Forensic Nurs* 5(1):49–50, 2009.

Williams DL: Is there a case for paternalism in forensic nursing? *J Forensic Nurs* 3(2):93–94, 2007.

Winfrey ME, Smith AR: The suspiciousness factor: critical care nursing and forensics. *Crit Care Nurs Q* 22(1):1, 1999.

World Health Organization: Responding to intimate partner violence and sexual violence against women: WHO clinical and policy guidelines. Available at http://www.who.int/reproductivehealth/publications/violence/9789241548595/en/. Accessed April 9, 2015, 2013.

# 45

# The Nurse in the Faith Community

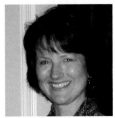

## Lisa M. Zerull, PhD, RN

Dr. Lisa M. Zerull provides leadership for faith-based services including faith community nursing and chaplaincy at Valley Health System in Winchester, Virginia, and serves as adjunct clinical faculty at Shenandoah University's School of Nursing. She teaches undergraduate clinical courses in addition to involvement with the educational preparation of faith community nurses since 1995. Dr. Zerull also has been a faith community nurse in her home congregation of Grace Evangelical Lutheran Church since 1996. Currently the editor for *Perspectives*, a newsletter for faith community nurses supported by the Church Health Center (Memphis, TN), Dr. Zerull is also an author and frequent conference presenter regionally, nationally, and internationally. Her research interests include nursing history, outcome measures of faith community nursing, and youth career exploration of the health professions.

## ADDITIONAL RESOURCES

Ⓔ **Evolve Website http://evolve.elsevier.com/Stanhope**
- *Healthy People 2020*
- WebLinks
- Quiz
- Case Studies

- Glossary
- Answer to Practice Application
- Resource Tools
  - Resource Tool 45.A: Resources for Faith Community Nursing

## OBJECTIVES

*After reading this chapter, the student should be able to do the following:*

1. Define faith community nursing and wholistic health promotion.
2. Examine the historical roots of nursing and healing ministries as well as professional issues and future development of faith community nursing.
3. Relate models of faith community nursing to the scope and standards of practice for faith community nursing.
4. Develop awareness of the nurse's role within faith communities for spiritual care, health promotion, and disease prevention.
5. Differentiate between spirituality and religiosity.
6. Use the nursing process in a faith community to assess, implement, and evaluate programs for healthy congregations using *Healthy People 2020* leading health indicators.

## KEY TERMS

## INTRODUCTION

Faith community nursing or parish nursing is a recognized nursing specialty practice in the community setting, yet is frequently overlooked when creative strategies are needed for improving the health of individuals and the larger community. According to Balboni et al (2013), only 12% to 14% of nurses report receiving spiritual care training as part of their nursing education. Nurses often confuse religious practice or religiosity, with spirituality and may neglect patients' spiritual needs (O'Brien, 2011). Whereas religiosity relates to "a person's beliefs and behaviors associated with a specific religious tradition or denomination" (O'Brien, 2011), spirituality is "an individual's attitudes and beliefs related to transcendence (God) or to the nonmaterial forces of life and nature" (O'Brien, 2011). Thus additional education in spiritual care to distinguish between the two and to provide an understanding of faith community nursing is needed.

Faith community nurses work in close relationship with individuals, families, and faith communities to coordinate programs and services that significantly affect health, healing, and wholeness (Dandridge, 2014; Sheehan et al, 2013; Bulechek et al, 2013, ANA/HMA, 2012; Solari-Twadell and Hackbarth, 2010). Faith community nurses balance knowledge and skill in their role to facilitate the faith community as it becomes a caring place—a place that is a source of health and healing for all members of the community. Many nurses are drawn to faith community nursing because it encourages the expression of spirituality as a part of health and healing. Others are drawn to this specialty practice out of vocational calling (Murphy and Walker, 2013; O'Brien, 2011).

Faith community nurses address health concerns of individuals, families, and groups of all ages. Like other communities, the members of faith communities experience birth and death; acute and chronic illness; growth and development; stress or dependency concerns; challenges from life transitions; and decisions regarding healthy lifestyle choices. Serving as good stewards of resources, faith community nurses encourage partnering with community health agencies as well as lay and professional church leaders to arrive at creative responses to

health issues and to develop health-promoting and spiritually healing activities. The nurse serves the faith community by focusing on the needs of the individual parishioner and the overall faith community with special attention given to spiritual needs.

## RATIONALE FOR FAITH COMMUNITY NURSING AS VIABLE COMMUNITY HEALTH MODEL

Early chapters in Parts 1 and 2 of this text familiarize the reader with the historical, economic, social, political, environmental, and ethical perspectives and influences on health care. The health care delivery system is challenged to work within parameters of tighter financial constraints while addressing patients' complex health concerns and also responding to federal mandates for expensive automated systems (i.e., electronic health records) that span the continuum of care. Current health care reform reflects a shift in health care delivery to a more comprehensive wellness-focused program. Faith community nurses are well positioned to provide lower cost and wholistic community-based care for vulnerable and underserved populations as well as collaborate with care providers (Horton et al, 2014; Sheehan et al, 2013; Shillam et al, 2013).

After major hospitalizations, clients may return to their homes very sick with few, if any, care providers available. Caregivers are faced with the multiple tasks of managing finances, maintaining family responsibilities, and learning care-giving skills. Fragmented care and inadequate caregiver training and availability are problems for the disenfranchised, underserved, and uninsured, as well as for economically well-situated and better-educated persons. Families are challenged to seek the best ways to meet the multiple demands of young children, teens, and aging parents whether living in metropolitan, suburban, or rural areas.

Consumer demand for involvement in health care decisions continues to increase, and society emphasizes individual responsibility for health. Simultaneously, consumers have increased interest in their own well-being and have expressed needs for health information to be available in a variety of formats (Beacom and Newman, 2010). In addition to consumer interest and a heightened awareness of responsibility for one's own health, health care providers and managed care systems have found it financially advantageous for individuals to remain healthy and minimize unnecessary access to care. Consumers struggle to cope with the challenges of rising costs of care, decreasing reimbursement, and the complex health system demands on individuals and families.

The traditional health care delivery model will not meet the burgeoning needs of the future. The skills of professional nurses, such as faith community nurses, will become more important with the provision of health care services in nontraditional settings (Horton et al, 2014; O'Brien, 2011; Djupe, 1992). It is important to differentiate the unique practice of faith community nursing from other community-based specialty practices. Faith community nursing shares many similarities with home health, hospice, and public health nursing—promoting health in the community setting; however, it is set apart from other community-based nurses by its wholistic approach and care of the spirit. Nursing care is also shaped and guided by the faith community's traditions, rites, and rituals.

A primary focus of all nurses in the last few decades has been to coordinate care and to link health care providers, groups, and community resources as the client tries to understand diverse health plans. Negotiating with individuals, agencies, and community partnerships within the complex maze of the broader health care environment demands a knowledgeable and seasoned professional. Nurses are aware of the necessity of collaborative practices and the formation of partnerships to care for groups and individuals throughout the life span. These nurses recognize the need for diverse ways to address health promotion and disease prevention at all levels. They advocate for healthy lifestyle choices in exercise, nutrition, substance use, and stress management. Nurses realize that information and guidance must be available via media, in schools, workplaces, faith communities, and residential neighborhoods. Faith community nurses need to partner with others such as health care institutions and federal agencies as they serve populations in faith communities (Horton et al, 2014) to help improve health outcomes.

## DEFINITIONS IN FAITH COMMUNITY NURSING

Faith community nursing is defined by the American Nurses Association as a specialized practice of professional nursing that focuses on the intentional care of the spirit as well as on the promotion of holistic health and prevention or minimization of illness within the context of a faith community (ANA/HMA, 2012). The ANA describes the development of a specialty practice in nursing as nurses expanding their practice to include the knowledge and skills necessary to meet the needs of patients requiring specialty care. Specialization involves focusing on nursing practice in a specific area, identified from within the whole field of professional nursing and in collaboration with specialty nursing organizations such as the Health Ministries Association (HMA), the membership organization for faith community nurses. Additionally, the ANA delineates the components of professional nursing practice that are essential for

any particular specialty. As the specialty evolves, the valuable contributions of nurses begin to distinguish them from other care providers (Hamric et al, 2013).

This has been true for the evolution of parish nursing. Early on, nurses involved with spiritual care struggled to find a workable definition for the role. Concerns were raised about nurses calling themselves parish nurses without any formal education—simply a nurse license and a willingness to serve their congregation. In order to validate the ministry of parish nurses to that of a recognized nursing specialty, all would need the foundation of a basic preparation with special focus on spiritual care. Following much dialogue and work to validate the specialty practice, parish nursing was recognized as a nursing specialty by the American Nurses Association (ANA/HMA, 2012).

With the 2005 revision of the *Scope and Standards of Practice*, the nurse title changed from parish nurse to faith community nurse. The new title was adopted to be more inclusive of diverse faith traditions and in response to international considerations (Patterson and Slutz, 2011). Parish nurse was the original title chosen by Granger Westberg in the 1980s as a theological choice because it connoted service to the congregation and also the wider community within a geographical area. The word "parish" can mean *congregation* and also *geographical area served by a congregation*. Additional titles for nurses working out of faith communities include parish nurse, congregational nurse, health ministry nurse, crescent nurse or health and wellness nurse (ANA/HMA, 2012, p. 7).

The faith community nurse is a licensed registered nurse "with well-developed clinical and interpersonal skills, a strong personal religious faith, and a desire or felt call to serve the needs of a faith community" (O'Brien, 2011, p. 335). With additional education in spiritual care of self, individuals, and groups, the faith community nurse works out of the congregational setting (Slutz and Wehling, 2013). It is expected that the professional registered nurse possesses competence in practice resulting from his/her application of knowledge, skills, and experience, functions with a deep understanding of the faith community's traditions, and fully integrates *care of the spirit* with care of the body and mind (ANA/HMA, 2012; O'Brien, 2011; Slutz and Wehling, 2013). The assumptions that underlie faith community nursing are as follows:

1. Health and illness are human experiences.
2. Health is the integration of the spiritual, physical, psychological, and social aspects of the health care consumer to create a sense of harmony with self, others, the environment, and a higher power.
3. Health may be experienced in the presence of disease or injury.
4. The presence of illness does not preclude health nor does optimal health preclude illness.
5. Healing is the process of integrating the body, mind, and spirit to create wholeness, health, and a sense of well-being when the health care consumer's illness is not cured.

While the majority of nurses serve Christian congregations in the United States, this specialty practice is found in many diverse faith traditions and has grown in its international outreach. Today, there are approximately 15,000 faith community

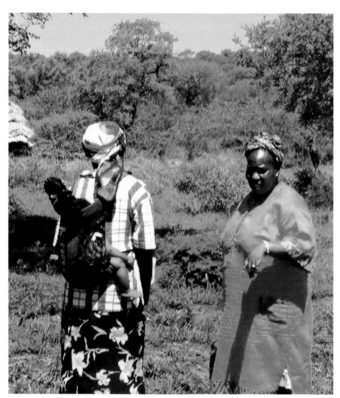

FIG 45-1 Parish nurse in rural Swaziland, Africa, making a home visit.

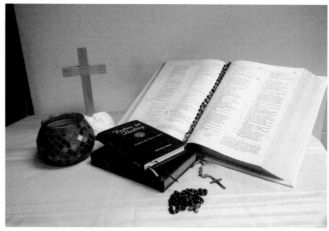

FIG 45-2 Religious symbols, images, rituals, and sacred places are significant to ministry.

nurses serving in a variety of faith settings including synagogues, temples, and mosques across the United States and in 23 countries around the world such as Canada, Australia, New Zealand, Germany, Swaziland (see Figure 45-1), Ukraine, and Pakistan (Daniels, 2014). This number is a conservative estimate based on the number of nurses who report taking an IPNRC-affiliated foundations course in faith community nursing and does not reflect the individuals who have completed nonaffiliated IPNRC programs or who practice without additional education in the specialty area (IPNRC, 2014).

Faith communities, also referred to as congregations, are organizations of groups, families, and individuals who share common values, beliefs, religious doctrine, and faith practices that influence their lives, such as a church, homeless shelter, synagogue, temple, or mosque, and that function as a patient system, providing a setting for faith community nursing (ANA/HMA, 2012, p. 108). Faith communities are found all over the world wherever individuals gather for the common purpose of worship, fellowship, the giving and receiving of love, grace, and hope, as well as the invitation, not obligation, to participate in the rites and rituals of a faith tradition (Figure 45-2). Some common examples include baptism, devotions, communion, reading of scripture, prayer, and singing. The important role of the faith community in a person's life is amplified with the recognition that it is one of the only institutions with a connection to an individual from birth through death. While many recognize and receive spiritual care support in the congregation, there may not be a conscious awareness of the church being an ideal place for health promotion of body and mind (Mauk and Schmidt, 2004).

Health ministries are visible activities, programs, and rituals of faith organized around health and healing of the congregation's membership and offered by the faith community nurse, clergy, layperson, or community resource. Health ministries may be informal or more specifically planned and encompass a gamut of activities including home visitation, providing meals for families in crisis or upon return home after hospitalization, quilting circles, grief support groups, and prayers for healing services (Figure 45-3) to name a few (Patterson, 2012; Patterson, 2013; Church Health Center, 2013; Hale and Koenig, 2004). Evidence suggests that health ministries potentially improve the health outcomes of all members of the faith community, including various ethnicities at higher risk for chronic disease (Horton et al, 2014; Asomugha et al, 2011). As an active member of the health ministry team, the faith community nurse emphasizes health promotion and models a visible healing presence to members of the congregation.

Faith community nurses respond to health and wellness needs of individuals, groups, and populations and are partners with the faith community in fulfilling the mission of health ministry and intentional spiritual care of its members. The faith community serves persons across the life span, infants through older adults. This may include active and less-active members, as well as those confined to home or living in institutional settings. Individuals or groups may be found in a geographic area near the congregational setting, or in a common cultural community. These individuals or groups may not be affiliated members of the faith community; however, services may be extended to those beyond the congregational setting, such as a food pantry, blood pressure screenings, transportation, and warm meals for those in need (Monay et al, 2010).

According to the ANA Scope and Standards of Practice for all nurses (ANA/HMA, 2012), spiritual care is part of all nursing practice and acknowledges a person's sense of meaning and purpose in life, which may or may not be expressed through formal religious beliefs and practices. It is also described as a distinct type of care defined by acts of listening, compassionate presence, open-ended questions, prayer, use of religious objects, talking with clergy, guided visualization,

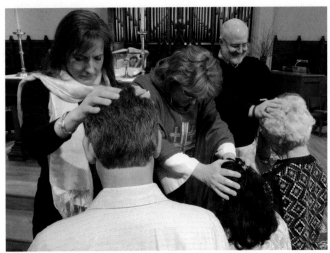

FIG 45-3 Prayers for healing service with ritual of laying on of hands.

### BOX 45-1   Nursing Interventions Classification

#### Core Interventions for Faith Community Nursing

- Abuse Protection Support
- Active Listening
- Anticipatory Guidance
- Caregiver Support
- Coping Enhancement
- Crisis Intervention
- Culture Brokerage
- Decision-Making Support
- Emotional Support
- Environmental Management: Community
- Family Integrity Promotion
- Family Support
- Forgiveness Facilitation
- Grief Work Facilitation
- Guilt Work Facilitation
- Health Care Information Exchange
- Health Education
- Health Literacy Enhancement
- Health System Guidance
- Hope Inspiration
- Humor
- Listening Visits
- Medication management
- Presence
- Referral
- Religious Addiction Prevention
- Religious Ritual Enhancement
- Relocation Stress Reduction
- Self-Care Assistance: IADL
- Socialization Enhancement
- Spiritual Growth Facilitation
- Spiritual Support
- Surveillance
- Sustenance Support
- Teaching: Group
- Teaching: Individual
- Telephone Consultation
- Touch
- Values Clarification

From Bulechek G, Dochterman J, Butcher H et al: Core interventions for nursing specialty areas: Faith community nursing. In *Nursing Interventions Classification (NIC)*, ed 6. St. Louis, 2013, Mosby, p. 429.

contemplation, meditation, conveying a benevolent attitude, or instilling hope (Chan, 2010; Puchalski and Ferrell, 2010). Spiritual care is helping the patient make meaning out of his/her experience or find hope (Murphy and Walker, 2013). Unique to faith community nursing as a specialty nursing practice is the primary focus on care of the spirit, with *spirit* defined as the core of a person's being. Box 45-1 provides a detailed listing of the core interventions for care of the spirit performed by faith community nurses. The compassionate and intentional healing presence of a spiritually mature nurse with individuals or groups is vital to addressing spiritual care needs.

Spiritual care is much different from religious care. Whereas religious care stems from the doctrine, rites, and rituals of a specific denomination or set of beliefs, spiritual care is unique to the individual's purpose in life, the fulfilling of that purpose and living it wholeheartedly. In most denominations, religion creates a nurturing environment where groups gather for worship or defined activity and in which spirituality emerges and grows. Nurses in secular health care may not give priority to spiritual care due to lack of time (Chan, 2010) or a reluctance to address spiritual care for fear of "stirring things up that they will not know how to address" (Jackson, 2011, p. 4), or crossing professional boundaries (Carr, 2010). With faith community nursing, intentional spiritual care is expected and appreciated. One nurse differentiated her experiences in providing hospital care versus faith community nursing care: "I have always thought of my nursing care as being whole person in nature; however in secular settings, I had to *ask permission* to care for the spiritual needs of my patients, whereas in the congregational setting, spiritual care *is expected*. It is a rare interaction with a parishioner where prayer, a gentle touch or warm embrace are not a part of my nursing care!" (Erbach, 2005).

Holistic/wholistic care relates to the relationship between body, mind, and spirit in a constantly changing environment and involves caring for the soul in a special kind of engagement that goes beyond seeing the physical patient but includes observation of the entire patient (Dossey and Keegan, 2013). The faith community nurse, supported by members of the congregation, assesses, plans, implements, and evaluates holistic care programs. The process of operationalizing holistic care is enhanced by an active wellness committee or health cabinet comprised of congregation members or congregants who may or may not be health professionals (e.g., doctors, therapists, social workers) and who are fully engaged in health ministry (Patterson, 2003; Chase-Ziolek, 2005; Westberg, 1990). The committee is most effective when members represent the broad spectrum of the life of the church. An active wellness committee provides leadership and influence throughout the faith community; ideas come not from one individual but are generated out of a committee structure (McNamara, 2006; Patterson, 2003; Westberg, 1990). The faith community nurse uses the collective knowledge and skills of this collaborative group to provide comprehensive and effective services. The outcome is a caring congregation that understands the strong link between faith and health and supports healthy, spiritually fulfilling lives. Resources for faith community nursing can be found on this book's Evolve website.

## HISTORICAL PERSPECTIVES

### Faith Communities

Throughout history, the church has been an integral part of the health, healing, and social well-being of a community. From its earliest days, churches have provided Christian nurturance and care of the marginalized: "At the core of every major faith tradition stands an explicit commitment to be with the sick, the poor, the alienated, the marginal, the wounded, and the dying. The commitments are very old, but the implications are ever new" (Gunderson, 2006, p. 1).

In the roots of many faith traditions are concerns for justice, mercy, and the need for spiritual and physical healing (Zerull, 2010). The appeal for caring, the healing of diseases, and acknowledging periods of illness and wellness is universal. Religion plays an important role in the lives of many individuals. Research suggests that individuals and families are inclined to turn to religion or spiritual counsel during stressful life events such as illness, crisis or death (Koenig et al, 2012). Seventy percent of Americans identify with a personal God, and an additional 12% believe in a higher power (Kosmin and Keysar, 2008). The relationship between spirituality, religion, and health is an important topic for nursing research. An important aspect of living out one's spirituality and religion is being a part of a community of faith from birth to death, throughout wellness and illness. Whether participating as individuals or as families, all benefit from association with a supportive faith community or congregation through enhanced happiness, peace, hope, and purpose (Koenig, 2009).

Dating back to apostolic times, the biblical reference to Phoebe (Romans 16:1-2) exemplifies the tradition of health and healing within a congregation as well as the important role of women serving in the church. In addition, many Old Testament accounts and healing stories in the New Testament provide additional faith foundations (Psalms 106, 107, 113; Mark; Luke; Acts). The charge of the early Christian church was to preach, teach, and heal. The church provided access to services such as shelter and food; the church tended to wounds and offered comfort and safety. Through the centuries, nuns, deacons, and deaconesses from the Christian tradition provide continuing examples of persons combining faith and health in the care of the sick. Although healing has been a primary mission, many churches have gotten away from that mission and relegated that mission to health care institutions. Somehow along the way, the body and soul got divided in our thinking. Medicine provides care to the physical body and the mind, whereas the church cares for the soul (Lounsbury, 1990).

The origins of wholeness and salvation are derived from similar concepts of *sodzo* (Greek) and *shalom*, or wholeness. These terms and harmony in health are common to most faith communities. Writings in Christian and Jewish sources address the individual and community relationships with God as the source for a wise use of resources of self, environment, and one's community. Hygiene, health, and healing were a part of the Holiness Code of Leviticus. Throughout history, health existed at the center of the interaction between one's creator and humankind. The integration of faith and health within the caring community results in beneficial outcomes (Brown et al, 2009). Persons who encounter physical and emotional illness and who are able to call upon their faith beliefs and religious traditions are able to increase coping skills and realize spiritual growth (O'Brien, 2011).

Individuals draw on their faith traditions and previous learning experiences, as well as accept support from family and friends to interpret brokenness, disasters, joys, births, deaths, illness, and recovery. Encouraging growth in faith beliefs and honoring traditions and rituals of the faith community brings individuals, families, and congregations into closer connection with their creator. The consolation of sacred liturgies, religious rituals, sacred space, and communal events aids the grieving and the healing process; they also affirm transcendent life (O'Brien, 2011; Dossey et al, 2013).

Some of the major Christian faith communities in the late nineteenth and early twentieth centuries used missionaries to develop multipurpose activities in communities, which included health activities and education along with religious messages. Hospitals were built in the United States and abroad targeting underserved populations. As political and economic forces changed through the years, health ministry strategies of faith communities have altered their approaches. Some faith groups have identified with community development efforts to help empower people to meet their needs for food, education, a clean environment, social support, and primary health care. Congregations have also recognized the need to increase awareness in several areas, including one's personal responsibility for healthy choices; the escalating cost of health care and the need for cost containment; the increasing numbers of the uninsured and underserved; the issues of domestic violence and substance abuse; childhood obesity; and the ever-increasing dilemma of interpreting the complex changes within the health care delivery system.

The governing bodies of various faith communities have supported health and wellness efforts by endorsing statements related to health and wellness (Evangelical Lutheran Church, 2014; LCMS, 2014). The Presbyterian Church (2012) is cited as an example of a long-standing tradition of encouraging members to be good stewards or responsible managers of body, mind, the environment, and total resources. In 2012 Presbyterian Church representatives met with key others and First Lady Michelle Obama at the White House to identify opportunities for faith groups to increase and promote wellness and healthy lifestyle options in their congregations, implement more health and fitness activities, and urge state-level policy changes (Presbyterian Church USA, 2012). Similar efforts exist in the Episcopal Church USA, the United Church of Christ, the Catholic Church, and other large denominations.

## Parish/Faith Community Nursing

Nursing has had a long history of association with churches and denominations, namely the Catholic Sisters and Protestant Deaconesses who promoted health and cared for the sick, the poor, the fallen and the unbelieving (Fliedner, 1870; Doyle, 1929). Likewise, parish or faith community nurses have followed that same tradition for more than three decades by working out of the church setting to promote whole person health–ministering to body, mind and spirit of parishioners from the time of birth through the end of life.

In 1984, the concept of parish nursing was introduced to churches in the Chicago, Illinois area by Lutheran chaplain Granger Westberg (1913-1999) as way of expanding existing health ministries and providing another link between faith and

BOX 45-2    **Timeline of Faith Community Nursing**

- 1983 Pilot program with a nurse running a wellness clinic out of the congregation setting—Our Saviour Lutheran Church, Tucson, AZ
- 1984 Parish Nurse Program partnership begun with six congregations and Lutheran General Hospital, Park Ridge, IL
- 1986 Lutheran General Hospital establishes a Parish Nurse Resource Center to share information about health ministry and parish nursing with others.
- 1987 First Westberg Parish Nurse Symposium is held and Granger Westberg publishes book *The Parish Nurse*. Parish Nurse Resource Center becomes the *National* Parish Nurse Resource Center.
- 1989 Health Ministries Association began in Iowa.
- 1991 Marquette University offers eight-day parish nurse education program titled the *Wisconsin Model*, a curriculum later modified to become the *Foundations of Faith Community Nursing* course.
- 1995 Lutheran General merges with Evangelical Health Systems Corporation to create Advocate Health Care. National Parish Nurse Resource Center becomes the *International* Parish Nurse Resource Center.
- 1997 American Nurses Association recognizes parish nursing as a specialty practice.
- 1998 First Scope and Standards for parish nursing practice released. Parish Nurse Preparation Curriculum is published.
- 1999 Parish Nurse Coordinator Curriculum is published. Death of Granger Westberg (July 1913-February 1999).
- 2002 IPNRC transfers assets from Advocate Health System to the Deaconess Foundation, St. Louis, MO.
- 2004 World Forum for Faith Community Nursing is formed with 22 members from Australia, Canada, South Korea, Swaziland, and U.S.
- 2005 ANA partners with HMA for scope and standards revisions—title changed from parish nurse to faith community nurse.
- 2011 IPNRC transfers assets from Deaconess Foundation, St. Louis, MO to the Church Health Center, Memphis, TN. The 25th Annual Westberg International Parish Nurse Symposium is held.
- 2012 Faith community nurse scope and standards 2nd edition published.
- 2014 American Nurses Credentialing Center (ANCC) launches faith community nursing certification through portfolio. *Foundations of Faith Community Nursing* curriculum revised.

health. See Box 45-2, Timeline of Faith Community Nursing. Westberg described parish nursing as a way for the church to reclaim its traditional role in healing (1990). Having previous experience with setting up holistic health centers out of churches, Westberg fully understood that hospitals and physicians deal with illness, yet there is a need for preventative medicine and wellness in the community and churches fit right in (1990). He also recognized that it was nurses who could have the largest impact on the delivery of whole person care within a congregation, using the nurse's broad background of health promotion, education spiritual care and social work (Westberg, 1985).

Westberg's rejuvenation of parish nursing in the 1980s built on the strengths of his previous work and focused on the nurse–clergy team working with individuals and their families. Nurses used their professional knowledge, skills, and experience to listen to the spoken and unspoken concerns of individuals resulting in whole person care provision with spiritual care

central to the relationship. By 1984, Westberg partnered with Lutheran General Hospital (Park Ridge, IL—now known as Advocate Health) on a pilot project with six Chicago-area congregations that included four Protestant and two Roman Catholic communities (Solari-Twadell and McDermott, 2006). These partnerships established the first institutionally-based paid parish nurse program between a health system and churches in the U.S. (Westberg and McNamara, 1987). Other historical, social, and economic factors contributed to the implementation and subsequent success of parish nursing. They included the timing of Westberg's parish nurse proposal to Lutheran General, the graying of America, the growing focus on partnerships in health care, empowerment of the consumer and the desire for a focus on whole person health care combined with obvious gaps in community follow-up care.

As the contemporary parish nurse movement grew, information was spread by advocates of whole person health. This resulted in the establishment of a Resource Center (IPNRC) in 1986 to provide information, printed literature, and news of emerging parish nurse programs across the U.S., both paid and unpaid. Basic education to prepare nurses and through the collaborative efforts of health system, educators, and the IPNRC, a foundational course was designed. As noted in the timeline, the IPNRC moved from Illinois, to Missouri and now its current home with the Church Health Center in Memphis, Tennessee. Throughout its tenure, the work of the IPNRC focused on the provision and promotion of education, research, and support through curriculum, resources and continuing education opportunities.

## FAITH COMMUNITY NURSING PRACTICE

As in the early history of the development of public health nursing in the United States, faith community nurses found that health promotion services were needed for persons across the life span, particularly in underserved urban and rural areas. Nurses identified gaps in the delivery of service. They found that congregants residing in communities that offered access to adequate health services also requested and benefited from health counseling and health promotion services at all levels of prevention. The following Levels of Prevention box provides an overview of levels of prevention for older adult health.

Faith community nurse services emphasized health promotion and disease prevention and provided the benefits of holistic care through the supportive, caring faith community. Nurses acknowledged the inner strength and spirituality of persons and groups to increase healing. The nurses developed effective skills in negotiation, collaboration, and leadership. They also honed astute nonverbal and verbal communication skills. They embraced the vital role of families for healthy outcomes, and parish nurses knew that community support augmented the interventions chosen by individuals and families. Working with the congregation as the population group, faith community nurses attempt to include in the wellness programs those persons who are less vocal or visible in the community of faith. The spiritual dimension of health was and is optimized by complementing the nursing role with pastoral care.

## LEVELS OF PREVENTION

### Older Adult Health

**Primary Prevention**

- Hold classes for older adults on healthy eating including food selection, preparation, and increasing socialization opportunities at mealtimes for widows/widowers.
- Promote and encourage age-appropriate activities that include daily physical exercise with increased focus on improved balance related to muscle strength, proprioception, and coordination.
- Encourage a variety of activities of individual and group interest and discourage extended inactivity.
- Encourage healthy snacks and meals for older adult gatherings and activities.
- Write faith community newsletter articles targeting topics of interest to older adults (e.g., recommended annual screenings, signs and symptoms of heart attack and stroke, medication management, Medicare benefits, etc.).
- Provide an eyeglasses drive for missions reminding older adults to get vision checks by an eye doctor at least every 1 to 2 years, and update glasses or contact lenses when vision changes.
- Provide support groups based on needs and interests (e.g., grief support/bereavement; low vision; transitions to long-term care/retirement community; Alzheimer caregivers; adults living with disabilities; etc.).
- Coordinate medication management opportunities such as inviting a pharmacist to assist in a medication review after worship.
- Initiate a walk for fun program (e.g., Walk to Emmaus).
- Host a community health fair offering resources related to whole person health.

**Secondary Prevention**

- Provide health assessment and counseling during home visits for health promotion such as visits after a hospitalization.
- When making home visits, identify safety concerns and make suggestions such as eliminating throw rugs, decreasing clutter, decreasing use of extension cords, and moving heat sources from flammable products such as oxygen.
- Using an attitudinal/behavioral risk survey, identify factors influencing health behaviors.
- Be available for health counseling for older adults before and after activities.

**Tertiary Prevention**

- Collaborate closely with ministerial team about sessions that deal with healthy nutrition, exercise with injury prevention guidelines, health concerns related to being overweight, and advantages of maintaining a healthy weight, and support, stress management, and improved quality-of-life sessions.
- Follow up and monitor health care provider's plan of care for older adults challenged with chronic disease such as diabetes, hypertension, and depression; provide education, support, and spiritual care.
- Facilitate a faith-based activities program for aging in place.
- Discuss in older adult gatherings the need for loving, caring friends and the support needed for mental health and overall well-being.

From U.S. Department of Health and Human Services: *Healthy People 2020*. Washington, DC, 2013, USDHHS.

## Profile of the Faith Community Nurse

The practice of the faith community nurse is governed by (1) the Nurse Practice Act of the state in which the nurse practices; (2) *Nursing: Scope and Standards of Practice* (ANA, 2010); (3) *Faith Community Nursing: Scope and Standards of Practice* (ANA/HMA 2012); and (4) *Code of Ethics with Interpretive Statements* (for nurses) (ANA, 2001). According to the International Parish/Faith Community Nurse Resource Center located in Memphis, Tennessee (Church Health Center, 2013), the suggested requirements to be a faith community nurse include the following:

- Active registered nurse license in the state of practice
- Baccalaureate degree or higher in nursing with experience in community nursing preferred
- Completion of a foundational education course in faith community nursing
- Specialized knowledge of the spiritual beliefs and practices of the faith community
- Personal spirituality maturity in practice
- Should be organized, flexible, self-started, and a good communicator

The majority of nurses choosing to become specialized in faith community nursing are experienced and have been in practice for several years. A large survey of faith community nurses (*n* = 1161) across the United States yielded the following description:

- Average age = 55 years
- 89% female
- 32% prepared at baccalaureate level in nursing, 24% prepared at the diploma level, 14% prepared at the associate's level, 12% hold a master's in nursing
- 68% serve as unpaid staff in towns (47%), cities (42%), and metro areas (11%)
- Majority are from Christian faith traditions with only 2% of the sample Jewish; 25%, Lutheran; 23%, Roman Catholic; 16%, Methodist
- 17% have membership in the American Nurses Association (Solari-Twadell, PA, 2006)

Because many faith community nurses practice within their own congregation, they are considered to be a known and trusted resource. By virtue of relationship, congregants access the services of the faith community nurse with a high comfort level and awareness that information shared will be kept confidential by the nurse professional. Faith community nurses are well aware of the beliefs, faith practices, and level of spiritual maturity of the members served, and they link these with health and healing (O'Brien, 2011).

Many faith community nurses function in a part-time capacity and serve as salaried or unpaid staff. Some nurses are responsible for services for several faith communities, whereas others engage in faith community nursing as part of a full-time commitment in other capacities. For example, a nurse might be employed part-time as a public health nurse and part-time as a faith community nurse in the same community. Alternatively, a nurse employed full-time in an acute care setting may spend

## KEY POINTS

- Faith community nurse services respond to health, healing, and wholeness within the context of the faith community. Although the emphasis is on health promotion and disease prevention throughout the life span, the spiritual dimension of nursing is central to the practice. The focus of the practice is on the "intentional care of the spirit."
- Spiritual care is different from religious care and is an expected component of nursing care in the faith community setting. Note that spiritual assessment and care can also be provided outside of a congregational setting.
- Faith community nursing evolved from the historical roots of healing traditions in faith communities; early public health nursing efforts with individuals, families, and populations in the community; and more recently the professional practice of nursing.
- The faith community nurse partners with the wellness committee and volunteers to plan programs that address health-related concerns within faith communities.
- The usual functions of the faith community nurse include health counseling and teaching for individuals and groups, facilitating linkages and referrals to congregation and community resources, advocating and encouraging support resources, and providing spiritual care.
- Faith community nurses collaborate to plan, implement, and evaluate health promotion activities considering the faith community's beliefs, rituals, and polity. *Healthy People 2020* objectives and health indicators offer effective frameworks for health ministry efforts of wellness committees and basic to partnering for programs.
- Nurses in congregational or institutional models enhance health ministry programs of faith communities when carefully chosen partnerships are formed within the congregation, with other faith communities, and with local health and social community organizations.
- Nurses working as faith community nurses must obtain foundational and ongoing educational and skill preparation to be accountable to those served.
- Faith community nurses document care interventions offered to individuals and groups, in addition to tracking and reporting program statistics and outcomes to validate and sustain the professional practice.
- Nurses are encouraged to consider innovative approaches to creating caring communities. These may be in individual faith communities; among several faith communities in a single locale, regionally or internationally; or in partnership with other organizations and institutions.
- To sustain oneself as a faith community nurse who provides spiritual care to support individuals, families, and communities in the healing and wholeness process, the nurse must be diligent to take time for self-care and renewal.

## CLINICAL DECISION-MAKING ACTIVITIES

1. Contact the local organization of faith communities (such as the Council of Churches or health system) to see if there is faith community nursing in your area. If so, make contact and arrange to spend a day with a nurse.
   A. Interview the nurse about the faith community nurse role functions. Contrast the nurse's answers to what you learned in this chapter.
   B. Ask how the faith community nurse standards of practice are integrated into the practice. How can you verify the answer?
   C. If possible, spend time in a variety of faith communities. Compare and contrast urban and rural settings, different faith traditions, and nontraditional settings.
2. Discuss with classmates the similarities and differences between home health care nursing, school nursing, public health nursing, and faith community nursing. Compare your answers.
3. Choose a *Healthy People 2020* indicator to implement in a faith community setting. Discuss plans for implementing the objective and evaluating the outcomes with the faith community nurse and wellness committee. What data did you use to develop a plan for implementation? How did you choose your population? How did you evaluate the outcomes of your goals and activities?
4. Interview a clergy member of a local church, temple, or mosque in your area (preferably with someone with a different background than your own). Ask the individual to elaborate on traditions of faith, health, and healing connections. Consider how you might be able to meet the unique needs of that faith community.
5. Visit a senior citizen daycare center and speak with participants about important events in their lives. Do they refer to rituals from faith traditions? Ask them about their connections to faith communities during their lives.
6. With classmates, interview a youth group leader and nurse in a local faith community about the concern of preventing risky behaviors among youths. What perspectives of this concern would the faith community staff need to consider?

# REFERENCES

American Heart Association: *EmPowered to Serve Faith-based Roundtable*, 2014. Available at http://powertoendstroke.org/events-ets.html. Accessed March 23, 2014.

American Holistic Nurses Association: *Holistic Nursing: Scope and Standards of Practice*. Washington, D.C., 2000, updated 2007, ANA.

American Nurses Association: *Code of Ethics with Interpretive Statements* (for nurses), 2001. Available at http://www.nursingworld.org/MainMenuCategories/EthicsStandards/CodeofEthicsforNurses/Code-of-Ethics.pdf. Accessed September 27, 2014.

American Nurses Association: *Holistic Nursing: Scope and Standards of Practice*. Silver Spring, MD, 2007, ANA.

American Nurses Association: *Nursing: Scope and Standards of Practice*. Silver Spring, MD, 2010, ANA.

American Nurses Association and Health Ministries Association (ANA/HMA): *Scope and Standards of Practice of Parish Nursing Practice*. Washington DC, 1998, American Nurses Publishing.

American Nurses Association and Health Ministries Association (ANA/HMA): *Faith Community Nursing: Scope and Standards of Practice*. Silver Spring, MD, 2005, ANA.

American Nurses Association and Health Ministries Association (ANA/HMA): *Faith Community Nursing: Scope and Standards of Practice*, ed 2. Silver Spring, MD, 2012, ANA.

American Nurses Credentialing Center: *ANCC Certification through Portfolio General Handbook*, 2013. Available at http://www.nursecredentialing.org/CertificationPortfolio-ApplicationHandbook.pdf. Accessed April 9, 2014.

American Nurses Credentialing Center: *Faith Community Nursing Certification through Portfolio*, 2014. Available at http://www.nursecredentialing.org/Certification/NurseSpecialties/FaithCommunityNursing. Accessed April 7, 2014.

Asomugha CN, Derose KP, Lurie N: Faith-based organizations, science, and the pursuit of health. *J Health Care Poor Underserved* 22(1):50–55, 2011.

Austin SA, Brennan-Jordan N, Frenn D, et al: Defy diabetes: a unique partnership with faith community/parish nurses to impact diabetes. *J Christ Nurs* 30(4):238–243, 2013.

Austin S, Brooks PS, Gleen LM, et al: *Nurses Legal Handbook*, ed 5. Philadelphia, PA, 2004, Lippincott Williams & Wilkins.

Balboni MJ, Sullivan A, Amobi A, et al: Why is spiritual care infrequent at the end of life? Spiritual care perceptions among patients, nurses and physicians and the role of training. *J Clin Oncol* 31(4):461–467, 2013.

Beacom AM, Newman SJ: Communicating health information to disadvantaged populations. *Fam Community Health* 2:152–162, 2010.

Bokinskie J, Kloster P: Effective parish nursing: Building success and overcoming barriers. *J Christ Nurs* 25(1):20–25, 2008.

Brown A, Coppolla P, Giacona M, et al: Faith community nursing demonstrates good stewardship of community benefit dollars through cost savings and cost avoidance. *Fam Community Health* 32(4):330–338, 2009.

Brown AR, Yore J: Documenting health ministry using available technology: the Henry Ford Macomb FCN/health ministry documentation and reporting system. *Perspectives (Montclair)* 12(3):8–9, 2013.

Bulechek G, Dochterman J, Butcher H, et al: Core interventions for nursing specialty areas: faith community nursing. In *Nursing Interventions Classification (NIC)*, ed 6. St. Louis, 2013, Mosby.

Burkhart L, Androwich I: Measuring the domain completeness of the nursing interventions classification system in parish nurse documentation. *Comput Inform Nurs* 22:72–82, 2004.

Carr TJ: Facing existential realities: exploring barriers and challenges to spiritual nursing care. *Qual Health Res* 20(10):1379–1392, 2010.

Cassimere M, Slutz M: The role of the faith community nurse coordinator. In *Faith Community Nurse Coordinator Manual: A Guide to Creating and Developing Your Program*. Memphis, 2013, Church Health Center.

Catanzaro A, Meador K, Koenig H, et al: Congregational health ministries: a national study of pastors' views. *Public Health Nurs* 24(1):6–17, 2006.

Centers for Disease Control and Prevention: *Chronic Diseases and Health Promotion*, August 13, 2012. Available at http://www.cdc.gov/chronicdisease/overview/index.htm. Accessed March 29, 2014.

Centers for Disease Control and Prevention: *Resources for Faith-based and Community Organizations*, 2014. Available at http://www.cdc.gov/flu/nivw/community.htm. Accessed March 23, 2014.

Chan MF: Factors affecting nursing staff in practicing spiritual care.

*J Clin Nurs* 19(15–16):2128–2136, 2010.

Chase-Ziolek M: *Health, Healing and Wholeness*. Cleveland, 2005, The Pilgrim Press.

Church Health Center: Health promoters lead congregations into healing. *Church Health Read* 3(1):14, 2013.

Dandridge R: Faith community/parish nurse literature: exciting interventions, unclear outcomes. *J Christ Nurs* 31(2):100–106, 2014.

Daniels M: The world forum for parish and faith community nursing ministries. *Perspectives (Montclair)* 13(1):1–3, 2014.

Djupe AM: *Looking Back: The Parish Nurse Experience*. Report to the W.K. Kellogg Foundation, Park Ridge, IL, 1992, National Parish Nurse Resource Center of Lutheran General Health System.

Dossey BM, Keegan L: *Holistic Nursing: A Handbook for Practice*, ed 6. Burlington, MA, 2013, Jones & Bartlett.

Doyle A: Nursing by religious orders in the United States: part VI—Episcopal sisterhoods 1845–1928. *Am J Nurs* 29(12):1466–1484, 1929.

Durbin N: *Interview*, January 11, 2006, interview DS 2013, transcript, Lisa Zerull Private Papers, Winchester, Virginia.

Durbin NLR, Cassimere M, Howard C, et al: *Faith Community Nurse Coordinator Manual: A Guide to Creating and Developing Your Program*. Memphis, 2013, Church Health Center.

Erbach M: *Interview*, October 10, 2005, transcript, Lisa Zerull Private Papers, Winchester, Virginia.

Evangelical Lutheran Church: *Mission*, 2014. Available at http://www.elca.org/About/Mission. Accessed April 12, 2014.

Fliedner T: *Some Account of the Deaconess Work in the Christian Church*. Kaiserswerth, Germany, 1870, Sam Lucas, p 26.

Gunderson G: Parish Nurse Ministry in Faith Community Nursing: A Specialty Practice of Professional Nursing. In *Pamphlet*. Park Ridge, IL, 2006, Advocate HealthCare.

Hale WD, Koenig HG: *Healing Bodies and Souls: A Practical Guide for Congregations (Prisms)*. Minneapolis, 2004, Augsburg Fortress Press.

Hamric AB, Hanson CM, Tracy MF, et al: *Advanced Practice Nursing: An Integrative Approach*, ed 5. St. Loius, MO, 2013, W.B. Saunders Co.

Hickman J: *Faith Community Nursing*. New York, 2006, Lippincott Williams & Wilkins.

Hodge DR, Limb GE: A Native American perspective on spiritual assessment: the strengths and limitations of a complementary set of assessment tools. *Health Soc Work* 2:121–131, 2010.

Horton SEB, Alvear EE, Horton DL: Health ministry partnerships: creating a habit for health. *J Christ Nurs* 31(1):28–33, 2014.

International Parish Nurse Resource Center: *Conversation with Maureen Daniels, faith community nurse specialist with the Church Health Center and IPNRC resource*, March 30, 2014.

Jackson C: Addressing spirituality: a natural aspect of holistic care. *Holist Nurs Pract* 25(1):3–7, 2011.

Jacob S: Planning for FCN Foundations Curriculum Revisions. In *Perspectives* 12(2):8–9, 2013.

Johnson EJ, Testerman N, Hart D: Teaching spiritual care to nursing students: an integrated model. *J Christ Nurs* 31(2):94–199, 2014.

Koenig HG: *Spirituality and Patient Care*. Philadelphia, 2002, Templeton Foundation Press.

Koenig HG: *Religion and Mental Health: A Review of Previous Research*. Durham, NC, August 2009. Paper presented at the Summer Research Workshop on Spirituality and Health.

Koenig HG, King DE, Carson VB: *Handbook of Religion and Health*, ed 2. Oxford, 2012, Oxford University.

Kosmin B, Keysar A: *American Religious Identification Survey*. Hartford CT, 2008, Trinity College.

Lounsbury P: Nurse ministry hails as first year ends: six others expected to join. *Evening Sentinel* August 31:1c, 1990.

Lutheran Church Missouri Synod: *Health Ministry*, 2014. Available at http://www.lcms.org/health. Accessed April 12, 2014.

Mauk KL, Schmidt NK: *Spiritual Care in Nursing Practice*. Philadelphia, 2004, Lippincott, Williams & Wilkins, p 12.

Mayernik D: Faith community nursing in the accountable care era: documentation of interventions demonstrates improved health outcomes. *Perspectives (Montclair)* 12(3):6–7, 2013.

McCloskey JC, Bulechek GM: *Nursing Interventions Classification (NIC): Iowa Interventions Project*. St Louis, 2000, Mosby.

McNamara JW: *Health & Wellness: What Your Faith Community Can Do*. Cleveland, 2006, Pilgrim Press.

Monay V, Mangione CM, Sorrell-Thompson A, et al: Services delivered by faith community nurses to individuals with elevated blood pressure. *Public Health Nurs* 27(6):537–543, 2010.

Murphy LS, Walker MS: Spirit-guided care: Christian nursing for the whole person. *J Christ Nurs* 30(3):144–152, 2013.

National Heart, Lung and Blood Institute: *Faith-based Toolkit*, 2014. Available at http://www.nhlbi.nih.gov/educational/hearttruth/materials/faith-based-toolkit.htm. Accessed March 23, 2014.

O'Brien ME: *Spirituality in Nursing: Standing on Holy Ground*, ed 4. Sudbury, MA, 2011, Jones and Bartlett.

Patterson DL: *The Essential Parish Nurse.* Cleveland, 2003, The Pilgrim Press.

Patterson D: *Get My People Going: On a Journey Toward Wellness.* Memphis, TN, 2012, Church Health Center.

Patterson D: Top ten ways to improve the health of a congregation. *Church Health Read* 3(1):5, 2013.

Patterson D, Slutz M: Faith community/parish nursing: what's in a name? *J Christ Nurs* 28(1):31–33, 2011.

Presbyterian Church USA: *Presbyterians, Other Faith Leaders Meet with White House Chef: Group Discusses Campaign to Combat Childhood Obesity Epidemic*, 2012. Available at http://www.pcusa.org/news/2012/5/31/presbyterians-other-faith-leaders-meet-white-house/. Accessed April 12, 2014.

Puchalski C: *FICA Spiritual History Tool of the George Washington Institute for Spirituality and Health*, 2014. Available at http://smhs.gwu.edu/gwish/clinical/fica/spiritual-history-tool. Accessed April 11, 2014.

Puchalski C, Ferrell B: *Making Health Care Whole: Integrating Spirituality into Patient Care.* West Conshohocken, PA, 2010, Templeton.

Robert Wood Johnson Foundation: *Chronic Care: Making the Case for Ongoing Care.* Princeton, NJ, 2010, Robert Wood Johnson Foundation, p 16. Available at: http://www.rwjf.org/content/dam/farm/reports/reports/2010/rwjf54583. Accessed September 26, 2014.

Sheehan A, Austin SA, Brennan-Jordan N, et al: Defy diabetes: impact on faith community/parish nurses teaching healthy living classes. *J Christ Nurs* 30(4):244–246, 2013.

Shillam CR, Orton VJ, Waring D, et al: Faith community nurses & brown bag events help older adults manage meds. *J Christ Nurs* 30(2):90–96, 2013.

Slutz M, Wehling B: Foundation of faith community nursing practice. In *Faith Community Nurse Coordinator Manual: A Guide to Creating and Developing Your Program.* Memphis, 2013, Church Health Center.

Solari-Twadell PA: The emerging practice of parish nursing. In Phyllis Ann Solari-Twadell PA, McDermott MA, editors: *Parish Nursing: Promoting Whole Person Health Within Faith Communities.* Thousand Oaks, CA, 1999, Sage Publications, pp 3–24.

Solari-Twadell PA: Uncovering the intricacies of the ministry of parish nursing practice through research. In Solari-Twadell PA, McDermott MA, editors: *Parish Nursing: Development, Education, and Administration.* St Louis, 2006, Elsevier, p 22.

Solari-Twadell PA, Hackbarth DP: Evidence for a new paradigm of the ministry of parish nursing practice using the Nursing Intervention Classification System. *Nurs Outlook* 58(2):69–75, 2010.

Solari-Twadell PA, McDermott MA, editors: *Parish Nursing: Development, Education, and Administration.* St Louis, 2006, Mosby.

Solari-Twadell PA, McDermott MA, Matheus R: Education for parish nursing: assuring congregational health and wholeness for the twenty-first century. *Perspect Parish Nurs Pract* 5(3):1–2, 1997.

The Joint Commission: *Comprehensive Accreditation Manual for Hospitals: The Official Handbook.* Chicago, 2013, Joint Commission Resources.

Timmons S: African American church health programs: what works? *J Christ Nurs* 1:100–106, 2010.

U.S. Department of Health and Human Services: *Healthy People 2020.* Washington, DC, 2013, USDHHS.

Weis D, Schank MJ: Use of a taxonomy to describe parish nurse practice with older adults. *Geriatr Nurs* 21:125–131, 2000.

Westberg GE: *Presentation on 12 September 1985*, Westberg Collection, Loyola University at Chicago University Archives, Box 1, folder 3, 1.

Westberg GE: *The Parish Nurse: Providing A Minister of Health for Your Congregation.* Minneapolis, 1990, Augsburg Press.

Westberg GE, McNamara JW: *The Parish Nurse: How To Start a Parish Nurse Program in Your Church.* Park Ridge, IL, 1987, Parish Nurse Resource Center.

Zerull LM: *Nursing Out of the Parish: A History of the Baltimore Lutheran Deaconesses 1893–1911*, Dissertation 2010.

Zerull LM, Solari-Twadell PA: Administration of parish nursing: describing the roles. In Solari-Twadell PA, McDermott MA, editors: *Parish Nursing: Development, Education, and Administration.* St Louis, 2006, Mosby.

# 46

# Public Health Nursing at Local, State, and National Levels

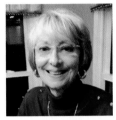

*Lois A. Davis, RN, MSN, MA*

Lois A. Davis began her public health career in 1977 in Eastern Kentucky with the Breathitt County Health Department, where she worked with the Appalachian population in a variety of public health preventive programs. She expanded her role in public health as a school nurse and initiated a program to reduce teen pregnancy in the Breathitt County Schools. She worked in community mental health and understands the importance of community partnerships. Lois spent three years in South America and afterwards fulfilled a desire to assist migrant health populations and the underserved. She is currently the public health nursing manager at the Lexington–Fayette County Health Department in Lexington, Kentucky, where she serves as the Maternal–Child Health Coordinator, and directs several community services programs, including HANDS, school health, and health equity and education. She has functioned as incident commander for preparedness exercises and operations lead for real events, such as special needs shelters during ice storms. At the state level, Lois serves on the Nurse Executive Council, where she helps define public health protocols and public health nursing competencies for local health department nurses. Lois has served on the board of the Bluegrass Community Health Center, a HRSA Federally Qualified Health Center, for ten years. Additionally, she has served as an adjunct faculty member and on advisory boards for the University of Kentucky College of Nursing, Eastern Kentucky University, and Midway College. She has precepted numerous nursing students and is passionate about preventive health.

## ADDITIONAL RESOURCES

(e) **Evolve Website http://evolve.elsevier.com/Stanhope**
- Healthy People 2020
- WebLinks—Of special note, see the links for these sites:
  - Council on Linkages Between Academia and Public Health Practice Core Public Health Competencies
  - Community-Campus Partnerships for Health Principles of Partnership
  - National Association of County and City Health Officials
  - Public Health Nursing Section of the American Public Health Association
  - Association of State and Territorial Health Officials
  - Nurse-Family Partnership Program

- Quiz
- Case Studies
- Glossary
- Answers to Practice Application
- Resource Tool 46.A: Core Competencies and Skill Levels for Public Health Nursing
- Appendixes
  - Appendix F.1: Essential Elements of Public Health Nursing
  - Appendix F.2: American Public Health Association Definition of Public Health Nursing
  - Appendix F.3: American Nurses Association Scope and Standards of Practice for Public Health Nursing

## OBJECTIVES

*After reading this chapter, the student should be able to do the following:*

1. Define public health, public health system, public health nursing, and local, state, and national roles.
2. Identify trends in public health nursing.
3. Provide examples of public health nursing roles.
4. Differentiate the emerging public health issues that specifically affect public health nursing.
5. Describe the principles of partnerships.
6. Identify educational preparation of public health nurses and competencies necessary to practice.

## KEY TERMS

federal public health agencies, p. 995
incident commander, p. 1006
local public health agencies, p. 995
partnerships, p. 994
public health, p. 994

public health nursing, p. 994
public health programs, p. 994
state public health agency, p. 995
*—See Glossary for definitions*

All of public health is built on partnerships. Public health programs are designed with the goal of improving a population's health status. They go beyond the administration of health care of individuals to a primary focus on the health of populations. Public health programs include community health assessment and interventions based on assessment results, analysis of health statistics, public education, outreach, case management, advocacy, professional education for providers, disease surveillance and investigation, emergency preparedness and response, compliance to regulations for some institutions/agencies and school systems, and follow-up of populations. Examples of follow-up care include communicating with persons with active, untreated tuberculosis, pregnant women who have not kept prenatal visits, and parents of underimmunized children. Public health programs are frequently implemented by the development of partnerships or coalitions with other providers, agencies, and groups in the location being served. Community-Campus Partnerships for Health (CCPH) defines partnerships as "a close mutual cooperation between parties having common interests, responsibilities, privileges and power" (CCPH Board of Directors, 2013). Partnerships are built on trust, mutual respect, and the sharing of power.

Box 46-1 presents principles of partnership within a public health system. Public health nurses are skilled at developing, sustaining, and evaluating community-wide partnerships. Public health nurses are involved in these activities in various ways depending on the public health agency (local, state, or federal) and the identified needs. Public health nurses may be the partnership facilitator or a member of the partnership representing their agency.

Public health is not a branch of medicine; it is an organized community approach designed to prevent disease, promote health, and protect populations. It works across many disciplines and is based on the scientific core of epidemiology (IOM, 1988, 2003). Governmental agencies at the local, state, and federal levels are partners in the public health system that must work together to develop and implement solutions that will improve a community's health. Figure 46-1 represents the diverse and complex network of individuals and agencies making up the public health system (CDC, 2005). This public health system may include public, private and voluntary entities such as the local health department, businesses, and civic associations. Public health nurses partner with interprofessional teams of people within the public health areas (Figure 46-2), in other human services and public safety agencies, and in community-based organizations. The health of communities is

---

### BOX 46-1   Principles of Partnership

Community-Campus Partnerships for Health (CCPH) involved its members and partners in developing the following "principles of good practice" for community partnerships:

1. The Partnership forms to serve a specific purpose and may take on new goals over time.
2. The Partnership agrees upon mission, values, goals, measurable outcomes and processes for accountability.
3. The relationship between partners in the Partnership is characterized by mutual trust, respect, genuineness, and commitment.
4. The Partnership builds upon identified strengths and assets, but also works to address needs and increase capacity of all partners.
5. The Partnership balances power among partners and enables resources among partners to be shared.
6. Partners make clear and open communication an ongoing priority in the Partnership by striving to understand each other's needs and self-interests, and developing a common language.
7. Principles and processes for the Partnership are established with the input and agreement of all partners, especially for decision making and conflict resolution.
8. There is feedback among all stakeholders in the Partnership, with the goal of continuously improving the Partnership and its outcomes.
9. Partners share the benefits of the Partnership's accomplishments.
10. Partnerships can dissolve, and when they do, need to plan a process for closure.
11. Partnerships consider the nature of the environment within which they exist as a principle of their design, evaluation, and sustainability.
12. The Partnership values multiple kinds of knowledge and life experiences.

From Community-Campus Partnerships for Health (CCPH) Board of Directors: Position Statement of Authentic Partnerships. *Community-Campus Partnerships for Health, 2013.* Available at https://ccph.memberclicks.net/principles-of-partnership. Accessed May 13, 2015.

---

a shared responsibility that requires a variety of diverse and often nontraditional partnerships. A critical partnership that shapes public health nursing practice in the United States is the interaction of local, state, and federal public health agencies.

## ROLES OF LOCAL, STATE, AND FEDERAL PUBLIC HEALTH AGENCIES

In the United States, the local-state-federal partnership includes federal agencies, the state, tribal and territorial public health

goal of LA

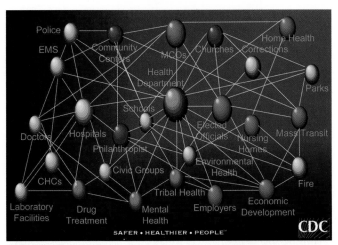

FIG 46-1 Centers for Disease Control and Prevention (CDC): *The National Public Health Performance Standards, An Overview, slide 9,* 2005. Available at http://www.cdc.gov/od/ocphp/nphpsp/Presentationlinks.htm.

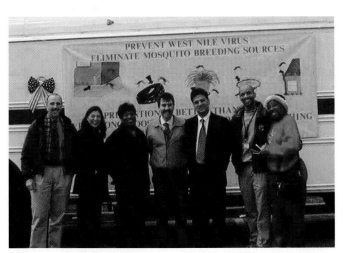

FIG 46-2 Public health nurses work on multidisciplinary teams that include environmental health specialists to increase public awareness about strategies to prevent transmission of West Nile virus. (Courtesy Arlington County Department of Human Services/Public Health Division, Arlington, VA.)

agencies, and the 2500 local public health agencies (ASTHO). The interaction of these agencies is critical to effectively leverage precious resources, both financial and personnel, and to protect and promote the health of populations. Public health nurses employed in all of these agencies work together to identify, develop, and implement interventions that will improve and maintain the nation's health.

Federal public health agencies develop regulations that implement policies formulated by Congress, provide a significant amount of funding to state and territorial health agencies for public health activities, survey the nation's health status and health needs, set practices and standards, provide expertise that

facilitates evidence-based practice, coordinate public health activities that cross state lines, and support health services research (IOM, 2003). The U.S. Department of Health and Human Services (USDHHS) and the Environmental Protection Agency (EPA) are the federal agencies that most influence public health activities at the state and local levels (see Chapter 3). The USDHHS includes the Centers for Disease Control and Prevention (CDC), the Health Resources and Services Administration (HRSA), the Agency for Healthcare Research and Quality (AHRQ), and the Food and Drug Administration (FDA). The USDHHS is the agency that facilitates development of the nation's *Healthy People* objectives (USDHHS, 2010).

In the United States, states hold primary responsibility for protecting the public's health. Each of the states and territories has a single identified official state public health agency that is managed by a state health commissioner. The structure of state public health agencies varies. Some states require that the state health commissioner be a physician. A growing number of states do not limit the position to physicians but rather require specific public health experience. California, Maryland, Iowa, Oregon, Washington, and Michigan are examples of states that focus on public health experience as a requirement for the state health commissioner position. Public health nurses have been appointed to the state health commissioner positions in a number of states: California, Oregon, Washington, and Michigan. The Association of State and Territorial Health Officials defines the state public health agency as the organizational unit of the state health officer, who works in partnership with other government agencies, private enterprises, and voluntary organizations to ensure that services essential to the public's health are provided for all populations. State public health agencies are responsible for monitoring health status and enforcing laws and regulations that protect and improve the public's health. In addition to state funds appropriated by state legislatures, these agencies receive funding from federal agencies for the implementation of public health interventions, such as communicable disease programs, maternal and child health programs, chronic disease prevention programs, and injury prevention programs. The agencies distribute federal and state funds to the local public health agencies to implement programs at the community level, and they provide oversight and consultation for local public health agencies. State health agencies also delegate some public health powers, such as the power to quarantine, to local health officers.

Local public health agencies have responsibilities that vary depending on the locality, but they are the agencies that are responsible for implementing and enforcing local, state, and federal public health codes and ordinances and providing essential public health programs to a community. The goal of the local public health department is to safeguard the public's health and to improve the community's health status. The health department's authority is delegated by the state for specific functions. The duties of local health departments vary depending on the state and local public health codes and ordinances and the responsibilities assigned by the state and local governments. Usually, the local public health department provides for the administration, regulatory oversight, public health, and environmental services for a geographic area. The National Association of County and City Health Officials' (NACCHO) operational definition of a local health department provides a description of the basic public health protections people in any community, regardless of size, can expect from their local health department. The description of local health departments includes the systems, competencies, frameworks, relationships, and resources that enable public health agencies to perform their core functions and essential services. Infrastructure categories encompass human, organizational, informational, legal, policy, and fiscal resources (NACCHO, 2014). A sample of these standards can be found in Box 46-2. As with state health departments, some states require that local health directors be physicians, whereas other states focus on public health experience. For example, public health nurses in Maryland, Kentucky, Illinois, Washington, Wisconsin, and California have held local health director positions.

### BOX 46-2 Local Public Health Agency Functions

The following are selected standards by selected essential public health service performed by local public health agencies:

**Essential Public Health Service 1: Monitor Health Status to Identify Community Health Problems**
- Obtain data that provide information on the community's health.
- Develop relationships with local providers and others in the community who have information on reportable diseases and other conditions of public health interest and facilitate information exchange.
- Conduct or contribute expertise to periodic community health assessments in order to develop a comprehensive picture of the public's health.
- Integrate data with other health assessment and data collection efforts conducted by the public health system.
- Analyze data to identify trends and population health risks.

**Essential Public Health Service 4: Mobilize Community Partnerships to Identify and Solve Health Problems**
- Engage the local public health system in an ongoing, strategic, community-driven, comprehensive planning process to identify, prioritize, and solve public health problems; establish public health goals; and evaluate success in meeting the goals.
- Promote the community's understanding of, and advocacy for, policies and activities that will improve the public's health.
- Develop partnerships to generate interest in and support for improved community health status, including new and emerging public health issues.

**Essential Public Health Service 7: Link People to Needed Personal Health Services and Ensure the Provision of Health Care When Otherwise Unavailable**
- Engage the community to identify gaps in culturally competent, appropriate, and equitable personal health services, including preventive and health promotion services, and develop strategies to close the gaps.
- Support and implement strategies to increase access to care and establish systems of personal health services, including preventive and health promotion services, in partnership with the community.
- Link individuals to available, accessible personal health care providers.

From National Association of County and City Health Officials: *Operational Definition of a Functional Local Health Department*, 2014. Available at http://www.naccho.org. Accessed August 23, 2014.

The majority of local, state, and federal public health agencies will be involved in the following:
- Collecting and analyzing vital statistics (Chapter 12)
- Providing health education and information to the population served (Chapter 16)
- Receiving reports about and investigating and controlling communicable diseases (Chapter 13)
- Planning for and responding to natural and man-made disasters and emergencies (Chapter 23)
- Protecting the environment to reduce the risk to health (Chapter 10)
- Providing some health services to particular populations at risk or with limited access to care (local public health agencies, guided by state and federal policies and goals and community needs) (Chapters 27-38).
- Conducting community assessments to identify community assets and gaps (Chapter 18)
- Identifying public health problems for at-risk and high-risk populations (Chapter 18)
- Partnering with other organizations to develop and implement responses to identified public health concerns (Chapters 17,18, 20, and 25)

Public health nurses practice in partnership with each other at the local, state, and federal levels and with other public health staff, other governmental agencies, and the community to safeguard the public's health and to improve the community's health status. Public health agency staffs include physicians, nutritionists, environmental health professionals, health educators, various laboratory workers, epidemiologists, health planners, and paraprofessional home visitors and outreach workers. Community-based organizations include the American Red Cross, free clinics, Head Start programs, daycare centers, community health centers, hospitals, senior centers, advocacy groups, churches, academic institutions, and businesses. Other governmental agencies include the fire/emergency services department, law enforcement agencies, schools, parks and recreation departments, and elected officials. Changes in local, state, and federal governments affect public health services, and public health nursing has to develop strategies for dealing with these changes. Public health nurses facilitate community assessments to identify emerging public health concerns within communities and, based on results of community assessments, help develop programs to provide needed services.

## HISTORY AND TRENDS IN PUBLIC HEALTH

A person born today can expect to live 30 years longer than a person born in 1900. Medical care accounts for 5 years of that increase. Public health practice, resulting in changes in social policies, community actions, and individual and group behavior, is responsible for the additional 25 years of that increase (USDHHS, 2010). Historically, public health nurses were valued by and important to society and functioned in an autonomous setting. They worked with populations and in settings that were not of interest to other health care disciplines or groups. Much public health service was delivered to the poor and to women and children, who did not have political power or voice. During

*7 priorities 21st century*

the course of the twentieth century, public health responsibilities expanded beyond communicable disease prevention, occupational health, and environmental health programs to include reproductive health, chronic disease prevention, and injury prevention activities. As a result of Medicaid-managed care, many public health agencies were no longer providing personal health care services. Public health agencies began to shift emphasis from a focus on primary health care services to a focus on core public health activities such as the investigation and control of diseases and injuries, community health assessment, community health planning, and involvement in environmental health activities. As the twentieth century came to a close, developments in genetic engineering, the emergence of new communicable diseases, prevention of bioterrorism and violence, and the management and disposal of hazardous waste were emerging as additional public health issues (CDC, 1999). The Institute of Medicine (IOM, 2003) identified the following seven priorities for public health in the twenty-first century:

- Understand and emphasize the broad determinants of health.
- Develop a policy focus on population health.
- Strengthen the public health infrastructure.
- Build partnerships.
- Develop systems of accountability.
- Emphasize evidence-based practice.
- Enhance communication.

Public health activities at the beginning of the twenty-first century were shaped by the September 11, 2001, terrorist attacks of the World Trade Center, the Pentagon, and a field in Pennsylvania, in which thousands were murdered. However, public health nursing activities at the federal, state, and local levels were even more dramatically affected by a series of anthrax exposures that occurred shortly after the terrorist attacks. In addition to anthrax exposures in Florida and New York, one month after the attacks of September 11, thousands of workers at the Brentwood Post Office and the Senate Building in Washington, DC, were exposed to an especially virulent strain of anthrax from a contaminated letter. These exposures required public health nurses to rapidly establish mass medication distribution clinics, while also responding to frightened calls from community members and requests for information from the media. The anthrax exposures alerted policy makers to the weakening public health infrastructure required to respond to bioterrorism events. As society grapples with the upheaval created by the reality of a bioterrorism event, public health nurses learn to leverage existing authority and expertise to ensure that all critical issues threatening the public's health are addressed. The shift of funding to support bioterrorism response efforts has the potential of weakening existing important public health programs. Nurses are well positioned to actively participate in policy decisions that will ensure that a public health infrastructure able to prevent and respond to bioterrorism will be strengthened and maintained within the context of general communicable disease surveillance and response. Public health nurses are facing issues such as unprecedented influenza, tetanus, and childhood vaccine shortages and emerging infections, such as SARS and the influenza A virus (H1N1)

pandemic, that compete with bioterrorism activities for resources. One of these issues presented itself in the fall of 2009 and spring of 2010 when the world grappled with the lack of enough vaccine to prevent the virus from spreading across the world. (See later discussion.)

During the twentieth century, public health nurses were a major force in the nation, achieving immunization rates that accounted for the dramatic decrease in measles. A policy brief issued by All Kids Count (2000, p. 1) stated, "in 1941, more than 894,000 cases of measles were reported in the U.S. In 2013, preliminary data indicated that just 159 cases were reported—a reduction of 99.9%." However, the general public is not well informed about how this immunization activity was accomplished or about its effect on improving health and lowering health care costs (CDC, 2013). Public health nurses' difficulty in explaining the value of ongoing prevention activities can result in a decrease in resources required to ensure adequate surveillance and containment of communicable disease outbreaks. For public health services to receive adequate funding, it is necessary for the public and the government to be aware of the benefits provided to a community by public health nurses. Public health nurses must be at the table, as advocates and experts, when issues are being discussed and decisions are being made to make certain that public health programs are provided for the populations at risk. For example, as the incidence of active tuberculosis (TB) cases decreases, officials will consider shifting funds for TB control to other efforts. Public health nurses at the national, state, and local levels work together to educate officials about the importance of continuing funding for surveillance and containment efforts if the lower TB incidence rates are to be maintained. A recent public health concern is the unaccompanied immigrant children crossing the Mexican borders with no medical records. Efforts are being made to provide TB tests and to start immunizations at clinics near the border before the children migrate to other states and enter school. Public health nurses working in schools are challenged with surveillance of the immigrant students to assure the health and safety of the indigenous students and the population of the community.

The twenty-first century public health nurse is working to develop a public health system able to monitor and detect suspicious trends and respond rapidly to prevent widespread exposure, whether the result of a deliberate or a natural epidemic. A prime example of emerging infectious diseases is severe acute respiratory syndrome (SARS), caused by a virus that brought illness and death to many in 2003. The disease spread quickly from China to other countries, being transported by airline passengers traveling internationally. The novel H1N1 influenza A virus pandemic provides another example of a natural epidemic that required a rapid, intensive, long-term response from public health nurses at the federal, state, and local levels. In 2009, the world was alerted to a new rapidly spreading influenza A virus (H1N1) when Mexico declared a state of emergency and closed schools and congregations in public settings in response to outbreaks of respiratory illness and increased reports of clients with influenza-like illness in several areas of the country (CDC, 2009). The first U.S. human cases of H1N1 were identified in April 2009 in California and Texas. On October 24, 2009, President Barack Obama declared H1N1 a national emergency in the United States. Public health nurses throughout the country shifted their activities to support the response to H1N1. Public health nurses who usually worked in areas such as family health services or school health services rapidly had to shift their focus to the H1N1 response. Family health service clinics and home-visiting services were either cancelled or scaled back to free up public health nurse time to respond to the emerging pandemic. More recent examples of diseases that have been monitored closely by public health nurses and officials are Middle Eastern Respiratory Syndrome (MERS) and Ebola virus. In the spring of 2014, the United States confirmed its first case of MERS-CoV, a corona virus, first reported in Saudi Arabia in 2012 (CDC, 2014a). The Ebola virus epidemic in African countries is being watched carefully by the public health officials and preventive measures are being taken to protect populations (see Chapter 13 for more on the Ebola virus outbreak in the United States).

## SCOPE, STANDARDS, AND ROLES OF PUBLIC HEALTH NURSING

In 1920 C. E. A. Winslow defined public health as "the science and art of preventing disease, prolonging life and promoting health and efficiency through organized community effort" (Turnock, 2010, p. 10). This definition is still used in public health textbooks because it focuses on the relationship between social conditions and health across all levels of society. The IOM defines public health practice as "what we as a society do collectively to assure the conditions in which people can be healthy" (IOM, 2003, p. 28). Reflecting these definitions, the Public Health Nursing Section of the American Public Health Association defined public health nursing as "the practice of promoting and protecting the health of populations using knowledge from nursing, social and public health sciences" (APHA, 2013, p. 1). The American Nurses Association (ANA) adds that public health nursing is a population-focused practice that works to promote health and prevent disease for the entire population. Public health nursing is a specialty practice of nursing defined by scope of practice and not by practice setting (APHA, 2013).

Additional knowledge, skills, and aptitudes are necessary for a nurse to go beyond focusing on the health needs of the individual to focusing on the health needs of populations (see Chapters 1 and 18). This additional knowledge distinguishes the public health nurse from other nurses who are practicing in the community setting. Public health nursing practices arise from knowledge gained from the physical and social sciences, psychological and spiritual fields, environmental areas, political arena, epidemiology, economics, community organization, public health ethics, community-based participatory research, and global health. The Quad Council of Public Health Nursing Organizations identified eight principles (Box 46-3) that distinguish the public health nursing specialty from other nursing specialties. Although other nurses may practice some or all of these eight principles, they are not incorporated as a core

---

**BOX 46-3   Tenets of Public Health Nursing**

The following eight tenets of public health nursing distinguish public health nursing from other nursing specialties, and are included in the *Scope and Standards of Public Health Nursing Practice* of the American Nurses Association (2013).

1. Population-based assessment, policy development, and assurance processes are systematic and comprehensive.
2. All processes must include partnering with representatives of the people.
3. Primary prevention is given priority.
4. Intervention strategies are selected to create healthy environmental, social, and economic conditions in which people can thrive.
5. Public health nursing practice includes an obligation to reach out to all who might benefit from an intervention or service.
6. The dominant concern and obligation is for the greater good of all the people or the population as a whole.
7. Stewardship and allocation of available resources supports the maximum population health benefit gain.
8. The health of the people is most effectively promoted and protected through collaboration with members of other professions and organizations.

From American Public Health Association, Public Health Nursing Section: *The Definition and Practice of Public Health Nursing: A Statement of Public Health Nursing Section.* Washington, DC, 2013, American Public Health Association.

---

foundation of the practice in other specialties. Public health nurses always adhere to all eight principles of public health nursing (APHA, 2013).

A variety of settings and a diversity of perspectives are available to nurses interested in developing a career in public health nursing. Public health nurses working at the federal, state, and local levels integrate community involvement and knowledge about the entire population with clinical understandings of the health and illness experiences of individuals and families in the population. They translate and articulate the health and illness needs of diverse, often vulnerable individuals and families in the population to planners and policy makers. As advocates, public health nurses help members of the community voice their problems and aspirations. Public health nurses are knowledgeable about multiple evidence-based strategies for intervention, from those applicable to the entire population, to those for the family and the individual. Public health nurses are directly engaged in the interprofessional activities of the core public health functions of assessment, assurance, and policy development. In any setting, the role of public health nurses focuses on the prevention of illness, injury, or disability, as well as the promotion and maintenance of the health of populations (APHA, 2013).

Public health nurses deliver services within the framework of ever-constricting resources coupled with emerging and complex public health issues. This requires the efficient, equitable, and evidence-based use of resources. The *Guide to Community Preventive Services* is a resource used by public health nurses to help determine which interventions to use (CDC, 2014b). This guide provides recommendations about the effectiveness of selected health promotion/disease prevention guidelines. Box 46-4 presents selected Task Group recommendations. The *National Public Health Performance Standards Program*

## BOX 46-4  How To Use Evidence to Determine Interventions

Selected Task Force on Community Preventive Services Recommendations: Vaccine-Preventable Diseases

| Recommendation | Interventions |
|---|---|
| **Enhancing Access to Vaccination Services** | |
| Recommended (strong evidence) | Expanding access in medical offices or public health clinics |
| Recommended (strong evidence) | Reducing out-of-pocket expenses |
| Recommended (sufficient evidence) | Vaccination programs in WIC settings |
| Recommended (sufficient evidence) | Home visits |
| Recommended (sufficient evidence) | Vaccination programs in schools |
| Insufficient evidence to determine effectiveness | Vaccination in childcare centers |
| **Increasing Community Demand for Vaccines** | |
| Recommended (strong evidence) | Client reminder/recall systems |
| Recommended (strong evidence) | Multicomponent interventions that include education |
| Recommended (sufficient evidence) | Vaccination requirements for childcare, school, and college attendance |
| Insufficient evidence to determine effectiveness | Clinic-based education only |
| Insufficient evidence to determine effectiveness | Client or family incentives |
| Insufficient evidence to determine effectiveness | Client-held medical records |
| Insufficient evidence to determine effectiveness | Community-wide education only |

From Centers for Disease Control and Prevention: *The Guide to Community Preventive Services*, 2014b. Available at http://www.thecommunityguide.org/index.html. Accessed May 24, 2014.

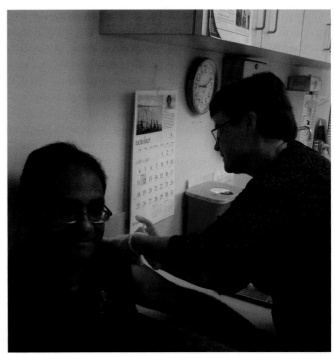

**FIG 46-3** Public health nurses protect the population's health by providing immunizations. (Courtesy Arlington County Department of Human Services/Public Health Division, Arlington, VA.)

(CDC, 2015), a federal, state, and local partnership, has developed evaluation instruments that can be used to collect and analyze data on the programs provided through state and local public health systems. The instruments link with the 10 essential services of public health that define the core functions of public health (see Chapter 1) and help public health nurses at state and local health departments identify which essential services are met and which need additional resources.

Public health nurses make a significant difference in improving the health of a community by monitoring and assessing critical health status indicators such as immunization levels (Figure 46-3), infant mortality rates, and communicable diseases. On the basis of their assessment and in partnership with the community, public health nurses advocate for evidence-based interventions to respond to negative health status indicators. For example, a community assessment may indicate that a significant percentage of children have hemoglobin levels below 11 mg/dL. The public health nurse will know that additional information such as blood lead levels will be needed in order to implement an appropriate intervention. Public health accreditation is being encouraged at the federal level by the

Public Health Accreditation Board (PHAB, 2014), for local and state health departments to meet specific standards of practice. Community health assessments and community health improvement plans are required components for each local health department. Community partnerships are imperative for the community health assessment and plan to be a meaningful and effective tool. Public health nurses are knowledgeable about resources and agencies within the community that can be partners in the accreditation process. Public health nurses can lead the accreditation process in their communities.

Public health's shift from being the primary care provider of last resort to developing partnerships to meet the health promotion and disease prevention needs of populations has raised concerns about available health care for the uninsured and underinsured. The public health nurses' role in this ongoing shift in health care delivery is still being developed for many agencies. Public health nurses retain responsibility for assuring that all populations have access to affordable, quality health care services. They accomplish this by advocating for legislation that promotes universal health care, such as increased funding for community health centers and expansion of Medicaid eligibility criteria; and by forming partnerships with hospitals, free clinics, and other organizations to guarantee health care for all populations in the community. Case management at the community level is a renewed effort in public health nursing. Through case management activities, public health nurses link populations with needed health care providers, as well as social services providers (see Chapter 22).

Uninsured individuals seek services on a sliding payment scale from such sources as university or public hospital clinics, neighborhood health centers, nurse-managed clinics, or community-based free clinics. Public health nurses serve as a bridge between these populations and the resource needs for this at-risk group by approaching health care providers on behalf of individuals seeking medical/health services and by keeping the needs of this population on the political agenda. Frequently, low-income populations or populations with multiple chronic illnesses lack the knowledge and skills to negotiate the complex health care system. This population needs education and training in identifying their problems, approaches to self-care, and illness prevention strategies and lifestyle choices that will have an effect on their health. The public health nurse understands barriers these populations confront, such as transportation issues, language barriers, cultural differences, and difficulty understanding and following health care provider instructions.

Although vulnerable populations have always benefited from public health nursing services, the populations that are most acutely in need of public health nursing services have changed dramatically over the last couple of decades. Of particular concern are the number of young women and their partners who are substance abusers and have risky behaviors that put their pregnancy or children at high risk of injury or abuse. Public health nurses at the federal, state, and local levels have developed innovative, collaborative approaches to prepare staff to work effectively with this population. Public health nurses can cultivate community partnerships to help address the needs of this population.

## EVIDENCE-BASED PRACTICE

The Nurse-Family Partnership home visitation program provides rigorously defined nurse home visits to first-time low-income mothers. It is an evidence-based public health program that has been rigorously evaluated in three randomized, controlled trials. Results demonstrated improvements in birth outcomes, prenatal health, child development, school readiness, and academic achievement, and reductions in child abuse and neglect and early childhood injuries. A recent study examined the effects of these nurse home visits on 594 urban mothers' birth spacing, partner relationships, and government spending. The study design was a randomized, controlled trial.

Results demonstrated that mothers receiving the nurse home visits, compared with the control group, experienced less role impairment from drug and alcohol use (0.0% vs 2.5%, $P = .04$) and longer partner relationships (59.58 vs 52.67 months, $P = .02$). It also demonstrated that over the 12-year study period, government spent less per year on Medicaid, food stamps, and Aid to Families with Dependent Children and Temporary Assistance for Needy Families for mothers receiving nurse home visits than the control group ($8772 vs. $9797, $P = .02$).

### Nurse Use
On March 23, 2010, President Obama signed into law health care reform legislation that included $1.5 billion in funding for evidence-based home visitation to states over 5 years. Nurses can change outcomes for first-time low-income mothers by rigorously implementing the Nurse-Family Partnership model.

From Olds DL, Kitzman HJ, Cole RE, et al: Enduring effects of prenatal and infancy home visiting by nurses on maternal life course and government spending: Follow-up of a randomized trial among children at age 12 years., *Arch Pediatr Adolesc Med* 164(5):419–424, 2010.

## ISSUES AND TRENDS IN PUBLIC HEALTH NURSING

The discovery and development of antibiotics in the 1940s, coupled with immunization programs and improvements in sanitation, contributed to the decrease in infectious disease–related morbidity and mortality during the twentieth century (CDC, 1999). Twenty-first century issues facing public health nursing include increasing rates of drug resistance to community-acquired pathogens, societal issues such as health reform legislation, access to affordable housing, racial and ethnic disparities in health outcomes, behaviorally influenced issues (such as chronic diseases, violence in society, and substance abuse), emerging infections (such as SARS and H1N1 influenza), and unequal access to health care. Community assessments need to reflect the factors that affect the populations the public health nurse serves.

For example, a major twenty-first century public health challenge is emerging infections resulting from drug-resistant organisms. The widespread, often inappropriate, use of antimicrobial drugs has resulted in loss of effectiveness for some community-acquired infections such as gonorrhea, pneumococcal infections, and tuberculosis and in increasing rates of drug resistance in community-acquired pathogens such as *Streptococcus pneumoniae*, *Escherichia coli*, and *Salmonella* spp. The rise in antimicrobial resistance in community and health care settings is causing alarm among public health leaders, nurses, and infectious disease experts. "Staph" infections caused by methicillin-resistant *Staphylococcus aureus* (MRSA) have received increasing attention in recent years. MRSA is a type of staph bacteria that has developed resistance to certain antibiotics, including methicillin and other more common antibiotics such as oxacillin, penicillin, and amoxicillin (CDC, 2010a). Public health nurses are building partnerships, providing education, and making surveillance a top priority to prevent the spread of antimicrobial-resistant infections. Public health nurses can influence this trend by objecting to inappropriate use of antibiotics by providers and educating individuals, families, health care providers, elected officials, and the community about the dangers of misuse and overuse of antibiotics (CDC, 2010b).

Societal issues such as welfare and health insurance reform will influence a population's ability to obtain preventive health services either because of limited health care providers accepting government-sponsored health care coverage or because the low-wage jobs they take do not allow time off for health care. When child care is an issue for the welfare mother returning to work, consideration must be given to effects on the individual, family, community, and population. Public health nurses assess the problem and determine what is wrong with a system that forces parents to go to work so they can be removed from welfare roles but that does not provide for child care. The question to be answered by a nurse is "What will it take to change the system?"

Partnerships and collaboration among groups are much more powerful in making change than the individual client and public health nurse working alone. As another example, the depressed, nonfunctional mother in need of counseling is a significant public health concern because the mother's, children's, and family's needs are not being met. Frequently, the problem may not be obvious to the health professional who sees this woman for the first time. Public health nurses have special preparation to help them both identify the individual's problem and look at its effects on the broader community. In this example, the children may grow to be adults with mental health problems, and the community mental health services will need to be able to handle the increase in this population. Children may become violent adults, resulting in a need for more correctional facilities. Mothers may need additional mental health services. Children may be absent from school often and may not be able to contribute to society. They may be nonproductive in the workplace because absence from school leads to lack of skills. One problem of the single individual can place great burdens on the community.

The IOM (2002) reported that disparities in health care treatment accounted for some of the gaps in health outcomes between racial and ethnic groups. This report found that minorities received lower-quality health care than white people, regardless of insurance status, income, and severity of the condition. Public health nurses work as case managers and at the policy level to promote equal access to health care, including health literature and spoken services that reflect the community in which the services are being delivered (see Chapter 8). The public health nurse working directly as a case manager or in a clinic setting or in the community can promote ethnicity-friendly services by partnering with other community agencies such as interpreter services. Identifying and alerting the community to gaps in available services can facilitate equal access to health care. For example, some communities may appear to have an adequate number of pediatricians to meet the community's needs. However, a community assessment may reveal that the community is home to a high number of children who rely on Medicaid as payment for services, or to families whose primary language is not English. Matching this information with the pediatrician population may reveal that none of the pediatricians accept Medicaid as payment for services, or they all deliver services in English only.

Population-focused public health nursing requires that public health nurses consider social determinants of health including social and environmental factors that influence the health of communities, families, and individuals. For example, a public health nurse providing communicable disease control services for the homeless population or the refugee population will also work for policies that ensure affordable housing. A public health nurse providing case management services for a new teen mother will include ensuring that the mother returns to school; has safe, affordable housing; and has safe child care available while she attends school. The Nurse-Family Partnership Program (2010) is an example of a model program that considers the social determinants of health.

## MODELS OF PUBLIC HEALTH NURSING PRACTICE

In response to the IOM (1988) report that described public health in a state of disarray and the need for all federal public

health agencies to work to identify core public health functions, public health nurses have worked to develop models of practice that will operationalize the role of public health nursing. This section presents examples of models developed by local and state departments of health. These models also serve as examples of the important work that can be accomplished by local, state, and federal partnerships.

In Virginia, a statewide committee led an examination of the role of public health nursing in the context of increasing public expectation of accountability and the shift of public health nursing emphasis from clinical services to population-focused services. Their work resulted in a document that identifies public health nursing roles within the framework of the core public health functions (see Chapter 1). The work identifies the educational needs of staff that would prepare them to function effectively in the changing public health arena. Essential elements of the role were identified. These essential elements are being implemented through multiprofessional public health teams. The document includes a matrix that demonstrates the relationship of the public health functions defined by the essential elements to the public health nursing roles at the local level, as well as the role of the state in this responsibility (see Appendix F.1).

The Public Health Nursing Section of the Minnesota Department of Health (2001) developed a framework called the Intervention Wheel that defines public health nursing interventions by level of practice (see Chapter 9). Public health nurses deliver services within a framework of core interventions. The three levels of public health nursing practice are systems, community, and individual/family. The model identifies 17 population-based public health interventions delivered by public health nurses. It also identifies population-based interventions as those that do the following:

- Focus on entire populations possessing similar health concerns or characteristics
- Are guided by an assessment of health status
- Consider the broad determinants of health, such as housing, income, education, cultural values, and community capacity
- Consider all levels of prevention, with primary prevention a priority
- Consider all levels of practice (community, system, and individual/family) (see Appendix F.1)

The public health nursing practice model of Los Angeles County Department of Health describes public health nursing practice as population based. It synthesizes the 10 essential services of public health practice, principles identified by the Quad Council of Public Health Nursing Organizations and the Minnesota Department of Health, PHN Section and tenets of the ANA *Scope and Standards of Public Health Nursing Practice.* It includes the following criteria:

- Focuses on entire populations possessing similar health concerns or characteristics
- Relies upon an assessment of population health status
- Considers the broad determinants of health
- Considers all levels of prevention, with a preference for primary prevention
- Considers all levels of practice: individual/family-focused practice, community-focused practice, and systems-focused practice
- Reaches out to all who might benefit, not focusing on just those who present themselves
- Demonstrates a dominant concern for the greater good of all the people (the interest of the whole taking priority over the best interest of the individual or group)
- Creates healthy environmental, social, and economic conditions in which people can thrive (Los Angeles County Department of Public Health/Public Health Nursing, 2007)

## EDUCATION AND KNOWLEDGE REQUIREMENTS FOR PUBLIC HEALTH NURSES

The Council on Linkages Between Academia and Public Health Practice (2014) examined a decade of work to identify a list of core public health competencies that represent a set of skills, knowledge, and attitudes necessary for the broad practice of public health. Initially adopted in 2001, the core competencies were revised and adopted unanimously by the Council in June 2009. The accomplishments of the Council on Linkages not only include developing the Core Competencies for Public Health Professionals to guide curriculum and workforce development, but also include promoting public health systems research to increase understanding of and improve public health infrastructure as well as focusing the field on evidence-based strategies to improve worker recruitment and retention and combat emerging worker shortages. The Council is located in Washington, DC, and is staffed by the Public Health Foundation. A list of member organizations is located at http://www.phf.org/link/membership.htm.

The competencies are built around the Essential Public Health Services. This is the only consensus set of core competencies in public health that apply to all practicing public health professionals. They capture the cross-cutting competencies necessary for all disciplines that work in public health, including public health nurses, physicians, environmental health specialists, health educators, and epidemiologists. The competencies are applied to three tiers. A detailed list of core competencies by job category and skill level is available. The core public health competencies have been applied to public health nursing (see the web links on the Evolve website for both items).

> ## LINKING CONTENT TO PRACTICE
>
> The core public health competencies are divided into the following eight domains. The content related to the domains can be found in the chapters noted.
> 1. Analytic assessment skills: Chapters 1, 9, 15, 17, 18, and 27 to 38
> 2. Basic public health sciences' skills: Chapters 3, 6, 8, 10, 12 to 14, 19, 23 to 26
> 3. Cultural competency skills: Chapters 4 and 7
> 4. Communication skills: Chapters 16 and 22
> 5. Community dimensions of practice skills: Chapters 18, 20, 21, and 41 to 45
> 6. Financial planning and management skills: Chapter 5
> 7. Leadership and systems thinking skills: Chapter 40
> 8. Policy development/program planning skills: Chapters 8 and 25

In addition to being skilled in the areas of epidemiology, analytic assessment skills, environmental health, health services administration, cultural sensitivity, and social and behavioral science, the twenty-first century public health nurse must be competent in areas such as community mobilization, risk communication, genomics, informatics, community-based participatory research, policy and law, global health, and public health ethics (ANA, 2007).

Many of these core public health competencies are provided by public health nurses who have learned these skills in the workplace while gaining knowledge through years of practice. Rapid changes in public health are providing a challenge to public health nurses in that there is neither the time nor the staff to provide the on-the-job training needed to learn and upgrade skills and knowledge of staff. Nurses with baccalaureate or master's preparation are needed to provide a strong public health system (see Chapter 1). In 2007 and again in 2013 the ANA revised the 1999 *Scope and Standards of Public Health Nursing Practice* to reflect the increasing complexity and rapid changes faced by public health nurses. The revised standards include those that are expected of all baccalaureate degree nurses, the entry level into public health nursing practice, and the standards of the advanced practice public health nurse prepared at the master's level (APHA, 2013).

## NATIONAL HEALTH OBJECTIVES

Since 1979 the U.S. Surgeon General has worked with local, state, and federal agencies; the private sector; and the U.S. population to develop objectives for preventing disease and promoting health for the nation. These objectives are revisited every 10 years. In 2009 proposed *Healthy People 2020* objectives were released for public comment (see the *Healthy People 2020* box).

 **HEALTHY PEOPLE 2020**

### *Selected National Health Objectives Related to the Public Health Infrastructure*

- PHI-1: Increase the proportion of federal, tribal, state, and local public health agencies that incorporate core competencies for public health professionals into job descriptions and performance evaluations.
- PHI-4: Increase the proportion of 4-year colleges and universities that offer public health or related majors and/or minors.
- PHI-13: Increase the proportion of tribal, state, and local public health agencies that provide or assure comprehensive epidemiology services to support essential public health services.
- PHI-14: Increase the proportion of state and local public health jurisdictions that conduct performance assessment and improvement activities in the public health system using national standards.
- PHI-15: Increase the proportion of tribal, state, and local public health agencies that have implemented a health improvement plan and increase the proportion of local health jurisdictions that have implemented a health improvement plan linked with their state plan.

From U.S. Department of Health and Human Services: *Healthy People 2020: National Health Promotion and Disease Prevention Objectives,* 2010. Available at http://www.healthypeople .gov/hp2020/objectives/TopicAreas.aspx. Accessed May 13, 2015.

State health departments help set local goals using the *Healthy People 2020* objectives as a framework. Knowing that public health departments do not have the resources to accomplish these goals independently, collaboration is essential to quality nursing practice and is encouraged at the local level with existing groups. New partnerships are developed related to specific goals. Communities develop coalitions to address selected objectives, based on community needs, to include all of the local community stakeholders such as social services, mental health, education, recreation, government, and businesses. Membership varies from community to community depending on that community's formal and informal structure. The groups join the coalition for a variety of reasons. For example, businesses see the value of developing a productive workforce that will be of importance to them and the community in the future.

Public health nurses help clients identify unhealthy behaviors and then help them develop strategies to improve their health. Some of the behaviors addressed by public health nurses are tobacco use, physical activity, and obesity, all of which affect quality and years of healthy life. Public health nurses also organize the community to conduct community health assessments to identify where health disparities exist and to target interventions to address those disparities. For example, community health assessments may disclose that certain populations are at higher risk for asthma, diabetes, low immunization rates, high cigarette smoking behavior, or exposure to environmental hazards.

Some *Healthy People 2020* communicable disease areas of focus are vaccine-preventable infectious diseases, emerging antimicrobial resistance, tuberculosis infection and disease, and levels of human immunodeficiency virus (HIV), acquired immunodeficiency syndrome (AIDS), and sexually transmitted infections. To help clients reduce their risk of acquiring a communicable disease, public health nurses provide clients with instructions on the use of barrier methods of contraception and information on the hazards of multiple sexual partners and street drug use. Obtaining a complete sexual history on all clients coming to the health department for services takes special skills but is essential to determine the behaviors that have brought the client to the local health department. Education of young persons before they become sexually active has helped reduce the incidence of some sexually transmitted diseases in this population.

## FUNCTIONS OF PUBLIC HEALTH NURSES

Public health nurses have many functions depending on the needs and resources of an area (Figure 46-4). Advocate is one of the many roles of the public health nurse. As an advocate, the public health nurse collects, monitors, and analyzes data and works with the client to identify and prioritize needed services, whether the client is an individual, a family, a community, or a population. The public health nurse and the client then develop the most effective plan and approach to take, and the nurse helps the client implement the plan so that the client can become more independent in making decisions and obtaining the services needed. At the community and population levels, public health nurses promote healthy behaviors, safe water and air, and sanitation. They advocate for healthy policies at the local, state, and federal levels that will develop healthy communities (see Chapter 8).

Legislation is a public health tool used to ensure the health of populations. Implemented with extreme concern for the balance between individual rights and community rights, public policy is a critical function for the public health nurse. Examples of legislation that has successfully improved the health of populations are required immunizations for school entry, seat belt use, smoke-free environments, and bicycle and motorcycle helmet use.

Case management is a major role for public health nurses (see Chapter 22). The 2010 health reform legislation will increase the importance of the case management role as newly insured clients attempt to link with health care providers and the Nurse-Family Partnership program (2010) is expanded.

# Public Health Nursing Roles

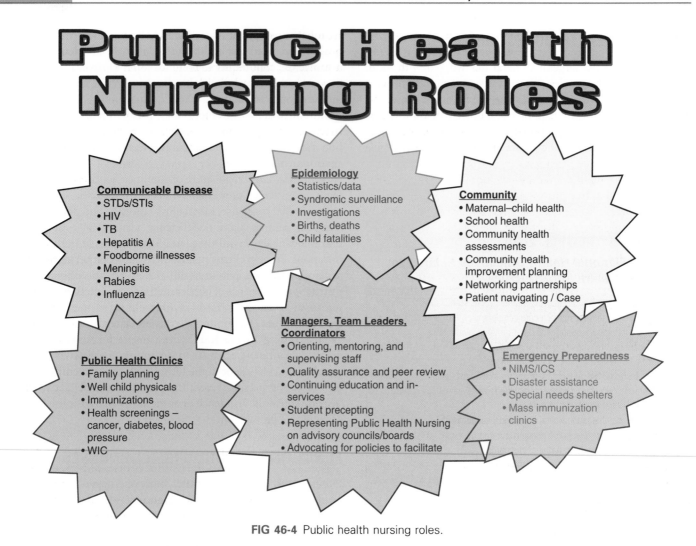

**Communicable Disease**
- STDs/STIs
- HIV
- TB
- Hepatitis A
- Foodborne illnesses
- Meningitis
- Rabies
- Influenza

**Epidemiology**
- Statistics/data
- Syndromic surveillance
- Investigations
- Births, deaths
- Child fatalities

**Community**
- Maternal–child health
- School health
- Community health assessments
- Community health improvement planning
- Networking partnerships
- Patient navigating / Case

**Public Health Clinics**
- Family planning
- Well child physicals
- Immunizations
- Health screenings – cancer, diabetes, blood pressure
- WIC

**Managers, Team Leaders, Coordinators**
- Orienting, mentoring, and supervising staff
- Quality assurance and peer review
- Continuing education and in-services
- Student precepting
- Representing Public Health Nursing on advisory councils/boards
- Advocating for policies to facilitate

**Emergency Preparedness**
- NIMS/ICS
- Disaster assistance
- Special needs shelters
- Mass immunization clinics

**FIG 46-4** Public health nursing roles.

Public health nurses use the nursing process of assessing, planning, implementing, and evaluating outcomes to meet clients' needs. Clear and complex communications are frequently an important component of case management. Other health and social agency providers may not be familiar with the home and community living conditions that are known to the public health nurse. It is the nurse who sees the living conditions and who can tell the story for the client or assist the individual, family, or community with the telling of their story. Case managers assist clients in identifying the services they need the most at the least cost. They also assist communities and populations in identifying and linking with services that will increase the overall population health status.

Public health nurses are a major referral resource. They maintain current information about health and social services available within the community. They know what resources will be acceptable to the client within the social and cultural norms for that group. The nurse educates clients to enable them to use the resources and to learn self-care. Nurses refer to other services in the area, and other services refer to the public health nurse for care or follow-up. For example, the mother and new baby may be referred to the public health nurse for postnatal care with postpartum home visit follow-up.

Assessment of literacy is a large part of public health nursing. Many individuals are limited in their ability to read, write, and communicate clearly. The public health nurse has to be culturally sensitive and aware of the specific areas of unique problems of clients, such as financial limitations that may in turn limit educational opportunities. Frequently, when a person goes to a physician's office, clinic, or hospital, they are clean and neatly dressed. The assumption is made that when they nod at the health care provider it means that they understand what has been said. This is frequently not the case, but the client is embarrassed to admit that he or she does not understand what has been said. Being illiterate does not mean a person is mentally slow. It is important for the public health nurse to follow up on the many contacts the individual or family has with medical, social, and legal services to clarify what is understood and to find an answer to the questions that have not been asked by the client or answered by the services.

The public health nurse is an educator, teaching to the level of the client so that information received is information that can be used. Patience and repetitions over time are necessary to develop trust and to enable the client to use the relationship with the nurse for more information. As educator, the public health nurse identifies community needs (e.g., playground safety, hand hygiene, pedestrian safety, safe-sex practices) and develops and implements educational activities aimed at changing behaviors over time.

Public health nurses are direct primary caregivers in many situations, both in the clinic and in the community. Where the public health nurse provides primary care is determined by community assessment and is usually in response to an identified gap to which the private sector is unable to respond, coupled with an assessment of the impact of the gap in services on the health of the population. Examples include prenatal services for uninsured women, free or low-cost immunization services for targeted populations, directly observed therapy for clients with active tuberculosis, and treatment for sexually transmitted infections.

Public health nurses ensure that direct care services are available in the community for at-risk populations by working with the community to develop programs that will meet the needs of those populations. Currently, no system of outreach service in the medical models of care addresses the multiple needs of high-risk populations. High-risk populations frequently do not understand the medical, social, educational, or judicial system and the professional languages, codes of behavior, or expected outcomes of these services. Clients need a case manager, a health educator, an advocate, and a role model to enable them to benefit from these services and to teach them how to avoid complex and expensive problems in the future. The local public health nurse fills these roles and many more for this population. These are examples of the difficult clinical issues that public health nurses face in making ethical and professional decisions.

The public health nurse's role is unique and essential in many situations. Access to homes gives the nurse information that usually cannot be gathered in the hospital or clinic setting. The public health nurse learns to ask intimate questions creatively and to seek information that will facilitate case management and provide the clinical and social care needed, including other community resources. Careful attention must be paid to privacy and confidentiality in delivering public health nursing services. The credibility of the nurse and the agency depends on the professional handling of the public health information of each and every staff member.

When a disaster (see Chapter 23) occurs, public health nurses at the local, state, and federal levels have multiple roles in assessing, planning, implementing, and evaluating needs and resources for the different populations being served. Whether the disaster is local or national, small or large, natural or manmade, public health nurses are skilled professionals essential to the team. As a health care facility, the local public health department has a disaster plan, as well as a role in the local, regional, and state disaster plans. Public health nurses' roles include providing education that will prepare communities to cope with disasters and professional triage for local shelters, conducting enhanced communicable disease surveillance, planning and implementing mass dispensing sites, working with environmental health specialists to ensure safe food and water for disaster victims and emergency workers, and serving on the local emergency planning committee. Their presence may be

required in other regions of the state or country to provide official public health nursing duties in a time of crisis, such as a hurricane, that requires a lengthy period of recovery. Each governmental jurisdiction has an emergency plan. The public health agency is expected to provide planning and staffing during a disaster. These local emergency preparedness plans may be multigovernmental, which requires coordination between communities. Public health nurses have a critical role in ensuring that emergency preparedness plans address the special needs of vulnerable populations such as those with disabilities, or low-income populations who lack the resources to maintain the recommended 3- to 5-day supply of food and medication.

Essential and unique roles for public health nurses exist in the area of communicable disease control. Public health nursing skills are necessary for education, prevention, surveillance, and outbreak investigation. Public health nurses can find infected individuals; notify contacts; refer; administer treatments; educate the individual, family, community, professionals, and populations; act as advocates; and in general be state-of-the-art resources to reduce the rate of communicable disease in the community (see Chapters 13, 14, and 24). The communicable disease role is one of the most important roles for public health nursing during disasters. During the terrorist attacks on September 11, 2001, the SARS outbreak, and the novel H1N1 pandemic, public health nurses at the federal, state, and local levels immediately implemented active enhanced surveillance activities and prepared for implementation of mass dispensing sites. Information about communicable diseases seen at the local level was passed on to the state public health agency and finally to the CDC. At each step, the data were analyzed for evidence of unusual disease trends.

When October 2001 alerts from the CDC began presenting information about a photo editor in Florida who had been hospitalized with inhalation anthrax, public health nurses and hospital infection control practitioners throughout the nation increased activity. Public health response to disasters requires that resources be redirected temporarily from other programs while maintaining programs that will prevent additional outbreaks. Therefore, public health nurses not normally involved in communicable disease activities can be shifted to this function. The exposures resulting from the anthrax-tainted letters presented unprecedented public health challenges. The Washington, DC, anthrax exposures resulted in thousands of possible work-related exposures, five cases of inhalation anthrax in the region, and two deaths over a period of months. Public health at the federal, state, and local levels was looked to for coordinated leadership and answers to a situation in which experience was limited and answers were uncertain.

With the first Ebola virus outbreak in the United States in Dallas, public health workers were case finding, that is, identifying contacts with the person presenting with Ebola virus. After contacts were identified, they were visited to assess them for symptoms of Ebola virus. In addition, public health workers were going door to door to see if anyone had been exposed to the virus through the identified contacts of the patient. The purpose in case finding is to be able to treat all who have symptoms to reduce the risk of a massive outbreak of a disease (CDC, 2014c).

Although communicable disease control is a core public health service, the role of the public health nurse as incident commander in a widespread public health emergency is a new role (see Figure 46-5). Issues such as how to conduct mass treatment in response to a bioterrorism event, which jurisdiction is in charge, how to communicate uncertain information to the public, and who should take antibiotics for how long had to be rapidly resolved across jurisdictional and agency lines. The anthrax exposures are typical of the nature of public health emergencies. They unfold as the communicable disease moves through communities.

Public health nurses are essential partners in disaster drills. In Virginia, an electrical company has a nuclear plant that requires annual multijurisdictional disaster drills. These disaster planning and practice sessions are an opportunity for local public health nurses to get to know other agencies' representatives and to let them know what public health nursing can offer. Because public health nurses are out in the communities and have assessment skills, they are essential in evaluating how the disaster was handled and making suggestions about how future events might be managed. To be most effective as disaster responders, public health nurses have to be a part of the team *before* an emergency. Knowing what type of disaster is likely to occur in a community is essential for planning. Types of disasters vary from place to place, but there is a history of past events and how they were handled, as well as resources and training from regional, state, and federal agencies. Public health nurses can help educate the public about the individual responsibilities

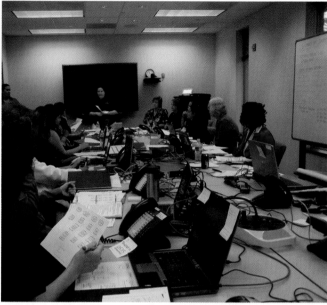

FIG 46-5 Public health nurses respond to community-wide disease outbreaks within the framework of the incident command structure. (Courtesy Arlington County Department of Human Services/Public Health Division, Arlington, VA.)

and preparations that can be in place both for the person and for the community. The Levels of Prevention box presents additional examples of public health nurses' functions by level of prevention. Public health nurses at the local, state, and federal levels work in partnership to accomplish each function.

---

### 📖 LEVELS OF PREVENTION

*Public Health Nursing*

**Primary Prevention**
- Partnering with the community to conduct a community health assessment to identify community assets and gaps
- Partnering with the community to develop primary prevention programs in response to identified gaps
- Providing information about safe-sex practices
- Providing individual and community-based education to increase knowledge and modify perceptions of risks
- Educating daycare centers and families about the dangers of lead-based paint
- Educating daycare centers, schools, and the general community about the importance of hand hygiene to prevent transmission of communicable diseases
- Inspecting daycare centers, nursing homes, and hospitals to ensure client safety and quality of care
- Providing immunizations
- Advocating for issues such as mandatory seat belt legislation, smoke-free environments, and universal access to health care
- Providing no-charge infant car seats accompanied by classes in use of safety seats
- Identifying environmental hazards such as housing quality, playground safety, pedestrian safety, and product safety hazards, and working with the community and policy makers to mitigate the identified hazards

- Developing social networking interventions to modify community norms related to sexual risk behaviors, condom use, and abstinence
- Larvaciding against mosquitoes in areas frequented by populations 55 years of age and over
- Working with communities to develop citizen emergency preparedness plans

**Secondary Prevention**
- Identifying and treating clients in a sexually transmitted disease clinic
- Identifying and treating clients with TB infection and disease in a TB clinic
- Providing directly observed therapy (DOT) for clients with active TB
- Conducting lead screening activities for children
- Conducting contacting/tracing for individuals exposed to a client with an active case of TB or a sexually transmitted disease
- Conducting ongoing disease surveillance for communicable diseases and implementing control measures when an outbreak is identified
- Implementing screening programs for genetic disorders/metabolic deficiencies in newborns; breast, cervical, and testicular cancer; diabetes; hypertension; and sensory impairments in children, and ensuring follow-up services for clients with positive results
- Conducting syndromic surveillance to ensure early identification of victims of an influenza epidemic or bioterrorism event
- Providing low-cost antibiotics for treatment of Lyme disease

## LEVELS OF PREVENTION—cont'd

### Public Health Nursing

- Conducting enhanced surveillance for novel influenza virus infection among travelers with severe unexplained respiratory illness returning from affected countries
- Establishing mass dispensing clinics for antibiotic distribution in response to a bioterrorism event or influenza pandemic

#### Tertiary Prevention

- Providing case management services that link clients with chronic illnesses to health care and community support services

- Providing case management services that link clients identified with serious mental illnesses to mental health and community support services
- Educating at rehabilitation centers to help clients with stroke optimize their functioning
- Establishing an alternative treatment site for victims of a smallpox epidemic

From U.S. Department of Health and Human Services: *Healthy People 2020: National Health Promotion and Disease Prevention Objectives*, 2010. Available at http://www.healthypeople.gov/hp2020/objectives/TopicAreas.aspx. Accessed May 13, 2015.

## QSEN FOCUS ON QUALITY AND SAFETY EDUCATION FOR NURSES

### Public Health Nursing at Local, State, and National Levels

#### Targeted Competency

**Teamwork and Collaboration** – function effectively within nursing and interprofessional teams, fostering open communication, mutual respect, and shared decision making to achieve quality patient care.

Important aspects of teamwork and collaboration include:

- **Knowledge:** Describe scopes of practice and roles of health care team members.
- **Skills:** Integrate the contributions of others who play a role in helping patient/family achieve health goals.
- **Attitudes:** Respect the unique attributes that members bring to a team, including variations in professional orientations and accountabilities.

#### Teamwork and Collaboration Question

Your state has recently been awarded funding from the Centers for Disease Control and Prevention to prevent the spread of viral hepatitis through increased testing, improving access to care, and strengthening surveillance to detect viral hepatitis transmission and disease. You are the Director of Nursing for the State Public Health Department and currently serve on the Infectious Disease

Prevention (IDP) committee. The IDP committee has been given the responsibility to determine how to best utilize this new funding to effectively meet the objectives of the grant. Consider the following:

- As the Director of Nursing for the State Public Health Department, what is your role in addressing this initiative at the state level? How would your role change if you were a public health nurse working at the local health department?
- In addition to nursing, give examples of other professionals who likely serve on the IDP committee with you. Describe the role for each professional for this committee?
- Identify local and state organizations in your community that would you recommend that the IDP committee collaborate with to develop and implement a response to identified
- Through this grant, your state is addressing several objectives in the Healthy People 2020 focus area of Immunization and Infectious Diseases. Go to the Healthy People 2020 website and identify which specific objectives would apply to this initiative.

Prepared by Lisa Turner, PhD, RN, PHCNS-BC , Assistant Professor, Berea College Nursing Program, Berea, Kentucky.

## PRACTICE APPLICATION

A retirement community in a small town reported to the local health department 24 cases of severe gastrointestinal illness that had occurred among residents and staff of the facility during the past 24 to 36 hours. It was determined that the ill clients became sick within a short, well-defined period, and most recovered within 24 hours without treatment. The communicable disease outbreak team, composed of public health nurses, public health physicians, and an environmental health specialist, was called to respond to this possible epidemic.

How should they respond to this situation? (Refer to Chapter 12 for help in answering this question.)

A. Call the Centers for Disease Control and Prevention and ask for help with surveillance.
B. Send all the ill persons in the retirement community to the hospital.
C. Evaluate the agent, host, and environmental relationships to determine the cause of the problem.
D. Close the dining room and find another source to provide food to the residents.

**Answers can be found on the Evolve site.**

## KEY POINTS

- Local public health departments are responsible for implementing and enforcing local, state, and federal public health codes and ordinances while providing essential public health services.

- The goal of the local health department is to safeguard the public's health and improve the community's health status.
- State health departments hold primary responsibility for promoting and protecting the public's health.

## KEY POINTS—cont'd

- Public health nursing is the practice of promoting and protecting the health of populations using knowledge from nursing and social and public health sciences.
- Public health is based on the scientific core of epidemiology.
- Marketing of public health nursing is essential to inform both professionals and the public about the opportunities and challenges of populations in public health care.
- A driving force behind public health nursing changes is globalization that allows rapid transmission of emerging infections and the expectation that public health nurses will be active partners in emergency preparedness activities.

- Some of the roles public health nurses function in are advocate, case manager, referral source, counselor, educator, outreach worker, disease surveillance expert, community mobilizer, and disaster responder.
- Public health nurses have an important role in conducting community assessments including partnering with the community to collect and analyze data, developing community diagnosis, and implementing evidence-based interventions.
- Public health nurses base interventions on identified health status of populations and their related determinants of health.

## CLINICAL DECISION-MAKING ACTIVITIES

1. What are some of the various roles of the public health nurse in the local, state, and federal public health systems? Contrast the roles. Explain why they may be different from one another.
2. How can public health nurses prepare themselves for change? Illustrate what you mean.
3. What can today's public health nurses learn from the past practice of public health nurses? How can you verify your answer?
4. Describe collaborative partnerships that public health nurses have developed. How do partnerships help solve public health problems?
5. What are some external factors that have an effect on public health nursing? How can you deal with the complexities of these factors?

6. What are core functions used by public health nurses as they plan interventions? Do these functions make sense to you? Explain.
7. If you were a public health nurse for a day, what would you like to accomplish? Why? Is your answer supported by evidence? Be specific.
8. How would you determine the most pressing public health issue in your community? Gather several points of view from key leaders in the community.
9. Give an example of a policy change or an effect from the work of public health nurses. How did this policy make a difference in client health outcomes?

## REFERENCES

All Kids Count: *Policy Brief – Sustaining Financial Support for Immunization Registries.* Decatur, GA, 2000, All Kids Count.

American Nurses Association: *Public Health Nursing: Scope and Standards of Practice.* Silver Springs, MD, 2007/2013, ANA.

American Public Health Association, Public Health Nursing Section: *The Definition and Practice of Public Health Nursing: A Statement of Public Health Nursing Section.* Washington, DC, 2013, American Public Health Association.

Centers for Disease Control and Prevention (CDC): Achievements in public health, 1900-1999. *MMWR* 48:621–629, 1999.

Centers for Disease Control and Prevention (CDC): The National Public Health Performance Standards, An Overview, slide 9, 2005. Available at: http://www.cdc.gov/od/ocphp/nphpsp/Presentationlinks.htm.

Centers for Disease Control and Prevention: Outbreak of swine-origin influenza A (H1N1) virus infection—Mexico, March–April 2009. *MMWR* 58(17):467–470, 2009. Available at: http://www.cdc.gov/mmwr/preview/mmwrhtml/mm5817a5.htm. Accessed March 20, 2011.

Centers for Disease Control and Prevention: MRSA, 2010a. Available at: http://www.cdc.gov/mrsa/index.html. Accessed March 25, 2011.

Centers for Disease Control and Prevention: Antibiotic/Antimicrobial Resistance Campaign, 2010b. Available at: http://www.cdc.gov/drugresistance/campaigns.html. Accessed March 25, 2011.

Center for Disease Control and Prevention: Control of infectious diseases-measles. *MMWR* 2013. Available at: CDC.gov. Accessed on 9/25/2014.

Centers for Disease Control and Prevention: MERS-CoV, 2014a. Available at: http://www.cdc.gov/coronavirus/mers/. Accessed May 13, 2015.

Centers for Disease Control and Prevention: The Guide to Community Preventive Services, 2014b. Available at: http://www.thecommunityguide.org/index.html. Accessed May 24, 2014.

Centers for Disease Control and Prevention: Cases of Ebola diagnosed in the United States, 2014c. Available at: http://www.cdc.gov/vhf/ebola/outbreaks/2014-west-africa/united-states-imported-case.html. Accessed May 13, 2015.

Centers for Disease Control and Prevention: The National Public Health Performance Standards (Homepage), 2015. Available at: http://www.cdc.gov/nphpsp/. Accessed May 13, 2015.

Community-Campus Partnerships for Health (CCPH) Board of Directors: Position Statement of Authentic Partnerships. *Community-Campus Partnerships for Health* 2013. Available at: https://ccph.memberclicks.net/principles-of-partnership. Accessed May 13, 2015.

Council on Linkages Between Academia and Public Health Practice: *Core Competencies for Public Health Professionals.* Washington, DC, 2014, PHF. Available at: http://www.phf.org/link/corecompetencies.htm. Accessed May 26, 2014.

Institute of Medicine: *The Future of Public Health.* Washington, DC, 1988, National Academies Press.

Institute of Medicine: *Unequal Treatment: Confronting Racial and Ethnic Disparities in Health Care.* Washington, DC, 2002, National Academies Press.

Institute of Medicine: *The Future of Public Health in the 21st Century*. Washington, DC, 2003, National Academies Press.

Los Angeles County Department of Public Health-Public Health Nursing: Public Health Nursing Practice Model, 2007. Available at: http://publichealth.lacounty.gov/phn/index.htm. Accessed March 20, 2011.

National Association of County and City Health Officials: Operational Definition of a Functional Local Health Department, 2014. Available at: http://www.naccho.org. Accessed August 23, 2014.

Nurse-Family Partnership Program: 2010. Available at: http://www.nursefamilypartnership.org/. Accessed June 3, 2010.

Olds DL, Kitzman HJ, Cole RE, et al: Enduring effects of prenatal and infancy home visiting by nurses on maternal life course and government spending: follow-up of a randomized trial among children at age 12 years. *Arch Pediatr Adolesc Med* 164(5):419–424, 2010.

Public Health Accreditation Board: Public health accreditation standards, 2014. Available at: PHAB.org. Accessed on 9\25\2014.

Public Health Nursing Section, Minnesota Department of Health: *Public Health Interventions—Applications for Public Health Nursing Practice*. St Paul, MN, 2001, Department of Health, APHA.

Turnock BJ: *Public Health: What It Is and How It Works*, ed 3. Sudbury, MA, 2010, Jones and Bartlett.

U.S. Department of Health and Human Services: Healthy People 2020: National Health Promotion and Disease Prevention Objectives, 2010. Available at: http://www.healthypeople.gov/hp2020/objectives/TopicAreas.aspx. Accessed May 13, 2015.

# APPENDIXES

# Resource Tools Available on the Evolve Website

| Resource Tool # | Resource Tool Title |
| --- | --- |
| 3.A | Declaration of Alma Ata |
| 4.A | Millennium Development Goals Report 2014 |
| 5.A | Select Major Historical Events Depicting Financial Involvement of Federal Government in Health Care Delivery |
| 5.B | Schedule of Clinical Preventive Services |
| 10.A | Recommendations from the President's Cancer Panel |
| 14.A | Resources on Sexually Transmitted Diseases |
| 21.A | Factors Influencing the Success of Collaboration |
| 21.B | The Evolution of Nursing Centers |
| 21.C | Nursing Center Positions |
| 21.D | Outline of Essential Elements in Nursing Center Development |
| 21.E | WHO Priorities for a Common Nursing Research Agenda |
| 21.F | Template for Research in Nursing Centers |
| 27.A | Family Systems Stressor-Strength Inventory |
| 27.B | Case Example of Family Assessment |
| 27.C | List of Family Assessment Tools |
| 29.A | Injury Prevention in Children |
| 29.B | Common Behaviors of the School-Age Child and Adolescent |
| 29.C | Developmental Characteristics: Summary for Children |
| 29.D | Feeding and Nutrition Guidelines for Infants |
| 29.E | Immunization Schedule for Children and Adolescents: Range of Ages for Routine Immunizations |
| 29.F | Immunization Schedule for Children Not Immunized in the First Year of Life |
| 29.G | Immunizations: General Recommendations |
| 29.H | Summary of Rules for Childhood Immunization |
| 30.A | Lifestyle Assessment Questionnaire |
| 30.B | A Health Risk Appraisal for Older Adults |
| 31.A | The Living Will Directive |
| 31.B | Assessment Tools for Communities with Special Needs Members |
| 31.C | Assessment Tools for Families with Special Needs Members |
| 31.D | Assessment Tools for Special Needs Members |
| 34.A | Resources for the Nurse Working with Migrant Farmworkers |
| 37.A | Smoking Cessation Resources |
| 37.B | Useful Web Resources |
| 37.C | Common Drugs of Abuse |
| 41.A | Home Health Patient Tracking Sheet |
| 41-B | The Living Will Directive |
| 43.A | Recommended Adult Immunization Schedule |
| 45.A | Resources for Faith Community Nursing |
| 46.A | Quad Council Competencies for Public Health Nurses |

# Program Planning and Design

Program planning is a process of outlining, designing, contemplating, and deliberating to develop actions to accomplish desirable goals and attain desirable outcomes.

## PLANNING PROCESS

The successful program requires a lot of planning before implementation. The following need to be considered:
1. Who is in charge?
2. Who should be involved?
3. When is the best time to plan?
4. What data are needed?
5. Where should planning occur?
6. Will there be resistance?
7. Where will resistance come from?
8. Who will be early adopters?

Failing to plan can result in the inability to have a program that is viable and that will attain the goals and outcomes.

## TIMETABLE

Timetables are very important to the success of planning. Two methods often used by planners are the following:
- Program Evaluation and Review Techniques (PERT)
- GANTT

### PERT

The PERT method requires the planner to do the following:
- State the goal.
- List in sequence all the steps and activities for each step to accomplish the goal.
- Target dates for accomplishing each step are set.
- Diagram the process for easy use.

### Student Activity

1. Go to literature and find a PERT application and diagram.
2. Draw a diagram of your program plan or a hypothetical one.
3. Be prepared to submit with end of module assignment.

### GANTT

A GANTT chart is also a flow diagram that can be used to map out the activities needed to be accomplished so that one can maintain a timeline to achieve the goal. The GANTT chart looks much like a calendar.

### Student Activity

1. Go to the literature and find a GANTT chart that has been applied to a project.
2. Complete a GANTT chart of the activities related to each objective in your project that are stated to meet the goal or do a hypothetical one.
3. Be prepared to submit at the end of the module.

## PEOPLE PLANNING

To have a successful plan one needs to involve the clients who are to be served by the program. Others to be involved are the following:
- Administrators
- Staff (providers)
- Other key stakeholders

## REASONS

- Develop ownership
- Develop commitment
- Develop pride
- Develop understanding of problems
- Brainstorm
- Generate ideas

## DATA PLANNING

To have a successful program one must collect data on the following:
- Demographics of clients
- Disease statistics
- Vital statistics
- Existing similar programs
- Successes and barriers of similar programs
- Socioeconomic/environmental support
- Political issues

### Student Activity

1. Find a source of data for one of the above categories.
2. Explain why it is a good data source for your program.

## PERFORMANCE PLANNING

Some programs, called projects are planned for a one-time-only event. Most programs are planned to be ongoing.

1. Question: Are problems that programs address usually solved?
   a. Explain your answer and give an example.
2. The following should be considered in planning for performance:
   a. Staff is the most expensive resource in planning.
   b. For efficiency, programs should be planned as ongoing activities.
   c. A 6-month start-up and a 5-year budget should be developed.
   d. Long-term commitment of resources to a program is essential.
   e. Planners must develop marketing tools, policies and procedures, and job descriptions before implementation.
   f. Organizational structures including committees need to be drafted.
   g. Community partners and advisory board should be planned and contacted for agreement to serve.

### Priority Planning

1. Plan programs for the greatest need and the best potential for making a difference.
2. Available resources to accomplish goal no. 1 must be sought. If resources are not available, the program plan is time wasted.
3. Be a comprehensive planner.
4. Complete ongoing needs assessments to determine community changes.
5. Prioritize the greatest needs.
6. Plan new programs or change existing ones for goal no. 5.

### Plan for Measurable Outcomes

1. Collect baseline data on the problem and the target population.
2. Analyze needs assessment.
3. Look at incidence and prevalence of problems.
4. Look at available services currently addressing the problem.
5. Determine the impact of the current services, using SWOT.

### Evaluation Planning

1. This must begin with the needs assessment.
2. Plan for process evaluation.
3. Plan for summative evaluation.
4. Develop a timeline for evaluation to occur.
5. Develop systems for records and data collection and choose evaluation instruments.

### Questions to be Answered

1. Do you have the right people doing the planning?
2. Do you have the essential data for planning?
3. Is this the right time to plan this program?'
4. Why should evaluation occur?
5. Who should do it?

6. What data should be gathered?
7. Should evaluation occur?

### Planning Models

1. Choose a model for planning your program.
2. Two models developed for program planning by the Centers for Disease Control and Prevention are PATCH and APEX.

### Student Activity

1. Read about these two models.
2. Briefly explain how these models can be applied to program planning.
3. Briefly explain the model you have chosen for planning. Include the following:
   a. Definition
   b. Goal
   c. Model elements
   d. Planning process

## MISSION

All programs will want to have a Mission Statement. Elements of a Mission Statement should include the following:
- Name of agency
- Name of program
- Who program serves
- Purpose of program
- Program goal
- Services offered

### Student Activity

Write a Mission Statement for your program.

## VISION

A Vision Statement is a brief one- or two-sentence statement that expresses the impact this program will have.

### Student Activity

Write a Vision Statement for your program.

## WORKSHEET FOR WRITING THE PHILOSOPHY

### Questions for Discussion

What are our community's values and beliefs about health?

What is the purpose of our program?

What is our position on community involvement and responsibility for health?

What is our role in providing leadership?

## Worksheet for Finding and Overcoming Obstacles

Goal:


Forces working against reaching goal (barriers/obstacles/challenges):


Forces working for reaching goal (existing resources/strengths):


Approaches to overcome obstacles:

## WORKSHEET FOR WRITING OBJECTIVES

Health Issue:


Goal:


Objectives (write the most important objectives first):

1.


2.


3.


4.

## CHECKLIST FOR PROGRAM PLANNING AND IMPLEMENTATION

1. Have you established a community advisory group with:
   ___ Representation of your targeted groups
   ___ The ability to provide valuable links with the community
   ___ Skills and resources that will be useful to the program

2. Have you identified community needs and concerns by way of:
   ___ Surveys/questionnaires
   ___ Focus groups
   ___ Public meetings or forums
   ___ Interested party analysis

3. Have you determined the community's priorities, taking into account:
   ___ Historical conditions
   ___ Traditional practices
   ___ Political and economic conditions

4. Have you developed program goals and objectives?
   ___ Yes
   ___ No

5. Have you decided on program strategies that:
   ___ Fit with the resources and needs of the community
   ___ Consider the beliefs, values, and practices of the community
   ___ Reflect field testing
   ___ Dispel health misconceptions
   ___ Change behavior
   ___ Change the environment

6. To implement your program, have you:
   ___ Prepared a timeline for program implementation
   ___ Listed people to be involved, and resources needed
   ___ Hired staff (preferably from the community)
   ___ Developed linkages with other community agencies, as appropriate
   ___ Planned to carry out an evaluation

7. Have you chosen appropriate methods and questions for:
   ___ Process evaluation
   ___ Outcome evaluation

## REFERENCES

Green LW, Kreuter M: *Health Program Planning: an Education and Ecological Approach*, ed 4. New York, 2004, McGraw-Hill.

Issel LM: *Health Program Planning and Evaluation: a Practical, Systematic Approach for Community Health*, ed 3. Boston, 2014, Jones and Bartlett.

Posavac EJ: *Program Evaluation: Methods and Case Studies*, ed 8. Boston, MA, 2010, Prentice Hall.

Veney J, Kaluzny A: *Evaluation and Decision Making for Health Service Programs*. Englewood Cliffs, NJ, 2005, Prentice Hall.

Form C

## The HEALTHIER PEOPLE NETWORK, Inc.

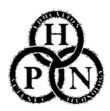

*. . . linking science, technology, & education to serve the public interest . . .*

### IDENTIFICATION NUMBER

The health risk appraisal is an educational tool, showing you choices you can make to keep good health and avoid the most common causes of death (for a person of your age and sex). This health risk appraisal is **not** a substitute for a check-up or physical exam that you get from a doctor or nurse; however, it does provide some ideas for lowering your risk of getting sick or injured in the future. It is NOT designed for people who already have HEART DISEASE, CANCER, KIDNEY DISEASE, OR OTHER SERIOUS CONDITIONS; if you have any of these problems, please ask your health care provider to interpret the report for you.

### DIRECTIONS:
To get the most accurate results, **answer as many questions as you can.** If you do not know the answer leave it blank.

*The following questions must be completed or the computer program cannot process your questionnaire:*

*1. SEX    2. AGE    3. HEIGHT    4. WEIGHT    15. CIGARETTE SMOKING*

**Please write your answers in the boxes provided.** ☞ (Examples: ☒ or ⟨ 98 ⟩)

| | | |
|---|---|---|
| 1. | SEX | 1 ☐ Male    2 ☐ Female |
| 2. | AGE | ☐ Years |
| 3. | HEIGHT (Without shoes) (No fractions) | ☐ Feet  ☐ Inches |
| 4. | WEIGHT (Without shoes) (No fractions) | ☐ Pounds |
| 5. | Body frame size | 1 ☐ Small<br>2 ☐ Medium<br>3 ☐ Large |
| 6. | Have you ever been told that you have diabetes (or sugar diabetes)? | 1 ☐ Yes    2 ☐ No |
| 7. | Are you now taking medicine for high blood pressure? | 1 ☐ Yes    2 ☐ No |
| 8. | What is your blood pressure now? | ☐ / ☐ <br>Systolic (High Number)/Diastolic (Low Number) |
| 9. | If you do not know the numbers, check the box that describes your blood pressure. | 1 ☐ High<br>2 ☐ Normal or Low<br>3 ☐ Don't Know |

Form C

| 10. | What is your TOTAL cholesterol level (based on a blood test)? | ☐ mg/dl |
|---|---|---|
| 11. | What is your HDL cholesterol (based on a blood test)? | ☐ mg/dl |
| 12. | How many cigars do you usually smoke per day? | ☐ cigars per day |
| 13. | How many pipes of tobacco do you usually smoke per day? | ☐ pipes per day |
| 14. | How many times per day do you usually use smokeless tobacco? (Chewing tobacco, snuff, pouches, etc.) | ☐ times per day |
| 15. | **CIGARETTE SMOKING** <br><br> How would you describe your cigarette smoking habits? | 1 ☐ Never smoked ☛ Go to 18 <br> 2 ☐ Used to smoke ☛ Go to 17 <br> 3 ☐ Still smoke ☛ Go to 16 |
| 16. | **STILL SMOKE** <br><br> How many cigarettes a day do you smoke? <br><br> ☛ **GO TO QUESTION 18** | ☐ cigarettes per day ☛ Go to 18 |
| 17. | **USED TO SMOKE** <br><br> a. How many years has it been since you smoked cigarettes fairly regularly? <br><br> b. What was the average number of cigarettes per day that you smoked in the 2 years before you quit? | ☐ years <br><br> ☐ cigarettes per day |
| 18. | In the next 12 months, how many thousands of miles will you probably travel by each of the following? (NOTE: U.S. average = 10,000 miles)    a. Car, truck, or van: <br><br> b. Motorcycle: | ☐ ,000 miles <br><br> ☐ ,000 miles |
| 19. | On a typical day, how do you USUALLY travel? (Check one only) | 1 ☐ Walk <br> 2 ☐ Bicycle <br> 3 ☐ Motorcycle <br> 4 ☐ Sub-compact or compact car <br> 5 ☐ Mid-size or full-size car <br> 6 ☐ Truck or van <br> 7 ☐ Bus, subway, or train <br> 8 ☐ Mostly stay home |
| 20. | What percent of time do you usually buckle your safety belt when driving or riding? | ☐ % |
| 21. | On the average, how close to the speed limit do you usually drive? | 1 ☐ Within 5 mph of limit <br> 2 ☐ 6-10 mph over limit <br> 3 ☐ 11-15 mph over limit <br> 4 ☐ More than 15 mph over limit |
| 22. | How many times in the last month did you drive or ride when the driver had perhaps too much alcohol to drink? | ☐ times last month |
| 23. | How many drinks of an alcoholic beverage do you have in a typical week? <br><br> ☛ **MEN GO TO QUESTION 33** | (Write the number of each type of drink) <br> ☐ Bottles or cans of beer <br> ☐ Glasses of wine <br> ☐ Wine coolers <br> ☐ Mixed drinks or shots of liquor |

Form C

## WOMEN ONLY

| | |
|---|---|
| 24. At what age did you have your first menstrual period? | [ ] years old |
| 25. How old were you when your first child was born? | [ ] years old   (If no children, write 0) |
| 26. How long has it been since your last breast x-ray (mammogram)? | 1 ☐ Less than 1 year ago<br>2 ☐ 1 year ago<br>3 ☐ 2 years ago<br>4 ☐ 3 or more years ago<br>5 ☐ Never |
| 27. How many women in your natural family (mother and sisters only) have had breast cancer? | [ ] Women |
| 28. Have you had a hysterectomy operation? | 1 ☐ Yes<br>2 ☐ No<br>3 ☐ Not sure |
| 29. How long has it been since you had a pap smear test? | 1 ☐ Less than 1 year ago<br>2 ☐ 1 year ago<br>3 ☐ 2 years ago<br>4 ☐ 3 or more years ago<br>5 ☐ Never |
| ★30. How often do you examine your breasts for lumps? | 1 ☐ Monthly<br>2 ☐ Once every few months<br>3 ☐ Rarely or never |
| ★31. About how long has it been since you had your breasts examined by a physician or nurse? | 1 ☐ Less than 1 year ago<br>2 ☐ 1 year ago<br>3 ☐ 2 years ago<br>4 ☐ 3 or more years ago<br>5 ☐ Never |
| ★32. About how long has it been since you had a rectal exam?<br><br>☞ **WOMEN GO TO QUESTION 34** | 1 ☐ Less than 1 year ago<br>2 ☐ 1 year ago<br>3 ☐ 2 years ago<br>4 ☐ 3 or more years ago<br>5 ☐ Never |

## MEN ONLY

| | |
|---|---|
| ★33. About how long has it been since you had a rectal or prostate exam?<br><br>☞ **MEN CONTINUE ON QUES. 34** | 1 ☐ Less than 1 year ago<br>2 ☐ 1 year ago<br>3 ☐ 2 years ago<br>4 ☐ 3 or more years ago<br>5 ☐ Never |
| ★34. How many times in the last year did you witness or become involved in a violent fight or attack where there was a good chance of a serious injury to someone? | 1 ☐ 4 or more times<br>2 ☐ 2 or 3 times<br>3 ☐ 1 time or never<br>4 ☐ Not sure |
| ★35. Considering your age, how would you describe your overall physical health? | 1 ☐ Excellent<br>2 ☐ Good<br>3 ☐ Fair<br>4 ☐ Poor |

★ Questions with a star symbol are not used by the computer to calculate your risks; however, answering these questions may help you plan a more healthy lifestyle.

Form C

| | |
|---|---|
| ★36. In an average week, how many times do you engage in physical activity (exercise or work which lasts at least 20 minutes without stopping and which is hard enough to make you breathe heavier and your heart beat faster)? | 1 ☐ Less than 1 time per week<br>2 ☐ 1 or 2 times per week<br>3 ☐ At least 3 times per week |
| ★37. If you ride a motorcycle or all-terrain vehicle (ATV), what percent of the time do you wear a helmet? | 1 ☐ 75% to 100%<br>2 ☐ 25% to 74 %<br>3 ☐ Less than 25%<br>4 ☐ Does not apply to me |
| ★38. Do you eat some food every day that is high in fiber, such as whole grain bread, cereal, fresh fruits or vegetables? | 1 ☐ Yes    2 ☐ No |
| ★39. Do you eat foods every day that are high in cholesterol or fat, such as fatty meat, cheese, fried foods, or eggs? | 1 ☐ Yes    2 ☐ No |
| ★40. In general, how satisfied are you with your life? | 1 ☐ Mostly satisfied<br>2 ☐ Partly satisfied<br>3 ☐ Not satisfied |
| ★41. Have you suffered a personal loss or misfortune in the past year that had a serious impact on your life? (For example, a job loss, disability, separation, jail term, or the death of someone close to you.) | 1 ☐ Yes, 1 serious loss or misfortune<br>2 ☐ Yes, 2 or more<br>3 ☐ No |
| ★42a. Race | 1 ☐ Aleutian, Alaska native, Eskimo or American Indian<br>2 ☐ Asian<br>3 ☐ Black<br>4 ☐ Pacific Islander<br>5 ☐ White<br>6 ☐ Other<br>7 ☐ Don't know |
| ★42b. Are you of Hispanic origin, such as Mexican-American, Puerto Rican, or Cuban? | 1 ☐ Yes    2 ☐ No |
| ★43. What is the highest grade you completed in school? | 1 ☐ Grade school or less<br>2 ☐ Some high school<br>3 ☐ High school graduate<br>4 ☐ Some college<br>5 ☐ College graduate<br>6 ☐ Post graduate or professional degree |

Name _____

Address _____

City _____ State ___ ___ Zip ___ ___ ___ ___ ___

(Note: Name and address are optional, depending on how your report will be returned to you. If you wish to remain anonymous, copy your Identification Number onto a receipt form. You can then use this receipt to claim your computerized report.)

# The
# HEALTHIER PEOPLE NETWORK, Inc.

## Participant's Guide to Interpreting the
## HEALTH RISK APPRAISAL REPORT

Unhealthy habits lead to early death or chronic illness. Every year, 1.3 million people in the United States die prematurely from conditions which could be prevented or delayed. This Health Risk Appraisal may help you avoid becoming one of these statistics by giving you a picture of how your health risks relate to your particular characteristics and habits.

## WHAT IS A HEALTH RISK APPRAISAL?

The Health Risk Appraisal is an estimation of your risk of dying in the next ten years from each of 42 causes of death. The twelve most important of these are printed individually on your report. The others are grouped together and printed as "All Other". These risks are calculated by a computer program which compares your characteristics to national mortality statistics using equations developed by epidemiologists. This Health Risk Appraisal does not tell you how long you will live, nor does it diagnose or treat disease.

## RISK FACTORS

Most chronic diseases develop slowly in the presence of certain risk factors. Risk factors are either controllable or uncontrollable. Controllable risk factors include lifestyle habits that you can change such as smoking, exercise, diet, stress and weight. Uncontrollable risk factors include items such as your age and sex, and the health history of your family.

The Health Risk Appraisal uses both controllable and uncontrollable risk factors in calculating health risks. Your focus, however, should be on controllable risk factors.

To help you decide which controllable risk factors to concentrate on, the Health Risk Appraisal identifies your controllable risk factors for each cause of death. Your report gives you an idea of their relative importance by indicating the number of risk years you could gain by controlling these factors.

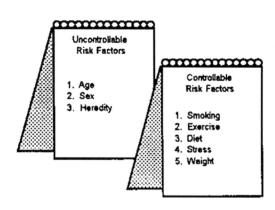

To identify your personal risks, to see what the numbers on your report mean, and to learn which risk factors you need to control, turn the page.

# Participant's Guide to Interpreting the Health Risk Appraisal Report Form

An example using a 48 year old woman: 5'7", 250 mg/dl cholesterol, 160/95 BP, 30 cigarettes/day, 9 drinks/week, seat belt use 15%, drives 4,000 mi/yr, menarche 13 yrs, 1st child at 32

| ❶ | YOUR RISK AGE | NOW 68.91 | TARGET 60.82 | ← Risks are elevated due to diabetes and family breast cancer |

Mrs. Lopez ❻
Female Age 48

THIS REPORT CONTAINS ESTIMATES DUE TO MISSING ITEMS, INCLUDING THE FOLLOWING ❼
Cigars per day. Pipes smoked per day. Smokeless tobacco.

Many serious injuries and health problems can be prevented. Your Health Risk Appraisal lists factors you can change to lower your risk. For causes of death that are not directly computable, the report uses the average risk for a person of your age and sex.

| MOST COMMON CAUSES OF DEATH | NUMBER OF DEATHS IN NEXT 10 YEARS FOR 1000 WOMEN AGE 48 | | | MODIFIABLE RISK FACTORS |
|---|---|---|---|---|
| | ❷ YOUR GROUP | ❸ TARGET | ❹ POPULATION AVERAGE | |
| Heart Attack | 104 | 22 | 5 | Avoid Tobacco Use, Blood Pressure, Cholesterol Level, ❽ HDL Level, Weight |
| Breast Cancer | 42 | 42 | 5 | A Low-Fat Diet and Regular Exercise Might Reduce Risk |
| Diabetes Mellitus | 21 | 21 | 1 | Control Your Weight and Follow Your Doctor's Advice |
| Stroke | 19 | 5 | 2 | Avoid Tobacco Use, Blood Pressure |
| Lung Cancer | 13 | 7 | 5 | Avoid Tobacco Use |
| Emphysema/Bronchitis | 2 | <1 | 1 | Avoid Tobacco Use |
| Kidney Failure | 2 | 2 | <1 | " |
| Colon Cancer | 1* | 1* | 1 | A High-Fiber and Low-Fat Diet Might Reduce Risk |
| Ovary Cancer | 1* | 1* | 1 | Get Regular Exams |
| Pancreas Cancer | 1 | 1 | 1 | Avoid Tobacco Use |
| Cirrhosis of Liver | 1 | 1 | 1 | Continue to Avoid Heavy Drinking |
| All Other | 21 | 19 | 20 | * = Average Value Used |
| TOTAL: | 228 | 122 | 46 | Deaths in Next 10 Years Per 1,000 Women, age 48 |

| For Height 5'7" and Large Frame, 175 pounds is about 20% Overweight. Desirable Weight Range: 139-153    ❾ |

| GOOD HABITS ❺ | TO IMPROVE YOUR RISK PROFILE: | RISK YEARS GAINED ❿ |
|---|---|---|
| + Regular pap tests | - Quit smoking <estimate> | 3.57 |
| + Safe driving speed | - Lower your blood pressure | 1.88 |
| | - Lower your cholesterol | 1.56 |
| | - Improve your HDL level | .92 |
| | - Bring your weight to desirable range | .13 |
| | - Always wear your seat belts | .03 |

Total Risk Years you could gain = 8.09 ⓫

**1** Your **RISK AGE** compares your total risk from all causes of death to the total risk of those who are your age and sex. It gives you an idea of your risks compared with the population average in terms of an age. Your **TARGET** risk age indicates what your risk age would be if you made the changes recommended below.

**2** The numbers in the **YOUR GROUP** column refer to the number of predicted deaths for each cause of death in the next 10 years from among 1,000 people who have habits and characteristics just like you.

**3** The numbers in the **TARGET** column refer to those predicted to die in the next 10 years from among 1,000 people who have characteristics just like you, but who have adopted the habits recommended below in the **TO IMPROVE YOUR RISK PROFILE** box.

**4** The numbers in the **POPULATION AVERAGE** column refer to the national average of deaths in 10 years for people of your same sex and age.

**5** This box lists your **GOOD HABITS**. Congratulations!

**6** Your I.D., sex and actual age is here.

**7** If you did not answer items on the questionnaire which are used for calculations, these missing items will be listed here. The computer substitutes national average values for the items you left blank and calculates your risks with these numbers.

**8** Beside each cause of death are listed the modifiable risk factors which your questionnaire responses indicate you need to work on. The list is specific for you unless you have none of the risk factors or if there are no known risk factors for a cause of death. In this case, a short statement of general advice related to risk reduction is printed.

**9** Your **DESIRABLE WEIGHT RANGE** is based on your height and frame size.

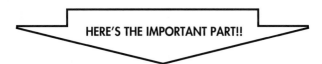

HERE'S THE IMPORTANT PART!!

**10** In this box is our prescription to lengthen your life and a prediction of how many **RISK YEARS** you can expect to gain by adopting these health habits.

**11** The **TOTAL RISK YEARS** you could gain by making these habit changes are printed here. This is also the difference between your **Risk Age Now** and your **Target Age**. Also important are the recommendations on page 2.

Page 2 of your report lists some **ROUTINE PREVENTIVE SERVICES** that are specific for people of your age and sex. The report also lists some **GENERAL RECOMMENDATIONS FOR EVERYONE**. For the 48 year old woman used in this example, the following messages were printed:

| ROUTINE PREVENTIVE SERVICES FOR WOMEN YOUR AGE | GENERAL RECOMMENDATIONS FOR EVERYONE |
|---|---|
| Blood Pressure and Cholesterol test<br>Pap Smear test<br>Breast cancer screening (check with your doctor or clinic)<br>Rectal exam (or Sigmoidoscopy)<br>Eye exam for glaucoma<br>Dental Exam<br>Tetanus-Diphtheria booster shot (every 10 years) | * Exercise briskly for 15-30 minutes at least<br>  three times a week.<br>* Use good eating habits by choosing a variety<br>  of foods that are low in fat and high in fiber.<br>* Learn to recognize and handle stress - get<br>  help if you need it. |

The standard report can also print health education messages.

## HEALTH RISK APPRAISAL LIMITS

Health Risk Appraisal is an educational tool. It does not take into consideration whether or not you already have a medical condition and it does not consider rare diseases and other health problems which are not fatal but can limit your enjoyment of life, such as arthritis.

Health Risk Appraisal does not predict when you will die or specifically what diseases you might get. It does tell you, however, your chances of getting a disease relative to a large group of people your age and sex, who answered the questionnaire just as you did.

Health Risk Appraisal does take into consideration lifestyle factors which account for a large number of premature deaths. When you become familiar with your particular risks, you can then do something about them!

## CHOOSING A HABIT TO WORK ON

Health Risk Appraisal is intended to encourage you to work on habits you can change by showing you which behaviors should have top priority. If you can't change the behavior that is at the top of your list (the one that would give the largest number of **RISK YEARS GAINED**), try to concentrate on changing the next highest one. You don't have to change your entire lifestyle overnight. In fact, trying to change too many habits at once is probably the quickest way to become discouraged and fail.

## MAKE A PLAN FOR CHANGING HABITS

Make a plan for changing the habit you choose as your first priority, write it down and keep it in sight. Be prepared for temptation! Observe the time, situation, or place that most often triggers your unhealthy habit and be ready to combat it when it appears. Let family and friends know of your goals and ask for their encouragement.

## REWARD YOURSELF

Rewards are an important part of changing behavior. Give yourself a reasonable reward when you accomplish your goal. Don't eat half a gallon of ice cream after losing 10 pounds! Choose a healthy and enjoyable reward and you'll be on the road to good health!

# 2013 State and Local Youth Risk Behavior Survey

This survey is about health behavior. It has been developed so you can tell us what you do that may affect your health. The information you give will be used to improve health education for young people like yourself.

DO NOT write your name on this survey. The answers you give will be kept private. No one will know what you write. Answer the questions based on what you really do.

Completing the survey is voluntary. Whether or not you answer the questions will not affect your grade in this class. If you are not comfortable answering a question, just leave it blank.

The questions that ask about your background will be used only to describe the types of students completing this survey. The information will not be used to find out your name. No names will ever be reported.

Make sure to read every question. Fill in the ovals completely. When you are finished, follow the instructions of the person giving you the survey.

***Thank you very much for your help.***

## DIRECTIONS

- Use a #2 pencil only.
- Make dark marks.
- Fill in a response like this: Ⓐ Ⓑ ● Ⓓ
- If you change your answer, erase your old answer completely.

1. How old are you?
   - Ⓐ 12 years old or younger
   - Ⓑ 13 years old
   - Ⓒ 14 years old
   - Ⓓ 15 years old
   - Ⓔ 16 years old
   - Ⓕ 17 years old
   - Ⓖ 18 years old or older

2. What is your sex?
   - Ⓐ Female
   - Ⓑ Male

3. In what grade are you?
   - Ⓐ 9th grade
   - Ⓑ 10th grade
   - Ⓒ 11th grade
   - Ⓓ 12th grade
   - Ⓔ Ungraded or other grade

4. Are you Hispanic or Latino?
   - Ⓐ Yes
   - Ⓑ No

5. What is your race? (**Select one or more responses.**)
   - Ⓐ American Indian or Alaska Native
   - Ⓑ Asian
   - Ⓒ Black or African American
   - Ⓓ Native Hawaiian or Other Pacific Islander
   - Ⓔ White

6. How tall are you without your shoes on?
   Directions: Write your height in the shaded blank boxes. Fill in the matching oval below each number.

   Example

   | Height | | Height | |
   |---|---|---|---|
   | **Feet** | **Inches** | **Feet** | **Inches** |
   | 5 | 7 | | |
   | 3 | 0 | 3 | 0 |
   | 4 | 1 | 4 | 1 |
   | ● | 2 | 5 | 2 |
   | 6 | 3 | 6 | 3 |
   | 7 | 4 | 7 | 4 |
   | | 5 | | 5 |
   | | 6 | | 6 |
   | | ● | | 7 |
   | | 8 | | 8 |
   | | 9 | | 9 |
   | | 10 | | 10 |
   | | 11 | | 11 |

7. How much do you weigh without your shoes on?
   Directions: Write your weight in the shaded blank boxes. Fill in the matching oval below each number.

   Example

| Weight | | |
|---|---|---|
| Pounds | | |
| 1 | 5 | 2 |
| ⓪ | ⓪ | ⓪ |
| ● | ① | ① |
| ② | ② | ● |
| ③ | ③ | ③ |
| | ④ | ④ |
| | ● | ⑤ |
| | ⑥ | ⑥ |
| | ⑦ | ⑦ |
| | ⑧ | ⑧ |
| | ⑨ | ⑨ |

| Weight | | |
|---|---|---|
| Pounds | | |
| | | |
| ⓪ | ⓪ | ⓪ |
| ① | ① | ① |
| ② | ② | ② |
| ③ | ③ | ③ |
| | ④ | ④ |
| | ⑤ | ⑤ |
| | ⑥ | ⑥ |
| | ⑦ | ⑦ |
| | ⑧ | ⑧ |
| | ⑨ | ⑨ |

**The next 5 questions ask about safety.**

8. **When you rode a bicycle** during the past 12 months, how often did you wear a helmet?
   - Ⓐ I did not ride a bicycle during the past 12 months
   - Ⓑ Never wore a helmet
   - Ⓒ Rarely wore a helmet
   - Ⓓ Sometimes wore a helmet
   - Ⓔ Most of the time wore a helmet
   - Ⓕ Always wore a helmet

9. How often do you wear a seat belt when **riding** in a car driven by someone else?
   - Ⓐ Never
   - Ⓑ Rarely
   - Ⓒ Sometimes
   - Ⓓ Most of the time
   - Ⓔ Always

10. During the past 30 days, how many times did you **ride** in a car or other vehicle **driven by someone who had been drinking alcohol?**
   - Ⓐ 0 times
   - Ⓑ 1 time
   - Ⓒ 2 or 3 times
   - Ⓓ 4 or 5 times
   - Ⓔ 6 or more times

11. During the past 30 days, how many times did you **drive** a car or other vehicle **when you had been drinking alcohol?**
   - Ⓐ I did not drive a car or other vehicle during the past 30 days
   - Ⓑ 0 times
   - Ⓒ 1 time
   - Ⓓ 2 or 3 times
   - Ⓔ 4 or 5 times
   - Ⓕ 6 or more times

12. During the past 30 days, on how many days did you **text or e-mail** while **driving** a car or other vehicle?
   - Ⓐ I did not drive a car or other vehicle during the past 30 days
   - Ⓑ 0 days
   - Ⓒ 1 or 2 days
   - Ⓓ 3 to 5 days
   - Ⓔ 6 to 9 days
   - Ⓕ 10 to 19 days
   - Ⓖ 20 to 29 days
   - Ⓗ All 30 days

**The next 11 questions ask about violence-related behaviors.**

13. During the past 30 days, on how many days did you carry **a weapon** such as a gun, knife, or club?
   - Ⓐ 0 days
   - Ⓑ 1 day
   - Ⓒ 2 or 3 days
   - Ⓓ 4 or 5 days
   - Ⓔ 6 or more days

14. During the past 30 days, on how many days did you carry **a gun?**
   - Ⓐ 0 days
   - Ⓑ 1 day
   - Ⓒ 2 or 3 days
   - Ⓓ 4 or 5 days
   - Ⓔ 6 or more days

15. During the past 30 days, on how many days did you carry a weapon such as a gun, knife, or club **on school property?**
   - Ⓐ 0 days
   - Ⓑ 1 day
   - Ⓒ 2 or 3 days
   - Ⓓ 4 or 5 days
   - Ⓔ 6 or more days

16. During the past 30 days, on how many days did you **not** go to school because you felt you would be unsafe at school or on your way to or from school?
   - Ⓐ 0 days
   - Ⓑ 1 day
   - Ⓒ 2 or 3 days
   - Ⓓ 4 or 5 days
   - Ⓔ 6 or more days

17. During the past 12 months, how many times has someone threatened or injured you with a weapon such as a gun, knife, or club **on school property**?
    - (A) 0 times
    - (B) 1 time
    - (C) 2 or 3 times
    - (D) 4 or 5 times
    - (E) 6 or 7 times
    - (F) 8 or 9 times
    - (G) 10 or 11 times
    - (H) 12 or more times

18. During the past 12 months, how many times were you in a physical fight?
    - (A) 0 times
    - (B) 1 time
    - (C) 2 or 3 times
    - (D) 4 or 5 times
    - (E) 6 or 7 times
    - (F) 8 or 9 times
    - (G) 10 or 11 times
    - (H) 12 or more times

19. During the past 12 months, how many times were you in a physical fight in which you were injured and had to be treated by a doctor or nurse?
    - (A) 0 times
    - (B) 1 time
    - (C) 2 or 3 times
    - (D) 4 or 5 times
    - (E) 6 or more times

20. During the past 12 months, how many times were you in a physical fight **on school property**?
    - (A) 0 times
    - (B) 1 time
    - (C) 2 or 3 times
    - (D) 4 or 5 times
    - (E) 6 or 7 times
    - (F) 8 or 9 times
    - (G) 10 or 11 times
    - (H) 12 or more times

21. Have you ever been physically forced to have sexual intercourse when you did not want to?
    - (A) Yes
    - (B) No

22. During the past 12 months, how many times did someone you were dating or going out with physically hurt you on purpose? (Count such things as being hit, slammed into something, or injured with an object or weapon.)
    - (A) I did not date or go out with anyone during the past 12 months
    - (B) 0 times
    - (C) 1 time
    - (D) 2 or 3 times
    - (E) 4 or 5 times
    - (F) 6 or more times

23. During the past 12 months, how many times did someone you were dating or going out with force you to do sexual things that you did not want to do? (Count such things as kissing, touching, or being physically forced to have sexual intercourse.)
    - (A) I did not date or go out with anyone during the past 12 months
    - (B) 0 times
    - (C) 1 time
    - (D) 2 or 3 times
    - (E) 4 or 5 times
    - (F) 6 or more times

**The next 2 questions ask about bullying. Bullying is when 1 or more students tease, threaten, spread rumors about, hit, shove, or hurt another student over and over again. It is not bullying when 2 students of about the same strength or power argue or fight or tease each other in a friendly way.**

24. During the past 12 months, have you ever been bullied **on school property**?
    - (A) Yes
    - (B) No

25. During the past 12 months, have you ever been **electronically** bullied? (Count being bullied through e-mail, chat rooms, instant messaging, websites, or texting.)
    - (A) Yes
    - (B) No

**The next 5 questions ask about sad feelings and attempted suicide. Sometimes people feel so depressed about the future that they may consider attempting suicide, that is, taking some action to end their own life.**

26. During the past 12 months, did you ever feel so sad or hopeless almost every day for **two weeks or more in a row** that you stopped doing some usual activities?
    - (A) Yes
    - (B) No

27. During the past 12 months, did you ever **seriously** consider attempting suicide?
    - (A) Yes
    - (B) No

28. During the past 12 months, did you make a plan about how you would attempt suicide?
    - (A) Yes
    - (B) No

29. During the past 12 months, how many times did you actually attempt suicide?
    - (A) 0 times
    - (B) 1 time
    - (C) 2 or 3 times
    - (D) 4 or 5 times
    - (E) 6 or more times

## GHB

A depressant approved for use in the treatment of narcolepsy, a disorder that causes daytime "sleep attacks." *For more information, see the* Club Drugs Drug Facts.

| Street Names | Commercial Names | Common Forms | Common Ways Taken | DEA Schedule |
|---|---|---|---|---|
| G, Georgia Home Boy, Goop, Grievous Bodily Harm, Liquid Ecstasy, Liquid X, Soap, Scoop | Gamma-hydroxybutyrate or sodium oxybate (Xyrem®) | Colorless liquid, white powder | Swallowed (often combined with alcohol or other beverages) | I |

### POSSIBLE HEALTH EFFECTS

| | |
|---|---|
| Short-term | Euphoria, drowsiness, decreased anxiety, confusion, memory loss, hallucinations, excited and aggressive behavior, nausea, vomiting, unconsciousness, seizures, slowed heart rate and breathing, lower body temperature, coma, death. |
| Long-term | Unknown. |
| Other Health-related Issues | Sometimes used as a date rape drug. |
| In Combination with Alcohol | Nausea, problems with breathing, greatly increased depressant effects. |
| Withdrawal Symptoms | Insomnia, anxiety, tremors, sweating, increased heart rate and blood pressure, psychotic thoughts. |

### TREATMENT OPTIONS

| | |
|---|---|
| Medications | Benzodiazepines |
| Behavioral Therapies | More research is needed to find out if behavioral therapies can be used to treat GHB addiction. |

## Hallucinogens

Drugs that cause profound distortions in a person's perceptions of reality, such as ketamine, LSD, mescaline (peyote), PCP, psilocybin, salvia, DMT, and aya-huasca. For more information, see the Hallucinogens and Dissociative Drugs Research Report.

## Heroin

An opioid drug made from morphine, a natural substance extracted from the seed pod of the Asian opium poppy plant. For more information, see the Heroin Research Report.

| Street Names | Commercial Names | Common Forms | Common Ways Taken | DEA Schedule |
|---|---|---|---|---|
| Brown sugar, China White, Dope, H, Horse, Junk, Skag, Skunk, Smack, White Horse; *With OTC cold medicine and antihistamine:* Cheese | No commercial uses | White or brownish powder, or black sticky substance known as "black tar heroin" | Injected, smoked, snorted | I |

### POSSIBLE HEALTH EFFECTS

| | |
|---|---|
| Short-term | Euphoria; warm flushing of skin; dry mouth; heavy feeling in the hands and feet; clouded thinking; alternate wakeful and drowsy states; itching; nausea; vomiting; slowed breathing and heart rate. |
| Long-term | Collapsed veins; abscesses (swollen tissue with pus); infection of the lining and valves in the heart; constipation and stomach cramps; liver or kidney disease; pneumonia. |
| Other Health-related Issues | Pregnancy: miscarriage, low birth weight, neonatal abstinence syndrome. Risk of HIV, hepatitis, and other infectious diseases from shared needles. |
| In Combination with Alcohol | Dangerous slowdown of heart rate and breathing, coma, death. |
| Withdrawal Symptoms | Restlessness, muscle and bone pain, insomnia, diarrhea, vomiting, cold flashes with goose bumps ("cold turkey"), leg movements. |

### TREATMENT OPTIONS

| | |
|---|---|
| Medications | • Methadone<br>• Buprenorphine<br>• Naltrexone (short and long-acting forms) |
| Behavioral Therapies | • Contingency management, or motivational incentives<br>• 12-Step facilitation therapy |

## Inhalants

Solvents, aerosols, and gases found in household products such as spray paints, markers, glues, and cleaning fluids; also nitrites (e.g., amyl nitrite), which are prescription medications for chest pain. For more information, see the Inhalants Research Report.

| Street Names | Commercial Names | Common Forms | Common Ways Taken | DEA Schedule |
|---|---|---|---|---|
| Poppers, snappers, whippets, laughing gas | Various | Paint thinners or removers, degreasers, dry-cleaning fluids, gasoline, lighter fluids, correction fluids, permanent markers, electronics cleaners and freeze sprays, glue, spray paint, hair or deodorant sprays, fabric protector sprays, aerosol computer cleaning products, vegetable oil sprays, butane lighters, propane tanks, whipped cream aerosol containers, refrigerant gases, ether, chloroform, halothane, nitrous oxide | Inhaled through the nose or mouth | Not scheduled |

### POSSIBLE HEALTH EFFECTS

| | |
|---|---|
| Short-term | Confusion; nausea; slurred speech; lack of coordination; euphoria; dizziness; drowsiness; disinhibition, light-headedness, hallucinations/delusions; headaches; sudden sniffing death due to heart failure (from butane, propane, and other chemicals in aerosols); death from asphyxiation, suffocation, convulsions or seizures, coma, or choking. Nitrites: enlarged blood vessels, enhanced sexual pleasure, increased heart rate, brief sensation of heat and excitement, dizziness, headache. |
| Long-term | Liver and kidney damage; bone marrow damage; limb spasms due to nerve damage; brain damage from lack of oxygen that can cause problems with thinking, movement, vision, and hearing. Nitrites: increased risk of pneumonia. |
| Other Health-related Issues | Pregnancy: low birth weight, bone problems, delayed behavioral development due to brain problems, altered metabolism and body composition. |
| In Combination with Alcohol | Nitrites: dangerously low blood pressure. |
| Withdrawal Symptoms | Nausea, loss of appetite, sweating, tics, problems sleeping, and mood changes. |

### TREATMENT OPTIONS

| | |
|---|---|
| Medications | There are no FDA-approved medications to treat inhalant addiction. |
| Behavioral Therapies | More research is needed to find out if behavioral therapies can be used to treat inhalant addiction. |

## Ketamine

A dissociative drug used as an anesthetic in veterinary practice. Dissociative drugs are hallucinogens that cause the user to feel detached from reality. For more information, see the Hallucinogens and Dissociative Drugs Research Report.

| Street Names | Commercial Names | Common Forms | Common Ways Taken | DEA Schedule |
|---|---|---|---|---|
| Cat Valium, K, Special K, Vitamin K | Ketalar® | Liquid, white powder | Injected, snorted, smoked (powder added to tobacco or marijuana cigarettes), swallowed | III |

### POSSIBLE HEALTH EFFECTS

| | |
|---|---|
| Short-term | Problems with attention, learning, and memory; dreamlike states, hallucinations; sedation; confusion and problems speaking; loss of memory; problems moving, to the point of being immobile; raised blood pressure; unconsciousness; slowed breathing that can lead to death. |
| Long-term | Ulcers and pain in the bladder; kidney problems; stomach pain; depression; poor memory. |
| Other Health-related Issues | Sometimes used as a date rape drug. Risk of HIV, hepatitis, and other infectious diseases from shared needles. |
| In Combination with Alcohol | Increased risk of adverse effects. |
| Withdrawal Symptoms | Unknown. |

### TREATMENT OPTIONS

| | |
|---|---|
| Medications | There are no FDA-approved medications to treat addiction to ketamine or other dissociative drugs. |
| Behavioral Therapies | More research is needed to find out if behavioral therapies can be used to treat addiction to dissociative drugs. |

## LSD

A hallucinogen manufactured from lysergic acid, which is found in ergot, a fungus that grows on rye and other grains. LSD is an abbreviation of the scientific name, *lysergic acid diethylamide.* For more information, see the Hallucinogens and Dissociative Drugs Research Report.

| Street Names | Commercial Names | Common Forms | Common Ways Taken | DEA Schedule |
|---|---|---|---|---|
| Acid, Blotter, Blue Heaven, Cubes, Microdot, Yellow Sunshine | No commercial uses | Tablet; capsule; clear liquid; small, decorated squares of absorbent paper that liquid has been added to | Swallowed, absorbed through mouth tissues (paper squares) | I |

### POSSIBLE HEALTH EFFECTS

| | |
|---|---|
| Short-term | Rapid emotional swings; distortion of a person's ability to recognize reality, think rationally, or communicate with others; raised blood pressure, heart rate, body temperature; dizziness and insomnia; loss of appetite; dry mouth; sweating; numbness; weakness; tremors; enlarged pupils. |
| Long-term | Frightening flashbacks (called Hallucinogen Persisting Perception Disorder ([HPPD]); ongoing visual disturbances, disorganized thinking, paranoia, and mood swings. |
| Other Health-related Issues | Unknown. |
| In Combination with Alcohol | May decrease the perceived effects of alcohol. |
| Withdrawal Symptoms | Unknown. |

### TREATMENT OPTIONS

| | |
|---|---|
| Medications | There are no FDA-approved medications to treat addiction to LSD or other hallucinogens. |
| Behavioral Therapies | More research is needed to find out if behavioral therapies can be used to treat addiction to hallucinogens. |

## Marijuana (Cannabis)

Marijuana is made from the hemp plant, *Cannabis sativa.* The main psychoactive (mind-altering) chemical in marijuana is delta-9-tetrahydrocannabinol, or THC. For more information, see the Marijuana Research Report.

| Street Names | Commercial Names | Common Forms | Common Ways Taken | DEA Schedule |
|---|---|---|---|---|
| Blunt, Bud, Dope, Ganja, Grass, Green, Herb, Joint, Mary Jane, Pot, Reefer, Sinsemilla, Skunk, Smoke, Trees, Weed; Hashish: Boom, Gangster, Hash, Hemp | Various brand names in states where the sale of marijuana is legal | Greenish-gray mixture of dried, shredded leaves, stems, seeds, and/or flowers; resin (hashish) or sticky, black liquid (hash oil) | Smoked, eaten (mixed in food or brewed as tea) | I |

### POSSIBLE HEALTH EFFECTS

| | |
|---|---|
| Short-term | Enhanced sensory perception and euphoria followed by drowsiness/relaxation; slowed reaction time; problems with balance and coordination; increased heart rate and appetite; problems with learning and memory; hallucinations; anxiety; panic attacks; psychosis. |
| Long-term | Mental health problems; chronic cough; frequent respiratory infections. |
| Other Health-related Issues | Youth: possible loss of IQ points when repeated use begins in adolescence. Pregnancy: babies born with problems with attention, memory, and problem solving. |
| In Combination with Alcohol | Increased heart rate, blood pressure; further slowing of mental processing and reaction time. |
| Withdrawal Symptoms | Irritability, trouble sleeping, decreased appetite, anxiety. |

### TREATMENT OPTIONS

| | |
|---|---|
| Medications | There are no FDA-approved medications to treat marijuana addiction. |
| Behavioral Therapies | • Cognitive-behavioral therapy (CBT) <br> • Contingency management, or motivational incentives <br> • Motivational Enhancement Therapy (MET) <br> • Behavioral treatments geared to adolescents |

## MDMA (Ecstasy/Molly)

A synthetic, psychoactive drug that has similarities to both the stimulant amphetamine and the hallucinogen mescaline. MDMA is an abbreviation of the scientific name, *3,4-methylenedioxy-methamphetamine*. For more information, see the MDMA (Ecstasy) Abuse Research Report.

| Street Names | Commercial Names | Common Forms | Common Ways Taken | DEA Schedule |
|---|---|---|---|---|
| Adam, Clarity, Eve, Lover's Speed, Peace, Uppers | No commercial uses | Colorful tablets with imprinted logos, capsules, powder, liquid | Swallowed, snorted | I |

### POSSIBLE HEALTH EFFECTS

| | |
|---|---|
| Short-term | Lowered inhibition; enhanced sensory perception; confusion; depression; sleep problems; anxiety; increased heart rate and blood pressure; muscle tension; teeth clenching; nausea; blurred vision; faintness; chills or sweating; sharp rise in body temperature leading to liver, kidney, or heart failure and death. |
| Long-term | Long-lasting confusion, depression, problems with attention, memory, and sleep; increased anxiety, impulsiveness, aggression; loss of appetite; less interest in sex. |
| Other Health-related Issues | Unknown. |
| In Combination with Alcohol | May increase the risk of cell and organ damage. |
| Withdrawal Symptoms | Fatigue, loss of appetite, depression, trouble concentrating. |

### TREATMENT OPTIONS

| | |
|---|---|
| Medications | There is conflicting evidence about whether MDMA is addictive. There are no FDA-approved medications to treat MDMA addiction. |
| Behavioral Therapies | More research is needed to find out if behavioral therapies can be used to treat MDMA addiction. |

## Mescaline (Peyote)

A hallucinogen found in disk-shaped "buttons" in the crown of several cacti, including peyote. For more information, see the Hallucinogens – LSD, Peyote, Psilocybin, and PCP Drug Facts.

| Street Names | Commercial Names | Common Forms | Common Ways Taken | DEA Schedule |
|---|---|---|---|---|
| Buttons, Cactus, Mesc | No commercial uses | Fresh or dried buttons, capsule | Swallowed (chewed or soaked in water and drunk) | I |

### POSSIBLE HEALTH EFFECTS

| | |
|---|---|
| Short-term | Enhanced perception and feeling; hallucinations; euphoria; anxiety; increased body temperature, heart rate, blood pressure; sweating; problems with movement. |
| Long-term | Unknown. |
| Other Health-related Issues | Unknown. |
| In Combination with Alcohol | Unknown. |
| Withdrawal Symptoms | Unknown. |

### TREATMENT OPTIONS

| | |
|---|---|
| Medications | There are no FDA-approved medications to treat addiction to mescaline or other hallucinogens. |
| Behavioral Therapies | More research is needed to find out if behavioral therapies can be used to treat addiction to hallucinogens. |

## Methamphetamine

An extremely addictive stimulant amphetamine drug. For more information, see the Methamphetamine Research Report.

| Street Names | Commercial Names | Common Forms | Common Ways Taken | DEA Schedule |
|---|---|---|---|---|
| Crank, Chalk, Crystal, Fire, Glass, Go Fast, Ice, Meth, Speed | Desoxyn® | White powder or pill; crystal meth looks like pieces of glass or shiny blue-white "rocks" of different sizes | Swallowed, snorted, smoked, injected | II |

### POSSIBLE HEALTH EFFECTS

| | |
|---|---|
| Short-term | Increased wakefulness and physical activity; decreased appetite; increased breathing, heart rate, blood pressure, temperature; irregular heart beat. |
| Long-term | Anxiety, confusion, insomnia, mood problems, violent behavior; paranoia, hallucinations, delusions, weight loss, severe dental problems ("meth mouth"), intense itching leading to skin sores from scratching. |
| Other Health-related Issues | Pregnancy: premature delivery; separation of the placenta from the uterus; low birth weight; lethargy; heart and brain problems. Risk of HIV, hepatitis, and other infectious diseases from shared needles. |
| In Combination with Alcohol | Masks the depressant effect of alcohol, increasing risk of alcohol overdose; may increase blood pressure and jitters. |
| Withdrawal Symptoms | Depression, anxiety, tiredness. |

### TREATMENT OPTIONS

| | |
|---|---|
| Medications | There are no FDA-approved medications to treat methamphetamine addiction. |
| Behavioral Therapies | • Cognitive-behavioral therapy (CBT)<br>• Contingency management or motivational incentives<br>• The matrix model<br>• 12-Step facilitation therapy |

## Over-the-counter Cough/Cold Medicines (Dextromethorphan or DMX)

Psychoactive when taken in higher-than-recommended amounts. For more information, see the Cough and Cold Medicine Abuse Drug Facts.

| Street Names | Commercial Names | Common Forms | Common Ways Taken | DEA Schedule |
|---|---|---|---|---|
| Robotripping, Robo, Triple C | Various (many brand names include "DM") | Syrup, capsule | Swallowed | Not scheduled |

### POSSIBLE HEALTH EFFECTS

| | |
|---|---|
| Short-term | Euphoria; slurred speech; increased heart rate, blood pressure, temperature; numbness; dizziness; nausea; vomiting; confusion; paranoia; altered visual perceptions; problems with movement; buildup of excess acid in body fluids. |
| Long-term | Unknown. |
| Other Health-related Issues | Breathing problems, seizures, and increased heart rate may occur from other ingredients in cough/cold medicines. |
| In Combination with Alcohol | Increased risk of adverse effects. |
| Withdrawal Symptoms | Unknown. |

### TREATMENT OPTIONS

| | |
|---|---|
| Medications | There are no FDA-approved medications to treat addiction to over-the-counter cough/cold medicines. |
| Behavioral Therapies | More research is needed to find out if behavioral therapies can be used to treat addiction to over-the-counter cough/cold medicines. |

## PCP

A dissociative drug developed as an intravenous anesthetic that has been discontinued due to serious adverse effects. Dissociative drugs are hallucinogens that cause the user to feel detached from reality. PCP is an abbreviation of the scientific name, *phencyclidine*. For more information, see the Hallucinogens and Dissociative Drugs Research Report.

| Street Names | Commercial Names | Common Forms | Common Ways Taken | DEA Schedule |
|---|---|---|---|---|
| Angel Dust, Boat, Hog, Love Boat, Peace Pill | No commercial uses | White or colored powder, tablet, or capsule; clear liquid | Injected, snorted, swallowed, smoked (powder added to mint, parsley, oregano, or marijuana) | I, II |

### POSSIBLE HEALTH EFFECTS

| | |
|---|---|
| Short-term | Delusions, hallucinations, paranoia, problems thinking, a sense of distance from one's environment, anxiety. |
| | Low doses: slight increase in breathing rate; increased blood pressure and heart rate; shallow breathing; face redness and sweating; numbness of the hands or feet; problems with movement. |
| | High doses: lowered blood pressure, pulse rate, breathing rate; nausea; vomiting, blurred vision; flicking up and down of the eyes; drooling; loss of balance; dizziness; violence; suicidal thoughts; seizures, coma, and death. |
| Long-term | Memory loss, problems with speech and thinking, depression, weight loss, anxiety. |
| Other Health-related Issues | PCP has been linked to self-injury. |
| | Risk of HIV, hepatitis, and other infectious diseases from shared needles. |
| In Combination with Alcohol | Increased risk of coma. |
| Withdrawal Symptoms | Headaches, sweating. |

### TREATMENT OPTIONS

| | |
|---|---|
| Medications | There are no FDA-approved medications to treat addiction to PCP or other dissociative drugs. |
| Behavioral Therapies | More research is needed to find out if behavioral therapies can be used to treat addiction to dissociative drugs. |

## Prescription Opioids

Pain relievers with an origin similar to that of heroin. Opioids can cause euphoria and are often used nonmedically, leading to overdose deaths. For more information, see the Prescription Drug Abuse Research Report.

| Street Names | Commercial Names (Common) | Common Forms | Common Ways Taken | DEA Schedule |
|---|---|---|---|---|
| Captain Cody, Cody, Lean, Schoolboy, Sizzurp, Purple Drank; *With glutethimide:* Doors & Fours, Loads, Pancakes and Syrup | Codeine (various brand names) | Tablet, capsule, liquid | Injected, swallowed (often mixed with soda and flavorings) | II, III, V |
| Apache, China Girl, China White, Dance Fever, Friend, Goodfella, Jackpot, Murder 8, Tango and Cash, TNT | Fentanyl (Actiq®, Duragesic®, Sublimaze®) | Lozenge, sublingual tablet, film, buccal tablet | Injected, smoked, snorted | II |
| Vike, Watson-387 | Hydrocodone or dihydrocodeinone (Vicodin®, Lortab®, Lorcet®, and others) | Capsule, liquid, tablet | Swallowed, snorted, injected | II |
| D, Dillies, Footballs, Juice, Smack | Hydromorphone (Dilaudid®) | Liquid, suppository | Injected, rectal | II |
| Demmies, Pain Killer | Meperidine (Demerol®) | Tablet, liquid | Swallowed, snorted, injected | II |
| Amidone, Fizzies With MDMA: Chocolate Chip Cookies | Methadone (Dolophine®, Methadose®) | Tablet, dispersible tablet, liquid | Swallowed, injected | II |
| M, Miss Emma, Monkey, White Stuff | Morphine (Duramorph®, Roxanol®) | Tablet, liquid, capsule, suppository | Injected, swallowed, smoked | II, III |
| O.C., Oxycet, Oxycotton, Oxy, Hillbilly Heroin, Percs | Oxycodone (OxyContin®, Percodan®, Percocet®, and others) | Capsule, liquid, tablet | Swallowed, snorted, injected | II |
| Biscuits, Blue Heaven, Blues, Mrs. O, O Bomb, Octagons, Stop Signs | Oxymorphone (Opana®) | Tablet | Swallowed, snorted, injected | II |

*Continued*

## Prescription Opioids—cont'd

### POSSIBLE HEALTH EFFECTS

| | |
|---|---|
| **Short-term** | Pain relief, drowsiness, nausea, constipation, euphoria, confusion, slowed breathing, death. |
| **Long-term** | Unknown. |
| **Other Health-related Issues** | Pregnancy: Miscarriage; low birth weight; neonatal abstinence syndrome. |
| | Older Adults: Higher risk of accidental misuse or abuse because many older adults have multiple prescriptions, increasing the risk of drug-drug interactions, and breakdown of drugs slows with age; also, many older adults are treated with prescription medications for pain. |
| | Risk of HIV, hepatitis, and other infectious diseases from shared needles. |
| **In Combination with Alcohol** | Dangerous slowing of heart rate and breathing leading to coma or death. |
| **Withdrawal Symptoms** | Restlessness, muscle and bone pain, insomnia, diarrhea, vomiting, cold flashes with goose bumps ("cold turkey"), leg movements. |

### TREATMENT OPTIONS

| | |
|---|---|
| **Medications** | • Methadone |
| | • Buprenorphine |
| | • Naltrexone (short- and long-acting) |
| **Behavioral Therapies** | Behavioral therapies that have helped treat addiction to heroin may be useful in treating prescription opioid addiction. |

## Prescription Sedatives (tranquilizers, depressants)

Medications that slow brain activity, which makes them useful for treating anxiety and sleep problems. For more information, see the Prescription Drug Abuse Research Report.

| Street Names | Commercial Names (Common) | Common Forms | Common Ways Taken | DEA Schedule |
|---|---|---|---|---|
| Barbs, Phennies, Red Birds, Reds, Tooies, Yellow Jackets, Yellows | Barbiturates: pentobarbital (Nembutal®), phenobarbital (Luminal®) | Pill, capsule, liquid | Swallowed, injected | II, III, IV |
| Candy, Downers, Sleeping Pills, Tranks | Benzodiazepines: alprazolam (Xanax®), chlorodiazepoxide (Limbitrol®), diazepam (Valium®), lorazepam (Ativan®), triazolam (Halicon®) | Pill, capsule, liquid | Swallowed, snorted | IV |
| Forget-me Pill, Mexican Valium, R2, Roche, Roofies, Roofinol, Rope, Rophies | Sleep Medications: eszopiclone (Lunesta®), zaleplon (Sonata®), zolpidem (Ambien®) | Pill, capsule, liquid | Swallowed, snorted | IV |

### POSSIBLE HEALTH EFFECTS

| | |
|---|---|
| **Short-term** | Drowsiness, slurred speech, poor concentration, confusion, dizziness, problems with movement and memory, lowered blood pressure, slowed breathing. |
| **Long-term** | Unknown. |
| **Other Health-related Issues** | Sleep medications are sometimes used as date rape drugs. |
| | Risk of HIV, hepatitis, and other infectious diseases from shared needles. |
| **In Combination with Alcohol** | Further slows heart rate and breathing, which can lead to death. |
| **Withdrawal Symptoms** | Must be discussed with a health care provider; barbiturate withdrawal can cause a serious abstinence syndrome that may even include seizures. |

### TREATMENT OPTIONS

| | |
|---|---|
| **Medications** | There are no FDA-approved medications to treat addiction to prescription sedatives; lowering the dose over time must be done with the help of a health care provider. |
| **Behavioral Therapies** | More research is needed to find out if behavioral therapies can be used to treat addiction to prescription sedatives. |

## Prescription Stimulants

Medications that increase alertness, attention, energy, blood pressure, heart rate, and breathing rate. For more information, see the Prescription Drug Abuse Research Report.

| Street Names | Commercial Names (Common) | Common Forms | Common Ways Taken | DEA Schedule |
|---|---|---|---|---|
| Bennies, Black Beauties, Crosses, Hearts, LA Turnaround, Speed, Truck Drivers, Uppers | Amphetamine (Adderall®, Benzedrine®) | Tablet, capsule | Swallowed, snorted, smoked, injected | II |
| JIF, MPH, R-ball, Skippy, The Smart Drug, Vitamin R | Methylphenidate (Concerta®, Ritalin®) | Liquid, tablet, chewable tablet, capsule | Swallowed, snorted, smoked, injected, chewed | II |

### POSSIBLE HEALTH EFFECTS

| | |
|---|---|
| Short-term | Increased alertness, attention, energy; increased blood pressure and heart rate; narrowed blood vessels; increased blood sugar; opened-up breathing passages. |
| | High doses: dangerously high body temperature and irregular heartbeat; heart failure; seizures. |
| Long-term | Heart problems, psychosis, anger, paranoia. |
| Other Health-related Issues | Risk of HIV, hepatitis, and other infectious diseases from shared needles. |
| In Combination with Alcohol | Masks the depressant action of alcohol, increasing risk of alcohol overdose; may increase blood pressure and jitters. |
| Withdrawal Symptoms | Depression, tiredness, sleep problems. |

### TREATMENT OPTIONS

| | |
|---|---|
| Medications | There are no FDA-approved medications to treat stimulant addiction. |
| Behavioral Therapies | Behavioral therapies that have helped treat addiction to cocaine or methamphetamine may be useful in treating prescription stimulant addiction. |

## Psilocybin

A hallucinogen in certain types of mushrooms that grow in parts of South America, Mexico, and the United States. For more information, see the Hallucinogens and Dissociative Drugs Research Report.

| Street Names | Commercial Names | Common Forms | Common Ways Taken | DEA Schedule |
|---|---|---|---|---|
| Little Smoke, Magic Mushrooms, Purple Passion, Shrooms | No commercial uses | Fresh or dried mushrooms with long, slender stems topped by caps with dark gills | Swallowed (eaten, brewed as tea, or added to other foods) | I |

### POSSIBLE HEALTH EFFECTS

| | |
|---|---|
| Short-term | Hallucinations, altered perception of time, inability to tell fantasy from reality, panic, muscle relaxation or weakness, problems with movement, enlarged pupils, nausea, vomiting, drowsiness. |
| Long-term | Risk of flashbacks and memory problems. |
| Other Health-related Issues | Risk of poisoning if a poisonous mushroom is accidentally used. |
| In Combination with Alcohol | May decrease the perceived effects of alcohol. |
| Withdrawal symptoms | Unknown. |

### TREATMENT OPTIONS

| | |
|---|---|
| Medications | It is not known whether psilocybin is addictive. There are no FDA-approved medications to treat addiction to psilocybin or other hallucinogens. |
| Behavioral Therapies | More research is needed to find out if psilocybin is addictive and whether behavioral therapies can be used to treat addiction to this or other hallucinogens. |

## Salvia

A dissociative drug that is an herb in the mint family native to southern Mexico, *Salvia divinorum*. Dissociative drugs are hallucinogens that cause the user to feel detached from reality. For more information, see the Hallucinogens and Dissociative Drugs Research Report.

| Street Names | Commercial Names | Common Forms | Common Ways Taken | DEA Schedule |
|---|---|---|---|---|
| Magic mint, Maria Pastora, Sally-D, Shepherdess's Herb, Diviner's Sage | Sold legally in most states as *Salvia divinorum*. | Fresh or dried leaves | Smoked, chewed, or brewed as tea | Not Scheduled (but labeled drug of concern by DEA and illegal in some states) |

### POSSIBLE HEALTH EFFECTS

| | |
|---|---|
| Short-term | Short-lived but intense hallucinations; altered visual perception, mood, body sensations; mood swings, feelings of detachment from one's body; sweating. |
| Long-term | Unknown. |
| Other Health-related Issues | Unknown. |
| In Combination with Alcohol | Unknown. |
| Withdrawal Symptoms | Unknown. |

### TREATMENT OPTIONS

| | |
|---|---|
| Medications | It is not known whether salvia is addictive. There are no FDA-approved medications to treat addiction to salvia or other dissociative drugs. |
| Behavioral Therapies | More research is needed to find out if salvia is addictive, but behavioral therapies can be used to treat addiction to dissociative drugs. |

## Steroids (Anabolic)

Man-made substances used to treat conditions caused by low levels of steroid hormones in the body and abused to enhance athletic and sexual performance and physical appearance. For more information, see the Anabolic Steroid Abuse Research Report.

| Street Names | Commercial Names (Common) | Common Forms | Common Ways Taken | DEA Schedule |
|---|---|---|---|---|
| Juice, Gym Candy, Pumpers, Roids | Nandrolone (Oxandrin®), oxandrolone (Anadrol®), oxymetholone (Winstrol®), stanozolol (Durabolin®), testosterone cypionate (Depo-testosterone®) | Tablet, capsule, liquid drops, gel, cream, patch, injectable solution | Injected, swallowed, applied to skin | III |

### POSSIBLE HEALTH EFFECTS

| | |
|---|---|
| Short-term | Headache, acne, fluid retention (especially in the hands and feet), oily skin, yellowing of the skin and whites of the eyes, infection at the injection site. |
| Long-term | Kidney damage or failure; liver damage; high blood pressure, enlarged heart, or changes in cholesterol leading to increased risk of stroke or heart attack, even in young people; aggression; extreme mood swings; anger ("roid rage"); paranoid jealousy; extreme irritability; delusions; impaired judgment. |
| Other Health-related Issues | Males: shrunken testicles, lowered sperm count, infertility, baldness, development of breasts, increased risk for prostate cancer.<br>Females: Facial hair, male-pattern baldness, menstrual cycle changes, enlargement of the clitoris, deepened voice.<br>Adolescents: Stunted growth.<br>Risk of HIV, hepatitis, and other infectious diseases from shared needles. |
| In Combination with Alcohol | Increased risk of violent behavior. |
| Withdrawal Symptoms | Mood swings; tiredness; restlessness; loss of appetite; insomnia; lowered sex drive; depression, sometimes leading to suicide attempts. |

### TREATMENT OPTIONS

| | |
|---|---|
| Medications | Hormone therapy |
| Behavioral Therapies | More research is needed to find out if behavioral therapies can be used to treat steroid addiction. |

## Synthetic Cannabinoids ("K2"/"Spice")

A wide variety of herbal mixtures containing man-made cannabinoid chemicals related to THC in marijuana but often much stronger and more dangerous. Sometimes misleadingly called "synthetic marijuana" and marketed as a "natural," "safe," legal alternative to marijuana. For more information, see the Spice ("Synthetic Marijuana") Drug Facts.

| Street Names | Commercial Names | Common Forms | Common Ways Taken | DEA Schedule |
|---|---|---|---|---|
| K2, Spice, Black Mamba, Bliss, Bombay Blue, Fake Weed, Fire, Genie, Moon Rocks, Skunk, Smacked, Yucatan, Zohai | No commercial uses | Dried, shredded plant material that looks like potpourri and is sometimes sold as "incense" | Smoked, swallowed (brewed as tea) | I |

### POSSIBLE HEALTH EFFECTS

| | |
|---|---|
| Short-term | Increased heart rate; vomiting; agitation; confusion; hallucinations, anxiety, paranoia; increased blood pressure and reduced blood supply to the heart; heart attack. |
| Long-term | Unknown. |
| Other Health-related Issues | Use of synthetic cannabinoids has led to an increase in emergency room visits in certain areas. |
| In Combination with Alcohol | Unknown. |
| Withdrawal Symptoms | Headaches, anxiety, depression, irritability. |

### TREATMENT OPTIONS

| | |
|---|---|
| Medications | There are no FDA-approved medications to treat K2/spice addiction. |
| Behavioral Therapies | More research is needed to find out if behavioral therapies can be used to treat synthetic cannabinoid addiction. |

## Tobacco

Plant grown for its leaves, which are dried and fermented before use. For more information, see the Tobacco/Nicotine Research Report.

| Street Names | Commercial Names | Common Forms | Common Ways Taken | DEA Schedule |
|---|---|---|---|---|
| None | Multiple brand names | cigarettes, cigars, bidis, hookahs, smokeless tobacco (snuff, spit tobacco, chew) | Smoked, snorted, chewed, vaporized | Not Scheduled |

### POSSIBLE HEALTH EFFECTS

| | |
|---|---|
| Short-term | Increased blood pressure, breathing, and heart rate. |
| Long-term | Greatly increased risk of cancer, especially lung cancer when smoked and oral cancers when chewed; chronic bronchitis; emphysema; heart disease; leukemia; cataracts; pneumonia. |
| Other Health-related Issues | Pregnancy: miscarriage, low birth weight, premature delivery, stillbirth, learning and behavior problems. |
| In Combination with Alcohol | Unknown. |
| Withdrawal symptoms | Irritability, attention and sleep problems, increased appetite. |

### TREATMENT OPTIONS

| | |
|---|---|
| Medications | • Bupropion (Zyban®)<br>• Varenicline (Chantix®)<br>• Nicotine replacement (gum, patch, lozenge) |
| Behavioral Therapies | • Cognitive-behavioral therapy (CBT)<br>• Self-help materials<br>• Mail, phone, and Internet quit resources |

# Friedman Family Assessment Model (Short Form)

Before using the following guidelines in completing family assessments, two words of caution. First, not all areas included below will be germane for each of the families visited. The guidelines are comprehensive and allow depth when probing is necessary. The student should not feel that every sub-area needs to be covered when the broad area of inquiry poses no problems to the family or concern to the health worker. Second, by virtue of the interdependence of the family system, one will find unavoidable redundancy. For the sake of efficiency, the assessor should try not to repeat data, but to refer the reader back to sections where this information has already been described.

## IDENTIFYING DATA

1. Family Name
2. Address and Phone
3. Family Composition (see table)
4. Type of Family Form
5. Cultural (Ethnic) Background
6. Religious Identification
7. Social Class Status
8. Family's Recreational or Leisure-Time Activities

## DEVELOPMENTAL STAGE AND HISTORY OF FAMILY

9. Family's Present Developmental Stage
10. Extent of Developmental Tasks Fulfillment
11. Nuclear Family History
12. History of Family of Origin of Both Parents

## ENVIRONMENTAL DATA

13. Characteristics of Home
14. Characteristics of Neighborhood and Larger Community
15. Family's Geographic Mobility
16. Family's Associations and Transactions with Community
17. Family's Social Support Network (Ecomap)

## FAMILY STRUCTURE

18. Communication Patterns
    Extent of Functional and Dysfunctional Communication (Types of recurring patterns)
    Extent of Emotional (Affective) Messages and How Expressed
    Characteristics of Communication within Family Subsystems
    Extent of Congruent and Incongruent Messages
    Types of Dysfunctional Communication Processes Seen in Family
    Areas of Open and Closed Communication
    Familial and External Variables Affecting Communication
19. Power Structure
    Power Outcomes
    Decision-Making Process
    Power Bases
    Variables Affecting Family Power
    Overall Family System and Subsystem Power
20. Role Structure
    Formal Role Structure
    Informal Role Structure
    Analysis of Role Models (Optional)
    Variables Affecting Role Structure
21. Family Values
    Compare the Family to American or Family's Reference Group Values and/or Identify Important Family Values and Their Importance (Priority) in Family
    Congruence Between the Family's Values and the Family's Reference Group or Wider Community
    Congruence Between the Family's Values and Family Member's Values
    Variables Influencing Family Values
    Values Consciously or Unconsciously Held
    Presence of Value Conflicts in Family
    Effect of the Above Values and Value Conflicts on Health Status of Family

## FAMILY FUNCTIONS

22. Affective Function
    Family's Need-Response Patterns
    Mutual Nurturance, Closeness, and Identification
    Separateness and Connectedness
23. Socialization Function
    Family Child-Rearing Practices
    Adaptability of Child-Rearing Practices for Family Form and Family's Situation
    Who Is (Are) Socializing Agent(s) for Child(ren)?
    Value of Children in Family
    Cultural Beliefs That Influence Family's Child-Rearing Patterns

Social Class Influence on Child-Rearing Patterns

Estimation About Whether Family Is At Risk for Child-Rearing Problems and, if so, Indication of High-Risk Factors

Adequacy of Home Environment for Children's Needs to Play

24. Health Care Function

Family's Health Beliefs, Values, and Behavior

Family's Definitions of Health-Illness and Their Level of Knowledge

Family's Perceived Health Status and Illness Susceptibility

Family's Dietary Practices

Adequacy of Family Diet (Recommended 24-hour food history record)

Function of Mealtimes and Attitudes Toward Food and Mealtimes

Shopping (and its planning) Practices

Person(s) Responsible for Planning, Shopping, and Preparation of Meals

Sleep and Rest Habits

Physical Activity and Recreation Practices (not covered earlier)

Family's Drug Habits

Family's Role in Self-Care Practices

Medically Based Preventive Measures (Physicals, eye and hearing tests, and immunizations)

Dental Health Practices

Family Health History (Both general and specific diseases—environmentally and genetically related)

Health Care Services Received

Feelings and Perceptions Regarding Health Services

Emergency Health Services

Source of Payments for Health and Other Services

Logistics of Receiving Care

## FAMILY STRESS AND COPING

25. Short- and Long-Term Familial Stressors and Strengths

26. Extent of Family's Ability to Respond, Based on Objective Appraisal of Stress-Producing Situations

27. Coping Strategies Utilized (Present/past)

Differences in Family Members' Ways of Coping

Family's Inner Coping Strategies

Family's External Coping Strategies

28. Dysfunctional Adaptive Strategies Utilized (Present/past; extent of usage)

## FAMILY COMPOSITION FORM

| Name (Last, First) | Gender | Relationship | Date and Place of Birth | Occupation | Education |
| --- | --- | --- | --- | --- | --- |
| 1. (Father) | | | | | |
| 2. (Mother) | | | | | |
| 3. (Oldest child) | | | | | |
| 4. | | | | | |
| 5. | | | | | |
| 6. | | | | | |
| 7. | | | | | |
| 8. | | | | | |

From Friedman MM, Bowden VR, Jones EG: *Family nursing: research, theory, and practice*, ed. 5. Stamford, CT, 2003, Prentice Hall.

# Instrumental Activities of Daily Living (IADL) Scale

Name _____  Rated by _____  Date _____

**1. Can you use the telephone**
without help, ........................................................... 3
with some help, or .................................................. 2
are you completely unable to use the telephone? .... 1

**2. Can you get to places beyond walking distance**
without help, ........................................................... 3
with some help, or .................................................. 2
are you completely unable to travel unless special arrangements are made? .... 1

**3. Can you go shopping for groceries**
without help, ........................................................... 3
with some help, or .................................................. 2
are you completely unable to do any shopping? ...... 1

**4. Can you prepare your own meals**
without help, ........................................................... 3
with some help, or .................................................. 2
are you completely unable to prepare any meals? ... 1

**5. Can you do your own housework**
without help, ........................................................... 3
with some help, or .................................................. 2
are you completely unable to do any housework? .... 1

**6. Can you do your own handyman work**
without help, ........................................................... 3
with some help, or .................................................. 2
are you completely unable to do any handyman work? .... 1

**7. Can you do your own laundry**
without help, ........................................................... 3
with some help, or .................................................. 2
are you completely unable to do any laundry at all? .... 1

**8a. Do you take medicines or use any medications?**
Yes (If yes, answer Question 8b.) ........................... 1
No (If no, answer Question 8c.) ............................... 2

**8b. Do you take your own medicine**
without help (in the right doses at the right time), ... 3
with some help (if someone prepares it for you and/or reminds you to take it), or .... 2
are you completely unable to take your own medicine? .... 1

**8c. If you had to take medicine, could you do it**
without help (in the right doses at the right time), ... 3
with some help (if someone prepared it for you and/or reminded you to take it), or .... 2
would you be completely unable to take your own medicine? .... 1

**9. Can you manage your own money**
without help, ........................................................... 3
with some help, or .................................................. 2
are you completely unable to manage money? ......... 1

From Philadelphia Geriatric Center, Philadelphia, PA. Used with permission.

# Comprehensive Older Persons' Evaluation

---

Name (print): _____ Date of visit: _____

Chief complaint: _____

---

Today, I will ask you about your overall health and function and will be using a questionnaire to help me obtain this information. The first few questions are to check your memory.

**Preliminary Cognition Questionnaire:** Record if answer is correct with (+); if answer is incorrect with (−).

1. What is the date today? _____
2. What day of the week is it? _____
3. What is the name of this place? _____
4. What is your telephone number or room number?
   Record answer: _____
   If subject does not have phone, ask:
   What is your street address? _____
5. How old are you? Record answer: ____ _____
6. When were you born? Record answer from records if patient cannot answer: ____ _____
7. Who is the president of the United States now? _____

8. Who was the president just before him? _____
9. What was your mother's maiden name? _____
10. Subtract 3 from 20 and keep subtracting from each new number until you get all the way down _____
    Total errors: ____

If more than 4 errors, ask 11. If more than 6 errors, complete questionnaire for informant.

11. Do you think you would benefit from a legal guardian, someone who would be responsible for your legal and financial matters? Do you have a living will? Would you like one?
    a. no
    b. has functioning legal guardian for sole purpose of managing money—describe:
    c. has legal guardian
    d. yes

---

From Pearlman R: Development of a functional assessment questionnaire for geriatric patients: the comprehensive older persons evaluation, *J Chronic Disease* 40(56): 85S–94S, 1987.

Comprehensive Older Persons' Evaluation—cont'd

**Demographic Section:**

1. Patient's race or ethnic background—record: _____

2. Patient's gender (circle)    male    female

3. How far did you go in school?
   a. post-graduate education
   b. four-year degree
   c. college or technical school
   d. high school complete
   e. high school incomplete
   f. 0-8 years

**Social Support Section:** Now there are a few questions about your family and friends.

4. Are you married, widowed, separated, divorced, or have you never been married?
   a. now married
   b. widowed
   c. separated
   d. divorced
   e. never married

5. Who lives with you? (circle all responses)
   a. spouse
   b. other relative or friend—specify: _____
   c. group living situation (non-health)
   d. lives alone
   e. nursing home, number of years: _____

6. Have you talked to any friends or relatives by phone during the last week?
   a. yes
   b. no

7. Are you satisfied by seeing your relatives and friends as often as you want to, or are you somewhat dissatisfied about how little you see them?
   a. satisfied—skip to #8
   b. dissatisfied—ask A
      A. Do you feel you would like to be involved in a Senior Citizens Center for social events, or perhaps meals?
         1. no
         2. is involved—describe: _____
         3. yes

8. Is there someone who would take care of you for as long as you needed if you were sick or disabled?
   a. yes—Skip to C
   b. no—Ask A
      A. Is there someone who would take care of you for a short time?
         1. yes—Skip to C
         2. no—Ask B
      B. Is there someone who could help you now and then?
         1. yes—Ask C
         2. no—Ask C
      C. Who would we call in case of an emergency?
         Record name and telephone: _____
         _____

**Financial Section:** The next few questions are about your finances and any problems you might have.

9. Do you own, or are you buying, your own home?
   a. yes—skip to #10
   b. no—ask A
      A. Do you feel you need assistance with housing?
         1. no
         2. has subsidized or other housing assistance
         3. yes—describe: _____
      B. What type of housing did you have prior to coming here?

10. Are you covered by private medical insurance, Medicare, Medicaid, or some disability plan? (Circle all that apply)
    a. private insurance—specify and skip to #11:
       _____
    b. Medicare
    c. Medicaid
    d. disability—specify and ask A:
       _____
    e. none
    f. other—specify: _____
       A. Do you feel you need additional assistance with your medical bills?
          1. no
          2. yes

11. Which of these statements best describes your financial situation?
    a. my bills are no problem to me—skip to #12
    b. my expenses make it difficult to meet my bills—ask A
    c. my expenses are so heavy that I cannot meet my bills—ask A
       A. Do you feel you need financial assistance such as: (circle all that apply)
          1. food stamps
          2. social security or disability payments
          3. assistance in paying your heating or electrical bills
          4. other financial assistance?
             describe: _____

**Psychological Health Section:** The next few questions are about how you feel about your life in general. There are no right or wrong answers, only what best applies to you.
Please answer yes or no to each question.

12. Is your daily life full of things that keep you interested? _____

13. Have you, at times, very much wanted to leave home? _____

14. Does it seem that no one understands you? _____

15. Are you happy most of the time? _____

16. Do you feel weak all over much of the time? _____

17. Is your sleep fitful and disturbed? _____

18. Taking everything into consideration, how would you describe your satisfaction with your life in general at the present time?
    a. good
    b. fair
    c. poor

19. Do you feel you now need help with your mental health; for example, a counselor or psychiatrist?
    a. no
    b. has—specify: _____
    c. yes

**Physical Health Section:** The next few questions are about your health.

20. During the past month (30 days), how many days were you so sick that you couldn't do your usual activities, such as working around the house or visiting with friends? _____

21. Relative to other people your age, how would you rate your overall health at the present time?
    a. excellent—skip to #22
    b. very good—skip to #22
    c. good—ask A
    d. fair—ask A
    e. poor—ask A
       A. Do you feel you need additional medical services such as a doctor, nurse, visiting nurse or physical therapy?
          1. doctor
          2. nurse
          3. visiting nurse

Comprehensive Older Persons' Evaluation—cont'd

    4. physical therapy

    5. none

**22.** Do you use an aid for walking, such as a wheelchair, walker, cane or anything else? (circle aid usually used)

    a. wheelchair

    b. other—specify: _____

    c. visiting nurse

    d. walker

    e. none

**23.** How much do your health troubles stand in the way of your doing things you want to do?

    a. not at all—skip to #24

    b. a little—ask A

    c. a great deal—ask A

      A. Do you think you need assistance to do your daily activities; for example, do you need a live-in aide or choreworker?

        1. live-in aide

        2. choreworker

        3. has aide, choreworker or other assistance—describe:

        _____

        4. none needed

**24.** Have you had, or do you currently have, any of the following health problems? (if yes, place an "X" in appropriate box and describe; medical record information may be used to help complete this section.)

| | HX | Current | Describe |
|---|---|---|---|
| a. Arthritis or rheumatism? | | | |
| b. Lung or breathing problem? | | | |
| c. Hypertension? | | | |
| d. Heart trouble? | | | |
| e. Phlebitis or poor circulation problems in arms or legs? | | | |
| f. Diabetes or low blood sugar? | | | |
| g. Digestive ulcers? | | | |
| h. Other digestive problem? | | | |
| i. Cancer? | | | |
| j. Anemia? | | | |
| k. Effects of stroke? | | | |
| l. Other neurological problem? specify: _____ | | | |
| m. Thyroid or other glandular problem? specify: _____ | | | |
| n. Skin disorders such as pressure sores, leg ulcers, burns? | | | |
| o. Speech problem? | | | |
| p. Hearing problem? | | | |
| q. Vision or eye problem? | | | |
| r. Kidney or bladder problems, or incontinence? | | | |
| s. A problem of falls? | | | |
| t. Problem with eating or your weight? specify: _____ | | | |
| u. Problem with depression? specify: _____ | | | |
| v. Problem with your behavior? specify: _____ | | | |
| w. Problem with your sexual activity? | | | |
| x. Problem with alcohol? | | | |
| y. Problem with pain? | | | |
| z. Other health problems? specify: _____ | | | |

Immunizations: _____

_____

_____

**25.** What medications are you currently taking, or have been taking, in the last month? (May I see your medication bottles?) (If patient cannot list, ask categories a-r and note dosage and schedule, or obtain information from medical or pharmacy records and verify accuracy with the patient.)

Allergies: _____

| | Rx (Dosage and Schedule) |
|---|---|
| a. Arthritis medication | _____ |
| b. Pain medication | _____ |
| c. Blood pressure medication | _____ |
| d. Water pills or pills for fluid | _____ |
| e. Medication for your heart | _____ |
| f. Medication for your lungs | _____ |
| g. Blood thinners | _____ |
| h. Medication for your circulation | _____ |
| i. Insulin or diabetes medication | _____ |
| j. Seizure medication | _____ |
| k. Thyroid pills | _____ |
| l. Steroids | _____ |
| m. Hormones | _____ |
| n. Antibiotics | _____ |
| o. Medicine for nerves or depression | _____ |
| p. Prescription sleeping pills | _____ |
| q. Other prescription drugs | _____ |
| r. Other nonprescription drugs | _____ |

**26.** Many people have problems remembering to take their medications, especially ones they need to take on a regular basis. How often do you forget to take your medications? Would you say you forget often, sometimes, rarely, or never?

    a. never

    b. rarely

    c. sometimes

    d. often

**Activities of Daily Living:** The next set of questions asks whether you need help with any of the following activities of daily living.

**27.** I would like to know whether you can do these activities without any help at all, or if you need assistance to do them. Do you need help to: (If yes, describe, including patient needs.)

| | Yes | No | Describe (include needs) |
|---|---|---|---|
| a. Use the telephone? | | | |
| b. Get to places out of walking distance? (using transportation) | | | |
| c. Shop for clothes and food? | | | |
| d. Do your housework? | | | |
| e. Handle your money? | | | |
| f. Feed yourself? | | | |
| g. Dress and undress yourself? | | | |
| h. Take care of your appearance? | | | |
| i. Get in and out of bed? | | | |
| j. Take a bath or shower? | | | |
| k. Prepare your meals? | | | |
| l. Do you have any problem getting to the bathroom on time? | | | |

**28.** During the past six months, have you had any help with such things as shopping, housework, bathing, dressing and getting around?

    a. yes—specify: _____

    b. no

Signature of person completing the form:

_____

## Comprehensive Occupational and Environmental Health History

### WORK HISTORY

1. List your current and past longest held jobs, including the military:

| Company | Dates Employed | Job Title | Known Exposures |
|---|---|---|---|
| | | | |
| | | | |
| | | | |

2. Do you work full-time?    NO ___    YES ___    How many hours per week? ___

3. Do you work part-time?    NO ___    YES ___    How many hours per week? ___

4. Please describe any health problems or injuries that you have experienced in connection with your present or past jobs:

5. Have you ever had to change jobs because of health problems or injuries?    YES ___    NO ___
   If yes, describe: Did any of your co-workers experience similar problems?

6. In what type of business do you currently work?

7. Describe your work (what you actually do):

8. Have you had any current or past exposure (through breathing or touching) to any of the following?

   __acids                __alkalies               __coal dust             __mercury              __silica powder
   __chlorinated          __chloroprene            __lead                  __radiation            __welding fumes
     naphthalenes         __isocyanates            __phenol                __vibration            __carbon tetrachloride
   __halothane            __perchloroethylene      __trichloroethylene     __beryllium            __fiberglass
   __PBBs                 __TDI or MDI             __asbestos              __ethylene dibromide   __noise (loud)
   __styrene              __ammonia                __cold (severe)         __methylene chloride   __solvents
   __alcohols             __chromates              __manganese             __rock dust            __x-rays
   __chloroform           __ketones                __phosgene              __vinyl chloride
   __heat (severe)        __pesticides             __trinitrotoluene       __cadmium
   __PCBs                 __toluene                __benzene               __ethylene dichloride
   __talc                 __arsenic                __dichlorobenzene       __nickel

9. Did you receive any safety training about these agents?    YES ___    NO ___
   Explain:

10. Are you involved in any work processes such as grinding, welding, soldering, or polishing that create dust, mists, or fumes?
    YES ___    NO ___
    If yes, describe:

11. Did you use any of the following personal protective equipment when exposed?

    __boots               __respirator             __welding mask
    __gloves              __sleeves                __glasses/goggles
    __shield              __earplugs/muffs
    __coveralls           __safety shoes

12. Is your work environment generally clean?   YES ____   NO ____
    If no, describe:

13. What ventilation systems are used in your workplace?

14. Do they seem to work? Are you aware of any chemical odors in your environment (if so, explain)?

15. Where do you eat, smoke, and take your breaks when you are on the job?

16. Do you use a uniform or have clothing that you wear only to work?   YES ____   NO ____

17. How is your work clothing laundered (at home, by employer, etc.)?

18. How often do you wash your hands at work and how do you wash them (running water, special soaps, etc.)?

19. Do you shower before leaving the worksite?   YES ____   NO ____

20. Do you have any physical symptoms associated with work?   YES ____   NO ____
    If yes, describe:

21. Are other workers similarly affected?   YES ____   NO ____

## HOME EXPOSURES

1. Which of the following do you have in your home?
   __air conditioner            __fireplace          __electric stove
   __central heating (gas or oil)     __air purifier        __woodstove

2. In approximately what year was your home built?

3. Have there been any recent renovations?   YES ____   NO ____
   If yes, describe:

4. Have you recently installed new carpet, purchased new furniture, or refinished existing furniture?   YES ____   NO ____
   If yes, explain:

5. Do you use pesticides around your home or garden?   YES ____   NO ____
   If yes, describe:

6. What household cleaners do you use? (List most common and any new products you use.)

7. List all hobbies done at your home:

8. Are any of the agents listed earlier for work exposures encountered in hobbies or recreational activities?
   YES ____   NO ____

9. Is any special protective equipment or ventilation used during hobbies?   YES ____   NO ____
   Explain:

10. What are the occupations of other household members?

11. Do other household members have contact with any form of chemicals at work or during leisure activities?
    YES ____   NO ____
    If yes, explain:

12. Is anyone else in your home environment having symptoms similar to yours?   YES ____   NO ____
    If yes, explain briefly:

## COMMUNITY EXPOSURES

1. Are any of the following located in your community?
   __industrial plant     __major source of air pollution     __waste site
   __landfill     __toxic spill     __other_____

2. What is your source of drinking water?
   __private well     __public water source     __other

3. Are neighbors experiencing any health problems similar to yours?    YES ___    NO ___
   If yes, explain:

## KEY OCCUPATIONAL AND ENVIRONMENTAL HEALTH QUESTIONS TO BE ASKED WITH ALL HISTORIES

1. What are your current and past longest held jobs?

2. Have you been exposed to any radiation or chemical liquids, dusts, mists, or fumes?    YES ___    NO ___

3. Is there any relationship between current symptoms and activities at work or at home?    YES ___    NO ___

From Pope AM, Snyder MA, Mood LH, editors: *Nursing, health, and environment: strengthening the relationship to improve the public's health,* Washington, DC, 1995, National Academy Press.

# Motivational Interviewing

Motivational interviewing (MI) is a collaborative strategy to promote behavioral change in clients and families. Clients and families are encouraged to set goals for making health changes, and the process allows the nurse to address ambivalence toward change and strengthen the client or family's commitment to behavioral change.

The core tenets of MI recognize the client and family as the experts who have the ability to make a change based on personal choices. The nurse provides a **collaborative** environment that supports change and has the client or family **share** their perceptions and knowledge about the behavior under discussion. The nurse then affirms the client or family's **autonomy** to make choices for change about the behavior.

There are four principles central to the spirit of MI to guide the nurse:

- *Expressing empathy* to communicate an understanding of the client or family's perspective
- *Rolling with resistance* and avoiding arguing with the client or family when ambivalence or unwillingness to change occurs
- *Supporting self-efficacy,* which is supporting the client's or family's confidence that change can be made
- *Developing discrepancy* is guiding the client or family when inconsistencies occur between current behavior and desired behavioral goals

The key components to interactions with clients and families during MI are guided by the acronym OARS:

- *Open-ended questions:* these questions allow the client or family to express their thoughts and share their personal experiences. It allows the nurse to develop a fuller understanding of barriers to change and individual values.
- *Affirmations of what the client and/or family says:* the nurse affirms the client or family's ability to change and how the behavior change is congruent with their values and goals.
- *Reflective listening:* this is the hallmark of MI. The nurse restates what the client or family shares and allows for clarifying what the client or family means to say or feels. This is an opportunity to focus on moving the client or family closer to behavioral change.
- *Summaries of the conversation and decisions made:* the nurse summarizes the MI session and the goals set by the client or family and reinforces the plan for change.

"Change" in health behavior is the overall goal of MI, and using strategies that promote movement toward change is important within the context of MI. This includes supporting statements expressing a desire for change, addressing perceived barriers to change, and having the confidence to make behavioral changes. Focus on linking the desired behavioral change to the client's or family's personal values, abilities, and goals. Developing small, achievable goals may be more attainable and less overwhelming for some clients and families in the beginning. Nurses can then continue to use MI in future interactions to promote progression in healthy behaviors.

Adapted from:

Lundahl B, Moleni T, Burke BL, Butters R, Tollefson D, Butler C, Rollnick S: Motivational interviewing in medical care settings: A systematic and meta-analysis of randomized controlled trials, *Patient Education and Counseling, 92*(2): 157–168, 2013.

Miller WR, Rollnick S: *Motivational interviewing—helping people change*, ed. 3, New York, NY, 2013, The Guilford Press.

Motivational Interviewing: Resources for clinical, researchers, and trainers. Available at http://www.motivationalinterview.org. Accessed May 13, 2015.

## EXAMPLES OF PUBLIC HEALTH NURSING ROLES AND IMPLEMENTING PUBLIC HEALTH FUNCTIONS

This document is intended to clearly present the role of public health nurses in Virginia as members of the multidisciplinary public health team in a changing health care environment. The following matrices present the role of public health nursing in Virginia. The following definitions were used to develop these matrices.

**Essential Element** is taken from the National Association of City and County Health Officials' (NACCHO's) document *Blueprint for a Healthy Community.* The following public health essential elements are used as a framework to present the role of public health nursing in Virginia:

- Conducting Community Assessments
- Preventing and Controlling Epidemics
- Providing a Safe and Healthy Environment
- Measuring Performance, Effectiveness, and Outcomes of Health Services
- Promoting Healthy Lifestyles
- Providing Targeted Outreach and Forming Partnerships

- Providing Personal Health Care Services
- Conducting Research and Innovation
- Mobilizing the Community for Action

*Public Health Function* is defined as a broad public health activity needed to ensure a strong, flexible, accountable public health structure. It may require a multidisciplinary team to carry out.

*Public Health Nurse Role* is the activity the public health nurse is responsible for, either alone or as a member of a team, to accomplish the stated public health function. This can be the public health nurse at the local level or at the state level.

*State Role* is what public health nurses need from the state level to do their jobs (e.g., policy, aggregate data, training). This refers to any Central Office program or staff, not just nurses.

A process was implemented that would involve all public health nurses in Virginia. Although this lengthened the timeline to completion, it will ensure that the final document represents a consensus developed through creative open dialogue.

From National Association of City and County Health Officials: *Blueprint for a healthy community: a guide for local health departments,* Washington, DC, 1994, The Association.

**ESSENTIAL ELEMENT 1: Conduct Community Assessment:** Systematically collecting, assembling, analyzing, and making available health-related data for the purpose of identifying and responding to community- and state-level public health concerns and conducting epidemiologic and other population-based studies.

| Public Health Function | PHN Roles | State Roles |
|---|---|---|
| Develop frameworks, methodologies, and tools for standardizing data collection and analysis and reporting across all jurisdictions and providers. | • Provide, review, and comment on proposed methodologies and tools for data collection.<br>• Field-test tools and methods. | • Collaborate with professional organizations and academic and governmental institutions to develop and test tools and methods.<br>• Provide educational opportunities in areas of and use of tools.<br>• Work with local-level agencies to standardize definitions, data collected, etc., across jurisdictions and among all stakeholders (schools, community-based organizations, and private providers). |
| Collect and analyze data. | • Collaborate with the community to identify population-based needs and gaps in service.<br>• Analyze data and needs, knowledge, attitudes, and practices of specific populations.<br>• Identify patterns of diseases, illness, and injury and develop or stimulate development of programs to respond to identified trends. | • Provide aggregated data to the local level in a timely and accurate manner.<br>• Provide census tract–level aggregated data to the local level.<br>• Provide national and state comparisons to be used with local data to obtain trends and assist localities in documenting need, progress, etc., to attain standard outcomes. |

**ESSENTIAL ELEMENT 2: Preventing and Controlling Epidemics:** Monitoring disease trends and investigating and containing diseases and injuries.

| Public Health Function | PHN Roles | State Roles |
|---|---|---|
| Develop programs that prevent, contain, and control the transmission of diseases and danger of injuries (including violence). | • Provide community-wide preventive measures in the form of health education and mobilization of community resources.<br>• Ensure isolation/containment measures when necessary.<br>• Ensure adequate preventive immunizations.<br>• Implement programs that control the transmission of diseases and danger of injuries during disasters. | • Work with local jurisdictions to develop tools such as videos, PSAs, and/or posters that local jurisdictions can use.<br>• Work with local jurisdictions to develop disaster plans for the control of the transmission of diseases and danger of injuries during disasters.<br>• Facilitate state-level partnerships that promote health, healthy lifestyles, and wellness (individual and family). |
| Develop regulatory guidelines for the prevention of targeted diseases. | • Implement regulatory measures.<br>• Implement OSHA Guidelines for Blood Borne Pathogens and the Prevention of the Transmission of TB in Health Care Settings. | • In partnership with localities, develop regulatory guidelines.<br>• Serve as clearinghouse or source of information. |

**ESSENTIAL ELEMENT 3: Providing a Safe and Healthy Environment:** Maintaining clean and safe air, water, food, and facilities both in the community and in the home environment.

| Public Health Function | PHN Roles | State Roles |
|---|---|---|
| Develop methods/tools for collection and analysis of health-related data (occurrence of mortality and morbidity relating to both communicable and chronic diseases, injury registries, sentinel event establishment, environmental quality, etc.). | • Provide reporting guidelines and consultation regarding disease prevention, diagnosis, treatment, and follow-up of cases/contacts to physicians and institutions (emergency department, university and secondary school student health, prisons, industries, etc.).<br>• Conduct/participate in community needs assessments to determine customer/provider knowledge deficits and perceptions of need.<br>• Provide education to individuals, providers, targeted populations, etc., in response to knowledge deficits, disease outbreaks, toxic waste emissions, etc.<br>• Provide individual follow-up/case management of communicable diseases that are transmitted by air, water, food, and fomites (TB, hepatitis A, salmonella, staphylococcus, etc.). | • Develop standard methodology and tools for collection and analysis of health-related data.<br>• Provide training in area of data collection and analysis.<br>• Evaluate activities and outcomes of interactions.<br>• Work in partnership with localities to develop program based on data analysis needs. |
| Develop programs that promote a safe environment in the home. | • Provide childhood lead poisoning screenings and follow-up.<br>• Teach clients to inspect homes for safety violations and toxic substances and to practice safe behaviors; assist families to access/use available resources/safety devices.<br>• Assess/teach regarding safe food selection, preparation, and storage.<br>• Train/supervise volunteers/auxiliary personnel in performance of the above tasks.<br>• Teach families that all men, women, and children have a right to a safe environment free of physical or mental abuse. | • Provide consultation and technical assistance to state/local organizations regarding laws and regulations that protect health and ensure safety.<br>• In partnership with localities, develop and evaluate educational programs. |
| Develop programs that promote a safe environment in the workplace. | • Provide consultation in implementation of OSHA regulations relating to occupational exposure to diseases.<br>• Provide educational program related to healthy lifestyles (smoking cessation, back protection, etc.).<br>• Ensure provision of screenings for individuals to determine baselines and occurrence of infectious diseases and preventable deterioration of health and function: hearing, back soundness, lung capacity, RMS indicators, PPDs, etc.<br>• Assist in policy/practice development to address prevention of the above.<br>• Provide immunizations. | • Monitor and assist localities to implement prevention activities.<br>• Assist localities in developing and evaluating educational programs.<br>• Monitor outcomes of screening activities and evaluate interventions. |

## ESSENTIAL ELEMENT 3: Providing a Safe and Healthy Environment—cont'd

| Public Health Function | PHN Roles | State Roles |
| --- | --- | --- |
| Develop programs that promote a safe environment in the school setting. | • Provide consultation on implementation of OSHA regulations relating to occupational exposure to diseases.<br>• Provide educational programs related to healthy lifestyles (smoking cessation, etc.).<br>• Ensure provision of screenings for students to determine baselines and occurrence of infectious disease and preventable deterioration of health and function.<br>• Assist in policy/practice development to address prevention of the above.<br>• Provide immunizations. | • Develop guidelines that ensure accountability in meeting standards set forth.<br>• Ensure that policy is developed to protect children in the school environment.<br>• Monitor immunization status of children and provide immunizations during outbreaks and evaluate activities. |
| Develop programs that promote a safe environment in the community. | • Identify population clusters exhibiting an unhealthy environment; provide consultation/group education regarding preventive measures.<br>• Participate in development of local disaster plans to ensure provision of safe water, food, air, and facilities.<br>• Respond in time of natural disasters such as floods, tornadoes, and hurricanes.<br>• Participate in developing plans for shelter management during disasters, especially "Special Needs" shelters that may require nursing staff. | • In times of disaster, facilitate availability of resources across jurisdictions.<br>• Have a statewide plan.<br>• Ensure that localities have developed plans to protect the public in time of national and/or other disasters.<br>• Coordinate efforts statewide.<br>• Assist localities in responding.<br>• Evaluate efforts. |
| Develop and issue standards that guide regulations and mandate policy and program development. | • Survey worksites, schools, institutions, etc., for compliance to regulations that protect health and ensure safety. | • Develop a systematic evaluation tool for collection of data to measure trends. |
| Develop protocols to ensure accountability of all health care providers, public and private. | • Provide technical assistance (i.e., interpretation, implementation, and evaluation processes). | • Assist localities in developing standards to mandate accountability. |
| Provide inservice to all providers of health care services. | • Share and implement knowledge gained in inservices. | • Provide consultation/technical assistance to localities. |

## ESSENTIAL ELEMENT 4: Measuring Performance, Effectiveness, and Outcomes of Health Services: Monitoring health care providers and the health care system to identify gaps in service, deteriorating health status indicators, effectiveness of interventions, and accessibility and quality of personal and population-wide health services.

| Public Health Function | PHN Roles | State Roles |
| --- | --- | --- |
| Promote competency in public health issues throughout the health delivery system.<br><br>Collect data. | • Provide educational and technical assistance in areas such as case management and appropriate treatment and control of communicable diseases to the community.<br>• Participate in data collection with a target population.<br>• Ensure that the data collection system supports the objectives of programs serving the community by participating in the design and operation of data collection systems.<br>• Collect data via surveys, polls, interviews, focus groups that will enable assessment of the community's perception of health status and understanding how the system works and how to obtain service needs. | • Develop appropriate regulatory, educational, and technical assistance programs.<br>• Provide technical assistance and training to local health department for local forecasting and interpretation of data.<br>• Work with localities (health districts, private providers, other state and local agencies) to develop standard data elements and definitions across jurisdictions and among all stakeholders, especially for consistency in coding of population-based data.<br>• Identify data collection and analytic issues related to monitoring the impact of health system changes such as costs and benefits of record linkage, strategies for ensuring confidentiality, and strategies for analyzing trends in health within a broader social and economic context.<br>• Advocate for uniform data collection from all managed care plans so that outcomes and health trends can be analyzed and tracked and sentinel events reported. |

**ESSENTIAL ELEMENT 4: Measuring Performance, Effectiveness, and Outcomes of Health Services—cont'd**

| Public Health Function | PHN Roles | State Roles |
|---|---|---|
| Analyze data to ensure accurate diagnosis of health status, identification of threats to health, and assessment of health service needs. | • Participate in a systematic approach to convert data into information that will identify gaps in service at the local and state level and will lead to action.<br>• Monitor health status indicators to identify emerging problems and facilitate community-wide response to identified problems.<br>• Facilitate data analysis as part of a local collaborative effort. | • Develop a systematic, integrated statewide approach to converting data into information that directs action.<br>• Ensure that resources, such as hardware and software, to analyze data are available at the local level.<br>• Work with localities (health districts, private providers, other state and local agencies) to address issues related to variable access to technology, confidentiality issues.<br>• Educate and train currently employed public health nurses in areas of epidemiology and population-based services. |
| Monitor health status indicators for the entire population and for specific population groups and/or geographic areas. | • Identify target populations that may be at risk for public health problems such as communicable diseases, unidentified and untreated chronic diseases.<br>• Conduct surveys or observe targeted populations such as preschools, childcare centers, and high-risk census tracks to identify health status.<br>• Monitor health care utilization of vulnerable populations at the local and regional level. | • Develop methodology for identification, measurement, and analysis of key indicators of health care utilization of vulnerable populations. |
| Monitor and assess availability, cost-effectiveness, and outcomes of personal and population-based health services. | • Identify gaps in services (e.g., a neighborhood with deteriorating immunization rates may indicate lack of available primary care services).<br>• Ensure that all receive the same quality of care, including comprehensive preventive services.<br>• Monitor the impact of health system reforms on vulnerable populations.<br>• Evaluate the effectiveness and outcomes of care.<br>• Plan interventions based on the health of the overall population, not just for those in the health care system.<br>• Identify interventions that are effective and replicable. | • Develop analyses that demonstrate the cost-effectiveness of investment in public health services.<br>• Develop protocols and technical assistance for ensuring accountability of Medicaid managed care plans and other government-funded plans for service delivery and overall health status of their covered populations.<br>• Identify standard theoretical, methodological, and measurement issues that are specific to population subgroups for monitoring the impact of health system changes on vulnerable populations. |
| Disseminate information. | • Disseminate information to the public on community health status, including how to access and use services appropriately.<br>• Disseminate information to other health care providers regarding gaps in services or deteriorating health status indicators. | • Ensure a mechanism for public accountability of performance and outcomes through public dissemination of information and in particular ensure that underservice, a risk inherent in capitated plans, is measurable through available data.<br>• Ensure that information is provided to communities, local health departments, managed care plans, and other appropriate state agencies. |

**ESSENTIAL ELEMENT 5: Promoting Healthy Lifestyles:** Providing health education to individuals, families, and communities.

| Public Health Function | PHN Roles | State Roles |
|---|---|---|
| Promote informed decision making of residents about things that influence their health on a daily basis. | • Exert influence through contact with individuals and community groups.<br>• Accept and issue challenge of healthy lifestyles to all contacts.<br>• Reinforce and reward positive informed decisions made for healthy lifestyles. | • Develop and monitor standards for the changes to determine changes in behavior. |
| Promote effective use of media to encourage both personal and community responsibility for informed decision making. | • Be a resource for the community.<br>• Gather data and address findings as appropriate.<br>• Work with community groups to promote accurate information for healthy lifestyle through the media.<br>• Use current information and other agency's resources to maximize information accessible to the public. | • Assist localities to provide current information to community organizations and other state organizations.<br>• Serve as a resource for localities and work with media. |
| Develop a public awareness/ marketing campaign to demonstrate the importance of public health to overall health improvement and its proper place in the health delivery system. | • Provide education to special groups (e.g., local politicians, school boards, PTAs, churches, civic groups, news media) regarding the benefits of preventive health. | • Develop training activities to assist localities in marketing. |
| Develop public information and education systems/ programs through partnerships. | • Provide educational sessions/programs to public regarding components of healthy lifestyles.<br>• Access grants/other funding sources to promote healthy lifestyle decisions (e.g., cervical and breast cancer prevention, bike helmets, hypertension).<br>• Provide/promote teaching for individuals and families at every opportunity (home, clinic, community settings). | • Assist localities in developing and evaluating educational programs.<br>• Assist localities in funding.<br>• Hold regional/state training sessions.<br>• Evaluate outcomes and plan ongoing educational systems/ programs. |

**ESSENTIAL ELEMENT 6: Providing Targeted Outreach and Forming Partnerships:** Ensuring access to services, including those that lead to self-sufficiency, for all vulnerable populations and ensuring the development of culturally appropriate care.

| Public Health Function | PHN Roles | State Roles |
|---|---|---|
| Ensure accessibility to health services that will improve morbidity, decrease mortality, and improve health status outcomes. | • Provide family-centered case management services for high-risk and hard-to-reach populations that focus on linking families with needed services.<br>• Improve access to care by forming partnerships with appropriate community individuals and entities.<br>• Increase influence of cultural diversity on system design and on access to care, as well as on individual services rendered.<br>• Ensure that translation services are available for the non–English-speaking population.<br>• Participate in ongoing community assessment to identify areas of concern and above needs for rules.<br>• Provide outreach services that focus on preventing epidemics and the spread of disease, such as tuberculosis and sexually transmitted diseases. | • Provide funds in cooperation with locality.<br>• Ensure policy development that includes case management and is culturally sensitive.<br>• Provide adequate ongoing continuing education for staff (especially in areas common to all localities).<br>• Participate in state-level contract development to ensure that contracts with health plans require and include incentives for health plans to offer and deliver preventive health services in the minimum benefits package.<br>• Educate financing officials about the roles of public health both in performing core public health services and in ensuring access to personal health services. |

**ESSENTIAL ELEMENT 7: Providing Personal Health Care Services:** Providing targeted direct services to high-risk populations.

| Public Health Function | PHN Roles | State Roles |
| --- | --- | --- |
| Provide direct services for specific diseases that threaten the health of the community and develop programs that prevent, contain, and control the transmission of infectious diseases. | • Plan, develop, implement, and evaluate: <br> • Sexually transmitted disease services <br> • Communicable disease services <br> • HIV/AIDS services <br> • Tuberculosis control services <br> • Develop and implement guidelines for the prevention of the above targeted diseases. | • Establish standards/criteria for personal health care. <br> • Work with local health departments to assist in developing infrastructure and management techniques to facilitate record-keeping and appropriate financial monitoring and tracking systems, which enable local health departments to enter into contractual arrangements for preventive health and primary care services. |
| Provide health services, including preventive health services, to high-risk and vulnerable populations (e.g., the uninsured working poor), and in geographic areas where primary health care services are not readily accessible or available in a privatized setting. | • Provide coordination, follow-up, referral, and case management as indicated. <br> • Integrate supportive services (such as counseling, social work, nutrition) into primary care services. <br> • Assess existing community medical capacity for referral and follow-up. | • Continue to work at the state and local level to build capacity of primary and preventive health services, particularly in traditionally underserved areas, to ensure availability to providers and primary care sites essential to primary care access. |

**ESSENTIAL ELEMENT 8: Conducting Research and Innovation:** Discovering and applying improved health care delivery mechanisms and clinical interventions.

| Public Health Function | PHN Roles | State Roles |
| --- | --- | --- |
| Ensure ongoing prevention research relating to biomedical and behavioral aspects of health promotion and prevention of disease and injury. <br> Implement pilot or demonstration projects. | • Develop outcome measures. <br> • Identify research priorities for target communities and develop and conduct scientific and operations research for health promotion and disease/injury prevention. <br> • Develop and implement linkages with academic centers, ensuring that clients and populations who participate in research projects benefit as a result of the research. | • Provide training in area of measuring program effectiveness. <br><br> • Support evaluations and research that demonstrate the benefits of public health, as well as the consequences of failure to support public health interventions. |

**ESSENTIAL ELEMENT 9: Mobilizing the Community for Action:** Providing leadership and initiating collaboration.

| Public Health Function | PHN Roles | State Roles |
| --- | --- | --- |
| Provide leadership to stimulate development of networks or partnerships that will ensure the availability of comprehensive primary health care services to all, regardless of ability to pay. <br> Initiate collaboration with other community organizations to ensure the leadership role in resolving a public health issue. | • Advocate for improved health. <br> • Disseminate health information. <br> • Build coalitions. <br> • Make recommendations for policy implementation or revision. <br><br> • Facilitate resources that manage environmental risk and maintain and improve community health. <br> • Provide information for a community group working on impacting policy at the local, state, or federal level. <br> • Use results of community health assessments to stimulate the community to develop a plan to respond to identified gaps in service. | • Facilitate the establishment and enhancement of statewide high-quality, needed health services. <br> • Administer quality improvement programs. <br> • Use information-gathering techniques of assessment to assist policy/legislature activities to develop needed health services and functions that require statewide action or standards. <br> • Recommend programs to carry out policies. |

# American Public Health Association Definition of Public Health Nursing

## THE DEFINITION AND PRACTICE OF PUBLIC HEALTH NURSING

### 2013

### Acknowledgments

This statement was developed by the Public Health Nursing Definition Document Task Force under the direction of the leadership of the Public Health Nursing Section of the American Public Health Association. The statement was adopted by the Public Health Nursing Section Council at the American Public Health Association Annual Meeting on November 5, 2013. The Task Force gratefully acknowledges the valuable assistance of individuals who contributed comments and recommendations throughout the development of this document.

### Public Health Nursing Definition Document Task Force

| | |
|---|---|
| Betty Bekemeier, Co-chair | Tessa Walker Linderman, Co-chair |
| Jo Anne Bennett | Shawn Kneipp |
| Martha Bergren | Kirk Koyama |
| Janet Braunstein Moody | Pam Kulbok |
| Marjorie Buchanan | Lauren Lawson |
| Laura Debiasi | Kathlynn Northrup-Snyder |
| Joyce Edmonds | Sue Stroschein |
| Alexandra Garcia | |

Recommended citation:

American Public Health Association, Public Health Nursing Section (2013). The definition and practice of public health nursing: A statement of the public health nursing section. Washington, DC: American Public Health Association.

November 11, 2013

## THE DEFINITION AND PRACTICE OF PUBLIC HEALTH NURSING

A Statement of the APHA Public Health Nursing Section

2013

This document updates the 1996 American Public Health Association Public Health Nursing Section definition statement and affirms the original definition.[1]  This statement addresses some of the evolving economic, health, political, and societal trends that shape the context of public health nursing practice.

### Definition
***Public health nursing is the practice of promoting and protecting the health of populations using knowledge from nursing, social, and public health sciences.***

Public health nursing is a specialty practice within nursing and public health.  It focuses on improving population health by emphasizing prevention, and attending to multiple determinants of health.  Often used interchangeably with community health nursing, this nursing practice includes advocacy, policy development, and planning, which addresses issues of social justice.  With a multi-level view of health, public health nursing action occurs through community applications of theory, evidence, and a commitment to health equity.  In addition to what is put forward in this definition, public health nursing practice is guided by the American Nurses Association *Public Health Nursing: Scope & Standards of Practice* [2] and the Quad Council of Public Health Nursing Organizations' *Core Competencies for Public Health Nurses.*[3]

### Elements of Practice
Key characteristics of practice include 1) a focus on the health needs of an entire population, including inequities and the unique needs of sub-populations; 2) assessment of population health using a comprehensive, systematic approach; 3) attention to multiple determinants of health; 4) an emphasis on primary prevention; and 5) application of interventions at all levels—individuals, families, communities, and the systems that impact their health.[4]

*Public Health Nursing Perspective*
Public health nursing aims to improve the health outcomes of all populations.  Applying their clinical knowledge and expertise in health care from an ecological perspective, public health nurses acknowledge the complexity of public health problems and the contextual nature of health—including cultural, environmental, historical, physical, and social factors.  Public health nurses apply systems-level thinking[5,6] to assess the potential or actual assets, needs, opportunities, and inequities of individuals, families, and populations and translate this assessment into action for public good.

*Public Health Nursing Activities and Practice Settings*
Public health nursing activities comprise the domains depicted by the *Public Health Intervention Wheel* and the *10 Essential Public Health Services.*[7,8]  These activities include community collaboration, health teaching, and policy development, in response to priorities derived from ongoing, comprehensive population focused assessment.  Public health nurses are members and leaders of interprofessional teams in diverse settings and in many different types of agencies and organizations including all levels of

November 11, 2013

government, community-based and other nongovernmental service organizations, foundations, policy think tanks, academic institutions and other research settings. Increasing numbers of public health nurses work in global health in an effort to promote global responsibility and connectivity. Public health nurses that work with individuals and families do so within the context of a population focus—applying a systems perspective to factors that impact health.

*Determinants of Health*
Eliminating population health disparities by addressing multiple determinants that lead to poor health is a national goal.[9] Public health nurses are in a position to provide leadership through public policy reform efforts, community-building, and system-level change.[10] Environmental, physical, and social determinants explain most health disparities in the United States.[11,12,13,14,15] Socioeconomic disadvantages such as poverty, low levels of education, and belonging to a racial or ethnic minority group, are more robust risk factors of poor health than a lack of access to health care or predominantly genetic factors of disease.[16,17,18] While the discipline of nursing was founded on improving environmental conditions to facilitate health at the bedside,[19] public health nurses focus on improving population health in the environments where people live, work, learn, and play.

**Opportunities & Challenges**
Adherence to public health nursing's key characteristics requires that the practice must evolve to address current societal needs. Public health nursing has faced multiple challenges over its history while engaging in leadership opportunities that have shaped nursing practice, addressing environmental and social justice issues, affecting population health, and exploring health promotion concepts. One example is the Patient Protection and Affordable Care Act (ACA).[20] The ACA has greatly altered the landscape for health care and health improvement in the U.S., creating the potential for new public health nursing roles and responsibilities. The ACA includes goals to 1) improve the individual health care experience; 2) reduce the cost of health care; and 3) improve the health of populations. With their positions embedded within communities, public health nurses are vital to the interprofessional teams needed to assure that all people have equitable access to high quality care and healthy environments through health system reform.[21] Their assessment skills, primary prevention focus, and system-level perspectives can assure that local and state needs are met, services and programs are coordinated, and communities are engaged.

Public health nurses are prepared to lead efforts that align emerging systems of care for population health improvement, health promotion, risk reduction, and disease prevention efforts that are within the nucleus of a reformed health system. Fewer public health nursing positions and decreased public health funding influence leadership roles and access to health care in communities.[22] Within the context of health care reform these challenges offer opportunities to emphasize a strong, well-educated public health nursing workforce to lead and carry out system coordination and change at local, state, national, and international levels.[23]

An emerging health care model that requires public health nursing leadership is the integration of primary care and public health.[24] Primary care and public health share a focus on prevention, population health, transitional care, and care coordination across settings to promote health through collaboration. With a unique focus from individuals and families to populations and systems, public health nurses are well

November 11, 2013

positioned to integrate new health system models and meet the demands of an ever-changing health system.[25]

**Public Health Nursing Education**

The baccalaureate degree in nursing (BSN) is recommended for entry-level public health nurses.[26] *The Essentials of Baccalaureate Education for Professional Nursing Practice* emphasize fundamental concepts for public health nursing practice such as clinical prevention, population health, health care policy, finance, and regulatory environments, and interprofessional collaboration.[27] The graduate is prepared to conduct community assessments and apply the principles of epidemiology among other competencies.

Nurses with a master's degree or higher, and with specialization in population health, demonstrate the knowledge and skills required for leadership positions. Competencies include mastery of interprofessional collaboration, health policy and advocacy, population assessment, prevention strategies, and program planning and evaluation.[28] The doctor of nursing practice (DNP) degree, with a public health emphasis, has emerged in the last decade, and provides the foundation for advanced practice in executive leadership, systems development, and the translation of research into practice. The doctor of philosophy (PhD) and other research-focused doctoral degrees remain the preparation for public health nurses to develop the science relevant to public health nursing and to generate the evidence needed to guide practice. In some states a public health nursing certification is needed to signify a nurse's specific competence and expertise in public health nursing. National advanced public health nursing certification is available via portfolio assessment through American Nurses Credentialing Center.

**Summary**

Public health nurses provide leadership for emerging advances in population health and health care—particularly in terms of addressing health inequities. Equipped with a baccalaureate degree or higher, public health nurses are prepared to address multiple determinants of health and participate fully in the challenges of attaining and maintaining population health. With a scope of practice that includes community-building, health promotion, policy reform, and system-level changes to promote and protect the health of populations; public health nurses have an essential role and responsibility as leaders in health improvement and promoting health equity.

---

[1] American Public Health Association, Public Health Nursing Section. (1996). Definition and role of public health nursing: A statement of the public health nursing section. Washington, DC; Author.

[2] American Nurses Association. (2013). *Public health nursing: Scope and standards of practice. (2nd ed.),* Washington, DC: American Nurses Publishing.

[3] Quad Council of Public Health Nursing Organizations. (2011). Core competencies for public health nurses. Washington, DC: Quad Council of Public Health Organizations.

[4] Keller, L.O., Schaffer, M., Lia-Hoagberg, B., Strohschein, S. (2002). Assessment, program planning, and evaluation in population-based public health practice. *Public Health Management Practice,* 8 (5), 31-32.

November 11, 2013

# F.3 APPENDIX

# American Nurses Association Scope and Standards of Practice for Public Health Nursing

## STANDARDS OF CARE

### Standard 1. Assessment

The public health nurse collects comprehensive data pertinent to the health status of populations.

### Standard 2. Population Diagnosis and Priorities

The public health nurse analyses the assessment data to determine the diagnoses or issues.

### Standard 3. Outcomes Identification

The public health nurse identifies expected outcomes for a plan specific to the population or situation.

### Standard 4. Planning

The public health nurse develops a plan that prescribes strategies and alternatives to attain expected outcomes.

### Standard 5. Implementation

The public health nurse implements the identified plan.

### Standard 5A: Coordination of Care

The public health nurse coordinates care delivery.

### Standard 5B. Health Teaching and Health Promotion

The public health nurse employs multiple strategies to promote health and a safe environment.

### Standard 5C: Consultation

The public health nurse provides consultation to influence the identified plan, enhance the abilities of others, and effect change.

### Standard 5D. Prescriptive Authority

Not applicable

### Standard 5D. Regulatory Activities

The public health nurse participates in applications of public health laws, regulations, and policies.

### Standard 6. Evaluation

The public health nurse evaluates progress toward the attainment of outcomes.

## STANDARDS OF PROFESSIONAL PERFORMANCE

### Standard 7. Ethics

The public health nurse practices ethically.

### Standard 8. Education

The public health nurse attains knowledge and competency that reflect current practice.

### Standard 9. Evidence-Based Practice and Research

The public health nurse integrates evidence and research findings into practice.

### Standard 10. Quality of Practice

The public health nurse contributes to quality nursing practice.

### Standard 11. Communication

The public health nurse communicates effectively in a variety of formats in all areas of practice.

### Standard 12. Leadership

The public health nurse demonstrates leadership in the professional practice setting and the profession.

### Standard 13. Collaboration

The public health nurse collaborates with the population and others in the conduct of nursing practice.

### Standard 14. Professional Practice Evaluation

The public health nurse evaluates her or his own nursing practice in relation to professional practice standards and guidelines, relevant statutes, rules, and regulations.

## Standard 15. Resource Utilization

The public health nurse utilizes appropriate resources to plan and provide nursing and public health services that are safe, effective, and financially responsible.

## Standard 16. Environmental Health

The public health nurse practices in an environmentally safe, fair, and just manner.

## Standard 17. Advocacy

The public health nurse advocates for the protection of the health, safety, and rights of the population.

---

From American Nurses Association: *Public health nursing: Scope and standards of practice*, Washington, DC, 2013, American Nurses Publishing.

## The Health Insurance Portability and Accountability Act (HIPAA): What Does It Mean for Public Health Nurses?

Public Health Nursing Practice—definition: a specialty practice within nursing and public health. Practice focuses on improving population health by emphasizing prevention, and attending to multiple determinants of health. Practice includes advocacy, policy development, and planning, which addresses issues of social justice. With a multi-level view of health, public health nursing action occurs through community applications of theory, evidence, and a commitment to health equity. The goal is to prevent disease and disability and promote and protect the health of the community as a whole.

### EXPLANATION

- Federal privacy standards were created by the Department of Health and Human Services (USDHHS) to protect patients' medical records and other health information provided to health plans, doctors, hospitals, and other health care providers.
- These standards took effect on April 14, 2003.
- Standardization of electronic transactions, and the elimination of inefficient paper forms, will save the health care industry more than $29 billion in the next 10 years.

### PRIVACY RULE

- Protects the confidentiality of individually identifiable health information, whether it is on paper, in computers, or communicated orally.
- Protected health information (PHI) is the name for this individually identifiable health information.
- Limits the ways that health plans, pharmacies, hospitals, and other covered entities can use patients' personal medical information.

### PATIENT PROTECTIONS

- Patients should be able to see, obtain copies, and make corrections to their medical records.
- Patients should receive a notice from health care providers regarding how their personal medical information may be used by them and their rights under the privacy regulation. Patients can restrict this use.
- Limits have been set on how health care providers can use individually identifiable health information. Doctors, nurses, and other providers can share information needed to treat a patient. For purposes other than medical care, personal health information generally may not be used.
- Pharmacies, health plans, and other covered entities must obtain an individual's authorization before disclosing patient information for marketing purposes.

### PUBLIC HEALTH SERVICES AND PHI

Overview: Although protection of health information is important, PHI is used for the public good by health officials to identify, monitor, and respond to disease, death, and disability among populations. Examples of ways PHI is used include public health surveillance, program evaluation, terrorism preparedness, outbreak investigations, direct health services, and public health research. Public health authorities have taken precautions in the past to protect the privacy of individuals and will continue to do so under HIPAA. The privacy rule, however, still permits PHI to be shared for important public health purposes.

### PERMITTED PHI DISCLOSURES TO A PUBLIC HEALTH AUTHORITY

#### Without Authorization

- Reporting of disease, injury, and vital events
- Conducting public health surveillance, investigations, and interventions
- Reporting child abuse or neglect to a public health or other government authority legally authorized to receive such reports
- To a person subject to jurisdiction of the Food and Drug Administration (FDA) concerning the quality, safety, or effectiveness of an FDA-related product or activity for which that person has responsibility
- To a person who may have been exposed to a communicable disease or may be at risk for contracting or spreading a disease or condition, when legally authorized to notify the person as necessary to conduct a public health intervention or investigation
- To an individual's employer, under certain circumstances and conditions, as needed for the employer to meet the requirements of the Occupational Safety and Health Administration, Mine Safety and Health Administration, or similar state law

# HIPAA AND NURSING RESEARCH

## Definitions

*Covered entity:* a health plan, a health care clearinghouse, or a health care provider who transmits any health information in electronic form.

*Individually Identifiable Health Information* (IIHI): information about an individual regarding his or her physical or mental health; the provision of health care; or the payment for the provision of health care; and which identifies the individual.

It is the covered entity's obligation not to disclose the information improperly when a researcher seeks data that includes PHI.

A covered entity can disclose IIHI for research purposes under any of the following conditions:

1. The IIHI pertains only to deceased persons.
2. The IIHI can be examined for reviews preparatory to research if it is not removed from the covered entity.
3. Information that has been de-identified can be disclosed; this information is no longer considered IIHI and thus not covered by HIPAA.
4. Data must be disclosed as part of a limited data set if the researcher has a data use agreement with the covered entity.
5. The researcher has a valid authorization from the research subject to disclose IIHI.
6. An IRB or privacy board has waived the authorization requirement.

## Creating Data

Researchers may also be creating IIHI. If the researcher is part of a covered entity, any PHI obtained by any means is covered by HIPAA, and the researcher and his or her institution are bound by HIPAA regulations. Most universities with nursing schools will be hybrid entities (i.e., some parts of the university are a covered entity and some are not). Researchers should check their institution's policies.

## Disclosing Data

Nurse researchers should be aware that sharing data with colleagues and students may constitute disclosures of IIHI and they should conform to HIPAA regulations. In this case, the researcher is the holder of the IIHI and can disclose it only under appropriate conditions:

1. Patients agree to specific disclosures in the initial authorization.
2. Former patients sign an additional authorization.
3. An IRB or privacy board waives the need for authorization.
4. The holder allows the colleague to review the data to prepare a research protocol if the colleague takes no information away.
5. A holder enters the data in a limited data set and signs a data use agreement with the recipient.
6. A holder de-identifies the data and shares it freely.

Page numbers followed by "*f*" indicate figures, "*t*" indicate tables, and "*b*" indicate boxes.

**1073**

## Healthy People 2020

**Vision** — A society in which all people live long healthy lives

**Overarching goals**
- Achieve health equity, eliminate disparities, and improve the health of all groups
- Eliminate preventable disease, disability, injury, and premature death
- Promote healthy development and healthy behaviors across every stage of life
- Create social and physical environments that promote good health for all

**Foundation measures**

General health status:
- Life expectancy
- Healthy life expectancy
- Year of potential life lost
- Physically and mentally unhealthy days
- Self-assessed health status
- Limitation of activity
- Chronic disease prevalence

Health-related quality of life and well-being
- Physical, mental, and social health–related quality of life
- Well-being/satisfaction
- Participation in common activities

Determinants of health
- A range of personal, social, economic, and environmental factors that influence health status are known as the determinants of health. They include things such as biology, genetics, individual behavior, access to health services, and the environment in which people are born, live, learn, play, work, and age.

Disparities
- Race/ethnicity
- Gender
- Physical and mental ability
- Geography

**Focus areas**
- Access to health services
- Adolescent health
- Arthritis, osteoporosis, and chronic back conditions
- Blood disorders and blood safety
- Cancer
- Chronic kidney disease
- Dementias, including Alzheimer's disease
- Diabetes
- Disability and health
- Early and middle childhood
- Educational and community-based programs
- Environmental health
- Family planning
- Food safety
- Genomics
- Global health
- Health communication and health information technology
- Health-related quality of life and well-being
- Hearing and other sensory or communication disorders
- Heart disease and stroke
- Human immunodeficiency virus
- Immunization and infectious disease
- Injury and violence prevention
- Lesbian, gay, bisexual, and transgender health
- Maternal, infant, and child health
- Medical product safety
- Mental health and mental disorders
- Nutrition and weight status
- Occupational safety and health
- Older adults
- Oral health
- Physical activity
- Preparedness
- Public health infrastructure
- Respiratory diseases
- Sexually transmitted diseases
- Sleep health
- Social determinants of health
- Substance abuse
- Tobacco use
- Vision

Guidance is also provided on how to implement *Healthy People 2020* in the community via MAP-IT, which refers to the steps of: mobilize, assess, plan, implement, and track. In the *MAP-IT Guide to Using Healthy People 2020 in Your Community*, instructions are provided for ways to implement each of the five steps. See http://www.healthypeople.gov/2020/default/aspx for details about *Healthy People 2020*.